Occupational and Environmental Health

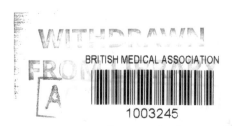

Occupational and Environmental Health

Recognizing and Preventing Disease and Injury

Seventh Edition

Edited by

Barry S. Levy
David H. Wegman
Sherry L. Baron
Rosemary K. Sokas

with the assistance of
Heather L. McStowe

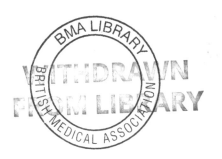
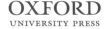

OXFORD
UNIVERSITY PRESS

OXFORD
UNIVERSITY PRESS

Oxford University Press is a department of the University of Oxford. It furthers
the University's objective of excellence in research, scholarship, and education
by publishing worldwide. Oxford is a registered trade mark of Oxford University
Press in the UK and certain other countries.

Published in the United States of America by Oxford University Press
198 Madison Avenue, New York, NY 10016, United States of America.

© Oxford University Press 2018

Fourth edition published by 2000
Fifth edition published by 2006
Sixth edition published by 2011
Seventh edition published by 2018

Library of Congress Cataloging-in-Publication Data
Names: Levy, Barry S., editor. | Wegman, David H., editor. | Baron, Sherry, L. editor. |
Sokas, Rosemary K., editor.
Title: Occupational and environmental health : recognizing and preventing disease and injury /
edited by Barry S. Levy, David H. Wegman, Sherry L. Baron, Rosemary K. Sokas, with the assistance of Heather L. McStowe.
Other titles: Occupational health (Levy) Description: Seventh edition. | Oxford ; New York : Oxford University Press, [2018] |
Includes bibliographical references and index.
Identifiers: LCCN 2017012926 (print) | LCCN 2017014701 (ebook) |
ISBN 9780190662684 (updf) | ISBN 9780190662691 (epub) | ISBN 9780190662677 (pbk. : alk. paper)
Subjects: | MESH: Occupational Diseases—prevention & control | Occupational Exposure—prevention & control |
Environmental Exposure—prevention & control | Occupational Health | Environmental Health
Classification: LCC RC963 (ebook) | LCC RC963 (print) | NLM WA 440 |
DDC 616.9/803—dc23
LC record available at https://lccn.loc.gov/2017012926

9 8 7 6 5 4 3 2

Printed by Sheridan Books, Inc., United States of America

Contents

SECTION III. HAZARDOUS EXPOSURES

SECTION IV. ADVERSE HEALTH EFFECTS

SECTION V. AN INTEGRATED APPROACH TO PREVENTION

Preface

Occupational and environmental health problems profoundly affect health and safety at the individual, family, community, national, and global level. All of us, as health and safety professionals, have important roles to play in recognizing and preventing these problems. We believe that a solid understanding of the core concepts of occupational and environmental health informs and empowers health and safety professionals to play these roles effectively.

The seventh edition of this textbook is intended to support health and safety professionals as well as students in the health professions in recognizing and preventing occupational and environmental diseases and injuries in individuals and populations. It is also intended to provide them with an understanding of the contexts in which these diseases and injuries occur. Although our focus is primarily on occupational and environmental health in the United States, we believe that this book will be useful to practitioners and students in health and safety professions throughout the world.

Dramatic changes continue to impact both occupational and environmental health, such as recognition of new workplace health hazards, the changing nature of work, global climate change, and the increasingly recognized vulnerabilities of children to hazardous exposures. In addition, dramatic changes continue to impact how we obtain, analyze, communicate, and use information for practice, prevention, research, advocacy, and policy development.

Along with the rapidly changing landscape, important relationships between occupational health and environmental health are increasingly recognized. For example, environmental health problems frequently originate in the workplace, and work-related hazards, environmental degradation, poverty, and social injustice are often interrelated. This textbook aims to reflect these developments and to enable readers to prepare themselves to recognize and prevent occupational and environmental diseases and injuries in a changing world.

We have extensively updated chapters from the sixth edition, continuing to emphasize aspects of both occupational and environmental health. In addition, we have added new chapters on climate change, children's environmental health, liver disorders, kidney disorders, and a global perspective on occupational health and safety.

All of the chapters in this book address ways in which health and safety professionals can recognize and prevent occupational and environmental health problems. Effectively addressing these problems calls for health and safety professionals to collaborate with people throughout society—business and labor leaders, government officials and representatives of nongovernmental organizations, educators and journalists, and, most importantly, workers and community members at risk of developing these problems. By engaging with others in partnerships and coalitions, we believe that readers will be able to translate the information in this book into policy and action to prevent disease, injury, and premature death and to promote health, safety, and quality of life.

The Editors
July 2017

Acknowledgments

We greatly appreciate the assistance and support of many people in the development of the seventh edition of *Occupational and Environmental Health*. We thank the many chapter authors, whose work is appropriately credited within the text. In addition, there have been many other people working behind the scenes, whom we deeply appreciate.

We acknowledge Heather McStowe for her excellent work in preparing the manuscript and communicating with the many contributors to the book.

We are grateful for the outstanding work and support of Chad Zimmerman and Chloe Layman at Oxford University Press and Rajeswari Balasubramanian at Newgen Knowledge Works.

The illustrative materials throughout the book reinforce key points and provide additional insights. We call special attention to the work of Earl Dotter, who provided many outstanding photographs to illustrate a wide range of occupational and environmental health issues, and Nick Thorkelson, who contributed creative drawings that provide fresh perspectives. We are also grateful for the photographic contributions of Aaron Sussell, David Parker, Marvin Lewiton, Nick Kaufman, and Frank Wenzel.

We express our deep appreciation to our families for their ongoing support.

Finally, we thank the many students, colleagues, workers, community members, and occupational and environmental health educators, researchers, governmental officials, advocates, and others, who, over the years, have broadened—and continue to broaden—our understanding of occupational and environmental health.

The Editors

About the Editors

The following section briefly describes the editors, who also edited earlier editions of this book.

Barry S. Levy, MD, MPH, is an occupational and environmental health physician and epidemiologist who is an Adjunct Professor of Public Health at Tufts University School of Medicine and a consultant in occupational and environmental health. He has co-edited 18 other books on occupational and environmental health, climate change, war and terrorism, and social injustice and authored more than 200 journal articles and book chapters. He previously worked as an epidemiologist at the Centers for Disease Control and Prevention, as a professor and director of the Occupational Health Program at the University of Massachusetts Medical School, and as a director of international health programs and projects. He has served as president of the American Public Health Association.

David H. Wegman, MD, MSc, is a physician epidemiologist engaged for 45 years in public health research and practice on the health and safety of working people. He is Professor Emeritus, Department of Work Environment, University of Massachusetts Lowell, and Adjunct Professor, Harvard T.H. Chan School of Public Health. He previously served on the faculty of the UCLA School of Public Health. Dr. Wegman currently directs chronic kidney disease research in Central America. He serves as Vice-President of the Alpha Foundation for Improvement of Mine Safety and Health. In addition, he consults to the Occupational Health Surveillance Program of the Massachusetts Department of Public Health and serves on committees and two boards of the National Academies of Sciences, Engineering, and Medicine.

Sherry L. Baron, MD, MPH, is a Professor of Occupational and Environmental Health at the Barry Commoner Center for Health and the Environment and the Department of Urban Studies at Queens College of the City University of New York (CUNY). She is also an affiliated faculty member of the CUNY Graduate School of Public Health and Health Policy. She previously worked for 25 years as a medical epidemiologist at the National Institute for Occupational Safety and Health (NIOSH) and served as the NIOSH coordinator for occupational health disparities. Her current interests focus on performing research on the intersection of work and health for low-wage and immigrant workers and on developing community-based programs to improve health.

Rosemary K. Sokas, MD, MOH, is Professor and Immediate Past Chair, Department of Human Science of the School of Nursing and Health Studies at Georgetown University. She has previously served on the faculty of the University of Pennsylvania and the George Washington University schools of medicine and the University of Illinois at Chicago School of Public Health, where she directed the Division of Environmental and Occupational Health Sciences. She has served as Associate Director for Science at NIOSH and directed the Office of Occupational Medicine of the Occupational Safety and Health Administration. Her research interests include occupational health disparities, evaluation of intervention effectiveness, and participatory action research among high-risk, low-wage workers.

Contributors

Aaron Aber, BS
University of Maryland
aaronjaber@gmail.com

Dean B. Baker, MD, MPH
Professor of Medicine, Epidemiology,
    and Public Health
Center for Occupational and
    Environmental Health
University of California, Irvine
Irvine, CA
dbaker@uci.edu

Stephen S. Bao, PhD, CPE, CCPE
Senior Epidemiologist
Washington State Department of Labor
    & Industries
Olympia, WA
baos235@lni.wa.gov

Sherry L. Baron, MD, MPH
Professor of Occupational and
    Environmental Health
Barry Commoner Center for Health and
    the Environment
Department of Urban Studies
Queens College
City University of New York
New York, NY
Sherry.Baron@qc.cuny.edu

Bruce P. Bernard, MD, MPH
Captain, U.S. Public Health Service
Chief Medical Officer
Hazard Evaluations and Technical
    Assistance Branch
National Institute for Occupational
    Safety and Health
Cincinnati, OH
bpb4@cdc.gov

Margit L. Bleecker, MD, PhD
Director
Center for Occupational and
    Environmental Neurology
Baltimore, MD

David C. Byrne, PhD
Research Audiologist
Captain, U.S. Public Health Service
National Institute for Occupational
    Safety and Health
Cincinnati, OH
zne2@cdc.gov

John Cardarelli II, PhD, CHP, CIH, PE
Captain, U.S. Public Health Service
Health Physicist
Environmental Protection Agency
CBRN Consequence Management
    Advisory Team
Erlanger, KY
Cardarelli.John@epa.gov

Dawn N. Castillo, MPH
Director
Division of Safety Research
National Institute for Occupational
    Safety and Health
Morgantown, WV
dnc0@cdc.gov

Jennifer M. Cavallari, ScD, CIH
Assistant Professor, Community
    Medicine and Health Care
Department of Community Medicine
University of Connecticut School of
    Medicine
Farmington, CT
cavallari@uchc.edu

Martin G. Cherniack, MD, MPH
Professor of Medicine
University of Connecticut School of
    Medicine
Farmington, CT
cherniack@uchc.edu

BongKyoo Choi, ScD, MPH
Assistant Professor
Center for Occupational and
    Environmental Health
Environmental Health Sciences
    Graduate Program
School of Medicine
University of California, Irvine
Irvine, CA
b.choi@uci.edu

David C. Christiani, MD, MPH, MS
Director
Environmental and Occupational
    Medicine and Epidemiology Program
Harvard T. H. Chan School of
    Public Health
Professor of Medicine
Harvard Medical School
Boston, MA
dchris@hsph.harvard.edu

Sadie Costello, PhD
Assistant Researcher
Environmental Health Sciences Division
School of Public Health
University of California, Berkeley
Berkeley, CA
sadie@berkeley.edu

Maryann M. D'Alessandro, PhD
Director, National Personal Protective
    Technology Laboratory
National Institute for Occupational
    Safety and Health
Pittsburgh, PA
bpj5@cdc.gov

Juan C. Dapena, MD
Undersea Medical Officer
U.S. Navy
Silverdale, WA
juan.dapena@navy.mil

Gary A. Davis
Davis & Whitlock, PC
Asheville, NC
gadavis@enviroattorney.com

Letitia Davis, ScD
Former Director
Occupational Health Surveillance
    Program
Massachusetts Department of
    Public Health
Cambridge, MA
Lkdavis49@gmail.com

Lisa Delaney, MS, CIH
Associate Director for Emergency
  Preparedness and Response
National Institute for Occupational
  Safety and Health
Atlanta, GA
lkd2@cdc.gov

Denny Dobbin, MSc, CIH
Chapel Hill, NC
rddobbin@att.net

Marnie Dobson, PhD
Assistant Adjunct Professor
Center for Occupational and
  Environmental Health
School of Medicine
University of California, Irvine
Irvine, CA
mdobson@uci.edu

Ellen A. Eisen, ScD
Professor and Head
Environmental Health Sciences Division
School of Public Health
University of California, Berkeley
Berkeley, CA
eeisen@berkeley.edu

Bradley Evanoff, MD, MPH
Richard and Elizabeth Henby Sutter
  Professor of Occupational and
  Environmental Medicine
Director
Division of General Medical Sciences
School of Medicine
Washington University
St. Louis, MO
bevanoff@wustl.edu

Jeffrey J. Fadrowski, MD, MHS
Associate Professor of Pediatrics
Associate Pediatric Residency Program
  Director
Division of Pediatric Nephrology
Johns Hopkins University School of
  Medicine
Baltimore, MD
jfadrow1@jhmi.edu

Jeffery A. Foran, PhD
Professor and Chair
Department of Environmental Studies
California State University, Sacramento
Sacramento, CA
jeffery.foran@csus.edu

Linda M. Frazier, MD, MPH
Philadelphia, PA
Lfrazier151@comcast.net

**Deborah Barkin Fromer, MT
  (ASCP), MPH**
New York, NY
db.fromer@gmail.com

Michael Gochfeld, MD, PhD
Professor Emeritus
Clinical Research and Occupational
  Medicine
Environmental and Occupational
  Health Sciences Institute
Rutgers University
Piscataway, NJ
mg930@eohsi.rutgers.edu

Amaryl Griggs
Undergraduate in Environmental
  Studies
California State University, Sacramento
Sacramento, CA
amarylgriggs@csus.edu

Carisa Harris-Adamson, PhD, CPE
Assistant Professor
Department of Medicine
University of California, San Francisco
Director
UCSF/UCB Ergonomics Research &
  Graduate Training Program
Richmond, CA
Carisa.Harris-Adamson@ucsf.edu

Craig W. Hedberg, PhD
Division of Environmental Health
  Sciences
School of Public Health
University of Minnesota
Minneapolis, MN
hedbe005@umn.edu

Mauricio Hernández-Ávila, MD, MPH, PhD
Dean
National Institute of Public Health
   of Mexico
Cuernavaca, Morelos, Mexico
mhernan@insp.mx

Bernard G. Jaar, MD, MPH
Assistant Professor
Division of Nephrology
Department of Medicine
Johns Hopkins School of Medicine
Welch Center for Prevention,
   Epidemiology and Clinical Research
Johns Hopkins Medical Institutions
Baltimore, MD
bjaar@jhmi.edu

Richard J. Jackson, MD, MPH
Berkeley, CA
dickjackson@ucla.edu

Peter W. Johnson, PhD
Professor
Department of Environmental and
   Occupational Health Sciences
University of Washington
Seattle, WA
petej@uw.edu

W. Monroe Keyserling, PhD
Professor
Departments of Industrial and
   Operations Engineering and
   Environmental Health Science
University of Michigan
Ann Arbor, MI
wmkeyser@umich.edu

Ann M. Krake, MS, REHS, CSP
Captain, U.S. Public Health Service
Chief, Safety and Occupational Health
U.S. Army Corps of Engineers—
   Northwestern Division
Portland, OR
Ann.M.Krake@usace.army.mil

Anthony D. LaMontagne, ScD, MA, MEd
Professor of Work, Health & Wellbeing
Director, Centre for Population Health
   Research
School of Health & Social Development
Deakin University
Melbourne, Australia
tony.lamontagne@deakin.edu.au

Philip J. Landrigan, MD, MSc
Dean for Global Health
Professor of Pediatrics and
   Environmental Medicine
Icahn School of Medicine at Mount Sinai
New York, NY
philip.landrigan@mssm.edu

Paul A. Landsbergis, PhD, EdD, MPH
Associate Professor
Department of Environmental and
   Occupational Health Sciences
School of Public Health
SUNY Downstate Medical Center
Brooklyn, NY
paul.landsbergis@downstate.edu

Robert Laumbach, MD, MPH, CIH
Associate Professor
Department of Environmental and
   Occupational Health
Rutgers School of Public Health
Environmental and Occupational
   Health Sciences Institute
Piscataway, NJ
laumbach@eohsi.rutgers.edu

Barry S. Levy, MD, MPH
Adjunct Professor
Department of Public Health and
   Community Medicine
Tufts University School of Medicine
Sherborn, MA
blevy@igc.org

Amy K. Liebman, MPA, MA
Director
Environmental and Occupational Health
Migrant Clinicians Network
Salisbury, MD
aliebman@migrantclinician.org

Jane A. Lipscomb, PhD, RN
Professor
School of Nursing
University of Maryland
Baltimore, MD
lipscomb151@gmail.com

Boris D. Lushniak, MD
Dean and Professor
School of Public Health
University of Maryland
College Park, MD
lushniak@umd.edu

John May, MD
Jane Forbes Clark Professor of Clinical
    Medicine and Epidemiology
Columbia University
Research Scientist
Bassett Healthcare Network
Cooperstown, NY
john.may@bassett.org

John D. Meeker, ScD, CIH
Professor
Environmental Health Sciences
Associate Dean for Research
School of Public Health
University of Michigan
Ann Arbor, MI
meekerj@umich.edu

Thais C. Morata, PhD
Coordinator
NORA Manufacturing Sector Council
National Institute for Occupational
    Safety and Health
Cincinnati, OH
tcm2@cdc.gov

Crystal M. North, MD
Division of Pulmonary and Critical
    Care Medicine
Massachusetts General Hospital
Boston, MA
cnorth@mgh.harvard.edu

Marie S. O'Neill, PhD
Associate Professor
Departments of Environmental Health
    Sciences and Epidemiology
School of Public Health
University of Michigan
Ann Arbor, MI
marieo@umich.edu

Jonathan A. Patz, MD, MPH
Director
Global Health Institute
Professor
Nelson Institute
Center for Sustainability and the Global
    Environment (SAGE)
Department of Population Health
    Sciences
University of Wisconsin – Madison
Madison, WI
patz@wisc.edu

John Piacentino, MD, MPH
Associate Director for Science
National Institute for Occupational
    Safety and Health
Washington, DC
gjt4@cdc.gov

Timothy J. Pizatella, MS
Deputy Director
Division of Safety Research
National Institute for Occupational
    Safety and Health
Morgantown, WV
tjp2@cdc.gov

Jorma H. Rantanen, MD, PhD
Professor
Director General Emeritus
Finnish Institute of Occupational Health
Visiting Scientist
Department of Public Health/
    Occupational Health
University of Helsinki
Helsinki, Finland
jorma.h.rantanen@gmail.com

Dori B. Reissman, MD, MPH
Associate Administrator
World Trade Center Health Program
National Institute for Occupational
   Safety and Health
Captain, U.S. Public Health Service
Washington, DC
dvs7@cdc.gov

Horacio Riojas-Rodríguez, MD, PhD
Director of Environmental
   Health
National Institute of Public Health
   of Mexico
Cuernavaca, Morelos, Mexico
hriojas@insp.mx

Cora Roelofs, ScD
CR Research/Consulting
Boston, MA
cora_roelofs@uml.edu

Bonnie Rogers, DrPH
Director
North Carolina Occupational Safety
   and Health Education and Research
   Center and Occupational Health
   Nursing Program
UNC Gillings School of Public Health
The University of North Carolina at
   Chapel Hill
Chapel Hill, NC
Rogersb@email.unc.edu

Isabelle Romieu, MD, MPH, ScD
Montpellier, France
iromieu@gmail.com

Kenneth D. Rosenman, MD
Chief of the Division of Occupational
   and Environmental Medicine
Professor of Medicine
Michigan State University
East Lansing, MI
Ken.Rosenman@hc.msu.edu

Mark Russi, MD, MPH
Medical Director
Wellness and Employee
   Population Health
Yale-New Haven Health System
Professor
Medicine and Epidemiology
Yale University
New Haven, CT

Peter Schnall, MD, MPH
Clinical Professor of Medicine
Center for Occupational and
   Environmental Health
University of California, Irvine
Irvine, CA
pschnall@workhealth.org

Ken Silver, DSc, SM
Associate Professor of
   Environmental Health
Department of Environmental Health
East Tennessee State University
Johnson City, TN
silver@mail.etsu.edu

Rosemary K. Sokas, MD, MOH
Professor and Immediate Past Chair
Department of Human Science
School of Nursing and Health Studies
Georgetown University
Washington, DC
sokas@georgetown.edu

Kerry Souza, ScD, MPH
Epidemiologist
Division of Surveillance, Hazard
   Evaluations, and Field Studies
National Institute for Occupational
   Safety and Health
Washington, DC
ksouza@cdc.gov

Emily A. Spieler, JD
Hadley Professor of Law
Northeastern University
Boston, MA
e.spieler@neu.edu

Nancy A. Stout, EdD
Morgantown, WV
nancystout@comcast.net

Loren C. Tapp, MD, MS
Medical Officer
Hazard Evaluations and Technical
    Assistance Branch
National Institute for Occupational
    Safety and Health
Cincinnati, OH
let7@cdc.gov

Gregory R. Wagner, MD
Department of Environmental Health
Harvard T.H. Chan School of
    Public Health
Boston, MA
Gwagner@hsph.harvard.edu

Elizabeth Ward, PhD
Former Senior Vice President,
    Intramural Research
American Cancer Society
Atlanta, GA
eward04@gmail.com

Virginia M. Weaver, MD, MPH
Associate Professor
Departments of Environmental Health
    and Engineering and Medicine
Associate Faculty Member
Welch Center for Prevention
    Epidemiology and Clinical Research
Bloomberg School of Public Health
Johns Hopkins University
Baltimore, MD
vweaver1@jhu.edu

David H. Wegman, MD, MSc
Professor Emeritus
Department of Work Environment
University of Massachusetts Lowell
Adjunct Professor
Harvard T.H. Chan School of
    Public Health
Cambridge, MA
David_Wegman@uml.edu

Laura S. Welch, MD
Medical Director
CPWR—The Center for Construction
    Research and Training
Silver Spring, MD
lwelch@cpwr.com

Gavin H. West, MPH
Research Analyst
CPWR—The Center for Construction
    Research and Training
Silver Spring, MD
gwest@cpwr.com

Sacoby Wilson, PhD, MS
Assistant Professor
Director, Community Engagement,
    Environmental Justice, and Health
Maryland Institute for Applied
    Environmental Health
School of Public Health
University of Maryland – College Park
College Park, MD
swilson2@umd.edu

Disclaimer

Authors' statements are independent of the institutions, agencies, or organizations with which they are affiliated.

Frequently Used Abbreviations

ANSI	American National Standards Institute
ATSDR	Agency for Toxic Substances and Disease Registry
BLL	blood lead level
BLS	Bureau of Labor Statistics
CDC	Centers for Disease Control and Prevention
CFOI	Census of Fatal Occupational Injuries
CT	computed tomography
EPA	Environmental Protection Agency
IARC	International Agency for Research on Cancer
ILO	International Labour Organization
IPCC	Intergovernmental Panel on Climate Change
ISO	International Organization for Standardization
MRI	magnetic resonance imaging
MSHA	Mine Safety and Health Administration
NCEH	National Center for Environmental Health
NIEHS	National Institute of Environmental Health Sciences
NIH	National Institutes of Health
NIOSH	National Institute for Occupational Safety and Health
NTP	National Toxicology Program
OSHA	Occupational Safety and Health Administration
PEL	permissible exposure limit
ppb	parts per billion
PPE	personal protective equipment
ppm	parts per million
REL	recommended exposure limit
SDS	safety data sheet
STEL	short-term exposure limit
TLV®	Threshold Limit Value
TWA	time-weighted average, usually averaged over an 8-hour work shift
WHO	World Health Organization

SECTION I
INTRODUCTION

1

Occupational and Environmental Health Challenges and Opportunities

Barry S. Levy, David H. Wegman, Sherry L. Baron, and Rosemary K. Sokas

Occupational and environmental health comprises the recognition, diagnosis, treatment, and prevention of illnesses, injuries, and other adverse health conditions resulting from hazardous environmental exposures in the workplace, the home, and the community. Multidisciplinary in nature, occupational and environmental health is a component of both clinical care and public health.

THE WIDE SPECTRUM OF CHALLENGING SITUATIONS

There are many challenging situations for occupational and environmental health, as illustrated by the following examples:

A 2-year-old girl, during a routine well-child checkup, is found to have an elevated blood lead level of 20 μg/dL. As part of her care and to prevent further adverse effects of lead, what needs to be done to determine if the source of the lead is deteriorating lead-containing paint in her home, the water supply in her community, or her father's work in a smelter?

A pregnant woman, who works as a laboratory technician, is regularly exposed to organic solvents at work. Should her nurse-midwife recommend that she change her job because of this exposure? How should the nurse-midwife address other toxic exposures, such as mercury in the fish that this woman regularly eats?

The wife of an asbestos-exposed pipefitter develops a pleural mesothelioma. How likely is it that this disease was caused by her washing her husband's dusty workclothes for many years? Can she or her family receive any compensation from her husband's employer or the companies that manufactured the asbestos to which they were exposed?

An oncologist observes an unusual cluster of 10 bladder cancer cases in a small town. To whom should she report this observation? Should she request an investigation to determine if some or all of these cases were due to a hazardous exposure that should be controlled?

Several members of a family, who live a half-mile from a hazardous waste site, smell odors from the site and report that they are experiencing headaches, dizziness, nausea, and other symptoms. As their primary care physician, what should you do?

The owner of a small nail salon is concerned about the possible health effects of chemicals used there. Where can she obtain helpful information and other resources?

These are but a few of the many occupational and environmental health challenges facing health-care practitioners, all of whom need to recognize and help prevent occupational and environmental health problems.

Many hazardous exposures occur simultaneously in the workplace and the ambient environment, including in the following situations:

- Contamination of ambient air and surface water near a chemical factory, whose workers are also exposed to hazardous substances
- Application by agricultural workers of pesticides that may contaminate surface water and groundwater
- Inadvertent transport of lead, asbestos, and other hazardous substances from the workplace to home on workers' clothes, shoes, skin, and hair.

While the workplace and the ambient environment present many hazards, as reflected throughout this book, they also provide many benefits that potentially contribute to health and well-being. The workplace provides opportunities for people to advance their knowledge and skills, contribute to society, and financially support themselves and their families. The environment provides opportunities for exploration and learning, recreation and relaxation, and communing with nature and appreciating the ecological context in which we live.

EVOLUTION OF OCCUPATIONAL HEALTH AND ENVIRONMENTAL HEALTH

Occupational health and environmental health evolved along separate—but often related—tracks. Hippocrates recognized the importance of air quality for health, although he was concerned only with the few Greeks who were "citizens"—not for the slaves or the free workers who supported them. Pliny the Elder recognized the ill effects of lead on slaves who painted ships in the Roman Empire in the first century A.D.; however, the use of lead in making cookware, sweetening foods, and souring vintages has persisted for 2,000 years. Occupational hazards were not addressed systematically until 1700, when Bernardino Ramazzini, an Italian physician, published *De Morbis Artificum Diatriba* (*On the Diseases of Workers*). Evolution of these related fields continued in the 20th century. Starting in the 1920s, Alice Hamilton, an American physician and colleague of the social reformer Jane Addams, pioneered occupational health as a specialty of public health and preventive medicine. In the 1960s, Rachel Carson, an American biologist and ecologist, focused public attention on the wide impact of hazardous agricultural chemicals in her landmark book, *Silent Spring*.

During the past 50 years, extraordinary developments in science, technology, legislation, public health, and social empowerment have led to much progress in both occupational health and environmental health. During this period, there have been more frequent interactions between these two fields and increasing recognition of fundamental areas of overlap in occupational and environmental health research as well as in community- and workplace-based interventions.

Historically, knowledge about adverse health effects of toxic environmental exposures in people has primarily resulted from research on occupational exposures. Workers have been more intensely exposed to specific known hazards than community residents and may have been exposed in the same workplaces throughout their work careers. By contrast, nonoccupational exposures to community residents have been more difficult to characterize and track, and individuals move from one community to another. Although community exposures are generally lower than occupational exposures, they occur throughout the day and night, rather than being confined to work shifts. In addition, community exposures may affect people who are too young, too old, too sick, or too disabled to work. And community exposures may include different routes of exposure than occupational exposures. Therefore, scientific findings from occupational health research alone cannot protect the general population from environmental exposures.

THE U.S. WORKFORCE

Table 1-1 lists the numbers of workers on nonfarm payrolls in the United States by major

Table 1-1. Employees on Nonfarm Payrolls by Major Industry Sector, Seasonally Adjusted, United States, May 2017

Industry Sector	Size of Workforce (in millions)
Services	65.2
Professional and business services	20.6
Educational services	3.6
Healthcare and social assistance	19.4
Leisure and hospitality	15.9
Other services	5.7
Government	22.3
Wholesale and retail trade	21.7
Manufacturing	12.4
Financial activities	8.4
Construction	6.9
Transportation and warehousing	5.1
Information	2.7
Mining and logging	0.7
Utilities	0.6
Total	146.1

Source: Bureau of Labor Statistics, U.S. Department of Labor. Available at: http://www.bls.gov/news.release/empsit.t17.htm. Accessed June 20, 2017.

industry sector. In recent decades in the United States, the percentage of workers in the manufacturing sector (Figure 1-1) has decreased and the percentage of workers in the service sector (Figure 1-2) has increased. This change means that occupational health practitioners are responding to a different mix of hazards and resultant illnesses and injuries. For example, the increasing number of workers in healthcare are more likely to face biological hazards (Chapter 13) compared to manufacturing workers.

CATEGORIES OF HAZARDS

Occupational and environmental hazards can be categorized as:

1. *Safety hazards*, which result in injuries through the uncontrolled transfer of energy to vulnerable recipients from sources such as electrical, thermal, kinetic, chemical, or radiation energy. Examples include unsafe playground equipment; loaded firearms in the home; causes of motor-vehicle or bicycle crashes; unprotected electrical sources and equipment; work at heights without fall protection; cluttered homes, leading to slips, trips, and falls; unguarded machinery in operation; and work in unshored trenches. (See Chapter 19.)

2. *Health hazards*, which result in acute illnesses or chronic disorders (Chapters 20 through 28):

   a. *Chemical hazards*, including heavy metals, such as lead and mercury; pesticides; organic solvents, such as benzene and trichloroethylene; and many other chemicals. Since 1979, approximately 85,000 chemicals have been, at some point, in commercial use in the United States;[1] however, the vast majority have not been adequately tested for adverse health effects.[2] (See Chapter 11.)

   b. *Physical hazards*, such as excessive noise, vibration, extremes of temperature and pressure, and ionizing and nonionizing radiation. (See Chapters 12A through 12D.)

   c. *Biomechanical hazards*, such as heavy lifting and repetitive or forceful movements, that cause musculoskeletal disorders, such as chronic low back pain and carpal tunnel syndrome (Figure 1-3). (See Chapters 8 and 20.)

   d. *Biological hazards*, such as hepatitis B virus and hepatitis C virus, the tubercle bacillus, and many other microorganisms that may be transmitted through direct contact, air, water, or food (Figure 1-4). (See Chapter 13.)

   e. *Psychosocial hazards*, including (i) socioeconomic stressors, such as discrimination, income inequality, migration or immigration status, and unemployment, and (ii) job and organizational stressors, such as excessive demands on and low control by workers, job insecurity, and inadequate job training and retraining opportunities (Figures 1-5 and 1-6). (See Chapter 14.)

MAGNITUDE OF PROBLEMS

Occupational and environmental disorders occur frequently, but the accuracy of morbidity and mortality data varies widely. For example,

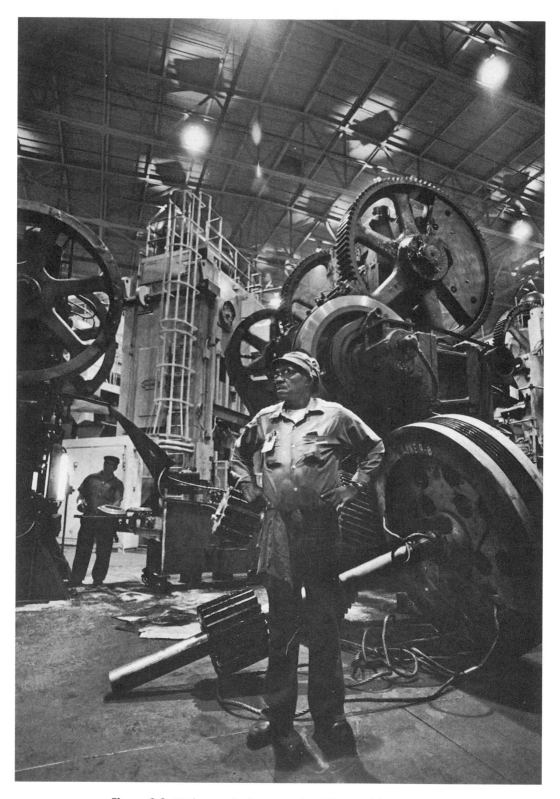

Figure 1-1. Worker at a wheel stamping plant. (Photograph by Earl Dotter.)

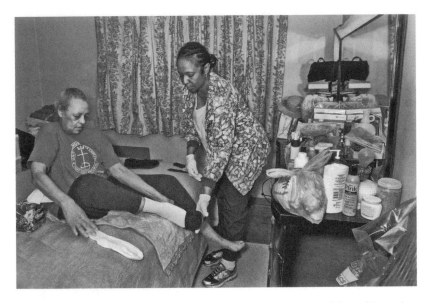

Figure 1-2. Home care worker with homebound patient. (Photograph by Earl Dotter.)

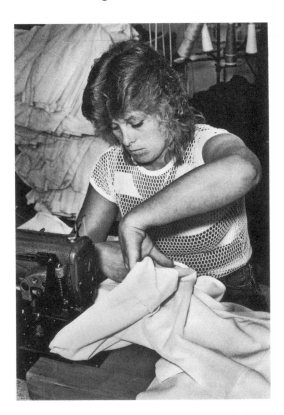

Figure 1-3. Garment workers are at increased risk of musculoskeletal disorders. (Photograph by Earl Dotter.)

Occupational Injuries and Illnesses

Mandated systems for counting injuries and illnesses at work offer some estimates of the adverse health impacts of employment. These systems provide useful information on trends, but generally not accurate information on magnitude because of underreporting.[3,4] (See Chapter 6.) In the United States in 2015, government reporting systems indicated that 4,836 workers died from occupational injuries—on average, about 13 a day—the highest number since 2008.[5] These systems also estimated that approximately 50,000 workers die from work-related illnesses each year—although this estimate was based on very limited data.[6,7] In 2015, employers reported approximately 2.9 million nonfatal workplace injuries and illnesses in private industry (3.0 cases per 100 equivalent full-time workers) and 722,000 in state and local government; about half of injured workers took time away from work or were transferred or placed on work restrictions.[8] In 2015, an estimated 2.7 million workers were treated in emergency departments for work-related injuries, resulting in 113,000 in-patient hospital admissions.[9] (See Chapter 19.) In low- and middle-income countries (LMICs), the rates of fatal and nonfatal occupational injuries and illnesses have been much higher than in the United States. (See Chapter 35.)

population-based data on fatal injuries are generally thought to be more accurate than data on chronic occupational and environmental illnesses.

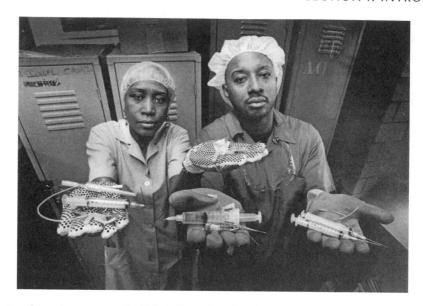

Figure 1-4. Laundry workers are exposed to biological hazards, such as sharps in soiled bed linens. (Photograph by Earl Dotter.)

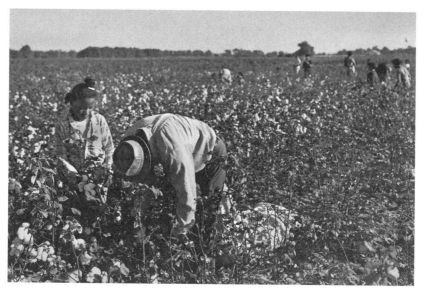

Figure 1-5. Migrant workers picking cotton face many challenges because of their minority status, poverty, inadequate education, and lack of information on and inadequate control over the agrochemicals to which they are exposed. (Photograph by Earl Dotter.)

Work-related injuries and illnesses are costly. In 2014, employers in the United States spent an estimated $91.8 billion on workers' compensation insurance costs.[10] However, this amount represents only part of all work-related injury and illness costs borne by employers, workers, and society overall—largely because the costs of many injuries and most illnesses are shifted to other health insurance systems. Thousands of workers become temporarily or permanently disabled from work-related injuries in the United States each day, but only a small percentage of them receives workers' compensation.

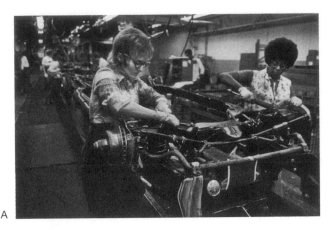
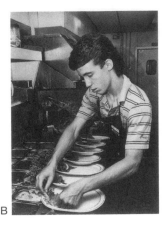

A   B

Figure 1-6. Workers exposed to occupational stressors, such as fast-paced work, include (A) assembly-line workers, and (B) short-order cooks. (Photographs by Earl Dotter.)

Table 1-2. Subjects of Environmental Health Objectives for 2020, United States

Subjects	Subtopics
Outdoor Air Quality	Air Quality Index
	Alternative modes of transportation for work
	Airborne toxins
Water Quality	Safe drinking water
	Waterborne disease outbreaks
	Water conservation
	Safety of beaches for swimming
Toxics and Waste	Elevated blood lead levels in children
	Risks posed by hazardous waste sites
	Pesticide exposures
	Toxic pollutants released into the environment
	Recycling of municipal solid waste
Healthy Homes and Healthy Communities	Indoor allergens
	Radon mitigation
	School policies to promote healthy and safe physical school environments
	Lead-based paint and related hazards
	Housing with physical problems
Infrastructure and Surveillance	Exposure to heavy metals, pesticides, and other hazardous chemicals in the environment
	Information systems for environmental health
	Monitoring for environmentally related diseases
Global Environmental Health	Global burden of disease due to poor water quality, sanitation, and insufficient hygiene

Source: Available at: https://www.healthypeople.gov/2020/topics-objectives/topic/environmental-health. Accessed January 2, 2017.

Environmental Health Hazards

The scope of environmental health hazards is broad, as partially reflected in the subjects of the environmental health objectives for the United States for 2020 (Table 1-2).

Outdoor air pollution remains a widespread environmental and public health problem, causing chronic impairment of the respiratory and cardiovascular systems, cancer, and premature death (Figure 1-7; see also Chapter 15). The Environmental Protection Agency (EPA), under the provisions of the Clean Air Act, set health-based standards (the National Ambient Air Quality Standards) for six "criteria air pollutants": particulate matter, ground-level ozone,

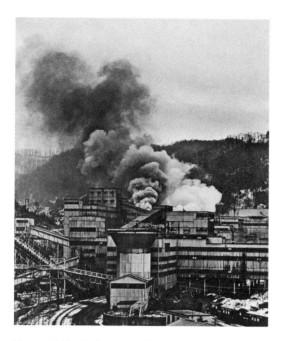

Figure 1-7. Outdoor air pollution from a coal-cleaning plant. (Photograph by Earl Dotter.)

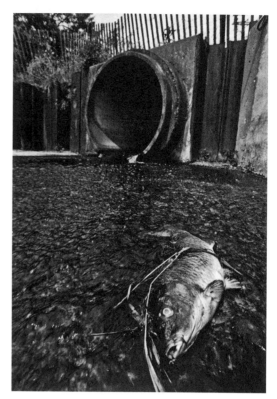

Figure 1-8. Water pollution from a plant that manufactured bleached white paper. (Photograph by Earl Dotter.)

sulfur dioxide, lead, nitrogen dioxide, and carbon monoxide. More than 100 million people in the United States reside in "nonattainment areas," locations that do not meet one or more of these standards.[11] Motor vehicles and electrical power plants account for much ambient air pollution.

Water quality continues to be a problem from both point sources, such as industrial sites, and nonpoint sources, such as agricultural runoff (Figure 1-8; see also Chapter 16). Toxic and hazardous substances, in addition to posing health problems for exposed workers, may also cause health problems to people exposed where they live and elsewhere. Hydraulic fracturing (fracking) to release petroleum and natural gas from shale, a process that is increasingly used in the United States to enhance the energy supply, is also raising concerns about water quality. Other concerns about fracking include noise from the extraction process, increased heavy equipment traffic, increased frequency of earthquakes, and the adverse impact of continued reliance on fossil fuels on global climate change.

Children are at increased risk for many environmental health problems because (a) their neurological and other systems are still in development, (b) they absorb substances and metabolize them differently than adults, and (c) they may be at risk for increased exposure from hand-to-mouth activity or improper storage of chemicals. (See Chapter 30.) Other environmental health hazards include poor indoor air quality (Chapter 15), lead-based paint (Figure 1-9), lead-contaminated drinking water, household cleaning products, mold, radon, and electrical and fire hazards. Many environmental hazards are present in homes; for example, over 90% of toxic exposures reported to poison control centers in the United States occur in the home environment.

Environmental Illnesses and Injuries

There are fewer data on the occurrence of environmental disorders than occupational disorders. For some environmentally related disorders in the United States, such as childhood lead poisoning, there are extensive data from screening

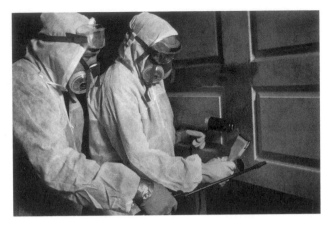

Figure 1-9. Lead abatement workers. (Photograph by Earl Dotter.)

programs, which in 2015 showed that 11,681 (0.5%) of the 2.4 million tested children under 6 years of age had blood lead levels (BLLs) that were 10 μg/dL or higher, and 79,955 (3.3%) had BLLs that were 5 μg/dL or higher.[12] However, since most of those tested were likely at elevated risk of lead exposure, these results cannot be projected to estimate the total U.S. burden of excessive lead exposure on children. Data on pesticide poisoning are very limited; many cases go unreported because of the nonspecificity of symptoms and occurrence of pesticide poisoning not related to agriculture. In 2014 in California, the state with the most extensive reporting system for pesticide poisoning, 74% of the 1,073 reported cases were due to non-agricultural pesticide use.[13]

In contrast, there are extensive data available to estimate the numbers of acute injuries in the home, on the road, and in other nonoccupational settings due to various causes, such as motor vehicles and firearms. In the United States in 2014, fatal unintentional injuries (135,928) were the fourth leading cause of death, accounting for 5.2% of deaths nationwide.[14,p.5] In 2014, there were 42,032 deaths due to unintentional poisoning, 33,736 motor vehicle traffic deaths, 31,959 unintentional fall deaths, and 461 unintentional firearm deaths (of a total of 33,594 firearm deaths).[14,p.87]

There is substantial respiratory morbidity and mortality related to outdoor and indoor air contaminants. In the United States in 2014, the prevalence of asthma in children was 8.6% and, in adults, 7.4%.[15] Environmental causes of asthma include outdoor air pollution, environmental tobacco smoke, and many allergens, including those disproportionately associated with substandard housing, such as mold and cockroach antigen (Chapter 22).

Under-recognition or Underreporting of Illnesses and Injuries

Many occupational and environmental health problems escape detection because of several factors (Figure 1-10):

1. Many problems do not come to the attention of health professionals, employers, and others and therefore are not included in data collection systems. A worker or community resident may not recognize a health problem as being occupationally or environmentally related; some workers may be afraid of possible retaliation and job loss if they recognize or report an occupational illness or injury. Educating workers and community residents about hazards, such as with workplace and community-based right-to-know programs, helps to improve recognition of disorders caused by occupational or environmental exposures. Although federal regulations prohibit retaliation against workers for reporting hazards or outcomes, rigorous enforcement of these regulations depends, in part, on labor unions and other worker advocacy organizations.

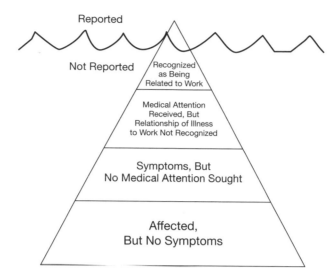

Figure 1-10. Most occupational and environmental disorders are below the surface.

2. Many health problems that *do* come to the attention of physicians, employers, and others are not recognized as occupationally and environmentally related. Recognition of occupational and environmental disorders is often difficult because of the long period between initial exposure and onset of symptoms (or time of diagnosis), making cause-and-effect relationships difficult to determine in groups or individuals. Recognition is also difficult because many people are exposed to multiple occupational and environmental hazards.

3. Some health problems that *are* recognized by health professionals, employees, or others as occupationally or environmentally related are not reported because the association with the workplace or other environments is not certain or because reporting requirements are not enforced. For example, only a few states require that physicians report cases of pesticide poisoning. (See Chapter 6.) One approach to address this problem at the federal level has been providing public access to information.

In addition, many occupational and environmental health problems that *are* reported are not adequately investigated and controlled because

of limited resources, inadequate development and enforcement of regulations, and opposition by those who are legally and/or financially responsible for the development and/or persistence of these problems.

CONTEXT

Occupational and environmental health problems can be understood in social, ecological, economic, political, and historical contexts. Those whose actions determine the broader structural context include workers, employers, representatives of business and labor organizations, community residents, members of environmental nongovernmental organizations, officials of government agencies and international organizations, educators and trainers, researchers, journalists, and representatives of foundations. These "actors" play multiple roles, rely on various sources of power and support, have specific strengths and vulnerabilities, and engage in complex sets of interactions with each other in multiple ways. Health and safety professionals and many other actors are engaged in the recognition, assessment, treatment, and prevention of occupational and environmental health problems within this broad context.

RECOGNITION AND PREVENTION

The first and most important step in diagnosis and treatment of an occupational or environmental illness or injury is the recognition that it is potentially caused by an occupational or environmental exposure. Recognition focuses both on (a) detecting occupational and environmental illnesses and injuries in symptomatic and asymptomatic individuals (Chapter 4), and (b) conducting public health surveillance in populations to detect individual cases and overall trends of illness and injury (Chapter 6).

Prevention consists of:

- *Primary prevention*: Preventing illnesses and injuries before they occur
- *Secondary prevention*: Identifying and treating health problems as early as possible, often before symptoms have developed or permanent impairment has occurred
- *Tertiary prevention*: Implementing interventions to arrest the progress of established diseases, injuries, or their consequences, including disability.

A useful paradigm to identifying opportunities for prevention and designing preventive measures is the public health model of host, agent, and environment. First, some preventive measures focus on a host or hosts—workers or community residents; these measures include education and training, providing immunizations or post-exposure prophylaxis, monitoring personal exposures, screening for early detection of disease, and use of personal protective equipment. Second, some preventive measures focus on the agent (hazard), such as an asbestos-containing product, and restricting or banning its production or use in order to reduce exposure. And third, some preventive measures focus on the environment, including engineering measures, such as local exhaust ventilation to remove airborne hazards in the workplace, placement of sound-barrier walls alongside highways to reduce noise in adjacent neighborhoods, and urban planning to create more green space or bicycle lanes. (See Chapters 4 and 8.)

CHANGING NATURE OF WORK AND THE WORKFORCE

Major changes in work structure have occurred in recent years, including company mergers, automated production, and outsourcing. In the United States, there have been significant changes within industries. For example, within agriculture, the number of poultry, beef, and pork producers has decreased while the size of these producers has grown. The number of family farms has decreased while the number of concentrated animal feeding operations, with large-scale production and mechanized processes, has increased—causing concerns about exploitation of workers, animal welfare, environmental contamination from concentrated waste, and production of greenhouse gases. Meat packaging and poultry processing plants have relocated near large producers, and the demographics of their workers has typically been transformed from relatively highly paid, unionized, mostly white workers to immigrant Latino workers who face poor working conditions, receive low pay, change jobs often, and infrequently belong to labor unions. In addition, one-third of those working in meat-processing plants are contingent workers, who work for subcontracting agencies and perform such tasks as cleaning and maintenance. Although these workers often face occupational hazards, workers' compensation systems and Occupational Safety and Health Administration (OSHA) standards often fail to address their needs. Similarly, many unauthorized immigrants work under informal work arrangements or as day laborers—without adequate legal protection. Reliance on contingent workers and outsourced work occurs throughout the U.S. economy, from healthcare to manufacturing to information technology. (See Chapter 2.)

During the past four decades in the United States, there has been a shift in the economy, with many more jobs created in the service sector than in manufacturing. This shift has resulted from both transfer of manufacturing to LMICs and developments in engineering technology that have produced increased efficiencies within manufacturing. Advances in information technology and in automation and robotics have reduced the number of jobs in the service and manufacturing sectors that pay good wages and provide health benefits and paid leave. There are not enough worker training and retraining programs available to help displaced workers learn the skills that they need in order to find employment in higher-technology industries.[16]

Accompanying these changes have been changes in the nature of work due to the *fissured workplace*, in which businesses, including large corporations, are not serving as direct employers of their workers but rather subcontracting work to smaller companies where competition can be harsh and the quality of jobs is low. In doing so, these companies typically avoid paying appropriate benefits to workers and tend to ignore occupational health and safety.[17] These nonstandard work arrangements have profound impacts on worker health and safety.[18] The presence of multiple levels of this type of subcontracting creates confusion regarding which businesses or other entities are responsible for protecting the health and safety of workers. As a result, wages have been declining, benefits have been eroding, workplace health and safety have not been adequately protected, and income inequality has continued to widen. Other major changes have included an increased number of women working outside the home; therefore, there have been increased needs both for professionals in child care and elder care and service-sector workers, such as in fast-food restaurants. Women are working in many of the jobs created by these needs.[19]

Another development has been the aging of the workforce, in parallel with the aging of the U.S. population. This development has been coupled with changing patterns of retirement, partly due to changes in retirement benefits. In 2016, almost 20% of people 65 years of age and older were working—the highest proportion since before Medicare was enacted in 1965.[20] Older workers are living longer, needing income, often like their jobs, and are often appreciated by employers who recognize what older workers can offer. From a health and safety perspective, older workers bring experience and expertise to the job, but they have to accommodate or adjust to gradual physiological and cognitive changes that accompany aging, they may face age discrimination, and they sustain more severe outcomes when injuries occur.[21]

Specific needs that have arisen from the changing nature of work and the workforce include (a) integrating family health with work schedules, recognizing that work-related stresses extend to the home environment, and (b) accommodating workers who have significant skills but reduced physical capacity, visual acuity, or other impairments. Advances in healthcare have increased the numbers of workers with functional limitations who are able to contribute to society and have the right to work, a right protected by the Americans with Disabilities Act. All of the challenges posed by the changing nature of work and the workforce can be met by preventive measures that are supported by laws and regulations, employment policies, education and research, and public health and clinical practice. (See Chapters 2, 3, and 10.)

Advances in Technology

In addition to transforming the workplace through robotics, advances in technology have introduced new potentially hazardous substances, such as nanomaterials, that are contaminating the workplace and the ambient environment (Chapter 8). Technological innovation has also led to important advances in occupational and environmental health research. For example, new methods can facilitate identification of potential workplace hazards, including new and improved assays to determine the possible carcinogenicity of substances and to measure concentrations of hazardous substances or their metabolites in body fluids (Chapter 21). In addition, advances in technology have introduced potentially hazardous substances or their metabolites in body fluids.

Promoting a Healthy Workforce

Work-related factors, such as wages, hours of work, and access to paid or unpaid sick leave, in addition to hazardous and stressful work environments, impact the well-being of workers, their families, and their communities. Recently, there has been broader acknowledgement that the workplace can contribute to health problems in ways that were previously not recognized as "work-related," such as contributing to sleep disorders, cardiovascular disease, obesity, and anxiety and depression. The NIOSH Total Worker Health® Program is advancing research to create prevention recommendations that employers and others can use to develop workplace policies, programs, and practices that improve worker health and well-being.[22]

Occupational and Environmental Health Services and Primary Healthcare

Despite limited resources and infrastructure, some safety-net primary care providers are exploring ways to integrate occupational and environmental health services with primary medical care and with a broader range of public health services. Although some successes have been achieved with this approach, there remains much untapped potential in fully achieving this integration. Electronic health records (EHRs) provide new opportunities to integrate occupational health information. For example, through clinical decision support systems, EHRs can deliver specific information related to diagnosing occupational asthma and to managing work-related factors, such as shift work, that can present challenges to management of diabetes.

EVOLVING ROLES OF GOVERNMENT

Governmental regulatory and research agencies in occupational health and those in environmental health have evolved over decades, generally with limited connection between agencies in these two fields. With the passage of laws that established the Mine Safety and Health Administration in 1969 and OSHA and the EPA in 1970, the federal government took an active role in setting and enforcing standards for a safe and healthful workplace and a safe and healthful ambient environment. (See Chapter 3 and parts of Chapters 15 through 18.) After promulgation of standards (regulations) in the 1970s, legal and political challenges slowed the setting of new standards and federal budget cuts often limited enforcement of existing standards. To help accomplish their core missions, regulatory agencies engage in outreach and technical assistance, such as OSHA's free On-site Consultation Program for small businesses and its provision of small grants for health and safety training. Important responsibilities in occupational health and environmental health are assumed by state and local government agencies, which vary considerably in size, resources, and levels of activity. These agencies closely interact with their counterparts at the federal level.

There are separate federal research agencies in occupational health, including the National Institute for Occupational Safety and Health, the National Center for Environmental Health, the Agency for Toxic Substances and Disease Registry, and the National Institute of Environmental Health Sciences. The EPA's Office of Research and Development also supports and conducts environmental health research. Over time, research has broadened to include community-based participatory research, which addresses environmental justice and related issues.

LIABILITY

Some workers, barred from suing their employers under workers' compensation laws, have filed *third-party lawsuits* (product-liability lawsuits) as a means of redress for occupational disease associated with specific agents or technologies; some community residents exposed to environmental hazards have also filed similar lawsuits (Chapter 3). Although these lawsuits may direct more attention to prevention, this approach may be cumbersome and outcomes may not be equitable. In recent years, plaintiffs and their attorneys have found it increasingly difficult to recover damages in such lawsuits for a variety of reasons, including federal and state court decisions as well as state laws that have restricted expert testimony or otherwise limited these lawsuits.

ENVIRONMENTAL JUSTICE

Attention to environmental justice has grown, with the recognition that disparities in environmental exposures between high-income and low-income communities partially account for differences in health status among communities. The Environmental Justice Movement is comprised of organizations and people representing low-income and minority individuals who oppose placement of hazardous waste sites and polluting facilities in their communities. It has transformed the Environmental Movement from a campaign of middle-class people concerned about ecological issues to a grassroots movement of poor and working-class communities concerned mainly about preserving their health. Many environmental health professionals work with urban sociologists, economists, community activists, and others to develop programs to reduce or eliminate environmental disparities that contribute to health disparities. (See Chapter 2.)

THE BUILT ENVIRONMENT

Many people spend most of their time in or on "the built environment," which includes homes, offices, industrial facilities, schools, roadways, sidewalks, parks, and even vehicles. All of these environments can increase or reduce risks for injuries; acute illnesses, such as exacerbations of asthma; and chronic disorders, such as obesity and diabetes. These environments also shape social, economic, and psychological well- being. Designing environments to promote physical activity, including walking, climbing of stairs, bicycling, and other forms of active transport, is a documented tool for public health improvement. (See Chapter 34.)

CLIMATE CHANGE

Climate change—or, more accurately, global climate disruption—is creating profound environmental consequences and adverse health effects. Environmental consequences include warmer temperatures and longer, more frequent, and more severe heat waves; extremes of precipitation, leading to droughts and floods; and sea-level rise, leading to more storm surges, coastal erosion, and saltwater incursion onto farmland and into groundwater. Direct adverse health

effects include heat-related disorders; respiratory and allergic disorders; vector-borne, water-borne, and foodborne infectious diseases; and injuries from extreme weather events. Indirect adverse health effects arise from food insecurity, distress migration, and collective violence that may be caused, or contributed to, by climate change. All of these consequences of climate change can cause mental health problems, including anxiety, depression, and posttraumatic stress disorders. Within the United States, the impact of climate change is greater on poor communities and on other vulnerable populations. Globally, high-income countries, which emit the most greenhouse emissions, tend to suffer the least from the consequences of climate change, and LMICs, which emit far lower levels of greenhouse emissions, tend to suffer the most. (See Chapter 29.)

NEW DIRECTIONS FOR RESEARCH

While extensive research continues on possible associations between hazardous exposures and illness, injury, and premature death, researchers are broadening the focus to new areas, including:

- The social determinants of health, investigating how these factors impact the health of workers and community residents
- Engaging community members to evaluate prevention programs on problems such as lead poisoning, childhood asthma, and physical fitness.

Emerging fields of research are exploring how *beneficial* "exposures" at work or in the natural environment may produce specific beneficial outcomes:

- How personal interaction with the natural environment may be associated with improved health and well-being[23,24]
- How positive aspects of worksite organization, such as opportunities for training or supportive supervision, may be associated with positive outcomes, such as improved mental health or reduced cardiovascular mortality.[25,26]

ECONOMIC GLOBALIZATION

The growth of multinational corporations, reduction in trade barriers, and development of regional treaty arrangements, such as the North American Free Trade Agreement, and global organizations, such as the World Trade Organization, have had a substantial adverse impacts on occupational and environmental health. In many LMICs, multinational corporations have exploited workers by employing them in jobs that have low wages and few benefits, offer little or no training or upward mobility, and expose them to health and safety hazards. Some regional trade agreements have included occupational and environmental health protections that have generally been poorly implemented and inadequately monitored. (See Chapter 35.)

ADDITIONAL CHALLENGES FOR LMICs

Low- and middle-income countries, which comprise two-thirds of all countries and include the vast majority of people globally, face additional challenges, as described briefly next.

Export of Hazard

High-income countries often export their most hazardous industries, hazardous materials (such as banned or restricted pesticides), and hazardous wastes—as well as tobacco products—to LMICs, where laws and regulations concerning these substances are more lax or nonexistent and where people may be less aware of these hazards.

Transnational Problems

Occupational and environmental health problems in LMICs often involve multiple countries in the same region, requiring transnational or regional approaches to problems, such as development and implementation of transnational standards.

Inadequate Infrastructure and Human Resources

In LMICs, there are far fewer adequately trained personnel to recognize, diagnose, treat, and prevent occupational and environmental health problems. Governments and other sectors of society have fewer resources to devote to occupational and environmental health, and labor unions, facing other challenges such as low wages and high unemployment, often give little attention to occupational health and safety.

Relationship Between the Workplace and the Home Environment

In LMICs, where so many people work in or near their homes, the distinction between the workplace and the home environment is blurred. As a result, family members may often be exposed to workplace hazards, such as lead and pesticides.

Economic Development

Governments of LMICs often give high priority to economic development, sometimes even higher priority than to the health of their citizens. In the context of economic development, industrialization, and urbanization, there is often pressure to overlook occupational and environmental health issues, given limited resources and the fear that attention to these issues may drive away potential international investors or employers. Similarly, workers desperate for jobs in economies with high unemployment rates are unlikely to complain about health and safety hazards at work once they are employed. In addition, many children are forced to leave school in order to work, often in hazardous jobs. (See Chapter 35.)

SOCIAL AND ETHICAL QUESTIONS

Serious social and ethical questions have been raised over the allegiance of occupational and environmental physicians who are employed by management; workers' and communities' "right to know" about occupational and environmental hazards; confidentiality of workers' medical records maintained by employers; restriction of female workers of childbearing age from certain jobs; and other contentious issues. Some of the questions concerning these subjects may eventually be answered by labor–management and community–company interactions and by the decisions of government bodies—courts, legislatures, and executive agencies. For example, the U.S. Supreme Court found that so-called "fetal protection" policies that excluded women of reproductive age from industrial jobs, where men were permitted to work, illegally discriminated on the basis of gender.[27,28]

Ethics and ethical analyses help provide guides for action that are consistent; justifiable by appeal to commonly held values, principles, or roles; and able to withstand close moral scrutiny.[29] Conflict and disagreement are common in many aspects of occupational and environmental health. Difficult questions often arise, such as the following: What degree of risk should trigger action? What are the costs and benefits of regulating use of a substance or of screening workers for early detection of disease? How safe is safe enough? To what information are exposed workers or community residents entitled? How should decisions that impact health, environmental protection, and economic development be made? Not all aspects of the conflicts implied by these questions are ethical in nature, but most have some underlying ethical or moral dimension.[30] Occupational and environmental health professionals can refer to codes of ethics and other ethics guidelines of their professional organizations, including the American College of Occupational and Environmental Medicine, the American Association of Occupational Health Nurses, the American Board of Industrial Hygiene, the American College of Epidemiology, and the International Commission on Occupational Health—all of which are available on the Internet.

DISCIPLINES AND CAREERS IN OCCUPATIONAL AND ENVIRONMENTAL HEALTH SCIENCES

Identification and remediation of threats to the environment is a stewardship responsibility for us all. For those who work in clinical care or public health, there is a wide range of career options that span the physical, biologic, and social sciences as well as communications, policymaking, and other fields. A key challenge is communicating effectively across disciplines to develop collaboration for safe, healthful, and sustainable environments for future generations.

Almost all healthcare providers encounter occupational and environmental health issues. The American College of Graduate Medical Education recognizes the specialty of preventive medicine, which includes three areas of expertise: public health and general preventive medicine, occupational medicine, and aerospace medicine. Physicians who choose to specialize in any of these areas may wish to become certified by the American Board of Preventive Medicine. (For criteria for certification, access the board's website, http://www.abpm.org.) The American College of Occupational and Environmental Medicine is a primary professional association for physicians engaged in the practice of occupational and environmental medicine.

For those who wish to specialize in occupational and environmental health nursing, there are certificate programs, advanced degree programs for nurse practitioners that offer the Master of Science in Nursing (MSN), and doctoral programs, which include the Doctor of Philosophy (PhD) degree for those interested in research and the Doctor of Nursing Practice (DNP), an advanced professional practice degree. The American Association of Occupational Health Nurses is the primary professional association for occupational health nurses.

Physicians' assistants are midlevel practice professionals who are trained typically in an applied master of science degree program. They form the practice core for several large occupational health programs in industry and in the Veterans Administration health system.

Other healthcare professions important to the field of environmental and occupational health include audiology, physical therapy and rehabilitation, clinical psychology, clinical social work, and optometry. Occupational health psychologists apply psychology to improving the quality of work life and to protecting and promoting the safety, health, and well-being of workers.

A wide range of environmental health science programs are available at levels ranging from community colleges to postgraduate doctoral programs, with credentialing (based on education, experience, and certifying examinations) available for registered environmental health specialists, sanitarians, environmental health technicians, food-safety professionals, hazardous-substance professionals, and others.

Engineering and public health programs overlap in the training of industrial hygienists and environmental engineers, who provide primary prevention through exposure assessment as well as design and implementation of interventions. Radiation physicists and biologists address a specific aspect of environmental and occupational exposure assessment and prevention.

Safety professionals have education in engineering disciplines, often with additional management training. Bachelor's, master's, and doctoral degree programs are available. Public health practitioners are also trained through Master of Public Health degree and other programs.

Research into any of the occupational and environmental health sciences can form the basis for a doctoral program that focuses on advancement of scientific knowledge. These sciences include toxicology, epidemiology, environmental chemistry, systems engineering, sociology, psychology, and anthropology. Communications science, including social marketing and journalism, represents an important related area of study and practice. Environmental law, economics, policy, urban planning, and environmental management are other important areas of work. Finally, ecology, agronomy, chemistry, physics, and geology, which do not directly address human health impacts, are nevertheless critical to understanding the environment and human impact on it. These disciplines provide additional career opportunities related to occupational and environmental health.

REFERENCES

1. Denison R. We don't know how many chemicals are in use today. We should know. EDF Health, July 13, 2015. Available at: http://blogs.edf.org/health/2015/07/13/we-dont-know-how-many-chemicals-are-in-use-today-we-should-know/. Accessed January 3, 2017.
2. U.S. Environmental Protection Agency. Final Contaminant Candidate List 3 chemicals: Identifying the universe. August 2009. Available at: https://www.epa.gov/sites/production/files/2014-05/documents/ccl3_chemicals_universe_08-31-09_508_v3.pdf. Accessed January 3, 2017.
3. Fagan KM, Hodgson MJ. Under-recording of work-related injuries and illnesses: An OSHA priority. Journal of Safety Research 2017; 60: 79–83.
4. Ruser JW. Examining evidence of whether BLS undercounts workplace injuries and illnesses. Monthly Labor Review, August 2008.
5. Bureau of Labor Statistics. Census of fatal occupational injuries—Current and revised data. Available at: https://www.bls.gov/iif/oshcfoi1.htm. Accessed January 1, 2017.
6. Steenland K, Burnett C, Lalich N, et al. Dying for work: The magnitude of U.S. mortality from selected causes of death associated with occupation. American Journal of Industrial Medicine 2003; 43: 461–482.
7. Leigh JP. Economic burden of occupational injury and illness in the United States. Milbank Quarterly 2011; 89: 728–772.
8. Bureau of Labor Statistics. Employer-reported workplace injuries and illnesses—2015. October 27, 2016. Available at: http://www.bls.gov/news.release/pdf/osh.pdf. Accessed January 1, 2017.
9. National Institute for Occupational Safety and Health. Unpublished data, 2016. (Cited in Centers for Disease Control and Prevention Workers' Memorial Day—April 28, 2016. Morbidity and Mortality Weekly Report 2016; 65: 389.)
10. National Academy of Social Insurance. Press release: Workers' compensation benefits as a share of payroll continue to decline even as employer costs rise. October 5, 2016. Available at: https://www.nasi.org/press/releases/2016/10/press-release-workers%E2%80%99-compensation-benefits-share-payrol. Accessed January 1, 2017.
11. U.S. Environmental Protection Agency. Summary nonattainment area population exposure report. September 22, 2016. Available at: https://www3.epa.gov/airquality/greenbook/popexp.html. Accessed January 2, 2017.
12. Centers for Disease Control and Prevention. Lead: CDC's national surveillance data (1997–2015). Available at: https://www.cdc.gov/nceh/lead/data/national.htm. Accessed January 1, 2017.
13. California Environmental Protection Agency. Summary of results from the California Pesticide Illness Surveillance Program—2014. Sacramento: California Environmental Protection Agency, December 14, 2016, p. 1.

14. Kochanek KD, Murphy SL, Xu J, Tejada-Vera B. Deaths: Final data for 2014. National Vital Statistics Reports 2016; 65: 1–122.

15. Centers for Disease Control and Prevention. Asthma: Most recent asthma data. Available at: https://www.cdc.gov/asthma/most_recent_data.htm. Accessed January 1, 2017.

16. Talbot D. "Tectonic shifts" in employment. MIT Technology Review, December 20, 2011.

17. Weil D. The fissured workplace: Why work became so bad for so many and what can be done to improve it. Cambridge, MA: Harvard University Press, 2014.

18. Howard J. Nonstandard work arrangements and worker health and safety. American Journal of Industrial Medicine 2017; 60: 1–10.

19. Urquhart M. The employment shift to services: Where did it come from? Monthly Labor Review, U.S. Department of Labor, April 1984.

20. Steverman B. "I'll never retire": Americans break record for working past 65. Bloomberg News, May 13, 2016. Available at: https://www.bloomberg.com/news/articles/2016-05-13/-i-ll-never-retire-americans-break-record-for-working-past-65. Accessed January 20, 2017.

21. National Center for Chronic Disease Prevention and Health Promotion. Older employees in the workplace: Issue brief no. 1, July 2012. Atlanta: Centers for Disease Control and Prevention.

22. National Institute for Occupational Safety and Health. Fundamentals of total worker health approaches: Essential elements for advancing worker safety, health, and well-being (DHHS [NIOSH] Publication Number 2017-112). December 2016. Available at: https://www.cdc.gov/niosh/docs/2017-112/. Accessed January 30, 2017.

23. Wang D, Lau KK, Yu RH, et al. Neighbouring green space and all-cause mortality in elderly people in Hong Kong: A retrospective cohort study. Lancet 2016; 388: S82.

24. Dadvand P, Sunyer J, Alvarez-Pedrerol M, et al. Green spaces and spectacles use in schoolchildren in Barcelona. Environmental Research 2017; 152: 256–262.

25. Milner A, Krnjack L, LaMontagne AD. Psychosocial job quality and mental health among young workers: A fixed-effects regression analysis using 13 waves of annual data. Scandinavian Journal of Work, Environment & Health 2017; 43: 50–58.

26. Kivimäki M, Ferrie JE, Brunner E, et al. Justice at work and reduced risk of coronary heart disease among employees: The Whitehall II Study. Archives of Intern Medicine 2005; 165: 2245–2251.

27. United States Supreme Court. United Auto Workers, et al. v. Johnson Controls, Inc., 499 U.S. 187, 111 S. Ct. 1196, 113 L. Ed. 2d 158 (1991).

28. Clauss CA, Berzon M, Bertin J. Litigating reproductive and developmental health in the aftermath of UAW versus Johnson Controls. Environmental Health Perspectives 1993; 101(Suppl 2): 205–220.

29. Beauchamp TL, Childress JF. Principles of biomedical ethics. New York: Oxford University Press, 1983.

30. Rest KM. Ethics in occupational and environmental health. In: BS Levy, DH Wegman (eds.). Occupational health: Recognizing and preventing work-related disease (3rd ed.). Boston: Little, Brown and Company, 1995, pp. 241–258.

FURTHER READING

Selected Books

Baxter PJ, AW T-C, Cockcroft A, et al. (eds.) Hunter's diseases of occupations (10th ed.). Boca Raton, FL: CRC Press, 2010.
A classic textbook on occupational diseases.

Burgess W. Recognition of health hazards in industry: A review of materials and processes (2nd ed.). New York: John Wiley & Sons, 1995.
An excellent summary of industrial hazards and how things work.

Frumkin H (ed.). Environmental health: From global to local (3rd ed.). San Francisco, CA: Jossey Bass, 2016.
A comprehensive introductory textbook.

Hamilton A. Exploring the dangerous trades: An autobiography. Boston: Little, Brown, 1943. (Also published by OEM Press in 1995.)
A classic historical reference.

Hathaway GJ, Proctor NH. Proctor and Hughes' chemical hazards of the workplace (5th ed.). Hoboken, NJ: John Wiley & Sons, 2004.
Brief summaries of many chemical hazards, including basic information about their chemical, physical, and toxicologic characteristics; diagnostic criteria; treatment; and medical control measures.

LaDou J, Harrison R (eds.). Current occupational and environmental medicine (5th ed.). New York: McGraw-Hill Medical, 2014.
A clinically focused guide on common occupational and environmental illnesses.

Rom WN, Markowitz SB (eds.). Environmental & occupational medicine (4th ed.). Philadelphia: Wolters Kluwer/Lippincott Williams & Wilkins, 2007.

An excellent, comprehensive, in-depth reference on occupational and environmental medicine.

Stellman JM (ed.). Encyclopaedia of occupational health and safety (5th ed.). Geneva: International Labor Organization, 2012.
An online multidisciplinary book on occupational hazards and disorders and related subjects.

Stave GM, Wald PH (eds.). Physical and biological hazards of the workplace (3rd ed.). Hoboken, NJ: John Wiley & Sons, 2016.
A practical reference on the diagnosis, treatment, and control of these hazards.

Selected Periodical Publications

Occupational and Environmental Health

American Journal of Industrial Medicine, published monthly by Wiley-Liss, Inc.

American Journal of Public Health, published monthly by the American Public Health Association

Environmental Health Perspectives, published monthly by the National Institute of Environmental Health Sciences

Journal of Occupational and Environmental Medicine, the journal of the American College of Occupational and Environmental Medicine, published monthly by Wolters Kluwer Health/ Lippincott Williams & Wilkins

New Solutions: A Journal of Occupational and Environmental Health Policy, published quarterly by SAGE Publications

Occupational and Environmental Medicine, the journal of the Faculty of Occupational Medicine of the Royal College of Physicians of London, published monthly by the BMJ Publishing Group, Ltd.

Scandinavian Journal of Work, Environment & Health, published every other month by the Nordic Association of Occupational Safety and Health

Occupational Health Nursing

American Association of Occupational Health Nurses Journal, published monthly by the American Association of Occupational Health Nurses

Occupational and Environmental Hygiene

Journal of Occupational and Environmental Hygiene, published monthly by the American Industrial Hygiene Association and ACGIH

Annals of Work Exposures and Health, the journal of the British Occupational Hygiene Society, published every other month by Oxford University Press

Occupational Safety

Professional Safety, published monthly by the American Society of Safety Engineers

Journal of Safety Research, published monthly by the National Safety Council and Elsevier

Accident Analysis & Prevention, published monthly by Elsevier

Injury Prevention, the official journal of the Society for Advancement of Violence and Injury Research, published every other month by BMJ

Occupational Ergonomics

Applied Ergonomics: Human Factors in Technology and Society, published every other month by Elsevier

Ergonomics, the journal of the Ergonomics Society, published monthly by Taylor & Francis

Human Factors: The Journal of the Human Factors and Ergonomics Society, published by SAGE Publications

International Journal of Industrial Ergonomics, published monthly by Elsevier

Occupational Health Psychology

Journal of Occupational Health Psychology, published quarterly by the American Psychological Association

General News and Scientific Update Publication

BNA Occupational Safety & Health Reporter, published weekly by the Bureau of National Affairs

2

Occupational and Environmental Health Equity and Social Justice

Cora Roelofs, Sherry L. Baron, Sacoby Wilson, and Aaron Aber

CASE 1

A 21-year-old African-American man who had graduated from high school and completed the Job Corps federal job training program applied for dozens of jobs. When he was not hired, he wondered if racial discrimination was a factor. Unable to find steady work, he went to a temporary services agency and found a job at a rum factory. Excited, he called his mother to tell her the good news. He asked her to drive him to a store to buy the required uniform, including steel-toe boots, and to the factory for a 15-minute orientation before the 3 pm start of his first shift. He then took a photo of himself in his workclothes and orange safety vest and texted it to his fiancée. Less than 2 hours later, he was dead. He had been sent to clean out broken bottles that were clogging a machine that stacked boxes on a pallet. While he was out of sight, another worker started the machine, crushing him to death. When the Occupational Safety and Health Administration (OSHA) investigated the incident, the agency found that it was similar to many others: temporary workers with little or no safety training, but wanting to prove themselves to gain permanent employment, had been fatally injured during the first few days at a hazardous job. Neither the temporary agency nor the site employer took responsibility for safety.[1]

CASE 2

Several physicians discovered that many children from a poor rural area in North Carolina near industrial hog operations were having diarrhea. Several of their parents were also having gastrointestinal symptoms, especially after heavy rains. They and other residents complained to the local health department about odors and rainwater runoff from the hog operations. The health department found high levels of *Escherichia coli* and fecal coliforms in residential well water—up to 1,000 times higher than maximum contaminant levels set by the Environmental Protection Agency (EPA). Using online mapping tools, some high school students found that the hog operations were near poor and African-American neighborhoods.

Health equity is a fundamental principle of social justice and human rights. According to the Centers for Disease Control and Prevention (CDC), health equity "is achieved when every person has the opportunity to 'attain his or her full potential' and no one is 'disadvantaged from achieving this potential because of social position or other socially determined circumstances.'"[2]

Low-income people and people of color are more likely to encounter chemical, physical, and biological hazards and psychosocial stressors in their communities and at work—an example of health *inequity*.[3] Neighborhood environmental stressors include air pollution, water contamination, hazardous wastes, unhealthful land uses (such as for incinerators and landfills), and inadequate health-promoting facilities (such as parks and bicycle lanes). Disparities in work-related exposures arise from disproportionate employment in hazardous jobs—compounded by workplace discrimination, ineffective prevention and training, and restructuring of the workplace, creating less secure jobs.

OCCUPATIONAL HEALTH EQUITY

In 1911, a fire occurred in the Triangle Shirtwaist Factory in New York City, killing 145 of the 600 workers, who were mostly young immigrant women. Many of the exit doors had been locked by factory owners to prevent workers from stealing items. In Hamlet, North Carolina, 80 years later, 25 workers trapped behind locked fire doors were killed and 55 workers were injured in a fire at a poultry-processing plant; most of the workers were African Americans. Workers today have much in common with these workers: They experience hazardous working conditions. Many do not speak English. Many have limited education and limited job skills. Many belong to minority groups disparaged by others. And many are imperiled by inadequate government action to assure safe and healthful working conditions.[4]

Almost 17 million workers (16% of all private-sector workers) in 2010 were employed in hazardous jobs where work-related injuries and illnesses occur twice as often than in other (safer) jobs.[5] Immigrant, minority, and low-wage workers with limited employment options are disproportionately employed in the most hazardous jobs. Understanding how and why these disparities exist provides insights for improving occupational health equity.

Changing Nature of Work

The U.S. poultry-processing industry today illustrates how industrial restructuring has contributed to occupational health inequity. Poultry

processing workers experience extremely high rates of injuries—close to 50% higher than all private-industry workers in 2015. These injuries include disabling repetitive strain injuries, such as carpal tunnel syndrome, and amputations. As consumer preference for chicken has increased, poultry plants have become larger and more mechanized, line speeds have increased, and work tasks no long require skilled workers. Poultry processing jobs are now predominantly concentrated in five southern states because companies find "an ample supply of nonunion, lower-wage workers" who are willing to work in these unskilled jobs.[6] Poultry processing workers are disproportionately African-American and Latino immigrants, reflecting both the historic concentration of African-American workers in the South and the increasing flow of Latino immigrant workers into southern states where they can find jobs. (See Figure 2-1.)

In North Carolina, Latino immigrant and African-American poultry-processing workers face more work hazards compared to other similar workers in their communities. Latino immigrant poultry workers report less opportunity to control how they do their work, experience more psychological demands, use more awkward postures and repetitive motions, and feel that management is not committed to safety, compared to other Latino immigrant manual-labor workers in their community.[7] Similarly, African-American female poultry-processing workers in a different region of North Carolina are three times as likely to have a musculoskeletal disorder (MSD) and three times as likely to report diminished physical health–related quality of life, compared to other African-American female low-wage workers in their community. Despite their higher injury rates, these women also feel reluctant to report their injuries because, as one woman commented, "There are 300 people in line behind me for my job."[8]

David Weil, former director of the Wage and Hours Division of the U.S. Department of Labor, describes the current workplace as "fissured"—with employers increasingly using contractors and subcontractors for hiring, evaluation, pay, supervision, training, and coordination of workers.[9] As a result, job insecurity has increased,

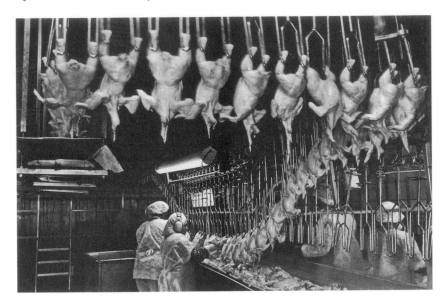

Figure 2-1. Workers processing chickens on an assembly line. Minority workers and women are overrepresented in entry-level jobs like this one, in which safety and health hazards are prevalent. Twenty-five workers in a similar chicken-processing plant died in 1991, when few workers were able to escape a fire that swept through the plant because the employer had locked most of the exit doors. (Photograph by Earl Dotter.)

real wages and benefits have declined, and fewer workers are represented by labor unions. Although hard to estimate, as many as 18% of U.S. workers are employed in these nonstandard work arrangements and are called temporary, contract, contingent, and, more recently, "gig" or "app-based" workers.[10,11]

By employing workers in nonstandard jobs, companies decrease labor costs, reduce employment during periods of low production, and avoid providing workers with benefits, such as health insurance and pensions.[12] These attributes that make temporary workers attractive to employers also often make temporary work more hazardous. Work-related injuries and illnesses among temporary workers are associated with increased workloads, longer working hours, decreased training, and breakdowns in workplace communication.[10,13] Temporary workers also have less knowledge of their work environment, less job training, and difficulties raising concerns about working conditions and getting their views heard by management. While many workers face unsafe production pressures, temporary workers often feel pressure to "cut corners" in hopes of securing permanent employment.

Temporary work usually involves complex employment relationships between the temporary employment agency, the worksite supervisor, and the worker. Employers report confusion over who is responsible for health and safety—the temporary agency (which does not have control over worksite conditions) or the person who is directly supervising the worker at the workplace (but is not the worker's legal employer). Recognizing this complexity, OSHA has recently issued guidance that clearly delineates shared and joint responsibility for health and safety between temporary agencies and host employers.[14] For example, the staffing agency is required to purchase any required personal protective equipment (PPE), but the host employer is responsible for informing the agency about what PPE is required.

Informal workers (who comprise the *underground economy*) represent a category of temporary workers. In the United States, there are over 100,000 day laborers, each of whom waits every workday on a street corner or at a hiring center, seeking temporary employment in construction, landscaping, agriculture, cleaning, or moving and hauling.[15] Like other contingent workers, informal workers have high rates of work-related injuries. Immigrants who lack legal authority to work in the United States (*undocumented immigrants*) frequently work in informal employment arrangements in which they face hazardous conditions. Undocumented workers report less knowledge of their rights to a safe workplace and significant fear of employer retaliation if they were to report hazards.[16]

Workplace Injustice

CASE 3

In 1930, a subsidiary of a large corporation contracted with a construction firm to dig a 3-mile tunnel, the Gauley Bridge, through a stone mountain in West Virginia to divert the New River and build a hydroelectric energy plant. This 2-year project employed thousands of workers, at least 75% of whom were African Americans, in a county whose population was 85% Caucasian. Many of these African-American workers came from Alabama, Virginia, North Carolina, and South Carolina, where work was hard to find then (during the Great Depression) and to whom the hourly wage of $0.30 to $0.60 was acceptable.

The rock through which the workers drilled had some of the highest known content of crystalline silica. To complete the job quickly, the company chose to use minimal water to suppress dust levels. One year after the project began, the local newspaper published a story commenting on "the unusually large number of deaths among the colored laborers. The deaths total about 37 in the past two weeks." Although the initial deaths were attributed to African-American workers' poor nutritional habits and unusual susceptibility to pneumonia, it soon became clear that they were dying of acute silicosis. As many as 581 of the 922 African-American workers who worked in the tunnels for at least 2 months may have died.[17] (See Chapter 22 for a discussion of silicosis.)

Although the blatant discrimination that is described in this case is far less common today, disparities persist. For example, in Michigan between 1985 and 2010, the incidence rate of silicosis over age 40 among African-American men was 8.5 per 100,000, compared to 1.6 per 100,000 for white men.[18]

Workplace injustice, including abuse, mistreatment, discrimination, and harassment, is associated with mental and physical health problems.[19–21] Workplace discrimination, based on race, gender, age, or sexual preference, occurs in many forms, including preferential hiring, firing, and job placement, as well as coworker and supervisor hostility. (See Chapter 14.) This discrimination is manifest in the wage and the unemployment gaps between African-American and white workers. Since 1976, the unemployment rate for blacks has consistently remained about twice that of whites, regardless of educational attainment. African-American households earn 40% less than white households. Black African Americans are only slightly less likely today to live in poverty than they were in 1976.[22]

Racial and ethnic discrimination is prevalent in many workplaces in the United States.[23,24] Experiencing racial insults, both at work and elsewhere, and unfair treatment at work have been associated with mental health disorders among workers and their families.[25,26]

Beyond its psychological toll, workplace discrimination may lead to differential exposure to chemical and physical hazards at work. *Job-placement discrimination* can mean that less-favored workers are assigned to more hazardous work tasks. For example, a study of immigrant poultry workers found an association between retaliatory behavior by supervisors and a 10% to 30% increase in adverse health outcomes. Workers reported that native-born workers were given easier and cleaner jobs and that undocumented immigrants were more frequently asked to work unpaid overtime or, if they refused, were assigned unpleasant tasks.[27]

Another form of discrimination is *workplace segregation*, in which one group of workers disproportionately works in certain jobs with a greater risk of psychosocial stress. African Americans, especially those in the middle class, who perceive that they are in a "black job" experience greater psychological distress.[28] African-American and white workers, who worked in jobs where more than 20% of the employees were African-American, reported poor or fair

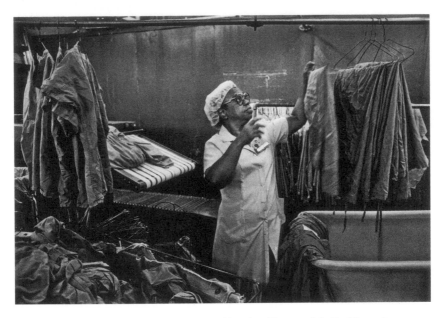

Figure 2-2. Worker in a commercial laundry. (Photograph by Earl Dotter.)

overall health more often, even after adjusting for demographic factors, income, and education.[29] This segregation is most apparent in many lower-status jobs, where workers lack power and are disproportionately exposed to hazardous conditions.[13] (See Figure 2-2.) For example, three of the six largest occupation groups—with more than 1 million workers each—that have the highest injury rates are disproportionately African-American and Hispanic; maids and housekeepers are predominantly female and disproportionately Hispanic; health aides are predominantly female and disproportionately African-American; and manual laborers are predominantly male and disproportionately African-American and Hispanic.[30]

CASE 4

A young man, in search of a job, crossed the border from his native Mexico to the United States. He had a cousin living in Los Angeles, who told him that construction jobs were easy to obtain. Once he arrived, he found a job working as a sandblaster for a small construction company. The company did not ask for any official documents and paid him informally in cash ("under the table"). Although the sandblasting created a lot of dust, his employer gave him no respiratory protection. To avoid breathing too much dust, he tied a bandana around his face, as farmworkers in his small home town in rural Mexico had done when they sprayed pesticides. He earned a good income and regularly sent money back to his family in Mexico. However, after a few years doing this job, he began to cough and wheeze. When he barely had enough energy to make it through the workday, he saw a doctor who diagnosed him with advanced silicosis. Unable to work and without medical insurance or knowledge of workers' compensation insurance, he returned to Mexico and died a few years later.

Many foreign-born immigrant workers (Figure 2-3) face challenges at work that negatively impact their health:

- They are often targets of racism and other forms of discrimination.[31]
- They are more likely to be employed in service, natural-resources, construction, maintenance, production, transportation, material-moving, and other high-risk occupations.
- Limited English-speaking ability, low job skills, and little education make many vulnerable to employers who exploit them.

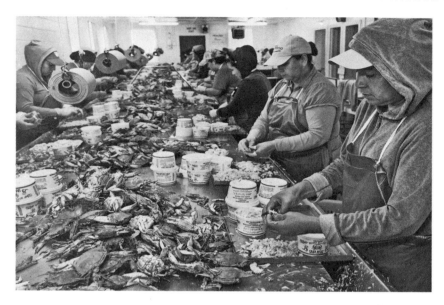

Figure 2-3. Crab pickers working as "guest workers" in Maryland. (Photograph by Earl Dotter.)

- They are less likely to be informed about their rights to a safe workplace and less likely to be provided appropriate PPE.[12,32]
- They are less likely to be aware of OSHA protections.
- They are more likely to work for employers who underreport injuries and illnesses.[33]
- They are more likely to be targeted by Immigration and Customs Enforcement if they are injured on the job.[34]

Approximately 11 million unauthorized immigrants reside in the United States, 8 million of whom are in the labor force. Unauthorized immigrants may be at high risk for work-related injuries and illnesses because their immigration status and their need for money drive them to take hazardous jobs. They are more likely to be employed as agricultural or construction laborers and less likely to report hazards.[16,35,36]

CASE 5

The manager of a sausage factory reviewed the factory's annual injury logs and noted that female employees were more likely to develop MSDs than men. He recalled reading in a trade magazine that women are more likely to develop carpal tunnel syndrome, and he

therefore attributed their relatively higher injury rate to biological factors. A union safety representative also reviewed these injury records and decided to investigate further. He inspected the sausage-finishing station, where several of the injuries had occurred, and observed women lifting 40-pound racks of sausages onto a shelf that was designed for much taller workers. After a short discussion, he learned that these women had previously worked in evening-shift jobs, which were less stressful ergonomically, but they had recently switched to day-shift jobs, in order to be home when their children returned from school. In order to prevent more injuries, the manager worked with the union safety representative and the workers to redesign the shelf to avoid lifting hazards.

This case illustrates how female workers may face discrimination at work. The design of a work station may be ergonomically optimal for the average male stature, but it may require significant reaching and awkward postures for short female workers, causing them to have more ergonomic stresses and increased risk of injury. In addition, female workers and their partners experience stress due to conflicts between work and family responsibilities. For low-wage female workers, many of whom are single mothers, the challenge of balancing their roles as wage earners and as mothers is often especially stressful.

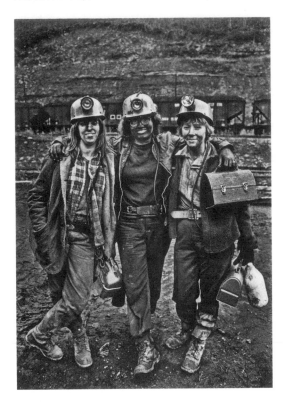

Figure 2-4. Women coal miners. (Photograph by Earl Dotter.)

Women—and people who do not conform to typical gender norms—may be harassed or bullied with adverse effects on their mental and physical health and safety at work. Sexual harassment of women workers includes gender stereotyping, sexist jokes, and demeaning behavior. This and other forms of gender discrimination can lead to inequities at work:

- Women are overrepresented in service occupations, such as nursing assistants, that have high injury rates.
- In jobs where they are underrepresented, like construction and mining jobs (Figure 2-4), women may feel the need to prove themselves in ways that put them at increased risk of injury.[37]
- Women are at higher risk than men to be exposed to violence at work.[38]
- Women may suffer because male physical norms are the bases for exposure standards and PPE may not be available for women (or men) of small stature.[37,39]

- Overall, women earn less than men. Among low-wage workers who are African-American or Hispanic, this income gap is even greater.[40]

Inadequate Government Protection

Government regulations and social-safety-net programs have not reduced many of the inequities described previously. Many OSHA standards on specific workplace hazards have become outdated, and the number of OSHA inspectors is inadequate to enforce standards. (See Chapter 3.)

Some workers, including farm workers (Chapter 32A), domestic workers (such as house cleaners and home care workers), and, in many states, public employees, are often excluded from coverage by OSHA. The Fair Labor Standards Act of 1938 enabled the U.S. Department of Labor to establish regulations limiting work hours and prohibiting work after 7 PM on school nights for children under age 16 and regulations prohibiting children under age 18 (or under 16 in agricultural work) from performing certain tasks, such as operating power-driven woodworking equipment. However, these regulations are frequently violated.[41]

OSHA enforces regulations in part by conducting inspections in response to worker complaints. Nonunion workers, immigrant workers, and workers with limited English-language skills face barriers in making complaints or participating in inspections. When OSHA requests input on new regulations or strengthens existing ones, these workers are often not represented.

Low-income workers without health insurance who are injured at work often have to pay for their medical expenses. As one study found, Hispanic construction workers are half as likely as non-Hispanic white construction workers to be covered by workers' compensation for a work-related injury and four times more likely to pay out-of-pocket expenses—on average, almost $2,000.[42]

Low-wage workers also have less paid sick leave. In 2015, for workers whose wages were in the bottom quartile, only 41% had access to paid sick leave.[43] When, as a result, ill or injured workers come to work (instead of staying at home)—a situation known as *presenteeism*—they and their

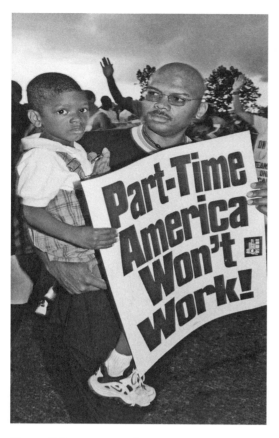

Figure 2-5. Part-time workers, like this man holding his son, often work for low wages and little or no benefits in precarious work situations. (Photograph by Earl Dotter.)

coworkers may suffer. Low-wage workers without paid sick leave are also less likely to take time off from work to care for themselves or sick family members.[44] When children with, for example, upper respiratory infections then go to school, they can spread these infections to other children. Without paid sick leave to care for an ill family member, a worker may be distracted and suffer a serious injury.[45] (See Figure 2-5.)

ENVIRONMENTAL HEALTH EQUITY

CASE 6

A father from a small community on the outskirts of a city testified in court about how, for the previous 15 years, a landfill near his property had adversely affected his health, his family members' health, and the quality of life in his neighborhood. He had smelled odors from the landfill and, when the wind blew in his direction, he experienced headaches, a bad cough, and burning of his eyes, nose, and throat. He heard noise from trucks bringing garbage to the landfill and saw rats in the woods near the landfill and buzzards flying overhead. He did not understand why more was not being done to monitor the landfill. His family members and many neighbors were sick. For 15 years, they complained to the local health department and the state environmental protection agency. They learned from the EPA that tests of local well water 20 years before indicated that the groundwater was not safe for consumption; it contained high levels of metals and other contaminants that can cause cancer, birth defects, and neurological disorders. The EPA recommended that anyone who lived within 2 miles of the landfill not drink well water and use the closest publicly-regulated drinking water system or drink only bottled water.

During testimony from town officials, the man learned that city officials knew about this contamination long before and had provided alternate water sources to well-to-do people living near the landfill but not to poor people, immigrants, or people of color. When the judge questioned town officials about their actions, they stated that they disseminated public notices and held stakeholder meetings but no one from the man's neighborhood had responded.

This case is not unique. For over 20 years, researchers have demonstrated that many low-income populations, communities of color, immigrant communities, and other underserved populations and marginalized and disenfranchised groups live in neighborhoods that experience disproportionate risks from exposure to environmental hazards. These hazards include many noxious land uses, such as landfills, incinerators, publicly owned treatment works (such as sewer and water treatment plants), industrial animal operations, hazardous waste sites, chemical factories, power plants, heavily trafficked roadways, and other locally unwanted land uses.[46-54] The cumulative impact of environmental injustice, due to the spatial concentration of environmental hazards, factories, and noxious land uses, leads to increases in adverse health outcomes and community stress as well as lower quality of life and community sustainability. (See Chapters 15, 16, and 18.)

In the 1980s, the Environmental Justice Movement arose to address the disproportionate burden of environmental exposures on low-income and minority communities.[46,47] It raised awareness of the many environmental and health issues that they faced and asked the federal government to respond. Two groundbreaking studies provided the initial evidence that supported claims of grassroots activists who had been fighting against environmental injustice in many places across the United States.

The first study, by the General Accounting Office in 1983, *Siting of Hazardous Waste Landfills and Their Correlation with Racial and Economic Status of Surrounding Communities*, examined the distribution of landfills in EPA Region IV (eight southeastern states); it found that (a) most residents in 75% of communities containing large hazardous waste landfills were African-American and (b) African Americans were overrepresented in communities with waste sites.[55]

The second study, by the Commission for Racial Justice of the United Church of Christ in 1987, *Toxic Waste and Race in America*, demonstrated that (a) in ZIP codes without a toxic facility, less than 12% of the residents were persons of color; (b) in those with only one toxic facility, 24% of the residents were persons of color; and (c) in those with multiple toxic facilities or one of the five largest landfills, 38% of residents were persons of color.[56] The study found that 60% of African-Americans and Hispanics resided in communities with toxic waste sites.

The *Toxic Wastes and Race at Twenty* report, a follow-up to the 1987 study that was released in 2007, provided additional evidence about the disproportionate burden on disadvantaged populations of environmental hazards, industrial facilities, and unhealthy land uses.[52] The report demonstrated that, nationally, people of color are approximately three times more likely to live in neighborhoods that host a commercial hazardous waste facility than whites. The study found that (a) more African Americans, Hispanics, and Asians reside in neighborhoods

that "host" toxic facilities than in "non-host" neighborhoods and (b) in metropolitan areas, more poor people live in host neighborhoods than non-host neighborhoods.

There is now a large body of literature on environmental justice, which has documented the disproportionate burden on poor populations, people of color, and other disadvantaged groups of environmental hazards, including unhealthy land uses (such as hazardous waste sites and landfills), refineries and petrochemical plants, other industrial facilities, and major highways.[46,47,49]

Environmental Injustice

CASE 7

At a community meeting in a poor segregated neighborhood, its primarily Latino, African-American, and Asian residents discussed government plans to build another highway in the neighborhood. The neighborhood already had much motor-vehicle traffic and associated air pollution, causing asthma and other respiratory problems for many residents. During summers, many "ozone-alert" days made children and elderly residents stay inside, and heat waves caused many hospitalizations for heat stroke and other disorders. Residents complained of diesel smoke from trucks that drove through the neighborhood and transit and school buses that idled throughout the day.

A Department of Transportation official at the meeting stated that an environmental impact assessment projected that the planned highway would not increase air pollution. Town officials stated that the new highway could help promote economic development and attract new industries, businesses, and consumer traffic. A local physician reported that many of his young patients had asthma and many of his adult patients, especially those who lived near bus stops and highway exit ramps, were experiencing respiratory and cardiovascular problems. Some residents, who lived near an incinerator that released airborne pollutants, observed that the building of highways in the neighborhood had been accompanied by the construction of polluting factories.

Asthma, a prime example of health disparities resulting from environmental injustice,[49] is more prevalent among people of color than white people. (See Chapter 22.) CDC has documented the following disparities in asthma in the United States:[57]

- In 2014, the asthma prevalence rate for Puerto Ricans (16.5%) was more than twice the rate for all Hispanics (6.7%) and significantly higher than the rate for whites (7.6%) and African Americans (9.9%).
- The asthma prevalence rates for Hispanic children (8.5%) and African-American children (9.9%) were higher than the rate for white children (7.6%). The rate for Puerto Rican children (23.5%) was significantly higher than for any other racial/ethnic group.
- In 2010, the rate of hospital inpatient discharges for asthma was 29.9 per 10,000 for African Americans and 8.7 per 10,000 for whites.
- In 2014, the asthma mortality rate for African Americans was 25.4 per million, compared to the rates for whites (8.8 per million) and Hispanics (7.7 per million).

Multiple factors likely account for higher rates of asthma among people color:

- Residence in areas with high exposure to fine particulate matter ($PM_{2.5}$)
- A high burden of social stressors, including unstable employment and community violence[58]
- Limited access to quality medical care.

Studies have demonstrated the relationship between environmental hazards and adverse pregnancy outcomes as well as disorders of children. For example, residential proximity to environmental hazards increases the risks for preterm birth, low birthweight, and birth defects, as well as childhood cancer and autism.[59,60]

Residential Segregation

Residential segregation leads to disproportionate exposure to environmental risk factors—physical, social, and economic—that adversely affect health and lead to health disparities in both urban and rural areas.[46–49] In many urban areas, social, economic, and political forces along with historical patterns of community development, disinvestment, industrialization, and zoning and planning (including for highway development and expansion) have segregated populations of color in impoverished communities that have few resources and increased environmental risks.[46,47] *Redlining* (a discriminatory practice by which banks and insurance companies refuse or limit loans, mortgages, or insurance within specific geographic areas, especially inner-city neighborhoods) and other forms of institutional discrimination have also contributed to segregation of disadvantaged populations.[48,50,51] In these communities, relatively few municipal services are available, infrastructure has deteriorated, and the physical and natural environments have been eroded.[58] Many segregated populations are exposed to high levels of *criteria air pollutants*, such as carbon monoxide, particulate matter (PM), sulfur dioxide, and oxides of nitrogen, released from vehicles and factories in or near these neighborhoods.[49] (See Chapter 15.) Exposure to these pollutants can cause lung cancer or nonmalignant respiratory disorders, such as asthma.[46,47,49] For example, studies in metropolitan areas with black–white segregation have shown that African Americans are exposed to higher levels of sulfur dioxide, PM, and ozone.[2,47] In addition, segregation is associated with (a) greater exposure of populations of color to hazardous air pollutants and (b) increased risk of cancer, even after controlling for socioeconomic status.

Segregated communities are characterized by concentrated poverty, limited economic infrastructure, and low-quality social services and medical care. These factors act synergistically to raise levels of stress, increase vulnerability, and limit capacity of burdened populations to overcome disease and increase health status.[46–49]

Community Planning and Development

Many factors have contributed to inequitable development in urban, suburban, and rural areas in the United States, including suburbanization (population movement from within cities to the rural-urban fringe, which leads to urban sprawl), discriminatory housing policies, segregation, massive highway construction, deindustrialization, and poor zoning and planning.[48,50] As a result, many areas have been divided by race, ethnicity, and socioeconomic status, creating environmental injustice. The segregation and spatial variation in planning and development in communities with different racial, ethnic, and socioeconomic composition have arisen from conditions and policies in different time periods. These conditions and policies have included *Jim Crow policies* in the South—state and local laws enacted between 1876 and 1965 that mandated racial segregation in all public facilities with a supposedly "separate, but equal" status for African Americans. They limited access for non-whites to low-interest home loans and they enabled exclusionary zoning, racial covenants, and redlining.[50] The uneven nature of community planning, zoning, and development has led to *fragmentation* (the division of metropolitan areas into multiple smaller municipal districts); *gentrification* (the restoration of run-down urban areas by the middle class, resulting in the displacement of low-income residents); and sprawl and the spatial concentration of environmental hazards and unhealthy land uses in communities affected by environmental injustice. Spatial fragmentation and gentrification have limited sustainable economic development, which, in turn, has adversely affected the quality of schools, housing, transportation, civic engagement, and social climate. (See Chapter 34.)

Although zoning and planning are sometimes perceived as objective processes, they actually are highly political, class-conscious practices. Early in the 20th century, zoning became widespread in the United States because it effectively regulated land use, making it difficult or impossible for less affluent people to cross community boundaries. For example, in New York City, zoning was a social and political process, in which much of Bronx, Brooklyn, and Queens was zoned as unrestricted, which promoted—for economic reasons—development of hazardous industrial facilities in poor and working-class areas.[61] Zoning and race were closely related. For example, the Bronx had the highest concentration of poor and minority residents as well as large increases in areas zoned for manufacturing,

which exposed nearby residents to disproportionate amounts of environmental toxicants. In contrast, more affluent Manhattan had the greatest decrease in manufacturing. This zoning pattern also occurred in Chicago, Atlanta, Detroit, Los Angeles, and other U.S. cities.

New movements in planning and community development, including *new urbanism* (an urban-design movement that focuses on the development of walkable communities) and *smart growth* (an urban planning approach that focuses on concentrated growth; mixed-use development; and compact, walkable, pedestrian-friendly, transit-oriented neighborhoods to reduce sprawl and improve neighborhood sustainability) have been adopted by planners, local government officials, architects, and environmental organizations to improve health, sustainability, and quality of life in neighborhoods, towns, and cities. (See Chapter 34.) These movements have not gone far enough in addressing environmental injustice and social inequalities, and they may lead to more segregation, gentrification, and uneven planning, zoning, and development.[48,50] For example, the adverse social, economic, environmental, and health impacts of urban revitalization on disadvantaged populations are evident in the destruction of core urban neighborhoods in large cities and displacement of underserved and disadvantaged residents. Therefore, economically advantaged populations, who benefitted disproportionately from suburbanization, may benefit disproportionately from new revitalization efforts, while historically disadvantaged populations may be adversely affected.[50] Without equity-based policies, the elimination of environmental injustice and health disparities in disadvantaged communities through new forms of planning and community development may not occur.

Inequitable zoning, planning, and community development contribute to lack of access to basic amenities, such as sewer and water infrastructure, good housing, parks, green space, recreational facilities, and pedestrian-friendly residential environments in rural areas and small towns.[48,50,51,62] The problems of unjust transportation planning and urban sprawl have been studied in Atlanta,[63,64] revealing how transportation inequities can contribute to environmental injustice and public health problems.

There is also a high concentration of *pathogenic infrastructure*, such as fast-food restaurants, liquor stores, and check-cashing facilities, in poor neighborhoods and communities of color in southern states and large cities.[65,66]

The Built Environment

CASE 8

A mother of three children attended a parent–teacher association meeting at a local junior high school to find out more information about its new garden. Her children had come home after school a few weeks before excited about a new school program in which students would have physical activity and eat organic produce from the school's garden or the local farmers' market. At the meeting, the mother was shocked to learn that the program was established because of high rates of obesity and diabetes among students. Two of her children were overweight and one had been diagnosed with diabetes at age 10. A local professor stated that her neighborhood was a *food desert*, with no supermarkets or grocery stores and fresh fruits and vegetables available only at a gas station's convenience store. The professor stated that the neighborhood had poor access to mass transit, preventing residents from having access to supermarkets in other locations, but an excessive number of fast-food restaurants. The mother recalled how often she bought her children hamburgers and French fries from a nearby fast-food restaurant.

In response to the professor's assertions, a community leader stated that the neighborhood was not a food desert, but rather that it had been impacted by environmental injustice and *food apartheid*. She said she had been working for 20 years to try to bring about better community development and more supermarkets, but that politicians countered that the neighborhood could not support a supermarket or even a medium-sized grocery store. However, she noted that some progress had been made in turning empty lots into community gardens and cleaning up many of the parks.

The lack of positive and health-promoting features in the built and social environments, which contributes to health inequalities, is a major concern for communities affected by environmental injustice.[48] For example, low-income neighborhoods, urban neighborhoods, and neighborhoods that are predominantly African-American have less access to supermarkets than wealthier neighborhoods, suburban neighborhoods, and those that are predominantly white.[65] The presence of supermarkets is associated with better diets and lower rates of overweight, obesity, and hypertension. In many segregated and fragmented areas, the lack of health-promoting food resources creates a food desert, which is made worse by limited transportation opportunities for local residents. Many of these poor segregated communities do not have access to personal vehicles or reliable public transit, which limits access to distant supermarkets. These environmental restraints and overabundance of food outlets in convenience stores and gas stations adversely affect diet, lifestyle, and risks for obesity, cardiovascular disease, and diabetes.[48,50] (See Chapter 34.)

Poor neighborhoods and communities of color impacted by environmental injustice are also less likely to have access to opportunities for physical activity, including green space, parks, and recreational facilities.[66] Even when there are facilities, other factors, such as poor neighborhood aesthetics and safety, limit physical activity in these neighborhoods. Limited access to medical care and lower quality of care adversely affect health and increase disparities in disadvantaged neighborhoods.[58] Being both disadvantaged and medically underserved means that residents are likely to have higher rates of chronic illnesses, drug abuse, mental health problems, unhealthful behaviors, lower childhood immunization rates, and more hospitalizations for preventable diseases than people living elsewhere. In addition, poor and minority communities impacted by environmental injustice are overburdened by health-restricting infrastructure with *environmental pathogens*.[48] Poor and minority communities have more access to fast-food restaurants and stores selling alcohol and tobacco and are more frequently targeted by advertisements for fast food, alcohol, and tobacco.

The local environment in disadvantaged communities, especially those affected by environmental injustice, has adverse impacts on quality of life, lifestyles, and behaviors. Taken together, the differential burden of increased exposure to environmental pathogens and decreased access to health-promoting resources have important implications for promoting public health and addressing environmental health disparities in these communities. The presence of environmental pathogens in a community can limit the ability of agencies to promote public health because these pathogens may create community stress or promote negative health behaviors. In addition, these pathogens may act as sources of pollution. And, because these communities have little or no access to health-promoting infrastructure, such as parks, open space, and healthcare facilities, policies to reduce environmental health disparities may be unsuccessful.

APPROACHES TO DECREASING OCCUPATIONAL AND ENVIRONMENTAL HEALTH INEQUITIES

Occupational and environmental health inequities are difficult to reduce, given the complex social, political, and economic forces that have created and sustained them. Successful interventions often require developing partnerships with community-based and other organizations that develop knowledge and insights about the problems and commitment to creating sustainable change.

Labor Unions

Labor unions have been important partners for occupational health practitioners and researchers in improving workplace safety and health. Many unions have health and safety staff who help members understand the hazards they are facing and work with managers to improve conditions. Unions help members engage in employer health and safety programs through joint labor-management health and safety committees and provide safety training through jointly funded programs. Occupational health practitioners have assisted labor unions in training workers to be knowledgeable and active members of these committees, such through the Worker Occupational Safety and Health Training and Education Program, funded by the California workers' compensation program. Unions have helped establish federal funding for the medical surveillance and compensation of workers who have experienced extreme work-related exposures. The Black Lung Compensation Program for disabled miners, the Energy Employees Occupational Illness Compensation Program, and the 9/11 World Trade Center Worker Health Program are examples of such surveillance and compensation programs. Unions also partner with researchers to investigate problems. A study showing that hotel housekeeping workers had high rates of back injuries due to heavy lifting, helped the workers' union negotiate workload reductions, which reduced the occurrence of back injuries.[67]

Worker Centers

The growing number of immigrant workers and their advocates, including faith-based organizations, have established community-based worker centers. Although these centers are not recognized as workers' representatives for the purposes of collective bargaining, as labor unions are, they organize and advocate for better working conditions. For example, the CLEAN Carwash Campaign has integrated occupational and environmental health issues into its campaign to combat wage theft and raise the minimum wage among the 10,000 mostly immigrant "carwasheros" in Los Angeles.[68] As another example, student interns in the national Occupational Health Internship Program worked with worker centers to interview workers, research chemical hazards, and support an outreach program to prevent heat-related illnesses and inform outdoor workers of their rights under state law to water, shade, and rest breaks.[69] In some cases, worker centers have formed national alliances to advocate for policy changes at the state and federal level. One such alliance is the National Domestic Workers Alliance, which has advocated for state laws supporting the rights of domestic workers. Several states have enacted "bills of rights" for domestic workers, guaranteeing them written contracts, workers' compensation coverage, maternity leave, and/or other rights, such as adequate time and conditions for sleeping.[70,71]

COSH Groups

State and regional coalitions for occupational safety and health (COSH groups) bring together academics, unions, worker centers, and public health professionals to provide technical assistance to workers; to advocate at the state level for better protections; and to honor workers who have died on the job by organizing Workers Memorial Day events. The Teens Lead @ Work project of the Massachusetts Coalition for Occupational Safety and Health, in collaboration with the Massachusetts Department of Public Health, trains teens to do peer-to-peer health and safety training. Working teens organized through Teens Lead @ Work successfully advocated for stronger child labor laws to enable the state attorney general to fine employers who place teen workers at risk.

Public Health Association

The Occupational Health and Safety (OHS) Section and the Environment Section of the American Public Health Association address equity and social justice issues at its annual meeting, through policy development, recognition of outstanding contributions to advancing health equity, and student mentoring. The OHS Section developed a curriculum for teaching about occupational health equity in colleges and schools of public health, which has been posted online.[72]

Community Empowerment Projects

An effective approach to increase health equity is *community-based participatory research* (CBPR), in which community groups, with their grassroots activism, resources, and local knowledge and expertise, collaborate with scientists to address local issues.[73-77] This approach allows for the research process to be action-oriented, thereby increasing and sustaining the community's capacity to address health equity issues as well as increasing civic engagement by minority and low-income stakeholders.[76,77] By creating a shared responsibility for research, this approach brings equality to the relationships between local and scientific experts and ensures that community-driven research is locally relevant. Many CBPR projects also emphasize the role and participation of community youth, which creates an intergenerational pipeline of community leaders knowledgeable about local health and social justice issues.

El Puente and the Watchperson Project, two community-based organizations in Brooklyn, have engaged in community-driven research to address asthma and risks from subsistence fish diets. Each organization has built its capacity to collect locally relevant data, working in partnership with EPA scientists, and to receive training in data-collection methods. Similarly, the West End Revitalization Association, a community-based environmental justice organization in Mebane, North Carolina, has developed a community–university partnership with researchers and students, primarily from the University of North Carolina at Chapel Hill. Community participants have received training on data-collection methods to build community capacity to address health disparities related to sewer and water infrastructure.[76,77]

REFERENCES

1. *A day's work* [Documentary film]. David M. Garcia and Dave DeSario, Executive Producers, 2015.
2. Centers for Disease Control and Prevention. CDC's Healthy Communities Program: Attaining health equity. Available at: https://www.cdc.gov/nccdphp/dch/programs/healthycommunitiesprogram/overview/healthequity.htm. Accessed June 8, 2017.
3. Adler N, Steward J, Cohen S, et al. Reaching for a healthier life: Facts on socioeconomic status and health in the U.S. The John D. and Catherine T. MacArthur Foundation Research Network on Socioeconomic Status and Health, 2007. Available at: http://www.macses.ucsf.edu/downloads/reaching_for_a_healthier_life.pdf. Accessed February 20, 2017.
4. Campbell R, Levenstein C. Fire and worker health and safety: An introduction to the special issue. New Solutions 2015; 24: 457–468.
5. Steege AL, Baron SL, Marsh SM, et al. Examining occupational health and safety disparities using national data: A cause for continuing concern. American Journal of Industrial Medicine 2014; 57: 527–538.

6. The Pew Charitable Trusts. The business of broilers: The high cost of putting a chicken on every grill, December 20, 2013. Available at: http://www.pewtrusts.org/en/research-and-analysis/reports/2013/12/20/the-business-of-broilers-hidden-costs-of-putting-a-chicken-on-every-grill. Accessed February 20, 2017.

7. Cartwright MS, Walker FO, Newman JC, et al. One-year incidence of carpal tunnel syndrome in Latino poultry processing workers and other Latino manual workers. American Journal of Industrial Medicine 2014; 57: 362–369.

8. Lipscomb H, Kucera K, Epling C, Dement J. Upper extremity musculoskeletal symptoms and disorders among a cohort of women employed in poultry processing. American Journal of Industrial Medicine 2008; 51: 24–36.

9. Weil D. Fissured workplace: Why work became so bad for so many and what can be done to improve it. Cambridge, MA: Harvard University Press, 2017.

10. Howard J. Nonstandard work arrangements and worker health and safety. American Journal of Industrial Medicine 2017; 60: 1–10.

11. U.S. Government Accountability Office. Contingent workforce: Size, characteristics, earnings, and benefits, April 20, 2015. Available at: http://www.gao.gov/assets/670/669766.pdf. Accessed February 20, 2017.

12. Virtanen M, Kivimäki M, Joensuu M, et al. Temporary employment and health: A review. International Journal of Epidemiology 2005; 34: 610–622.

13. Landsbergis PA, Grzywacz JG, LaMontagne AD. Work organization, job insecurity, and occupational health disparities. American Journal of Industrial Medicine 2014; 57: 495–515.

14. Occupational Safety and Health Administration. Recommended practices: Protecting temporary workers, 2014. Available at: https://www.cdc.gov/niosh/docs/2014-139/pdfs/2014-139.pdf. Accessed February 20, 2017.

15. Seixas NS, Blecker H, Camp J, Neitzel R. Occupational health and safety experience of day laborers in Seattle, WA. American Journal of Industrial Medicine 2008; 51: 399–406.

16. Flynn MA, Eggerth DE, Jacobson CJ. Undocumented status as a social determinant of occupational safety and health: The workers' perspective. American Journal of Industrial Medicine 2015; 58: 1127–1137.

17. Cherniack, M. The Hawk's Nest Incident: America's worst industrial disaster. New Haven, CT: Yale University Press, 1986.

18. Stanbury M, Rosenman KD. Occupational health disparities: A state public health-based approach. American Journal of Industrial Medicine 2014; 57: 596–604.

19. Okechukwu CA, Souza K, Davis KD, de Castro AB. Discrimination, harassment, abuse, and bullying in the workplace: Contribution of workplace injustice to occupational health disparities. American Journal of Industrial Medicine 2014; 57: 573–586.

20. Fleming PJ, Villa-Torres L, Taboada A, et al. Marginalisation, discrimination and the health of Latino immigrant day labourers in a central North Carolina community. Health and Social Care in the Community 2017; 25: 527–537.

21. Slopen N, Williams DR. Discrimination, other psychosocial stressors, and self-reported sleep duration and difficulties. Sleep 2014; 37: 147–156.

22. National Urban League. 2016 state of black America: Locked out: Education, jobs, and justice. Available at: http://soba.iamempowered.com/. Accessed February 20, 2017.

23. Byrd DR. Race/ethnicity and self-reported levels of discrimination and psychological distress, California, 2005. Preventing Chronic Disease 2012; 9: 120042. doi:http://dx.doi.org/10.5888/pcd9.120042.

24. Chavez LJ, Ornelas IJ, Lyles CR, Williams EC. Racial/ethnic workplace discrimination: Association with tobacco and alcohol use. American Journal of Preventive Medicine 2015; 48: 42–49.

25. Williams DR, Mohammed SA. Discrimination and racial disparities in health: Evidence and needed research. Journal of Behavioral Medicine 2009; 32: 20–47.

26. Krieger N. Discrimination and health inequities. International Journal of Health Services: Planning, Administration, Evaluation 2014; 44: 643–710.

27. Marín AJ, Grzywacz JG, Arcury TA, et al. Evidence of organizational injustice in poultry processing plants: Possible effects on occupational health and safety among Latino workers in North Carolina. American Journal of Industrial Medicine 2009; 52: 37–48.

28. Forman TA. The social psychological costs of racial segmentation in the workplace: A study of African Americans' well-being. Journal of Health and Social Behavior 2003; 44: 332–352.

29. Chung-Bridges K, Muntaner C, Fleming LE, et al. Occupational segregation as a determinant of US worker health. American Journal of Industrial Medicine 2008; 51: 555–567.

30. Baron S. Nonfatal work-related injuries and illnesses—United States, 2010. Morbidity and Mortality Weekly Report 2013; 62: 35–40.

31. Roelofs C, Sprague-Martinez L, Brunette M, Azaroff, L. A qualitative investigation of Hispanic construction worker perspectives on factors impacting worksite safety and risk. Environmental Health 2011; 10: 84.

32. Cummings KJ, Kreiss K. Contingent workers and contingent health: Risks of a modern economy. JAMA 2008; 299: 448–450.

33. Committee on Education and Labor. Hidden Tragedy: Underreporting of workplace injuries and illnesses. 2008. Available at: https://www.bls.gov/iif/laborcommreport061908.pdf. Accessed February 20, 2017.

34. Grabell M, Berkes H. They got hurt at work. Then they got deported. ProPublica and National Public Radio. August 16, 2017. Available at: https://www.propublica.org/article/they-got-hurt-at-work-then-they-got-deported. Accessed August 25, 2017.

35. AFL-CIO. Immigrant workers at risk: The urgent need for improved workplace safety and health policies and programs. 2005. Available at: http://www.coshnetwork.org/sites/default/files/Immigrants%20at%20Risk%20AFL%20CIO.pdf. Accessed February 20, 2017.

36. Trujillo-Pagán N. Hazardous constructions: Mexican immigrant masculinity and the rebuilding of New Orleans. In: C Johnson (ed.). The neoliberal deluge: Hurricane Katrina, late capitalism, and the remaking of New Orleans. Minneapolis, MN: University of Minnesota Press, 2011.

37. Goldenhar LM, Sweeney MH. Tradeswomen's perspectives on occupational health and safety: A qualitative investigation. American Journal of Industrial Medicine 1996; 29: 516–520.

38. Bureau of Labor Statistics. Nonfatal occupational injuries and illnesses requiring days away from work, 2015. Available at: https://www.bls.gov/news.release/osh2.nr0.htm. Accessed February 12, 2017.

39. Onyebeke LC, Papazaharias DM, Freund A, et al. Access to properly fitting personal protective equipment for female construction workers. American Journal of Industrial Medicine 2016; 59: 1032–1040.

40. Platt J, Prins S, Bates L, Keyes K. Unequal depression for equal work? How the wage gap explains gendered disparities in mood disorders. Social Science & Medicine 2016; 149: 1–8.

41. Runyan CW, Schulman M, Dal Santo J, et al. Work-related hazards and workplace safety of U.S. adolescents employed in the retail and service sectors. Pediatrics 2007; 119: 526–534.

42. Dong X, Ringen K, Men Y, Fujimoto A. Medical costs and sources of payment for work-related injuries among Hispanic construction workers. Journal of Occupational and Environmental Medicine 2007; 49: 1367–1375.

43. Bureau of Labor Statistics. Employee benefits in the United States—March 2016. Available at: https://www.bls.gov/news.release/pdf/ebs2.pdf. Accessed February 20, 2017.

44. Scherzer T, Rugulies R, Krause N. Work-related pain and injury and barriers to workers' compensation among Las Vegas hotel room cleaners. American Journal of Public Health 2005; 95: 483–488.

45. Siqueira CE, Gaydos M, Monforton C, et al. Effects of social, economic, and labor policies on occupational health disparities. American Journal of Industrial Medicine 2014; 57: 557–572.

46. Morello-Frosch R, Lopez R. The riskscape and the color line: Examining the role of segregation in environmental health disparities. Environmental Research 2006; 102: 181–196.

47. Morello-Frosch R, Jesdale B. Separate and unequal: Residential segregation and estimated cancer risks associated with ambient air toxics in U.S. metropolitan areas. Environmental Health Perspectives 2006; 114: 386–393.

48. Wilson SM. An ecologic framework to address environmental justice and community health issues. Environmental Justice 2009; 2: 15–24.

49. Gee GC, Payne-Sturges D. Environmental health disparities: A framework integrating psychosocial and environmental concepts. Environmental Health Perspectives 2004; 112: 1645–1653.

50. Wilson SM, Hutson M, Mujahid M. How planning and zoning contribute to inequitable development, neighborhood health, and environmental injustice. Environmental Justice 2008; 1: 211–216.

51. Wilson SM, Heaney CD, Cooper J, Wilson OR. Built environment issues in unserved and underserved African-American neighborhoods in North Carolina. Environmental Justice 2008; 1: 63–72.

52. Bullard RD, Mohai P, Saha R, Wright B. Toxic wastes and race at twenty, 1987–2007: A report prepared for the United Church of Christ Justice & Witness Ministries. 2007. Available at: https://www.nrdc.org/sites/default/files/

toxic-wastes-and-race-at-twenty-1987-2007.pdf. Accessed February 20, 2017.

53. Bullard RD. Unequal protection: Environmental justice and communities of color. San Francisco: Sierra Club Books, 1994.

54. Bryant B (ed.). Environmental justice: Issues, policies and solutions. Washington, DC: Island Press, 1985.

55. U.S. General Accounting Office. Siting of hazardous waste landfills and their correlation with racial and economic status of surrounding communities. 1983. Available at: http://archive. gao.gov/d48t13/121648.pdf. Accessed February 20, 2017.

56. Commission for Racial Justice, Union Church of Christ. Toxic wastes and race in the United States: A national report on the racial and socioeconomic characteristics of communities with hazardous waste sites. 1987. Available at: https://www.nrc.gov/docs/ML1310/ ML13109A339.pdf. Accessed February 20, 2017.

57. Centers for Disease Control and Prevention. Most recent asthma data. Available at: https:// www.cdc.gov/asthma/most_recent_data.htm. Accessed February 20, 2017.

58. Williams DR, Collins C. Racial residential segregation: A fundamental cause of racial disparities in health. Public Health Reports 2001: 404–416.

59. Ritz B, Wilhelm M, Hoggatt KJ, Ghosh JK. Ambient air pollution and preterm birth in the environment and pregnancy outcomes study at the University of California, Los Angeles. American Journal of Epidemiology 2007; 166: 1045–1052.

60. Ritz B, Yu F, Frui, S. Ambient air pollution and risk of birth defects in Southern California. American Journal of Epidemiology 2002; 155: 17–25.

61. Sze J. Noxious New York: The racial politics of urban health and environmental justice. Cambridge, MA: MIT Press, 2007.

62. Lindsey G, Maraj M, Kuan S. Access, equity and urban greenways: An exploratory investigation. Professional Geographer 2001; 53: 332–346.

63. Bullard RD. Growing smarter: Achieving livable communities, environmental justice, and regional equity. Cambridge, MA: MIT Press, 2007.

64. Houston D, Wu J, Ong P, Winer A. Structural disparities of urban traffic in southern California: Implications for vehicle-related air pollution exposure in minority and high poverty neighborhoods. Urban Affairs Quarterly 2004; 26: 565–592.

65. Morland K, Wing S, Diez Roux A. Neighborhood characteristics associated with the location of food stores and food service places. American Journal of Preventive Medicine 2002; 22: 23–29.

66. Taylor WC, Hepworth JT, Lees E. Obesity, physical activity, and the environment: Is there a legal basis for environmental injustices? Environmental Justice 2008; 1: 45–48.

67. Lee PT, Krause N. The impact of a worker health study on working conditions. Journal of Public Health Policy 2002; 23: 268–285.

68. UCLA Labor Center. CLEAN Carwash Campaign. Available at: http://www.labor.ucla. edu/what-we-do/labor-studies/research-tools/ campaigns-and-research/clean-carwash-campaign/. Accessed February 20, 2017.

69. Delp L, Riley K, Jacobs S, et al. Shaping the future: Ten years of the occupational health internship program. New Solutions 2013; 23: 253–281.

70. Gaydos M, Hoover C, Lynch JE, et al. A health impact assessment of California Assembly Bill 889: The California Domestic Work Employee Equality, Fairness, and Dignity Act of 2011. May 2011. Available at: http://www.pewtrusts.org/ ~/media/assets/2011/05/01/health_impact_ assessment_ab_8891.pdf. Accessed February 20, 2017.

71. National Domestic Workers Alliance. Available at: https://www.domesticworkers.org/home. Accessed February 13, 2017.

72. UCLA Labor Occupational Safety and Health Program. Work & health equity curriculum. Available at: http://losh.ucla.edu/resources-2/ work-health-equity-module/. Accessed February 13, 2017.

73. Israel BA, Eng E, Schulz AJ, et al (eds.). Methods in community-based participatory research. San Francisco: Jossey-Bass, 2005.

74. O'Fallon LR, Dearry A. Community-based participatory research as a tool to advance environmental health sciences. Environmental Health Perspectives 2002; 110: 155–159.

75. Corburn J. Street science: Community knowledge and environmental health justice. Cambridge, MA: MIT Press, 2005.

76. Heaney CD, Wilson SM, Wilson OR. The West End Revitalization Association's community-owned and managed research model: Development, implementation, and action. Progress in Community Health Partnerships 2007; 1: 339–349.

77. Wilson SM, Wilson OR, Heaney CD, Cooper C. Use of EPA collaborative problem-solving

model to obtain environmental justice in North Carolina. Progress in Community Health Partnerships 2007; 1: 327–338.

FURTHER READING

UCLA Labor Occupational Health Program. Work & health equity curriculum. Available at: http://losh.ucla.edu/resources-2/work-health-equity-module/. Accessed February 20, 2017.
Useful materials for teaching undergraduates and graduate students about occupational health equity.

Michaels D. Adding inequality to injury: The costs of failing to protect workers on the job. U.S. Occupational Safety and Health Administration, 2015. Available at: https://www.dol.gov/osha/report/20150304-inequality.pdf. Accessed February 20, 2017.
A critically important report by the director of OSHA at the time.

Special Issue: Achieving health equity in the workplace. American Journal of Industrial Medicine 2014; 57: 493–614.
This special issue includes a series of research and review articles on health equity in the workplace.

Benach J, Muntaner C, Santana V. Employment conditions and health inequalities: Final report to the WHO Commission on Social Determinants of Health, Employment Conditions Knowledge Network, 2007. World Health Organization. Available at: http://www.who.int/social_determinants/resources/articles/emconet_who_report.pdf.
This comprehensive report provides a global overview of the contribution of working conditions to worldwide health inequalities.

Morello-Frosch R, Lopez R. The riskscape and the color line: Examining the role of segregation in environmental health disparities. Environmental Research 2006; 102: 181–196.
This paper provides an excellent example of research demonstrating how segregation concentrates economic disadvantage and environmental risks. The authors examine links between racial residential segregation and estimated ambient air exposures to toxic substances and their associated cancer risks, using modeled concentration estimates from the EPA.

Wilson SM, Heaney CD, Cooper J, Wilson OR. Built environment issues in unserved and underserved African-American neighborhoods in North Carolina. Environmental Justice 2008; 1: 63–72.
This article describes built-environment issues that burden communities of color in North Carolina. The authors use a case study from Mebane, North Carolina, to describe how neighborhoods of color in this small town have been impacted by environmental injustice through the denial of basic amenities, especially sewer and water services, and overburdened by unhealthy land uses through inequities in the use of extraterritorial jurisdiction and annexation statutes.

Bullard RD, Mohai P, Saha R, Wright B. Toxic wastes and race at twenty, 1987–2007: A report prepared for the United Church of Christ Justice & Witness Ministries. 2007. Available at: https://www.nrdc.org/sites/default/files/toxic-wastes-and-race-at-twenty-1987-2007.pdf. Accessed February 20, 2017.
This report, essential reading on environmental justice in the United States, discusses exposure disparities at the regional, state, and local level using data on hazardous waste sites. It includes various tools to assess disparities in exposure to, and body burden of, toxic substances among demographic groups.

3

The Roles of Government in Protecting and Promoting Occupational and Environmental Health

Gregory R. Wagner and Emily A. Spieler

This chapter describes a conceptual framework for the roles and responsibilities of government to mitigate occupational and environmental hazards and thereby protect individuals from resultant injury, illness, or death. The focus is on U.S. governmental agencies, but the framework is relevant to other countries, especially those with democratic forms of government. The general principles described are applicable to both occupational and environmental risks, but the specific examples are drawn primarily from the workplace.

From the beginning of recorded history, people have organized themselves into groups of varying size and complexity—from families, to tribes, to nation-states, to multi-state nations, and ultimately into transnational alliances. People organized to protect against external threats and to improve the chance that individuals within the group and the group itself can survive and thrive in challenging and potentially hostile environments. Modern governments act to provide services and protect citizens and other residents from external and internal threats, including threats to public health and welfare.

The preamble to the U.S. Constitution, for example, states: "We the People of the United States, in Order to form a more perfect Union, establish Justice, insure domestic Tranquility, provide for the common defence, promote the general Welfare, and secure the Blessings of Liberty to ourselves and our Posterity, do ordain and establish this Constitution for the United States of America." It is this power of the state that underlies laws and policies designed to regulate occupational and environmental hazards.

The scope of government action varies depending on the nature of the challenge and the surrounding economic, political, and social forces. Consider the following examples:

- A worker in a small foundry is concerned about loud noise, heat, and dust. He has recently heard about the cancer risk from silica exposure but does not know if this is something he should worry about. This is the best job available to him, and he does not want to "rock the boat."
- The parent of a child with asthma is worried that stagnant air and exhaust fumes from nearby highways trigger attacks. The family lives in the northeastern United States and has heard that some of the air pollutants

they inhale come from coal-burning power plants in states to the west.

- A coal mine operator in the midwestern United States is concerned that restrictions on power plants burning coal will force him out of business and his 120 employees out of work.
- A family that owns a small dry-cleaning business learns that the solvent they use to clean clothes will soon be unavailable because of government restrictions. All substitutes are more expensive and would require investment in new equipment. All of their savings are invested in their business. They do not know how to address this problem.

In the first two examples, the individuals are incapable of acting effectively to resolve their concerns adequately. Collective action, often in the form of government intervention, is needed to provide protection for the worker or for the child. This governmental action may be taken at the local, state, or national level. The third and fourth examples illustrate the competing concern that these same government interventions intended to protect the health of the public as a whole may also have adverse effects on specific individuals or businesses. Some businesses may close, with workers losing their jobs; services and goods may become more expensive.

Democratically elected governments do not take action without justification. Elected representatives and governmental agencies have the responsibility to investigate the interests of stakeholders and to understand their concerns and needs, to protect vulnerable people who may not be able to protect themselves, and to attempt to optimize the results of any action – or, alternatively, to justify any decision not to act. Governments are expected—and often legally required—to follow the principles of fairness, nondiscrimination, constraint, and accountability. In public health, laws and policies generally attempt to balance individual and corporate rights against the best collective public health outcome. In this sense, the law serves both as an important tool for achieving public health objectives and, at times, as an obstacle. The right of workers to a safe working environment—or of residents to a safe community—may be compromised or balanced against competing rights of employers and businesses to due process and

protection from excessive government intrusion, rights established by the U.S. Constitution.

Preventive measures to protect health can be developed or implemented by any branch or level of government. In the United States, the federal government has three co-equal branches, each with separate (but interactive) powers and responsibilities:

- The *legislative branch* enacts legislation (laws) and provides resources (through taxation and budget allocation) to implement the laws. In the federal government, this branch is the Congress, which consists of the Senate and the House of Representatives. In occupational health, the most important federal laws are the Occupational Safety and Health Act (OSH Act) and the Mine Safety and Health Act (MSH Act). In environmental health, the most important federal laws include the Environmental Protection Act, the Clean Water Act, the Safe Drinking Water Act, the Clean Air Act, and the Toxic Substances Control Act.
- The *executive branch*, which in the federal government consists of the President and the executive (Cabinet) agencies, is responsible for implementing the laws enacted by Congress and signed by the President. The President can also veto (not sign) a law passed by Congress; if Congress does not override the veto with a supermajority vote, the law will not go into effect. The executive branch can propose legislation and budgets to the Congress. Federal executive agencies include the Department of Labor (in which the Occupational Safety and Health Administration [OSHA] and the Mine Safety and Health Administration [MSHA] are located), the Environmental Protection Agency (EPA), and the Department of Health and Human Services. These executive branch agencies develop regulations (also known as standards or rules) for implementing the laws and enforcing the standards.
- The *judicial branch* (the judiciary) interprets the law. The federal courts determine whether laws passed by Congress are consistent with the U.S. Constitution, and whether actions by executive agencies to implement these laws are consistent with the U.S. Constitution and with the laws as they are passed by Congress.

Box 3-1. Alignment of Political Forces
for Protective Legislation

The passage of the federal Coal Mine Health and Safety Act in 1969 was one of the best examples of the alignment of political forces resulting in protective legislation. Coal mining has always been both unsafe and unhealthy. But coal mining takes place out of sight and out of the consciousness of most Americans—in rural, sparsely populated, and, often, economically depressed areas.

This invisibility changed when, in 1968, a fire and explosion ripped through the Farmington Coal Mine near Fairmont, West Virginia, trapping and ultimately killing 78 miners. For weeks, national television news programs covered this tragedy, with daily pictures and stories documenting the anxiety of miners' families—and eventually their grief when rescue attempts were abandoned.

This recognition of the hazards of coal mining came at a time of social and political activism—supporting the Civil Rights Movement and opposing the Vietnam War. In addition, coal miners, supported by the work of public health professionals, had been organizing demonstrations to bring attention to the disabling, life-threatening lung diseases afflicting coal miners. The result was the passage of comprehensive legislation to protect and compensate coal miners, establish medical surveillance, and promote prevention-focused research.

State and local governments also have similar branches. Laws and regulations vary widely among states and among local government jurisdictions. State legislatures may pass laws pertaining to occupational and environmental health as long as they are consistent with federal laws. (See section on Federalism.)

At any level of government, the development and implementation of new laws, regulations, or other policies require recognition of the existence of a problem, available solutions, financial resources to address the problem, and the popular and political will to act. Without these elements, action will not likely be taken.[1] The passage of the Coal Mine Health and Safety Act of 1969 illustrates this alignment. (See Box 3-1.)

FRAMEWORKS FOR GOVERNMENT ACTION

Governments have a variety of tools to improve prevention of occupational and environmental illnesses and injuries. Once a problem is identified and a commitment is made to address it, people within the government consider options for interventions. Their objective, as a rule, is to prevent disease or injury in the least coercive and most economical manner possible. Government options, ranging from the least to the most coercive, are described in the following sections.

Disseminating Information

The least costly action for a government may be to disseminate existing information to those who can take useful action. This process may take the form of information releases through the news media and social media; targeted distribution to individuals, employers, or communities affected by the problem; or participation in public meetings or scientific conferences.

The government can, for example, simply make administrative data, such as injury and illness reports, results of worksite inspections, or data on air and water quality, available to anyone who knows how to access these data through governmental agency websites and portals. Federal data are available at www.data.gov. Health and medical publications by government scientists and others can be accessed through the National Library of Medicine. The effectiveness of this kind of passive dissemination depends both on the willingness of the government to make information available, on people's knowledge that the information exists, and on their skills and access to tools that enable the target audience to utilize the information.

Governments may also send messages about specific issues to particular stakeholders. The underlying assumption of this type of *awareness campaign* is that informed stakeholders who can take action are more likely to act if they better understand the issue and the consequences of inaction. For example, MSHA's annual press releases, mailings to mine facilities, and postings to websites remind miners and operators at underground coal mines of the increased risk of mine roof falls during the late fall and early winter.

Governments may also alert the public to enforcement actions that have been taken against entities that have violated rules. For example, they may provide information to the public about the nature of violations, harms caused, and fines and other actions it has taken to punish a violator. This public communication informs other actual or potential violators that they too might be held accountable and have their reputations tarnished. This strategy, sometimes called *public shaming*, has been shown to be effective in modifying employer behavior.[2]

Generating and Communicating New Information

Government agencies can generate—and then disseminate—new information by conducting or supporting research or by gathering and performing new analyses of existing data. For example, the National Institute for Occupational Safety and Health (NIOSH), established by the same legislation that created OSHA, is charged with developing new information about occupational hazards and the methods for controlling them. NIOSH conducts research, financially supports nongovernmental research, and makes recommendations to OSHA, state government agencies, employers, workers, and others on the best approaches to recognize and control workplace hazards. The EPA, the National Center for Environmental Health (part of the Centers for Disease Control and Prevention), and the National Institute of Environmental Health Sciences (part of the National Institutes of Health) conduct and support research on environmental hazards. Other government agencies, such as the Department of Energy, may support research that can be used to inform the public about occupational and environmental health and safety hazards. The results of all relevant scientific research inform government decisions concerning new and existing regulations and other policies.

Providing Guidance and Advocating for the Establishment of Improved Norms

Government agencies routinely communicate nonenforceable guidelines or recommendations to reduce risk based on the best available information. For example, NIOSH is legislatively mandated to develop and update recommended exposure limits for toxic substances found in workplaces. While these guidelines do not set legally-enforceable limits, they nevertheless provide information to employers and workers about risks that may be inadequately regulated (either because there is no rule or because new information has shown that the legal limit is not adequately protective) and ways in which these risks can be reduced.

Many agencies charged with health protection also produce and communicate recommendations for improved practices. For example, OSHA and NIOSH have jointly issued guidance for protecting workers in hot environments. The EPA has issued many guidance documents advising employers and communities on ways to comply with environmental regulations. While guidelines are not legally enforceable, a government agency can encourage establishment of new norms of exposure or activity and facilitate voluntary implementation of preventive measures by issuing guidelines (recommendations). In addition, government agencies may sometimes issue guidelines when there is sufficient information to encourage action on a significant problem, but there are barriers to developing formal regulations.

The government may also certify the adequacy of certain protective approaches. For example, NIOSH tests respiratory protective devices, classifies them, and certifies that specific models perform as advertised in the environments where they are intended to be used. Individuals or companies can use this certification to determine what equipment to purchase and use for protection against workplace hazards. When regulations mandate use of respiratory protection, only certified respirators may be used.

Providing Incentives for Health Protective Actions

The government may establish incentives for employers to voluntarily adopt measures for protection of health. For example, the OSHA Voluntary Protection Program encourages employers to develop and implement comprehensive health and safety management programs relevant to their industry and enterprise.

Tax policy is frequently used to encourage voluntary adoption of societally-desirable practices. For example, businesses and individuals may be given subsidies in the form of credits against taxes if they spend money on solar panels for generation of clean energy or on more efficient heating or air-conditioning systems. Favorable tax treatment may encourage the purchase of new, safer equipment. The tax code may provide incentives for specific actions without penalizing those who cannot—or choose not to—take advantage of the incentives.

Establishing and Enforcing Standards and Regulations

Formal enforceable regulations, which are promulgated by the executive agencies, are essential tools for reducing occupational and environmental health and safety risks. Without regulations, employers and businesses may not have sufficient motivation and may lack adequate financial incentive to reduce these risks. For example, much of the cost of occupationally related deaths and disabilities is externalized from workplaces, and the costs are borne by entities other than the employer.[3,4]

Effective regulatory intervention requires all of the following:

1. A law that sets out the principles and justification for regulation
2. An agency with expertise to decide what hazards warrant intervention and to develop specific rules governing intervention
3. Enforcement methods to ensure adequate compliance with both general and specific regulatory requirements
4. Dissemination of information to affected parties regarding the regulatory requirements
5. Protection of workers or community members who initiate and participate in enforcement activities.

Because establishing regulations (standard setting) and implementing them (inspection and enforcement) are central to the federal government's role in preventing occupational and environmental illnesses and injuries, the following section describes this approach in detail.

THE U.S. REGULATORY SYSTEM

Occupational Safety and Health

The two primary federal laws governing occupational safety and health are the OSH Act,[4] which covers general industry, and the MSH Act,[5] which covers coal, metal, and non-metal mining as well as quarrying. Other federal laws govern health and safety in specific industries, including railroads, trucking, nuclear energy, and agriculture (for pesticide use).

The Occupational Safety and Health Act

Until 1970, there was no comprehensive federal law concerning occupational safety and health in general industry. Early in the 20th century, the U.S. Supreme Court even limited the right of states to regulate working conditions. But the understanding of the federal government's powers changed during the first half of the 20th century. A broader interpretation of the Interstate Commerce Clause of the U.S. Constitution meant that Congress could enact federal laws in a wide variety of areas, including occupational and environmental health. In response to growing public concern about workplace hazards, in 1970 Congress passed, and President Richard Nixon signed, the OSH Act. Congress justified the law on economic grounds, noting that occupational injuries and illnesses impose a substantial burden on interstate commerce with lost production, wage loss, medical expenses, and payment for disability compensation.

The OSH Act expresses a lofty goal:

To assure safe and healthful working conditions for working men and women; by authorizing enforcement of the standards developed under the Act; by assisting and encouraging the States in their efforts to assure safe and healthful working conditions; by providing for research, information, education, and training in the field of occupational safety and health; and for other purposes.

The Act also states that any regulation pertaining to toxic materials or harmful physical agents must assure, to the extent feasible, that no workers will suffer impairment of health or functional capacity even if they have regular exposure to a hazard for their entire working lives.

The OSH Act established two agencies: OSHA to develop regulations (standards) and enforce the law and NIOSH to perform research and provide OSHA with scientifically based recommendations. OSHA promulgates regulations that cover specific hazards and issues orders (citations) to employers who are not in compliance with the law. The OSH Act created a separate adjudicatory body, the Occupational Safety and Health Review Commission (OSHRC), to settle disputes when employers challenge OSHA enforcement actions. The OSH Act permits enforcement of OSHA regulations by state agencies in certain circumstances. (See the later discussion of federalism to understand the interaction between federal and state government agencies.)

The primary focus of OSHA is the responsibility of employers to maintain safe workplaces. To comply with the law, every employer has two primary duties: (a) to furnish each employee employment and a place of employment that are "free from recognized hazards that are causing or are likely to cause death or serious physical harm" (in compliance with the General Duty Clause) and (b) to comply with occupational safety and health standards promulgated by OSHA. Employees also must comply with regulations relevant to their own individual actions and conduct.

Even if there is no specific standard that regulates a hazard, the General Duty Clause obliges employers to provide safe workplaces. Because the process of setting standards (promulgating regulations or making rules) is very slow, the General Duty Clause has special significance. OSHA can cite employers under the General Duty Clause for hazards not covered by other regulations and for more generalized serious hazards.

OSHA may develop a standard when an assessment demonstrates that a hazard is (a) sufficiently widespread and (b) causes illnesses or injuries that can be reduced or controlled by methods that are technologically and economically feasible. OSHA promulgates permanent standards, interim standards, and emergency temporary standards.

When the OSH Act was passed, it authorized the initial issuance of interim standards,

without adhering to the formal rulemaking procedure required for new permanent standards. These interim standards, known as *consensus standards*, were based on existing recommendations from professional organizations or existing rules developed under old laws. In 1971, OSHA promulgated 4,400 federal consensus standards under this rulemaking authority. The interim standards remained in effect until revoked or revised using the procedure for new permanent standards. OSHA's power to set interim standards expired in 1973. Because OSHA has had difficulty in issuing permanent standards, many of these initial standards are still in effect.

Since 1973, OSHA has been authorized to issue only permanent standards or emergency standards and must meet strict substantive and procedural requirements. In order to issue a permanent standard, OSHA must demonstrate all of the following:

1. The targeted hazard, if left unregulated, would pose a significant risk of injury or death. In developing standards, OSHA, in response to judicial decisions, has decided not to propose new standards without scientific evidence that shows that workers exposed to the substance or hazard for their working lifetimes will experience at least a one-in-a-thousand (0.1%) risk of death or serious harm.

2. The proposed change (such as reduction in exposure or change in workplace design) will result in a demonstrable reduction in this risk.

3. The imposed regulation is based on the best available scientific information.

4. The proposed regulation is both technically and economically feasible. (Economic feasibility focuses on the viability of an entire industry, not individual employers in that industry.)

Permanent standards, particularly those that regulate toxic substances, are often quite complex. They set exposure limits, identify specific methods for hazard control, and mandate required training of workers. Several health standards also require medical monitoring to try to identify workers with excessive exposure or subclinical disease and provide them with therapeutic or preventive interventions. (For example, the OSHA lead standard provides for temporary transfer for workers who have elevated blood lead levels to jobs with lower or no lead exposure.)

To issue a *permanent standard*, OSHA must follow a strict administrative process, set out in the Administrative Procedures Act, which requires:

1. Publication of an initial intent to engage in rulemaking
2. Publication of the proposed standard
3. A sufficient period for the agency to receive comments and hold public hearings
4. Finally, promulgation of the final rule, including the agency's justification and responses to the comments.

Standards are then subject to rigorous judicial review if challenged by an affected party. Every recent OSHA and MSHA standard has been challenged by businesses, business associations, or unions. The judicial review process can be lengthy. (Some of the steps in the standard-setting process are illustrated in Figure 3-1.)

Without conducting hearings or using advisory committees, OSHA may issue a *temporary emergency standard*, which is effective immediately upon publication. To do so, OSHA must show that "employees are exposed to grave danger from exposure to substances or agents determined to be toxic or physically harmful or from new hazards" and that the standard "is necessary to protect employees from such danger." A temporary emergency standard can be in effect only for 6 months. OSHA has, since 1971, issued only nine temporary standards, five of which were rescinded when they were successfully challenged in court.

Enforcement

All federal health and safety laws are based on the concept of *preinspection compliance*. The laws assume that employers will comply in order to prevent illnesses and injuries—not that the agencies will be able to inspect every employer before an illness or injury occurs or that deterrence will be achieved by punishment after it occurs.

OSHA is not required to inspect the workplaces of every employer. Fines for violations

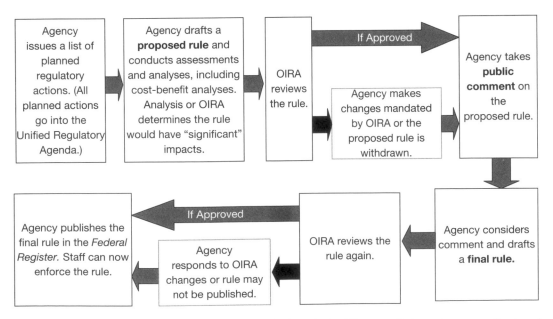

Figure 3-1. Steps in federal rulemaking for significant rules (over $100 million annually in costs or new policy issues). *Note.* OIRA, Office of Information and Regulatory Affairs. (Project on Government Oversight.)

are relatively low, and criminal sanctions are limited. The OSHA inspection force is also very small compared to the breadth of its jurisdiction; there are 2,200 federal and state inspectors (compliance officers) responsible for the health and safety of 130 million workers, employed at more than 8 million worksites in the United States—about one for every 59,000 workers. According to one analysis, OSHA is able to inspect each U.S. workplace about once a century, on average, with current staffing levels.[6] Given these constraints, expecting and requiring employers to comply with the OSH Act *before* or in the absence of an inspection is the only possible approach that will result in effective prevention.

OSHA is empowered to enter and inspect workplaces, to levy civil penalties, and to bring criminal actions against employers for failing to comply with either specific standards or the General Duty Clause. Compliance officers from OSHA's regional and district offices, located throughout the United States, inspect workplaces to determine if employers are in compliance with all applicable standards and the General Duty Clause. OSHA's operating procedures are set out in its field operations manual, which includes guidelines for selecting workplaces to be inspected and procedures for inspections, preparation of citations, and assessment of penalties.

The OSH Act established the following general priorities for inspections:

1. Imminent danger investigations
2. Investigations of fatalities and catastrophes involving three or more employees
3. Investigations of complaints
4. Targeted or programmed inspections, generally in industries where there is particular concern due to especially high rates of injuries or toxic exposures
5. Follow-up inspections (to ensure that an employer has achieved full compliance after prior inspections). These inspections may receive higher priority in high-risk industries or when the employer is a repeat violator.

When conducting an OSHA inspection, the compliance officer first presents credentials to the employer and then conducts an inspection tour of the facility (a *walkaround*). If the employer refuses to allow the inspector to enter, OSHA will seek an administrative search warrant from a federal district court; administrative search warrants are routinely issued. The employer has a right to accompany the inspector on the walkaround. An employee representative may also participate in the walkaround, although inspections are not invalidated by the lack of an employee representative and employers are not required to pay workers for their time spent on walkarounds. In general, workers assert their rights to participate in walkarounds more frequently in workplaces that are unionized.

After the inspection, the compliance officer convenes a closing conference to discuss safety and health conditions and possible violations. The inspector then returns to the OSHA regional or district office and confers with supervisors to determine what, if any, citations will be issued. All citations provide details regarding the specific violations, any proposed penalties, and the time limits (*abatement periods*) for the employer to correct the violations. Penalties depend on the seriousness of the violation. OSHA can bring criminal charges in certain circumstances for willful violations of standards.

If an imminent danger is present at the facility, the compliance officer will inform the employees and the employer. Although OSHA cannot immediately stop any work, OSHA may seek an order from a federal district court requiring the employer to eliminate the imminent danger. The on-site compliance officer has no authority to stop any work, no matter how dangerous, without a court order.

An employer has the right to challenge any aspect of a citation within 15 working days. In contrast, employees and their representatives have limited rights; if the employer does not challenge the citation, employees can only challenge the duration of the abatement period. However, if the employer challenges the citation, the employees' representative may request formal involvement in the proceedings that follow. Administrative law judges within OSHRC hold hearings on employer challenges to citations, and the Commission rules on appeals of these judges' decisions. Appeals of Commission decisions go to a U.S. Circuit Court of Appeals.

The employer has no obligation to abate a hazard during any pending challenge to the citation. Citations are therefore often settled for reduced penalties in order to induce the employer to address the hazard at the workplace more quickly.

Voluntary Consultations

Given the vast number of workplaces and the shortage of OSHA inspectors, several administrative programs seek voluntary compliance with OSHA regulations. On-site consultation services, funded by OSHA, are provided free of charge; priority is given to small businesses and companies in hazardous industries.

OSHA also operates two programs that give special privileges to approved employers including exempting them from OSHA programmed inspections. Its Voluntary Protection Program recognizes employers that have implemented effective safety and health management systems and maintain injury and illness rates below national averages for their industries. Its Safety and Health Achievement Recognition Program recognizes small businesses that operate "exemplary" injury and illness prevention programs.

Workers' Rights under the OSH Act

Under the OSH Act, workers have several rights, including:

- Protection from retaliation for raising concerns about safety or notifying their employers about injuries
- Exemptions from being fined for violations of the Act found on workplace inspections
- Limited rights to participate in inspections and appeals of citations against employers
- The right to participate, personally or through their unions, in the public process for development of new standards.

Mine Safety and Health

Underground mining has long been recognized as extremely hazardous. Federal safety and health regulation of mining began earlier than in general industry. Multiple mining disasters resulted in progressively stronger attempts by the federal government to improve mine safety. Starting in 1941, federal mine inspectors were given a legal right to enter mines, and, in 1947, the first legally enforceable federal mine safety regulations were authorized by Congress.

Over time, authority to regulate safety grew as did the mandate to inspect and enforce regulations. Responding to increasing public concerns about the health and safety of coal miners, Congress passed the Coal Mine Safety and Health Act of 1969. The Act established more stringent requirements, including financial penalties for violations of regulations; a limit to coal mine dust exposure; and a health surveillance program for coal miners. The Act also mandated regular inspection of all mines and created a federal compensation system for victims of severe lung disease from coal mine dust ("black lung" disease). In 1977, after a mine disaster in Kentucky caused 27 deaths, Congress strengthened mine safety laws by passing the Federal Mine Safety and Health Act (the Mine Act), which consolidated responsibility for regulating and inspecting coal mines as well as metal mines and rock quarrying in MSHA. The Mine Act expanded the rights of miners to request inspections when they identified hazardous conditions and improved miners' protection from retaliation for expressing concerns about safety or health. The Act also enabled MSHA to impose severe penalties on mine operations with a "pattern of violations" indicating an unwillingness to comply with mining safety laws.

The administrative and adjudicative structure of MSHA is similar to that of OSHA. Appeals of citations go to the Mine Safety and Health Review Commission, a separate agency similar to OSHRC.

Reflecting the widely held view that mines are more dangerous than other workplaces, the Mine Act is stronger than the OSH Act in several ways:

- It provides for mandatory comprehensive inspections of all mines: four times a year for all underground mines, twice a year for all surface mines.
- Inspectors have on-site authority to shut down an operation if it poses an imminent danger to workers.
- Workers who accompany inspectors on walkarounds must be paid for their time.

- Fines are higher than in general industry.
- Employers must abate hazards immediately, even if they appeal citations or fines.
- Protection for workers against retaliation is stronger, including an immediate right to reinstatement if they are discharged, as long as their claims are not viewed as "frivolous."
- State agencies can establish parallel mine safety programs that do not displace any federal regulatory or enforcement programs.

Environmental Health

In the United States, interest in environmental protection arose from a commitment to the preservation of unspoiled areas of wilderness (generally for recreational purposes) and a desire to protect people from health threats posed by toxic contamination of air, water, and soil. Historically, regulatory authority to protect the environment had been spread among multiple federal and state agencies, without coordination or sufficient attention to a scientific foundation for environmental policy.

In the 1960s, growing attention to the threat of toxic pollutants, in part sparked by the book *Silent Spring* by Rachel Carson, drew attention to the hazards posed by DDT and other pesticides and encouraged environmental and political movements that advocated for increased environmental protections.[7] In response, President Nixon proposed and Congress passed the National Environmental Policy Act of 1969 to improve coordination of environmental policy formation, regulation, and scientific research. The stated goals of the Act were to:

- Fulfill the responsibilities of each generation as trustee of the environment for succeeding generations
- Assure for all Americans safe, healthful, productive, and esthetically and culturally pleasing surroundings
- Attain the widest range of beneficial uses of the environment without degradation, risk to health or safety, or other undesirable and unintended consequences
- Preserve important historic, cultural, and natural aspects of our national heritage, and maintain, wherever possible, an environment that supports diversity and variety of individual choice
- Achieve a balance between population and resource use, which will permit high standards of living and a wide sharing of life's amenities
- Enhance the quality of renewable resources and approach the maximum attainable recycling of depletable resources.

The Act established the Environmental Planning Council and mandated broad responsibilities for assessing the environmental impact of federal government activities. The Act was soon followed by a reorganization of federal agencies, resulting in the consolidation of responsibilities related to health protection from environmental pollution into the EPA. President Nixon, in proposing the creation of the EPA, said it was needed to:

- Establish and enforce environmental protection standards consistent with national environmental goals
- Conduct research on the adverse effects of pollution and on methods and equipment for controlling it, gather information on pollution, and use this information for strengthening environmental protection programs and recommending policy changes
- Assist others, through grants, technical assistance, and other means, in arresting pollution of the environment
- Assist the Council on Environmental Quality in developing and recommending to the president new policies for the protection of the environment.

The EPA is responsible for enforcement of several laws relating to environmental protection, including the Clean Air Act (see Chapter 15), the Clean Water Act, and the Safe Drinking Water Act (see Chapter 16), as well as laws governing hazardous wastes (see Chapter 18) and protection of endangered species. (Details of these laws are described in the cited chapters.)

CONSTRAINTS ON GOVERNMENT ACTIONS

Government actions attempt to balance a range of conflicting social, political, and economic interests. Although the potential for the federal government to protect against occupational and environmental hazards is broad, there are substantial constraints, both within and external to the government. Mandatory inclusion of stakeholder input to priority setting, regulation, and actions provides transparency but also reduces government decision latitude.

Budgetary and Other Legislated Constraints

The executive branch proposes budgets, but the legislative branch, through taxes and fees, raises and allocates money for all government activities. Executive agencies, such as OSHA, MSHA, and EPA, may only spend money on programs specifically authorized by legislation, and they cannot spend more money than they are allocated. In addition, Congress can restrict spending on specific activities that appear to be within the domain of particular agencies. The legislative budgeting process can result in limitations on agency actions in two ways. First, the budget may be inadequate to support some activities. For example, OSHA's budget is insufficient to hire and train enough compliance officers to inspect all workplaces. Second, Congress may restrict the use of funds for specific purposes that would appear to be within the agency's powers. For example, Congress does not permit OSHA to use authorized funds for routine inspections of agricultural worksites, thereby limiting the protection of agricultural workers. Small businesses employing fewer than 10 people are also exempted from routine inspections.

The Congressional Review Act (CRA) allows Congress to review and override regulations that have been legally developed and issued. For example, in 2001, Congress nullified a comprehensive occupational ergonomics rule that was issued by OSHA; since then, OSHA has been precluded from developing a new standard to protect workers from ergonomic hazards. This was the only time the CRA was used prior to 2017, when it was employed to overturn several federal regulations, including an OSHA regulation that had clarified OSHA's ability to cite employers for failure to maintain records of injuries and diseases for the 5 years prior to an inspection.

The Office of Information and Regulatory Affairs (OIRA), established by a Presidential executive order, exerts the primary constraint within the executive branch on agencies developing and issuing regulations. OIRA assures that government activities and demands on citizens are not burdensome. The executive order mandated OIRA involvement in all rule-making and set out the following guiding philosophy:

- Federal agencies should promulgate only regulations that are required by law, necessary to interpret the law, or made necessary by compelling public need, such as material failures of private markets to protect or improve public health and safety or the environment.
- In deciding whether and how to regulate, agencies should assess all costs and benefits of available regulatory alternatives, including the alternative of not regulating. Both quantifiable and qualitative measures of costs and benefits should be considered.
- In choosing among alternative regulatory approaches, agencies should select those approaches that maximize net benefits (including potential economic, environmental, public health and safety, and other advantages; distributive impacts; and equity), unless a statute requires another regulatory approach.[8]

Compliance with this executive order means that all proposals from executive agencies to issue regulations pass through OIRA for review and approval before being made public (Figure 3-1). OIRA may refuse permission to issue a rule because of insufficient justification, excessive cost, or a belief that the issuing agency has not been sufficiently thorough in exploring alternatives to the proposed regulation. Proposed rules that pass OIRA review are then made available for a period of public comment, after which agencies revise or abandon the proposed rules. Any revised rules must be approved again by OIRA before being issued. The result of this often-lengthy deliberative process is that OSHA infrequently issues regulations, and those regulations that it does issue take many years to develop.[9]

PUBLIC ENGAGEMENT IN THE REGULATORY PROCESS

Throughout the regulatory process, there are many opportunities for public engagement to either encourage or oppose government actions. Individuals and organizations may informally ask government agencies to pay attention to their specific concerns. If they are unsatisfied, they may formally petition agencies to take action. Agencies are obligated to publish a *regulatory agenda*, identifying the regulations that they are considering or developing and the status of their work on these regulations. Members of the public may comment on the published agenda to encourage agencies to accelerate or slow action.

Agencies frequently make formal *requests for information*, asking individuals, organizations, and other government agencies to provide information relevant to developing a regulation in order to assure that they are acting, as legally mandated, on the best available information. Organizations and individuals may interact with OIRA during the regulatory process to try to ensure that their concerns are being addressed.

Once a regulation is formally proposed, there is a public comment period, during which individuals and organizations are encouraged to submit comments on the proposal. Each of the comments is reviewed by the agency and must be considered and addressed in the framing of the final regulation.

Organizations or individuals who believe that they will be adversely affected by a regulation can seek judicial review, if they feel that the proper procedures were not followed by the agency in developing the regulation.

There are formally established independent federal advisory committees, such as the Advisory Committee on Construction Safety and Health, the National Advisory Committee on Occupational Safety and Health, the Mine Safety and Health Research Advisory Committee, and the Clean Air Scientific Advisory Committee, which provide advice to the regulatory agencies. Agencies may also establish ad hoc advisory committees to focus on a specific hazard or in response to petitions requesting rulemaking. Representatives of stakeholder organizations also have frequent informational meetings with staff members of regulatory agencies in order to remain current regarding regulatory and enforcement policies and scientific developments.

FEDERALISM AND THE ROLE OF STATE AND LOCAL GOVERNMENTS

The concept of *federalism* guides and constrains the actions of the U.S. government in addressing occupational and environmental threats. The federal government's ability to act is framed by the U.S. Constitution. Whatever powers are not specifically granted to the federal government are held by the states. As the understanding and interpretation of federal powers broadened through the 20th century, the balance between federal authority on the one hand and state and local authority on the other has evolved.

The federal government's authority to regulate occupational and environmental health is largely derived from the Interstate Commerce Clause of the Constitution. Regulated activity therefore must, in some way, involve activities that cross state boundaries. Today, because of the interconnectedness of the economy and the nature of commerce, the reach of the federal government is deep and broad. However, the federal government may also delegate some of its regulatory and enforcement powers to states. This somewhat complex relationship plays out differently under the different federal laws.

The OSH Act provides that states may develop their own state plans, apply for federal approval, and then enforce the OSH Act, *replacing* the enforcement structure of the federal government described previously. Currently, 26 states have approved state plans, of which 21 cover both private-sector and public-sector (government) workers; the remaining five states cover public-sector workers only. State plans for the private sector must be at least as protective as the OSH Act requirements. These states can also enact and enforce laws or regulations that are more protective than the federal requirements; this has been done in some states, including California and Washington.

In addition, if the federal government does not create a regulation concerning a hazard, states without approved state plans retain the right to regulate that hazard within their own borders. The OSH Act allows any state to create its own standards if there is no federal standard to govern a workplace hazard or practice.

Sometimes the federal government will promulgate a standard after states have regulated the same hazard or issue; states that do not have approved state plans then lose their authority to regulate in this specific area. For example, many states passed "right-to-know" laws that required companies to provide information to employees. After OSHA developed a national right-to-know regulation (the Federal Hazard Communication Standard), however, state right-to-know laws were no longer enforceable. Tensions between federal OSHA and states can occur when pre-existing state laws have been more (or less) protective than a new federal standard.

The federal–state relationship under the MSH Act operates under a different model. States are entirely free to regulate the mining industry, with no effect on the federal program; state laws and their implementation exist in parallel to the federal system. Therefore, an underground mine may be inspected four times a year by the federal government but may also be subject to inspections, citations, and fines from a state agency.

Under the federal environmental statutes, much of the implementation and enforcement is delegated to the states. States may apply national standards, but (with a few exceptions) states can opt to set stricter standards than those required by federal law. Some states, reacting to concerns about climate change, have developed more aggressive environmental programs than the national program. For example, in California, the Clean Energy and Pollution Reduction Act of 2015 strengthened targets for renewable energy, requiring California to obtain half its electrical power from renewable sources by the end of 2030. (See Chapter 29.)

States may also allow counties, cities, and towns to pass their own ordinances. The "home-rule" powers of local government are always delegated by state governments to local governments. A state legislature can grant or take away powers of a local government. In general, home rule allows local governments to protect the public and regulate property use. Local zoning and construction regulations may result in improved environmental protection. Construction permitting can create barriers for companies with poor safety or environmental records to obtain permits. State and local ordinances, which are subject to home-rule limitations, may restrict use of toxic materials, require labeling and communication where hazards are present, and otherwise provide targeted protections against recognized local threats.

WHEN PREVENTION FAILS

Failures of prevention may result in illnesses or injuries. Workers' compensation programs, which operate primarily at the state level, generally provide partial wage replacement as well as payment for medical and rehabilitative services for workers with work-related illnesses or injuries. These programs are complex and vary substantially from one state to another.[10]

Several federal laws provide compensation to targeted groups of workers. In general, these laws were passed because of major gaps in state compensation laws and significant political pressure. These laws include:

- The Federal Black Lung Benefits Act, which provides compensation for totally-disabled coal miners suffering from coal workers' pneumoconiosis ("black lung")
- The Energy Employees Occupational Illness Compensation Program Act, which provides compensation for civilian workers in the nuclear weapons industry
- The September 11th Victim Compensation Fund and the James Zadroga 9/11 Health and Compensation Act, both of which provide compensation and medical care to victims of the 9/11 attacks on the World Trade Center

- The Radiation Exposure Compensation Act, which provides compensation for illnesses and injuries related to atmospheric testing of nuclear weapons and work in the uranium industry.

There are also federal compensation programs for federal government workers, longshore and harbor workers, and railroad workers in interstate commerce.

There are no comparable programs to provide compensation or care for individuals harmed by environmental hazards. In general, individuals or communities seeking compensation because of harms caused by environmental hazards must pursue their claims through other legal actions, including court proceedings. The cost and complexity of these proceedings are a substantial barrier to action by individuals or communities seeking restitution.

Other laws that target a more general population may provide protections to people with occupationally or environmentally caused illnesses or injuries. All individuals with substantial impairments may be protected under the Americans with Disabilities Act or analogous state laws. These laws guarantee the right to be free from discrimination and the right to reasonable accommodation at work.

In addition, health-relevant work-related policies are affected by laws and regulations related to wages, hours of employment, child labor, benefits, and policies affecting work leave. Labor-management regulations affect the extent to which workers have a voice in limiting workplace hazards. Some regulations protect whistleblowers who identify problems from reprisal or discrimination or reward them for identifying problems in the conduct of government activity. Financial reporting regulations can bring the attention of investors to the poor environmental record of companies, which, in turn, may encourage or force the companies to improve.

Government agencies can respond to major failures of prevention. For example, MSHA conducts comprehensive investigations of mine disasters to determine which of its own policies and practices should change to reduce the likelihood of future similar disasters. After the Upper Big Branch Mine Disaster in 2010, which killed 29 miners, MSHA conducted a comprehensive 2-year investigation, which involved the public release of thousands of pages of documents and ultimately resulted in numerous changes in agency practices and regulations. The EPA, OSHA, and NIOSH conducted investigations of the Deepwater Horizon oil-drilling disaster in the Gulf of Mexico in 2010, which resulted in the deaths of 11 workers and extensive environmental contamination. In response to these kinds of events, legislators often convene hearings to determine whether laws or regulations need to be strengthened.

CONCLUSION

In developing and implementing actions to protect the public from occupational and environmental hazards, the government performs a balancing act. Interventions take place within ever-changing social, economic, legal, and political environments that result, over time, in greater or lesser senses of urgency and support for action. When there is alignment of a sense of urgency, shared recognition of a problem worth addressing, probable solutions, and the resources (both inside and outside the government) to take effective action, the government may move forward. In moving ahead, the actions that the government may take range from information dissemination, to research, to development and distribution of guidelines for improved practices, to providing incentives for health protective actions, to the development and enforcement of regulations.

Under federal laws, agencies are given broad enforcement powers to advance the public health policies written into their enabling statutes. But there may be substantial barriers to action: There may not be adequate support for a regulatory intervention; the political climate may not be conducive to stronger enforcement; scientific evidence may not be adequately compelling or publicly accepted to justify regulations; the proposed interventions may not be viewed as economically or technologically feasible; and the specific proposed regulation may not be a priority when weighed, by OIRA, against other regulations being issued by other agencies unrelated to occupational or environmental health. Facing these kinds of barriers, government agencies often work to employ the least coercive action in order to put nongovernmental actors in a better position to protect occupational or environmental health.

Improvements in these fields do not rest on government intervention alone. In particular, public health professionals and the public overall can promote and encourage improvements in worker and community protection, and can support the government in fulfilling its public protection responsibilities.

REFERENCES

1. Kingdon JW. Agendas, alternatives, and public policies (2nd ed.). New York: Longman Publishing Group, 2011.
2. Johnson MS. Regulation by shaming: Deterrence effects of publicizing violations of workplace safety and health laws. September 29, 2016. Available at: http://kenan.ethics.duke.edu/regulation/files/2016/09/johnson_osha_press_releases_091216.pdf. Accessed January 14, 2017.
3. Occupational Safety and Health Administration. Adding inequality to injury: The costs of failing to protect workers on the job, 2015. Available at: https://www.dol.gov/osha/report/20150304-inequality.pdf. Accessed August 25, 2017.
4. Occupational Safety and Health Act of 1970, 29 U.S.C. § 651 et seq. Available at: https://www.osha.gov/pls/oshaweb/owadisp.show_document?p_table=oshact&p_id=2743. Accessed August 25, 2017.
5. Federal Mine Safety and Health Act, 30 U.S.C. § 801 et seq. Available at: https://www.fmshrc.gov/sites/default/files/response.pdf. Accessed August 25, 2017.
6. AFL-CIO. Death on the job, the toll of neglect: A national and state-by-state profile of worker safety and health in the United States (23rd ed.). Available at: http://www.aflcio.org/content/download/126621/3464561/version/1/file/DOTJ2014.pdf. Accessed January 14, 2017.
7. Carson R. Silent spring. New York: Houghton Mifflin, 1962.
8. Office of the President. Executive Order 12866: Regulatory Planning and Review. Federal Register Vol. 58, No. 190, October 4, 1993. Available at: https://www.archives.gov/files/federal-register/executive-orders/pdf/12866.pdf. Accessed August 25, 2017.
9. U.S. Government Accountability Office. Multiple challenges lengthen OSHA's standard setting. (GAO-12-330). April 2012. Available at: http://www.gao.gov/assets/590/589825.pdf. Accessed January 20, 2017.
10. Boden LI, Spieler EA. Workers' compensation. In: Béland D, Howard C, Morgan KJ (Eds.). *The Oxford Handbook of U.S. Social Policy*. New York: Oxford University Press, 2014. pp. 451–468.

SECTION II

RECOGNITION, ASSESSMENT, AND PREVENTION

4

Recognizing and Preventing Occupational and Environmental Disease and Injury

Rosemary K. Sokas, Barry S. Levy, David H. Wegman, and Sherry L. Baron

The occupational and environmental history of an individual is central to recognizing the relationship of an illness or injury to occupational or environmental exposures or other factors. There are three main reasons for clinicians to obtain a patient's occupational and environmental history:

- To identify whether or not an established exposure-outcome association accounts for a specific illness or injury or its exacerbation, enabling immediate implementation of measures to prevent further damage to the individual and other workers or community members.[1,2] In addition, by obtaining a history, a clinician can rule out (or rule in) other causative and contributory factors.
- To identify a previously unrecognized cause for an illness or injury. In this situation, a search and review of the medical literature for further evidence of a suspected association can be critically important. Perspectives articulated by Austin Bradford Hill can help guide a review of the evidence.[3] (See appendix at the end of this chapter.)
- To obtain information about patients' lives by understanding their work, home, and community environments. When clinicians understand patients' lives, they are in the best position to recommend measures to prevent a recurrence or exacerbation of the illness or injury, to provide anticipatory guidance, and to establish a therapeutic alliance.[4] Clinicians may make recommendations to reduce fall hazards in the home or exposure to respiratory allergens and irritants.[5,6] They may also improve treatment plans for their patients with insulin-dependent diabetes who work night shifts, since irregular hours tend to disrupt management of blood glucose.

The following cases illustrate situations where clinicians did not initially obtain an occupational and environmental history:

1. An emergency medicine physician diagnosed acute alcohol intoxication in a machinist who developed loss of balance at work.
2. A family nurse practitioner correctly diagnosed carpal tunnel syndrome in a garment worker who had finger numbness and weakness but attributed this disorder to her rheumatoid arthritis.

3. An internist diagnosed the worsening chronic cough of a man working at a bottle-making factory as a side effect of his antihypertensive medication.

4. A psychologist attributed a young boy's learning difficulties in school to attention deficit hyperactivity disorder.

5. A pediatrician concluded that a young girl's asthma exacerbation was caused by a viral infection.

In each of these cases, the facts fit together and resulted in a coherent story, leading each clinician to recommend a specific therapeutic and preventive regimen. But, in each case, the clinician made an inadequate or incorrect diagnosis because of a common oversight—failure to take an occupational and environmental history. Taking an occupational and environmental history would have helped to make the following diagnoses and determine their causes:

1. The first patient had acute central nervous system intoxication caused by exposure to organic solvents at work.

2. The garment worker's carpal tunnel syndrome may have been partially caused or exacerbated by strenuous repetitive movements that she performed with her hands and wrists hundreds of times an hour.

3. The man working in the bottle-making factory had worsening of his chronic cough because of occupational exposure to hydrochloric acid fumes.

4. The young boy had lead poisoning from hand-to-mouth exposure to dust from eroding lead-containing paint in his home.

5. The young girl had exacerbation of her asthma caused by allergy to mold resulting from water damage in the basement of her home.

Without an occupational and environmental history, the opportunities for making the correct diagnosis and providing appropriate treatment and preventive measures are missed. Although a physical examination and laboratory tests may raise suspicion or help confirm that an illness or injury is related to occupational or environmental factors, identification of an occupational or environmental health problem depends most importantly on the occupational and environmental history (Figure 4-1).

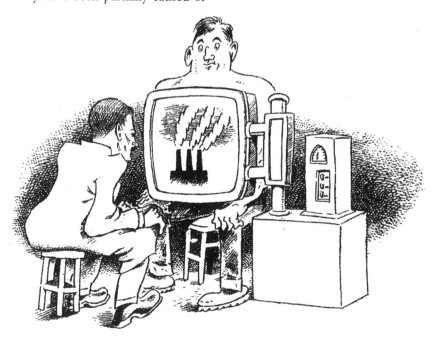

Figure 4-1. Physicians and other health professionals have a vital role in recognizing occupational and environmental disease. Contrary to this drawing, there is no simple test. The suspicion and the determination of work-relatedness depend primarily on a carefully obtained occupational and environmental history. (Drawing by Nick Thorkelson.)

WHAT QUESTIONS TO ASK

All primary care and specialty clinicians will encounter patients with illnesses or injuries associated with work, home, or community exposures. Sometimes these illnesses and injuries may result *only* from an occupational or environmental exposure. However, many illnesses and injuries are caused by multiple factors. Recognizing the role of occupational, environmental, and other exposures, sometimes acting in combination, can lead to preventive opportunities that should be included in patient management. Patient information obtained from self-administered questionnaires and from interviews conducted by support staff can supplement information obtained directly by clinicians.

A comprehensive set of questions in the occupational and environmental history is shown in Table 4-1. Although it is obtained primarily by clinicians, the occupational and environmental history is also elicited by epidemiologists, other researchers, and other health and safety professionals. The extent and level of detail of the history depends on the degree of suspicion that occupational or environmental factors may have caused or contributed to a patient's illness or injury. All patients presenting with new complaints should be asked if they think that their health problems might be associated with a workplace or other environmental exposure. Further elaboration of each of the key parts of the occupational and environmental history may be helpful, especially when (a) the patient raises concerns about potential exposures, (b) the clinician needs to evaluate further exposures of concern, (c) organ systems that are commonly associated with exposure are adversely affected, or (d) the diagnosis remains unclear.

Table 4-1. Outline of the Occupational and Environmental History

Components	Specific Questions and Issues
Description of all jobs held	Obtain information on employers, details of jobs, and starting and ending dates of each job.
	Ask about second jobs, work in the home as a homemaker or parent, military service, and part-time and summer jobs, including jobs while a student.
	Ask worker to describe typical work shift.
	Ask worker to simulate performance of work tasks by demonstrating body movements associated with them. (Visiting the workplace may be necessary.)
	Obtain information on routine tasks as well as unusual and overtime tasks, such as cleaning out tanks or cleaning up spills.
Exposures	Ask about chemical, physical, biomechanical, biological, and psychosocial exposures at work.
	Start with open-ended questions, such as "What have you worked with?"
	Follow with specific questions, such as "Were you ever exposed to lead or other heavy metals? To solvents? To asbestos?"
	Obtain safety data sheets for workplace chemicals.
	Ask about tasks performed in adjacent areas of the workplace that may contribute to a worker's exposure.
	Ask about unusual incidents, such as spills of hazardous materials, work in confined spaces (Figure 4-2), use of new substances, and changed processes at work.
	Quantify exposures to the extent feasible, usually by estimating concentration and determining duration of exposure and route of entry.
	Check for the presence of protective engineering systems and devices, such as ventilation systems, and whether they seem to function adequately.
	Check for the use of personal protective equipment, such as gloves, workclothes, masks, respirators, and hearing protectors.
	Ask about eating, drinking, and smoking in the workplace (Figure 4-3).
	Ask about handwashing and showering at work, changing of workclothes, and who cleans the workclothes.
Timing of symptoms	What is the time course of symptoms in relation to exposures?
	When do symptoms begin and end in relation to work shifts?
	Are symptoms present during weekends and vacation periods?
	Are symptoms related to certain processes, work tasks, or work exposures?

(continued)

Table 4-1. (Continued)

Components	Specific Questions and Issues
Symptoms among coworkers	Are there other workers at the same workplace or in similar jobs elsewhere who have the same symptoms or illnesses? If there are people similarly affected, find out what they may share in common.
Present and prior residences	List all the places where you have lived and the periods when you lived at each place. Have you ever lived near any of the following: (a) an industrial facility that may be polluting the air, surface water, groundwater, or soil; (b) a hazardous waste site; and (c) a farm where herbicides, insecticides, or other pesticides may have been applied.
Jobs of household members	Ask if workplace contaminants, such as lead, may have been brought into the home. Ask if children have been brought to the worksite, such as occurs frequently in farm work.
Environmental tobacco smoke	Do you share your home, car, or other environment with a smoker?
Lead exposure	Have you ever lived in a home built before 1978? Have you known anyone who has had lead poisoning? Is lead present in pipes in your home or supplying water to your home? Is there imported pottery in your home? Do you use traditional (folk) medicines that may contain lead?
Home insulating, heating, and cooking	What type of fuel do you use for heating and cooking in your home? What type of insulation do you have in your home? Is your stove properly ventilated?
Household building materials	With what type of materials was your home built?
Home cleaning agents and other household products	What type of cleaning agents and other household products do you use in your home?
Presence of pests, mold, pets, dust in the home	Do you have dust mites or cockroaches in your home? Do you have growth of mold in your home? Is there evidence of water damage in your home? What type of carpeting do you have in your home and what carpet cleaners do you use? What pets do you have in your home?
Pesticide usage	What types of insecticides, herbicides, or other pesticides have you used in or near your home?
Water supply	What is the source of water for your home? If you have a private well, when was it last tested and what were the results?
Foodborne illness	What food was eaten in the time period just before onset of illness?
Renovation/remodeling	Has your home recently been renovated or remodeled?
Air contamination	Are you concerned about contamination or pollution of the air in or near your home?
Hobbies	What hobbies have you or other household members had? Are any of these hobbies associated with hazardous exposures?
Recreational history	Have you been exposed to any hazards in recreational activities, such as swimming in polluted water?
Travel	Have you had any recent travel?

For primary care clinicians or those engaged in managing chronic conditions, the occupational and environmental history should contain sufficient detail to understand how patients spend their workdays and to determine their exposure to health and safety hazards (Figures 4-2 and 4-3). Answers to questions about noise exposure at work or elsewhere, exposure to ultraviolet radiation from sunlight, and other exposures may lead clinicians to provide patients with anticipatory guidance for preventive measures, such as use of hearing protectors, sunscreen, or bicycle helmets. Clinicians should ask patients who are working if they have had physical examinations or screening (medical monitoring) tests, such as audiograms or

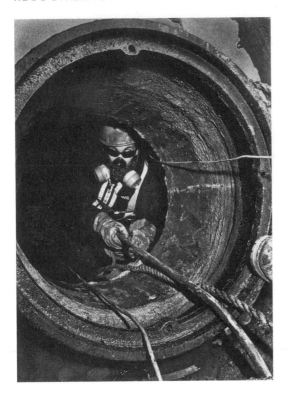

Figure 4-2. Many jobs require work in confined spaces, which can be lethal unless strict safety precautions are followed. (Photograph by Earl Dotter.)

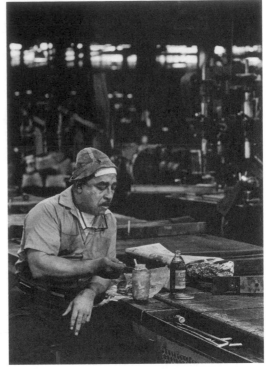

Figure 4-3. Workers who eat in the workplace may ingest toxic substances, which may be absorbed in the gastrointestinal tract. (Photograph by Earl Dotter.)

pulmonary function tests, performed on them at work. These exams and tests may provide helpful information and suggest the presence of specific hazardous occupational exposures.

In addition, workers should be asked if they suspect that their symptoms are related to identified exposures, if they work with any known hazards, and if other workers have similar problems. Workers concerned about potential chemical exposures can obtain from their employers Safety Data Sheets, which include detailed information about products used at work as well as hotlines and sometimes other sources of information and assistance. Information about other aspects of work, including working hours, supervisory support, and work–home life challenges, may provide clinicians with insights into patients' overall health.

A visit to the workplace can provide critically important information to supplement the history (Figure 4-4).

WHEN TO TAKE A MORE THOROUGH HISTORY

Respiratory Disorders

A detailed occupational and environmental history should be obtained for any patient with a significant respiratory illness. Any respiratory symptom can be potentially associated with occupational and environmental factors. Environmental factors, including outdoor and indoor air contaminants, account for much childhood asthma. Adult-onset asthma is frequently caused by work but not recognized as such.[7,8] More often, patients with pre-existing asthma may experience exacerbations of their asthma when exposed to sensitizers or to nonspecific irritants in the workplace. Although other chronic obstructive lung diseases are usually caused by cigarette smoking, they can be caused or significantly exacerbated by exposure to welding fumes, irritant gases, smoke, or dusts at work or in the ambient environment. (See Chapter 22.)

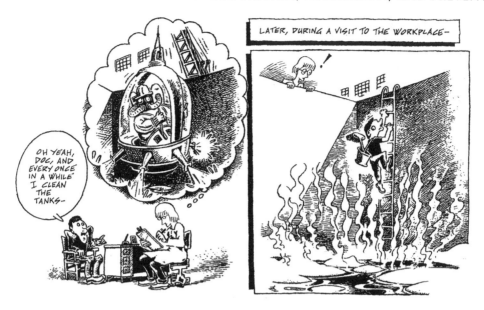

Figure 4-4. It is crucial to clearly understand working conditions and exposures. (Drawing by Nick Thorkelson.)

Skin Disorders

Skin disorders can impact both work and home life. The occupational and environmental history often helps to identify the responsible irritant, sensitizer, or other factor. Contact dermatitis, which accounts for about 90% of cases of work-related skin disorders, may be challenging to treat if the causative agent is not identified and exposure to it discontinued. (See Chapter 25.)

Hearing Impairment

Many cases of sensorineural hearing impairment are inaccurately attributed solely to aging (presbycusis). Millions are exposed to hazardous noise at work or elsewhere. Exposure to organic solvents also can cause hearing impairment. A focused occupational and environmental history should include all sources of exposure to loud noise (and loud music) and to organic solvents. Noise abatement, noise avoidance, and use of effective hearing protectors may prevent further hearing impairment. (See Chapter 12A.)

Musculoskeletal Disorders

Musculoskeletal disorders frequently are related to work. For example, work-related back disorders represent a major cause of days away from work. Because there are no tests or other procedures that can determine if back pain is related to work, determination of work-relatedness depends largely on the occupational and environmental history. Many cases of arthritis and tenosynovitis are caused or exacerbated by forceful and/or repetitive movements at work. Application of ergonomics—the study of the interactions among workers, their work environments, job demands, and work tasks—can help prevent many of these problems. (See Chapters 9 and 20.)

Cancer

As the number of chemicals in commercial use increases and as research increases our knowledge of their potential hazards, more carcinogens are being recognized. Sometimes the initial suspicion that a substance may be carcinogenic comes from reports of individual cases or clusters of cases, especially if the type of cancer is uncommon. Typically, occupational or environmental exposure to a carcinogen has begun—or occurred entirely—many years before a diagnosis of cancer is made. (See Chapter 21.)

Cardiovascular Diseases

The frequency or severity of symptoms of cardiovascular diseases may increase due to chemical factors, such as occupational exposure to nitrates or carbon disulfide, and environmental exposure to lead, carbon monoxide, or fine airborne particulate matter. (See Chapter 26.) Increasingly, the importance of occupational stress and life stressors, such as unemployment and underemployment, have been shown to increase risk of cardiovascular diseases. (See Chapter 14.)

Neurobehavioral Disorders

The possible association between neurobehavioral disorders and occupational and environmental factors is also often overlooked. An occupational and environmental history should be obtained whenever there is new onset of neurological symptoms or when a change in mental status or behavior has occurred. Peripheral neuropathy may be inappropriately attributed to diabetes, alcohol abuse, or "unknown etiology." Central nervous system depression may be inappropriately attributed to substance abuse. Behavioral abnormalities, which may be the first sign of occupational stress or childhood lead poisoning, may be attributed inappropriately to a psychosis, a personality disorder, or attention deficit hyperactivity disorder. More than 100 chemicals, including virtually all organic solvents, can cause central nervous system depression, and several neurotoxins, including arsenic, lead, mercury, and methyl n-butyl ketone, can produce peripheral neuropathy. Carbon disulfide exposure can cause symptoms that mimic a psychosis. And manganese can cause symptoms of parkinsonism. (See Chapter 23.) In addition, when workers face difficult working conditions or fear of job loss after an occupational injury or illness, chronic depression can develop, with adverse consequences for the worker and the worker's family.[9-11] Environmental concerns that make a person feel helpless or trapped may produce similar symptoms.

Liver Disorders

The liver is the major site for metabolism of chemicals. The association between alcohol and liver disease may lead a clinician to overlook occupational or environmental causes of liver disease, such as hepatitis C virus and organic solvents. (See Chapter 27.)

Kidney Disorders

As a major organ of excretion, the kidney is exposed directly to a wide range of toxic substances. Kidney disorders may be caused or exacerbated by occupational and environmental exposures to metals, solvents, medications, and other chemicals. Occupational and environmental factors are thought to contribute to the emergence of chronic kidney disease of unknown etiology among agricultural workers performing extreme physical exertion in hot weather in some countries. (See Chapter 28.)

Reproductive Disorders

Although little is known about the causes of many reproductive disorders, any reproductive system abnormality, such as reduced fertility or a congenital anomaly, should lead the clinician to take a complete occupational and environmental history. (See Chapter 24.)

Illnesses of Unknown Cause

A thorough occupational and environmental history should be obtained in cases when the cause is unknown or uncertain and when the diagnosis has not been clearly established.

High-Risk Working or Living Conditions

Workers in insecure jobs, those working in informal or precarious working arrangements, and undocumented workers are at increased risk of occupational injury and illness. Primary care clinicians in safety-net settings, such as Federally Qualified Health Centers, are likely to be the only source of occupational or environmental healthcare for their patients. Therefore, obtaining an occupational and environmental history may lead to life-saving preventive measures, such as providing patients working in hot environments with information about the need to drink enough water and to take frequent rest breaks.

RECOGNIZING OCCUPATIONAL OR ENVIRONMENTAL DISEASE CLUSTERS OR OUTBREAKS

The following two situations illustrate how accurately identifying the causal relationship between exposure and disease makes appropriate treatment and prevention possible.

SITUATION 1

Four hospitals in the same city simultaneously admitted eight cyanotic men with acute complaints, ranging from nausea and vomiting to seizures. Although the men were admitted to different hospitals, emergency health workers recognized that all of them worked at the same warehouse. A terrorist attack was suspected until a team of hazardous materials workers who were sent to the warehouse found there barrels of *p*-nitroaniline (PNA), which can cause serious illness or death after inhalation, skin absorption, or ingestion. Once the chemical was identified, the men were treated appropriately, and all of them survived. Health workers notified the Occupational Safety and Health Administration (OSHA), which sent inspectors to the warehouse, where they identified many lost opportunities for prevention, including failures to train workers as mandated, provide personal protective equipment, and implement appropriate safety measures. Occupational and environmental hygienists, toxicologists, and other health workers discovered that PNA had contaminated equipment and surfaces at the hospitals as well as in the workers' homes and cars, all of which required extensive decontamination that prevented additional cases among hospital personnel and patients' household contacts.[12]

SITUATION 2

In another town, several immigrant workers developed rapid onset of symptoms, which ranged in severity from weakness to leg paralysis. They were diagnosed with an inflammatory neuropathy. Although the workers saw different physicians, they all used the same interpreter, who noticed the similarity of their stories.

A public health investigation found that all of the affected workers performed the same specific task, harvesting pig brains using a forced-air hose. Preventive intervention involved changing work practices, both in the workplace of these workers and industrywide, to eliminate the exposure to aerosolized brain material—after which no further cases occurred.[13]

Both of these situations are unusual. But they illustrate the importance of promptly recognizing hazardous exposures and implementing appropriate treatment and preventive interventions. Situation 1 highlights the importance of workplace inspections for prevention and illustrates how prompt recognition of a responsible chemical can prevent secondary cases among hospital personnel and patients' household contacts. Situation 2 illustrates how an occupational and environmental history can provide information about a new cause of an occupational and environmental disease and promptly lead to elimination of exposures to prevent additional cases.

PREVENTION

Health and safety professionals anticipate and recognize hazards through systematic approaches. They also design, implement, and evaluate preventive measures at all levels of prevention (Figure 4-5):

Primary prevention: Preventing illnesses and injuries before they occur
Secondary prevention: Identifying and treating health problems as early as possible, often before symptoms have developed or permanent impairment has occurred
Tertiary prevention: Implementing interventions to arrest the progress of established diseases, injuries, or their consequences, including disability.

When properly planned and integrated, these approaches help to (a) control risks at the source, (b) identify new health problems as early as possible, (c) provide treatment and rehabilitation for patients, (d) prevent recurrent and new illnesses and injuries, (e) ensure appropriate economic compensation, and (f) help to discover new

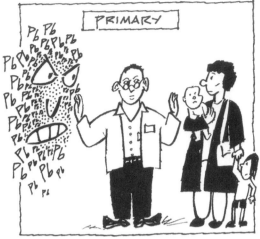

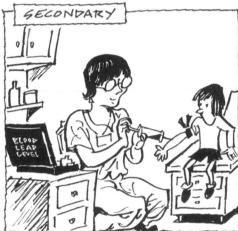

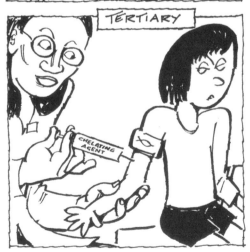

Figure 4-5. Illustrative examples of the levels of prevention: Primary prevention to prevent exposure of children to lead, secondary prevention to determine blood lead levels in children for early identification of excessive lead exposure, and tertiary prevention to treat children with very high blood lead levels. (Drawings by Nick Thorkelson.)

associations between occupational and environmental exposures and adverse health effects.

A public health approach to prevention aims to "move upstream"—to address the primary sources and underlying causes of health problems. The following sections describe primary prevention measures at the organizational level and the individual level. (See Table 19-3 in Chapter 19.)

Prevention at the Organizational Level

Substitution of a Hazardous Substance with a Safer One

Hazardous substances have often been substituted with substances of similar effectiveness that are safer and equally or less expensive. Synthetic vitreous fibers, such as fibrous glass, have been substituted for asbestos, for example. Caution is necessary, however, as substitute substances may later be found to be hazardous. Long ago, fire protection was enhanced by replacing flammable cleaning solvents with carbon tetrachloride. Then, carbon tetrachloride was found to be hepatotoxic and was repeatedly replaced by other chlorinated hydrocarbons—with each substitute thought to be less toxic. Each time, substitutions reduced certain risks but introduced new ones. Substitution of a known hazard with an unassessed substance can be problematic; it may require a long period of monitoring to determine the health effects of a substituted substance. There can be adverse effects or unanticipated benefits. An example of the latter is when substituting water-based solvents for perchloroethylene in industrial dry-cleaning of textiles eliminated exposure to a potential human carcinogen but also improved organization of dry-cleaning jobs and reduced ergonomic risk factors.

Substitution of a Hazardous Process with a Safer One

There are many ways in which substitution of a process can be accomplished, including:

- Mixing chemicals in closed bags or other containers to reduce dermal or inhalational exposures to hazardous substances
- Giving medications orally or by transdermal patches to reduce needlestick injuries among healthcare workers

- Implementing policies that promote use of mass transit or active transport (walking and bicycling)—rather than private vehicular travel—to decrease air pollution, emission of greenhouse gases, and vehicle crashes, thereby reducing illnesses and injuries, addressing climate change, and improving physical fitness
- Using wind power or solar energy to reduce air pollution from greenhouse gas emission from burning fossil fuels and to reduce safety risks from nuclear power plants
- Giving employees more control over their work to reduce occupational stress and associated disorders
- Implementing design features or programs in the built environment, such as bicycle-share programs, to reduce traffic and associated air pollution and to increase physical fitness.

Substitution requires careful attention to assure that any hazards associated with the new process are anticipated and controlled. For example, windmills do not create pollution, but they can introduce some occupational safety hazards that need to be anticipated and controlled. (See Figure 29-3 in Chapter 29.)

Installation of Engineering Controls and Devices

Often more feasible than substitution, this approach includes a wide range of options to reduce hazards by separating the hazard from the user or reducing the impact of the hazard, including:

- Installing airbags in motor vehicles
- Installing ventilation exhaust systems to remove hazardous dusts or fumes (Figure 4-6)
- Using jigs or fixtures that support pieces during machining or other work to reduce static muscle contractions while holding parts or tools
- Applying soundproof materials to reduce loud noise that cannot be engineered out of a work process or an ambient environment
- Installing tools on overhead balancers to eliminate torque and vibration transmitted to the hand
- Constructing enclosures to isolate hazardous processes
- Installing hoists to eliminate manual lifting of containers or parts
- Carefully maintaining aging equipment to reduce or eliminate (a) fugitive emissions

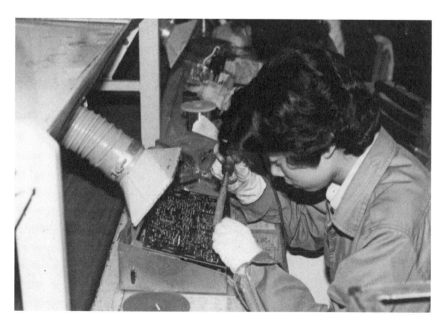

Figure 4-6. Local exhaust ventilation removes soldering fumes from the breathing zone of this worker. (Photograph by Barry S. Levy.)

from processes in closed systems, or (b) hazardous vibration

- Using scrubbers or other mechanisms to reduce emissions of airborne pollutants
- Maximizing fuel use by co-generating hot water from the heat exhaust from generation of electricity
- Treating wastewater effluent before discharge
- Installing safety partitions, cameras, and police-alert mechanisms in taxis to reduce violent assault of drivers.

Although installation of engineering controls and devices can be costly, it often saves money by reducing use of materials, decreasing generation of toxic and other wastes, reducing occurrence of illnesses and injuries, and increasing productivity. Often, engineering controls are not considered or implemented because employers are not aware of them.

Changes in Job Design, Work Practices, and Work Organization

These changes can reduce or eliminate risks associated with work. This type of preventive measure is almost always more effective than types that rely primarily on the changed behavior of workers. To be most effective, these changes should be developed through labor-management collaboration that gives workers a voice in illness and injury prevention programs.

Job redesign, which often combines engineering and administrative measures, aims to increase job content, make physical work less redundant or repetitive, and improve workers' individual or collective autonomy in decision-making. Changes in work organization, often integrated with job redesign, are directed at eliminating undesirable features in the structure of work processes. For example, a change from piece-rate to hourly-rate work reduces inappropriate physical and mental pressure on workers and decreases the occurrence of musculoskeletal disorders. (See Chapters 9, 14, and 20.)

Other Administrative Measures

There are a variety of less extensive changes in work practices that may reduce occupational hazards. For example, noisy or disruptive operations can be scheduled for time periods when fewer workers are present, and workplace procedures that eliminate or reduce handling cash may decrease the risk of robberies and assaults.

Prevention at the Individual Level

Education and Training

Education and training concerning occupational and environmental hazards is an essential aspect of health and safety programs. While it is important to convey information about adverse effects of potential exposures in individual clinical settings, most training and education occurs in group settings that educate and empower workers and community members. Participatory, popular-education approaches utilize learner-centered methods, which are designed to foster maximum participation and interaction and to empower participants to devise effective strategies for improving health and safety. They recognize that adults (a) bring much experience to the classroom that should be utilized and (b) learn more effectively by doing, rather than listening passively. Learners' experiences are incorporated into course material to expand their learning of new concepts and skills. Combining instructors' specialized knowledge and participants' direct experience leads to effective approaches to address future health and safety problems.

Examples of participatory teaching methods include:

1. *Speakouts* (large-group discussions): Participants share their experiences in relation to a specific hazard or situation.
2. *Brainstorming sessions*: The instructor provides a specific question or problem, to which participants provide responses that are recorded on a flipchart so that patterns and broad concepts can be identified.
3. *Buzz groups and report-back sessions* (small-group discussions or exercises): Each group of three to six participants discusses a specific problem, situation, or question, and then a spokesperson for each small group reports its findings to the larger group for further discussion.
4. *Case studies* (small-group exercises): Participants apply new knowledge and skills to explore solutions to a specific problem or situation.
5. *Discovery exercises*: Participants obtain items, such as OSHA injury logs for their

workplaces or Toxic Release Inventory records for their communities, or interview coworkers or neighbors about specific hazards. Information obtained is then brought to the classroom for discussion.

6. *Hands-on training*: The participants practice skills, such as by testing fit of respirators, simulating asbestos removal or hazardous waste clean-up, using OSHA injury logs to identify hazards in need of correction, or handling monitoring equipment.

7. *Hazard mapping*: Participants create maps of their workplaces or communities, locating hazards, including psychosocial and work-organization problems, and indicating their type, severity, and number of people potentially exposed. Maps enable participants to visually integrate existing knowledge with new knowledge and to use the maps to prioritize actions and resources for change.[14]

Understanding how people perceive risk is important. People often dread some outcomes, such as cancer, more than others, such as heart disease. People distinguish between risks that they perceive they can control and risks that only others can control. Providing information that restores some control to workers can be an important component of education and training.

Workers and community members should always be given complete information about hazards to which they may be exposed, by training courses, written materials, or warning signs (Figure 4-7) as well as ways that they can reduce their risk of illness and injury. When new materials, procedures, or equipment are introduced, workers should be trained on appropriate safety measures. Providing hazard and safety training should supplement, and not replace, other forms of hazard control, such as installing ventilation or implementing pollution-prevention measures. Training should build on life experiences and empower people to address and solve problems.

Personal Protective Equipment

Personal protective equipment (PPE) (Figure 4-8) is considered the least reliable form of protection, since it may be cumbersome or uncomfortable and it relies on the individual to use it correctly each time. However, it may be critically important. Health and safety specialists identify the need for PPE and the appropriate type of PPE, but clinicians may be asked to determine whether the worker is able to use the device without adverse health effects. Clinicians should be aware that PPE may sometimes cause problems, such as when ear plugs irritate the external auditory canal or protective gloves cause skin irritation or sensitization.

Screening and Surveillance

Screening (medical monitoring), which is a form of secondary prevention, seeks to identify disorders

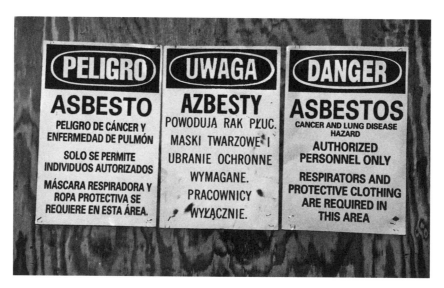

Figure 4-7. Warning signs, as illustrated in this photograph, should be in multiple languages, if appropriate. (Photograph by Earl Dotter.)

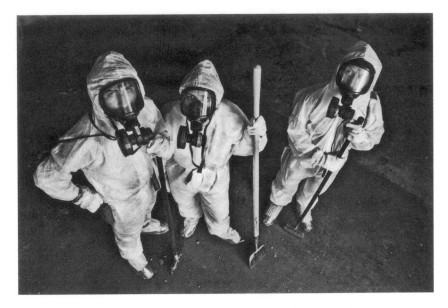

Figure 4-8. Workers with personal protective equipment. (Photograph by Earl Dotter.)

in asymptomatic individuals at an early stage when treatment and prevention may improve outcomes. Specific screening guidelines take into consideration risks and benefits. The Agency for Toxic Substances and Disease Registry has published criteria for determining the appropriateness of a medical monitoring program.[15]

Surveillance, in contrast to screening, is generally designed to obtain, analyze, and disseminate information on hazardous exposures or health outcomes that have already occurred in populations or groups of people. *Exposure surveillance* (also known as *hazard surveillance* and *risk surveillance*) describes and tracks known hazards to identify opportunities for preventive measures and to evaluate the effectiveness of these measures. For workers at risk of illness due to some specific workplace hazards, such as lead, OSHA mandates surveillance by biological monitoring (with measurement of blood lead levels) and environmental monitoring (with measurement of airborne lead levels, see Figure 4-9). Disorders that have already occurred in populations or groups of people need to be counted and followed over time to maximize opportunities for prevention at both the individual and the population level. *Case-based surveillance* is designed to identify *sentinel health events*, individual cases of a disease that signal a breakdown in prevention.

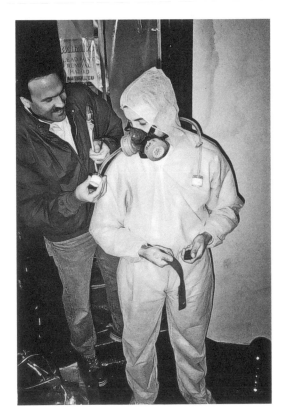

Figure 4-9. A NIOSH industrial hygienist prepares to sample a worker's lead exposure during a residential lead-based paint abatement project. (Photograph by Aaron Sussell.)

Population-based (or *rate-based*) *surveillance* is designed to identify trends in the occurrence of disorders, symptoms, or abnormalities in test results and clusters of cases, which may represent outbreaks of disease. (See Chapter 6.)

Tertiary Prevention

For individuals who have already suffered an occupational or environmental illness or injury, rehabilitation and other tertiary prevention measures can help them avoid complications and long-term disability. These measures include modifying work, home, and community environments to speed recovery and prevent recurrence of illness or injury.

OPTIONS FOR PREVENTIVE MEASURES

Once a probable case of occupational or environmental illness or injury has been identified, preventive measures should be implemented along with appropriate treatment. Failure to do so may lead to recurrence or worsening of the condition in the affected individual and additional cases among other workers or community residents. While therapeutic interventions can be provided in the clinical setting, most of the interventions that make worksites and communities healthier and safer occur outside of clinical settings and require collaboration with technical, legal, or other experts and active participation by affected individuals or groups. Clinicians are responsible for advising patients, providing appropriate treatment, and making recommendations or referring them for further assistance.

Advise the Patient

The clinician should always advise the patient concerning the nature and prognosis of an illness or injury, the likelihood that specific occupational or environmental factors caused or contributed to it, and appropriate preventive measures (Figure 4-10). Referral to one or more specialists may be necessary to explore the possibilities of engineering controls to remove the hazard, the need for PPE, or, in extreme

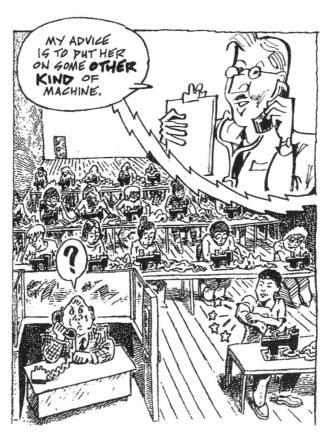

Figure 4-10. Advice to employees and employers should be practical. (Drawing by Nick Thorkelson.)

circumstances, changing jobs or moving to a different home. Given the devastating impact of dislocation for individuals and families, the clinician should consider engaging scientific, technical, and legal resources. Clinicians should inform patients about the probabilities of risks and benefits of various possible actions. For work-related injuries and illnesses, clinicians should inform patients that they will provide necessary medical information if the patient chooses to apply for workers' compensation for lost income and medical and rehabilitation expenses. (See Chapter 3.)

Affected workers may be reluctant to file a workers' compensation claim (or make a complaint to a government agency) for fear of job loss or other punitive action. Clinicians can reassure the patient of their ongoing support through what can be a contentious process and point out that a workers' compensation claim may lead the employer to assess the problem and implement effective preventive measures.

Additional Preventive Options for the Clinician

The clinician can choose one or more of the following three options, which may lead to preventive measures:

1. Contact the responsible party
2. Contact an appropriate government regulatory agency or public health agency
3. Obtain clinical, research, or other support.

Unless the situation is deemed an imminent danger to life and health, the clinician must first obtain the patient's consent before initiating any of these actions and should act in partnership with the patient.

Contact the Responsible Party

A clinician may report the problem to the responsible party, such as the patient's employer or landlord. This report can lead to preventive measures. Larger employers may have on-site health facilities as well as health and safety programs that can facilitate preventive measures. (See Chapter 10.) Many smaller employers do not have the staff to deal with reported problems adequately, but often they can obtain assistance from workers' compensation insurance

companies who employ health and safety experts to assist clients. Even small employers may have resources to hire occupational and environmental hygienists or other experts. However, cost concerns frequently limit employers' willingness to contact insurance companies or hire experts.

Discussions with an employer may enable a clinician to obtain useful information concerning exposures and the presence or potential of similar cases among other workers. Depending on the circumstance, the clinician may be able to arrange a visit to the patient's workplace to observe the possibly hazardous environment and to encourage managers to implement preventive measures.

A governmental resource that may be useful to employers who want to improve health and safety is the On-site Consultation Program, which is funded by OSHA and administered through state agencies or academic institutions. The program offers free assistance to employers with up to 250 employees. Once an employer initiates a request, the program provides health and safety consultants who will identify problems amenable to prevention and control measures. A health and safety evaluation by the program is not conducted by OSHA personnel and does not carry the threat of fines or other penalties. An evaluation does not result in a report to OSHA, except in rare and extreme circumstances. (Information for this program is available through https://www.osha.gov; under "Take action," click on "Request a free consultation.")

Contact an Appropriate Government Regulatory Agency or Public Health Agency

If an occupational or environmental illness or injury appears to be serious or may be affecting others in the same workplace, company, industry, or community (including in rental housing), the clinician should encourage the patient to consider filing a complaint with the appropriate governmental regulatory or public health agency. With the patient's approval, the clinician can offer to contact that agency. (See Chapter 3.) For workplace issues, the clinician can support or assist the patient with filing a complaint to OSHA or the Mine Safety and Health Administration (MSHA). Although OSHA and MSHA regulations include "whistleblower" protections for workers who file complaints against resultant discrimination by the employer, this protection is difficult to enforce and workers' fears of loss of job, earnings, or benefits are not unfounded. Despite these protections, employers have fired workers who have disorders possibly related to work. Clinicians should be familiar with relevant laws and regulations as well as resources that can provide useful information for their patients with work-related illnesses or injuries and should refer them for appropriate assistance. For example, clinicians should be aware that workers who do not file an "11(c)" antidiscrimination complaint within 30 days of discriminatory acts lose their rights. Workers who file complaints (or unions, for those workers who are union members) and their clinicians have the right to obtain findings of resultant OSHA workplace inspections.

OSHA establishes and enforces standards for hazardous exposures in the workplace and undertakes inspections in response to complaints from workers, physicians, and others. In about half of U.S. states, the program is implemented directly by federal OSHA; in the other states, a state agency—often the state department of labor—implements the program. A federal or a state OSHA program may inspect a workplace in response to a complaint. There is evidence that OSHA inspections help to protect workers without damaging the inspected company's financial status.[16]

OSHA does not cover workers who are self-employed. However, the definition of employment includes the ability to set the terms of work, and certain working arrangements—such as hiring day laborers (Chapter 2) or leasing trucks to operators and then establishing time requirements—violate these rules, placing workers at increased risk.

Since OSHA cannot regulate states, counties, or municipalities, public hospital workers, police officers, and other state and local government employees can only be protected by a state-based OSHA program. Several states have adopted state plans only for public-sector (government) employees, allowing federal OSHA to maintain responsibility for the private sector. The Occupational Safety and Health Act (OSH Act) created exemptions for worker health and safety for specific populations for which other federal agencies assert regulatory oversight. For example, within the Department of Transportation,

the Federal Aviation Administration sets and enforces standards for pilot medical requirements and the Federal Motor Carrier Safety Administration sets and enforces regulations for hours of work for interstate truck drivers. Similarly, because the Environmental Protection Agency has responsibility for regulating pesticides, it assumes responsibility for how pesticide applicators and field agricultural workers are to be protected from pesticide toxicity, through its Worker Protection Standard.

Information on how to file an OSHA complaint is available on the OSHA website, http://www.osha.gov. (Under "Take Action," click on "File a safety and health complaint.") Although the decision on whether to file a complaint rests with an individual worker, clinicians can help ensure that OSHA inspections are performed appropriately. Patients who do not have union representatives and do not want to file complaints directly may, in writing, designate healthcare providers or others as their representatives. The OSH Act directs OSHA to investigate complaints from employees or their representatives. OSHA will review all other complaints but will consider them "referrals," with less certainty that it will perform a worksite inspection.

Clinicians can assist their patients further by calling the OSHA area office and speaking directly to an inspector or supervisor. While this is not required, it will increase the likelihood that OSHA will respond quickly and seriously. Contact information for the OSHA area offices is available on the OSHA website. It is also important for clinicians to provide as much specific information as possible about the issues of concern. The OSH Act requires unannounced, on-site inspections only when there are reasonable grounds to believe that there is an imminent danger at a workplace or that a violation of an OSHA regulation threatens physical harm. Finally, if workers have U.S. Senators, Congressional representatives, or state legislators call OSHA on their behalf, their complaints are more likely to be seriously considered.[17]

Enforcement of environmental regulations is done at the state or local level. State departments of environmental protection enforce most environmental regulations. So, for example, people concerned about whether municipal incinerators are in compliance with regulations can contact these departments. Local departments of public health, consumer affairs, environmental protection, and zoning often enforce local regulations or ordinances concerning noise, construction-related dust, waste disposal, and other environmental hazards. Local residents can often access information on regulatory compliance via a "3-1-1" telephone number or online.

Local departments of public health and housing may be able to assist people with household environmental hazards in homes that they are renting or homes that are otherwise not under their control. For example, the Safe at Home project in Washington, DC, has assisted low-income or elderly residents by identifying fall hazards and provides up to $10,000 to reduce these hazards.[18] However, there are few such programs, and renters who complain may face eviction. Legal clinics in many law schools may also be able to assist tenants address environmental hazards. Local and state departments of health, environment, and sanitation may help address community environmental hazards.

Obtain Clinical, Research, or Other Support

The following governmental agencies, non-governmental networks, and professional associations can provide clinical, research, or other support:

- OSHA, in addition to inspecting worksites and enforcing regulations, offers a clinicians' web page that provides extensive information useful for occupational health practice. The web page links to other governmental and professional resources (https://www.osha.gov/dts/oom/clinicians/index.html).
- The EPA offers specific guidance to clinicians for a number of environmental hazards that impact human health, including preventive guidance concerning asthma and both indoor and outdoor air pollution. It also offers clinical guidance on caring for pesticide applicators and agricultural workers who are covered under the Agricultural Worker Protection Standard, and has produced a clinical manual for the recognition and treatment of pesticide poisoning. (See https://www.epa.gov/asthma/publications-about-asthma and https://www.epa.gov/pesticide-worker-safety.)

- The Association of Occupational and Environmental Clinics is a not-for-profit network of practitioners and clinics with expertise in occupational and environmental health. (More information is available at http://www.aoec.org.)
- Pediatric Environmental Health Specialty Units comprise a federally funded network of academic clinicians who provide to health professionals and the general public educational outreach and information about environmental health hazards that can affect children. They provide referrals to experts in occupational and environmental medicine, nursing, toxicology, allergy and immunology, neurodevelopment issues, and reproductive health. (More information is available at http://www.pehsu.net.)
- The Migrant Clinicians Network offers technical assistance and educational information to clinicians and health centers who care for migrant workers. It has an extensive online library of English and Spanish outreach materials addressing occupational and environmental hazards that disproportionately impact low-income workers and their families. (More information is available at http://www.migrantclinician.org.)
- Eighteen university-based Education and Research Centers (ERCs) across the United States, which are funded by the National Institute for Occupational Safety and Health (NIOSH), provide continuing education and professional outreach in core fields of occupational safety and health, including industrial hygiene, nursing, medicine, and safety. The ERCs are a useful source of academic expertise. They may be able to fund pilot research projects for preliminary investigation into new or emerging hazards. (More information is available at https://www.cdc.gov/niosh/oep/ercportfolio.html.)
- The Health Hazard Evaluation program of NIOSH can, on request, perform field evaluations, especially of unusual or poorly

understood occupational exposures and possibly related health outcomes. A request can be made by an employer, a labor union, or three or more current employees or their representatives. (More information is available at https://www.cdc.gov/niosh/hhe/request.html. See also Chapter 33.)

- The Agency for Toxic Substances and Disease Registry, within the Department of Health and Human Services, can address concerns about possible health effects from hazardous waste sites. It can also conduct investigations concerning hazardous exposures and health effects possibly related to these waste sites in response to clinicians, community residents, and others. (More information is available at https://www.atsdr.cdc.gov. See also Chapter 18.)

- Professional associations that focus some of their resources on occupational and environmental health, such as the American Public Health Association, the American Thoracic Society, the American Academy of Pediatrics, the American College of Physicians, and the American Nurses Association, can often provide helpful information.

- Labor and environmental organizations can also help. If the patient is a member of a labor union (as are about 34% of public-sector workers and about 6% of private-sector workers in the United States), information and support from that union may be available. Worker-oriented community-based organizations, such as coalitions for occupational safety and health (COSH) groups can also assist workers with occupational health and safety issues. Worker centers, many of which are affiliated with the National Day Labor Organizing Network or the Interfaith Worker Justice Network, can often assist workers with occupational health and safety as well as other labor issues.[19] (See Chapter 2.) Environmental nongovernmental organizations and community advocacy groups may provide information and support to community members suffering from environmentally related illnesses. (See Appendix.)

- State-level clinical assistance networks are present in two states. The Washington State Department of Labor and Industry sponsors six Centers of Occupational Health and Education in the state to provide technical assistance for clinicians and referrals for patients. (More information is available at http://www.lni.wa.gov/ClaimsIns/Providers/ProjResearchComm/OHS/default.asp?utm_source=shortmarketingurl&utm_medium=url&utm_campaign=COHE.) The New York State Department of Health manages the Occupational Health Clinic Network, which consists of 10 general occupational centers and one agricultural center that offer services to individual workers, businesses, and clinicians. (More information is available at https://www.health.ny.gov/environmental/workplace/clinic_network.htm).

REFERENCES

1. Bepko J, Mansalis K. Common occupational disorders: Asthma, COPD, dermatitis, and musculoskeletal disorders. American Family Physician 2016; 93: 1000–1006.
2. Taiwo OA, Mobo BHP, Cantley L. Recognizing occupational illnesses and injuries. American Family Physician 2010; 82: 169–174.
3. Hill AB. The environment and disease: Association or causation? Journal of the Royal Society of Medicine 1965; 58: 295–300.
4. Possner A. Trying not to miss the point. JAMA 2008; 300: 2836.doi:10.1001/jama.2008.877.
5. Toren K, Blanc PD. Asthma caused by occupational exposures is common: A systematic analysis of estimates of the population-attributable fraction. BMC Pulmonary Medicine 2009; 9: 7. doi:10.1186/1471-2466-9-7.
6. Tarlo SM, Lemiere C. Occupational asthma. New England Journal of Medicine 2014; 370: 640–649.
7. Walters GI, McGrath EE, Ayres JG. Audit of the recording of occupational asthma in primary care. Occupational Medicine (London) 2012; 62: 570–573.
8. Holness DL, Tabassum S, Tarlo SM, et al. Practice patterns of pulmonologists and family physicians for occupational asthma. Chest 2007; 132: 1526–1531.
9. Kim J. Depression as a psychosocial consequence of occupational injury in the US working population: Findings from the Medical

Expenditure Panel Survey. BMC Public Health 2013; 13: 303. doi:10.1186/1471-2458-13-303.

10. Asfaw A, Souza K. Incidence and cost of depression after occupational injury. Journal of Occupational and Environmental Medicine 2012; 54: 1086–1091.

11. Strunin L, Boden LI. Family consequences of chronic back pain. Social Science & Medicine 2004; 58: 1385–1393.

12. Fagan K, Sokas R, Grimes R, Sternes J. Paranitroaniline poisoning: A failure in basic prevention. Journal of Occupational and Environmental Medicine 2014; 56: 112–114.

13. Centers for Disease Control and Prevention. Investigation of progressive inflammatory neuropathy among swine slaughterhouse workers—Minnesota, 2007–2008. Morbidity and Mortality Weekly Report 2008; 57: 122–124.

14. Quinn MM, Lessin N. Effectively educating workers and communities (Textbox). In BS Levy, DH Wegman, SL Baron, RK Sokas (eds.). Occupational and environmental health: Recognizing and preventing disease and injury (6th ed.). New York: Oxford University Press, 2011, pp. 39–41.

15. Agency for Toxic Substances and Disease Registry. ATSDR's final criteria for determining the appropriateness of a medical monitoring program under CERCLA. Federal Register July 28, 1995; 60: 38840–38844.

16. Levine DI, Toffel MW, Johnson MS. Randomized government safety inspections reduce worker injuries with no detectable job loss. Science 2012; 336: 907–911.

17. Silverstein M. How to use the Occupational Safety and Health Administration (OSHA) (Textbox). In BS Levy, DH Wegman, SL Baron, RK Sokas (eds.). Occupational and environmental health: Recognizing and preventing disease and injury (6th ed.). New York: Oxford University Press, 2011, p. 47.

18. District of Columbia Office on Aging. Safe at Home Program for District Seniors. Available at: https://dcoa.dc.gov/release/safe-home-program-district-seniors. Accessed February 20, 2017.

19. Hernandez G, Kimmel L, Marshall B, et al. Bending towards justice: How Latino immigrants became community and safety leaders. 2014. Available at: http://www.cpwr.com/sites/default/files/publications/Bending%20Toward%20Justice.pdf. Accessed December 4, 2016.

APPENDIX TO CHAPTER

THE NINE PERSPECTIVES OF AUSTIN BRADFORD HILL

In 1965, Sir Austin Bradford Hill, a British statistician and epidemiologist put forward, in an address and a published paper, the following nine perspectives ("viewpoints") to help determine if an epidemiologic association is causal:

1. *Strength*: The magnitude of the association between exposure (or some other possible causative factor) and the disease (or other health outcome).

2. *Consistency*: Repeated observation of an association in different populations under different circumstances.

3. *Specificity*: A cause leads to a single effect, rather than multiple effects. (This perspective does not consider diseases with more than one cause.)

4. *Temporality*: The cause precedes the effect. (This is the only essential perspective in determining general causation.)

5. *Biologic gradient*: The presence of a unidirectional dose-response relationship between a possible causative factor and a health outcome.

6. *Plausibility*: The biologic plausibility of a hypothesis concerning the relationship between an exposure and a disease. (This perspective is dependent on current biological information.)

7. *Coherence*: A possible cause-and-effect association between an exposure and a disease does not conflict with knowledge about the natural history and biology of the disease.

8. *Experiment*: "Occasionally, it is possible to appeal to experimental, or semi-experimental, evidence." For example, removal of a hazardous exposure leads to decreased occurrence of a disease.

9. *Analogy*: In some circumstances, reasoning by analogy may be helpful.

(Adapted from: Hill AB. The environment and disease: Association or causation? Journal of the Royal Society of Medicine 1965; 58: 295–300.)

5

Epidemiology

Sadie Costello, Jennifer M. Cavallari, David H. Wegman,
Marie S. O'Neill, and Ellen A. Eisen

The goal of most epidemiological research is to develop and investigate hypotheses on the causal associations between specific exposures and adverse health effects in human populations. Environmental epidemiology focuses on the health consequences of exposures to hazards in the general environment through the environmental media of air, water, soil, or food. The related field of occupational epidemiology focuses on health consequences of workplace exposures to chemical, physical, and biological agents as well as psychological stressors.

The generation of hypotheses about specific exposures causing specific health outcomes is often guided by disease clusters, surveillance data, toxicological information, workplace investigations, or previous epidemiological studies. For example, a hypothesis was generated by the report to a state health department of eight workers employed at a microwave popcorn manufacturing plant who had bronchiolitis obliterans, a rare and debilitating lung disease.[1] An epidemiological study, which included medical evaluations and occupational hygiene surveys, found excess rates of lung disease and lung function abnormalities among workers at the plant compared to the general population. Analysis of these data suggested that inhalation of a volatile butter-flavoring ingredient may have been the cause, prompting an industry-wide evaluation of this exposure and pulmonary health effects.

The study hypothesis identifies both the health outcome(s) and the exposure(s) of interest. The health outcome may be an indicator of biological function, injury, or disease and may range in clinical severity from preclinical, asymptomatic disease, to physician-diagnosed disease or injury, to death. A variety of data sources can provide information on health outcomes. These include death certificates, medical records, questionnaires, and direct measurements of physiologic function, such as blood pressure or pulmonary function.

Exposure assessment, defined as the estimation of exposure to specific hazards in a well-defined population, is critical to the validity of an environmental or occupational epidemiological study. The process of exposure assessment includes identification of existing exposure monitoring data, collection of additional exposure data, and characterization of both duration and intensity (concentration) of exposure, taking into consideration variation over time and place.

In tandem with generating a hypothesis about the association of the health outcome(s) and exposure(s), an epidemiologist identifies the population of interest (the target population), about which conclusions are to be drawn. Characteristics of the target population may be implied by the hypothesis. For example, for environmental epidemiology studies, the target populations are groups of people in the general population, and, for occupational epidemiology studies, the target populations are groups of workers. As another example, for studies of the respiratory effects of air pollution among children, age group is a characteristic of the target population.

All epidemiological investigations utilize standard epidemiological measures to describe and quantify disease occurrence and associations between exposures and health outcomes. Descriptive studies provide and analyze data on the incidence, prevalence, or mortality of disease or injury by time, place, and person. Some studies evaluate the impact of a public health intervention, such as fluoridation of drinking water in a community or a new ventilation system in a workplace. Identifying the appropriate epidemiological measure depends on the study design used to investigate the exposure–health outcome relationship. The randomized control trial design is the "gold standard" for research on the efficacy and safety of medical care; however, most environmental or occupational exposures do not lend themselves to randomization. Thus, the gold standard for observational epidemiologic investigations is the cohort study design. Alternative designs discussed in this chapter include case-control, cross-sectional, and ecologic study designs. Identifying a target population, choosing the right study design, establishing appropriate eligibility and recruitment criteria, and properly collecting and analyzing the data are all critical to produce valid results. Two types of error may lead to incorrect study results: random error and systematic error. *Random error*, defined as the portion of variation in a measurement that has no apparent connection to any other measurement or variable, affects the precision of the estimated exposure–response relationship in a study. *Systematic error*, defined as error that is consistently wrong in a specific direction (often due

to a recognizable source), can result in biased or invalid estimation of the exposure-response relationship. One way to understand the difference between these two types of error is to consider an infinitely large study; random error would be completely eliminated, but systematic errors might remain.

The three sources of systematic error are:

- *Selection bias*, due to the way subjects are enrolled or retained
- *Information bias*, due to the way study variables are measured
- *Confounding bias*, due to the failure to separate out the effect of exposure from the effect of an extraneous factor.

Systematic error should be evaluated both before a study is begun and later during analysis and interpretation of results.

In order to understand how environmental and occupational exposures affect health outcomes, epidemiologists consider exposure assessment (characterizing and quantifying exposure), outcome measures (measures of disease occurrence), and the analytic tools of epidemiology (measures of effect and association, epidemiologic study designs, precision and validity, and interpretation of epidemiological studies). These are the subjects of the sections that follow.

CHARACTERIZING AND QUANTIFYING EXPOSURE

Assigning an accurate and precise exposure to individuals or groups is a critical component of epidemiological investigations. It is challenging for two reasons. First, environmental exposures are seldom constant in time or space. Exposure to environmental air pollution, noise, and green space can vary dramatically, even within a brief period of time or short distance. Occupational exposures also vary over time due to job changes or modifications in processes, materials, or ventilation. Second, data on person-level exposures are seldom available over long time periods, because of prohibitive cost or because studies are often performed years after exposure has occurred. Epidemiologists must find alternative ways of measuring exposure based on available data and resources. For example, epidemiologists used historical pesticide-use reports, land-use maps, and geographic information system software to retrospectively assign 25 years of exposure to specific pesticides from agricultural applications near the home in a case-control study of Parkinson disease in California.[2]

The choice of an appropriate exposure measure is largely dependent upon the disease of interest and the presumed causal path between exposure and disease. Measures of exposure, or the quantity of a substance external to the body, are often characterized by intensity or concentration as well as duration. In studies of short-term or acute disorders, current exposures or exposures over short recent time periods are measured. In contrast, studies of chronic disease typically focus on long-term exposures. In environments that are fairly constant over time, current exposure may be a reasonable surrogate for past exposure.

Exposure Metrics

When information is available, recent or long-term exposure is quantified for groups or individuals. Measures of exposure should incorporate the intensity, frequency, and duration of exposure most appropriate to the health outcome being studied. Exposure estimates are improved when formal exposure assessment has been performed based on judgments of potential exposure or measurements of actual exposure.

In the workplace, a complete occupational history includes documentation of time spent in specific jobs together with information on gaps in employment, such as prolonged sick leaves, periods of layoff, and military leaves (Chapter 4). Estimates of cumulative workplace exposure rely on compilation of current and historical industrial hygiene data and interviews of workers about the history of changes, such as in production processes and exposure controls. Workplace exposure monitoring programs can provide historic data on exposure levels for individuals or areas over time. These representative measurements, combined with work histories, provide measures of exposure intensity and frequency that can be integrated to estimate cumulative exposure for each worker.

To calculate cumulative exposure to an occupational hazard, estimated exposure levels are weighted by the number of years in successive jobs and summed over all jobs held by each worker. For some chronic diseases, exposure that occurred years ago may be assumed to be biologically equivalent to exposure that occurred last year. Weighting schemes that are more complex should be based on specific biologic hypotheses about the relative importance of different exposure patterns. For example, exposures in the distant past may be weighted more heavily than those in the recent past for diseases such as silicosis, for which irreversible changes are believed to accumulate gradually over many years.

In contrast to workplace-based studies, cumulative exposure is rarely estimated in community-based studies. In air pollution studies, for example, information on residential address is often used to account for geographic (spatial) variation in exposure to air pollution using data from existing Environmental Protection Agency air monitors. Air pollution exposure is usually based on current residence, even when cumulative exposure is biologically relevant. For some outcomes, current residence may provide adequate information. For example, researchers studying birth outcomes take advantage of maternal residence, which is routinely collected on birth certificates. The address listed on the birth certificate may be a good proxy for residence during the 9 months of pregnancy. In contrast, associations of lung cancer mortality with air pollution derived from the address at the time of death are probably not credible since the address at death is not a good estimate of lifelong residence. If historic residence data were available, a credible air pollution metric could be derived.[3] Assigning long-term exposure to an environmental pollutant, such as particles in the air or disinfection by-products in drinking water, requires knowledge of residential history and/or consumption habits over a long period of time. This information is rarely publicly available but can be obtained from surveys, questionnaires, water treatment practices, or environmental monitoring.

Quantified exposures—permitting continuous rather than categorical or nonordinal estimates of actual or potential exposures—are advantageous in epidemiological studies because they allow estimation of exposure–response relationships, providing information on the level or quantity of exposure that produces a specific health outcome.

Biological Monitoring

An alternative method of evaluating exposure is biological monitoring to estimate dose—the amount of a substance that has entered the body. Evaluation of individuals with biomarkers—toxic agents or their metabolites in blood, urine, hair, nails, or exhaled air—sometimes improves estimation of dose. Biological monitoring can complement environmental monitoring because it accounts for exposures from multiple routes of absorption: inhalation, skin absorption, and ingestion. For example, the blood lead level has been used in epidemiologic studies of workers and children because it integrates recent absorption from both inhalation and ingestion. Another advantage of biomarkers is that they may reflect exposure over specific time intervals. For example, in studies of the health effects of chronic lead exposure, X-ray fluorescence of bone provides a more relevant biomarker of exposure than blood lead level because it estimates the accumulated body burden of lead, reflecting long-term exposure. Although biological monitoring tests do not exist for many hazardous substances, biological monitoring is being used to measure damage at the molecular level, such as oxidative stress or inflammation. Such biomarkers allow mechanisms of biologic effects to be explored. New and improved measures of the burden of toxic agents on the body continue to be developed. For example, newly developed metrics, such as epigenetic changes, are being used to evaluate how occupational and environmental exposures may affect health.[4]

MEASURES OF DISEASE OCCURRENCE

Incidence and *prevalence*, two epidemiological measures used to quantify disease occurrence, are standard variables used to measure disease frequencies.

Incidence

Incidence measures the occurrence of new cases of disease over a specified time period. The term *risk* is used to describe an individual's probability of developing a disease. On a population level, the risk (probability) of a specific disease is referred to as the *cumulative incidence*. It is based on the number of new cases occurring in a given population during a specified period of time:

$$\text{Cumulative incidence} = \frac{\text{Number of new cases}}{\substack{\text{Total population at risk} \\ \text{during the specified} \\ \text{time period}}}$$

For example, an investigation of 1,157 workers in a coated fabrics plant identified 68 cases of peripheral neuropathy over a 1-year period.[5] Only 50 affected workers had onset of this disease during the previous year; 18 of the 68 prevalent cases had onset more than 1 year before. Therefore, the population at risk for development of a new case within the past year was: 1,157 − 18 = 1,139. The 18 workers who already had the disease at the beginning of the study period are excluded from both the numerator and denominator, as incidence only refers to the onset of new cases. Because the number of new cases in that period was 50, the plant-wide annual incidence proportion was as follows:

$$\frac{50}{1,139} = 4.4 \text{ per 100 workers}$$

The *incidence rate* uses the same numerator as the incidence proportion but a different denominator. The denominator incorporates the concept of person-time, usually expressed in units of person-years. This denominator takes into account not only the number of at-risk persons but also the length of time during which each participant was at risk for development of the specific disease. An example of how to calculate the contribution of a single worker to a person-years denominator is illustrated in Figure 5-1. The incidence rate can be thought of as the "speed" at which new cases arise in a population per unit of time.

$$\text{Incidence rate} = \frac{\text{Number of new cases}}{\text{Sum of person-time at risk in a year}}$$

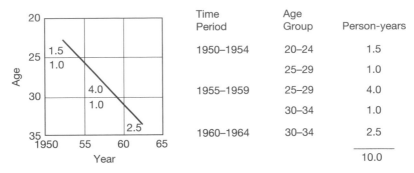

Time Period	Age Group	Person-years
1950–1954	20–24	1.5
	25–29	1.0
1955–1959	25–29	4.0
	30–34	1.0
1960–1964	30–34	2.5
		———
		10.0

Figure 5-1. Person-years experienced by a worker entering a follow-up program at age 23 years 6 months in mid-1952 and leaving in mid-1962. (Source: Adapted from Monson RR. Occupational epidemiology [2nd ed.] Boca Raton, FL: CRC Press, 1989, p. 79.)

Prevalence

While the incidence rate assesses the frequency of disease onset, *prevalence* is a measure of disease status. The simplest quantity, known as *point prevalence*, is the ratio between the number of cases present and the size of the population at risk at a single point in time:

$$\text{Point prevalence} = \frac{\text{Number of cases}}{\text{Population at risk}}$$

Unlike incidence, which is based on new cases during a given time period, prevalence is based on the number of cases at one point in time. To interpret the public health significance of the situation previously described of 68 peripheral neuropathy cases in a coated fabrics plant,[5] one needs a denominator. The total plant population was 1,157. Therefore, the point prevalence was as follows:

$$\frac{68}{1,157} = 5.9\%$$

To determine whether this prevalence was excessive, the prevalence in the plant had to be compared with the prevalence in the general population or some other appropriate comparison group. Two limitations of point prevalence are that (a) it does not distinguish between old and new cases and (b) it does not take into account the amount of time a person has had a disease. Diseases of short duration may have a low prevalence, even if their incidence rate is high; in contrast, diseases of long duration,

even if their incidence rate is low, may have a high prevalence. Because prevalence is a reflection of both incidence rate and disease duration, it may therefore be misleading. It is best suited for measuring the burden of chronic disease; it is poorly suited for studying the causes of disease.

MEASURES OF EFFECT AND ASSOCIATION

The goal of environmental and occupational epidemiology is most often to estimate the causal effect of the exposure of interest on a health outcome. Ideally, epidemiologists could follow a group of exposed people over time to find out who developed the health outcome of interest and then, magically, rewind time, un-expose all those same people (keeping everything else about them the same), and follow them again to find out who developed the outcome of interest. The causal effect of exposure is defined by the comparison (ratio or difference) of disease occurrence between the exposed and non-exposed follow-up periods. Winding back time is clearly impossible, so the idea that we could follow the same people twice over is referred to as *counterfactual* because it is counter to the facts of nature. Therefore, most studies compare the occurrence of health outcomes between a group of exposed and a different group of non-exposed people. Quantitative estimates for comparisons are discussed in the next section.

Rate Ratio and Risk Ratio

The *rate ratio* is designed to communicate the relative importance of an exposure by comparing the rate in an exposed population with that in an otherwise comparable non-exposed population. Often the term *relative risk* is broadly used to refer to either an incidence rate ratio or a risk ratio (a ratio of cumulative incidences). In their simplest forms, a rate ratio is the ratio of two rates while a risk ratio is the ratio of two probabilities (Table 5-1). In the case of the fabrics plant, the suspect neurotoxin was in the print department, so it was possible to create a within-plant comparison. Of the 1,139 disease-free workers in the plant, 169 worked in the print department and 34 of these workers had onset of peripheral neuropathy during the past year, resulting in the following annual incidence rate:

$$\frac{34}{169} = 20.1 \text{ per 100 workers}$$

Among the remaining 970 workers, there were 16 new cases, resulting in the following incidence proportion during the 1-year period:

$$\frac{16}{970} = 1.6 \text{ per 100 workers}$$

Therefore, the incidence risk ratio was:

$$\frac{20.1}{1.6} = 12.6$$

When examining different diseases or the effects of different hazards, relative risks can be compared directly. For example, the relative risk of lung cancer in heavy smokers compared with nonsmokers is very large (32.4), whereas that for cardiovascular disease is small (1.4). This finding suggests that smoking is more potent as a lung carcinogen than as a cardiotoxic agent.

Rate and Risk Difference

Whereas the risk and rate *ratios* are measures of the potency of the hazard, the incidence rate and risk *differences* measure the magnitude of the disease burden in the population that is ascribed to the exposure under study. This concept is especially useful in studies of an occupational or environmental health hazard when an exposure is generally one of several possible causes of a specific disease. The incidence risk difference or prevalence difference is calculated by subtracting the prevalence of the disease in the non-exposed population from that in the exposed population (Table 5-1). Likewise, the incidence rate difference is calculated by subtracting the incidence rate of the disease in the non-exposed population from that in the exposed population. In the coated fabrics plant, the annual incidence rate per 100 workers in the non-exposed population (1.6) is subtracted from the rate in the exposed population (20.1) to yield an incidence rate difference of 18.5 per 100 workers per year—the rate of disease attributed to the exposure.

The concept of risk difference is illustrated by the impact of cigarette smoking on health. Table 5-2 shows that the smoking-attributable risk for lung cancer (2.20 per 1,000) is smaller than the smoking-attributable risk for cardiovascular disease (2.61 per 1,000). The risk difference takes account of both the potency of the disease-causing factor and the magnitude of the disease in the population. Despite the lower relative risk of cardiovascular disease due to smoking, the larger attributable risk indicates that, in a population, reduction of smoking leads to a greater reduction in the occurrence of cardiovascular disease than lung cancer.

Interpreting Rates

Crude Rates

When rates are calculated without consideration of factors such as age or calendar year,

Table 5-1. Derivation of Risk Ratio and Risk Difference*

Disease	Exposure		Total
	Present	Absent	
Present	a	c	a + c
Absent	b	d	b + d
Total	a + b	c + d	a + b + c + d

* Calculations:
Exposed disease prevalence = a/(a + b)
Non-exposed disease prevalence = c/(c + d)
Risk ratio (prevalence ratio) = a/(a + b) ÷ c/(c + d)
Attributable risk (prevalence difference) = a/(a + b)–c/(c + d)

Table 5-2. Relative and Attributable Risk of Death among British Male Physicians from Selected Causes Associated with Heavy Cigarette Smoking

Cause of Death	Death Rate*		Relative Risk	Attributable Risk
	Nonsmokers	Heavy Smokers[†]		
Lung cancer	0.07	2.27	32.4	2.20
Other cancers	1.91	2.59	1.4	0.68
Chronic bronchitis	0.05	1.06	21.2	1.01
Cardiovascular disease	7.32	9.93	1.4	2.61
All causes	12.06	19.67	1.6	7.61

* Number of deaths per 1,000 per year.
† Smokers of 25 or more cigarettes per day.

Table 5-3. Age Effect on Incidence of Myocardial Infarction in a Hypothetical Population*

Location	Workers <45 years			Workers ≥45 years			All Workers			
	Cases	Population at Risk	Age-Specific Incidence Rate	Cases	Population at Risk	Age-Specific Incidence Rate	Cases	Population at Risk	Crude Incidence Rate	Age-Adjusted Incidence Rate[†]
Factory 1	4	400	10.0	18	600	30.0	22	1,000	22.0	18.0
Factory 2	10	800	12.5	10	200	50.0	20	1,000	20.0	27.5

* The incidence rate is expressed as new myocardial infarctions occurring in a 10-year period of observation per 1,000 population.
† Based on age distribution summed for Factory 1 and Factory 2.

they are referred to as *crude rates*. Crude rates can be misleading. For example, if the exposed group includes a high proportion of older people and disease incidence increases with age, then observed differences in crude rates may only reflect differences in age.

Stratum-specific Rates

Stratum-specific rates are calculated for homogeneous subgroups of a population that are defined by age, gender, or other specific factors. Sometimes an elevated rate of disease exists only in one subgroup, such as people aged 35 to 44 years.

Externally Adjusted Rates

Although specific rates can sometimes provide valuable information, it is cumbersome to compare many specific rates. Methods have been developed for estimating a single summary rate that takes account of differences in the distribution of population characteristics, such as age. Such rates are known as *externally adjusted*

rates or *standardized rates*. Two types of external adjustment are commonly used: *direct adjustment*, in which rates in the study population are weighted by person-time distribution across age categories in an external reference population, and *indirect adjustment*, in which rates in a reference population are weighted by person-time distribution in an external study population. These methods are illustrated with examples of adjustment for age in Table 5-3. For a further description of these types of adjustment, see the Appendix at the end of this chapter.

EPIDEMIOLOGIC STUDY DESIGNS

Epidemiologic studies are conducted to measure disease occurrence and to identify associations between exposures and health outcomes. There are several different designs, each with strengths and weaknesses. Cross-sectional, cohort, and case-control designs are those that are most often used. Choice of the appropriate study design

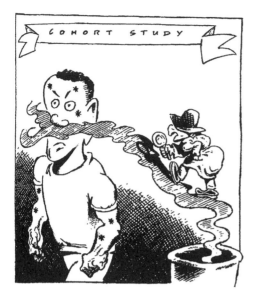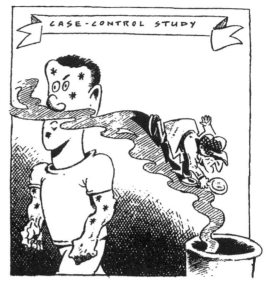

Figure 5-2. One way to envision a cohort study is that it investigates from exposure to health outcomes. In contrast, one way to envision a case-control study is that it investigates from health outcome to exposures. (Drawing by Nick Thorkelson.)

depends upon several factors, including the research question, data and resources available, and the feasibility of the study. (See Figure 5-2.)

Cross-Sectional Studies

A cross-sectional study examines the association between exposure and a health outcome at one single point, or short period, in time. The study population includes all subjects in the population of interest who are present at the time of data collection. Study populations may be derived from population surveys, such as the National Health and Nutrition Examination Survey (NHANES), population lists such as from a driver's license registry or other public records, and lists of labor union members or workers employed in a given industry. Analyses are performed either by comparing the outcome between subgroups defined by exposure status or by comparing exposure between subgroups defined by disease status. Exposure can be classified (a) dichotomously, such as exposed versus non-exposed; (b) categorically, such as low, medium, and high; or (c) as a continuous measurement. Exposure classification can be based on current or lifetime exposure. The following is an example of a cross-sectional study:

The association between environmental lead exposure and blood pressure was investigated in a cross-sectional study based on data from NHANES II, a general health survey based on a representative sample of the U.S. population. The study population was restricted to the white males age 40 through 59. Considering both blood pressure and lead exposure as continuous variables, researchers found that subjects with higher blood lead levels had higher levels of both systolic and diastolic blood pressure. These associations were statistically significant in linear regression models (a statistical approach used to estimate the relationship between dependent variable y and predictor variables x), after adjusting for known risk factors for high blood pressure, including age, body mass index, nutritional factors, and measures of blood chemistry.[6]

Cross-sectional studies are frequently done when investigating risks in the workplace and the general environment. Compared to studies based on other designs, cross-sectional studies generally cost less and take less time to perform. By questionnaire and by direct measurement, they can simultaneously collect information on demographic parameters; exposures; personal habits, such as smoking and diet; past medical history; and current health status.

Cross-sectional studies have several important limitations. The primary disadvantage is that it may be difficult to determine whether exposure preceded disease because information on both is obtained at the same time. Although it may be possible to obtain date of diagnosis and timing of exposure to help establish temporality, cross-sectional studies rarely provide compelling evidence for a causal effect. In addition, they are less appropriate for investigating causal relations because they are often based on prevalent, rather than incident, cases of disease. Prevalence is a poor proxy for incidence, especially for diseases of short duration. A related limitation in working populations is that cross-sectional studies oversample workers with long duration of employment and undersample workers with short duration of employment. Occupational cross-sectional investigations based on current workers employed at the time of study do not include workers who have left work and those who are absent from work, some of whom may have the disease being studied. Absence of less healthy workers may result in an underestimate of the association of interest due to the "healthy worker effect." (See section on Healthy Worker Bias.)

Cohort Studies

In a cohort study design, the study population is identified as those who are at risk for developing the disease of interest. These individuals are divided into groups based on their exposure levels and monitored over time to measure the occurrence of adverse health outcomes. A conceptually important feature of a cohort study is that participants are followed for the outcome starting at the time of their first exposure. A cohort study is analogous to a randomized control trial in which people are recruited, then assigned an exposure and followed for the outcome.[7] Deviation from this feature can alter the interpretation of the results from the study. (See a detailed explanation in the "Healthy Worker Bias" section.) The incidence of adverse health outcomes is observed in the exposed group and compared with that in a non-exposed, reference group. Cohort studies are either retrospective, in which the cohort is defined at some point in the past and monitored to the present, or prospective, in which the cohort is defined at present and monitored into the future.

The cohort design is used to study risks associated with fatal and nonfatal health outcomes. Retrospective studies can be conducted if information on *past* health status is available, such as in existing medical records, a cancer registry or other disease registry, or death certificates. Some studies may require prospective study designs in which health data are collected directly by performing medical examinations, physiologic tests, or surveys of *current* health status. Longitudinal studies examine change in health status over time.

The following is an example of a *retrospective cohort morbidity* study:

A cohort of approximately 1,000 hospital nurses was studied to examine possible reproductive effects associated with use of sterilizing agents.[8] Questionnaires and medical records were used to collect information retrospectively about both exposure and pregnancy history as far back as 30 years. The frequency of spontaneous abortion among nurses currently using the sterilizing agents was only slightly higher than that for currently non-exposed nurses. A more striking difference was observed when results were stratified according to whether exposure to sterilizing agents had occurred during a previous pregnancy. Among those exposed, the rate of spontaneous abortion was 16%, compared with 6% among the non-exposed. Of the three specific sterilizing agents considered, ethylene oxide showed the strongest association with spontaneous abortion.

The following is an example of a *prospective cohort morbidity* study:

A cohort of 1,022 infants born in the Faroe Islands, an island group situated between the Norwegian Sea and the North Atlantic Ocean, was followed forward in time to investigate the possible neurobehavioral effects of prenatal exposure to methylmercury. The source of exposure was dietary and derived mostly from eating whale meat, a custom in this Nordic community. Batteries of neurophysiologic and neuropsychologic tests were administered to school children at about age 7. The exposure variables were biomarkers: mercury concentration in both cord blood and maternal hair. Mercury concentration in hair of subjects at 12 months of age was also measured. Neurophysiologic testing did not reveal any mercury-related abnormalities, but neuropsychological deficits in language, attention, and memory were related to prenatal exposure to mercury.[9]

Historically, a common type of cohort study has been the standardized mortality study, in which cause-specific mortality rates of the exposed cohort are compared with those of the general population, which is assumed to be non-exposed, using indirect standardization. Each comparison results in an approximation of relative risk, known as the *standardized mortality ratio* (SMR). If the number of deaths observed in the exposed cohort is equal to the number expected based on death rates in the standard population, the SMR equals 1.0, indicating neither an excess nor a deficit of risk. If the SMR is greater than 1.0, the data suggest an increased risk in the exposed population. Because workers are often healthier at hire than the general population and healthier workers tend to remain employed longer, workers are relatively healthier than the general population despite their occupational exposure. Therefore, the general population is an inappropriate reference population for a worker population and the SMR is typically a downwardly biased estimate of the relative risk (as discussed further in the "Healthy Worker Bias" section).

The following is an example of a *retrospective cohort mortality study* using the general population as the non-exposed group:

A cohort of autoworkers was studied to examine the relationships between exposure to metalworking fluids and specific causes of death.[10] All workers who had ever been employed in one of three Midwestern automobile manufacturing plants for at least 3 years prior to 1984 were included. Subjects were followed for vital status from 1941, the year Social Security records became available, through 1994. By the end of the follow-up period, almost 25% of the 46,400 subjects had died. When the observed number of deaths due to all causes combined was compared to the expected number, there was no obvious excess among white males (SMR = 1.0) and a slight deficit among African-American males (SMR = 0.9). For all cancers combined, the SMRs were 1.05 for white males and 0.95 for African-American males. When observed deaths due to specific cancers were compared to expected, slight excesses, with SMRs between 1.2 to 1.4, were found for leukemia and cancers of the esophagus, larynx, stomach, and liver among white males and for two of these same cancers, as well as pancreatic cancer, among African-American males (Table 5-4). When lifetime exposure to metalworking fluids was evaluated in an internal analysis using assembly workers without direct exposure as the reference, increasing risk for cancers of the esophagus, larynx, skin, and prostate was associated with increasing exposure.

Cohort studies have several advantages. First, the study population includes all subjects at risk, rather than a cross-sectional sample of workers employed at a specific point in time. Second, because the population is observed over time, the timing of the exposure relative to the outcome is known. Therefore, cohort studies using an internal reference group (non-exposed workers rather than the general population) can provide the strongest evidence for a causal relationship. The design is efficient for studying relatively common chronic diseases. Several specific causes of death or disease can be studied in the

Table 5-4. Standardized Mortality Ratios (SMRs) for Selected Cancers among White and African American Male Autoworkers

Cause of Death	White Males		African-American Males	
	Observed	SMR (95% CI)	Observed	SMR (95% CI)
All causes	13,105	1.01 (0.99–1.03)	1,882	0.86 (0.82–0.90)
All cancers	2,983	1.05 (1.01–1.09)	460	0.95 (0.86–1.04)
Esophagus	83	1.22 (0.97–1.51)	21	0.76 ((0.47–1.16)
Stomach	151	1.16 (0.98–1.36)	28	0.96(0.63–1.38)
Pancreas	143	0.99 (0.83–1.16)	36	1.50 (1.05–2.07)
Liver	78	1.42 (1.12–1.77)	16	1.31 (0.75–2.13)
Larynx	44	1.16 (0.85–1.56)	11	1.26 (0.63–2.25)
Lung	1,002	1.08 (1.02–1.15)	153	0.95 (0.80–1.11)
Prostate	261	1.06 (0.94–1.20)	55	0.98 (0.74–1.28)
Leukemia	147	1.34 (1.14–1.58)	15	1.28 (0.71–2.10)

Note. SMR = standardized mortality rate; CI = confidence interval.

same cohort study. In addition, detailed exposure assessment can be conducted.

Cohort studies have several limitations. For example, retrospective cohort studies typically rely on outcomes recorded for other purposes, such as disease diagnosis or cause of death, and therefore the endpoint is unlikely to be an early marker of disease. In addition, cohort studies: (a) are often expensive and time-consuming because information should be obtained on all members of the cohort and (b) usually include little information on lifestyle, socioeconomic status, and other determinants of health status because of the cost of obtaining detailed data on a large number of people.

Case-Control Studies

Case-control studies aim to achieve the same goals as cohort studies with a more efficient sampling design. In a case-control study, the investigator examines associations between exposures and a health outcome by comparing exposures of people who developed the health outcome (cases) with those of controls, a sample of nonaffected people in the same population. Exposure information is obtained only for cases and controls rather than the whole population as in a cohort study. The case-control design is especially well suited for infrequent and rare diseases, for cohort studies would have to be very large—and prohibitively expensive—to generate enough cases to study. Although case-control studies are limited to the study of a single health outcome, information can be collected on a wide variety of exposures.

There are three general types of case-control studies: (a) those that are nested within cohorts, (b) those that are population-based, and (c) those that are registry-based. In nested case-control studies, all cases of a specific disease are identified within the cohort, and controls represent a sample of the cohort without the disease. In a mortality study, disease status is generally based on death certificates; in a morbidity study, disease status is generally based on medical records. The nested-case control design is often used when an epidemiologist would like to collect more detailed information on cohort study participants, such as smoking history. It may be cost-prohibitive and logistically challenging to contact every member of a large cohort study to obtain smoking information but feasible and affordable to contact the cases and a sample of the controls.

In a *population-based case-control study*, all cases occurring in residents of a defined geographic area in a specific time period are included, and controls are selected from the same defined population. A major challenge in population-based case-control studies is to define the population that gave rise to the cases and obtain a nonbiased sample of controls from that population. This type of study is prone to selection bias if the controls selected for the study have a different exposure distribution than the defined population.

In a *registry-based case-control study*, reported cases of disease during a defined time period are identified from a registry, and controls are selected from the same registry. Although this is an easy study design to implement, it is difficult to define the population that gave rise to the cases in a registry and even more difficult to defend the claim that people with a different disease in the registry who are used as the controls have the same exposure distribution as the population that gave rise to the cases.

A conceptually important feature is that the controls selected for the study should have the opportunity to be cases in the study if they develop the disease of interest later during the defined time period. For example, in a nested case-control study, epidemiologists often choose controls for each case from among other cohort members who were *at risk to become a case at the time when the case was diagnosed*, including subjects who became cases later in the cohort study. This type of sampling, called *risk-set sampling*, can also be used in other types of case-control designs.

The effect measure typically estimated in a case-control study is the odds ratio (OR), which is a ratio of the odds of exposure among the cases compared with the odds of exposure among the controls. In Table 5-1, a/c is the odds of exposure among the cases, and b/d is the odds of exposure among the controls. If the controls were sampled using risk-set sampling, then the OR approximates the incidence rate ratio that is estimated in cohort studies. Interpretation of them is similar: When OR = 1, there is no excess or deficit of risk.

A case-control study need not include all cases within a defined population. Valid results may still be obtained when the case group includes only a sample of cases. The two main requirements for a case-control study to be valid are that (a) the controls be selected from the population from which cases were identified, and (b) both cases and controls be selected without prior knowledge of past exposure history. The following is an example of a *population-based case control study*:

Non-Hodgkin lymphoma has been associated with agricultural pesticide use in men, but little is known about risks in women. To address this lack of knowledge, National Cancer Institute investigators conducted a population-based case-control study in which cases were defined as incident cases of non-Hodgkin lymphoma among women residing in 66 counties in eastern Nebraska, diagnosed between 1983 and 1986 in area hospitals.[11] Controls were selected from female residents in the same counties, using random-digit dialing of telephone numbers. The study did not find increased risk due to living or working on a farm. Small risks were observed for women who personally handled insecticides (OR = 1.3) or chlorinated hydrocarbons (OR = 1.7), and women who personally handled organophosphate insecticides had a 4.5-fold increased risk (Table 5-5). Because non-Hodgkin lymphoma is a relatively infrequent disease with a long latency, a case-control study was more feasible than a cohort study.

The following is an example of a *nested case-control study*:

The risk of cancer due to exposure to pulsed electromagnetic fields was examined in a series of case-control studies, each focused on a different malignancy, nested in a cohort of electric utility workers.[12] Cases of a particular cancer were diagnosed at any time after entry into the cohort (beginning of employment as an electric utility worker) until the end of follow-up in 1988. Controls were chosen at random from sets of cohort members matched, by age and gender, to each cancer patient, from among those alive at the time of diagnosis of each case. Cumulative exposures were estimated up to the date of cancer diagnosis. Smoking information was obtained from company medical records. The study found no association between exposure to pulsed electromagnetic fields and cancers previously suspected of being associated with magnetic fields. However, the study found an association between cumulative exposure to pulsed electromagnetic fields and lung cancer (after adjusting for cigarette smoking history), with an OR of 3.1 in the highest exposure category.

The *case-crossover study* design is a variation of the case-control design. It is used to investigate transient risk factors that may trigger acute events. In a case-crossover study, all cases serve as their own controls by comparing exposures near the health event to exposures at a time when the event did not occur, either before or after. A case-crossover study is designed to investigate whether exposures immediately preceding the health event are different from those that typically occur.[13] Because cases serve as their own controls, the only extraneous factors that could explain both the exposure and the health outcome are confounding factors (see section on Confounding Bias below) that could change over time between the event and the control time period. The following is an example of a case-crossover study:

The association between exposure to vehicular traffic in urban areas and the triggering of an acute myocardial infarction (MI) was evaluated in a

Table 5-5. Non-Hodgkin Lymphoma, According to Insecticide Use among Women in Eastern Nebraska

Insecticide Class	Used on Farms			Personally Handled		
	Cases	OR	95% CI	Cases	OR	95% CI
Any insecticide	56	0.8	0.5–1.3	22	1.3	0.7–2.3
Chlorinated hydrocarbons	20	1.6	0.8–3.1	5	1.7	0.5–5.8
Organophosphates	14	1.2	0.6–2.5	6	4.5	1.1–17.9
Metals	3	1.6	0.3–7.5	0	–	–

Note. OR = odds ratio; CI =confidence interval.

case-crossover study in southern Germany.[14] A total of 691 cases were identified from individuals listed in a regional MI registry for whom (a) dates and times of MIs were known, (b) survival had been at least 24 hours after the MI, (c) the registry's standardized interview had been completed, and (d) information had been provided on factors that may have triggered the MI. Patient diaries were used to collect exposure data on activities during the 4 days preceding onset of symptoms. For each individual, the 4 days of data were divided into two periods of traffic exposure: a "case period" for the 6 hours prior to the onset of the MI and a control period for the 24 to 71 hours prior to the onset of the MI. The study found an association between exposure to traffic and the onset of an MI within 1 hour following exposure (OR, 2.92; 95% confidence interval, 2.22 to 3.83; $p < 0.001$). The MI patient's use of a car was the most common source of exposure to traffic. However, the study also found an association between time spent on public transportation and the onset of an MI 1 hour later.

The principal advantages of case-control studies, including case-crossover studies, are their relative simplicity and relatively low cost of studying diseases that do not occur frequently. Case-control studies are useful when multiple exposures are being explored as causes of a specific disease, such as bladder cancer. In contrast, cohort studies are useful when multiple diseases are hypothesized to be caused by a specific exposure, such as inorganic lead.

Case-control studies are more susceptible to biases than cohort studies (see section on Precision and Validity below). For example, if exposure information depends on self-reports, it may be recalled and reported differently by subjects with and without disease. In addition, the need to identify a control group from the same population that generated the cases often presents a challenge.

Ecologic Studies

In an ecologic study, the group -- rather than the individual -- is the unit of analysis. Ecologic studies require that information is available for both exposure and disease for an entire group, such as a class of students, or the entire population of a community, a state, or a nation. Disease rates and average exposures are compared either between different groups in different places at the same point in time or within the same group at different points in time. For example, an ecologic study in Spain used census-derived data on cancer mortality and information on water source, by municipality, to assess associations between chlorination of drinking water and both stomach and bladder cancer.[15]

Use of ecologic variables is common in environmental epidemiology because high-quality data often exist for a region but not for individuals in the region. For example, concentrations of air pollutants measured at the city or county level (ecologic measures) may be assigned to all individuals living in that city or county area and may be associated with health outcomes in individuals, as was done in a study of daily ozone levels and daily mortality in Mexico City.[16] A validation study found that outdoor particle measurements correlated reasonably well with personal particle exposure over time, supporting their use in longitudinal studies of air pollution and health.[17]

Studies using ecologic variables for both exposure and outcome may be more prone to the *ecologic fallacy*—the inappropriate inference of a causal effect at the individual level from data that are aggregated at the group level. For example, suicide rates were found to be higher in predominantly Catholic countries than in predominantly Protestant countries, suggesting that Catholics had higher suicide rates.[18] While possibly true, this finding could also be explained by Protestants in predominantly Catholic countries having higher suicide rates. In addition, some other variable unrelated to religion, such as unemployment, might be operating as a causal factor.

Ecologic data are properly interpreted as representing a contextual effect, such as living in neighborhoods with little green space or a high literacy rate. Although one needs to interpret ecologic studies with caution, ecologic studies can be used appropriately, such as in (a) developing hypotheses for further study, or (b) evaluating the effectiveness of an intervention by comparing disease rates in a target population before and after an intervention to the rates in a control population at the same two points in time.

Panel Studies

A panel study is similar to a cohort study in which a small group of individuals are followed prospectively over a short time period. Its goal is to investigate short-term health effects of environmental exposures that vary within a brief period. Repeated measures of exposure and health outcomes are obtained during the study period. For example, in environmental epidemiology, panel studies effectively examine acute health effects of air pollution. For example, a panel of 88 elderly men and women were recruited and, over a 24-hour period, monitored for heart rate variability (HRV).[19] Participants were monitored for 24-hour periods in three different seasons. Data on concentrations of particles in ambient air were available for each of these periods. This panel study found that particulate concentration in ambient air was associated with a decline in HRV, indicative of an adverse effect on the heart. In cohorts of workers, panel studies have examined the health effects of workplace exposures over short periods, ranging from a few hours to entire workweeks. In another panel study that monitored welders over a 24-hour period, an association was found between 4-hour average exposure to particles 2.5 μm or smaller ($PM_{2.5}$) and a decline in HRV.[20] Panel studies can collect much information on each individual studied. However, in panel studies with long observation periods, participants may leave before the studies are completed, which could result in bias.

PRECISION AND VALIDITY

The *precision* of an epidemiologic study is determined by the amount of random error (error arising from variability in the data that cannot be readily explained) that may contribute to the study results. Random error often arises due to chance. The precision of a study can be improved by increasing the size of the study population or by modifying the efficiency (reducing random error) of a study.

Careful consideration needs to be given to the validity, or lack of bias, of a study. The *validity* of a study is the degree to which the inferences drawn from a study are warranted when one considers the study methods and the characteristics of study participants.

The degree to which the inferences drawn from a study are warranted is determined largely by the absence of bias. Bias, which is a form of systematic error, can be distinguished from precision, which is related to random error. Reports of epidemiologic studies should provide sufficient information for readers to understand what potential sources of bias were present and how these biases were addressed. There are three types of bias: selection bias, information bias, and confounding bias.

Selection Bias

Selection bias results from biases in the selection of study participants as well as any loss to follow-up. Ideally, study participants reflect the same distributions of both exposure and health status as the population of interest. Selection bias may occur if participants are chosen into the study, or remain in the study, based on two conditions: their potential for, or level of, exposure (Condition A) *and* their health outcome status (Condition B).

In cohort studies in which all members of the cohort are followed for the outcome starting at the same time as their exposure began, selection bias can result from exposure-related loss to follow-up. *Loss to follow-up* describes the process of cohort subjects dropping out of study participation (possibly by moving out of the study area in environmental studies or leaving the workforce in occupational studies). As a result, there is no information on whether these subjects ever developed the outcome of interest. If the exposure causes people to drop out of the study (Condition A) *and* if the people who drop out of the study are more at risk for the outcome (Condition B), then loss to follow-up can result in selection bias.

In addition, selection bias may occur if the included subjects differ from the rest of the population by both exposure status and probability of experiencing the outcome. A subtle way in which selection into a cohort can bias the study is best understood in the context of occupational studies. A cohort study should start when people are first exposed. In occupational studies, this would be achieved if all workers who were ever employed are included in the cohort and followed from date of hire. Selection bias may occur if the epidemiologist defines the study population as anyone at work *at a specific point in time* (typically determined by when outcome data become available). Therefore, subjects who would have otherwise been eligible (if outcome data had been available earlier) are no longer eligible at the start of follow-up. In such a scenario, the epidemiologist has selected a group of survivors—workers who had not yet experienced the exposure-related health outcome. Unless the epidemiologist is interested in knowing if exposure causes disease among a group of workers who already did not get the disease, the study population is a biased sample of the target population. Loss to follow-up may sometimes be addressed using inverse censoring weighting (also known as inverse probability weighting), in which the inverse censoring weight is defined by the fraction: 1/Probability of being lost to follow-up. However, selection bias in general is not easily corrected in the analysis and is best avoided during the design and implementation of the study. If possible, workers should be followed for the outcome from their first day at work, and information about why they left work should be collected.

In case-control studies, which ideally contain all of the cases in a source population and a sample of the controls, Condition B is always met because health outcome status is an integral part of the eligibility criteria. Preventing selection bias in case-control studies is therefore accomplished by avoiding Condition A—ensuring that the selection of the controls is not influenced by exposure status.

Information Bias

Information bias, or *misclassification*, results from errors in the measurement of subjects' exposure or health outcome. Technically, *measurement error* refers to errors in measuring or assigning a continuous variable and *misclassification* refers to errors in measuring or assigning a binary or categorical variable. Although any study variable can be misclassified, this section focuses on misclassified exposure and outcome variables.

There are two types of misclassification. *Nondifferential misclassification* occurs as a result of either (a) misassignment of exposure status that occurs regardless of disease status or (b) misassignment of disease status that occurs regardless of exposure status. Nondifferential misclassification may occur when a health outcome is death from a specific cause that is ascertained from death records. Death records are imperfect, more so for some causes of death than others; in general, death certificates are more reliable for cancers than they are for nonmalignant chronic diseases. However, usually there is no reason to believe that a decedent's exposure status would influence the recorded cause of death.

Differential misclassification of an outcome may occur in the context of an occupational cohort study if workers with the highest exposure are more likely to be screened for the outcome of interest. In this case, there may be more false positives among the highly-exposed workers and more missed cases among lower-exposed workers. To avoid differential-outcome misclassification in cohort studies the investigators can be kept "blind" to exposure status during collection of outcome information, thereby randomly distributing any errors in collection of information from exposed and non-exposed subjects.

Nondifferential exposure misclassification may occur when the exposure is broadly defined. For example, a study on the health effects of pesticide exposures in utero may quantify *all* pesticide use, rather than exposure to organophosphate pesticides, which can adversely affect fetal development and growth. This problem is generally worse in retrospective studies because adequate documentation of historical exposures is more difficult. Since the classification of pesticide exposure is equally broad for all subjects, it is nondifferential. Nondifferential exposure misclassification generally attenuates an estimate of an exposure–disease association or obscures an actual exposure–disease association entirely.

Differential exposure misclassification, in which misassignment of exposure is related to disease status, can lead to the perception of a stronger or a weaker association than actually exists. In cohort studies, avoiding differential exposure misclassification is paramount, because the investigator often knows—and the subject always knows—disease status when past exposure information is being collected. A classic example of differential exposure misclassification in case-control studies is *maternal recall bias* in studies of birth outcomes when prenatal exposure data is collected by interview of mothers. If mothers of children with adverse birth outcomes are more likely to correctly remember—or possibly exaggerate—their prenatal exposures compared to mothers of unaffected (control) children, then exposure will be classified differentially by disease status. Therefore, in case-control studies, prevention of differential exposure misclassification depends on collecting data as objectively as possible.

Confounding Bias

Confounding, a central issue in epidemiological studies, occurs when the effect of the exposure of interest is mixed with the effect of another variable, leading to bias. A confounder meets all three of the following conditions:

- It is predictive of the health outcome in the absence of the exposure (Condition A).
- It is predictive of, or associated with, exposure in the population (Condition B).
- It is not caused by the exposure (Condition C).

For example, in a study comparing stomach cancer in coal miners and iron miners, chewing tobacco was considered to be a potential confounder because (a) it may be a cause of stomach cancer regardless of exposure, (b) it is more commonly used by coal miners, who are prohibited from smoking in coal mines, and (c) it is not caused by coal mining.

A conceptually important point is imbedded in Condition C: Confounders must not be on the causal pathway between the exposure and disease of interest or be a part of the pathogenic disease process. For example, a study of coal dust exposures and chronic obstructive pulmonary disease (COPD) should not control for reduced lung function, which is part of the pathogenic disease process. Reduced lung function is not a confounder, but it is likely to be an intermediate or mediating variable. In this example, controlling for lung function would block part of the effect that coal dust has on COPD. Therefore, not all risk factors for the outcome (Condition A) are confounders, nor should they all be controlled

for in data analyses. If exposure preceded the risk factor in time or could have caused the risk factor, then the risk factor fails to meet Condition C and is therefore not a confounder.

Confounding can be controlled either during the design phase of the study or the analysis of the data. To avoid confounding bias during the design phase, the population can be restricted to people with (or without) the potential confounder. For example, a study population may be restricted to include only nonsmokers if smoking is a predictor of the outcome and is also associated with exposure of interest—and would therefore be considered a potential confounder. In case-control studies, matching of study subjects on potential confounders during the design phase can facilitate control of confounding during the analysis. To control confounding in the earlier example of a study of stomach cancer, subjects could be matched on tobacco-chewing habits so that the proportion of tobacco chewers would be the same among cases and controls.

Stratification is the major approach to control of confounding during the analysis phase of cross-sectional, cohort, and case-control studies. A confounder, such as age, is used to define strata, such as 10-year age groups. The exposure–response association is then estimated in each stratum. Stratification, however, becomes problematic as the number of confounders increases, because the strata ultimately become too small to allow stable measures of risk. For example, if age, smoking, race, and gender must be controlled for simultaneously, there may be no non-smoking, 40- to 49-year-old, white females in the study population. In this case, stratification becomes an inadequate method of controlling confounding, and statistical modeling must be used to control confounding. Data analysis of most modern epidemiologic studies is based on regression models for the outcome as a function of exposure. Including a confounder along with exposure in the regression model is the most common way to control for confounding.

Healthy Worker Bias

The *healthy worker effect* (HWE) refers to a bias that arises in occupational epidemiology. Unless proper statistical methods are applied, the HWE will lead to biased results. Selection bias can occur at two time points, upon entering or leaving the workforce. Healthier individuals are more likely to seek and gain employment, which is often called the *healthy hire effect*. Conversely, less healthy workers are more likely to leave the workplace and more healthy workers are more likely to remain in the workplace, creating the *healthy worker survivor effect*. When either selection in or out of the workplace is associated with both health outcome and exposure, selection bias may occur.

As a result of self-selection, employed people are healthier than the general population, which includes older people, people who are chronically ill, and people who are otherwise unfit to obtain and maintain employment. The bias occurs if exposed workers are compared to the non-exposed general population because the two groups differ by underlying health status (an unmeasured confounder). As a result of this bias, studies of illness or death in working populations often find lower rates of chronic diseases than in the general population. In the mortality study of autoworkers described previously, the overall SMR for African-American males, expected to be 1.00, was only 0.86. Bias from the healthy hire effect is most often eliminated in the design of occupational studies by defining a non-exposed comparison group drawn from within the worker study population.

Healthy worker survivor effect, which can occur even when the exposed and non-exposed workers are from the same population, can develop when exposure causes some workers to feel ill from symptoms from the prodromal phase of disease, which causes both (a) reduction in their subsequent exposure (by job transfer or employment termination) and (b) eventual disease. As a result, the workers who terminate early both accumulate less exposure and are more likely to experience the health outcome of interest. Such a scenario results in the erroneous conclusion that less cumulative exposure is associated with worse health outcomes. One way to understand healthy worker survivor bias is that symptoms caused by earlier exposure are on the pathway to the ultimate health outcome, and therefore *should not* be treated as a confounder. On the other hand, symptoms are also predictive of subsequent exposure and therefore a confounder of subsequent exposure

and the eventual outcome and *should* be treated as a confounder. Symptoms are an example of a time-varying confounder affected by prior exposure. A class of sophisticated statistical methods, collectively referred to as *g methods*, have been developed to handle this type of data structure.[21] These enable one to draw causal inferences from appropriately analyzed observational studies.

INTERPRETATION OF EPIDEMIOLOGIC STUDIES

Results from observational epidemiologic studies are often criticized for producing mere statistical associations—rather than determining causation—between exposures and health outcomes. Randomized controlled studies provide stronger evidence for causality than observational studies, since confounding and some forms of selection bias are avoided. However, most of the questions in environmental or occupational epidemiology cannot be feasibly—or ethically—addressed with a randomized control trial.

Ultimately, the results from epidemiologic studies are used to guide the development of preventive measures to regulate exposures, to identify workers or communities at risk of disease, or to lead to further research. The interpretation of epidemiologic studies depends on several factors, including the strength of the association and the validity of the observed association (the extent to which bias is minimized). (See Box 5-1.) The strength of an association usually is measured by (a) the size of the risk or rate ratios in studies of discrete health outcomes, such as cancer, or (b) the magnitude of the difference between groups in studies of physiologic parameters, such as the forced expiratory volume in 1 second (FEV_1). Larger effect estimates are less likely to be erroneous due to systematic or random error.

The validity of results from observational data must be evaluated by examining for selection bias, misclassification, and confounding. Since all studies suffer from some problems with validity, one must judge whether biases could account for the findings of a study. If a study finds a positive association, one should consider biases that could account for this finding; similarly, when

---

Box 5-1. Guide for Evaluating Epidemiologic Studies

To assist health professionals in reading, understanding, and critically evaluating epidemiologic studies, the following questions should serve as a useful guide.

Collection of Data

1. What were the objectives of the study? What was the association of interest?
2. What was the primary outcome of interest? Was it accurately measured?
3. What was the primary exposure of interest? Was it accurately measured?
4. What type of study was conducted?
5. What was the study base? Consider the process of subject selection and sample size.
6. Selection bias: Was subject selection based on the outcome or the exposure of interest? Could the selection have differed with respect to other factors of interest? Were these likely to have introduced a substantial bias?
7. Misclassification: Was subject assignment to exposure or disease categories accurate? Were possible misassignments equally likely for all groups? Were these likely to have introduced a substantial bias?

8. Confounding: What provisions, such as study design and subject restrictions, were made to minimize the influence of external factors before analysis of the data?

Analysis of the Data

9. What methods were used to control for confounding bias?
10. What measure of association was reported in the study? Was this appropriate?
11. How was the stability of the measure of association reported in the study?

Interpretation of Data

12. What was the major result of the study?
13. How was the interpretation of this result affected by the previously noted biases?
14. How was the interpretation affected by any nondifferential misclassification?
15. To what larger population may the results of this study be generalized?
16. Did the discussion section adequately address the limitations of the study? Was the final conclusion of the paper a balanced summary of the study findings?

Source: Adapted from: Monson RR. Occupational epidemiology (2nd ed.). Boca Raton, FL: CRC Press, 1989.

---

a study fails to find an association, one should evaluate the potential for an attenuating bias.

Results of tests of statistical significance, such as p-values and/or confidence intervals, are presented along with estimates of the relative risk. These results contribute to interpretation of studies by providing a measure of stability of the reported associations. Statistical tests guide investigators in deciding whether to reject a null hypothesis. (For example, if the null hypothesis is that no association exists between the exposure and outcome, rejection of the null hypothesis implies that there is an association between exposure and outcome.) Rejection is based on a prespecified significance level, defined as the probability that the observed association could have occurred by chance alone (assuming that no effect is expected a priori). For example, a p-value of 0.07 indicates that the probability of observing an effect at least as large as the one actually observed is 0.07, given that no association truly exists. By convention, a significance level of $p < 0.05$ or $p < 0.01$ is most commonly used as the decision rule for rejecting the null hypothesis. A p-value can also be interpreted as a continuous measure of the degree of support the

data provide for a hypothesis. Confidence intervals provide more information than probability values alone because they provide both (a) the range of the magnitude of association consistent with the observed data and (b) a measure of the stability of the estimate of the magnitude of association.

The statistical power of a study to detect a true effect of a particular size depends on the background prevalence of the disease or exposure, the number of subjects in the study population, the length of follow-up, and the level of statistical significance required. Monitoring of a small cohort for a brief period can yield a false negative result. For this reason, when interpreting a negative study, one should examine whether the design precluded a positive finding. For example, a retrospective cohort study of formaldehyde exposure had only 80% power to detect a four-fold risk in nasal cancer mortality—despite having 600,000 person-years of observation—because nasal cancer has a very low background prevalence.[22] Formulas for calculating the statistical power associated with a given sample size are available in standard biostatistics and epidemiology textbooks.

One epidemiologic study alone cannot determine causality between an exposure and a health outcome. Careful assessment of multiple studies is needed to infer causation of a health outcome, based on multiple observational studies of an environmental or occupational exposure. In 1965, Sir Austin Bradford Hill proposed nine "perspectives" for reviewing a body of epidemiologic studies to determine whether or not there is a causal association between an exposure or some other factor and a disease or other health outcome (*general causation*).[23] These perspectives include strength of association, consistency (repeated observation of an association), specificity, temporality, biologic gradient (dose–response relationship), plausibility, coherence, experimental evidence, and analogy. Although temporality is the only necessary element for establishing causality using the Bradford Hill perspectives, each of the other perspectives contribute to the assessment of causality. (See Appendix to Chapter 4.)

REFERENCES

1. Kreiss K, Gomaa A, Kullman G, et al. Clinical bronchiolitis obliterans in workers at a microwave-popcorn plant. New England Journal of Medicine 2002; 347: 360–361.

2. Costello S, Cockburn M, Bronstein J, et al. Parkinson's disease and residential exposure to maneb and paraquat from agricultural applications in the Central Valley of California. American Journal of Epidemiology 2009; 169: 919–926.

3. Jerrett M, Burnett RT, Ma R, et al. Spatial analysis of air pollution and mortality in Los Angeles. Epidemiology 2005; 16: 727–736.

4. Rozek LS, Dolinoy DC, Sartor MA, Omenn GS. Epigenetics: Relevance and implications for public health. Annual Review of Public Health 2014; 35: 105–122.

5. Billmaier D, Yee HT, Allen N, et al. Peripheral neuropathy in a coated fabrics plant. Journal of Occupational Medicine 1974; 16: 668–671.

6. Pirkle JL, Schwartz J, Landis JR, et al. The relationship between blood lead levels and blood pressure and its cardiovascular risk implications. American Journal of Epidemiology 1985; 121: 246–258.

7. Hernan MA. Specifying a target trial prevents immortal time bias and other self-inflicted injuries in observational analyses. Journal of Clinical Epidemiology 2016; 79: 70–75.

8. Hemminki K, Mutanen P, Saloniemi I, et al. Spontaneous abortions in hospital staff engaged in sterilizing instruments with chemical agents. British Medical Journal 1982; 285: 1461–1463.

9. Grandjean P, Weihe P, White RF, et al. Cognitive deficit in 7-year-old children with prenatal exposure to methylmercury. Neurotoxicology and Teratology 1997; 19: 417–428.

10. Eisen EA, Bardin J, Gore R, et al. Exposure-response models based on extended follow-up of a cohort mortality study in the automobile industry. Scandinavian Journal of Work, Environment & Health 2001; 27: 240–249.

11. Zahm SH, Weisenburger DD, Saal RC, et al. The role of agricultural pesticide use in the development of non-Hodgkin's lymphoma in women. Archives of Environmental Health 1993; 48: 353–358.

12. Armstrong B, Theriault G, Guenel P, et al. Association between exposure to pulsed electromagnetic fields and cancer in electric utility workers in Quebec, Canada and France. American Journal of Epidemiology 1994; 140: 805–820.

13. Maclure M, Mittleman MA. Should we use a case-crossover design? Annual Review of Public Health 2000; 21: 193-221.

14. Peters A, von Klot S, Heier M, et al. Exposure to traffic and the onset of myocardial infarction. New England Journal of Medicine 2004; 351:1721–1730.

15. Morales Suarez-Varela MM, Llopis Gonzalez A, Tejerizo Perez ML, et al. Chlorination of drinking water and cancer incidence. Journal of Environmental Pathology, Toxicology and Oncology 1994; 13: 39–41.

16. O'Neill MS, Loomis D, Borja-Aburto VH. Ozone, area social conditions, and mortality in Mexico City. Environmental Research 2004; 94: 234–242.

17. Janssen NA, Hoek G, Brunekreef B, et al. Personal sampling of particles in adults: Relation among personal, indoor, and outdoor air concentrations. American Journal of Epidemiology 1998; 147: 537–547.

18. Durkheim E. Le suicide. Paris: F. Alcan, 1897. English translation by JA Spalding. Toronto: Free Press, Collier-MacMillan, 1951.

19. Pope CA 3rd, Hansen ML, Long RW, et al. Ambient particulate air pollution, heart rate variability, and blood markers of inflammation in a panel of elderly subjects. Environmental Health Perspectives 2004; 112: 339–345.

20. Magari SR, Hauser R, Schwartz J, et al. Association of heart rate variability with

occupational and environmental exposure to particulate air pollution. Circulation 2001; 104: 986–991.

21. Buckley JP, Keil AP, McGrath LJ, Edward JK. Evolving methods for inference in the presence of healthy worker survivor bias. Epidemiology 2015; 26: 204–212.

22. Blair A, Stewart P, O'Berg M, et al. Mortality among industrial workers exposed to formaldehyde. Journal of the National Cancer Institute 1986; 76: 1071–1084.

23. Hill AB. The environment and disease: Association or causation? Proceedings of the Royal Society of Medicine 1965; 58: 295–300.

FURTHER READING

Baker D, Nieuwenhuijsen M. Environmental epidemiology: Study methods and application. New York: Oxford University Press, 2008. *Well-organized, comprehensive text on epidemiologic approaches specific to environmental studies. Numerous examples guide the reader toward understanding and applying environmental epidemiologic methods.*

Checkoway H, Pearce NE, Kriebel D. Research methods in occupational epidemiology (2nd ed.). New York: Oxford University Press, 2004. *Very readable, comprehensive text on epidemiologic approaches specific to occupational studies. Numerous examples are provided to guide the reader in understanding both the simple and the complex issues that must be addressed.*

Olsen J, Merletti R, Snashall D, Vuylsteek K. Searching for causes of work-related diseases: An introduction to epidemiology at the work site. Oxford: Oxford Medical Publications, 1991. *A practical introduction to epidemiology for health professionals with no formal training in the discipline. It is written to assist professionals to better plan and carry out investigation of worksite health problems.*

Jewell NP. Statistics for epidemiology. Boca Raton, FL: Chapman & Hall/CRC Press, 2004. *Provides intuitive descriptions of the most important statistical methods in epidemiology and the skills to use them effectively.*

Rothman KJ. Epidemiology: An introduction. New York: Oxford University Press, 2002. *An engaging introductory epidemiology primer for those with little or no background in epidemiology.*

Rothman KJ, Greenland S, Lash TL. Modern epidemiology (3rd ed.). Philadelphia: Wolters Kluwer/Lippincott Williams & Wilkins, 2008. *Probably the best general text on epidemiologic methods designed both for the novice and the expert. Provides principles of epidemiology in substantial detail as well as the quantitative basis for the research methods. Particularly useful as a reference. Especially good chapters on ecologic studies and on environmental epidemiology.*

Steenland K, Savitz DA. Topics in environmental epidemiology. New York: Oxford University Press, 1997. *A survey of environmental health issues associated with different environmental media. While examining a number of different problems, the text provides an overview of important methodologic concerns, particularly exposure assessment and statistical methods.*

APPENDIX TO CHAPTER

ADJUSTMENT OF RATES

For purposes of illustration, adjusting for differences in age is examined in detail. Table 5-3 presents a hypothetical problem involving myocardial infarction occurrence in two viscose rayon factories. To compare the incidence of myocardial infarction, a summary rate is calculated for each factory. If crude rates were calculated, it would appear that workers in Factory 1 have a slightly greater risk. Comparison of these rates, however, ignores the rather striking difference in age distribution of the populations in the two factories. These can be taken into account by adjusting for age differences by either the direct method or the indirect method.

Direct Adjustment

The principle of direct adjustment is to apply the age-specific rates determined in the study groups to a set of common age weights, such as a standard age distribution. The selection of the standard is somewhat arbitrary, but often the sum of the specific age groups for the study groups is chosen. In Table 5-3, the standard population consists of 1,200 persons younger than 45 years and 800 persons 45 years or older. The specific rates are applied to this set of weights and then added to create an adjusted rate:

$$\text{Factory 1} = \frac{(.010 \times 1,200) + (.030 \times 800)}{2,000} = .018$$

$$\text{Factory 2} = \frac{(.0125 \times 1,200) + (.050 \times 800)}{2,000} = .0275$$

Not only is the magnitude of the rate of myocardial infarction affected by the adjustment procedure, but the rank order is reversed. If another age distribution had been selected as the standard, the standardized rates would change. For example, for 1,500 persons younger than 45 years and 500 age 45 or older, the rate for Factory 1 would become 0.015 and that for factory 2 would become 0.022. Although the absolute magnitudes of the two adjusted rates have no inherent meaning, the relative magnitudes do. While the size of the ratio will change slightly, it will be closely duplicated regardless of the weights. In these two examples of weighting, the ratios of the adjusted rates are 1.53 and 1.47.

Indirect Adjustment

In indirect adjustment, standard rates are applied to the observed weights or the distribution of specific characteristics, such as age, sex, or race, in the study populations. This provides a value for the number of cases (events) that would be expected if the standard rates were operating. The expected number of cases can be compared with the number actually observed for each study group in the form of a ratio. In Table 5-3, assume a national standard rate for myocardial infarction of 1 in 1,000 (0.001) for those younger than 45 years of age and 2 in 1,000 (0.002) for those 45 years or older. The expected number of cases in the two factories would then be as follows:

$$\text{Factory 1} = (.001 \times 400) + (.002 \times 600) = 1.6$$

$$\text{Factory 2} = (.001 \times 800) + (.002 \times 600) = 1.2$$

These expected values are compared with the observed values to calculate a standardized incidence ratio (SIR), as follows:

$$\text{Factory 1 SIR} = \frac{22}{1.6} = 13.8$$

$$\text{Factory 2 SIR} = \frac{20}{1.2} = 16.7$$

It is tempting to compare the two SIRs and calculate a ratio similar to that calculated for the directly standardized rates. However, a drawback of indirect standardization is that SIRs cannot be compared. Because the age distributions and age-specific rates are significantly different for the two factories, the resulting comparison of the two SIRs would not distinguish differences caused by a different disease incidence rate from differences caused by a different age distribution.

It is reasonable, then, to ask why indirectly standardized rates are used. One reason is that often only one population is being studied, so comparison with the general population experience is convenient and possibly the only reasonable comparison available. Probably of greater importance is the instability of observed rates. In the example presented here, if five rather than two age groups were used and it was also necessary to adjust for both race and sex, then the total number of subdivisions necessary would be $5 \times 2 \times 2 = 20$. With a maximum of 22 cases in either factory, several of the subdivisions would contain no cases and therefore have no reliable rate estimate. Even in the illustration provided, one case more or one case less among the group of younger workers in Factory 1 would have changed the age-specific incidence rate to 12.5 or 7.5, respectively—a very large difference.

6

Occupational and Environmental Health Surveillance

Letitia Davis and Kerry Souza

How many workers are fatally injured at work each year? In which industries and occupations are workers at highest risk of fatal injury?

How are environmental hazards changing temporally and spatially? Are these changes associated with changes in disease occurrence?

Which industries and workplaces should the Occupational Safety and Health Administration (OSHA) focus on to prevent amputations, noise-induced hearing loss, or musculoskeletal disorders?

Which communities should the state health department prioritize for prevention of childhood lead poisoning?

Public health surveillance provides data to help answer these and many other questions to protect the health of workers and communities. Surveillance is recognized as the cornerstone of public health practice that provides the foundation upon which to build successful prevention programs and to evaluate their impact. *Surveillance*, sometimes also called *tracking*, is defined as the "ongoing, systematic collection, analysis, interpretation of health data essential to the planning, implementation and evaluation of public health practice closely integrated with the timely dissemination of data to those who need to know for purposes of prevention."[1] (Figure 6-1.) Its key elements are:

- *Surveillance is ongoing*: Collection, analysis, interpretation, and dissemination of data are often continuous but can also be periodic, such as biannual surveys conducted to monitor trends. (However, cross-sectional studies and one-time surveys are not considered surveillance.)
- *Surveillance is systematic*: It involves using consistent methods over time.
- *Surveillance involves interpretation of findings*: It is not sufficient to simply generate data tables; surveillance programs must interpret data so that findings and their significance can be understood.
- *Dissemination of surveillance findings for the purpose of prevention*: Surveillance carries with it the responsibility for public health action. The final link in the surveillance chain is the actual application of the data to prevention. Findings and their interpretation must be promptly and appropriately disseminated to those who can use the information to take preventive action.

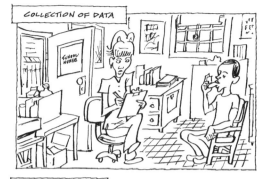

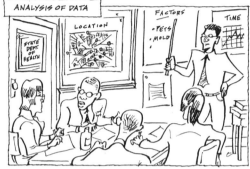

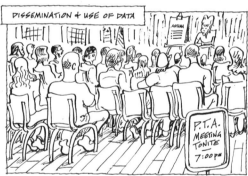

Figure 6-1. The three phases of surveillance. (Drawing by Nick Thorkelson.)

SURVEILLANCE IN OCCUPATIONAL AND ENVIRONMENTAL HEALTH

The overarching aim of occupational and environmental health (OEH) surveillance is to protect the health of workers and communities by providing information needed to target, design, and evaluate actions to control hazards and prevent occupational and environmental injuries and illnesses. It provides data used to inform public policy, regulatory and educational activities, development of safer technologies, and future research priorities. Specific objectives of surveillance are to:

- Document the nature, extent, and time trends of occupational and environmental injuries and illnesses
- Characterize the nature and distribution of OEH hazards and exposures—information that allows for interventions before injuries or illnesses occur
- Identify geographic locations, industries, specific workplaces, and occupations in which interventions are needed
- Identify emerging OEH problems that require investigation
- Generate hypotheses for etiologic research
- Evaluate the effectiveness of interventions.

Public health, in general, places special emphasis on addressing health needs of vulnerable populations. Therefore, another objective of OEH surveillance is to assess health risks by population characteristics, including race, ethnicity, age, and gender, in order to guide preventive measures to reduce health inequities. Surveillance findings can also be used to educate and mobilize the political and financial support of policymakers and the general public for necessary preventive actions.

OEH surveillance involves tracking many different types of hazards and health outcomes. A wide range of approaches and data sources are used, each with strengths and limitations. There is no single national surveillance system in occupational or environmental health but rather sets of different systems to meet different surveillance objectives.

Surveillance can be divided into two broad categories: *surveillance of health outcomes*, such as work-related injuries or childhood asthma, and *surveillance of hazards*, such as the presence of toxic substances in the workplace or drinking water. A subcategory of hazard surveillance is *exposure surveillance*, which provides more detailed information about intensity and duration of exposure to hazards. This may involve, for example, monitoring of individuals to assess exposure to a toxic agent, such as elevated levels of lead in the blood, or preclinical health effects. Surveillance of diseases caused by environmental or occupational hazards is especially challenging because (a) most of the diseases have many potential causes, and (b) there can be a substantial lag time between onset of exposure and onset of disease. In the United States, most occupational health surveillance systems focus on injuries and illnesses—not hazards. In environmental health surveillance, there is increasing focus on hazards in the environment.

Occupational and environmental health surveillance is conducted at national and state levels. National data are used to help determine national priorities and plan federal programs. However, relying solely on national data can obscure risks that are relevant to specific states or communities. In the United States, state government agencies—mainly in public health, labor, and environmental protection—often with financial and technical support from the federal government, play a central role in occupational and environmental surveillance. Many national surveillance systems rely on data sent to them by states. State health agencies have the legal authority to require disease and injury reporting, such as from physicians and laboratories, and to access a wide variety of health-related data. State agencies can also respond to local concerns by collaborating with city and county health departments, other agencies, and nongovernmental community organizations to translate surveillance findings into preventive action.

While public health surveillance is often thought of as a function of government, workplace-based tracking of injuries, illnesses, and hazards is also critical to protect worker and community health. Surveillance is recognized as an essential component of effective workplace injury and illness programs and environmental management programs.[2] Many large companies have extensive programs, some of which are mandated by law, for monitoring emissions to air and water and for tracking workplace hazards and exposures. OSHA requires many companies to maintain records of work-related injuries and illnesses. Some companies voluntarily go beyond required surveillance by tracking other indicators, including leading indicators such as "near misses," which

enables them to identify and control risks before illnesses and injuries occur.[3]

CASE-BASED AND POPULATION-BASED SURVEILLANCE IN OCCUPATIONAL HEALTH

Occupational health surveillance systems may be (a) case-based, providing detailed information—although often not complete and not representative—on individual cases of work-related injury or illness, and/or (b) population-based, generating representative data on the occurrence and distribution of work-related injuries and illnesses. Case-based surveillance is based on the concept of a *sentinel health event*—a case is a warning sign that prevention has failed and intervention may be warranted.[4] It involves the ongoing timely collection of data on cases, including personal identifying information, such as name and contact information, which allows for case follow-up. Case-based surveillance is usually implemented under the state's authority to require illness and injury reporting by physicians and other healthcare providers. Follow-up may be done to assure that the affected individual has received medical treatment, that hazards are controlled to protect other workers, and that opportunities are taken to improve scientific understanding of the hazard and the associated illness or injury.

Several states implement case-based surveillance of selected occupational disorders using the Sentinel Event Notification System for Occupational Risks (SENSOR), a model developed by the National Institute for Occupational Safety and Health (NIOSH).[5] Following this model, state programs identify sentinel cases of illness or injury from various data sources, such as mandatory case reports from healthcare providers, hospital records, and workers' compensation claims. Identified cases are assessed to see if they meet stringent case definitions. Results of summary data analyses, while not necessarily representative, are informative and useful for planning preventive measures. Data from several states are often aggregated to gain a broader perspective on a problem, such as work-related asthma. (See Box 6-1.)

Box 6-1. Data for Action: Work-related Asthma Data Influence Green Cleaning Standards

Data from California, Massachusetts, Michigan, and New Jersey, which conduct surveillance of work-related asthma, demonstrated that 12% of reported cases of work-related asthma between 1993 and 1997 were associated with cleaning products. About 20% of these workers were employed in jobs where cleaning was their primary task; the other 80% worked in non-cleaning jobs near areas being cleaned.[1] In response to these findings, these states recommended that chemicals known to cause asthma, such as formaldehyde and quaternary ammonium compounds, be prohibited from products certified by third-party environmental certification standards. They successfully worked with environmental certification organizations to include this prohibition in the revision of several environmental standards for institutional, industrial, and household cleaning products. These state-based surveillance programs are collaborating with schools and hospitals to adopt safer cleaning practices and products.

Reference

1. Rosenman KD, Reilly MJ, Schill DP, et al. Cleaning products and work-related asthma. Journal of Occupational and Environmental Medicine 2003; 45: 556–563.

(Adapted from Council of State and Territorial Epidemiologists. Putting data to work for worker safety and health: Success in the states. Available at: http://www.cste2.org/webpdfs/ohsuccessstories.pdf. Accessed November 21, 2016.)

In contrast, *population-based* (or *rate-based*) *surveillance* collects data that can be used to assess the nature and magnitude of a problem and to monitor trends in a population over time. It may involve collecting data on a *census*—all cases of an illness or injury—or a representative sample of cases. Population-based surveillance collects data on demographic characteristics, such as age and gender, and, ideally, type of industry or occupation—but does not necessarily collect personally identifying information on workers or employers. Population-based surveillance requires denominator information—such as the number of workers at risk for a specific injury or illness. The annual Survey of Occupational Injuries and Illnesses conducted by the Bureau of Labor Statistics is an example of a widely used population-based surveillance system.

Case-based and population-based approaches to surveillance are not mutually exclusive. Some of the most effective surveillance systems at the state level have attributes of both, identifying both sentinel health events (cases) for follow-up and representative summary data to understand the magnitude and distribution of the problem and to plan preventive measures. A combination of compelling case reports (stories) and summary data (statistics) is often most successful in raising awareness of the public and policymakers about a problem. The state-based surveillance system for elevated blood lead levels (BLLs) in adults, which has contributed to a substantial reduction of occupational exposure to lead over time, is an example of a system that generates both case reports and summary data.

NATIONAL SURVEILLANCE SYSTEMS FOR OCCUPATIONAL INJURIES AND ILLNESSES

The major U.S. national surveillance systems for occupational illnesses and injuries are the Census of Fatal Occupational Injuries (CFOI) and the Survey of Occupational Injuries and Illnesses (SOII). Both are population-based surveillance systems that are administered by the Bureau of Labor Statistics (BLS) in the U.S. Department of Labor, in collaboration with state labor departments or other state government agencies. CFOI, which has been implemented in all U.S. states since 1992, produces a complete count of all fatal occupational injuries in a timely manner. For a death to be counted, the person who died must have been self-employed, working for pay, or volunteering at the time of the event, engaged in a legal work activity, and present at the site of the incident as a job requirement. Homicides and suicides as well as unintentional injuries at work are included. To provide counts that are as complete as possible, CFOI uses multiple data sources, including death certificates, police reports, and news media reports, to identify, verify, and describe fatal occupational injuries. For each death, information is collected about the worker, the workplace, and the circumstances of the event. BLS provides training and resources to the states for data collection. States transmit the data to BLS, which compiles a national data set. National and state-level findings are reported annually.

The most comprehensive source of statistics on nonfatal work-related injuries and acute illnesses, SOII provides estimates of the numbers and rates of work-related injuries and illnesses, overall and by industry, nationally and for most states. For serious cases that involve one or more days away from work, SOII also provides more detailed data on the nature and circumstances of the injury or illness as well as characteristics of affected workers. Unlike other major public health surveillance systems, SOII collects data from workplaces, rather than from healthcare providers or facilities or from individuals at risk. BLS uses a scientific sampling approach to select employers that represent all industries and employers of all sizes. Selected employers are required to provide information on all work-related injuries and illnesses for which OSHA requires recordkeeping—those resulting in loss of consciousness, one or more days away from work, restricted work activities, transfer to another job, or medical treatment beyond first aid. As with CFOI, BLS provides training and resources to state agencies to collect SOII data. Data are transmitted to BLS. National and state-level surveillance reports, which are issued annually, are an important source of information used widely by government agencies, industries, labor unions, and others. However, SOII has several limitations:

- Excluded are self-employed, household workers and workers on farms with fewer than 11 employees, which together comprise about 14% of the total U.S. workforce.
- Injuries and illnesses that are not recorded by employers on OSHA logs or not reported by workers to their employers are not captured by SOII.
- SOII fails to capture most chronic occupational illnesses—physicians' failure to recognize occupational illnesses, the long latency periods for many occupational diseases, and the multifactorial nature of many of these diseases make tracking difficult by a workplace-based reporting system.
- Injuries are also underreported, probably by 20% to 50%, in SOII, and there is some evidence that reporting varies by worker and employer and by injury characteristics.[6-9] For example, immigrant workers, many of whom perform very hazardous tasks, may be reluctant to report their injuries because of fear of reprisal or job loss. (See Box 6-2.)
- Since SOII, like CFOI, is a population-based surveillance system, it does not allow for case-based follow-up to intervene in specific workplaces in order to protect others at risk or to learn more about factors contributing to injuries and illnesses.

A range of additional approaches are undertaken by federal and state agencies to address these surveillance gaps, as described next.

Box 6-2. Underreporting of Injuries in the Workplace

Multiple factors contribute to underreporting of work-related injuries. Some employers, especially in smaller workplaces, are unaware of or confused about OSHA recordkeeping requirements. Others do not have effective systems for documenting and recording injuries. Yet other employers intentionally avoid recording injuries because they want to avoid OSHA penalties, increases in workers' compensation premiums, or rejection as subcontractors due to poor safety records. In addition, workers often fail to report their injuries to their employers or file workers' compensation claims, especially if the injury is not serious, sometimes fearing retaliation by their employers if they report injuries. Workplace programs that punish workers for injuries or reward workers or their managers for good safety records can deter workers from reporting their injuries. In 2016, OSHA issued new recordkeeping regulations that specify that employer policies for reporting workplace injuries and illnesses must be reasonable and prohibit retaliation against employees who report a workplace injury or illness. Workplace safety programs should encourage workers to report injuries.

Box 6-3. State Health Data Sources Used for Occupational Health Surveillance

- Trauma registries
- Burn registries

Case Reports

- Healthcare providers
- Clinical laboratories
- Poison control centers

Administrative Data

- Hospital discharges
- Emergency department visits
- Hospital outpatient visits
- Emergency medical services
- Workers' compensation

State Registries

- Birth and death registries (vital records)
- Cancer registries
- Birth defect registries

Surveys

- State SOII data
- Behavioral Risk Factor Surveillance System
- Youth Risk Behavior System
- Other state health surveys

Other Sources

- News media searches
- OSHA and Coast Guard records
- Autopsy reports
- National Violent Death Reporting System

Potential New Sources

- All payer claims data
- Electronic health records
- Social media

STATE-BASED OCCUPATIONAL HEALTH SURVEILLANCE

State agencies have access to a wide variety of state data sources that can be used to identify local health and safety problems and help fill gaps in surveillance at the national level. (See Box 6-3.) State health and labor departments, many with funding from NIOSH, use these data sources to perform a variety of both case- and population-based surveillance activities. State government agencies can, in turn, collaborate with local intervention partners, such as trade associations, unions, worker centers, healthcare organizations, and OSHA and other government agencies, to address identified health and safety problems. In addition, occupational health programs within state health departments can partner with other public health programs to develop more comprehensive approaches to hazards, such as indoor air in schools, distracted driving, and infectious diseases, which can affect workers and the general public alike.

States rely on both data collected specifically for occupational surveillance, such as case reports of occupational health illnesses and injuries from physicians and existing administrative data sources, such as statewide emergency department data systems. States can also incorporate information about occupation and industry into other public health surveillance systems, such as state health surveys. Doing so

not only leverages use of these other surveillance resources for occupational health but can also enhance practice in other areas of public health by providing information about patterns of health outcomes and determinants of health, such as smoking behaviors or access to preventive health services, in relation to work.

With financial support from NIOSH, 26 states, in 2016, were using data from state data systems to generate information for a standardized set of occupational health indicators to track trends in occupational health.[10,11] Some states conduct more intensive surveillance focused on specific industries, populations, or health outcomes, such as fatal injuries, pesticide poisoning, carbon monoxide poisoning, occupational lung disease, and injuries to young workers, hospital workers, and truckers. Many of these systems combine data from several data sources. All of them include intervention and prevention activities to protect worker health.

PHYSICIAN AND LABORATORY REPORTING

Public health reporting laws enable state agencies to gather surveillance data, mainly on communicable diseases, with information about the affected individuals that allows for case follow-up. In 1874, physician reporting of disease to public health agencies began when Massachusetts established a voluntary reporting program in which physicians mailed a postcard every week to the state health department listing "prevalent" diseases. In 1893, Michigan became the first state to require physician reporting of specific diseases. By 1901, reporting of smallpox, tuberculosis, and cholera was legally required in all states. While communicable diseases still dominate the list of reportable conditions, 30 states also require healthcare providers to report to the state health department selected occupational disorders, such as work-related asthma, silicosis, and injuries to teen workers. These laws may also allow the health departments to follow up to obtain confidential medical information from healthcare providers and facilities when they identify possible cases using other data sources. Healthcare providers should become familiar with which, if any, occupational and environmental disorders are required to be reported in the states where they practice. Reporting these cases to the designated government agency is not a violation of the Health Insurance Portability and Accountability Act (HIPAA), which has specific exemptions of its privacy provisions related to public health reporting laws.[12]

While not all cases are reported, as required, these laws have been valuable in facilitating identification of new occupational risks. Recent examples include lung disease due to diacetyl exposure in food-flavoring industry workers and deaths from methylene chloride exposure in bathtub refinishers.

Mandatory reporting by clinical laboratories provides the foundation for yet other surveillance systems, such as those for identifying people with high BLLs. Most states require clinical laboratories to report to a state health agency results of BLL tests in both adults and children. Results at or above the reference level of 5 μg/dL indicate what is deemed to be excessive exposure, although any presence of lead in blood may be harmful. Since 1987, the NIOSH Adult Blood Lead Epidemiology and Surveillance (ABLES) program has provided financial support to states for adult blood lead surveillance. Participating states conduct follow-up of individual cases, based on BLLs, to assure adequate medical treatment and removal from exposure and to control exposures in order to protect others at risk. Some state health departments

collaborate with OSHA to conduct follow-up in workplaces where workers with elevated BLLs were exposed to lead. Summary data are used to monitor trends and to identify for outreach industries and communities with high levels. The ABLES program demonstrated a 50% decline in occupational lead exposure in the United States from 1994 through 2010.[13]

USE OF ADMINISTRATIVE DATA FOR OCCUPATIONAL HEALTH SURVEILLANCE

Data collected for administrative purposes, such as on hospital discharges, emergency department visits, and workers' compensation claims, contain useful information on occupational injuries and illnesses that can augment information from employer-based reporting. Data from hospitals include demographic, diagnostic, and cause-of-injury information but generally not information on work-relatedness of the disorder or industry or occupation of the affected worker. Diagnostic information for those conditions that, by definition, are likely caused by workplace exposures—such as silicosis—can be used to identify occupational cases. Payment information indicating that hospital charges were paid by a workers' compensation insurer can be used to identify other work-related cases in these data sets. Workers' compensation records provide more detailed information about the workplaces in which workers are injured or made ill.

Workers' compensation data have been used extensively for surveillance research and prevention in some states. The Safety and Health Assessment for Research and Prevention program in the state of Washington regularly reports on injury and illness data from the state's workers' compensation system. Ohio routinely uses workers' compensation data to identify state health and safety priorities. The Massachusetts Young Workers Project uses records of workers' compensation claims to identify injuries affecting workers under age 25. Information obtained in all these programs is used to plan worksite interventions. Findings, which are disseminated to employers, labor unions, schools, and state legislatures, have been used to promote policy

---

Box 6-4. Data to Action: Protecting Teens at Work in Massachusetts

Since the early 1990s, the Young Workers Project of the Massachusetts Department of Public Health has used multiple data sources, including emergency department records, workers' compensation claims, and burn registry reports, to track injuries to working teens—a population at high risk of being injured on the job. The project collaborates with multiple agency and community partners to address identified risks. Findings have been used to promote updates to the state child labor laws, require youth job training programs to provide health and safety training, and offer statewide outreach to teens, parents, teachers, and employers about protecting youth at work.

When the surveillance data revealed many burns in a large franchised restaurant chain, the project conducted worksite investigations and found that injured teens had changed coffee filters without realizing that coffee was still brewing in filters full of near-boiling water. When they pulled out the brew baskets, hot coffee slurry splashed on their hands and wrists causing second- and third-degree burns. The project presented data to corporate officials and recommended that the company work with its equipment suppliers to develop a safer coffee machine design. Subsequently, the company introduced a new coffee brewer with a funnel lock, which prevents the brew basket from being pulled out before the machine has completed brewing. This engineering solution—an example of prevention through design—could protect all workers, not just teens, in the company's 13,000 restaurants across the United States.

---

and practice changes and educational initiatives for worker safety and health. (See Box 6-4.)

Because workers' compensation laws and eligibility requirements vary among states, surveillance findings based on based on workers' compensation records cannot be readily compared among states. In addition, workers' compensation records are not representative of all workers with occupational injuries and illnesses because some workers are not covered by workers' compensation and some never submit claims or receive payments.[14] The NIOSH Center for Workers' Compensation Studies promotes the use of workers' compensation data to improve workplace safety and health. The Center develops new methods for coding, analyzing, and disseminating workers' compensation data; fosters research collaborations; and shares best surveillance and research practices among state agencies, research programs, and insurance companies who use these data.

SELECTED OTHER OCCUPATIONAL HEALTH SURVEILLANCE SYSTEMS

The NIOSH Fatality Assessment Control and Evaluation (FACE) program aims to prevent fatal occupational injuries by identifying underlying risk factors and developing and disseminating prevention recommendations. FACE is a collaborative program between NIOSH and seven states that NIOSH funds to conduct surveillance and investigations of select fatal occupational injuries. Each investigation results in a report, describing the event and recommendations to prevent similar incidents, which is disseminated, with related alerts, to businesses, labor unions, equipment manufacturers, and others. Overall, FACE provides in-depth information about the circumstances leading to deaths and compelling case studies that augment the CFOI statistics.

The National Electronic Injury Surveillance System, operated by the Consumer Product Safety Commission, collects data from a national sample of hospitals on emergency department visits for nonfatal injuries associated with consumer products and with work.

The Behavioral Risk Factor Surveillance System is a national health survey, conducted by telephone, of a representative sample of adults. Administered by state health departments in collaboration with the Centers for Disease Control and Prevention (CDC), it provides state- and national-level surveillance data. In 2016, about half of the states, with support from NIOSH, started collecting current occupation and industry of survey respondents, enabling assessment of health-related behaviors, health outcomes, and use of health services in relation to employment characteristics.

The National Health Interview Survey, conducted by the National Center for Health Statistics, is an annual health survey of representative sample of U.S. households. It collects basic employment information that is used to analyze the occurrence of chronic diseases by occupation and industry. Periodically, it collects national-level data on some occupational health outcomes and exposures.[15]

The National Occupational Respiratory Mortality System, maintained by NIOSH, is an interactive data system based on death certificate data for deaths caused by pneumoconiosis, malignant mesothelioma, hypersensitivity pneumonitis, and other respiratory disorders. It is used to evaluate trends in death rates for these diseases by occupation and industry.

Occupational health indicators are a group of well-defined surveillance measures of occupational health or risk status that are used by state health departments to track health problems over time (or among states) and guide preventive measures.[16] Developed by the Council of State and Territorial Epidemiologists, the list of recommended occupational health indicators is evolving, with new indicators being added over time as new issues emerge and as new data sources become available.[16]

OSHA requires employers to report, within hours, workplace fatalities and hospitalizations of three or more employees. In 2014, OSHA expanded reporting requirements to include all amputations, in-patient hospitalizations, and losses of an eye. OSHA receives about 30 reports of these severe injuries daily from about half of the states. OSHA uses this system to prioritize its enforcement and compliance-assistance activities. Summary data provide useful information on trends in severe injuries by industry and other variables.[17]

OSHA also requires employers in certain industries to maintain on-site logs of workplace injuries and illnesses. While the SOII collects information from these logs from a sample of employers every year, employers have not had to routinely submit their detailed log data to OSHA. In 2016, OSHA issued new regulations requiring employers to submit their OSHA log data to it electronically. The amount of data to be submitted varies, depending on size of the company and type of industry.

HEALTHY PEOPLE

Some of the *Healthy People* objectives for the United States, developed for each decade by government officials, researchers, and others, relate to occupational health and safety as well as environmental health.[18]

Disaster Surveillance

Recognizing the dangers confronted by response workers, the CDC-NIOSH Emergency Preparedness and Response Office has developed the Emergency Responder Health Monitoring and Surveillance system for monitoring these workers, before, during, and after deployment. (See Chapter 31.)

Hazard Surveillance

Hazard surveillance involves tracking health and safety hazards in the workplace, such as the presence and levels of toxic substances, noise, and ionizing radiation as well as, in farming communities, the prevalence of tractors lacking rollover protection.[19] Its aim is to identify opportunities to intervene and control hazards before illnesses or injuries occur.[20] Especially valuable is surveillance of health hazards, such as asbestos, that are associated with diseases with long latency periods. Hazard surveillance also provides information that can be used to generate hypotheses about potential associations between hazards and diseases that warrant further research.

There is no U.S. national system for surveillance of occupational hazards or exposures. In the past, NIOSH has conducted surveys to collect data on occupational exposures to chemical, physical, and biologic hazards from a sample of over 4,000 workplaces nationwide. Using survey data, it estimated the number of workers potentially exposed to each of thousands of hazardous substances, by industry and occupation.

OSHA maintains data, in the OSHA Information System database, on hazards and exposures collected during its investigations of workplaces. However, the information is limited to hazards regulated by OSHA at these workplaces. Some OSHA regulations require employers to conduct assessments of exposures to chemical and physical hazards, such as silica dust and noise. Data from these assessments, which may be used for internal hazard surveillance by these companies, are available to OSHA during its investigations but not to others. Data on hazards in the mining industry are collected and made publically available by the Mine Safety and Health Administration.

The Occupational Information Network (O*NET) program of the U.S. Department of Labor provides information useful for surveillance of some workplace hazards. The O*NET interactive online database contains information on hundreds of standardized and occupation-specific descriptors for over 900 occupations, including training requirements and types of tasks, tools, and technology used.

Additional data sources on environmental health hazards can help in monitoring potential occupational risks, including the Toxic Release Inventory, a publicly available Environmental Protection Agency database that contains information on toxic chemical releases and pollution prevention activities reported by industrial or federal facilities. Data from poison control centers have also been used to track exposures to both occupational and environmental hazards.

ENVIRONMENTAL HEALTH SURVEILLANCE

Environmental health surveillance provides information to plan and take action to prevent environmental illnesses and injuries. It involves monitoring of environmental hazards, ranging from toxic substances to extreme weather events, and associated illnesses and injuries.[21] State departments of public health and environmental protection, often with federal support, conduct environmental health surveillance with multiple data sources and various approaches. Data are used to guide state and local prevention activities and are sent to federal agencies, which use the data to set national environmental health priorities.

State departments of environmental protection and agriculture generally take the lead in collecting data, for regulatory and ecologic purposes, on environmental hazards, such as air pollutants and spills of hazardous substances. State health departments more frequently take the lead in tracking the impact of environmental hazards on human health. For example, state and some city health departments, with the support of the CDC Center for Environmental Health,

conduct surveillance of BLLs of children, relying on physician and laboratory reports of children with elevated BLLs. State and city health departments perform follow-up to ensure that affected infants and children receive appropriate medical treatment and that environmental measures are taken to reduce their lead exposure and prevent additional cases. As of 2016, there were 46 states reporting data to CDC as part of the Childhood Blood Lead Surveillance System. CDC also supports state-based surveillance of asthma through the Behavioral Risk Factor Surveillance System.

Some states also participate in the CDC National Biomonitoring Program to assess human exposures to toxic substances though air, water, food, soil, dust, and consumer products. This program measures environmental chemicals in human tissues and body fluids. In addition, the CDC collects representative national data on human exposures through the National Health and Nutrition Examination Survey.

State health departments collaborate with state environmental agencies to combine health and environmental data on illnesses that may have environmental causes, such as certain cancers, heart disease, and birth defects.[22] Methods and mapping tools based on geographic information systems are used extensively in this work.

The National Environmental Public Health Tracking Network, an interactive, multitiered, web-based system of integrated health, exposure, and hazard information from a wide variety of national, state, and city sources, aims to help identify associations between environmental factors and adverse health outcomes as well as elevated risks among vulnerable populations, such as children and older people. The CDC provides funds to many state and local health departments to implement local tracking networks to obtain data on environmental health indicators. These data improve the understanding of associations between environmental factors and diseases and assess unusual trends and events to help plan interventions to reduce risks.

Although occupational health and environmental health surveillance systems are almost always separate, there can be value in combining occupational and environmental health surveillance and including it within a holistic approach to public health surveillance.[23] Many of the hazardous substances to which workers are exposed are released into the environment through waste disposal, stack emissions, on workclothes, or in other ways, leading to family and community exposures. Other hazards, such as environmental (secondhand) tobacco smoke, cleaning products containing chemicals that cause asthma, lead exposures during home renovation, and extreme weather events, pose risks to both workers and the general public. In addition, some populations, such as low-income and minority individuals, are often exposed to hazards in both the ambient environment and at work. Some state OEH surveillance programs are collaborating by including data on occupational health indicators in the Environmental Public Health Tracking Network and collecting occupation and industry data in other public health surveillance systems, such as the Behavioral Risk Factor Surveillance System.

CONCLUSION

Changes in healthcare delivery, information technology, the workplace, and the environment provide new surveillance opportunities and challenges.[24] New initiatives include:

- Promoting the integration of occupation and industry data in electronic health records to improve both clinical care and population health
- Developing and using new methods and tools to conduct surveillance of workers and community members after natural disasters or terrorist events
- Using surveillance to understand the health effects of climate change (Chapter 29)
- Using information technology to enhance completeness, efficiency, and timeliness of data collection and reporting
- Developing and implementing new approaches for the early detection of disease outbreaks (syndromic surveillance) to mobilize rapid response
- Exploring approaches to documenting work-related health effects, given the changing nature of work relationships, such as the increase in short-term independent contractors and temporary workers as well as the increase in multi-employer worksites.

To address new challenges effectively, OEH surveillance programs will continue to rely on professionals from a wide range of disciplines—including epidemiology, medicine, nursing, industrial hygiene, safety, informatics, and health communication—and to provide rewarding opportunities to bridge the gap between science and practice to advance public health.

AUTHORS' NOTE

The findings and conclusions in this chapter are those of the authors and do not necessarily represent the views of the National Institute for Occupational Safety and Health, the Centers for Disease Control and Prevention, or the Massachusetts Department of Public Health.

REFERENCES

1. Thacker SB, Berkelman RL. History of public health surveillance. In: Halperin W, Baker EL (eds.). Public health surveillance. New York: Van Norstrand Reinhold, 1992.
2. Occupational Safety and Health Administration. OSHA Safety and Health Program Management Guidelines: November 2015 Draft for Public Comment. Available at: https://www.osha.gov/shpmguidelines/SHPM_guidelines.pdf. Accessed November 21, 2016.
3. National Safety Council. Transforming EHS performance measurement through leading indicators. Available at: http://www.nsc.org/CambpellInstituteandAwardDocuments/WP-Transforming-EHS-through-Leading-Indicators.pdf. Accessed November 21, 2016.
4. Rutstein DD, Mullan RJ, Frazier TM, et al. Sentinel health events (occupational): A basis for physician recognition and public health surveillance. American Journal of Public Health 1983; 73: 1054–1062.
5. Baker EL. Sentinel Event Notification System for Occupational Risks (SENSOR): The concept. American Journal of Public Health 1989; 79: 18–20.
6. Committee on Education and Labor. Hidden tragedy: Underreporting of workplace injuries and illnesses, 2008. Available at: http://www.bls.gov/iif/laborcommreport061908.pdf Accessed November 21, 2016.

7. Wuellner SE, Adams DA, Bonauto DK. Underreported workers' compensation claims to the BLS Survey of Occupational Injuries and Illnesses: Establishment factors. American Journal of Public Health 2016; 59: 274–289.

8. Ruser JW. Examining evidence on whether BLS undercounts workplace injuries and illnesses. Monthly Labor Review 2008: 20–32. Available at: https://www.bls.gov/opub/mlr/2008/08/art2full.pdf. Accessed January 9, 2017.

9. Azaroff LS, Levenstein C, Wegman D. Occupational injury and illness surveillance: Conceptual filters explain underreporting. American Journal of Public Health 2002; 92: 1421–1429.

10. National Institute for Occupational Safety and Health. State surveillance portfolio. Available at: http://www.cdc.gov/niosh/oep/statereports.html. Accessed November 21, 2016.

11. Thomsen C, McClain J, Rosenman K, Davis L. Indicators for occupational health surveillance. Morbidity and Mortality Weekly Report 2007; 56: 1–7.

12. U.S. Department of Health and Human Services. Health information privacy. Available at: http://www.hhs.gov/hipaa/for-professionals/special-topics/public-health/index.html. Accessed November 22, 2016.

13. National Institute for Occupational Safety and Health. Adult blood lead epidemiology and surveillance. Available at: http://www.cdc.gov/niosh/topics/ables/description.html. Accessed November 21, 2016.

14. Bonauto D, Fan J, Largo T, et al. Proportion of workers who were work-injured and payment by workers' compensation systems—10 states, 2007. Morbidity and Mortality Weekly Report 2010; 59: 897–900.

15. National Institute for Occupational Health: National health interview: Occupational health supplement. Available at: https://www.cdc.gov/niosh/topics/nhis/HIS. Accessed November 21, 2016.

16. Council of State and Territorial Epidemiologists. Occupational health indicators. Available at: http://www.cste.org/group/OHIndicators. Accessed November 21, 2016.

17. Michaels D. Year one of OSHA's Severe Injury Reporting Program: An impact evaluation. March 2016. Available at: https://www.osha.gov/injuryreport/2015.pdf. Accessed November 22, 2016.

18. U.S. Department of Health and Human Services, Office of Disease Prevention and Health Promotion. Healthy People 2020. Available at: https://www.healthypeople.gov/. Accessed November 21, 2016.

19. May JJ, Earle-Richardson G, Burdick PA, et al. Rollover protection on New York tractors and farmers' readiness for change. Journal of Agricultural Safety and Health 2006; 12: 199–213.

20. LaMontagne AD, Ruttenberg AJ, Wegman DH. Exposure surveillance: Exposure surveillance for chemical and physical hazards. In: Maizlish NA (ed.). Workplace health surveillance: An action-oriented approach. New York: Oxford University Press, 2000.

21. Thacker SB, Stroup DF, Parrish RG, Anderson HA. Surveillance in environmental public health: Issues, systems, and sources. American Journal of Public Health 1996; 86: 633–638.

22. Stanbury M, Anderson H, Blackmore C, et al. Functions of environmental epidemiology and surveillance in state health departments. Journal of Public Health Management and Practice 2012; 18: 453–460.

23. Levy BS. Toward a holistic approach to public health surveillance. American Journal of Public Health 1996; 86: 624–625.

24. Smith PF, Hadler JL, Stanbury M, et al. Blueprint version 2.0: Updating public health surveillance for the 21st century. Journal of Public Health Management and Practice 2013; 19: 231–239.

FURTHER READING

Azaroff LS, Levenstein C, Wegman D. Occupational injury and illness surveillance: Conceptual filters explain underreporting. American Journal of Public Health 2002; 92: 1421–1429.
A thoughtful examination of the many reasons for underreporting.

Centers for Disease Control and Prevention. CDC's vision for public health surveillance in the 21st century. Morbidity and Mortality Weekly Report 2012; 61; 1–39.
A forward-looking document.

Environmental Public Health Tracking. Journal of Public Health Management Practice 2015; 21(2 Suppl).
A valuable publication on environmental health surveillance.

National Institute for Occupational Safety and Health. Guidelines for minimum and comprehensive state-based public health activities in occupational safety and health. (DHHS [NIOSH] Publication No. 2008-148).

2008. Available at: https://www.cdc.gov/niosh/docs/2008-148/pdfs/2008-148.pdf.
Federal guidelines for state health departments and other agencies at the state level.

National Research Council: A smarter national surveillance system for occupational safety and health in the 21st century. Washington, DC: National Academies Press, 2017.
A comprehensive assessment of the state and the potential for occupational health surveillance in the United States.

Teutch, SM, Churchill RE (eds.) Principles and practice of public health surveillance. New York: Oxford University Press, 2000.
An essential book on the subject.

KEY WEBSITES

Centers for Disease Control and Prevention. National Environmental Public Health Tracking Network (NEPHTN). Available at: https://ephtracking.cdc.gov/showHome.action. Accessed December 4, 2016.
An interactive website with data on toxic chemicals and other hazards in the environment and chronic diseases and conditions from a variety of national, state, and city sources. Includes maps and charts and links to state-level NEPHTN websites.

Council of State and Territorial Epidemiologists. Environmental Health/Occupational Health/Injury. Available at: http://www.cste.org/?page=EHOHI. Accessed December 15, 2016.
A valuable website that includes information on standard measures of occupational health status of the population (occupational health indicators) for many states.

National Institute for Occupational Safety and Health. Worker health surveillance. Available at https://www.cdc.gov/niosh/topics/surveillance/. Accessed December 5, 2016.
An important source of information for data on worker health and safety from many different occupational health surveillance systems.

U.S. Department of Labor, Bureau of Labor Statistics. Injuries, illnesses and fatalities. Available at: http://www.bls.gov/iif/. Accessed December 5, 2016.
An important source of national and state statistics on fatal and nonfatal occupationally related injuries and acute illnesses. Includes findings from the Census of Fatal Occupational Injuries and the Survey of Occupational Injuries and Illnesses.

U.S. Department of Labor, Employment and Training Administration. O*NET Resource Center. Available at: http://www.onetcenter.org/overview.html. Accessed December 5, 2016.
An informative website that includes an interactive application, providing standardized descriptions of the characteristics of hundreds of occupations and skills required for those occupations.

U.S. Department of Labor, Occupational Health and Safety Administrations. OSHA recordkeeping and reporting requirements. Available at: https://www.osha.gov/recordkeeping/. Accessed December 15, 2016.
Detailed information on employer requirements for maintaining and reporting data on work-related injuries and illnesses to OSHA.

7

Toxicology

Robert Laumbach and Michael Gochfeld

*T*oxicology is the study of the harmful effects of chemicals, including drugs, on living organisms. Toxicologists explore these effects using methods ranging in scale from the entire organism to tissues, cells, and molecules. Toxicity is the ability of a chemical substance to cause harm to a living organism. Toxic chemicals range from very simple molecules, such as carbon tetrachloride, to large complex molecules, such as the toxins produced by many marine organisms. There are several terms for toxic chemicals: A *toxin* is a poisonous substance produced naturally by a living organism, such as animal venoms and many plant chemicals. A *toxicant* is a poisonous substance produced artificially by human activity. We use the terms *toxic chemical* and *toxic substance* interchangeably. The term *xenobiotic* refers to any chemical substance that is foreign to the body. (See Box 7-1 for definitions.)

All substances have the potential to be toxic, depending on the amount absorbed into the body (dose), the circumstances of exposure, and the sensitivity of the organism. Chemicals with recognized toxicity vary in potency (degree of toxicity), from highly potent toxins causing profound injury at low doses to less hazardous chemicals that only cause injury at extremely

high doses. A chemical that is highly toxic to one species may be only slightly toxic to another species that has more effective mechanisms for detoxifying or excreting the chemical or has genetic or biochemical factors that confer resistance to the toxic effects of the chemical. Toxicity may be apparent shortly after exposure or the harm may not be apparent until years after exposure.

This chapter covers basic principles of toxicology, including how chemicals enter and move through the body and how they exert pathophysiological effects on target organs. It describes several classifications of toxic chemicals, but it is neither a catalogue of toxic effects nor a compendium of individual toxic chemicals. (See also Chapter 11.)

Of the more than 80,000 chemicals in commerce, few have been adequately tested for toxicity. Even the Occupational Safety and Health Administration (OSHA) hazard communication standard, which requires employers to provide hazard warning container labels and safety data sheets, is made ineffective if basic information on the chemicals is not available.

All chemicals have properties or characteristics that are related to the source from which they

Box 7-1. Definitions

Aerosol: Either fine liquid droplets or solid particles dispersed in the air or other gaseous medium.

Bioavailability: The ability of a substance that enters the body to be liberated from its environmental matrix, especially soil or food, thereby gaining access to enter the body.

Biotransformation: Intermediary metabolism consisting of metabolic processes that change the structure of a chemical. It may increase (activate) or decrease (detoxify) the toxic properties of a chemical.

Carcinogenicity: The ability of a chemical to cause cancer. Carcinogens can be genotoxic chemicals that damage DNA, leading to unbridled cell replication (induction), or chemicals that enable induced cells to undergo rapid cell divisions (promotion).

Concentration: The level of a chemical present in an environmental medium or in a body organ or fluid.

Dose: The amount of a chemical that is absorbed into the body (absorbed dose), or the amount that reaches a target organ (target organ dose).

Effect dose 50% (ED_{50}): The dose of a chemical that produces a specified effect in 50% of the animals studied.

Exposure: Contact between a chemical in environmental media (air, water, soil, or food) and the human body, usually specified by concentration of the chemical in the medium and duration of contact.

Exposure pathway: How a chemical moves from a source, through a medium, and into contact with the body through a route of exposure.

Fumes: Very fine solid particles, usually generated when a heated vapor condenses.

Lethal dose 50% (LD_{50}): The dose of a chemical that causes death in 50% of the animals studied.

Lipophilic: A chemical (nonpolar) that is much more soluble in organic solvents than in water and can readily move through membranes and concentrate in lipid-rich tissues. (See *Polar and nonpolar compounds*.)

Mechanism: The way in which toxic substances act at the molecular and cellular level to cause morbidity and mortality.

Mutagenicity: The ability of a substance to damage genetic material either by disrupting chromosomal structure or changing the sequence of nucleotides in DNA.

Polar and nonpolar compounds: Polar compounds (such as many inorganic salts) tend to be soluble in water. Nonpolar compounds (many organic compounds) tend to be soluble in organic solvents, such as toluene and lipids, but have very low water solubility. The standard for describing this is the "octanol-to-water partitioning coefficient" (solubility in octanol, divided by solubility in water). Nonpolar compounds pass through the skin and cell membranes more readily than polar compounds. Polar compounds are more readily excreted in urine.

Route of exposure: How a chemical in an environmental medium can come in contact with the body (inhalation, ingestion, skin contact, injection).

Susceptibility: The vulnerability of an individual or population to be harmed by an agent. It is influenced by many factors, including age, sex, genetic polymorphisms, nutrition, prior exposure, and overall health status.

Teratogenicity: The ability to interfere with normal fetal development, resulting in birth defects.

Threshold dose: The lowest dose of a chemical that has a detectable effect. For any given chemical, each cellular, biochemical, physiologic, or clinical response may have a threshold dose. Some effects occur without a known threshold dose. Since susceptibility varies among animal species and among humans, the threshold dose is approximated. Threshold doses are often used to categorize or rank chemical toxicity.

Toxicity: The intrinsic ability of a substance to harm living cells or processes, organisms, or ecosystems.

Toxicodynamics: The physiologic mechanisms by which toxic substances are absorbed, distributed, metabolized, and excreted and the mechanisms of action on affected target molecules, orgenelles, and cells.

Toxicokinetics: Quantitative study of time course of absorption, distribution, metabolism, and excretion of a xenobiotic.

Xenobiotic: Any substance foreign to the body, including all synthetic chemicals as well as many pharmaceuticals and essential nutrients.

---

originate, their fate and transport in the environment, the circumstances under which they come in contact with a living organism, the routes of absorption into that organism, and their distribution, metabolism, storage, and excretion after entering the organism.

For a chemical to cause a toxic effect, it must follow a pathway from its source to the site of molecular interaction in the body. Toxic chemicals enter and move through environmental "media" (air, water, soil, and food) at various concentrations until they do one, or likely more, of the following:

- Contact a receptor individual
- Enter the body by inhalation, ingestion, or skin absorption
- Are absorbed into the bloodstream (uptake), reaching a certain concentration
- Undergo metabolism (which may enhance or reduce their toxicity)
- Are stored or excreted
- Are delivered to target organs and tissues, where they affect some molecular target, causing damage at the genetic, biochemical, cellular, and/or physiologic level.

Many toxic chemicals occur naturally, including many metals and their compounds, while others are anthropogenic or synthetic in origin, created deliberately or inadvertently through human activities. Among the most dangerous toxic chemicals are biocides, which are used deliberately for their toxic effects on certain forms of life. Some biocides are toxins, such as the pyrethrins extracted from plants in the daisy family.

The birth of toxicology is often ascribed to Paracelsus (1493–1541), who recognized that a substance that was harmless at a low dose could be toxic at a higher dose.[1] However, as early as 1500 B.C., natural venoms were used for therapeutic purposes. In medieval times, a variety of poisons, many of them of botanical origin, were found to have medicinal uses. Modern science emerged in the mid-1600s, but it was not until the 1850–1900 period that the chemical industry arose, especially for the development of dyes and paints. In the early 20th century, modern toxicology emerged, largely in the service of warfare, pest control, drug development, and food safety.

Toxicology has become a very broad interdisciplinary field of science, embracing virtually all aspects of biology and many aspects of chemistry. It has played an important role in the development of pharmaceuticals and pesticides, products in which toxic chemicals are used deliberately in relatively high concentrations. Industrial toxicology focuses on the toxicity of raw materials, intermediates, products,

and waste products. Workers directly involved in the manufacture, distribution, and use of chemical products may be exposed to chemicals at relatively high concentrations. Data generated by toxicologists play important roles in risk assessment and regulation. Areas of subspecialization within toxicology focus on organs (such as neurotoxicology), functions (such as behavioral toxicology), and organizational levels (such as genetic toxicology). Molecular toxicology is aimed at understanding the most basic level at which xenobiotics interact with organisms. Mechanistic toxicology explores the details of how xenobiotics cause damage at the molecular, biochemical, and cellular levels.

EXPOSURE

Hazardous materials, including both naturally occurring and anthropogenic (synthetic) chemicals, can contaminate environmental media, such as air, water, soil, dust, and food. Chemicals present in environmental media can come in contact with the human body by inhalation, ingestion, dermal contact, or, rarely, injection. In Table 7-1, an exposure matrix, each cell represents a potential exposure pathway. Table 7-2 similarly illustrates pathways that are important in residential or community exposures; in this case, soil ingestion by toddlers is often the most important pathway.

Figure 7-1 illustrates media that are potentially part of an exposure pathway from source

Table 7-1. Exposure Matrix for Occupational Exposure

	Air	Water	Soil/Dust	Food
Inhalation	Very important for occupational health	Volatilizes when cooking or showering	Both workplace and residential	Not a common pathway
Ingestion	Airborne deposition on foods or crops	A major residential pathway	Gardeners and workers who eat at work or without washing	A major residential pathway
Dermal	A few gases penetrate skin	Important for a few chemicals or mixtures	Some direct contact with workplace chemicals	Not a pathway
Injection	Not a pathway	Not a pathway	Some sharp solid objects can penetrate	Not a pathway

Source: Exposure matrix modified from M. Gochfeld (©). A matrix of routes and media of exposure for risk assessment scenarios. Piscataway, NJ: Environmental and Occupational Health Sciences Institute, 1991.

Table 7-2. Exposure Matrix for Residential or Community Exposure

	Air	Water	Soil/Dust	Food
Inhalation	Important for community air pollution or indoor contaminants	Volatilizes when cooking or showering	Fine dust particulates	Not applicable
Ingestion	Airborne deposition on foods or crops	A major residential pathway, particularly with private wells	Toddlers and gardeners	A major residential pathway for garden crops, wildlife, and fish
Dermal	A few gases penetrate skin	Important for a few chemicals or mixtures. Also for some household chemicals through direct contact	Some direct household chemicals or pesticides	Not a pathway
Injection	Not a pathway	Not a pathway	Some sharp solid objects can penetrate	Not a pathway

Source: Exposure matrix modified from M. Gochfeld (©). A matrix of routes and media of exposure for risk assessment scenarios. Piscataway, NJ: Environmental and Occupational Health Sciences Institute, 1991.

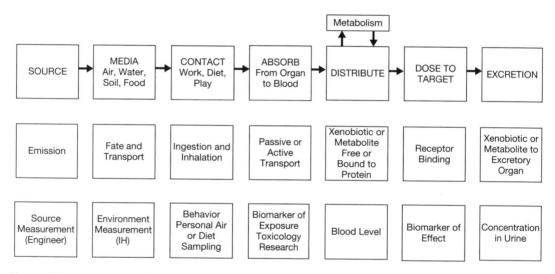

Figure 7-1. An exposure pathway from source through one or more environmental media, to contact, absorption, and distribution in the body, eventually reaching a target organ and excretory organs. Rectangles in the top row identify the components of the pathway. Rectangles in the middle row indicate the processes involved in each step along the pathway. Rectangles in the bottom row indicate what can be measured. (Used with permission of the Environmental and Occupational Health Sciences Institute.)

to exposure, to internal dose, to toxicokinetics to dose to the target organ. The dose to the target organ determines the health effect, but many factors intervene, including those governing (a) fate and transport in the environment; (b) efficiency of absorption into the body; and (c) metabolism, distribution, storage, and excretion of the chemical in the body. A number of factors can modify absorption; for example,

physical activity increases respiratory rate and therefore increases inhalation of contaminants.

Routes of Exposure

Routes of exposure are the ways that people can come in contact with chemicals. The four major routes of exposure are inhalation (breathing), ingestion (eating or drinking), dermal contact

(contact with the skin), and injection (direct penetration through the skin). After contact, chemicals may exert toxicity locally at the site of contact or more distally after absorption and distribution of the primary compound and/ or its metabolites within the body. Special sites of absorption include the mucous membranes of the eyes, nose, and mouth and the placenta. However, many chemicals to which humans are exposed do not enter the body.

Assessment of Exposure to Chemicals

Exposure assessment is the discipline that develops and applies measurement techniques and models to quantify human exposure to hazards in the home, community, and workplace. The task of measuring the amount or concentration of a substance in an environmental medium, such as by air sampling, is relatively straightforward, requiring appropriate collection and analytic instrumentation. For example, the degree of exposure to an airborne chemical can be determined by sampling the air in an individual's breathing zone near the nose and mouth. However, direct measurement of the amount of a chemical that contacts the body is challenging and usually requires extensive research. Therefore, methods have been developed to infer exposure by measuring biomarkers in biological samples, such as blood or urine. Biomarkers are especially useful for assessing exposure by multiple routes of exposure, but interpretation can be complicated by factors affecting differences in absorption, metabolism, distribution, and excretion (toxicokinetics) among individuals. Blood lead level is an example of a highly specific biomarker for exposure to lead. Similarly, exhaled ethanol, which is closely correlated with contemporaneous blood alcohol level, forms the basis of breath-testing of motorists suspected of intoxication.

Many absorbed organic compounds are present only transiently in the bloodstream before being metabolized or excreted. In such cases, measurement of a specific metabolite in urine may be useful for estimating exposure. For example, while benzene is rapidly metabolized and cleared from the blood after exposure, one of its metabolites, phenol, is excreted in the urine and may be a useful biomarker under some circumstances. However, there are other sources of urinary phenol, including some cough medicines. Therefore, urinary phenol is a sensitive, but not specific, biomarker of benzene exposure. Blood or urine concentrations of cotinine, a breakdown product of nicotine, are useful biomarkers of inhalation of cigarette smoke.

Time Course of Exposure and Toxicity

In addition to the total dose, the time course of exposure to a chemical can profoundly affect the observed toxic effects. Time courses of exposure can range from a one-time, acute, short-term exposure, lasting seconds to hours, to continuous or intermittent, chronic exposure lasting for most of the lifespan (Figure 7-2). Various nonspecific terms (acute, subacute, subchronic, and chronic) are used to characterize the duration of exposure in toxicology studies. *Acute exposure* usually refers to less than 1 day, *subacute exposure* to a few days, *subchronic exposure* to 1 to 3 months for rodent studies, and *chronic exposure* for longer, including lifelong, exposure. Subchronic exposure may also refer to approximately 10% of the lifespan. *Lifetime exposure* is about 2 years for rats and 40 to 70 years for humans. Despite the use of these discrete terms, there is a continuum in the duration and frequency of exposure, both in laboratory experiments on animals and in human life.

Most occupational exposures are intermittent, occurring only during working hours or while performing specific tasks during those working hours. The tradition of averaging exposures over an 8-hour period (as a time-weighted average [TWA]), ignores peaks that may exceed thresholds for acute injury. One of the central dogmas of toxicology, Haber's law, states that a toxic effect is a product of exposure concentration multiplied by duration of exposure. Under Haber's law, the following would have equivalent toxicity: 1 microgram per day for 100 days, 4 micrograms per day for 25 days, and 100 micrograms for 1 day. However, Haber's law operates over a very limited range, and it can be either useful or seriously misleading, depending on how it is applied. Consider the analogy of a person who has been prescribed a bottle of

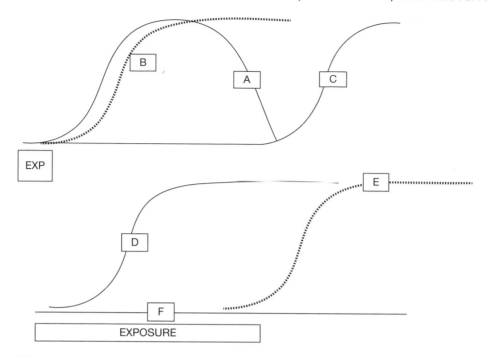

Figure 7-2. Time-course of exposure and response, showing acute versus chronic exposures as well as acute and chronic responses with both short and long latency demonstrated. Curves A, B, and C show responses to a single acute, high-level exposure. (A) An acute self-limited effect; (B) an acute and persistent effect; (C) a long-delayed effect beginning after a long latency following the acute exposure. Curves D, E, and F show response to a chronic, lower-level exposure. (D) A chronic condition arising shortly after onset of exposure, and probably idiosyncratic; (E) a chronic condition beginning after a long period of cumulative exposure; (F) no appreciable response even after long-term, low-level exposure. (Used with permission of the Environmental and Occupational Health Sciences Institute.)

30 pills to take once a day for a month. Taking all the pills on the first day gets the chore out of the way and, according to Haber's law, would be equivalent to one pill per day for a month; however, this could have very serious toxic consequences. Relationships among exposure concentrations, frequency, and duration are difficult to model, and there are relatively few studies that address this important topic. Therefore, in setting occupational exposure limits, the time factor is usually accounted for by either full-shift, 8-hour TWA standards, 15-minute short-term exposure limits (STELs), or ceiling limits not to be exceeded for any length of time. ACGIH publishes annual updates of its threshold limit values, which are based on 8-hour TWAs, and STELs. OSHA standards for air contaminants are called the *permissible exposure limits* (PELs).

The terms *acute* and *chronic* can refer to outcomes as well as exposure. There is usually a time lag between a dose and its effect, which is referred to as *latency*, defined as the period between the start of exposure and the appearance of disease. Apparent latency may become shorter when new diagnostic tests detect disease at earlier stages. Some latencies are only seconds in duration, such as the chemical asphyxiant effects of hydrogen sulfide, which at high concentrations can cause "knockdowns," in which an individual collapses after as little as one breath. At the other extreme, the latency between start of asbestos exposure and diagnosis of mesothelioma may be 50 years or longer. In general, the latency period for a carcinogen decreases as the cumulative dose of it increases. Long-term chronic exposure may reach a point where the cumulative dose has become sufficient to trigger an adverse health effect. In addition, an acute dose may cause damage that eventually causes an adverse health effect after a long latency. In general, the longer the latency, the more difficult it is to determine that a specific effect was caused by a specific exposure.

Reversible, Progressive, and Permanent Effects

A pathophysiological effect caused by a toxic chemical exposure may be reversible, permanent, or progressive. Once the exposure is removed, many toxic effects have some degree, often complete, of reversibility back to normal structure and function. Reversibility is a function of dose—that is, a change, such as neurologic or renal damage, may be reversible until it reaches a point where definite structural damage occurs. For example, methylmercury poisoning produces a variety of symptoms and signs, beginning with tingling sensations on the lips; progressing to visual, auditory, and gait impairments; and culminating in blindness, coma, convulsions, and death. The early changes are reversible, but complete recovery from blindness is not possible. In general, irreversible damage may persist without progressing, or it may progressively worsen as exposure continues. In some cases, damage, such as cancer, may progress even after the exposure has ceased.

Different organ systems have different capacities for repair. Death of a cell is not reversible, but almost all organs are capable of replacing damaged cells by regeneration, which is not always perfect. For example, after viral or toxic hepatitis, the liver regenerates, but the healing often results in cirrhosis because new liver cells have interposed fibrous tissue that compresses cells and interferes with function. Similarly, after lung injury, the healing process involves formation of fibrous tissue that eventually impairs respiratory function.

When DNA is damaged, there are repair enzymes capable of restoring the original sequence of nucleic acids, although the damage is not always corrected with complete accuracy. DNA repair mechanisms become less efficient in older people, and this is believed to be one of the factors associated with cancer rates increasing with age.

TOXICOKINETICS

Figure 7-3 summarizes the movement of substances from environmental media into and out

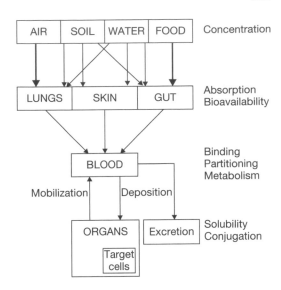

Figure 7-3. A multicompartment model of toxicant distribution showing the relationship among uptake, metabolism, distribution, storage, and excretion. (Used with permission of the Environmental and Occupational Health Sciences Institute.)

of various body compartments. *Toxicokinetics* (and *pharmacokinetics*, a related term) is the study of how much and how quickly a xenobiotic undergoes absorption, distribution, metabolism, and excretion. Distribution includes interchanges between blood and target, storage, and excretory organs. Toxicokinetic studies are used to determine the relationships between systemic exposure and the time course of dose to target organs and elimination from the blood and to assess relationships between exposures to animals and corresponding exposures to humans.

Toxicodynamics describes the physiologic mechanisms by which toxic substances are absorbed, metabolized, and excreted and the mechanism of action on affected target molecules, organelles, and cells. As researchers provide data on partitioning coefficients and metabolic rates, it becomes possible to develop models that predict how much of a chemical will circulate through each organ, using data on the perfusion rate (amount of blood delivered per minute). These are called *physiologically based pharmacokinetic* (PBPK) models, patterned after models that predict the fate of pharmaceutical agents in the body.

Absorption

Major pathways of absorption into the body include the respiratory tract, the gastrointestinal tract, and the skin. When the skin or mucous membranes (mucosa) lining the respiratory or gastrointestinal tract come in contact with a contaminated medium, there is an opportunity for transfer of contaminants across the skin or mucosa into the bloodstream. Chemicals have characteristic rates of absorption through the skin (usually relatively very low) and mucosa (often relatively high), depending on the chemical and physical attributes of the chemical, including its polarity, solubility, and size. Small, nonpolar compounds tend to be lipophilic and readily pass through membranes. The skin and mucosa prevent the ingress of most large, polar molecules. In addition, there are differences among organs. For example, elemental mercury is volatile at room temperature, and mercury vapor is readily absorbed through the lung; however, the same amount of elemental mercury, if swallowed, would pass through the intestinal tract with negligible absorption. In contrast, if methylmercury were ingested, there could be almost complete absorption.

The superficial linings of the skin, lungs, and gastrointestinal tract form barriers that retard the exchange of water and solutes between the environment and the extracellular and intracellular compartments. Material crosses membranes in various ways, by free diffusion (mainly of polar molecules), through small pores, and by transporter molecules (mainly for polar compounds).

Rates of absorption vary among individuals, based on age and other factors. For example, children can absorb about 50% of the lead they ingest, while adults absorb usually less than 10%. Women who have depleted iron stores absorb a much higher proportion of ingested cadmium than men or women with normal iron stores. Transporter molecules are specific carriers of certain toxics, and their presence and efficiency varies among people, in part due to genetic factors. Transporters serve a normal physiologic function; for example, metallothionein proteins regulate movement of zinc, an essential element, through the body. Cadmium, a xenobiotic, strongly binds to metallothionein, which carries

it to other organs, including the kidney, where it is excreted.

Crossing Membranes

To enter and move through the body, chemicals must cross various membranes. For example, in the lung a chemical must cross the membrane that separates the air in the alveolus from the blood in the adjacent capillary. Once in the bloodstream, the chemical may enter a metabolic organ, such as the liver; an excretory organ, such as the kidney; or a target organ. To reach these organs, the chemical must again pass through a capillary wall into interstitial space and then into contact with and/or through the membrane of target organ cells. Cell membranes are not inert "plastic bags" but rather dynamic, fluid structures of lipids and proteins, with different features in different cell types. Some substances pass mainly through membrane pores or channels; others are transported by transporter molecules; and some remain in the membrane, bound to receptors on the cell surface. Transportation via pores often involves passive diffusion along a gradient from higher to lower concentration. Active transport involves processes that use energy to move a substance through a membrane, against a concentration gradient with the aid of transporter molecules. In addition, membranes can be targets for chemicals that injure membranes by causing lipid peroxidation and alteration of membrane fluidity.

Inhalation Exposure and Absorption

Inhalation is the primary route of exposure in industrial workplaces and in other environments where airborne contaminants are of concern. A typical adult at rest may take about 12 breaths a minute, each with a tidal volume of about 500 ml (of which about 150 ml is the "dead space" of the upper airway). This amounts to 4.2 L (12×350 ml = 4,200 ml) per minute (about 6,000 L per day) of air exchange in the lung—6 m³ of air for a resting adult. With activity, both breathing rate and volume increase substantially, so that 20 m³ of air is used to estimate how much airborne contaminant a moderately active person would breathe in a day.

As air passes through the nose and upper airway, large particles (dusts) are trapped by nasal hairs or may be removed by impaction on the mucous membranes of the nasal passages and pharynx. For example, pollen grains, which are spherical and about 20 μm in size, are scrubbed out in the nasopharynx and do not enter the lungs.

Smaller particles enter the tracheobronchial tree, where they may land on the ciliated epithelium that lines the walls of larger airways. A thin layer of mucus covers the cilia; particles trapped in this mucus are swept upward by the rhythmic wave-like action of the cilia until they reach the throat, where they are usually swallowed but can also be expectorated. Air contaminants may interfere with this important defense mechanism against inhaled particles. For example, in vitro experiments show that a puff of tobacco smoke temporarily paralyzes this mucociliary escalator.

The trachea divides into two branches (main stem bronchi), and these divide again and again (about 27 generations) until the alveolar duct ends in the alveolus. The toxicity of particles may be related to physical properties, such as size and shape, as well as the toxicity of their chemical constituents. Particles that are deposited in the alveoli are likely to be engulfed by pulmonary macrophages, which secrete reactive compounds and enzymes that destroy many kinds of particles. Some particulates stimulate the macrophages to secrete cytokines, which invoke a local inflammatory response, followed by formation of a microscopic fibrous area, similar to scarring. Recurrent exposure to such substances may lead to progressive fiber deposition. Eventually, the elasticity of the lung may be compromised by interstitial fibrosis, leading to restrictive lung disease. (See Chapter 22.) Particles that are very small (ultrafine particles or nanoparticles) may not be recognized by macrophages and therefore may evade scavenging.

The size, shape, and density of a particle influence its aerodynamic diameter, which determines the efficiency with which particles in air entering the respiratory tract are deposited on various surfaces as they move from the nose and mouth to the distal alveoli. The *inhalable fraction* consists mainly of particles with aerodynamic diameters less than 100 μm. The *thoracic fraction* consists of inhaled particles that pass the larynx, mainly smaller than 10 μm. The *respirable fraction*, which may reach the alveoli, consists mainly of particles smaller than 4 μm. The Environmental Protection Agency (EPA) defines particles greater than 10 μm as supercoarse, from 2.5 to 10 μm as coarse, smaller than 2.5 μm as fine, and smaller than 0.1 μm as ultrafine. Engineered particles in the ultrafine size range are also referred to as nanoparticles. (See Box 8-2 in Chapter 8.) Particles smaller than 10 μm are designated as the PM_{10} fraction and particles smaller than 2.5 μm as the $PM_{2.5}$ fraction.

Physical properties also affect toxicity from inhalation of chemical vapors and gases. Highly water-soluble chemical vapors or gases are rapidly absorbed in the aqueous fluid that lines the airways, exerting toxic effects more proximally (in the upper airways), whereas less water-soluble vapors and gases are absorbed more distally (in the lower airways or alveoli). Water-soluble chemicals, such as ammonia, typically cause irritation of the upper airway, manifested as burning sensations in the nose and throat and cough. Chemicals with low water solubility, such as phosgene, reach the vulnerable surfaces of the alveoli, where they can induce severe injury and inflammation, leading to pulmonary edema (fluid accumulation), which may be delayed for 6 to 12 hours after exposure.

Dermal Absorption

The skin is a very effective barrier for many chemicals, but there are remarkably few data on skin absorption of chemicals. Some nonpolar compounds pass through the skin, while polar compounds do not. For example, methylmercury readily passes through intact skin and enters the bloodstream, whereas inorganic mercury compounds are not absorbed through the skin in any appreciable amount. The mucous membranes are less effective barriers. Both the skin and mucous membranes, including those of the eyes, can also be target organs.

A tragic example of dermal absorption occurred in a chemist, who died after 3 to 5 drops of dimethylmercury were spilled on her latex gloves. Unbeknownst to her—and apparently to the university health and safety officer—dimethylmercury quickly passes through latex gloves and is readily absorbed through the skin. Just a few drops contained a lethal dose.

Gastrointestinal Absorption

Chemicals may enter the body in the food we eat or the water or other liquids we drink. Contamination of drinking-water supplies from natural or anthropogenic sources has the potential to affect large populations. Risk assessment assumes a default value of 2 L per day to represent residential drinking water intake to a homebound adult. After ingestion, many nonpolar compounds readily pass through the wall of the gastrointestinal tract into the bloodstream. First, they are carried by the splanchnic circulation to the liver, where they may undergo metabolic activation or deactivation. From the liver, ingested nutrients and xenobiotics enter the venous circulation and are subsequently distributed throughout the body.

Transplacental Absorption

The placenta is a complex organ, with several cell layers, that provides oxygen and nutrients to the fetus, removes fetal waste products, and maintains pregnancy through secretion of hormones. The placenta provides active transport for necessary nutrients, such as vitamins, amino acids, calcium, and iron. Xenobiotics pass through the placenta mainly by passive diffusion, unless they are similar in structure to a transported substance. Although it is customary to speak of a placental barrier, there are many infectious agents (especially viruses) and chemicals that readily cross the placenta to reach the fetal circulation. Nonpolar compounds, such as methylmercury and polychlorinated biphenyls (PCBs), readily pass the placenta. Xenobiotics that are bound to proteins or are conjugated are less likely to cross the placenta.

Traversing the Blood–Brain Barrier

The blood–brain barrier, with its low permeability, restricts entrance of many compounds into the brain. It exists because capillary cells in the central nervous system (CNS) form a tight endothelial layer with few pores. There are also tightly wound glial cells that impede passage of chemicals into the brain from the circulation. In addition, the protein concentration in the CNS is lower than in other organ systems, restricting the amount of protein available to bind and transport xenobiotics. The blood–brain barrier is poorly developed at birth, and therefore fetuses and young infants are particularly vulnerable to toxicants that can harm the brain. Lipid-soluble methylmercury crosses the blood–brain barrier directly by diffusion, and inorganic mercury passes through the barrier, by binding to cysteine in the cell membranes.

Bioavailability Alters Absorption

Whereas absorption of a chemical is determined by its properties and the membrane being crossed, bioavailability refers to the properties of the matrix, especially for soil and food, which may bind a toxic compound and interfere with absorption. Even a chemical that is readily absorbed in pure form may not be absorbed from a particular environmental medium. The amount of absorption of any chemical depends on both (a) the absorptive capacity of the contact organ and (b) the bioavailability of the chemical in its environmental medium or matrix.[2] For example, soil characteristics affect binding of dioxin, altering its bioavailability, and hence absorption, and toxicity. The importance of bioavailability is illustrated by dioxin contamination in Times Beach, Missouri, and Newark, New Jersey. In the small town of Times Beach, dioxin-contaminated oil was used to suppress dust on dirt roads throughout the town, ultimately leading to an unprecedented buy-out of the entire town by the federal government and relocation of all of its residents in the early 1980s. In Newark, where Agent Orange, a herbicide contaminated with dioxin, had been manufactured at a factory on the Passaic River, leaks and fires had contaminated surface soil and river sediment with dioxin. The relatively sandy soil from Times Beach readily yielded dioxin when fed to animals by gavage (indicating high bioavailability); in contrast, dioxin was bound tenaciously to the oil-contaminated soil from Newark so that little could be extracted and absorbed in the gastrointestinal tract (indicating low bioavailability).

Distribution

Once a xenobiotic has entered the bloodstream, it is transported by the blood to many organs. Chemicals absorbed from the gastrointestinal tract are carried first to the liver through the portal circulation—sometimes referred to as the *first pass*, where they may undergo metabolic transformation prior to entry into the systemic circulation. In contrast, volatile chemicals absorbed through the lung enter the pulmonary circulation, returning to the left heart and entering the systemic circulation directly. Chemicals in the blood can be in unbound "free" form or bound to transporter molecules, which are usually proteins. Once a substance reaches the capillaries of an organ, its transfer into the extracellular fluid or into cells is partially governed by how strongly it is bound in the bloodstream.

Sequestration or Storage

A chemical or its metabolite circulating in the bloodstream can be distributed to many organs simultaneously—excretory organs, target organs, or storage organs. Chemicals may be stored for days, months, or decades in storage organs, usually while manifesting little evidence of harm. For example, lead is stored in bone, where it is probably fairly innocuous; lead exerts its primary toxic effects in the nervous system and other organ systems. Organochlorines, such as PCBs, are stored in fat. They generally do not harm fatty tissue, but if a person mobilizes fat rapidly, release of stored PCBs may lead to a potentially harmful, relatively acute, dose to sensitive target organs. Cadmium is stored mainly in the kidney, its primary target organ; even after exposure is terminated, the cadmium is eliminated from the kidney very slowly.

Distribution to Target Organs

Toxic chemicals in circulation are delivered to *target organs*, where their toxic effects occur. The *target organ dose* is the amount of the substance that enters the target organ. This dose depends on the blood perfusion rate of the organ and the movement of the substance from the blood across membranes into the organ, either by passive diffusion or by active-transport mechanisms. The diffusion rate, following Fick's Principle, is proportional to the concentration gradient, the membrane surface area, and a compound-specific coefficient (which depends on the octanol:water partitioning coefficient, with lipophilic compounds passing membranes more quickly than

hydrophilic ones). Theoretically, the diffusion coefficient is inversely related to the cube root of the molecular weight of the compound, with smaller molecules therefore passing through membranes more rapidly than large ones.

Any organ can be a target organ. The lungs and the skin are frequent target organs, because they are in close contact with environmental media. The liver and kidneys are also frequent target organs because of the characteristics of their blood supplies and the many metabolic and excretory processes that take place in these organs. Adverse effects of chemical exposures on the liver (hepatotoxicity) include hepatocellular injury, cholestatic injury, fatty liver, granulomatous disease, cirrhosis, and malignancies, including hepatocellular carcinoma and hepatic angiosarcoma. A wide variety of chemicals, including organic solvents, vinyl chloride monomer, arsenic, chlorinated pesticides, and infectious agents can adversely affect the liver. Adverse effects of chemical exposures on the kidneys include proximal tubule dysfunction or damage, immune-mediated glomerulonephritis, end-stage kidney disease, and malignancies of the kidney or bladder. A wide variety of chemicals, including cadmium and other heavy metals, organic solvents, and aniline dyes, can adversely affect the kidneys.

Metabolism

Metabolism consists of the chemical transformations of xenobiotics that have been absorbed into the body. Metabolism of xenobiotics is divided into Phase I and Phase II reactions. Phase I reactions are mainly oxidation or reduction that make the absorbed compound more water soluble (Figure 7-4). Phase I reactions include hydrolysis or hydroxylation, leading to epoxide formation and other outcomes. The cytochrome-P450 enzyme systems play major roles in Phase I reactions (see next section). Sometimes, the metabolite is less toxic (*detoxification*); in other cases, toxicity is increased (*bioactivation*). Some oxidized metabolites, often referred to as *reactive intermediates*, can "attack" cell membranes as well as intracellular membranes and macromolecules. Since metabolism of any compound is usually incomplete, varying proportions of the absorbed chemical and one

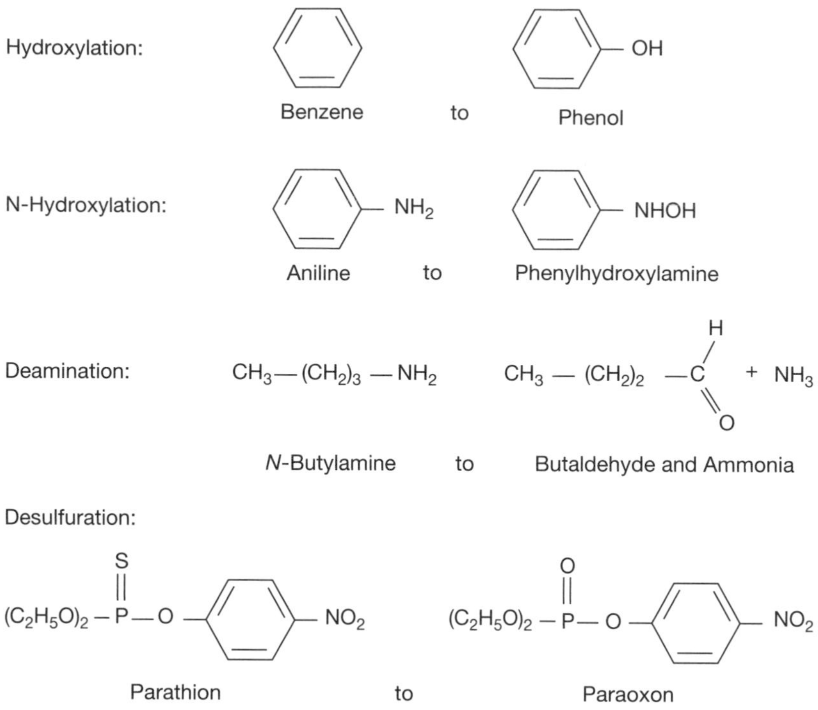

Figure 7-4. Examples of oxidation reactions in metabolism of several common industrial chemicals.

or more metabolites are often circulating at the same time. The ratio of the metabolite(s) to the parent compound in the blood is called the *metabolic ratio*, which is sometimes used to measure the efficiency of metabolism in humans.

Phase I Reactions

The most important Phase I metabolic enzymes are *cytochrome P-450s* (or *P450s*). Cytochrome P450s occur in many forms and in all organisms. An entire subdiscipline has arisen to study the classification of P450s and their variation among species and organs, the different substrates on which they act, their specificity (or lack thereof), and the metabolites they produce. Once known generically as *liver microsomal oxidases* or *mixed function oxidases*, various metabolic functions are now being assigned to specific P450s, a few of which are discussed next.

P450s are found in most tissues, although the greatest amount and variety occur in the liver. They have a general feature of adding oxygen to a substrate, forming a highly reactive epoxide or a less reactive hydroxide. Oxygen can be involved in breaking double bonds, cleaving esters, and in

dehalogenation reactions. As new forms of these enzymes have been discovered, they are assigned to major families and subfamilies. Much of the research on P450s has come from investigations of how drugs are metabolized. For example, the P450 that metabolizes caffeine is referred to as P450 1A2 (often abbreviated as CYP1A2).

The flavin-containing monooxygenases (FMOs) represent another family of oxidizing enzymes that are NADPH-dependent. They act on substrates containing nitrogen, phosphorus, or sulfur, such as amines, organophosphates, or thiols. The FMOs have various isoforms that are distributed differently among species and organs. FMO1 occurs at high levels in rat and rabbit liver, with low levels in mouse and human liver; FMO3 occurs at a high concentration in human and mouse liver but low concentrations in rat and rabbit liver. Liver cells of female mice have higher amounts of FM01 and FMO3 than do male mice.

Phase II Reactions

Phase II involves linking the toxic substance, or its Phase I metabolite, to a molecule that increases

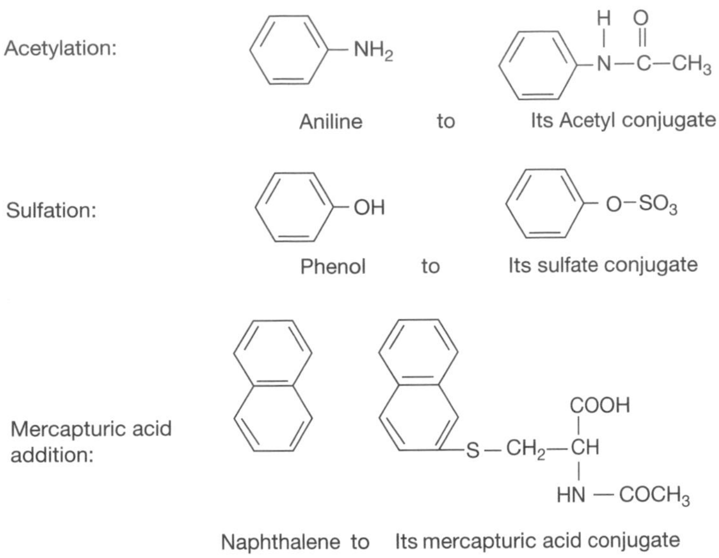

Figure 7-5. Examples of Phase II (conjugation) reactions.

its water soluble and facilitates its excretion in the urine. Phase II reactions link a metabolite to glucuronic acid, or add an acetyl, methyl, or sulfate radical. Phase II reactions include several important conjugation reactions. Metabolites from Phase I reactions can undergo conjugation with other molecules, which facilitates their transport and excretion in urine.

There are several types of conjugation reactions, among which conjugation to reduced glutathione (GSH) is especially common (Figure 7-5). This affects a wide range of electrophilic substrates and is accelerated by glutathione-S-transferase (GST) enzymes. Glucuronidation involves connecting the metabolite to glucuronic acid by various enzymes called glucuronosyltransferases that are found in various mammal tissues. The low-molecular-weight glucuronide complexes are excreted mainly in the urine, although some forms are excreted in the bile.

Sulfation is the major means of preparing phenol for excretion. It is also used for alcohols, amines, and other categories of chemicals. Sulfation and acetylation exemplify the sequential Phase I and Phase II metabolic reactions. Phenol and aniline can be metabolites of other toxins and then be conjugated and excreted. The addition of mercapturic acid (N-acetylcysteine) is a multistep process that proceeds through the addition of glutathione and subsequent cleavage

to cysteine derivatives. This reaction is extremely important in handling reactive electrophilic compounds that result from exogenous exposure or endogenous metabolic processes. Polycyclic aromatic hydrocarbons (PAHs) and polyhalogenated hydrocarbons are predominantly excreted in this manner.

Aromatic amines or hydrazines with a nitrogen atom can be metabolized by attaching acetate to the nitrogen (N-acetylation). This is accomplished by N-acetyltransferases (NATs) and serves as a major degradation pathway. There are at least three forms of NAT, and a deficiency in either activity or structure of NAT2 results in slow acetylation of certain drugs, such as isoniazid.

Examples of Metabolic Activation

An example of the importance of metabolic activation is the case of 1-methyl-4-phenyl-1,2,5,6-tetrahydropyridine (MPTP), an accidental by-product in the production of a designer narcotic. MPTP is oxidized by monoamine oxidase to MPP+, which is transported by the dopamine transporter and concentrates in dopaminergic neurons of the brain, where it inhibits cellular respiration and causes cell death. An MPTP-containing drug was sold "on the street" and many young adult users ingested dangerous levels and developed irreversible parkinsonism. Since this discovery, toxicologists have used MPTP to create animal models for research on parkinsonism.

Many chlorinated and aromatic hydrocarbons, such as vinyl chloride and trichloroethylene, undergo metabolic activation by formation of a reactive epoxide intermediate. The P450 system also metabolizes the analgesic acetaminophen to a quinone, which causes centrilobular necrosis of the liver. Acetaminophen is acted on by prostaglandin H synthase in the kidney, producing a nephrotoxic free radical. In the bladder, the prostaglandin H synthase system metabolizes a variety of aromatic amines into genotoxic metabolites that can induce bladder cancer. In rats, these same organic amines undergo N-hydroxylation in the liver and cause liver cancer.

Sites of Metabolism

A xenobiotic may undergo metabolic transformations in any organ, although metabolism of xenobiotics is one of the specialized functions of the liver. Metabolic enzymes are found in most tissues, including those at sites of initial contact with chemicals, such as the epithelium lining the respiratory and gastrointestinal tracts and the skin. The greatest variety and quantity of metabolic enzymes are in the liver. Within cells, these enzymes are found mainly in the microsomal component of the endoplasmic reticulum but also in the cytosol and other organelles. Certain xenobiotic compounds are metabolized by intestinal flora. Many of the metabolic responses begin with an oxidation step (Figure 7-4). Variability in P450 expression in different tissues is important, since significant metabolic activation or detoxification may occur in target tissues. Thus, CYP1A2 is expressed in the liver but not other organs, while CYP1A1 is low in the liver of most mammals but high in other tissues. Both are induced by PAHs and indoles. Since the two CYPs catalyze different reactions, a single substrate may follow different metabolic pathways in different tissues.

EXCRETION

Once a xenobotic and/or its metabolites are circulating in the bloodstream, they can be delivered to an excretory organ. Excretion is mainly through the urine and feces, but volatile compounds can be excreted primarily in exhaled breath or through the skin. Some substances that bind to keratin are eliminated in hair and nails. Many biomarker tests rely on measuring the concentration of a chemical in urine or exhaled breath. Many chemicals, especially those that are lipophilic, are readily transferred to breast milk, posing more of a hazard for an infant than its mother. Some compounds, particularly metals, concentrate in skin or hair and are lost through the natural sloughing of epidermal cells or hair growth. Substances that are water-soluble—or become water-soluble through conjugation—are excreted via the kidney; however, they may be toxic to the kidney or bladder because they are concentrated in these organs during urine production. Lipophilic substances or complexes may be secreted into bile and then excreted in the feces; some compounds excreted in the bile—in what is termed an *enterohepatic cycle*—may be reabsorbed in the intestine, thereby retarding excretion and enhancing toxicity.

The bloodstream delivers toxic substances to the renal glomerulus, where most are filtered with water and many other substances, forming the glomerular ultrafiltrate. Only cellular elements—large proteins such as albumin and substances bound to them—escape the filter and remain in the blood. Some of these may be secreted into the renal tubule. As the filtrate leaves the glomerulus and begins to pass down the tubule, the concentration of the toxic substance is similar to its concentration in the bloodstream. However, by the time the filtrate has traversed the tubular system and enters the collecting duct, about 99% of the water has been reabsorbed, so that the toxic substance is about 100 times more concentrated in the urine than in the blood. In this form, it is delivered to the bladder, where it may reside for hours before being eliminated. The liver also plays a prominent role in excretion by producing bile, which may incorporate nonpolar compounds that are not easily excreted by the kidney. Bile carries toxic compounds with it into the intestinal tract.

Biological Half-Life

The *biological half-life* for any compound is the amount of time it takes for half of an absorbed

TOXICOLOGY

129

dose to be eliminated from a tissue, organ, or the entire body. The biological half-life may be difficult to calculate, especially if there is ongoing exposure. Unlike the constancy of a radiological half-life, the excretion of a compound may be biphasic or even triphasic—that is, much of the dose can be eliminated rapidly in a few hours, and the remainder eliminated more slowly over days or weeks. The amount of a toxic substance that is circulating in the bloodstream at any time or the amount delivered to target organs represents a balance between the rates of (a) uptake and (b) excretion or storage. If exposure were terminated, the amount of the toxic substance in the body would gradually decrease. Some substances with short biological half-lives are rapidly excreted, while others with long biological half-lives tend to remain in the body for long periods. There can be substantial interindividual variation in the biological half-life of a given chemical. For example, cadmium may have a biological half-life ranging from a few years to many decades.

TOXICOLOGIC ENDPOINTS

Health professionals are concerned with identifying and preventing morbidity and mortality endpoints—ranging from transient skin lesions to death and involving molecular, biochemical, anatomic, physiologic, behavioral, or other effects. For example, Figure 7-6 shows a series of dose–response curves for different endpoints of methylmercury toxicity, reflecting a major poisoning episode in Iraq due to contaminated grain. For each endpoint, a separate dose–response curve can be drawn; these are nested from the least serious on the left, occurring at the lowest dose, to death on the right.

Traditionally, toxicologists have used the LD_{50}, the dose that kills 50% of organisms tested, for comparing the potency of different substances. The LD_{50} has also been used to assess the efficacy of antibiotics and pesticides. The potency of chemicals can be ranked on the basis of the LD_{50}. Other endpoints can be quantified the same way, yielding an ED_{50} (the dose that produces a particular effect in 50% of the organisms) or an ED_{10} (the dose that produces the effect in 10%). The ED_{10} is sometimes referred to as a benchmark

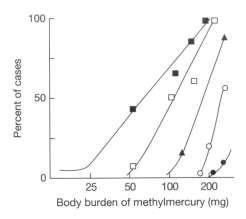

Figure 7-6. A series of dose–response curves for different endpoints of methylmercury toxicity reflecting a major poisoning episode from contaminated grain in Iraq. For each endpoint, a separate dose–response curve can be drawn, and these are nested from the least serious on the left (paresthesias occurring at the lowest dose) to death on the right, compared to the estimated body burden of methylmercury. Solid squares, paresthesias; open squares, ataxia; solid triangles, dysarthria; open circles, deafness; solid circles, death. (Used with permission of the Environmental and Occupational Health Sciences Institute. Based on data from Takizawa Y. Epidemiology of mercury poisoning. In Nriagu J [ed.]. The biogeochemistry of mercury in the environment. Amsterdam: Elsevier, 1979.)

dose. However, in assessing safety we are often interested in doses that affect only 1% or less of the population—the most sensitive people.

DOSE–RESPONSE CURVES

The *dose–response curve* describes how any particular response increases in frequency or intensity in an individual or population as the dose increases. Figure 7-7 represents a series of dose–response curves, with dose plotted on the x-axis and the response on the y-axis. Dose is usually measured as amount of chemical, such as in milligrams per kilogram of body weight. The y-axis may be the number of cells killed, the amount of a biomarker released, the number of animals affected, the percentage of people with a particular symptom, or the number who die. The most common dose–response curve has a sigmoid shape with three zones: subthreshold, rapid increase, and maximal effect or plateau.

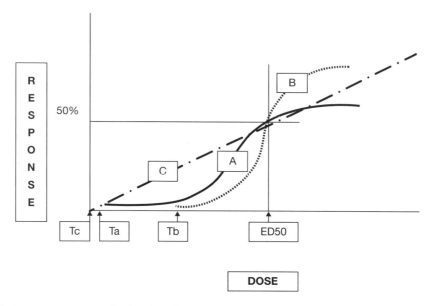

Figure 7-7. Dose–response curves for three hypothetical chemicals. Curves A and B are typical sigmoid curves differing in potency and efficacy. C is a linear, no-threshold curve presumed to be characteristic of the causation of cancer by ionizing radiation. B has a higher threshold than A. Thresholds are indicated by T. ED50 represents the dose corresponding to a 50% response. (Used with permission of the Environmental and Occupational Health Sciences Institute.)

The central portion of the dose–response curve can rise with varying degrees of steepness, reflecting the breadth of susceptibility between individuals in the exposed sample. A dose–response curve with a steeper rise indicates that there is less variation in susceptibility among exposed individuals.

Threshold Dose

Theoretically, a *threshold dose* is the lowest dose at which a toxic substance causes a toxic endpoint, usually in the most susceptible individual. Practically, the ability to establish and precisely estimate threshold doses is limited by several factors, including the size of the population sample and the number and range of different doses used in an experiment. For any given chemical and toxic endpoint, the threshold dose may vary, depending on conditions of exposure and the range of susceptibility among individuals in the sample. Thresholds must be defined in terms of a particular form of a chemical, time course of exposure, target population, and response. The threshold dose can be used as a basis for establishing guidelines or setting standards for acceptable risk.

Most toxicological experiments use at least three doses (including a zero-dose control), but relatively few studies use as many as five doses. Thus, estimation of the threshold dose is usually subject to considerable error, since it is very unlikely to correspond exactly to one of the doses used. Thus, dose-response experiments yield a *lowest observed adverse effect level* (LOAEL), which is the lowest dose above the control value at which the effect is detected. In some studies, this may correspond to the lowest dose tested. A *no observed adverse effect level* (NOAEL) is the lowest level above the zero control dose at which no effect can be detected. Both LOAELs and NOAELs are used in risk assessment and standard setting.

Although for most chemicals and most responses it is possible to estimate a threshold dose, this is not always achievable. Radiation carcinogenesis is generally assumed to follow a nonthreshold pattern. For childhood blood lead levels, there is no detectable NOAEL for neurobehavioral effects; some studies have found that the response slope is steeper in the 5 to 10 μg/dL range than above 10 μg/dL. Since the threshold is the dose below which no effect is detected, it is possible—and indeed likely—that earlier observations of putative threshold doses were due to the insensitivity of endpoint measurements, rather than to lack of adverse responses at those doses.

The *linear nonthreshold model* for low-dose extrapolation is based on the assumption that there is a direct relationship between dose and toxic response at any level of dose above a zero dose. A major controversy in toxicology is whether the linear nonthreshold model is an appropriate description of the dose–response relationship for chemical carcinogens. At present, this model is used for genotoxic carcinogens. In developing its risk assessments for cancer, the EPA uses a linearized multistage model to account for cancer arising not only from induction (chemical alteration of the genetic material) but also from factors governing promotion and proliferation.

Hormesis

A special issue in dose–response is hormesis, a phenomenon in which harmful substances, such as radiation, may have some beneficial effects at low doses (Figure 7-7).[3] This phenomenon of benefit and harm is best exemplified by pharmaceutical agents or nutrients, such as vitamin A and copper, which not only have a therapeutic (beneficial) threshold, but also a toxicological threshold. Ideally, these two thresholds are far apart. However, where they are close, indicating a small margin of safety, toxicity is more likely to occur at doses in the therapeutic range. Many drugs have been removed from the market, or never make it to market, because of a small margin of safety.

The concept of hormesis emerged from studies of ionizing radiation, where low doses of radiation have sometimes been associated with increased longevity in some organisms. However, the dose–responses curve for radiation-induced mutation and cancer are independent of any beneficial dose–response curve that might exist, and genetic damage can occur at doses below those postulated to give benefit. Proponents of hormesis argue that dose–response curves are often U-shaped. However, virtually all examples intended to illustrate hormesis use noncomparable endpoints and therefore are not true U-shaped curves. Critics

of linear low-dose extrapolation argue that it ignores hormesis. Hormesis is therefore highly controversial, including in the political context or in the regulation of chemicals. It has not been accepted that exposure standards should be based on hormesis.

BEYOND DOSE–RESPONSE RELATIONSHIPS: PREDICTING TOXICITY IN HUMAN INDIVIDUALS AND POPULATIONS

Dose–response relationships are fundamental to understanding and predicting the degree of toxicity of toxic substances. A general principle of toxicology relies on the extrapolation of dose–response relationships derived from animal studies to effects on humans. The biochemistry, physiology, and organ structure of humans is very similar to that of other mammals—and to vertebrates in general. Information needed to establish dose–response relationships in human beings comes mainly from animal studies and from epidemiological studies of workers exposed to relatively high levels of toxic substances. For some common industrial chemicals, studies of acute and chronic exposures among workers provide useful dose–response information. To estimate environmental effects, we customarily extrapolate from relatively high workplace exposures down to levels found in nonoccupational settings. For most industrial chemicals, however, data on adverse effects in humans are limited; therefore, we must rely on animal studies.

Variation in susceptibility among humans is an additional challenge in using dose–response information from animal studies to assess the toxicity of exposures to human populations. In most animal toxicity studies, genetically homogenous, inbred animal strains are used to reduce variability of responses. But results need to be extrapolated to genetically diverse humans who have a broader range of susceptibility. In human populations, responses to toxicants vary by age, gender, race/ethnicity, and individuals' genetic backgrounds. In addition, human populations may be exposed to a variety of other chemical substances as well as other factors, such as diet, psychosocial stress, and physical activity, which may enhance or reduce responses to toxic substances. In contrast, in dose–response laboratory experiments, environmental conditions are usually strictly controlled so that only the dose of the substance being tested is varied.

Many chronic diseases, such as cancer, heart disease, asthma, and diabetes, appear to result largely from interactions between the person's genetic material and environmental exposures. New so-called "omic" technologies allow for profiling of toxic responses at the levels of genes, gene transcription, protein expression, and metabolism of small molecules. Ultimately, these technologies may help us to understand complex gene–environment interactions and the effects of multiple stressors. For example, genomics (see later discussion) is the study of the human genome. By sequencing the entire DNA of entire genomes and parsing it into gene products, such as enzymes and modifiers (noncoding DNA), it may be possible to predict who will respond strongly to, or be resistant to, a particular xenobiotic, whether it is an industrial chemical or an anticancer drug.

Interspecies Differences in Response

Although the overall similarities in biochemistry and physiology among animals allow toxicologists to extrapolate between species, the well-established differences in response among species are equally important to understand. These differences have long been exploited in the development of biocidal agents that selectively target specific organisms, such as pesticides, fungicides, herbicides, and antibiotics. This biological diversity makes it difficult to use results of experiments performed in laboratory animals to predict, with a high degree of certainty, the toxicity of a substance in humans. For the most part, these differences are quantitative (matters of degree) rather than qualitative; however, even among similar species, large differences in toxic responses may be observed. For example, the LD_{50} for 2,3,7,8-tetrachlorodibenzo-p-dioxin (TCDD or dioxin) is more than 1,000 times larger in hamsters than in guinea pigs. Differences in toxicity may be due to differences in toxicokinetics and/or toxicodynamics. Most of the almost 100,000-fold difference in susceptibility to liver tumors

induced by aflatoxin B1 between rats and mice can be explained by differences in metabolism related to expression of cytochrome P450 and glutathione-S-transferase genes.[4] Better understanding of underlying biological mechanisms will contribute to improved accuracy in extrapolating from animals to humans.

Interindividual Differences in Response

Some individual differences in susceptibility are continuous, whereas others appear to be dimorphic. Males and females show significant differences in the expression of several metabolic enzymes, resulting in clinically significant differences in response to drugs.[5] Some P450 enzymes are sex-specific. For example, CYP1A1 protein and mRNA were detected in kidney and lung of female rats but not male rats.[6]

One person may be a heavy cigarette smoker who dies of lung cancer at age 50. Another person may by a heavy smoker who dies at age 90 of other causes. Which biological processes underlie these individual differences in susceptibility to the carcinogenic effects of tobacco smoke? Proteins—primarily enzymes, receptors, and transport proteins—drive toxicokinetic and toxicodynamic processes. The structure, function, and level of expression of these proteins are, in turn, determined, largely by the genes that code for these proteins. However, this is not the whole story. Previous or concurrent exposures to other chemicals and nonchemical stressors can cause variation in toxicity by several mechanisms.

Genetic Differences

The genomes of individual organisms are the complete sets of genetic information encoded in the sequence of bases in their DNA. An individual's genetic heritage is determined at conception. The human genome consists of about 3 billion nucleotide base pairs and includes about 20,000 genes. While the amount of genomic variation between individuals is remarkably small—about 0.1% between any two people—these differences underlie the uniqueness of each individual. A polymorphism is a genetic variant that, by convention, occurs in more than 1% of a population. More than 90% of human genetic variants are single nucleotide polymorphisms (SNPs), in which a single nucleotide (A, T, G, or C) differs within a DNA sequence. Other types of genetic variants include insertion or deletion of one or more nucleotides. The extent to which a given SNP or other variant will alter the expression of a gene is highly variable. If a SNP is in a noncoding region of the gene, it may be "silent." If a SNP is in a coding region and alters the amino acid sequence of the protein, it may change the activity of the protein product. Deletions and other variants may lead to nonfunctional proteins. Variants that do not alter amino acid sequence may affect expression by altering gene splicing or transcription-factor binding.

While some genetic variants cause "simple" genetic diseases, such as Huntington disease (inherited as an autosomal dominant condition), most genetic variants that contribute to disease only cause relatively small increases in risk of "complex" diseases. Sometimes referred to as Mendelian disorders—because high penetrance allows them to be tracked in families—these "simple" genetic diseases account for less than 5% of the human disease burden. Sickle cell anemia is an example of a genetic disease caused by a single base-pair substitution in the gene for the hemoglobin beta subunit, which alters a single amino acid in the protein. In contrast, multiple combinations of genetic variants, each making small contributions to disease risk, are believed to contribute to most of the human disease burden. Furthermore, gene–environment interactions are believed to be important in many diseases, such as asthma, in which individuals with a genetic susceptibility only manifest the disease after some presumed environmental exposure(s).

Polymorphisms in the genes that code for various P450 proteins have been shown to result in different metabolic phenotypes that may increase or decrease risk of toxic responses to particular chemical substances. For example, about 5% to 10% of Caucasians, and a smaller percentage of Asians, have a mutant CYP2D6 that was found to be inefficient at metabolizing the antihypertensive drug debrisoquine to its hydroxide form. The metabolic ratio, defined as:

$$\text{Metabolic ratio} = \frac{\text{Debrisoquine} - \text{OH}}{\text{Debrisoquine}}$$

can serve as a measure of metabolic efficiency. Those who are poor metabolizers of debrisoquine (with a low metabolic ratio) are also poor metabolizers of other substances acted on by CYP2D6.

For example, people whose CYP2D6 genotype makes them poor metabolizers of debrisoquine are at risk of various adverse drug reactions, whereas extensive metabolizers are at increased risk of lung cancer, probably because of carcinogenic metabolites they produce. CYP2D6-deficient people may be protected from certain environmentally caused cancers, such as lung, bladder, and liver cancer, because of their failure to activate certain pro-carcinogens.

Polymorphisms at the GST loci result in variable efficiencies of the Phase II conjugation reaction. Divalent cations, such as many metals, readily bind with sulfhydryl groups, including GSH. Exposure to mercury increases the activity of several enzymes involved in the synthesis of GSH and the reduction of oxidized glutathione. Conversely, acetaminophen depletes GSH levels in the liver. Both the depletion and the subsequent hepatotoxicity are inhibited by diallyl sulfone, a metabolite of garlic, which inhibits CYP2E1, the enzyme that activates acetaminophen.

Toxicogenetics and Toxicogenomics
Toxicogenetics is the study of individual differences in a single gene lead to different responses to toxicants. *Toxicogenomics* is the study of how multiple genes impact susceptibility to the toxicity of chemical substances. Profiling of macromolecules is an important measure of toxicant actions at the level of mRNA transcripts (*transcriptomics*), proteins (*proteomics*), and metabolites (*metabolomics*). These approaches can contribute to the understanding of individual differences in response to toxicants. Ultimately, these methods may lead to *personalized medicine*, in which approaches to the prevention, detection, and treatment of disease are tailored to an individual's risk profile and predicted response to interventions.[7] However, reaching this goal will require overcoming the computational and statistical challenges arising from huge quantities of data and enormous numbers of gene–gene and gene–environment interactions.

Over the past two decades, new omic technologies have been developed that allow for profiling and analysis of biological responses at the genetic, protein, and metabolite levels. Modern genetic methods, such as next generation sequencing, make it possible to quantitate the numbers of copies of genes coding for enzymes, receptors, and transport proteins involved in toxicokinetic and toxicodynamic processes. Modern genetic methods, such as high-throughput automated DNA sequencing, make it possible to document an individual's entire genome, although translating the findings to toxicology remain challenging.[4] With genomic technologies, thousands of genes, microRNAs, or alternatively spliced genes can be identified on a single gene chip (microarray). Microarrays consist of thousands of 150–200 micron spots of DNA bound to microscope slides in a known pattern. In *transcriptomics*, similar microarray technology enables the very efficient quantification of mRNA expression of thousands of genes simultaneously. The degree of hybridization of specific mRNA at each spot can be quantified with great sensitivity and specificity. At the level of protein expression, proteomic techniques for separating and identifying proteins are used to analyze the proteome—the proteins present in the cell or tissue at any one time. Within tissues, matrix-assisted laser desorption ionization is coupled with mass spectrometry to study the spatial distribution of small molecules, peptides, or proteins. Finally, metabolomic analysis of thousands of metabolic substrates, products, and cofactors in biological samples can now be achieved using nuclear magnetic resonance and mass spectrometry techniques.

Omics technologies enable researchers to obtain enormous amounts of information about genes, gene regulation, and responses to the environment among large samples of human populations. Two main approaches are used in attempts to unravel the complex gene–environment interactions that are believed to underlie most human disease. In targeted approaches, a limited number of hypotheses about associations are tested. For example, a specific gene that plays a role in the biochemical pathways involved in a disease may be identified and sequenced. Omics technologies have enabled newer, untargeted approaches that examine thousands of potential associations between genomes, epigenomes, metabolomes, environmental factors, and/or disease states and traits. For example, genome-wide association studies identify variation in a wide range of genes, examining numerous associations with a disease or trait.

Ethical Issues in Genetic Screening

In addition to technical difficulties, the potential application of genetic information to individualized risk assessment faces ethical challenges that are not unprecedented. In 1938, the geneticist J.B.S. Haldane suggested that someday genetic screening might allow identification of hypersusceptible workers—but he emphasized that in the meantime industrial hygiene controls were needed.[8] In 1967, H.E. Stokinger advocated, with limited success, genetic screening of workers for glucose-6-phosphate dehydrogenase deficiency, sickle cell anemia, and alpha-1-antitrypsin deficiency,[9] arguing that workers with these genetic conditions would be hypersusceptible to chemicals. Over the ensuing decade, some companies experimented with mandatory or voluntary genetic screening tests; however, like preemployment back X-rays, most were abandoned because of inadequate positive predictive value in the populations screened, high potential for discrimination, and inadequate cost-effectiveness. Genetic screening for susceptibility has resurfaced as a potential "preventive" approach, with completion of the Human Genome Project, and serious ethical and legal issues have been raised. Some states have legislated that genetic information cannot be used to deny health insurance or treatment, but they have not excluded its use in denying life insurance.

Epigenetics

Every somatic cell of an individual contains the entire genome of the individual. The turning "on" or "off" of specific genes results in the diversity of cell types in the body. Although some of these changes in gene expression are heritable in somatic or germ cell lines, they are not solely governed by the genetic makeup of an individual. *Epigenetics* describes the heritable changes in gene expression that are not coded in the DNA sequence. New discoveries indicate that epigenetic changes may be an important mode of action for toxic substances.

Known molecular mechanisms for epigenetic changes include DNA methylation, histone modification, and expression of noncoding RNAs. These regulatory mechanisms generally involve initiation and maintenance of the silencing of gene expression. Methylation of the promoter regions of genes silences them, and demethylation permits transcription. Cancer is a disease in which epigenetic changes are well established. (See Chapter 21.) Cancer cells are characterized by both global hypomethylation and regional hypermethylation of tumor suppressor genes. Recently, toxic substances have been shown to cause aberrations in DNA methylation. Cigarette smoke stimulates demethylation of genes involved in lung cancer metastasis. Epigenetic effects of other environmental exposures have recently been discovered. For example, exposure of pregnant Agouti mice to genistein, a phytoestrogen, results in methylation of a regulatory element for a gene that determines coat color, changing the coat color in the offspring. The extent to which epigenetic changes may be reversible is not yet clear.

Interactions between Multiple Exposures

Prior or concurrent exposures to other chemical and nonchemical stressors can lead to complex alterations in the response to a toxic substance. When an individual is exposed simultaneously to two or more chemicals or to a mixture of chemicals, a variety of interactions may occur, both outside and inside the body. These interactions are generally grouped into three categories: (a) independence and additivity, (b) synergism, and (c) antagonism.

If chemical A and chemical B each produce their effects independently of the other chemical, then there is no interaction. There is no interaction when chemicals affect different organs or produce different endpoints. Independence can occur when two chemicals follow different metabolic pathways, bind to different receptors, and do not compete. Additivity occurs when the two chemicals contribute to the same endpoint but show no interaction.

Synergism (or synergy)—a multiplicative effect—is of great practical importance, although there are remarkably few documented examples.

In synergism, two chemicals interact such that their combined effect on some endpoint is greater than would be expected from their independent dose–response curves. Chemical A may enhance the effect of chemical B, enhance its activation, or interfere with its degradation and excretion. The best documented example of synergism is based on a study of lung cancer in relation to smoking and occupational exposure to asbestos.[10] In some research, smoking increased lung cancer risk about 10 times; asbestos, about 5 times; and both, about 50 times.

Chemical A may reduce the effect of chemical B, if, for example, they compete for the same activating metabolic pathway or for the same receptor. Chemical A may inhibit the uptake of chemical B or its delivery to the target organ. If both A and B are activated by the same pathway, A may saturate the enzyme, preventing B from being activated. Or A may induce an enzyme, thereby enhancing the metabolism and elimination of B.

Hypersensitivity

Hypersensitivity is a special case of susceptibility induced by prior exposure to particular substances. Exposure to allergenic compounds will eventually sensitize some workers so that they respond immunologically, developing either dermal or respiratory symptoms. Some allergens, such as chromium, are potent sensitizers, quickly affecting a small proportion of people who contact them. A worker who becomes allergic to a particular chemical at work will often require relocation, as avoidance of the low levels of exposure that cause hypersensitivity reactions is usually difficult and desensitization therapy is seldom an option. However, if an allergen is encountered only infrequently and predictably, then engineering controls and/or special personal protective equipment may reduce exposure below an individual's response threshold.

Adaptation, Tolerance, and Hardening

At the opposite end of the spectrum are workers who show very little response to a chemical at a dose that would produce symptoms in most coworkers. In some instances, with repeat exposure, physiologic adaptation—the opposite of sensitization—occurs in the metabolism of the chemical or at the target organ. People who build up tolerance to a chemical no longer experience its acute effects, but they may accumulate enough exposure over time for chronic effects to develop. Work hardening is the deliberate process of allowing, or requiring, individuals to work in conditions of gradually increasing exposure so they build up tolerance. This process usually deals with physical stressors, such as extremes of temperature or physically demanding work. Work hardening has little if any role in managing exposures to toxic substances in the workplace. Adaptation and tolerance may limit the usefulness of relying heavily on workers' symptoms in evaluating exposures to toxic substances in the workplace.

MECHANISMS OF TOXICITY

Mechanism refers to the detailed, step-by-step process by which a toxic chemical causes damage, usually at the subcellular or molecular level. Knowledge of mechanisms is useful in risk assessment, such as in choosing between alternative extrapolation models for nongenotoxic, as opposed to genotoxic, carcinogens. Toxic substances can interact with different types of macromolecules, such as nucleic acids and proteins. They may bind to receptors, causing hyperactivation or inhibition of normal activation. The explosion of knowledge in cell and molecular biology, including the mapping of the human genome, gene expression and transcription, cell-cycle regulation, enzyme polymorphisms, cytokines, transcription factors, and cascades of signaling molecules, has greatly increased the opportunity to understand toxicological mechanisms.

Metabolic and Cellular Poisons

Chemicals, such as cyanide, that interfere with cellular respiration are among the oldest known poisons. A chemical may cause enzyme inhibition by binding to a site on an enzyme, altering its three-dimensional structure, and distorting its active site(s) so that it is no longer functional. Some chemicals alter the structure or function of intracellular membranes, such as membranes of the endoplasmic reticulum or the mitochondria. For many toxic substances, swelling of the mitochondria, with loss of detailed structure, is an early histological sign of damage. Other chemicals, such as the hemolysins of certain snake venoms, cause lysis of cells. Some chemicals, especially metals, may bind to the sulfhydryl groups of the cell membrane protein, disrupting its structure and increasing membrane fluidity.

Enzyme Induction and Inhibition

The body does not maintain a complete inventory of all the enzymes that it may need. Some constitutive enzymes are always present, but most enzymes must be induced by introduction of their substrate; it may take up to 24 hours before there is sufficient enzyme to metabolize a xenobiotic completely. During this period, the amount of enzyme in a cell may increase by several orders of magnitude. Some enzyme systems are highly specific and act only on a single substrate; others are nonspecific, catalyzing reactions on a wide range of substrates. Conversely, different substrates vary in their potency at inducing enzymes. Induction of some enzymes can be accomplished, although with different efficiencies, by a range of substrates. CYP1A2 is induced by a variety of PAHs. Before its identity was known, it was referred to as aryl hydrocarbon hydroxylase, as its induction was triggered by compounds that bound to the aromatic hydrocarbon (Ah) receptor. Enzyme induction plays an important role in detoxification and excretion of xenobiotics. However, sometimes the most important consequence of enzyme induction is the greatly accelerated bioactivation of compounds.

Enzyme inhibition is a common mode of action for toxic substances. Both cyanide and hydrogen sulfide interfere with the function of cytochrome oxidase, thereby inhibiting oxidative phosphorylation that is necessary for cellular respiration. Heavy metals, which have a strong affinity for sulfur in proteins, are able to break the disulfide bridges that confer the tertiary structure necessary for normal function. Yet, because of differences in their atomic radius, different metals tend to inhibit different enzymes. For example, several enzymes in the pathway for making hemoglobin, such as delta-aminolevulinic acid dehydratase, are inhibited strongly by lead but only weakly by mercury.

Receptors

Advances in receptor biology are proceeding rapidly. Many toxic effects involve the binding of a xenobiotic or metabolite to a receptor, usually on a cell membrane. Receptors vary in their degree of specificity. Many hormone effects are mediated by attachment of the hormone to a specific receptor. Some endocrine-active substances act by binding to a receptor without initiating the appropriate response, thereby antagonizing hormonal effects. The effects of TCDD (dioxin) are partially mediated by binding to the Ah receptor. Related substances that bind to the Ah receptor have effects similar to TCDD but with vastly different dose–response curves due, in part, to their binding affinity. In animal studies, dioxin binds to estrogen receptors in the breast tissue, interfering with normal estrogenic stimuli and possibly reducing the likelihood of estrogen-stimulated breast cancer.

During normal function, a signal molecule binds to a receptor and initiates a response. After the signal molecule is removed or released from the receptor, another signal molecule may interact with receptor, causing a sustained response. Toxic compounds may bind to the receptor and not release, thereby blocking any further impulses and responses. For example, acetylcholine is a neurotransmitter that is secreted from the presynaptic terminal of parasympathetic nerve cell junctions. It rapidly diffuses across the gap and binds to special receptors on the postsynaptic nerve terminal, initiating a nerve impulse. Acetylcholine is then immediately deactivated by acetylcholinesterase. Some chemicals block the enzyme and others bind irreversibly to the receptor, in both cases preventing further nerve transmission.

Oxidative Stress and Free Radicals

Oxygen, essential to aerobic life, may also be highly toxic, because of its ability to alter molecules and change their function. Many bioactivation reactions involve oxidation. Normally, there is a balance between oxidative and antioxidant reactions. Oxidative reactions play important roles in inflammation, aging, carcinogenesis, and other aspects of toxicity. Research is discovering an increasing number of toxicants for which oxidative stress is an important mechanism. For example, chromium increases the formation of superoxide anion and nitric oxide in cells and enhances DNA single-strand breaks.

Toxicologists speak of reactive oxygen species, which are highly reactive molecules containing oxygen. Oxygen can receive an electron and form superoxide anion radical, which can, in turn, react with hydrogen to form hydrogen peroxide, which reacts with free electrons and hydrogen ion to form water and a highly reactive hydroxyl radical:

$$O\text{-}O + e\text{-} \longrightarrow O\text{-}O\text{-·} \text{ (superoxide radical)}$$

$$O\text{-}O\text{·} + e\text{-} + H^+ \longrightarrow H\text{-}O\text{-}O\text{-}H \text{ (hydrogen peroxide)}$$

$$H\text{-}O\text{-}O\text{-}H + e\text{-} + H^+ \longrightarrow H_2O + \text{·}OH \text{ (hydroxyl radical)}$$

In the course of these reactions, the highly reactive free radicals, especially the hydroxyl radical, are available to attack macromolecules, initiating a variety of toxic effects. The superoxide anion radical is formed in many oxidation reactions, where oxygen acts as an electron receptor. In response to the potential harm these reactive oxygen species may cause, the body has evolved antioxidant defenses, including water-soluble vitamin C and lipid-soluble vitamins E and A. Superoxide dismutase, a metalloprotein, and glutathione-dependent peroxidases, in association with glutathione reductase, serve to scavenge free radicals. Catalase catalyzes the conversion of hydrogen peroxide to water and oxygen.

A new area of interest is oxidative damage to proteins through the binding of oxygen to various sites on the protein, forming protein carbonyls. Oxidizers, such as reactive oxygen species and nitric oxide, can bind to proteins, altering their configuration and activity. Much of the toxicity attributed to nitric oxide may be caused by peroxynitrite, which is formed by the reaction between nitric oxide and another free radical species, superoxide anion. Peroxynitrite causes oxidative damage to lipids, DNA, and proteins. In general, the amount of oxidation correlates with aging and, in some cases, disease severity. Although oxidation is clearly involved in many chronic disease processes, in most cases it is not clear to what extent it plays a causative role in pathogenesis or is a result of the disease process.

One of the consequences of the formation of free radicals is reaction with unsaturated lipids, including those in cell and organelle membranes, to form lipid peroxides, which, in turn, lead to cell damage and dysfunction. Peroxyl radicals, which are also formed during lipid peroxidation, can react with other unsaturated lipid molecules to initiate additional lipid peroxidation. This chain reaction, initiated by a single free radical, can lead to formation of multiple molecules of peroxide. Some cytotoxicity of chlorinated hydrocarbons, such as carbon tetrachloride, is mediated by peroxidation of membrane lipids, which can be caused by a variety of reactive oxygen species. An active area of research involves identifying naturally occurring and synthetic compounds that interfere with lipid peroxidation.

Effects on Signal Transduction

Cell cycles are regulated by molecules that serve as signals to activate certain genes or receptors that influence the expression of other genes. Signal transduction pathways typically alter gene expression or modify gene products, either enhancing or inhibiting their function. Many endogenous signal chemicals, such as hormones and xenobiotics, can alter gene expression by activating transcription factors, which, in turn, promote the transcription of certain genes.

Adduct Formation via Covalent Binding to Macromolecules

Many chemicals react with and covalently bind to proteins and nucleic acids, forming stable adducts. DNA-repair enzymes may remove DNA adducts, but some adducts persist long enough to cause mutations during DNA replication. Adducts have been linked to cancer induction, and DNA adducts have been investigated as possible markers of exposure to genotoxicants or carcinogens. (Interpretation of the frequency of adducts, however, is difficult, partly due to variable rates of DNA repair. Some adducts are repaired within hours, while others persist.) Smokers have higher levels of benzo(a)pyrene

adducts to DNA than nonsmokers. DNA-protein cross-linking is promoted by a variety of genotoxic chemicals, including hexavalent chromium. Quantification of specific adducts has improved understanding of toxic mechanisms, but it has not yet proven useful for primary or secondary prevention of disease. In general, further study is needed to validate relationships between adducts and exposure and disease.

Genotoxicity

Genetic damage to germ cells (ova and sperm) may be heritable in offspring. Damage to somatic cells is not heritable, but it may lead to induction of cancer. Various chemicals and ionizing radiation damage nucleic acid directly or interfere with chromosomal replication and cell division. For example, even in the absence of anthropogenic sources, people are constantly bombarded with ionizing radiation from natural terrestrial and cosmic sources, almost all of which is quickly repaired.

Mutagens are substances that cause point mutations (replacement of one base nucleotide with another), chromosomal damage (breakage or translocations), or interference with meiosis, mitosis, or cell division. A variety of tests can measure chromosomal aberrations, aneuploidy, sister chromatid exchange, translocation, micronucleus formation, glycophorin A, and T-cell receptor genes. New genetic techniques allow sequencing of genes and detection of changes at a specific codon (sequence of three nucleotides).

Genetic analysis can reveal changes, such as GC or AT base pair substitutions, deletions, or duplications at a single gene locus in individuals. The relative frequency of the different mutations is influenced by dose and the conditions of exposure. While GC substitutions are more common in nonsmokers, there is an increased frequency of AT substitutions in smokers. After radiotherapy, there is a substantial increase in rearrangements and deletions that can persist for several years.

Genotoxic chemicals may cause mutation in proteins called *proto-oncogenes*, producing a mutant oncogene that encodes for a modification of the natural protein product. Some changes, such as that in the Ras proto-oncogene, increase cell susceptibility to cancer. The p21 protein (so-called because it has a mass of 21,000 daltons) binds with a receptor on the inner cell membrane and mediates responses to growth factors). Mutation at codon 13 "locks" the protein into the active form such that it no longer responds to other cell signals. With signal transduction impaired, this permanent activation is associated with malignant transformation and proliferation.

Another important phenomenon is the role of *tumor suppressor genes*, such as p53. Mutant forms of p53 allow unbridled cell proliferation. "Knockout mice," which lack p53, develop cancer at an early age. Some patients with hepatocellular carcinoma have a specific mutation at the 249th codon of the p53. The same mutation also occurs in people exposed to aflatoxin B1, suggesting that the toxin may cause liver cancer by this highly specific mutation.

Carcinogenesis

Carcinogenesis typically involves three steps: initiation, promotion, and proliferation. Many carcinogens exert direct action on DNA and are referred to as genotoxic, but others seem to cause or allow cancer without a direct genotoxic mode of action. *Initiation* is the stage during which genotoxic damage occurs. *Promotion* is the stage during which initiated cells are induced to undergo cell division by certain promoter compounds. *Proliferation* is the stage when unbridled and uncontrolled cell division occurs, accompanied by growth of blood vessels that supply the growing tumor. (See Chapter 21.)

Some scientists believe that there must be a threshold dose for cancer as there is for other toxic responses. Others argue that single-molecular events, such as mutations, can lead to cancer, so that, in the absence of a demonstrable threshold dose, one must assume that there is no threshold dose for cancer. Still others believe that there are likely to be threshold doses for some, but not all, carcinogens. In the light of the uncertainty, some governmental regulatory agencies have concluded that it is prudent, in the absence of evidence to the contrary, to assume that there is no threshold dose for carcinogens.

Apoptosis

Apoptosis, or programmed cell death, is a necessary part of the life history of most cell types.

Activation of apoptosis leads to expression of proteins that prepare the cell to die. This is followed by phagocytosis of apoptotic cells. The important feature of this natural form of cell death, compared with cytotoxicity, is that the former proceeds without invasion of inflammatory cells. Apoptosis is an essential phenomenon during development, allowing the remodeling of tissues. Apoptosis also selectively eliminates cells with damaged DNA and counters the clonal expansion of neoplastic cells. Inhibition of apoptosis, such as by estrogens, allows mutations to accumulate and tumor proliferation to occur. Hormone-dependent tumors expand when the hormone inhibits apoptosis, while an antiestrogenic drug, such as tamoxifen, allows apoptosis to occur. Conversely, the tumor-promoter phenobarbital inhibits apoptosis. Some chemicals appear to inhibit apoptosis, thereby enhancing the proliferative phase of carcinogenesis. Some new approaches to cancer chemotherapy focus on exploiting apoptosis to destroy tumor cells.

Immunotoxicity

Immunotoxins act by activating or suppressing the immune system. Some alter the expression of immunoglobulins, while others affect lymphocytes. T lymphocytes mature in the thymus and are the main factor in cell-mediated immunity. B lymphocytes are responsible for producing antibodies (humoral immunity). T cells are classified by their surface antigens, and techniques exist for quantifying types and subtypes of different T populations to identify which functions are depressed. Some agents interfere with the production, function, or lifespan of T and B lymphocytes.

Substances known to interfere with the immune system include (a) polyhalogenated aromatic compounds, such as dioxins; (b) metals, including mercury; (c) pesticides; and (d) air pollutants, such as particulate matter and oxides of nitrogen and sulfur. Tobacco smoke has constituents that are immunotoxic. Mercury causes autoimmune damage and glomerulonephritis in rats due to depletion of the $RT6^+$ subpopulation of T-lymphocytes.

Sensitizers or allergens induce hypersensitivity immune responses in sensitized individuals. The main target organs are the skin and the respiratory system. Nickel and poison-ivy (Rhus) contact dermatitis are common examples of such skin sensitization. (See Chapter 25.) Sensitization of the airways to airborne allergens in the workplace can cause occupational allergic rhinitis or asthma. (See Chapter 22.)

Reproductive Effects

The processes of gametogenesis, fertilization, implantation, embryogenesis, and organogenesis, and postnatal development are complex and subject to many environmental insults. Major errors incompatible with life generally result in spontaneous abortion (miscarriage), which can be viewed as a quality-control procedure. All stages are vulnerable to chemical hazards, including the failure to form gametes, such as azoospermia, and formation of abnormal gametes. Dibromochloropropane (DBCP), which causes testicular toxicity, can eliminate or reduce the number of sperm in semen. (See Box 24-1 in Chapter 24.) Many other chemicals, such as lead, have also been implicated in toxicity to the male reproductive system, including interfering with spermatogenesis, semen quality, erection, and libido. The list of chemicals affecting the female reproductive system includes cancer chemotherapeutic agents, other pharmaceuticals, metals, insecticides, and various industrial chemicals. (See Chapter 24.)

Endocrine Disruptors

For more than a decade, there has been an intense research and policy focus on endocrine disruption. Endocrine disruptors can mimic hormones, leading to overactive endocrine functions, or can bind with high affinity to endocrine receptors, thereby inhibiting normal endocrine functions.[11] Chemicals can lead to overexpression or underexpression of genes governing hormone or receptor synthesis, and chemicals can exert effects on target tissues influencing their response. The potency of these compounds is influenced by environmental persistence and bioamplification, bioavailability, and binding affinities. Endocrine disruption was well-recognized by the 1970s, when the ability of DDT to alter estrogen metabolism through enzyme induction was described. Although major concerns were then raised regarding the effect of chemicals on human reproductive function, adverse effects in a wide range of animals have since been clearly demonstrated, including effects on development, maturation, and reproduction, as well as cancer.[12]

Phytoestrogens, compounds in plants that have estrogenic activity, include a group of isoflavonoid and lignin polycyclic compounds. While there is concern about their interference with reproduction and development, their beneficial features are being exploited. One isoflavonoid, coumesterol, antagonizes estrogen during embryonic development, leading to reproductive abnormalities in behavior and hormone function. Others, such as genistein, protect against (a) certain hormone-dependent breast cancers by competing with estrogens and (b) other cancers by inhibiting proliferation, differentiation, or the vascular supply. The bioengineered yeast estrogen screen was developed as a screen for the endocrine disruptor action of xenobiotics.

Teratogenesis

Development from conception to birth involves a remarkable sequence of carefully timed interactions among cells through chemical signals, which results in the differentiation of a few primordial embryonic cells into different tissues and organs. Cells multiply, migrate, connect, and often die, to be replaced by other cells—a necessary part of complex developmental biology. Chemicals may interfere with morphogenesis in varying ways. They may inhibit necessary signals or alter the timing of signals so that cells migrate and differentiate before the appropriate time. The effect of a particular chemical depends on the stage of embryogenesis and fetogenesis, as well as dose. Different chemicals cross the placental barrier with different efficiencies.

Chemicals may have no effect, produce subclinical alterations, or cause major birth defects or fetal death. For example, some effects on the developing nervous system from lead or methylmercury may disrupt the migration, maturation, and connections of nerve cells, leading to a viable infant with cognitive impairment. This impairment may only be apparent when the child has learning difficulties in school or is subjected to psychometric testing. Recognition of this phenomenon has given rise to the field of *behavioral teratology*, which focuses on studying the impact of fetal exposure to lead or alcohol on development and behavior.

Approximately 3% of live births have detectable congenital abnormalities, usually with no known cause. In general, the endpoint of toxic exposure prior to implantation is likely to be lethality. Exposures that cause toxicity during organogenesis can cause birth defects or embryolethality. Later in fetal life, toxic exposures can cause intrauterine growth retardation, fetal death, or functional changes that interfere with birth or postnatal development.

TOXICOLOGIC CONSIDERATIONS IN CLINICAL EVALUATION

Occupational and environmental exposures to toxic chemicals occur frequently, and adverse health effects are not rare. Clinicians are frequently confronted by patients who have symptoms that the patients ascribe to, or suspect are caused by, some chemical or event. It is easy for a clinician to be skeptical, especially when histories are complex and exposures uncertain. However, an initial high index of suspicion is often necessary to determine that an illness is caused by occupational or environmental factors. Many chemical exposures have both specific endpoints (such as bone marrow depression due to benzene) and nonspecific endpoints (such as lightheadedness due to benzene). Some effects are acute, whereas others develop only after long periods of exposure.

First, one must establish whether the reported symptoms are typical of, or even likely to be associated with, the putative exposure. If not, one is likely to look for a different causal explanation, which may often be a different chemical or biologic agent. *General causation* is the methodology of determining whether a specific chemical or other agent can cause a specific adverse health effect. (See Appendix to Chapter 4.)

Second, one must establish exposure. A careful history can often confirm exposure. (See Chapter 4.) If exposure is recent or ongoing, clinical testing may reveal a biomarker of exposure. In addition, environmental measurements can be made to document the presence of the chemical. However, often many months—and many physician visits—have passed before the

patient reaches a clinician who understands occupational and environmental disease. (By this time, the trail may be cold and only the history is available to provide information.) The clinician must then determine whether the specific individual's illness was due to this chemical (special causation).

For toxicity due to metals, one can often use chelation to help determine specific causation, given the propensity of metals to bind to sulfhydryl (–SH) groups. A variety of drugs with high concentrations of sulfur can be used to circulate through the body and bind any metal encountered. This can be used in a provocative mode to try to extract stored metal from prior exposures. A baseline urine measurement is obtained; then the chelator is administered (usually intramuscularly or intravenously, although some oral medications, such as DMSA, are now available). Urine is then measured, usually at 12-, 24-, and 72-hour intervals. If there is an excessive body burden of the metal, there should be a rapid increase in excretion of the metal, followed by a gradual return to baseline. Although chelation can be useful, it is more often misused by clinicians, who fail to obtain a baseline and then compare the concentration in the provoked urine to standard levels for unprovoked urine—resulting in false-positive results.

Biomarkers

A *biomarker* is a substance that can be measured, usually in blood or urine, to provide information about exposure or pathophysiologic responses to toxic substances (Box 7-2). There are numerous applications of biomarkers in estimating internal dose. They can be defined as endpoints in a dose–response assessment. Some biomarkers reflect exposure, some reflect damage, and some can identify susceptibility. DNA adducts are biomarkers of exposure to carcinogens or mutagens; the carcinogenic polyaromatic hydrocarbon, benzo[a]pyrene, forms a specific adduct with DNA. Although adduct formation is believed to be part of carcinogenesis, and smokers who have high exposure to benzo[a]pyrene have an increased rate of adduct formation, this marker has not had sufficient predictive value to support widespread use. Familiar biomarkers include blood lead level (a biomarker of exposure) and

---

Box 7-2. Illustrative Examples of Biomarkers

Biomarkers of Exposure (in Body Fluids)

Specific chemical agents, such as blood lead level

Metabolites, such as urinary hippuric acid, a metabolite of toluene

DNA adducts

Biomarkers of Effect

Male reproductive disorders

Sperm motility

Semen quality

Müllerian-inhibiting factor

Chromosomal aberrations

Female reproductive disorders

Chorionic gonadotropin assay

Urinary progesterone metabolites

Pulmonary disorders

Pulmonary function

Airway reactivity (challenge tests)

Pulmonary cytology

Immunology disorders

Immunoglobulin levels

Lymphocyte ratios (T and B cells)

T-helper cells

T-suppressor cells

Natural killer cells

Lymphocyte functional assays

T-cell-dependent antibody response

Plaque-forming assays

Lymphocyte proliferation tests

Interleukin-2 activity

Specific receptor expression assays

Macrophage/leukocyte respiratory burst response

Lead poisoning

Zinc or erythrocyte protoporphyrin

---

zinc protoporphyrin (a biomarker of effect from lead exposure). (The Committee on Biological Markers of the National Research Council has published monographs on markers in pulmonary toxicology, reproductive toxicology, urinary toxicology, and immunotoxicology.)

TOXICITY TESTING

A wide variety of systems and paradigms are used to test chemicals to predict their effects on human health or the environment. Under the Toxic Substances Control Act, new chemicals must undergo extensive safety testing. It is important to select the appropriate animal model or in vitro test system and to have well-chosen controls, which can include positive controls (those known to readily manifest a specific endpoint). Animal researchers need to choose the appropriate species, genetic strain, gender, and age as well as exposure route. The dosage schedule may be single or multiple. It may be acute, subchronic, or chronic. Duration of a study should be longer than the longest expected latency period. Dosages must be chosen to span the suspected threshold, if one is thought to exist. The route of administration should be relevant to natural conditions of exposure.

Toxicity testing must be subject to good quality-assurance and quality-control procedures. *Quality*

assurance includes using trained (and, in some cases, certified) personnel, buying and maintaining appropriate equipment and standards, maintaining laboratory hygiene and avoiding cross-contamination, documenting procedures, maintaining records, and participating in interlaboratory testing programs. *Quality control* refers to laboratory procedures of calibration using blanks and known standards, as well as running replicate samples and analyzing spiked samples (those to which a known quantity of a specific chemical has been added).

Good laboratory practices describe animal care, dosing, and data management. Many commercial laboratories have been found to have faulty laboratory procedures, especially for documenting exposure, side effects, and outcomes.

The National Toxicology Program (NTP), which is operated by the National Institute of Environmental Health Sciences, sponsors long-term rodent studies to detect the carcinogenic and other toxic properties of chemicals. Chemicals are selected on the basis of data needs of governmental agencies and in response to public input. The standard protocol utilizes two species (rat and mouse), both sexes, and a minimum of 50 individuals for each category, with oral dosing over a 2-year "lifespan." These 2-year bioassays can provide information on metabolism; genetic, reproductive, and developmental toxicity; and toxic effects on various organ systems. National Toxicology Program bioassays screen new chemicals for carcinogenic activity and classify them with respect to human carcinogenicity. However, their main application has been to provide tumor incidence data in risk assessment.

ANIMAL WELFARE AND ANIMAL RIGHTS

Animal studies have played an important role in human toxicology and in the development of drugs that are safe for humans and for animals as well. Advances in toxicology have included the exploration of alternative testing procedures, including reducing the number of animals, using animals other than mammals, and developing in vitro techniques. Toxicologists have become increasingly attentive to animal welfare, due to (a) the recognition that reducing stress for animals makes them more reliable subjects and (b) pressure from animal-rights activists, who assert that animals have intrinsic rights that, in the extreme, should protect them from any and all use in experimental research. The Animal Welfare Act, administered by the Animal and Plant Health Inspection Service of the U.S. Department of Agriculture, applies to all mammals, except mice and rats. Toxicologists generally agree that experimental animals should not be exposed to unnecessary stress, discomfort, or pain. Researchers using animals must consider animal-care guidelines. Most universities and other animal-testing organizations have animal-use committees that review all research protocols to minimize unnecessary stress and pain, inspect conditions under which animals are kept, and assure availability of veterinary care.

The concern over animal welfare reaches its peak when primates are used. Primates are expensive to acquire and maintain. Most primate studies can afford only a few animals that often live under unnatural and extremely stressful conditions. The capturing of many primates for medical research and industrial applications has had a drastic impact on the survival of several species in the wild.

The assumption that primates are the best models for humans makes sense, when cognitive performance is studied, but it does not take into account great differences in diet, since most primates are primarily herbivorous, or the importance of social organization. Thus, extrapolation from primates to humans is not always more appropriate than extrapolation from other animal models. Statistical interpretation of primate research is thwarted by small sample sizes, and, in some cases, by reuse of the same animals in sequential experiments. Over the past two decades, many primate laboratories have been closed, and, with few exceptions, primate research can be expected to play a diminishing role in future toxicological research.

ACKNOWLEDGMENT

The authors wish to thank Helmut Zarbl, PhD, and Lauren Aleksunes, PhD, for their contributions to preparation of this chapter.

REFERENCES

1. Gallo MA. History and scope of toxicology. In: Klaassen C (ed.). Cassarett and Doull's toxicology: The basic science of poisons (8th ed.). New York: McGraw Hill, 2013, pp. 3–11.

2. Umbreit TH, Hesse EJ, Gallo MA. Bioavailability and cytochrome P-450 induction from 2,3,7,8-tetrachlorodibenzo-P-dioxin contaminated soils from Times Beach, Missouri, and Newark, New Jersey. Drug and Chemical Toxicology 1988; 11: 405–418.

3. Douglas H. Science, hormesis and regulation. Human Experimental Toxicology 2008; 27: 603–607.

4. Eaton DL, Bammler TK, Kelly EJ. Interindividual differences in response to chemoprotection against aflatoxin-induced hepatocarcinogenesis: Implication for human biotransformation enzyme polymorphisms. Advances in Experimental Medicine and Biology 2001; 500: 559–576.

5. Gochfeld M. Sex differences in human and animal toxicology: Toxicokinetics. Toxicologic Pathology 2017; 45: 172–189.

6. Iba MM, Scholl H, Fung J, et al. Induction of pulmonary CYP1A1 by nicotine. Xenobiotica 1998; 28: 827–843.

7. Green E. Charting a course for genomic medicine from base pairs to bedside. Nature 2011; 470: 204–213.

8. Haldane JBS. Heredity and politics. New York: Norton, 1938.

9. Stokinger HE, Mountain JT. Progress in detecting the worker hypersusceptible to industrial chemicals. Journal of Occupational Medicine 1967; 9: 537–542.

10. Hammond EC, Selikoff IJ, Seidman H. Asbestos exposure, cigarette smoking and death rates. Annals of the New York Academy of Sciences 1979; 330: 473–490.

11. Colburn T, Dumanoski D, Myers TJ. Our stolen future. New York: Dutton, 1996.

12. Miyamoto J, Burger J. Implications of endocrine active substances for humans and wildlife. SCOPE/IUPAC Conference. Pure and Applied Chemistry 2003; 75: 1617–2615.

FURTHER READING

Agency for Toxic Substances and Disease Registry, Centers for Disease Control and Prevention. Toxicological profiles. Available at: http://www.atsdr.cdc.gov/toxpro2.html
Exhaustive monographs and reviews of over 200 chemicals most commonly found at "Superfund sites."

ACGIH. Threshold limit values for chemical substances and physical agents, & biological exposure indices. Cincinnati, OH: ACGIH, 2017. *Provides threshold limit values and short-term exposure limits for a long list of commonly encountered industrial chemicals. Updated biennially. The 1969 list was adopted as OSHA standards by reference, and OSHA has been able to update only a few.*

Barceloux DG. Medical toxicology of natural substances. Hoboken, NJ: Wiley, 2009. *A compendium on the toxicology of natural plant and animal toxins.*

Brooks S, Gochfeld M, Herzstein J, et al. Environmental medicine. St Louis, MO: Mosby, 1995. *Introduction to the clinical and exposure aspects of toxicology.*

Environmental Protection Agency. Integrated risk information system web site. Available at: http://www.epa.gov/iriswebp/iris/index.html *Reference doses and documentation of literature reviewed by the EPA.*

Greenberg MR, Hamilton P, McClusky GJ. Occupational, industrial, and environmental toxicology. St. Louis, MO: Mosby, 2003. *Valuable chapters on industrial chemicals.*

Klaassen CD (ed.). Casarett and Doull's toxicology: The basic science of poisons (8th ed.). New York: McGraw-Hill Education, 2013. *A textbook for toxicology students with detailed coverage of toxicokinetics and toxicodynamics and mechanisms of toxicity as well as organ systems and groups of chemicals.*

McQueen CA (ed.). Comprehensive toxicology (2nd ed.). Kidlington, UK: Elsevier, 2010. *A comprehensive 14-volume set reference on toxicology.*

Mendelsohn ML, Mohr LC, Peeters JP. Biomarkers: Medical and workplace applications. Washington, DC: Joseph Henry Press, 1998. *Many papers describing different applications and the strengths and limitations of biomarkers.*

National Institute for Occupational Safety and Health. NIOSH pocket guide to chemical hazards. Available at: http://www.cdc.gov/niosh/npg/npg.html. *Concise information on different toxicity levels recommended by NIOSH (more protective than OSHA standards), including levels Immediately Dangerous to Life and Health.*

National Institute for Occupational Safety and Health. NIOSH Publications and Products. Available at: http://www.cdc.gov/niosh/database.html *A collection of databases on toxicity, workplace hazards, industrial hygiene methods, and protective equipment.*

Plog BA, Quinlan PJ. Fundamentals of industrial hygiene (6th ed.). Itasca, IL: National Safety Council, 2012. *More than the fundamentals of industrial hygiene, including the anticipation, recognition, control, and evaluation of exposure to workplace hazards.*

Sheehan HE, Wedeen RP. Toxic circles: Environmental hazards from the workplace into the community. New Brunswick, NJ: Rutgers Press, 1993. *Eight detailed case studies on occupational toxicology problems.*

Sullivan JB, Krieger GR. Clinical environmental health and toxic exposures (2nd ed.). Philadelphia: Lippincott, 2001. *Readable chapters on toxicology with an emphasis on environmental exposures.*

8

Occupational and Environmental Hygiene

John D. Meeker

Occupational hygiene (industrial hygiene) is the environmental science of anticipating, recognizing, evaluating, and controlling health hazards in the working environment with the objectives of protecting workers' health and well-being and safeguarding the community at large. It encompasses the prevention of acute and chronic health conditions due to hazards posed by physical, chemical, and biological agents, as well as stress in the occupational environment and concern for the outdoor environment.

Environmental hygiene is the science of anticipating, recognizing, evaluating (including conducting surveillance), and controlling health hazards in the general environment with the objectives of protecting health and well-being for individuals and communities. Environmental hygiene, which is discussed in more detail later in this chapter, includes the traditional environmental health components of public health—such as sanitation, waste management, and controlling contamination of air, water, and soil—as well as the newer problems of trace residues of hazardous chemicals in drinking water and food (Chapters 16 and 17), global climate change (Chapter 29), and the built environment (Chapter 34).

An occupational hygienist, for example, determines the composition and concentrations of air contaminants in a workplace where there have been complaints of eye, nose, and throat irritation and determines whether the contaminant exposures exceed the Occupational Safety and Health Administration (OSHA) permissible exposure limit or other national limits. If the problem is new and appears to be the result of airborne materials, which might be determined in consultation with a physician or an epidemiologist, then the hygienist would be responsible for selecting (a) the techniques used to reduce or eliminate the exposure, such as installing exhaust ventilation around the source of the air contaminants and isolating it from the general work area, and (b) performing follow-up sampling to verify that the controls were effective.

Most occupational hygienists have earned either a bachelor's degree in science or engineering and/or a master of science degree in industrial hygiene. Occupational hygienists tend to specialize in specific technical areas because the scope of the field is wide. Occupational hygienists must work with physicians and/or nurses to develop comprehensive occupational health programs and with epidemiologists to perform research on adverse health effects. It has been traditional to separate occupational hygiene and occupational safety, but the recent trend has been to broaden the training for each discipline to include that of the other. This has led to the specialty of risk management for evaluating and controlling all types of workplace hazards. At present, occupational hygienists generally do not deal with mechanical hazards or job activities that can cause physical injuries, which are the responsibility of safety specialists. However, it is not uncommon for private companies to have a single individual responsible for both occupational hygiene and safety who has no formal training in either area. In some companies, there has also been a new trend for occupational hygienists to lead or be involved with environmental health and sustainability, worker wellness, product safety and stewardship, emergency and disaster planning and response, and even security.

Most occupational hygienists work for large companies, consulting firms, academic institutions, or governmental agencies. A small number work for labor unions. For whomever they work, occupational hygienists unfortunately are often located in organizational units where they have little organizational power to bring about necessary changes. For example, hygienists who work for labor unions may be restricted in their access to the workplace for sampling and exposure measurements, which can limit their ability to assess and control hazards.

The closeness of working relationships between occupational hygienists and physicians or nurses varies. Some have close collaborative activities with an extensive exchange of information, while others operate with nearly complete independence and have little more than formal contact. A physician who is familiar with the workplace, job activities, and health status of workers in all parts of the process may be very helpful in guiding the occupational hygienist in assessing environmental hazards and vice versa. Within a framework of multidisciplinary approaches, occupational hygienists and physicians should collaborate with safety specialists, workers in production units, staff members in personnel departments, worker representatives, and delegates of the health and safety committees. Where contact among these groups is minimal, many opportunities are lost for improving the effectiveness of health hazard control and the prevention of adverse effects. (See Chapter 10.)

Occupational hygiene should be integrated into an overall program for occupational health, without which the effectiveness of intervention strategies may be limited. An effective occupational hygiene program must have good working relationships with the production, personnel, and health and safety departments and strong support by upper management. Core activities of hazard anticipation, recognition, evaluation, and control must be well integrated with the day-to-day activities of the enterprise. There is no single organizational structure that is optimal.

ANTICIPATION, RECOGNITION, EVALUATION, AND CONTROL OF HAZARDS

Formal strategies for workplace assessment have not been well developed. However, the American Industrial Hygiene Association has published a monograph on exposure assessment, titled *A Strategy for Assessing and Managing Occupational Exposure* (see Further Reading), which is widely used in the United States.

In the European Union (EU), regulations now require workplace assessment to identify occupational hazards, but no formal mechanism has been established or validated to demonstrate its consistency. It is expected that EU regulations, when fully implemented, will be beneficial to small and medium-sized enterprises because they will create awareness and an expectation of controlling the problems identified.

In 2007, the EU began to implement REACH, an ambitious new regulation that addresses the *r*egistration, *e*valuation, *a*uthorization, and restriction of *c*hemical substances. (It is being phased in over an 11-year period ending in 2018.) Although not designed as an occupational health assessment, REACH aims to improve the safe handling of hazardous chemicals, requires manufacturers and importers of chemicals to compile more detailed information on the properties of substances and register this information in a centralized database, which is accessible to professionals and consumers. A requirement of

REACH is progressive substitution of the most hazardous chemicals once suitable alternatives are identified.

Anticipation

Anticipation of hazards has become an important responsibility of the occupational hygienist. Anticipation refers to the application and mastery of knowledge that permits the occupational hygienist to foresee the potential for disease and injury. The occupational hygienist should thus be involved at an early stage in planning of technology, process development, and workplace design. Consider the following example:

An electronics company was developing a new process for making computer chips. The process involved dissolving a photographic masking agent in toluene and then spraying the mask on a large surface covered with chips. The company's occupational hygienist noted that this would expose the workers to potentially high airborne levels of toluene. She suggested they substitute xylene, which has a lower vapor pressure, and modify the process to use smaller amounts of solvent, which would reduce the amount of hazardous waste generated by the process.

It is common that process engineers or industrial researchers will propose using hazardous materials or will not consider the interaction of the worker and the process or machine. Consequently, hygienists can prevent many problems that will be expensive to fix after installation by reviewing early plans and findings of pilot plant experiments.

Identification of hazards may be most easily accomplished using an overview of the production process that describes the complete flow from raw material to final product. Production can be subdivided into its component unit processes. In this stepwise fashion, the processes with hazards can be recognized, worker exposures evaluated, and exposures in nearby areas assessed. Examples of some common unit processes and their hazards are shown in Table 8-1. This general approach and the hazards of a wide range of common industrial processes are discussed in more detail in William Burgess's *Recognition of Health Hazards in Industry: A Review of Materials and Processes* (see Further Reading).

This approach can be illustrated by considering a small company that manufactures toolboxes from sheets of steel by a six-step process: (1) sheets of steel are cut into the specified shape, (2) sharp edges and burrs are removed by grinding, (3) sheets are formed into boxes with a sheet metal bender, (4) box joints are spot welded, (5) boxes are cleaned in a vapor degreaser in preparation for painting, and (6) boxes are painted in a spray booth. Production steps 2, 4, 5, and 6 use unit processes with known sources of airborne emissions, and their hazards (Table 8-1) should be evaluated. Exposures of workers involved with steps 1 and 3 may need to be evaluated because they may be located near enough to the operations with hazards to have significant exposure. Additional hazards may also be present depending on the specific processes and equipment used in the various steps. For example, worker exposures to nonionizing radiation and metal fumes may need to be considered if a high-powered laser is used to cut the steel in step 1. (See Chapter 12D.)

The design of job tasks and an individual's work habits can both have an important influence on exposures. For example, a furnace tender's exposure to metal fumes will depend on the length of tools used to scrape slag away from the tapping hole in the furnace and on the instructions for performing the task. Lack of adequate tools or sufficient operating instructions may cause excessive exposure to fumes emitted by molten materials. Similarly, the furnace tender, who is positioned close to the slag as it runs out of the furnace, may receive a much higher exposure to fume than a coworker who stands farther away from the molten slag. Therefore, an important part of an evaluation is the observation of work practices used in hazardous unit processes.

Recognition

Recognition of problems in a new or unfamiliar workplace generally requires that the occupational hygienist engage in collection of background information on production layout, processes, and raw materials. This usually begins with a visit to the workplace to become familiar with the production processes and their hazards. These visits are crucial for detecting unique aspects of the workplace that may strongly affect exposures.

Table 8-1. Common Unit Processes and Associated Hazards by Route of Entry*

Unit Process	Route of Entry and Hazard
Abrasive Blasting	
Surface treatment with high-velocity materials, such as sand, steel shot, pecan shells, glass, or aluminum oxide	Inhalation: silica, metal, and paint dust Noise
Acid/Alkali Treatments	
Dipping metal parts in open baths to remove oxides, grease, oil, and dirt	Inhalation: acid mist with dissolved metals
Acid pickling (with hydrochloric acid, nitric acid, sulfuric acid, chromic acid, or a mixture of nitric acid and hydrogen fluoride)	Skin contact: burns and corrosion, hydrofluoric acid toxicity Inhalation: nitrogen dioxide, acid mists
Molten caustic descaling	Inhalation: smoke and vapors Skin contact: burns
Blending and Mixing	
Powders and/or liquid are mixed to form products, or undergo reactions	Inhalation: dusts and mists of toxic materials Skin contact: toxic materials
Cleaning	
Application of cleansers, solvents, and strong detergents to clean surfaces and articles; and operation of devices to aid cleaning such as floor washers, waxers, polishers, and vacuums	Inhalation: dust, vapors Skin contact: defatting agents, solvents, strong bases
Crushing and Sizing	
Mechanically reducing the particle size of solids and sorting larger from smaller with screens or cyclones	Inhalation: dusts and mists of toxic materials Noise
Degreasing	
Removing grease, oil, and dirt from metal and plastic with solvents and cleaners	Inhalation: vapors Skin contact: dermatitis and absorption
Cold solvent washing (clean parts with ketones, cellosolves, and aliphatic, aromatic, and stoddard solvents)	Fire and explosion (if flammable) Metabolic: carbon monoxide formed from methylene chloride
Vapor degreasers (with trichloroethylene, methyl chloroform, ethylene dichloride, and certain fluorocarbon compounds)	Inhalation: vapors; thermal degradation may form phosgene, hydrogen chloride, and chlorine gases Skin contact: dermatitis and absorption
Electroplating	
Coating metals, plastics, and rubber with thin layers of metals, such as copper, chromium, cadmium, gold, or silver	Inhalation: acid mists, hydrogen cyanide, alkali mists, chromium, nickel, cadmium mists Skin contact: acids, alkalis Ingestion: cyanide compounds
Forging	
Deforming hot or cold metal by presses or hammering	Inhalation: hydrocarbons in smoke (hot processes), including polyaromatic hydrocarbons, sulfur dioxide, carbon monoxide, oxides of nitrogen, and metals sprayed on dies, such as lead and molybdenum Heat stress Noise
Furnace Operations	
Melting and refining metals; boilers for steam generation	Inhalation: metal fumes, combustion gases, such as sulfur dioxide and carbon monoxide Noise from burners Heat stress Cataracts from infrared radiation

(continued)

Table 8-1. (Continued)

Unit Process	Route of Entry and Hazard
Grinding, Polishing, and Buffing	
An abrasive is used to remove or shape metal or other material	Inhalation: toxic dusts from both metals and abrasives Vibration from hand tools Noise
Industrial Radiography	
X-ray or gamma ray sources used to examine parts of equipment	Radiation exposure
Machining	
Metals, plastics, or wood are worked or shaped with lathes, drills, planers, or milling machines	Inhalation: airborne particles, cutting oil mists, toxic metals, nitrosamines formed in some water-based cutting oils, endotoxin Skin contact: cutting oils, solvents, sharp chips Noise
Materials Handling and Storage	
Conveyors, forklift trucks are used to move materials to/from storage	Inhalation: carbon monoxide, exhaust particulate, dusts from conveyors, emissions from spills or broken containers
Mining	
Drilling, blasting, mucking to remove loose material, and material transport	Inhalation: silica dust, nitrogen dioxide from blasting, gases from mine can lead to low oxygen levels Explosion hazards from methane and airborne combustible dusts Vibration stress Heat stress Noise
Painting and Spraying	
Applications of liquids to surfaces, such as paints, pesticides, coatings	Inhalation: solvents as mists and vapors, toxic materials Skin contact: solvents, toxic materials
Repair and Maintenance	
Servicing malfunctioning equipment; cleaning production equipment and control systems	Inhalation: dusts, vapors, and gases from the operation Skin contact: grease, oil, solvents
Quality Control	
Collection of production samples, performance of test procedures that produce emissions	Inhalation: dusts, vapors, and gases Skin contact: solvents
Soldering	
Joining metals with molten lead or silver alloys	Inhalation: lead or cadmium particulate (fumes) and flux fumes
Welding and Metal Cutting	
Joining or cutting metals by heating them to molten or semi-molten state Arc or resistance welding Flame cutting and welding Brazing	Inhalation: metal fumes, toxic gases and materials, flux particulate Noise from burner Eye and skin damage from infrared and ultraviolet radiation

* Health hazards may also depend on the toxicity and physical form of the materials used. For further information, see Burgess WA. Recognition of health hazards in industry: A review of materials and processes (2nd ed.). New York: John Wiley & Sons, 1995.

Information is collected on:

- Types, composition, and quantities of substances and materials, including raw materials, intermediate products, and additives
- Design of work processes and tasks
- Emission sources
- Design and capacity of ventilation systems or other control measures.

Flow visualization with smoke tubes (glass tubes with a packing that produces dense white smoke when air is forced through it) can give qualitative information on effectiveness of local exhausts or process ventilation. Work practices, worker position relative to sources, and task duration can be recorded. Information can be collected on cleaning routines and performance as well as tidiness, often termed *housekeeping*, which are important determinants of exposure. Consider the following example:

Farmworkers were experiencing episodes of depressed blood cholinesterase levels from organophosphate exposure despite their observing the required waiting times before reentry into sprayed fields and wearing long-sleeved shirts and gloves to prevent skin contact. The pesticide had a very low vapor pressure so there was no significant inhalation exposure. However, it was known that environmental moisture decomposes this type of pesticide. Since the weather was very dry during these episodes, there was concern that the pesticide was not decomposing as rapidly as expected. Consequently, despite the skin protection, there could still be sufficient skin absorption of the pesticide to depress cholinesterase levels. Skin sampling with patches showed that fine dust was sifting through the cloth of the shirt sleeves and depositing much pesticide on workers' arms. The problem was solved by extending the standard reentry times.

If the initial appraisal cannot definitely rule out a hazard, a basic survey has to be performed to provide quantitative information about exposure of workers. Particular account has to be taken of tasks with high exposure. Sources of information are as follows:

- Earlier measurements
- Measurements from comparable installations or work processes

- Reliable calibrations or modeling based on relevant quantitative data
- Air sampling measurements to determine the range of exposures.

Sampling may show that sensory impressions underestimate or overestimate exposures; for example, the odor threshold for most solvents is well below the level at which they present a toxic exposure hazard.

If this information is insufficient to enable valid comparisons to be made with the limit values, a full-scale survey must be performed. The full-scale survey examines all phases of workplace activities—both normal activities and abnormal or infrequent ones, such as maintenance, reactor cleaning, or simulation of malfunctions. The survey activities may take several weeks or months in a complex manufacturing or chemical plant.

Evaluation

For the evaluation of recognized or suspected hazards, the hygienist uses techniques based on the nature of the hazards, emission sources, and the routes of environmental contact with the worker. For example, air sampling can show the concentration of toxic particulates, gases, and vapors that workers may inhale; skin wipes can be used to measure the degree of skin contact with toxic materials that may penetrate the skin; biological samples (blood or urine) can sometimes provide data where there are multiple routes of entry; and noise dosimeters record and electronically integrate workplace noise levels to determine total daily exposure. Both acute and chronic exposures should be considered in the evaluation because they may be associated with different types of adverse health effects.

The workplace is not a static environment: Exposures may change by orders of magnitude over short distances from exposure sources, such as welding, and over short time intervals because of intermittent source output or incomplete mixing of air contaminants. In addition, operations and materials used or produced commonly change, as do job titles and definitions. The nature of these changes and their possible effects on exposure and health must be recognized and taken into consideration by the occupational hygienist.

All monitoring programs for both acute and long-term problems should be structured with a clear focus on the individual's sources of exposures and the ultimate objective to estimate dose. Monitoring organized solely around compliance with today's standards will probably be unable to answer tomorrow's questions about hazards associated with personal exposures. Adverse health effects can be associated with exposures below regulatory standards that were set decades ago. The effects of environmental controls, such as ventilation and personal protective equipment that intervene between the emission source and the worker, must also be considered.

The occupational hygienist's decision on whether a hazard is present is based on three sources of information:

1. Scientific literature and various health-based exposure limits, such as (a) the threshold limit values (TLVs) of ACGIH, a set of consensus standards developed by occupational hygienists, toxicologists, and physicians from governmental agencies and academic institutions; (b) World Health Organization (WHO) recommendations; and (c) National Institute for Occupational Safety and Health (NIOSH) health-based recommended exposure limits for select agents (considered by OSHA in standard-setting processes).
2. The legal requirements of OSHA and regulatory agencies of other countries.[1] In many instances, OSHA limits are less stringent than TLVs because (a) TLVs are updated more often and (b) OSHA limits must also consider technical and economic feasibility of controlling the exposures below limits.
3. Problems identified by other health professionals who have examined exposed workers and evaluated their health status.

In cases where health effects are present but exposures do not exceed the TLVs, WHO or NIOSH recommended limits, or OSHA or other national requirements, prudent hygienists and others may conclude that there is a relationship between adverse health effects and workplace exposures if evidence supports such a relationship. Exposure limits are designed to prevent adverse effects in most exposed workers, but they are not absolute levels below which adverse effects cannot occur. The supporting data for many exposure limits are sometimes insufficient, out of date, or based too much on evidence of acute toxic effects and not enough on evidence of carcinogenicity, mutagenicity, teratogenicity, or other chronic or delayed-onset conditions.

Control

Once a hazard is identified and the extent of the problem evaluated, the hygienist next designs a control strategy or plan to reduce exposure to an acceptable level. Such controls may have two phases, an immediate response with personal protective equipment (PPE) to quickly reduce the hazard and an engineering follow-up to control the problem more effectively, including:

1. Changing the industrial process or the materials used to eliminate the source of the hazard, such as changing to clean technologies
2. Isolating the source and installing engineering controls, such as ventilation systems
3. Using administrative controls to limit the duration of exposure a worker receives, or, as a final resort, requiring the development of a formal program for the prolonged use of PPE. Administrative controls are less reliable because they depend on enforcement by managers and conscientious application by workers.

In designing control strategies, one should also consider the environmental impact (outside the occupational setting) of emissions, waste, storage, spills, and leaks. Action can be taken at the levels of processes, materials, components, systems, and the entire workplace. Education of workers and supervisors is essential. Both workers and supervisors must understand the nature of hazards and support efforts to control or eliminate the hazards. Implementation of control measures should be supervised and their efficacy evaluated.

CASE

Automobile manufacturers have been concerned about the hazards of coolants used in machining and grinding operations. Workers have complained of skin and inhalation problems associated with exposures to liquids splashed on their skin and to airborne mists that they breathe. In the past, controls were implemented based on hypotheses about causal factors, without investigations of specific causes for exposures. Some hypotheses were later found to be incorrect and control was incomplete, despite substantial expenditures. Inhalation exposures were only partially controlled by local exhaust ventilation and by enclosure of processes. Exposures were found to be associated with symptoms and reduced pulmonary function. Analysis of coolants revealed that safety data sheets (SDSs) were inaccurate, and the machining department did not know about some of the hazardous materials that were being used. Investigations are ongoing to determine what additional controls will be needed to further reduce the exposures, including substitution of components in coolants and better control of microbial contaminants with filtration and other techniques.

This case demonstrates that controlling hazards in large, complex manufacturing operations is very frequently a stepwise process. Control strategies are most effective when based on complete knowledge of the nature of problems.

After hazards are controlled, the hygienist may recommend a hazard surveillance program to ensure that controls remain adequate. Material components of inexpensive raw materials can change without notice, thereby generating problems. This type of environmental surveillance is most effective when performed with a medical surveillance program designed to detect subtle health effects that may occur at low levels of exposure.

The following sections illustrate how assessment and control techniques are utilized. The approach for toxic materials is used as a paradigm, which can also be used for other environmental hazards, including noise, vibration, ionizing and non-ionizing radiation, temperature extremes, poor lighting, and infectious agents.

TOXIC MATERIALS

Exposure Pathways

The health hazard of a given exposure to a toxic material depends on the toxicity of the substance and on the intensity and duration of contact with the substance. Thus, adverse effects can result from chronic low-level exposure to a substance or from a short-term exposure to a dangerously high concentration of it. However, the pharmacologic mechanisms for acute and chronic effects may differ. Occupational hygienists are concerned with both long-term, low-level exposures and brief acute exposures.

In assessing a given hazardous material, the hygienist determines the route of exposure by which workers contact it and by which it may enter their bodies. There are four major routes of exposure: (a) direct contact with skin or eyes; (b) inhalation, with absorption or deposition in the upper or lower respiratory tract; (c) inhalation of particulate substances, with deposition in the upper respiratory tract and subsequent ingestion; and (d) direct ingestion from eating or drinking. In the workplace, several concurrent routes of exposure may occur for a toxic substance.

Inhalation of airborne particulates, vapors, or gases is, by far, the most common route of hazardous occupational exposure and therefore occupies much of a hygienist's assessment and control activities. Skin absorption may be important if the substance is lipid soluble or the skin's barrier is damaged or otherwise compromised. Ingestion of contaminated food and drink is a problem, especially for particulate and liquid materials, whose degree of risk may depend on the worker's level of awareness of the hazard and personal hygiene habits and on the availability of adequate facilities for washing and eating at the workplace. Contamination of cigarettes with toxic materials and their subsequent inhalation is also a problem for some substances.

For example, workers handling lead ingots are exposed to a low-level hazard from ingesting small amounts of lead by eating contaminated food or by inhaling small amounts of lead fumes from contaminated cigarettes. However, workers refining lead at temperatures above 800°F are exposed to a serious hazard from inhaling large amounts of lead fume if they work close to unventilated refining kettles for several hours daily. Workers handling liquid nitric acid are exposed to the hazard of direct contact with the liquid on their skin, but they may also be exposed to a respiratory hazard from inhaling acid mist generated by an electroplating process that uses nitric acid. In these two examples, lead and nitric acid cause different types and magnitudes of hazards because their physical forms vary: for lead, solid material and small-diameter airborne particulates; for nitric acid, liquid material and airborne droplets.

Anticipation and Recognition

The first problem the hygienist faces in evaluating an unfamiliar workplace for toxic hazards is identification of toxic materials. In many cases, such as a lead smelter or pesticide manufacturing process, emission sources for toxic materials are clearly evident. But even in these examples some hazards may not be evident without a careful examination of an inventory of the chemicals to be used or in use in the facility, including raw materials, by-products, products, wastes, solvents, cleaners, and special-use materials. Workers in lead smelters can also be exposed to carbon monoxide, arsenic, and cadmium; pesticide workers can be exposed to solvents. Relatively nontoxic chemicals can be contaminated with highly toxic ones; for example, some chlorinated hydrocarbons historically used in weed killers, such as trichlorophenoxyacetic acid (2,4,5-T), may contain highly toxic dioxin, and, in some parts of the world, technical-grade toluene may contain highly toxic benzene. In some cases, toxic materials may not be hazardous to workers because exposures are adequately controlled.

Safety data sheets list the composition of commercial products. The United States and other countries recently began requiring a 16-section SDS as part of global harmonization efforts to classifying and labeling chemicals. Safety data sheets are available from manufacturers and can be useful for anticipation or recognition of hazards, but they are sometimes too general or out of date. Toxicity data on specific substances can also be obtained by literature searches or by searches of toxicity data indices.

Since exposure to toxic substances can occur by contamination of food, drink, or cigarettes, the hygienist determines whether (a) eating and drinking facilities are physically separated from the work area, (b) facilities for washing are close to eating areas, and (c) sufficient time is permitted for workers to use these facilities. Protective clothing and facilities for showering after a work shift should also be provided, where indicated, based on the type and level of exposures present in the workplace. Workers' understanding of hazards from toxic materials they are using must also be assessed. Finally, the hygienist determines whether there are rules prohibiting eating, drinking, and smoking in areas with toxic substances and whether these rules are being enforced.

Evaluation

Measurement Techniques

Direct-reading instruments have sensors that instantaneously detect air concentration of substances and often produce a reading on a dial or digital readout. Most direct-reading instruments can store data for 8-hour time profiles for later retrieval and display. All require careful calibration, adherence-to-use specifications and conditions, and maintenance to obtain accurate data. The detector tube is another type of direct-reading instrument often used in determining approximate concentrations of air contaminants. This simple device uses a small hand pump to draw air through a bed of reagent in a glass tube that changes color or develops a length of stain that is proportional to the concentration of a given gaseous air contaminant. The conventional tube is suitable for short-term sampling, such as for 10 minutes; however, short-term samples can misrepresent long-term average exposures. Tubes for 8-hour sample collection can measure time-weighted average (TWA) exposures. Short-term samples are typically used for screening purposes, such as during an initial walkthrough survey, or for acute hazards when peak or ceiling exposure levels need to be known; in contrast, TWA measurements are more useful for exposure scenarios when chronic hazards are of concern. Detector tubes are manufactured under strict quality control, and their degree of measurement uncertainty is specified. Consideration must always be given to interference from other substances, which usually is specified on the tube's data sheets.

Sample collectors that remove substances from the air for analysis in a laboratory may be a less expensive alternative to direct-reading instruments. Personal sampling is a common approach used by hygienists to obtain accurate and precise measurements of workers' exposures. Particulate contaminants are collected with filters, and gases and vapors are collected by solid adsorbents or liquid bubblers. The sampling apparatus is generally simple, consisting of a small air pump usually worn on a worker's belt, connected by tubing to a collector and attached to the worker's shirt at the neck (Figure 8-1). (Some gas and vapor collectors are passive, using diffusion instead of an air pump to move the contaminant into the sampler.) With the appropriate selection of a gas or particulate collector, or both combined in a sampling train, it is possible to measure the average concentration of an air contaminant in the worker's breathing zone during an 8-hour work shift.

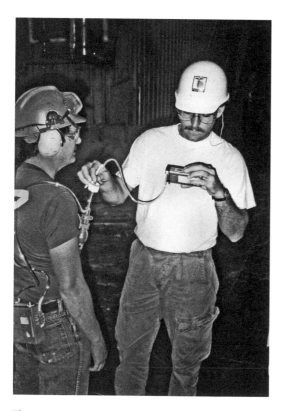

Figure 8-1. A NIOSH industrial hygienist checks the airflow rate of a personal sampling pump to measure a worker's formaldehyde exposure in a fiberboard manufacturing plant. (Photograph by Aaron Sussell.)

Collection devices for toxic particulates may capture either total dust—that is, all particle sizes that can enter the collector—or only the respirable dust—that is, only particles that can penetrate the terminal airways and alveolar spaces (less than 4 μm). Total particulate samples are collected if the toxic substance causes systemic health problems, as lead and pesticides do. Respirable dust samples are collected if the particulate causes a chronic pulmonary disease, such as coal worker's pneumoconiosis. The type of sampler should be matched to the route of entry, type of effect, and target tissue.

Charcoal and other sorbent material packed into tubes have been the most common collectors for gases and vapors; a small amount of charcoal inside a small glass tube acts as an activated surface that retains nonpolar materials, such as benzene. These collectors are commonly used to measure inhalation exposures to solvents, such as vapor exposures of printers. The specific methods for chemicals are discussed in detail in the *NIOSH Manual of Analytical Methods*.

Passive or badge-type samplers are much more convenient to use for gas and vapor sampling than collectors requiring air pumps, are relatively inexpensive, and have better worker acceptance because they weigh less than pumps. After the sampling period is completed, the cover is replaced on the badge, the total exposure time is noted, and it is sent to a laboratory for analysis. Several passive samplers have well-documented sampling rates. They may surpass active samplers in accuracy. Contamination from liquid splashes during use must be avoided.

Sampling Strategy

The hygienist must design a sampling strategy that takes into account the types of hazards, variations in exposure, routes of exposure, and the uses for the data, such as risk assessment or source evaluation and control. The approach should enable most efficient use of resources.[2] Personal measurements are designed to reflect the accumulation of exposure from a variety of sources that a worker may encounter during a work shift. In some cases, exposure may occur only during certain operations. Workers in adjacent areas not directly involved with the air contaminant of interest are frequently found to have significant exposures because the air contaminant drifts into their work areas. *Worst-case sampling* is the approach used when it is clear that high emissions from certain activities or sources will occur and it is decided that sampling will only be done during the period of highest exposure. This approach is used by OSHA.

Sampling strategies are designed to assess variability in exposures and factors associated with this variability. Variability in exposure levels can be large due to day-to-day variation in work pattern, production rate, and differences in a process. Differences in personal work habits, wind velocity, and wind direction also can cause large variations. The exposed populations should be subdivided into smaller, well-defined groups of workers performing identical or similar tasks. Properly selecting subgroups reduces within-group variability so that measurement resources can be concentrated on the highest exposed groups, although these may be difficult to identify a priori. Single samples are generally avoided because it is difficult to know what one sample value represents. In addition, because workers have different work habits and techniques, there frequently are differences in average exposures among workers.[3] Several replicate samples on multiple workers, from groups performing different tasks, may indicate how large these differences are and how much the assumption of uniform mean exposure within groups is violated.

In addition to personal sampling, the occupational hygienist also uses *fixed-location sampling*. In this strategy, the sampler is set at a given location that has some useful relationship to a source of exposure. This type of sampling is advantageous because it can enable determination of features of the exposure that would be difficult with personal samples. For example, a large sampler can be used to (a) determine the particle size distribution of airborne dust in a work area or (b) provide sufficient airborne material for detailed chemical analysis if the composition of the contaminants is not known. These samplers can be very useful for identifying and characterizing sources of exposure and assessing the effectiveness of engineering controls. One must carefully select the sampling location and strategy for fixed-location sampling. In some cases, a combination of personal and fixed-location samples is used to completely describe

a situation. For example, personal samples are used to describe the highly variable exposures of steel workers tending a blast furnace, while fixed-location samples measure exposures to the uniform, well-mixed air levels they experience while waiting in the lunchroom for their next job assignments (for 2 to 4 hours per work shift).

Some large plants use continuous multipoint sampling of gases and vapors with central analysis. The monitors can be linked to alarms, so that rapid action can be taken if concentrations exceed specified limits. Continuous monitoring at stationary sites should be part of a total quality management process when exposures are near the allowable limits.

In some workplaces, the most important route of exposure is skin contact. This route of exposure is difficult to evaluate with environmental sampling because even if the amount of skin contamination can be determined, it is not possible to know how much of the contaminant has already entered the body, or would enter, given sufficient time.[4] Two principal sampling approaches are employed:

1. Cloth patches with impermeable backing can be used to cover given locations of skin, such as the forehead, back of the neck, back of the hands, and forearms, to measure the amount of contamination per unit area that resulted during a period of exposure.
2. Wipe sampling can be performed, in which an area of skin is washed with an appropriate nontoxic solvent to determine the quantity of contamination remaining on the skin after a period of exposure.

Both of these techniques have been used to estimate pesticide exposures of agricultural workers. Addition of a fluorescent whitening agent to the pesticide as a tracer allows visualization of contamination. Additionally, wipe sampling on surfaces can be used as a method to detect and control indiscriminate distribution of toxic materials that workers may contact throughout the workplace. This type of sampling is also useful in estimating the exposure of one person relative to another or of one area relative to another. It is, however, difficult to know in absolute terms the quantity of contaminant that may penetrate the skin and cause an adverse health effect. Biologic monitoring is probably the best method for determining the intensity of skin exposures to a substance, if a biological monitoring test is available for the agent of interest.[5]

Some nonpolar substances, such as pesticides and solvents, may enter the body both via the respiratory tract and through skin contact. For these substances, both skin contact and air exposure must be evaluated to completely assess the risk. Biologic sampling that integrates these two routes of intake may be a practical necessity. Problems can be associated with biologic monitoring. First, some types of tests detect adverse effects, such as reduced red blood cell cholinesterase in pesticide-exposed workers, but they may show that excessive exposures have already occurred. Second, since there is a complex relationship between exposures and levels of compounds and metabolites in blood, urine, exhaled breath, and other biologic media, proper interpretation of biologic monitoring tests requires knowledge of the toxicokinetics of the specific agent and the temporal variations of a worker's exposure.[6] In many situations, biologic monitoring should only be used to verify that exposures have been controlled. Its use in detecting high exposures should be limited, such as when absorption is primarily through the skin.

It is almost never possible to evaluate ingestion as a route of exposure with sampling. Occasionally, samples of food and drink may be collected to assess the level of contamination; however, this type of exposure is likely to be extremely variable and episodic, so that occasional environmental sampling is usually an ineffective way of assessing exposure.

Exposure measurements on workers performing the same job under similar conditions commonly show substantial variation in mean exposure between workers. These differences are the primary limitation to what can be achieved with exposure controls. There are many reasons why differences might occur. First, individuals have differences in skill, training, and experience, which may lead them to perform a job with different techniques that affect personal exposure. Second, they may have differences in their level of concern about the hazards of the job and take more or fewer precautions to avoid exposure through the use of engineering controls or PPE. Differences among workers on these factors are generally assigned to "work practices" and dismissed. As a result, there has been little systematic investigation of the nature of these differences, especially the behavioral components, and effective ways for intervening to reduce exposures.

Control

In this section, the hierarchy of controls is described: substitution, limitation of release and build-up of contamination, and limitation of worker contact by various measures.

Substitution

Substances and materials that pose risks to impair health and safety should not be used if they can be substituted with something that is safer. There are several reasons why safer substitutes may not be used in a specific process, such as availability, cost, and effectiveness of the substitutes; however, in some instances, the failure to consider substitutes may simply stem from an attitude of "We have always done it this way." Substitution is part of the concept of toxics use reduction and waste management. *Toxics use reduction* is a formal programmatic approach to examining the materials being used and produced in a workplace, identifying the hazards associated with each, and then developing strategies to reduce the overall burden of toxic materials used or produced (More information can be found at http://www.turi.org/ or at https://www.osha.gov/dsg/safer_chemicals/index.html.) Potential benefits to health and safety have to be balanced against technological and economic consequences. This balance should include product properties, production process, environment, and reliability of supply. For example, toluene and xylene may be inexpensive, less-toxic replacements for benzene being used as a solvent, because they have similar chemical properties and may work as effectively as benzene. They also are less volatile and will produce fewer environmental emissions. Both are readily available commercially and unlikely to be affected by supply shortages. Regular auditing of use of substances and materials helps to identify opportunities for substitution and promotes ongoing toxics use reduction.

Limitation of Release and Build-up of Contamination

If substitution is not possible, then the next step is to attempt to control or limit releases and to prevent the buildup of toxic materials in the worker's environment. Local exhaust ventilation combined with source isolation will control process emissions. General room ventilation is used to prevent the buildup of hazardous concentrations in the work area from contaminants escaping local exhaust, from spills, or from fugitive emissions (from seals, valves, or pumps). An example of these two ventilation approaches is shown in Figure 8-2.

Local exhaust systems surround the point of emission with a partial or complete enclosure and attempt to capture and remove the emissions

before they are released into the worker's breathing zone. Figures 8-3 through 8-5 show several examples of local ventilation systems; various types, with differing degrees of effectiveness, are available. Unfortunately, it is not possible before installation to determine precisely the effectiveness of a particular system, although this is an area of active research. As a result, it is important to measure exposures and evaluate how much control has been achieved after a system is installed. Unless contaminant sources are

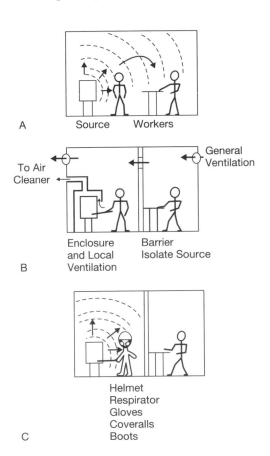

Figure 8-2. Examples of controls for airborne exposures: (A) Workers with primary and secondary exposure to source emissions. (B) Ventilation and source isolation to control exposures. (C) Personal protection and source isolation to control exposures. (Diagrams prepared by T.J. Smith, Harvard School of Public Health, Boston, Massachusetts.)

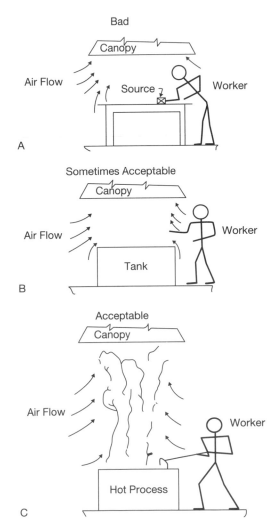

Figure 8-3. The proper use of a canopy hood, which does not allow the air contaminants to be drawn through the worker's breathing zone. The worker's location is crucial. (Source: National Institute for Occupational Safety and Health. The industrial environment: Its evaluation and control. Washington, DC: NIOSH, 1973; p. 599.)

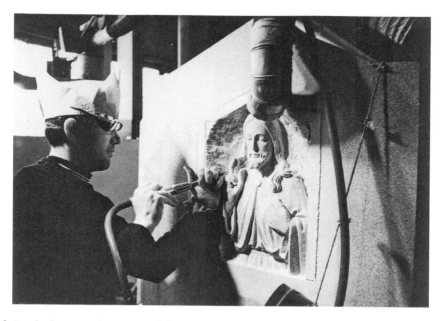

Figure 8-4. Local exhaust ventilation successfully captures dust produced by stone cutting. (Source: W.A. Burgess, Harvard School of Public Health, Boston, Massachusetts.)

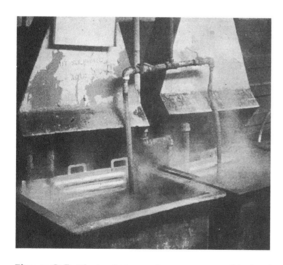

Figure 8-5. Electroplating workers are protected by local slot exhaust ventilation. (Source: W.A. Burgess, Harvard School of Public Health, Boston, Massachusetts.)

totally enclosed, collection will only capture a percentage of total emissions. Release of smoke from smoke tubes at the point of contaminant generation is a useful technique for visualizing the flow of air toward the exhaust. It may reveal if the distance to the exhaust is too large, if there are cross-drafts or strong air disturbances, or if the worker creates wakes, all of which greatly

reduce the collection efficiency. A good system may collect 80% to 99%, but a poor system may capture only 50% or less. Careful maintenance must be performed on the system to maintain efficiency. Poor maintenance is probably most responsible for system failures. It is also very important to reevaluate the system in the event of any additions, deletions, or other changes to the system or to the process it is being used to control.

The increasing cost of energy has made the practice of ventilating work areas with outside fresh air an increasingly expensive process; much work is being done on the design of systems that can recirculate decontaminated air or use heat exchangers so the heat value is not lost.

Limitation of Worker Contact

The third important approach to controlling exposures to toxic materials is to limit worker contact by (a) automating processes, (b) isolating processes using toxic materials from the remainder of the work area so that the potential for contact with these materials is limited (Figure 8-6), or (c) furnishing workers with PPE, such as respirators (dust masks or gas masks) or hoods or suits with externally

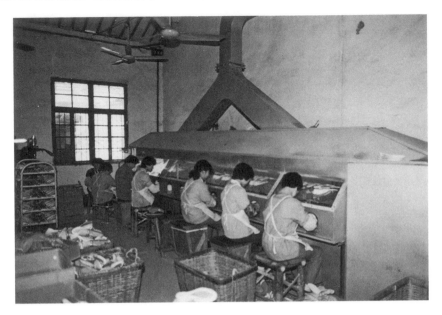

Figure 8-6. A glovebox enclosure system prevents solvent exposure to workers gluing shoes. (Photograph by Barry S. Levy.)

supplied air for controlling inhalation of toxic materials.

Many people mistakenly think that the use of respirators is a simple and inexpensive way to control exposure to toxic airborne materials. However, there is discomfort in wearing these masks, leading to poor worker acceptance, and a tight seal to the face is needed to achieve good protection, which reduces comfort and leads to variable levels of protection. There are extensive OSHA requirements for an adequate respirator program to ensure that the quality of devices is maintained and that workers are receiving adequate protection. The annual cost of a good respirator program for lead dust exposures is approximately $1,000 or more per worker. Fitting of respirators is also extremely important but often neglected; a poorly fitting respirator provides substantially less protection than expected because, even if the respirator filters are highly efficient, there can be inhalation of contaminated air around the edges of the face mask.

The use of rubber gloves and protective clothing does not automatically ensure that workers are protected adequately. Toluene and other aromatic solvents readily penetrate rubber gloves; thus, glove composition must be matched to the chemical nature of the substance. Similarly, long-sleeved shirts or coveralls may not prevent skin contact with toxic dusts because small dust particles can sift through the openings between threads in woven cloth.

A study demonstrated adverse health effects in orchard workers due to pesticide exposures, even though they had been wearing dust masks and long-sleeved work shirts.[7] Despite the shirts, their arms were covered with dust that contained pesticide residues. Even impermeable protective suits are difficult to seal to prevent migration of dust past cuffs and the neck opening. The suits also trap body heat and moisture, resulting in potential heat stress.

To limit contact with hazardous substances, protective clothing should be changed each day and not worn outside the work area, and workers should shower after each work shift. These practices also prevent workers from taking home hazardous materials on their workclothes, skin, and hair, thereby exposing family members and other household contacts.

Exposure can be partially decreased by administrative controls, such as scheduling workers to spend limited amounts of time in areas with potential exposure, possibly reducing their cumulative exposure below recommended guidelines; however, this practice may increase the total number of workers exposed to a hazard. While this approach may be effective in certain situations, it (a) requires good exposure data to demonstrate its effectiveness and the careful attention of supervisory personnel, (b) may be an inefficient use of workers, and (c) may be inappropriate for controlling exposures to carcinogens or teratogens.

Ideally, all of these control approaches should be used together to develop an overall control strategy that will address all aspects of exposure to toxic substances in a workplace. Short-term measures, such as extensive use of PPE, may be adopted immediately after a problem is recognized to allow time for developing engineering controls or process modifications that will provide better control over the long term. Despite their undesirable aspects, respirators may be the only effective control device for some exposures, such as those faced by maintenance or cleanup workers. (OSHA policy is to use respirators only as a last resort.)

An approach that has gained in popularity in recent decades is the concept of *control banding*, a more generalized approach for controlling hazardous exposures that was developed in the pharmaceutical industry in the 1980s to complement the traditional air sampling and analysis.[8] To assess risk associated with a task or process, control banding combines qualitative and/or semiquantitative information on the toxicity of an agent and the risk of increased exposures occurring. Based on this risk, each task or process is categorized into hazard "bands" within a facility that encompass broad categories of risk. Each hazard band is associated with a prescribed control strategy that is applied to all tasks or processes in a facility that fall within the band. Bands associated with higher risk are assigned to more stringent control strategies and assessment/reassessment procedures. This approach was designed to reduce time and toxicological expertise required in an occupational health unit in a workplace to assess risk, since hazards could be stratified into broad bands designed to protect workers from agents falling within a given band with a reasonable margin of safety. While there are many examples of successful implementation of this approach, one must properly rate the toxicity of an agent and account for exposure variability to ensure that this control strategy provides an adequate margin of safety.

NOISE PROBLEMS

Occupational exposure to excessive noise is an important problem that is evaluated and controlled, in part, by occupational hygienists. (See Chapter 12A.) Hygienists are trained to measure the intensity and quality of noise, assess its potential for producing damage, and devise means to control noise exposures. Two principal types of workplace noise, continuous and impact, have somewhat different techniques of evaluation and control. *Continuous noise* is produced by high-velocity airflow in compressors, fans, gas burners, and motors. Crushing, drilling, and grinding are important sources of continuous noise because much energy is used in a small space. *Impact noise* results from sharp or explosive inputs of energy into some object or process, such as hammering or pounding on metal or stone, dropping heavy objects, or materials handling.

During the evaluation of a workplace, a hygienist looks for sources of excessive noise, determines which workers are exposed, and then selects an evaluation strategy to clarify the nature and extent of the exposures. If the noise is continuous or almost continuous, a hand-held noise survey meter may be used to determine the noise levels at a worker's location. If the exposure involves impact noises, an electronic instrument that records and averages the high-intensity, but short-duration, pulses is used to characterize the source and exposures.

Typically, workers spend variable amounts of time exposed to noise sources and may work at different distances from noise sources, which will alter their exposures. Exposures may also vary because the output of noise sources may change over time. Therefore, the TWA exposure may not be easy to estimate, even though the sources may present clear potential for overexposure. This problem has been solved by the use of small noise dosimeters worn by workers, which electronically record sound levels and indicate average noise levels during work shifts. Dosimeters are very useful for describing average exposures; however, short-term exposure to high levels may be missed by dosimeters that determine average exposures, such as over an 8-hour period. Modern dosimeters store 8-hour (or longer) time traces, which can be displayed and linked to records of worker activities. A typical noise evaluation will include both assessment of the noise level at the source and dosimeter measurements of workers' noise exposure.

National requirements and TLV guidelines are used by the hygienist to evaluate noise data and decide whether a hazard is present. In addition to the hazard to hearing, a high noise level can significantly interfere with verbal communication, which may create another hazard by interfering with verbal warnings and worker detection of safety hazards, such as moving equipment. The OSHA standard for continuous noise for 8 hours is 90 dBA.* Higher levels are permitted for shorter periods of time. The OSHA standard allows levels of noise exposure that will protect some but not all workers from the adverse effects of workplace noise. The TLV for an 8-hour exposure to noise is 85 dBA, which is significantly lower than the 90 dBA OSHA standard for (continuous) noise.

Although techniques exist to obtain an overall TWA of noise exposures received in several different work settings, no techniques exist for assessing the hearing risks of combined exposure to both continuous and impulse noise. Many workers are exposed to both types of noise, such as brass foundry workers who are exposed to continuous noise from gas burners and to impulse noise from brass ingots dropping into metal bins from conveyors.

The strategies for controlling noise are similar to those used for toxic material control:

1. *Substitute*: Use another process or piece of equipment. For example, electrically heated pots for melting metal can be used instead of gas-heated pots to eliminate burner noise.
2. *Prevent or reduce release of noise*: Modify the source to reduce its output, enclose and soundproof the operation, or install mufflers or baffles. For example, noisy air compressors can be fitted with mufflers and placed in soundproofed rooms to control their noise; impact-absorbing materials can be installed to eliminate impulse noise from ingots dropping into a metal bin.
3. *Prevent excessive worker contact*: Provide PPE, such as earplugs or earmuffs, or provide a control booth.

As with toxic materials, the overall strategy to control exposures usually involves separate approaches for various aspects of the problem. It may be necessary to consult an acoustical engineer with advanced evaluation and engineering expertise to address complex noise problems. If engineering controls are not completely effective or are impractical, ear protectors may be required; however, the effectiveness of these devices is limited because sound may also reach the ear by bone conduction. A full-shift exposure above 120 dBA cannot be controlled adequately using earplugs or muffs.

RADIATION PROBLEMS

Radiation hazards are commonly first identified by occupational hygienists, but the responsibility for their evaluation and control overlaps among the occupational hygienist, the health physicist, and the radiation protection officer. (See Chapter 12D.) Exposure to ionizing radiation can be external (from X-ray machines or radioactive materials) or internal (from radioactive substances in the body). External exposures can be monitored instrumentally by several methods; the type of detector system chosen for a given problem depends on the nature of the ionizing radiation. Personal monitoring is commonly performed with badges of photographic emulsions, thermal luminescent materials, or induced radiation materials that will indicate the cumulative dose during the period the badge is worn. Data from these measurement systems can be used to construct relatively accurate estimates of tissue exposure. If there are also detailed supporting data on worker activities, sources of exposure and points of intervention can also be identified.

---

* dBA denotes decibels (units of sound intensity on a logarithmic scale) that are summed across frequencies using the "A" scale, which weights frequency in proportion to the human ear's sensitivity to sound (Chapter 12A).

Non-ionizing radiation is also an external exposure problem. This type of radiation includes a variety of electromagnetic waves, ranging from short-wavelength ultraviolet, to visible and infrared, to long-wavelength microwaves and radio waves. Exposures to ultraviolet, visible, and infrared radiation are measured with photometers of various types. Microwaves and radio waves can also be measured by several standardized techniques, but there is uncertainty over the exposure intensities required to produce adverse health effects. Lasers may also provide a source of exposure to varying regions of the non-ionizing radiation spectrum, depending on the power and lasing medium involved in a particular application.

Exposures to radioactive materials can be evaluated with similar methodology to that used for toxic substances. Personal air sampling, surface sampling, and skin contamination measurement can be used to quantify exposures by their route of contact or entry into the body. For example, personal air sampling in uranium mines can measure miners' exposure to respirable radioactive particles that will be deposited in their respiratory tracts. Internal levels of some radionuclides can be detected outside the body and measured directly if they emit sufficient penetrating radiation, such as gamma rays emitted from radioactive cobalt. However, most cannot be detected externally; the quantities of radioactive substances reaching sensitive tissues, such as the bone marrow, usually must be estimated by determining the worker's external exposures and making assumptions about the amount entering the body and being transported to the site(s) of adverse effects.

The Nuclear Regulatory Commission has set standards for allowable ionizing radiation exposures for both external and internal sources. These exposure limits can be used, like TLVs, to decide whether a given exposure presents a health risk. Radiation protection programs have strict requirements about techniques for handling radioactive materials and working with radiation sources. They also require extensive routine exposure monitoring and medical monitoring.

Exposure limits for non-ionizing radiation have been set by OSHA, based on published scientific data, the TLVs developed by the ACGIH, and standards developed by the American National Standards Institute. Equivalent limits have been developed by WHO and several countries (see Further Reading). The eyes and the skin are critical organs to be protected. Standards have been set for the most susceptible organs, such as the eyes. There is concern about reproductive hazards for these agents. Standards also have been developed for lasers based on ophthalmoscopic data and irreversible functional changes in visual responses. As with other types of standards, the numerical limits cannot be treated as absolute and the margin of safety is often uncertain.

Control of external ionizing and non-ionizing radiation exposures is achieved by minimizing the amounts of radiation used, isolating processes, shielding sources, using warning devices, interlocking door and trigger mechanisms to prevent accidental exposures, educating workers and supervisors about the hazards, and, if necessary, requiring use of PPE. Consider the following example:

An industrial X-ray machine used to check castings for flaws is placed in a separate room with extensive lead shielding, and it cannot be triggered when the door to the room is open. The room also has signs warning of a radiation hazard. A red warning light inside the room is lit for 30 seconds before X-rays are released so that a worker inside the room when the door is closed could activate an emergency override switch to prevent operation of the machine. All personnel working near the X-ray machine are required to wear film badges to monitor their accumulated radiation exposure.

Control of internal radiation exposures from radioactive materials is very similar to controls for toxic materials. The objectives are to use minimal amounts of radioactive materials; isolate the work areas; enclose any operations likely to produce airborne emissions; use work procedures that prevent or minimize worker contact with contaminated air or materials; have workers wear PPE to prevent skin contact, eye exposure, or inhalation of materials; monitor environmental contamination levels; and educate workers about the hazards. Careful supervision of work activities and monitoring of program implementation are required to provide adequate protection.

CONCERNS FOR THE FUTURE

Workplaces in heavy industry have been a concern of hygienists for many years, although this concern is somewhat less at present in the United States and Europe. However, as older technologies have been exported to developing countries, hygienists have been increasingly concerned because these countries seek the economic benefits of heavy industry without adequate resources to ensure worker health and safety.

In some high-income countries, there has been increasing concern about the office environment and the health effects associated with energy-efficient, tightly sealed buildings. There also is concern that, although hazards in large companies have been largely controlled, those in small and midsized companies have not been adequately controlled because these companies have fewer resources.

The scientific basis for occupational hygiene practice has been eroding because of limited research funding and a small number of researchers. Examination of the scientific literature in occupational hygiene shows it to be narrowly focused on limited issues. Internal research funded by companies is often not published because it may aid competitors or may raise liability concerns. Gaining access to workplaces for academic research has also become more difficult. There is a reluctance of employers to examine the hazards of their operations because of concerns about the costs of additional government regulation and legal liability for health claims from previously unrecognized hazards. As a result, there has been little development, updating, and refinement of exposure assessment methods, control technology, intervention strategies, or governmentally enforced exposure limits—despite extensive worldwide development of new materials, production technologies, biomedical and drug manufacturing, and other advances.

Occupational hygiene has not kept up with this development. Some occupational hygienists who are concerned about this situation have begun working to strengthen local research and to develop collaborative international research programs. Joint labor and management research programs supported by company funds have also become increasingly important sources of workplace access and research funding.

ENVIRONMENTAL HYGIENE

Environmental hygiene has much in common with occupational hygiene. There is considerable overlap in basic concepts and approaches for hazard recognition, exposure assessment, and source controls, especially for air pollution. The major difference is that the occupational hygienist works in a prescribed setting and with a generally healthy adult population. In contrast, the environmental hygienist covers the entire environment and all of the population, including young, older, and ill people, in addition to healthy adults. Exposures tend to be higher in occupational settings, but not always. Environmental transport of contaminants is usually more extensive in the outdoor environment than the workplace. Residents of an area will have both ambient exposures as well as exposures inside their homes and other buildings.

Source-Transport-Receptor Model

Environmental hygienists find it useful to organize approaches to environmental problems using the framework of the *source-transport-receptor model*. This model is a simple, yet powerful, representation of environmental exposures that has gained wide acceptance by environmental scientists (Figure 8-7). The *source* produces and releases emissions into the environment, such as airborne emissions from a power plant or toxic organic solvents released into groundwater by a waste dump. The source defines the composition and release rate of the emissions. Source sampling is very useful when it can be accomplished. Sometimes there are many small sources that are dispersed, such as individual vehicles in traffic and heating units in homes. Given knowledge about the source, we can identify what types of hazards might be present and what to measure. Environmental processes during transport of emissions include dispersion and dilution, photochemical reactions with sunlight, and removal by rain, adsorption to soil particles, and sedimentation. The main concern is

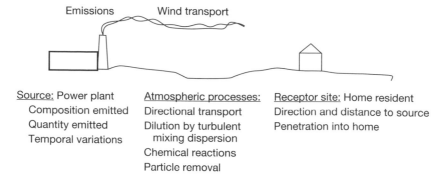

Source: Power plant
   Composition emitted
   Quantity emitted
   Temporal variations

Atmospheric processes:
Directional transport
Dilution by turbulent
   mixing dispersion
Chemical reactions
Particle removal

Receptor site: Home resident
Direction and distance to source
Penetration into home

Figure 8-7. Source-transport-receptor model for wind transport of emissions from a power plant to a home.

the composition and concentration of emissions reaching the receptor—the exposed person.

Major Problems

Air and water emissions from vehicular traffic, power plants, industrial operations (especially chemical manufacturing and mining), food sanitation, municipal and agricultural wastes, sewage, and solid waste are all major problems (Table 8-2). Usually, one must investigate the characteristics of a given source in detail to understand fully the hazards it presents. There is no simple summary that can adequately describe the complexity and variety of source releases. One should also consider the natural sources that may affect the background levels of an environmental contaminant.

EXPOSURE CHARACTERIZATION

A variety of methods are used by the Environmental Protection Agency (EPA) and other regulatory agencies to characterize common and dangerous exposures. These methods are based on (a) sample collection and analysis and, more commonly, (b) direct-reading instruments. The most important part of an evaluation is the sampling strategy, which specifies how, when, and where samples will be obtained and measurements performed. The goal is to define the magnitude of exposures, which can be highly variable among individuals and across time and space. Thus, a series of measurements must be made to define the distribution of exposures that

a person may have. For environmental problems, we generally measure contamination of air, water, food, and soil. There are also measurement techniques for noise, radiation, and other hazards.

Sampling Strategy

One of the most challenging aspects of environmental sampling is ensuring that samples are representative of exposure, since there are so many different sources of variation. Most importantly, time-activity patterns, which dictate one's duration of contact with environmental contaminants in a given microenvironment, can vary greatly within and among individuals—so one needs to consider what conditions may influence the difference between environmental and human exposures. For example, there can be important temporal variations on the scale of minutes, hours, days, weeks, months, seasons, and years and spatial variations on the scale of feet, yards, hundreds of yards, miles, and more. Contaminants in wells, streams, rivers, and lakes can vary dramatically, as can contaminants in individual food items and batches of food items. As a result, one needs to be clear about the exposure distribution one is attempting to characterize: Is it for healthy adults, children, elderly people, or ill people? for homes along a busy street, for a neighborhood, for a particular time period, or for a certain activity? Do we need to collect personal samples, or will fixed-location area samples alone be sufficient? If we wish to define the mean and standard deviation of an

Table 8-2. Major Sources of Environmental Emissions and Releases

Major Sources	Emissions–Contaminated Media	Route of Entry
Natural processes • Erosion • Vegetation and microbes • Volcanoes • Geothermal springs • Forest and grass fires • Storm runoff and floods • Sea spray • Radon	Airborne dusts, pollen, terpenes, ammonia, methane, sulfur dioxide, hydrogen sulfide Waterborne particles, dissolved carbon and metals, hydrogen sulfide, arsenic Soil contamination with metals, radon	Inhalation and ingestion
Power plants	Airborne ash, nitrogen oxides, metals — Sulfur oxides, arsenic from coal — Sulfur oxides, vanadium from oil Radionuclides in air and water from nuclear power	Inhalation and ingestion
Vehicle emissions • Traffic—cars, trucks, buses • Off road—trains, mining • Boats and ships	Airborne unburned fuel, nitrogen oxides, PAHs, particles, lead Secondary photochemical smog Waterborne hydrocarbons, lead in street runoff water Soil contamination with hydrocarbons, lead Ship ballast water releases of oil, organisms	Inhalation and ingestion
Home heating emissions—combustion	Particles, hydrocarbons, sulfur oxides, metals	Inhalation
Sewage systems • Human wastes • Small business wastes	Waterborne pathogens, nutrients, toxic chemicals, solvents, metals	Ingestion
Industrial activities • Chemical releases	Airborne contaminants (depend on the specific industry) Wastewater contaminants (depend on the specific industry)	Inhalation and ingestion

Note. PAHs = polynuclear aromatic hydrocarbons.

exposure, fewer samples are required than if we are trying to define the range or the probability of the highest values (the upper tail of the exposure distribution). If we are looking for exposures that exceed a legal limit, it may be necessary to use a strategy and methods defined by law or regulation. Therefore, the hygienist must have a well-developed set of questions to answer and a sampling strategy that will obtain answers as efficiently as possible.

Sample Collection

Each exposure media has different collection approaches (Table 8-3). Airborne particles may be collected on filters, impacted on surfaces, or electrostatically collected. Nonreactive gases can be collected in bags and bottles. Reactive gases may be collected in liquids using bubblers or treated substrates, such as filters or adsorbents.

Vapors, such as gasoline vapors, are gaseous, but their normal state is solid or liquid.

Consequently, they will readily condense on surfaces like the inside of collection bags, whereas gases will not. The preferred method for sampling vapors is with special materials in small holders, such as charcoal in tubes or reactants impregnated on papers or fibrous glass. The collection process may be either active, using a pump to draw air through the collector, or passive, using diffusion to bring the gaseous materials into the collector. Badge-type passive collectors are better accepted by subjects for personal sampling. Automated collectors may be used to collect a long series of air or water samples in a chosen fixed-station location, or instruments drifting with balloons to follow the removal of power-plant emissions by atmospheric reactions, or floating devices for monitoring ocean water in currents.

Table 8-3. Examples of Environmental Sampling and Analysis Methods for Common Contaminants

Media and Contaminant	Collection Method Examples	Analytical Method
Air—Metals (lead, cadmium)	Total metals—Membrane filter (0.2 μm pore size) and pump (4 liters per minute) Respirable particles—Use cyclone or impactor precollector before filter Direct analysis[a] by specific light scattering instrument	Acid digestion of filter and sample, AA, or inductively coupled plasma mass spectrometry measurement
Air—Organic vapors	Hydrocarbon vapors—charcoal in canister Pesticides—Tenax or XAD or other suitable resin	Strip vapors with solvent and GC analysis
Air—Reactive gases (ozone, ammonia, sulfur dioxide)	Collect on treated substrate; selective for gas Direct analysis by specific electrochemical instrument Direct analysis by specific colorimetric detector tubes	Specific reaction products; ion chromatography analysis
Air—Carbon monoxide	Collect in bag Direct analysis by specific electrochemical instrument	Gas sample injected for direct analysis by GC
Water—Metals (lead)	Collect sample[b] with acid cleaned polyethylene bottle (1 liter)	Free lead—Acidify water and AA analysis Total lead—perchlorate digestion then AA
Water—Microorganisms	Collect water in sterile bottle	Filter water; culture organisms on filter or directly culture water; digest filtered organisms and polymerase chain reaction (analysis
Food and soil—Pesticides	Collect food or soil sample[c] in chemically clean container	Macerate and prepare[d] food and soil; extract preparation with solvent; GC analysis

Note. AA = atomic absorption; GC = gas chromatography.

[a] Direct analysis is a real-time measurement with a very short averaging time, usually 1 minute or less. [b] A variety of components may need to be characterized to accurately represent a water contamination problem, such as organisms, suspended materials, or sediments. [c] Because food and soil are very heterogeneous, careful sampling strategies are needed to collect representative samples that indicate human exposures. [d] Food and soil are complex matrices and may require extensive preparation to prepare them for analysis.

Sample Analysis

Sampling media or containers are sent to a laboratory with experience performing the desired analyses. Accredited labs are best. If the data are to be used for determining compliance or legal proceedings, analyses for all regulated substances must follow the method given in regulations. If the measurements are to be used for a research project, where there is no accepted method for the substances of interest, then the investigator must work closely with the lab to ensure the validity of the data. Developing new methods to measure an environmental contaminant is a major undertaking, even for highly skilled environmental chemists. It is not unusual for the development and validation process to take several years.

In all cases, there must be detailed quality-control and quality-assurance plans, which should include lab and field blank samples, analysis of standards with each batch of samples, duplicate field samples, replicate analyses, and sometimes spiked blanks or spiked samples to verify that no problems occurred during field collection or lab analyses. More information about quality-assurance programs can be found in standard texts on environmental monitoring or publications by regulatory agencies.

DEFINING A HAZARD

Complaints

It is common for residents of an area to complain about odors, dust, and damage to materials from air pollutants. Likewise, they may complain about the odors, color, and opacity of water in ponds, lakes, streams, and rivers, and all of these problems in addition to the taste of drinking water. Any of these complaints may indicate a potential problem. In some cases, the problem is one of aesthetics, and, in others, it is a health risk. If the source of the poor quality can be identified, such as a chemical plant upwind or a sewage treatment plant upriver, then it may be possible to identify what might be contaminating the environment. Often the source is not known, but the odor or other characteristics may be identified. For example, in the past many private wells were contaminated with gasoline leaking from underground storage tanks, and the gasoline odor from the water was notable. Spills or accidental releases are most often noted by people living or passing nearby, and they may be the people most at risk.

Exposure Assessment Study

Where the resources are present, an exposure study may be conducted to define what contaminants are present and determine whether they exceed allowable exposure standards developed by the EPA, WHO, or other agencies. However, it is very difficult to determine what unknown agents are present in sampled media. Despite much interest in and development of untargeted laboratory analysis, there are no widely used, broad-spectrum methods that can readily determine (a) the components of substances such as the gunk scraped off the bottom of a pond or material obtained from an abandoned barrel left at a waste site or (b) the cause of an unpleasant odor in air, water, or food. In general, one must tell laboratory personnel what to measure, so they can choose appropriate methods. If a suitable, sample collection strategy is used, then exposure levels can be compared to exposure standards. When measured levels are less than the standard, it may mean that there is no hazard; however, if there are health complaints related to the exposure, the findings may also mean that the exposure standard has been set too high.

Epidemiologic Study

If there are local health complaints, such as by neighbors of a local industrial plant, then a small study may be conducted by the local health

department. A larger, full-scale epidemiological study may also be warranted in some cases. The water contamination problem in Woburn, Massachusetts, starting in the 1950s and ending in 1979 with the closure of contaminated wells, is a good example.[9,10] Excess leukemia in children was found to be associated with these wells. (See Box 18-1 in Chapter 18.) Other community studies have been launched to examine apparent unusual clusters of cases of disease. (See Chapter 5.)

CONTROL OF HAZARDS

The same processes used to control occupational exposures and waste emissions are also used in environmental controls. Elimination of the source is the only completely successful control approach. Sometimes it is possible to change the source or limit its output. Personal exposure controls are even less successful for general environmental hazards than they are for occupational hazards. Respirators and protective clothing are impractical and unreasonable for the general public. Although there is an active market for home and personal air cleaners, the amount of protection they can provide is limited; in addition, some of the electrostatic particle collectors will expose people to ozone, a hazardous gas. Therefore, emission controls at the source are the most common and effective way to deal with emissions from large or numerous sources.

EXAMPLES OF MAJOR ENVIRONMENTAL PROBLEMS

In this section, we consider some of the major types of environmental problems, their sources, transport phenomena, and characterization of exposures at the receptors.

Air Pollution

Daily variation in concentrations of airborne particulate matter less than 10 μm in diameter (PM_{10}) and/or less than 2.5 μm in diameter ($PM_{2.5}$) have been closely correlated, in many cities worldwide, with daily fluctuations in death rates—especially from respiratory and cardiovascular diseases. These effects occur even at low concentrations (20 to 200 µg/m³). Some, but not all, of those who have died have been people with pre-existing respiratory and cardiovascular diseases that would not have otherwise been fatal.

Environmental hygienists have been challenged to better define air pollution exposures associated with adverse health effects in the general population. Time-activity studies have followed the daily lives of children, young and middle-age healthy adults, older people, and ill people, while monitoring their exposures. Surprisingly, aside from children playing outdoors and people engaged in outdoor sports, most people in cities spend limited time outdoors during which they are exposed to urban air pollution. Indoor exposures account for much more of their time. Exposures to some general categories of air contaminants, such as oxides of nitrogen (NOx), can be higher inside homes than outdoors because there are sources of NOx indoors, such as gas-fired stoves. However, the outdoor levels of $PM_{2.5}$ permeate indoors. Therefore, even though some people do not spend much time outdoors, their indoor exposure—and their mortality rates—correlate with people who have had much exposure to outdoor $PM_{2.5}$. (See Box 8-1.)

Indoor and outdoor exposures may be qualitatively and quantitatively different if there are differences in strong emission sources in one place or the other. In some instances, aerosols generated inside homes may be less toxic than outdoors. For example, indoor $PM_{2.5}$ comes from reentrainment of dust and dirt tracked into homes or from vacuuming and sweeping, whereas outdoor $PM_{2.5}$ comes from combustion sources and atmospheric reaction products (smog). In that case, higher indoor exposures do not translate to higher risk. Some toxic outdoor air contaminants, such as some gases and small-diameter particles within $PM_{2.5}$, can readily penetrate into homes. However, highly reactive ozone in smog is found at lower concentrations indoors than outdoors because it reacts quickly with surfaces.

Once materials are released to the environment, there are several processes that operate to modify and remove them—processes that differ for particles and gases. Combustion processes can produce dense clouds of nanoparticles (0.01 to 0.1 µm), sometimes visible as smoke. These rapidly agglomerate into larger particles (~1 µm in diameter). As the particles become larger, they settle out of the air or are removed by impaction on surfaces of buildings and trees. During periods of high humidity, water-soluble particles will absorb water and may grow large enough to be removed by sedimentation and impaction on surfaces. Particles can also be removed by precipitation. Semi-volatile vapors of polynuclear aromatic hydrocarbons (PAHs), tars, and greases condense on ambient particles

---

Box 8-1. Assessing Indoor Air Pollution

In many cases, problems with indoor air quality cannot be characterized by a generally uniform clinical picture and a specific cause. These problems result from complex interactions among several factors, including air contaminants (including their odor), temperature, ventilation, air movement, illumination, noise, ergonomics, and psychological and social factors. Emerging complaints about indoor air quality should be assessed and controlled promptly. It is important to engage the affected individuals or groups in evaluating and addressing these complaints. Specific measures should include the following:

1. Checking whether operational conditions are normal for the HVAC and other systems
2. Determining the nature and magnitude of problem by using a standardized "sick building" questionnaire and/or structured interviews

3. Performing a technical survey to assess risk factors inherent in the use and operation of the building
4. Assessing construction materials, furniture, quality of cleaning, moisture damage and mold growth, temperature, air movement, and carbon dioxide concentration
5. Estimating degree of recirculation of air and possible contamination of intake air
6. Measuring ventilation efficiencies with tracer gas studies
7. Making a detailed assessment of contaminant sources and concentrations
8. Performing clinical examination of affected persons and additional occupational hygiene investigations, such as performing detailed chemical analyses of complex mixtures and assessing individual work habits to guide training interventions.

as hot combustion gases cool. Gaseous emissions can also undergo atmospheric reactions. Photochemical reactions of some hydrocarbons can produce nanoparticles. Sulfur dioxide from burning materials containing sulfur, such as coal and fuel oil, can be photochemically oxidized to sulfur trioxide, which reacts with water to form sulfuric acid, which absorbs water to form tiny droplets. Atmospheric ammonia reacts with the sulfuric acid to form ammonium sulfate. Some hydrocarbons will be oxidized to peroxides, aldehydes, and organic acids by ozone and other strong oxidants.

The hydrocarbons and nitrogen oxides released by vehicles in the summer can be photochemically converted to intense eye and upper respiratory irritants, especially highly reactive oxidants including ozone, under the action of ultraviolet radiation from the sun. The classic time pattern is as follows: Vehicle emissions during the morning rush hours are converted to afternoon smog, as occurs in Los Angeles, Denver, Houston, and other large cities. Although emission controls on cars, improved engines, and fuel and catalytic mufflers have all dramatically reduced emissions per car over the past three decades, the number of cars has dramatically increased during this period, especially in low- and middle-income countries. (See Chapter 15.)

Common Personal Sources

Although many personal items, such as cars, home heating units, barbeque grills, and power mowers, are minor sources of pollution, when taken together in large numbers in a city or an area where people are concentrated, they can contribute significantly to air pollution. Areas that have poor air flow, such as valleys, can have major episodes of ambient air pollution. Car and truck traffic accounts for much of the emissions in urban and suburban areas, including particulates containing elemental carbon, oils, grease, unburned fuel, and PAHs, as well as gases containing carbon monoxide, carbon dioxide, oxides of nitrogen, benzene, toluene, xylene, aldehydes, organic acids, and other volatile organic compounds.

Biological Sources

Biological hazards include pollens, airborne molds, bacteria (and related by-products, such as endotoxins from gram-negative bacteria), and other infectious agents. Seasonal allergies are a consequence of contact with pollens released by plants. Less familiar are releases by pine trees of terpenes (chemicals found in turpentine, a paint solvent). The haze in the Smoky Mountains in North Carolina is produced by the photochemical reaction of sunlight with the summertime releases of terpenes. This is supplemented by sulfuric acid aerosol from power plants in the Midwest burning high-sulfur coal. Natural decomposition of vegetation and dead animals by microorganisms produces several common air contaminants. Proteins are reduced to ammonia, nitrates, hydrogen sulfide, and sulfates. Organic carbon is ultimately reduced to methane under anaerobic conditions and carbon dioxide when there is sufficient oxygen; both methane and carbon dioxide are greenhouse gases that can be produced in large amounts not only by manmade sources but also by natural sources.

Natural Sources

Forest and grass fires, volcanoes, erosion, and sea spray produce large amounts of air contaminants across broad areas. Natural fires are dangerous due to both the destruction they cause and the large amounts of smoke they produce. Outdoor fires release many of the same combustion products that are found in emissions from cars, trucks, and other humanmade sources. Volcanoes release inorganic particles of ash and sulfur dioxide, producing hazardous conditions in broad areas downwind. The rare catastrophic eruptions, such as of Mount Pinatuba in the Philippines, can inject thousands of tons of ash and sulfur high into the stratosphere, which can remain airborne for a year or more and cause adverse health effects. Erosion produces soil particles, which can be entrained into the air if the soil is dry and dusty. Dust storms scour tons of dust into the air, exposing populations to very high dust levels. Coastal areas receive constant inputs of sea-salt aerosol from breaking waves and the nanoparticles of salt that are formed by bursting bubbles on the ocean.

Industrial Sources

Generally, these are point sources associated with local operations, such as power plants, chemical manufacturing facilities, and petroleum refineries. Most of these are required to meet governmental regulations on emissions. The specific emissions from these operations depend on the specific industry, which can be found in reference books and databases of governmental agencies in the United States and many European countries. Information is widely available for recognized hazards, such as the criteria pollutants defined by EPA and WHO,[11] but not for many new chemicals and materials. Small enterprises, such as foundries, auto repair, painting, small manufacturing, and recycling operations, can also be sources of local problems. Public health agencies must conduct continuous environmental surveillance to determine whether controls are effective and to detect problems if they are not. (See Chapter 15.)

Power plants are one of the most common industrial sources of airborne materials. They burn coal, oil, or natural gas, and some can switch between different fuels. They are major sources of carbon dioxide and oxides of nitrogen, and, depending on their fuel, they may also release large amounts of sulfur oxides (from coal and oil with sulfur); coal burning also releases mercury vapor and fine particles of ash that contain metals (lead and cadmium in coal, and vanadium in oil). Exposures will depend on wind direction and weather conditions.

Industrial operations run as designed most of the time. Unfortunately, there can be acute situations that result in large emissions. Spills of chemicals, fires, breakdowns of processing equipment, accidental releases, and failures of control systems can all produce massive emissions. In cases where the failure of a key part of the operation, such as a cooling system, will result in an explosion or a chemical release, a special system is usually in place to deal with a potential breakdown. One of the best examples of this is a nuclear power plant, which has back-up systems to maintain the flow of cooling water and control rods to limit the nuclear reaction. The few cases of malfunction are well known. One lesson from the Three Mile Island reactor accident in 1979 is that despite "fail-safe" engineering, unforeseen combinations of failures can still occur. Catastrophic breakdowns and accidents do occur, and disaster preparedness to minimize their effects is critical (Chapter 31).

Emission Controls

There are well-developed emission controls for nearly all of the common industrial processes that produce airborne waste products. Particles can be collected by filters, cyclone separators, electrostatic precipitators, and gases and can be removed by scrubbers and other specialized devices. Collection efficiency is never 100%. As a result, even if the proportion collected is 98%, as it is in some power-plant electrostatic precipitators, if the amount of particles produced is very large, then the amount that escapes collection can be large. Engineering controls used to minimize emissions must be well designed and carefully maintained to operate effectively. Assessment of these systems must be done by specialists. In general, elimination of waste production is a much more effective control strategy than removal of waste. Changes in processes and raw materials can sometimes eliminate problematic wastes, such as reducing residual amounts of sulfur in fuels.

Water Pollution

Problems with water pollution tend to be more localized than air pollution, although contamination of large watersheds can affect large populations. Water contaminants can take several forms: dissolved substances, such as salts, and gases; suspended particles, such as clay and organic matter that will settle out of the water; colloids, stable suspensions of very small particles that will not settle out; and floating substances, such as oils and grease. Oxygen content is one of the critical dimensions of water quality because it is necessary to sustain plants and animals in the water and sediments. Solubility of oxygen varies inversely with temperature; cold water holds more oxygen than warm water. The exchange of oxygen with the atmosphere is relatively slow, so conditions that either block the surface uptake or rapidly use up dissolved oxygen can create anaerobic conditions. Oil slicks block oxygen uptake. Large amounts of biological debris and organic carbon, such as from bacterial decay of vegetation and sewage, can deplete water of its oxygen. Then decay becomes anaerobic, which limits what can grow and creates odor and other problems. (See Chapter 16.)

Bioaccumulation

Accumulation and concentration of toxic chemical contaminants in the food chain is a serious problem for some substances, such as lipid-soluble materials with very low water solubility that are not broken down by natural biochemical processes or organisms in the environment. Biological transport into and out of organisms requires some water solubility, and Phase II metabolism of toxic materials, such as adding polar groups like –OH or –NH$_3$ to nonpolar hydrocarbons, increases their water solubility. The classic example of a substance that accumulates in biological systems is DDT. Since DDT has a low order of human toxicity, it was extensively sprayed to control mosquitoes and other insect pests in the 1940s and 1950s. Then, during the 1960s, it was found that populations of avian predators, such as fish-eating ospreys and eagles, were rapidly declining as a result of high losses of their eggs because the shells had become very fragile and easily broken. Rachel Carson brought this story to national attention in 1962 with her book *Silent Spring*. Researchers had found that trace concentrations of DDT in natural waters accumulated in the lipids of tiny plants. Small aquatic animals ate those plants, collected the lipids from many plants, and concentrated DDT into their own body fat. Small fish ate relatively large amounts of those small animals, further concentrating DDT in their fat. Medium-sized fish ate the small fish, and large fish ate the medium-sized fish. This concentrating process progressed up the food chain, with DDT becoming more concentrated at each step—as much as 10,000-fold relative to the starting concentration in the tiny plants. Finally, at the top of the food chain, the ospreys and eagles ate the large fish, whose fat now contained toxic levels of DDT. People who eat the contaminated fish can also accumulate high levels of DDT, polychlorinated biphenyls (PCBs), and other environmental chemicals.

A high degree of chemical stability and a low rate of metabolism are critical requirements for bioaccumulation. The stability of DDT and some other chemicals has allowed them to spread throughout the world so that even in the most remote places one can find DDT in the body fat of "top predators." Bioaccumulation also occurs for methylmercury, which is formed in aquatic sediments by bacterial methylation of inorganic mercury. Tuna and swordfish accumulate methylmercury, and when people eat these fishes they accumulate mercury in body fat, including in highly lipid neurological tissue. PCBs accumulate in fat, and some radioactive materials, such as strontium-90, bioaccumulate in bone.

Common Sources

The major sources of water pollution in high-income countries are storm runoff and sanitary waste water from cities, wastes from industries, runoff from agricultural land where fertilizers and pesticides are used, and runoff from concentrated animal-feeding operations. Large industrialized animal-feeding operations can produce as much fecal waste and urine as a small city. Fertilizers as well as animal and human wastes are major stimulants of plant growth in the receiving waters, leading to algae blooms. The bacteria decay of large amounts of organic wastes can strip the oxygen from the water, producing anaerobic conditions that kill fish and aquatic vegetation and lead to the growth of fungi, slug worms, and bacteria. This process has produced large "dead zones" in the Gulf of Mexico and other locations.

While large oil spills are catastrophic when they occur, they are rare. A larger problem is the discharging of contaminated bilge water from ship tanks. After a ship pumps out a liquid cargo, the empty tanks must be refilled with water to stabilize the ship. When the ship prepares to take on another cargo, it must pump out the water to make space for the new cargo. This constant filling and emptying of ship tanks is a major source of water pollution because the bilge water becomes contaminated with oil or other materials previously in the tanks. This procedure is also a common way that aquatic species are transferred from one area to another, where they may not be native.

Industrial waste releases have historically resulted in water-quality problems, from spills and accidental releases as well as routine releases. Specific hazards depend on the industry. Reference books on water pollution and toxic chemicals can help one identify which materials a given industry may commonly release and the problems they cause. Governmental regulations have greatly reduced the problems in areas where they are enforced. However, new industrial processes can produce wastes with unrecognized hazards.

There are natural cleaning processes that can lead to recovery in polluted waterways. Given sufficient time without further pollution, natural processes will remove the organic oxygen demand and lead to the return of plants and organisms that prefer clean, well-oxygenated conditions. Acidic and alkaline wastes will be neutralized. Toxic metal ions will be removed by complexation, in which insoluble complexes are formed and, by sedimentation, deposited. The bottom sediments will remain toxic but without much effect if they remain undisturbed.

Water Treatment

Drinking water treatment is directed toward removing floating particle contaminants and killing pathogens. Surface waters with minimal contamination are purified by (a) addition of chemicals, such as alum or ferric sulfate, that will cause any particles to stick together (flocculation); then (b) sediment to allow the big particles to deposit on the bottom of large tanks; and (c) filtration through beds of sand, which removes the fine particles. Following filtration, water is disinfected by adding chlorine, chloramines, or other bactericides until there is free bactericide in the water flowing to the customer. The free bactericide provides some residual protection against pathogens that might be introduced through breaks or problems in the distribution system. In places where there are mineral contaminants, such as iron or hydrogen sulfide, or hardness in the source water, additional chemical treatments can be used.

Drinking water treatment is directed toward bacterial contamination, which is generally not effective for viruses or toxic chemicals. Chlorination creates by-products, some of which are carcinogens, by oxidizing some trace organic chemicals found in surface water; however, many public health officials justify chlorination, stating that the risk from bacterial diseases far outweighs the small risk from these carcinogens, especially when their concentrations are very low. Some alternative treatment methods do not have this risk, but they are more expensive. There is little routine water-quality monitoring

for chemical hazards. There are small, expensive devices using reverse osmosis that can be used to purify personal drinking water, but they are impractical for wide use in areas where local drinking-water supplies are contaminated. (See Chapter 16.)

Sanitary wastewater treatment is also focused on (a) the presence of pathogenic bacteria and (b) the large amount of particulate organic matter that requires oxygen to decompose, known as the *biological oxygen demand* (BOD). Biological oxidation in standard sewage treatment plants is the current method of choice. Typically, raw sewage is filtered with coarse screens and passed through settling tanks to remove large particles that form sludge on the bottom of the tanks. The water phase is then aerated, which produces more particles and sludge. The bacteria are mostly collected in the sludge. The sludge is passed to an anaerobic digester, where more of the biological oxygen demand is removed and many of the bacteria are killed. The water continues to a trickle filter that has a bacterial biofilm (slime) on a solid phase to remove much of the remaining soluble organic waste, followed by a sand filter. In some cases, there is a final disinfection tank to minimize releases of viable organisms. These steps constitute tertiary treatment, which can remove almost 100% of suspended solids and approximately 99% of BOD. Additional steps, such as pH control, addition of complexing agents, and air stripping, can remove inorganic and volatile hydrocarbons. Many areas in low- and middle-income countries do not have any sewage treatment or only primary treatment to remove suspended solids. (See Chapter 16.)

The beneficial bacteria in digesters are vulnerable to releases of chemical wastes, as illustrated in the following case:

A chrome-plating shop dumped its acid bath directly into a sanitary sewer, leading to a shutdown of the Salem, Massachusetts, municipal treatment plant, with considerable hazard to workers. The strong acid and toxic metals killed the bacteria and produced a major release of hydrogen sulfide from the sludge and the anaerobic sludge digester. Fortunately, the plant workers escaped without harm when they were warned by alarms from sensors detecting high concentrations of hydrogen sulfide. Several weeks were needed to clean out the system and restart the treatment process, during which raw sewage went into Salem Harbor.

Food Contamination and Sanitation

Food animals and plants can become contaminated by ingestion or absorption of hazardous materials. They can also be contaminated externally by contact with contaminants. Bioaccumulation of aquatic contaminants can be a hazard to humans and other animals. Plants can absorb metals, such as lead and cadmium, from the soil. Pesticides can contaminate the surface of food. Many pesticides are biodegradable, but sufficient time and appropriate environmental conditions must occur to reduce pesticide residues to safe levels. Food crops are tested routinely for pesticide levels and other contaminants; there are strict requirements for allowable levels of pesticides in food, but only a tiny fraction of food crops is tested.

Animal carcasses are visually inspected for quality by government inspectors in many countries. However, the frequency and extent of chemical testing of food items is very limited. When testing is done, it is generally focused on detecting extensive contamination, so limited and localized contamination can easily pass undetected. Testing is expensive and adds to the complexity of the food distribution system for producers. Unless testing is performed by government agencies, it is likely to be very limited.

Contamination of food items by biological agents, such as bacteria and molds, is common and well recognized as a hazard. Most do not produce disease, but some infectious agents may be transmitted by food. Similarly, it is extremely difficult to prevent contamination of food by materials from rodents and insects. Consumers routinely reject food that has visible contamination or has been exposed to insects. Handling and preparing food under sanitary conditions can minimize contamination and subsequent adverse health effects. (See Chapter 17.)

Consumer Products

Adverse health effects can occur due to exposure to very low levels of chemicals used in consumer products. Biomarkers of exposure to common pesticides and chemicals used in consumer and personal care products can be detected in almost all people living in the United States.[12] Although detection of a chemical in the body does not alone prove that it is causing (or has caused) a toxic effect, widespread exposures to a population of even low levels of some chemicals might cause more cancer, birth defects, endocrine disruption, or other adverse health effects.

Solid Waste and Land Pollution

For centuries, people have disposed of many types of wastes in landfills, or "dumps." As populations have grown, especially in large cities, the amount of waste has become overwhelming, sparking recycling programs for paper products, plastics, metals, and petroleum products. As our consumer culture has grown, the composition of materials in landfills has broadened and has become more complex. Today's computer, cell phone, or tablet will be part of tomorrow's toxic waste because of its built-in obsolescence and its toxic components. Low- and middle-income countries (LMICs) are also experiencing these problems, due to increased consumption and high-income countries sending them toxic materials, such as used electronic equipment, for disposal.

Surface water and groundwater have been contaminated by runoff and leakage from improperly discarded wastes. Often unrecognized are the potential hazards from small amounts of toxic materials in homes, such as cadmium batteries, paint solvents, pesticides, and cleaners. It is easier to recognize industrial waste problems from large producers of waste. In high-income countries, strong regulations generally control releases of industrial wastes, and most large industrial companies reclaim and recycle wastes. However, small firms lack the knowledge about hazards and the resources to control them.

Nanotechnology and Nanomaterials

Nanotechnology is the manipulation of matter on a near-atomic scale to produce new structures, materials, and devices. Nanoscale materials include a wide range of elements, other chemicals, and materials that may be engineered to develop unique configurations or shapes, such as hollow tubes or spheres. At this small scale, nanomaterials may have different properties than the same materials at larger scales, such as greater strength, lighter weight, and greater chemical reactivity.

Nanotechnology has led to scientific advances and new applications in many areas, including materials science, consumer products, medicine, energy, and manufacturing. The global market for these materials is growing rapidly. However, rapidly expanding manipulation and use of nanomaterials has raised concerns, among workers and consumers, about exposure to the nanomaterials used in these applications. Traditional mass-based approaches to exposure assessment are likely not appropriate for nanomaterials; therefore, much recent research has focused on how best to measure and to characterize exposure to the wide range of nanomaterials. Much about the health and safety risks of nanomaterials remains unknown. However, research and regulatory agencies in the United States and elsewhere are investigating the potential for hazardous exposures and associated health effects in order to determine how best to regulate the production and use of these materials.

ACKNOWLEDGMENT

The author thanks Thomas J. Smith, PhD, for his important contributions to earlier versions of this chapter, which appeared in previous editions of this book.

REFERENCES

1. Occupational Safety and Health Administration, U.S. Department of Labor. General industry: OSHA safety and health standards (29 CFR 1910). Available at: http://www.osha.gov/. Accessed October 18, 2016.
2. Kromhout H. Design of measurement strategies for workplace exposures. Occupational and Environmental Medicine 2002; 59: 349–354.
3. Loomis D, Kromhout H. Exposure variability: Concepts and applications in occupational epidemiology. American Journal of Industrial Medicine 2004; 45: 113–122.
4. Scher DP, Sawchuk RJ, Alexander BH, Adgate JL. Estimating absorbed dose of pesticides in a field setting using biomonitoring data and pharmacokinetic models. Journal of Toxicology and Environmental Health, Part A-Current Issues 2008; 71: 373–383.
5. Vermeulen R, Stewart P, Kromhout H. Dermal exposure assessment in occupational epidemiologic research. Scandinavian Journal of Work, Environment & Health 2002; 28: 371–385.
6. Andersen ME. Toxicokinetic modeling and its applications in chemical risk assessment. Toxicology Letters 2003; 138: 9–27.
7. Spear RC, Poppendorf WJ, Spencer WF, Milby TH. Worker poisonings due to paroxone residues. Journal of Occupational Medicine 1977; 19: 411–414.
8. Zalk DM, Nelson DI. History and evolution of control banding: a review. Journal of Occupational and Environmental Hygiene 2008; 5: 330–346.
9. Cutler JJ, Parker GS, Rosen S, et al. Childhood leukemia in Woburn, Massachusetts. Public Health Reports 1986; 101: 201–205.
10. Durant JL, Chen J, Hemond HF, Thilly WG. Elevated incidence of childhood leukemia in Woburn, Massachusetts: NIEHS Superfund Basic Research Program searches for causes. Environmental Health Perspectives 1995; 103: 93–98.
11. U.S. Environmental Protection Agency. Criteria air pollutants: NAAQS table. Available at: https://www.epa.gov/criteria-air-pollutants/naaqs-table. Accessed January 12, 2017.
12. Centers for Disease Control and Prevention. Fourth national report on human exposure to environmental chemicals. Atlanta: Author, 2009.

FURTHER READING

ACGIH. Industrial ventilation (29th ed.). Cincinnati, OH: ACGIH, 2016.
Manual containing recommendations for the design and operation of ventilation systems to control air contaminants.
Anna DH (ed.). The occupational environment: Its evaluation, control, and management (3rd ed.), Volumes 1 and 2. Fairfax, VA: American Industrial Hygiene Association, 2011.
Burgess WA. Recognition of health hazards in industry: A review of materials and processes (2nd ed.). New York: John Wiley & Sons, 1995.
The classic source of much of the data in Table 8-1 and a highly recommended basic reference for all occupational health professionals. The hazards discussed are still highly relevant for industries that have been moved to LMICs.

Gardiner K, Harrington JM (eds.). Occupational hygiene (3rd ed.). Malden, MA: Blackwell, 2005.
A useful and comprehensive general reference on industrial hygiene. It provides a more European perspective.

Hocking, MB. Handbook of chemical technology and pollution control (3rd ed.). San Diego, CA: Academic Press, 2005.
A good technical source for gathering background information on basic industries and industrial processes and related pollution control technology.

Jahn SD, Bullock WH, Ignacio JS (eds.). A strategy for assessing and managing occupational exposures (4th ed.). Fairfax, VA: American Industrial Hygiene Association, 2015.
A valuable resource.

National Institute for Occupational Safety and Health. NIOSH publications and products. Available at: http://www.cdc.gov/niosh/pubs/default.html
This website features many different types of databases and information resources. The most popular databases include the International Chemical Safety Cards, the NIOSH Pocket Guide to Chemical Hazards, and NIOSHTIC-2. The NIOSH Manual of Analytical Methods can be obtained at this website.

Occupational Safety and Health Administration, U.S. Department of Labor. OSHA analytical methods manual, part I–organic substances Vol 1–3, 1990; part 2–inorganic substances, Vols. 1–2, 1991. Washington, DC: Author.
This manual is designed for the laboratory chemist and industrial hygienist. New methods are continuously being added and all can be found through the OSHA website: https://www.osha.gov/dts/sltc/methods/.

Perkins, JL (ed.). Modern industrial hygiene, Vol. 1: Recognition and evaluation of chemical agents (2nd ed.), 2008; Vol. 2: Biological aspects, 2003; Vol. 3: Control of chemical agents, 2012. Cincinnati, OH: ACGIH.

Rappaport SM, Kupper L. Quantitative exposure assessment. Lulu, Inc., 2011. Available at: http://www.lulu.com/.
While these two works contain much useful information, the former is difficult to follow in places and both require a strong background in statistics. They are important because they lay out the rationale for sampling strategies to determine compliance with OSHA's permissible exposure limits.

World Health Organization publications: Environment health, hazard assessment. Available at: http://www.who.int/publications/en/.
WHO has published a series of books and monographs on hazard assessment on broad topics, such as climate change, air and water pollution, risks to children, and specific agents, such as radon, organotin compounds, and trichloroethylene. These references contain relevant material about exposure standards in Europe and elsewhere.

9

Occupational Ergonomics: Promoting Safety and Health Through Work Design

W. Monroe Keyserling

*O*ccupational ergonomics is the holistic study of people at work to understand the complex interrelationships with their work environments (including facilities, equipment, furniture, and tools), job demands, and work methods. All work activities place physical, mental, and psychosocial demands on workers. If these demands are kept within reasonable limits, work performance will likely be satisfactory and workers' health and well-being will likely be maintained. However, if demands are excessive or poorly matched to the capabilities or expectations of workers, errors, injuries, and decrements in physical or mental health may occur.

Some work-related injuries, such as amputations, fractures, and burns, occur suddenly in association with overt events (such as entrapments, falls, collisions, and explosions), where the resulting energy exchange produces immediate and discernible tissue damage (Chapter 19). Other injuries, including many work-related musculoskeletal disorders (MSDs), are cumulative, resulting from low-level chronic exposures, such as repetitive and/or prolonged motions or awkward

postures, and the onset of symptoms can be delayed for years (Chapter 20).[1]

Occupational ergonomists evaluate work demands and the corresponding abilities of people to react and cope. The goal of an occupational ergonomics program is to maintain a safe work environment by designing organizational structures, facilities, furniture, equipment, tools, training, and job demands to be compatible with workers' attributes, such as size, strength, mobility, aerobic capacity, information-processing capacity, and expectations. A successful ergonomics program should simultaneously improve health and enhance productivity. Conversely, failure to consider ergonomics in the design of work environments and job demands can lead to increased risk of catastrophic events, sudden-onset injuries, and/or chronic MSDs.

ERGONOMIC APPROACHES

Ergonomic approaches can be applied to preventing errors, acute injuries, MSDs, and excessive fatigue and discomfort (Box 9-1).

Box 9-1. Ergonomic Approaches to Prevention

Preventing Sudden-Onset Injuries

- Designing a machine guard that allows a worker to operate equipment with smooth, comfortable, and time-efficient motions. This reduces inconveniences introduced by the guard and decreases the likelihood that it will be bypassed or removed, thus exposing the worker to mechanical hazards that may cause serious fatal or disfiguring injuries. A well-designed guard may also eliminate awkward postures that lead to MSDs in vulnerable body parts, such as the lower back, shoulders, and upper extremities.

- Evaluating the mechanics of human gait to determine forces acting between the floor surface and the sole of the shoe. This information is used to determine friction required to reduce the risk of a slip or fall. Falls can also be prevented by eliminating slip and trip hazards, such as puddles of oil on the floor, uneven floor surfaces, and changes in floor elevation. In situations where these hazards cannot be completely eliminated, ergonomic principles can enhance the ability of workers to perceive and react to these hazards by providing good lighting and contrasting surface colors.

- Designing warning signs for hazardous equipment and work locations so that workers take appropriate actions to avoid accidents. Warnings are particularly important for visitors, inexperienced workers, and contract workers, or if the hazards are hidden or subtle.

- Designing automated manufacturing systems so that individual machines can be easily isolated and locked out to a zero-energy state so that maintenance activities can be performed safety and without interrupting nearby machines. Design for maintenance should also allow easy access to critical components while concurrently guarding hazards to the greatest extent possible.

Preventing Musculoskeletal Disorders Caused by Overexertion or Overuse

- Evaluating lifting tasks to determine biomechanical strain on the lower back and designing lifting tasks to prevent back disorders.

- Evaluating workstation layouts to discover causes of postural stress. These include torso bending and twisting as well as overhead work with arms and hands. They also include implementing changes in workstation layout to eliminate awkward or sustained work postures that may lead to MSDs in the trunk and shoulders. Eliminating awkward postures may also reduce fatigue and enhance performance.

- Evaluating highly repetitive, manual assembly-line jobs and developing alternative hand tools and work methods to reduce the risk of cumulative trauma disorders of the upper extremities. These include tendonitis, epicondylitis, tenosynovitis, and CTS.

Preventing Excessive Fatigue and Discomfort

- Designing equipment and furniture of a computer workstation and associated tasks so that an operator can use a monitor, mouse, and keyboard for extended periods without experiencing visual fatigue or musculoskeletal discomfort. Discomfort in the back, neck, or upper extremities may be a precursor of potentially disabling problems, such as tendonitis or CTS.

- Evaluating the metabolic demands of a job performed in a hot, humid environment to develop a work–rest regimen that prevents heat stress.

- Establishing maximum work times for transportation workers, such as truck drivers and airline pilots, to reduce the risk of drowsiness, performance errors, and accidents caused by sleep deprivation.

Prevention through Design

Prevention through design is a process being promoted by the National Institute for Occupational Safety and Health (NIOSH)[2] and other agencies and professional organizations to prevent occupational injuries and illnesses by eliminating, or substantially reducing, hazards early in the job-design process and when existing jobs are modified or retrofitted. Prevention through design is intended to cover the entire life cycle of organizational structures, facilities, equipment, and processes, including conceptualization, construction, operation, maintenance, and dismantling and disposal. Ergonomists are an important part of the prevention through design team and consider a broad range of issues, including the following:

- *Physical ergonomics of production tasks*: Assuring that the physical demands of the job, such as force, posture, and energy expenditure, do not exceed the capability and capacity of workers.

- *Cognitive ergonomics of production tasks*: Assuring that the mental and information-processing demands of the job are matched to capabilities and expectations, thus reducing the likelihood of human error that could lead to injuries and other losses.

- *Ergonomics of maintenance tasks*: This includes (a) assuring that there is adequate physical space to safely perform maintenance activities in biomechanically efficient work postures, (b) designing tools that allow workers to perform maintenance tasks without exerting excessive force, and (c) designing lock-out and energy-control systems so that diagnosis and repair of equipment problems can be performed safely. In addition, developing robust preventive maintenance programs and standard operating procedures for diagnosis and repair reduces the likelihood of errors that may result in injury and extended production interruptions.

Accommodating Persons with Disabilities

The previous examples focus primarily on preventing situations and workplace exposures that could cause death, injury, discomfort, or fatigue. Ergonomic methods and principles can be used to assist workers with disabilities who may need special accommodations to work safely, effectively, and comfortably, such as the following:

- Fire alarms with strobe lights to warn people who are hearing impaired
- Computers equipped with voice-recognition hardware and software to accommodate persons who have lost the use of their hands, or where a traditional data-entry device (keyboard or mouse) may cause or aggravate an upper-extremity MSD
- Accommodations for older workers because many human capabilities, such as vision, hearing, balance, aerobic endurance, reaction time, and strength, begin to slowly decline starting at about age 40.

Universal design (sometimes called *inclusive design*) is the concept of designing the built environment, vehicles, and products to be usable by as many people as possible. Examples include curb cuts into sidewalks and "kneeling" buses with ramps to accommodate wheelchair users. Ergonomists also develop accommodations for people who have become disabled, working with physiatrists, psychologists, physical and occupational therapists, rehabilitation engineers, and other health professionals to create work environments and job demands that facilitate return to work.

The remainder of this chapter describes subdisciplines of ergonomics concerned with occupational safety and health.

COGNITIVE ERGONOMICS

Cognitive ergonomics (human factors engineering or engineering psychology) is concerned with the perceptual, information-processing, and psychomotor aspects of work. Engineering psychologists design displays, controls, procedures, software, equipment, warning signs, alarms, and general work environments to improve work performance and reduce human error that can lead to injuries and production and property losses. Common causes of human error include the following:

1. *Failure to perceive or recognize a hazardous condition or situation*: To react to a dangerous situation, a worker must first perceive that danger exists. Many workplace hazards are not easily perceived through vision, hearing, smell, or touch. Examples include excessive pressure inside a boiler, a fork truck or automatic guided vehicle (AGV) approaching from behind in a noisy factory, uneven flooring in a poorly lit room, and a sudden release of an odorless, colorless toxic gas. These situations require special displays or alarms. Boilers should be equipped with gauges that display internal pressure and audible alarms that activate when pressure exceeds safe limits. A simple display can be enhanced by trend information, indicating the direction and rate of pressure changes over time. To protect pedestrians, fork trucks and AGVs must have beepers and flashing lights that operate when the vehicle moves. Good lighting is required near trip hazards, and alarm systems should sound if toxic gases are released. Warning signs at locations with concealed hazards, such as confined-space entry points, enhance awareness so that appropriate preparation and prevention actions are taken. Piping systems should have signage to show contents and direction of flow.

2. *Failure in information-processing, situational awareness and/or decision-making processes*: Decision-making involves combining real-time information with existing knowledge and assumptions to provide a basis for action. Errors can occur when assumptions do not match reality. In 2013, a plane crashed during an attempted landing at San Francisco International Airport, resulting in three deaths and 187 injured passengers and crew members. A complete investigatory report on the crash was written by the National Transportation Safety Board (NTSB).[3] The pilot and copilot incorrectly assumed that the autopilot system was controlling airspeed. As a result, they did not adequately monitor instrumentation or recognize that the plane was descending too quickly. By the time they discovered their errors, it was too late to recover. The plane crashed into a sea wall, short of the runway. The NTSB determined that overreliance on automation, incorrect assumptions due to inadequate training, and poor situational awareness were factors that contributed to this crash.

3. *Failures in motor actions following correct decisions*: Following a decision, it is frequently necessary for a worker to perform a motor action, such as flipping a switch or adjusting a knob to control the status of a system or machine. Problems can occur if required actions exceed motor abilities. For example, the force required to adjust a control valve in a chemical plant should not exceed a worker's strength. Errors can occur if controls are not clearly labeled or if manipulation of controls causes unexpected responses. Switches that start potentially dangerous machinery or equipment should be guarded to prevent unintentional activation, by covering them, locking them in the "off" position during maintenance and other activities, or placing them in locations where they cannot be accidentally touched.

WORK PHYSIOLOGY

Physical work, such as walking, carrying, lifting, or gripping, occurs as the result of contractions of muscle. *Work physiology* is the branch of ergonomics concerned with the responses of the cardiovascular system, pulmonary system, and skeletal muscles to the metabolic demands of work. If demands exceed metabolic capacities, workers will likely experience excessive fatigue of a few muscles or their entire bodies.

Localized Muscle Fatigue

Local muscle fatigue is associated with work activities that require a body segment to perform static work, high-intensity work, or highly repetitive work. It may result from sustained awkward posture, such as when automobile mechanics flex their torsos while working in engine compartments or when electricians elevate their shoulders for prolonged periods when reaching overhead to install wires. In other instances, static work may involve short-duration, forceful exertions, such as using a tire iron to unfreeze a rusted lug nut when changing a tire. Local muscle fatigue may be an early indicator of work-related MSDs.

When a muscle contracts, internal blood vessels are compressed. Because vascular resistance increases with the level of muscle tension, the blood supply to the working muscle decreases. Without periodic relaxation, the demand for metabolic nutrients and oxygen exceeds the supply, and metabolic wastes accumulate. In the short term, ischemic pain, tremor, and reduced strength may occur; in the long term, injuries may occur.[3]

The general relationship between the intensity and duration of a static exertion was first described by Walter Rohmert in 1960 (Figure 9-1). A contraction of maximum (100%) intensity can be sustained for a few seconds; a contraction of 50% of maximum intensity for about 1 minute. To sustain a static contraction indefinitely, he recommended that exertion intensity be kept below 15% of the maximum.[4] A recent meta-analysis of 194 publications confirmed the basic shape of the Rohmert curve for lower extremity, trunk, and upper extremity muscle groups.[5] Figure 9-1 reflects time to exhaustion. Since workers should not exert themselves to the point of exhaustion, static work demands should stay below the curve. Sustained hand-grip exertions

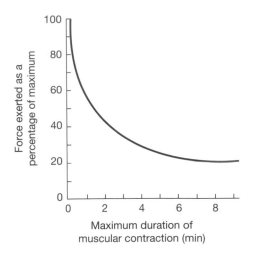

Figure 9-1. Maximum duration of a static muscle contraction for various levels of muscular contraction. (Source: Keyserling WM, Armstrong TJ. Ergonomics. In JM Last [ed.]. Maxcy-Rosenau public health and preventive medicine [12th ed.] Norwalk, CT: Appleton, Century, Crofts, 1986, pp. 734–750.)

as low as 10% of maximum strength can produce residual muscle fatigue after 24 hours.[6] Work activities should be designed so that static exertions are of limited duration and adequate recovery time is built into the job. Dynamic activities involving cyclical contraction and relaxation of working muscle are generally preferable to static work.

Dynamic Work and Whole-Body Fatigue

Whole-body dynamic work occurs when large skeletal muscle groups repeatedly contract and relax while performing a task. Common examples of dynamic work include walking on a level surface, pushing a loaded cart, climbing stairs, shoveling snow, and carrying a load.

The intensity of whole-body dynamic work is limited by the capacity of the respiratory and cardiovascular systems to deliver adequate supplies of oxygen and glucose to working muscles and remove products of metabolism. Whole-body fatigue occurs when the collective metabolic demands of working muscles throughout the body exceed this capacity. Symptoms of whole-body fatigue include shortness of breath, weakness in working muscles, and a general feeling of tiredness. These symptoms continue and

may increase until the work activity is stopped or decreased in intensity.

For extremely short durations of whole-body dynamic activity (generally 4 minutes or less), people can work at intensities equal to their aerobic capacities before a rest break is required. As the duration of work increases, the intensity must decrease. For a 1-hour work period, the average energy expenditure should not exceed 50% of the worker's aerobic capacity. For an 8-hour shift, the average energy expenditure should not exceed 33% of the worker's aerobic capacity.[7]

Aerobic capacity varies considerably within the population. Aerobic capacity peaks in the third decade (20 to 29 years) for both men and women. At age 20, average aerobic capacity is 15 kcal/min for untrained men and 11 kcal/min for untrained women. At age 50, these values decrease to 12 kcal/min for men and 8 kcal/min for women. By age 70, the values drop to 9 kcal/min for men and 6.5 kcal/min for women.[8] These are average values for each age- and-gender group and do not reflect the full range of variability among adults. This variability is an important consideration when evaluating ergonomic stress; a job that is relatively easy for a person with high aerobic capacity can be extremely fatiguing for a person with low capacity.

The prevention of whole-body fatigue is accomplished through good work design. The energy demands of a job should be sufficiently low to accommodate the adult working population, including persons with limited aerobic capacity. This can be accomplished by designing the workplace to minimize unnecessary body movements (excessive walking, carrying, or climbing) and providing mechanical assists, such as hoists or conveyors for handling heavy materials. If these approaches are not feasible, it may be necessary to provide rest allowances to prevent excessive fatigue, especially in hot, humid work environments due to the metabolic contribution to heat stress.

In establishing metabolic criteria for jobs that involve repetitive manual lifting, NIOSH recommends that the average energy expenditure during an 8-hour work shift should not exceed 3.5 kcal per minute.[9,10] Caution should be practiced when placing persons with low levels of physical fitness on metabolically strenuous jobs.*

To assess the potential for whole-body fatigue for a specific job, one must determine the energy expenditure rate by one of the following three methods:

1. *Table reference*: One can refer to extensive tables of the energy costs of various work activities. (The text by McArdle, Katch, and Katch cited in the Further Reading section provides tables describing the energy costs of many work tasks.)
2. *Indirect calorimetry*: One can estimate energy expenditure for a specific job by measuring a worker's oxygen uptake while performing the job.[8,11]
3. *Modeling*: One can analyze a job and break it down into fundamental tasks, such as walking, carrying, and lifting. Parameters describing each task can be inserted into equations to predict energy expenditure.[12]

There is no one best method for determining energy expenditure. The selection of a method is often a trade-off between (a) the availability of published tables or prediction equations for the specific work activities of interest and (b) the time and expenses associated with data collection for indirect calorimetry, which is necessary to obtain a precise measure of energy expenditure.

BIOMECHANICS

Biomechanics is concerned with the properties of tissue and its response to mechanical stresses. Some injury-causing mechanical stresses in the workplace are caused by overt, sudden-onset events, such as crushed foot bones caused by the impact of a dropped object. The hazards that produce these injuries can usually be controlled through safety engineering techniques. (See Chapter 19.) Other mechanical stresses are more subtle and often do not cause injuries that are immediately perceptible. Work-related

overexertion MSDs frequently affect the lower back, neck, shoulders, and upper and lower extremities. They include sprains, strains, tendonitis, bursitis, and carpal tunnel syndrome (CTS). Because these disorders can impair mobility, strength, tactile capabilities, and motor control, affected workers may be unable to perform their jobs. Primary risk factors for overexertion injuries and disorders include the following:

• Forceful exertions
• Sustained or awkward postures
• Localized mechanical contact stresses or compression
• Vibration
• Temperature extremes.

All of these risk factors are modified by repetition (frequency of exposure) to these risk factors and duration (total time of exposure to them).[13–21] Psychosocial factors in the work environment, such as monotony, autonomy, and social support from supervisors and colleagues, may act in synergy with primary risk factors, contributing to the development and/or aggravation of MSDs. (See Chapter 14.)

In addition to identifying the presence of these risk factors, ergonomic job analysis evaluates specific job attributes, such as workstation layout, production standards, incentive systems, work organization, and work methods—all of which affect the magnitude, frequency, and duration of worker exposure to these risk factors. This information needs to be obtained to design and implement job modifications effectively.

Forceful Exertions

Whole-body exertions, such as strenuous lifting, pushing, and pulling, can cause back pain and other injuries and disorders (Figure 9-2). Because the lifting and handling of heavy weights are the most commonly cited activities associated with occupational low back pain, NIOSH[9–10] and ACGIH[19] have issued guidelines for the evaluation and design of jobs that require manual lifting. These guidelines consider factors, such as lift frequency, work duration, workplace geometry, and posture, to establish the amount of weight that a worker can lift safely. Factors

---

* Aerobic capacity can be determined by measuring oxygen uptake and carbon dioxide production during a stress test. For additional information on measuring or estimating aerobic capacity, see the text by McArdle, Katch, and Katch in the Further Reading section.

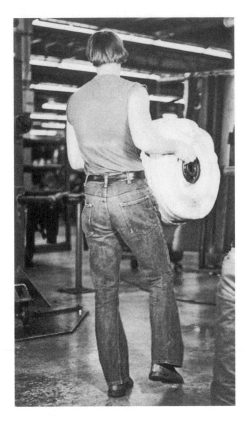

Figure 9-2. The load carried by this worker exceeds 50 kg (110 lbs.). A mechanical assist device, such as an overhead hoist, would reduce the risk of back injuries on this job. (Photograph by W. Monroe Keyserling.)

other than object weight play a significant role in the amount of force that workers can safely exert during lifting and other manual transfer tasks. Due to the effect of long moment arms, handling relatively light loads can stress muscles in the back and shoulder if loads are held at a long horizontal distance in front or to the side of the body (Figure 9-3).

The following approaches may help reduce the magnitude of forces exerted during whole-body exertions:

- Reduce the weight of lifted objects, such as by placing fewer parts in a tote bin or purchasing smaller bags of powdered or granular materials
- Reduce extended reach postures by removing obstructions that prevent a worker from getting close to the lifted object
- Use mechanical aids, such as conveyors, hoists, conveyors, and articulating arms, to assist a worker and/or eliminate the manual exertion (Figure 9-4).

Forceful exertions of the hands, such as cutting with knives or scissors, tightening screws, "snapping" together electrical connectors, and using the hands or fingers to sand or buff parts,

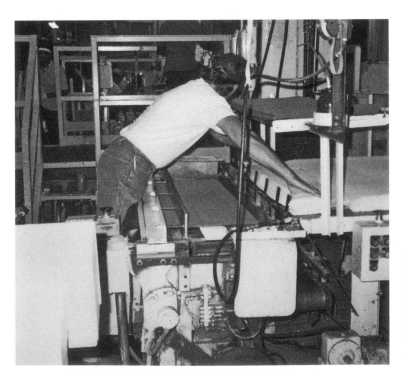

Figure 9-3. Although the lifted load is relatively light (approximately 8 kg), the combination of forward bending and lifting places a high load on the spine, increasing the risk of a back injury. (Photograph by W. Monroe Keyserling.)

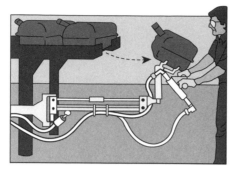
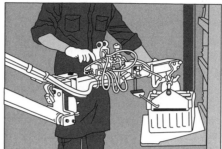

Figure 9-4. Mechanical assist devices can reduce or eliminate forceful exertions during manual materials handling activities such as lifting or carrying. (Courtesy of the University of Michigan and the UAW/Ford Joint National Committee on Health and Safety.) (Source: University of Michigan Center for Ergonomics. Fitting jobs to people: An ergonomics process. Ann Arbor: Regents of the University of Michigan, 1991.)

can cause upper-extremity disorders, such as tendonitis and CTS.[13–18,20] Factors that can increase forces exerted by the finger flexor and extensor muscles and tendons include pinch grips, heavy tools, poorly balanced tools, poorly maintained tools (such as dull knives or scissors), or low friction between a hand and a tool handle. Gloves may increase force requirements of some jobs due to reduced tactile feedback, reduced friction, or resistance of gloves to stretching or compression. Environmental conditions may also increase force requirements; for example, some rubber and plastic materials lose their flexibility when cold and become more difficult to shape or manipulate. The following approaches help reduce the forcefulness of hand exertions:

- Substitute power tools for manual tools (If a power tool is not feasible, redesign the manual tool to increase mechanical advantage or otherwise decrease required hand forces.)
- Suspend heavy tools with "zero-gravity" balance devices
- Treat slippery handles with friction-enhancing coatings to minimize slippage and reduce hand force
- Relocate the handle of an off-balance tool closer to the center of gravity or suspending the tool so that off-balance characteristics are minimized
- Use torque-control devices (reaction arms or automatic shut-offs) on power tools, such as air wrenches, nut runners, or screw drivers (Figure 9-5)

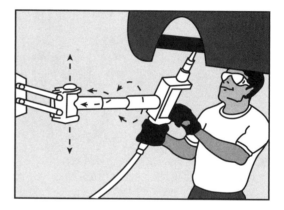

Figure 9-5. Torque control devices can substantially reduce the amount of force exerted when using air wrenches and similar tools. Note that the weight of the tool is also borne by the device, further reducing the force exerted by the worker. (Courtesy of the University of Michigan and the UAW/Ford Joint National Committee on Health and Safety.) (Source: University of Michigan Center for Ergonomics. Fitting jobs to people: An ergonomics process. Ann Arbor: Regents of the University of Michigan, 1991.)

- If high force is required to engage tightly fitting parts, improve quality control to achieve a better fit and/or use a lubricant to reduce friction
- Pre-warm rubber and plastic components if these become cold and unmalleable during storage.

Sustained or Awkward Posture

Awkward posture (positioning a joint at or near the limit of its range of motion) may cause transient discomfort and fatigue. Prolonged awkward

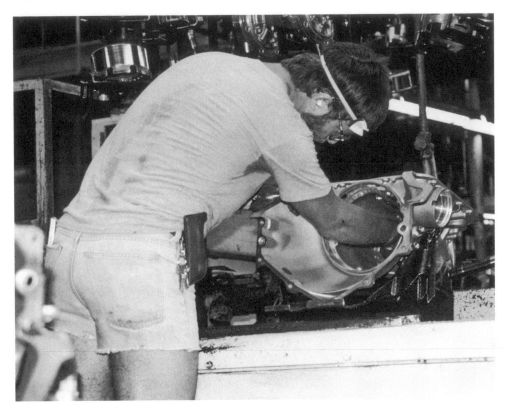

Figure 9-6. This assembly-line worker must twist and laterally bend his back in order to see his hands to install a part. (Photograph by W. Monroe Keyserling.)

postures may contribute to disabling injuries and disorders of musculoskeletal tissue and/or peripheral nerves. Awkward trunk postures (Figures 9-3 and 9-6) increase the risk of back injuries.[13,15–17,21] Raising the elbow above shoulder height or reaching behind the torso can increase the likelihood of MSDs in the neck and shoulders. The workers shown in Figure 9-7 must position their arms awkwardly due to poor workstation layout.

Most awkward postures of the trunk and shoulder result from excessive reach distances, such as bending into bins to place or retrieve parts, reaching overhead to high shelves and conveyors, or reaching overhead or in front of the body to activate machine controls. These postures can be eliminated through improved workstation layout. In general, workers should not reach below knee height or above shoulder height for prolonged periods. Horizontal-reach distances in front of the body should be limited in order to keep the trunk upright and the upper arms nearly parallel to the trunk. Where possible, workstations and equipment should offer

adjustability to accommodate workers of different body sizes using *anthropometry*, the branch of ergonomics concerned with designing facilities and equipment to accommodate populations of varying body dimensions. (See the textbook by Pheasant in the Further Reading section.)

Allowing workers to sit reduces fatigue and discomfort in the legs and feet and can increase the stability of the upper body, a necessity for highly precise manual tasks. However, prolonged sitting may lead to back pain. A well-designed work seat, such as one with good lumbar support and adjustability of the seat pan and backrest, enhances comfort and can reduce the risk of MSDs. Layouts that allow workers to alternate between standing and sitting postures are also desirable. Certain jobs, such as working at a moving conveyor line or in a job that requires constant movement among different workstations, cannot be performed while sitting. In situations where workers are required to stand for most of the work shift, antifatigue matting and shoe inserts have been shown to

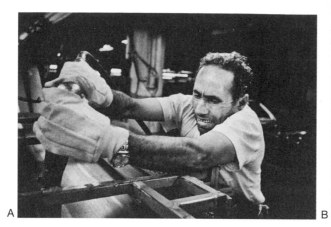
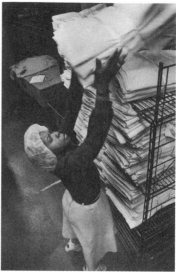

A   B

Figure 9-7. Both of these workers are at risk of MSDs: (A) The worker on this job exerts high hand force with elevated shoulders, increasing the risk of shoulder and upper extremity injuries. (B) This laundry worker is at increased risk of upper-extremity and back injuries as a result of a poorly designed work task. (Photographs by Earl Dotter.)

enhance comfort in the legs and lower back.[22] In addition, workers should be encouraged and allowed to sit during temporary production interruptions.

Awkward upper-extremity postures can occur at the shoulder (see previous discussion), elbow, or wrist. Jobs and tools should be designed to avoid frequent or prolonged activities that require forearm pronation or supination that approaches range-of-motion limits and/or wrist excursions, such as extreme flexion, extension, and radial or ulnar deviation. Jobs that involve precise alignment and positioning of parts and materials frequently require substantial wrist deviations. (See Figure 1-3 of garment workers in Chapter 1.)[13] Features of hand tools, such as the shape and orientation of handles, together with workstation layout (location and orientation of work surfaces), strongly influence wrist postures.

Localized Contact Stresses and Compression

Local mechanical stresses result from concentrated pressure during contact between body tissues and objects and tools and from compression of the plantar foot during sustained standing. The time to discomfort decreases as the magnitude of pressure increases; however, certain tissues tolerate compression better than others.[23]

Hand hammering (using the palm as a striking tool) is used in some manufacturing and maintenance tasks as a method for joining two parts. This activity, which can irritate nerves and other parts of the palm, can be avoided by using a mallet. Hand tools with hard, sharp, or small-diameter handles, such as knives, pliers, and scissors, can compress and irritate nerves and tendons in the palm and fingers. This problem can be controlled by padding and/or increasing the radius of curvature of handles. In some bench-assembly activities and office jobs, contact stresses result from resting forearms or wrists against a sharp, unpadded edge of a work bench. This problem can usually be controlled by rounding or padding the edge, or by providing a support for forearms and wrists.

Seated workstations that produce localized pressure on the posterior knee and thigh can impair circulation, causing swelling and discomfort in the lower legs, ankles, and feet. A common cause of this condition is a work seat that is too high, allowing the lower legs to dangle, producing concentrated compressive forces on tissues where the thighs contact the front edge of the seatpan. Solutions to this problem include adjustable seats and providing a footrest to partially support the weight of the legs.

Vibration

Exposure to whole-body vibration while driving or riding in motor vehicles, including fork trucks and off-road vehicles, may be a factor that increases the risk of back pain.[13,15] Because driving tasks are usually performed in a seated posture, most drivers are simultaneously exposed to two back pain risk factors. Driving over rough surfaces for prolonged periods, while sitting in a poorly suspended seat, can increase vibration exposure.

Localized vibration of the upper extremity (segmental vibration) can occur when using powered hand tools, such as screwdrivers, nut runners, grinders, jackhammers, and chippers. Segmental vibration may contribute to the development of hand-arm vibration syndromes, such as vibration white finger.[13,15] Careful selection of proper tools can help to reduce exposure. For example, an air wrench that uses an automatic shut-off system produces less exposure to vibration than a slip-clutch mechanism. Many manufacturers offer a variety of low-vibration hand tools. (See Chapter 12B.)

Temperature Extremes

Exposure to unusually hot or cold ambient temperatures can produce a variety of adverse health effects. In addition to considering the general thermal characteristics (air temperature, air movement, and relative humidity) of the workplace, one should consider temperature extremes that affect the hands. For example, handling extremely hot or cold parts may require the use of special gloves that increase the force requirements of the job. In jobs that involve the use of pneumatic tools, air from high-pressure lines and tool exhaust ports may be directed onto the hands, causing local chilling and reducing manual dexterity and tactile sensitivity. This exposure can be controlled by eliminating leaks and directing exhaust air away from the hands. (See Chapter 12C.)

Repetitive and Prolonged Activities

Biomechanical and physiological strains experienced by workers are related to cumulative exposure to all the risk factors discussed earlier in this chapter.[13–16,20,21] Because ergonomic risk factors are often related to specific work tasks, jobs that involve high repetition and/or duration, such as driving 5,000 screws a day on an assembly line or continuous word-processing in an office, typically involve higher exposures than nonrepetitive jobs, such as inspection work in a factory or a supervisory position in an office. Repetitiveness is not a risk factor limited to the upper extremity. For example, frequent lifting and repetitive and/or prolonged use of awkward trunk postures increase the risk of back pain.

Repetitiveness can often be measured or estimated using industrial engineering records and other work standards. For example, on an assembly line, repetitiveness may be a function of the line speed or the time allowed to complete one unit of work. For a clerk in a bank or insurance office, repetitiveness may be a function of the number of forms processed a day. For a supermarket checker, repetitiveness may be a function of the number of items scanned over the course of a work shift. Repetitiveness can also be measured using an observational technique, where the rapidity and intensity of hand motions are compared against benchmarks or a scale with verbal anchors.[24] (A verbal anchor is a word or phrase that describes the speed or urgency of the hand motions required to perform a job.) An ordinal scale with verbal anchors for describing the repetitiveness of hand-intensive work has been incorporated into an ACGIH threshold limit value for evaluating worker exposure to repetitive hand activities.[19] Additional techniques for assessing repetition, combined with other risk factors for distal upper-extremity MSDs include the Strain Index[25] and the Rapid Upper Limb Assessment.[26]

Two approaches to resolving problems of repetition and prolonged exertions are job enrichment and job rotation. The premise behind these approaches is to increase the overall variety of activities performed by a worker to reduce the repetitiveness of any specific stressful activity. While good in theory, these approaches may be very difficult to implement. Job enrichment and job rotation will not be feasible in workplaces where there are no "low-repetition" jobs to combine with the "high-repetition" jobs. Even in situations with a good mix of low- and high-repetition jobs, there may be other implementation barriers, such as increased learning time and seniority restrictions. In these situations, it may be necessary to establish a participative ergonomics program and to educate management and workers before attempting these interventions.

COMPONENTS OF AN ERGONOMICS PROGRAM

An effective ergonomics program starts with the commitment and involvement of management to provide the organizational resources and motivation to control ergonomic hazards in the workplace. Management must also perform regular reviews and evaluations of the program to assure program goals are met in a deliberate and timely manner. Because ergonomic programs focus on improving the complex interrelationships among workers and their jobs, employee involvement is essential to assuring the success of the program.[16]

An effective program should do all of the following:

- Review health and safety records, such as workers' compensation reports and OSHA logs, to identify patterns of overexertion injuries and illnesses. (In some instances, relevant cases may be underreported, making it difficult to establish direct links between outcomes and specific work exposures.)
- Supplement review of archival records with plant walkthroughs and interviews of workers, supervisors, and/or ergonomic teams[16-27]
- Improve recordkeeping so that overexertion injuries and disorders can be linked to specific jobs and workstations
- Train managers, engineers, and other workers to recognize ergonomic risk factors
- Proactively analyze jobs to identify worker exposures to risk factors that cause overexertion injuries and illnesses
- Design and, if necessary, redesign jobs to reduce or eliminate ergonomic risk factors

- Provide effective treatment and rehabilitation of injured workers to improve the possibility of a timely return to work.

Limited resources must be directed at those jobs with the greatest ergonomic problems. One approach for identifying high-hazard jobs is to analyze available medical, insurance, and safety records for evidence of high rates of overexertion disorders in certain departments, job classifications, or workstations. This approach is called *passive surveillance* because it relies on previously collected information. Passive surveillance may underestimate the true level of the problem. For example, at small plants that do not have in-plant medical services, workers may seek treatment from their personal physicians. Unless workers request coverage under the workers' compensation system, their complaints and associated treatment may not appear in any company records. *Active surveillance* is a more aggressive approach to identifying potential problems. It may include employee surveys to identify jobs associated with elevated rates of discomfort in the back, neck, shoulders, and upper extremities. It may also include interviews with supervisors and personnel managers to identify jobs with high turnover. If alternative employment opportunities exist, workers often seek relief by leaving jobs with unusually high physical stress before a cumulative trauma disorder develops.

Once high-risk jobs have been identified, the next step is to determine specific causes so that corrective actions can be taken. This activity involves job analysis to identify the various risk factors discussed previously, followed by developing engineering and/or administrative interventions to reduce or eliminate exposures. The appropriateness of an intervention will vary among and within facilities. Changes that are practical at one workstation may not be appropriate for others. Alternatives must be evaluated to determine the best strategy for resolving each problem. Most solutions will require fine-tuning to assure that they are acceptable to workers and accomplish the intended reductions in exposure. Follow-up job analyses should be performed to confirm that solutions are effective and that no new stresses have been introduced.

Follow-up health surveillance is also recommended to detect any changes in the pattern of injuries, illnesses, or employee complaints.

CONCLUSION

Occupational ergonomics is a multidisciplinary approach to workplace design, evaluation, and management. The goal of an occupational ergonomics program is to establish and maintain a safe work environment by assuring that job demands are compatible with workers' attributes, capacities, and expectations. Ergonomists collaborate with health professionals, engineers, managers, and workers to identify and ameliorate conditions that can lead to both sudden-onset injuries and chronic MSDs. A successful ergonomics program should simultaneously improve safety, health, and productivity.

REFERENCES

1. Keyserling W, Smith GS. A new look at Haddon's pre-event: Using process control concepts to model energy release in sudden-onset occupational injuries. Journal of Occupational and Environmental Health 2007; 4: 467–475.
2. National Institute for Occupational Safety and Health. The State of the National Initiative on Prevention Through Design (NIOSH Publication No. 2014-123). Cincinnati, OH: NIOSH, 2013.
3. Visser B, vanDieen, JH. Pathophysiology of upper extremity muscle disorders. Journal of Electromyography and Kinesiology 2006; 16: 1–16.
4. Rohmert W. Statische Haltearbeit des Menchen, Special issue of REFA-Nachrichten, 1960. Cited in Kroemer KHE, Grandjean E. Fitting the task to the human—a textbook of occupational ergonomics. London: Taylor & Francis, 1997.
5. Frey-Law LA, Alvin, KG. Endurance time is joint specific: A modelling and meta-analysis investigation. Ergonomics 2010; 53: 109–129.
6. Bystrom S, Fransson-Hall C. Acceptability of intermittent handgrip contractions based on physiologic response. Human Factors 1994; 36: 158–171.
7. Chengalur SN, Rodgers SH, Bernard TE. Kodak's ergonomic design for people at work (2nd ed.). New York: John Wiley & Sons, 2003.
8. McArdle WD, Katch FI, Katch VL. Exercise physiology: energy, nutrition, and human performance (8th ed.). Baltimore: Wolters Kluwer Health and Lippincott Williams and Wilkins, 2015.
9. Waters TR, Putz-Anderson V, Garg A, Fine LJ. Revised NIOSH lifting equation for the design and evaluation of manual lifting tasks. Ergonomics 1993; 36: 749–776.
10. Lu ML, Putz-Anderson V. Garg A, Davis KG. Evaluation of the impact of the revised National Institute for Occupational Safety and Health Lifting Equation. Human Factors 2016; 58: 667–682.
11. Astrand P, Rodahl K, Dahl HA, Stromme SB. Textbook of work physiology: Physiological bases of exercise (4th ed.). Champaign, IL: Human Kinetics, 2003.
12. Garg A, Chaffin DB, Herrin GD. Prediction of metabolic rates for manual materials handling jobs. American Industrial Hygiene Association Journal 1978; 39: 661–674.
13. National Institute for Occupational Safety and Health. Musculoskeletal disorders and workplace factors—a critical review of epidemiologic evidence for work-related musculoskeletal disorders of the neck upper extremity, and low back (NIOSH Publication No. 97-141). Cincinnati, OH: NIOSH, 1997.
14. Violante F, Armstrong T, Kilbom, A. Occupational ergonomics: Work related musculoskeletal disorders of the upper limb and back. London: Taylor & Francis, 2000.
15. National Research Council. Musculoskeletal disorders in the workplace: Low back and upper extremities. Washington, DC: National Academy Press, 2001.
16. European Agency for Safety and Health at Work (Podniece Z, ed.) Work-related musculoskeletal disorders: Prevention report. Luxembourg: Office for Official Publications of the European Communities, 2008.
17. McCauley-Bush P. Ergonomics: Foundational principles, applications, and technologies. Boca Raton, FL: CRC Press, Taylor & Francis Group, 2012.
18. Keyserling WM, Armstrong TJ, Punnett L. Ergonomic job analysis: A structured approach for identifying risk factors associated with overexertion injuries and disorders, Applied Occupational and Environmental Hygiene 1991; 6: 353–363.
19. ACGIH. 2016 TLVs and BEIs. Cincinnati, OH: ACGIH Worldwide, 2016.
20. Rempel D, Gerr F, Harris-Adamson C, et al. Personal and workplace factors and median nerve function in a pooled study of 2396

US workers. Journal of Occupational and Environmental Medicine 2015; 57: 98–104.

21. Punnett L, Fine LJ, Keyserling WM, et al. A case-referent study of back disorders in automobile assembly workers: The health effects of non-neutral trunk postures. Scandinavian Journal of Work, Environment & Health 1991; 17: 337–346.

22. Wiggermann N, Keyserling WM. Effects of anti-fatigue mats on perceived discomfort and weight shifting during prolonged standing. Human Factors 2013; 55: 764–775.

23. Wiggermann N, Keyserling WM. Time to onset of pain: Effects of magnitude and location of static pressures applied to the plantar foot. Applied Ergonomics 2015; 46A: 84–90.

24. Latko WA, Armstrong TJ, Foulke JA, et al. Development and evaluation of an observational method for assessing repetition in hand tasks. American Industrial Hygiene Association Journal 1997; 58: 278–285.

25. McAtamney L, Corlett E. RULA: A survey method for the investigation of work-related upper limb disorders. Applied Ergonomics 1993; 24: 91–99.

26. Moore JS, Garg A. The Strain Index: A proposed method to analyze jobs for risk of distal upper extremity disorders. American Industrial Hygiene Association Journal 1995; 56: 443–458.

27. Keyserling WM, Ulin SS, Lincoln AE, and Baker SP. Using multiple information sources to identify opportunities for ergonomic interventions in automotive parts distribution: A case study. American Industrial Hygiene Association Journal 2003; 64: 690–698.

FURTHER READING

Chaffin DB, Andersson GBJ, Martin BJ. Occupational ergonomics (4th ed.). New York: Wiley-Interscience, 2006.
This text discusses in detail the biomechanical basis of many occupational injuries and disorders, with special coverage of the lower back and upper extremities. Quantitative methods of job analysis are presented with numerous examples of ergonomic approaches to equipment, tool, and workstation design.

Kroemer KH, Grandjean, E. Fitting the task to the human: textbook of occupational ergonomics (5th ed.). London: Taylor & Francis, 1997.
A well-written survey text that covers all aspects of ergonomics. Chapters on fatigue, work physiology, anthropometry, biomechanics, and cognitive ergonomics provide an excellent introduction to these topics.

McArdle WD, Katch FI, Katch VL. Exercise physiology: Energy, nutrition, and human performance (8th ed.). Baltimore: Wolters Kluwer Health, Lippincott Williams and Wilkins, 2015.
This comprehensive textbook covers a wide range of issues in work and exercise physiology. Introductory chapters cover basic exercise physiology (nutrition, energy conversion during exercise, structure and function of the pulmonary, cardiovascular, and neuromuscular systems) while advanced chapters cover applied topics, such as measurement of human energy expenditure, training for muscle strength and aerobic power, and rehabilitation training programs. Appendices include comprehensive tables of energy expenditure costs of common household, occupational, and recreational activities.

McCauley-Bush P. Ergonomics: Foundational principles, applications, and technologies. Boca Raton, FL: CRC Press, Taylor & Francis Group, 2012.
This textbook provides general coverage of ergonomics with special emphasis on physical ergonomics. Primary topics include muscular anatomy and physiology, neuromuscular control of movement, fatigue, anthropometry, workplace design, hand-tool design, work-related MSDs, and job analysis methods. Secondary topics include sensory functions, design of displays, and design of warnings.

National Institute for Occupational Safety and Health. Applications manual for the revised NIOSH lifting equation. NIOSH Publication No. 94-110. Cincinnati, OH: NIOSH, 1994.
A "hands-on" users' guide for evaluating work activities that require manual lifting. Numerous examples demonstrate application of the 1991 Revised NIOSH Lifting Equation in a variety of work environments. The guide includes a brief summary of the scientific basis of the 1991 Lifting Equation with references to biomechanical, physiological, psychophysical, and epidemiological research. The text is supplemented with numerous illustrations and examples.

National Research Council. Musculoskeletal disorders in the workplace: Low back and upper extremities. Washington, DC: National Academy Press, 2001.
A comprehensive review of the scientific literature on the relationship between work and MSDs of the low back and upper extremities. Major sections include discussions of epidemiology, tissue pathology, biomechanics, and interventions. Summary tables provide descriptive synopses of key studies, and the list of references is extensive.

Pheasant S, Haslegrave C. Bodyspace: Anthropometry, ergonomics, and the design of work (3rd ed.). Boca Raton, FL: CRC Press/ Taylor & Francis Group, 2005.
This textbook provides comprehensive coverage of the anthropometric aspects of ergonomics. Introductory chapters describe methodologies for measuring and statistically summarizing human body dimensions. This is followed by an excellent presentation of how anthropometric principles are used to design furniture, equipment, and workstations in the home, office, and factory environments. Numerous examples, illustrations, and anthropometric tables make this text an indispensable reference book for both novice ergonomists and experienced ergonomic designers.

Salvendy G (ed.) Handbook of human factors and ergonomics (4th ed.). Hoboken, NJ: John Wiley & Sons, 2012.
This comprehensive volume, which covers physical, cognitive, and social ergonomics, is intended for both practitioners and researchers. Of special interest to occupational health specialists are chapters on anthropometry, workstation design, task analysis, personal protective equipment, occupational low back pain, upper-extremity MSDs, office ergonomics, illumination, mental workload, prevention of human error, and accident investigation.

Wickens CD, Lee JD, Liu Y, Gordon-Becker SE. An introduction to human factors engineering (2nd ed.). Upper Saddle River, NJ: Pearson/ Prentice Hall, 2004.
This textbook provides a good introduction to all aspects of ergonomics with special emphasis on cognitive ergonomics. Introductory chapters cover human sensory mechanisms, displays, cognition, decision-making, and design of controls. Advanced chapters cover a variety of topics, including human–computer interaction, human factors in transportation, usability testing, stress and work performance, and the role of human error in accidents.

10

Clinical Occupational and Environmental Health Practice

Bonnie Rogers

Occupational and environmental health (OEH) programs can range from those that are very comprehensive, offering a large array of services to the worker population, to those that provide focused services to meet mandatory regulatory requirements. In the United States, OEH programs are generally available at the workplace in larger companies, while mid-sized companies often outsource these services to OEH clinics and small employers may not provide any, or only limited, OEH programs. While employers need to determine the types of OEH programs that best meet their needs and those of their employees, the primary goals of these programs include the following:

- To identify and control work-related health and safety hazards and prevent occupational and environmental illness and injuries
- To provide healthcare and case management for work-related injuries and illnesses
- To facilitate worker job placement and monitor ongoing work compatibility within the context of physical and mental health capabilities
- To promote a healthy workforce.

These goals aim to benefit both employees and employers by improving health, morale, and productivity.

THE MULTIDISCIPLINARY APPROACH

Essential to the success of an OEH program are two elements: (a) a thorough assessment of the work and work environment to determine potential and actual work-related exposures and (b) continuous monitoring to prevent and control workplace hazards. These elements are complex, requiring knowledge and skills of many types of OEH specialists—occupational and environmental medicine physicians and nurses, safety specialists, occupational and environmental hygienists, ergonomists, and others.

There is great diversity among providers of OEH services. The training and experience of physicians who provide OEH services vary widely. Some occupational and environmental medicine physicians have completed occupational medicine residencies, but most have been trained in other specialties. About 20% are board-certified in occupational medicine.

Business and industry have traditionally provided the most employment in clinical occupational medicine. Physicians who work in upper management are more involved in policy issues, whereas those employed at the workplace are more involved in clinical care. Physicians also work for federal and state governmental agencies. In some cases, occupational medicine clinics are independent contractors that provide services to client companies. Some clinical occupational medicine units are in medical centers or medical schools, usually within departments of medicine, community medicine, public health, or family practice. Physicians may manage cases of illness or injury, evaluate patients for insurance companies (such as for disability impairment ratings), and participate in surveillance or medical monitoring programs.

Many physicians in other specialties also see patients with occupational illnesses and injuries. For example, patients with work-related injuries and musculoskeletal disorders may be treated by orthopedic surgeons or specialists in physical medicine and rehabilitation, and patients with occupational asthma may be treated by pulmonologists or allergists. Most cases of work-related injury or illness are seen by primary care or emergency medicine physicians.

Occupational and environmental healthcare is also provided by OEH nurses. Although not all nurses working in OEH are specialty trained, available training curricula include approved academic certificate programs, master's and doctoral degrees in occupational health nursing, and specialty continuing education. In addition, certified occupational health nurses have completed requisite work experience and educational training and have passed a certification examination.[1]

The OEH nurse practicing in the clinical setting will need to be familiar with occupational and environmental illnesses and injuries within the contexts of nursing practice and process and the exposures relevant to the workers served. For example, a major cause of occupational illnesses among production workers is exposure to toxic chemicals. The OEH nurse must be able to assess problems and provide treatment or refer injured or ill workers to the appropriate healthcare providers, when necessary. Nurses are often the only licensed health professionals at the worksite and often manage the functions of an OEH clinic, refer employees needing medical management to consulting physicians, and serve as case managers in managed care organizations and insurance companies.

Occupational and environmental hygiene is the environmental science of anticipating, recognizing, evaluating, and controlling health hazards in the work environment with the objectives of protecting workers' health and well-being and safeguarding the community at large. It encompasses the study of hazards posed by chemical agents, physical agents, biologic agents, and stress in the workplace and the general environment. (See Chapter 8.)

Hazard recognition requires skill in assessing the work and work environment and investigating health risks. A full-scale worksite assessment and walkthrough survey, which is a major component of the hazard recognition process, should be done in a multidisciplinary context.

Safety in the workplace is everyone's responsibility, and awareness of safety and health issues is critical to prevention of injuries. The principal responsibility of the safety professional is to design, implement, and evaluate strategies aimed at preventing and controlling workplace hazards and to train workers on job safety. The emphasis and commitment on safety starts with top management and extends, by example, throughout the organization to managers and frontline employees.

Ergonomics is concerned with job design and matching work to fit the capabilities of most workers. The design of the work environment should be flexible enough to consider the need for individual variation.[2,3] (See Chapter 9.)

The establishment of a workplace health and safety committee is vital to transforming health safety ideas into prevention and protection strategies—through policies, procedures, program development, and training about health and safety in the workplace. A workplace health and safety committee should include representatives of various levels of management, employees, an OEH physician and nurse, the safety manager, other healthcare professionals, and worker or union representatives. A health and safety plan with specific goals and objectives should be established by the committee, with input from employees and all levels of

---

Box 10-1. The Association of Occupational and Environmental Clinics Patient Bill of Rights

Many occupational and environmental medicine clinics are members of the Association of Occupational and Environmental Clinics (AOEC). As AOEC members, clinics are committed to providing quality healthcare and to help patients understand the nature of their illnesses and any health risks. Their primary obligation is their patients. They assure their patients that their medical care will be handled with compassion and strict confidence.

Patients at AOEC clinics have rights to the following:

1. To know and consent to all tests and procedures before they are performed
2. To know the results of all tests and procedures
3. To obtain a copy of your medical records, if requested
4. To obtain a list of contracts and grants that this clinic has with any organizations, such as government agencies, industries and companies, labor unions, or community groups.

AOEC clinics promise their patients to do the following:

1. Maintain records in strict confidence and not release them to anyone outside this clinic without patient's express written permission (A patient's filing of worker's compensation, health insurance, or legal claims may require release of records.)
2. Help obtain information about worker's compensation, Social Security, disability, and other health and welfare benefits, if requested
3. Provide information on OSHA rights, assist in getting a workplace inspection, and help improve workplace health and safety
4. Provide legal testimony of findings, if necessary
5. Declare any possible conflict of interest by providing patients with a list of the clinic's grants and contracts, if requested
6. Explain the results of all medical tests and procedures performed under the clinic's direction
7. Help the patient to understand the causes of the illness and health risks
8. Work with the patient to prevent future health problems.

---

management. All members of the occupational health and safety team play an integral role in identifying and managing workplace exposures and other hazards.

ETHICAL ISSUES RELATED TO CLINICAL OCCUPATIONAL AND ENVIRONMENTAL HEALTH PRACTICE

Ethical issues are encountered by OEH professionals in their practice. Because the environments in which they function can be characterized by competing goals and interests and differential power structures, thorny ethical issues frequently arise.

Ethical conflicts relate to a number of issues, including confidentiality of employee health records, potential hazardous workplace exposures, informed consent, conflicts of interest for healthcare providers, genetic screening, worker literacy and understanding, work organization, and return to work.[4] The American College of Occupational and Environmental Medicine has developed a code of ethics (seehttp://www.acoem/org/codeofconduct.aspx). All OEH professionals recognize that patients deserve quality care. The Association of Occupational and Environmental Clinics has developed a patient bill of rights, which can serve as a useful framework for providing quality care (Box 10-1). (See Chapter 1 for a further discussion of ethical issues.)

ASSESSING WORK AND THE WORK ENVIRONMENT: RESPONSIBILITIES FOR CLINICIANS

In OEH practice, clinicians need to be aware of work processes, work demands, and potential health and safety hazards. Understanding the specifics of job tasks and hazards as well as the relationship between those and previous illnesses and injuries to job demands enables clinicians to (a) determine if a task is likely to exacerbate a preexisting injury or illness in an individual worker and (b) identify aspects of job tasks that should be modified to reduce risks for all workers.

To provide well-informed, effective guidance on an individual's fitness to perform specific tasks, clinicians should routinely visit the workplace and view work processes. By doing so, clinicians can:

- Better understand the relationship between work processes and worker health
- Help determine work limitations and accommodations for individual workers

Box 10-2. Issues a Clinician Can View or Ask About During a Workplace Visit

Job titles and duties
Speed and volume of work
Adequacy of engineering controls, such as ventilation
Use of personal protective equipment
Other health and safety precautions
Presence of chemical, physical, and biological hazards
Presence of occupational stress
Noise levels
Preparedness for breakdowns, such as spills and other unintended releases of hazardous materials
Break times and break rooms
Personal hygiene practices, such as handwashing, showering, and cleaning of workclothes
Routine maintenance operations
Roles of contract laborers
Product packaging
Staffing levels
Shift rotation
Worker morale

- Develop a useful vocabulary concerning work tasks and processes
- Gain insights into the pace, protection, and demands of work assignments and related hazards
- Identify hazardous aspects of jobs that require modifications and implementation of preventive measures. (See especially Chapters 4, 8, and 9 for discussions of preventive measures.)

During workplace visits, clinicians can view and ask about many aspects of work (Box 10-2). Managers often expect clinicians visiting the workplace to discuss first-aid preparedness and smoking cessation programs, but these subjects should not dominate clinicians' visits.

OCCUPATIONAL AND ENVIRONMENTAL HEALTH CLINICAL VISITS

The most common types of OEH clinical services—preplacement evaluations, drug testing evaluations, specific work approvals, and fitness-for-duty and return-to-work evaluations—are described in this section.

Preplacement Evaluations

Preplacement evaluations, formerly termed "pre-employment physicals," were renamed with the enactment of the Americans with Disabilities Act (ADA) in 1990, which prohibits use of medical evaluation before employment is offered. Now, these evaluations yield clinical approvals for specific jobs or recommendations for necessary specific work accommodations. The ADA limits

which restrictions can be considered disqualifying and which must be accommodated. Important issues are whether or not a specific prohibited task is an "essential function of the job" and whether or not accommodating the restriction would involve "undue hardship" to the employer.

Experienced clinicians recognize that nearly all pertinent health and medical information required for clinical assessment is included in the patient's history. Since most illnesses are not diagnosed by physical exams or testing, employee candor is necessary to help identify medical conditions, such as asthma, coronary artery disease, low back pain, carpal tunnel syndrome, and epilepsy, that may require work accommodations. Employees should be fully informed about confidentiality rules governed by the Health Insurance Portability and Accountability Act (HIPAA), medical record disclosure policies, and ADA procedures relating to work accommodations.

Established and reliable confidentiality rules are required. While managers should inform workers that disclosure of relevant medical information to the healthcare provider is essential for appropriate job placement, workers should also be informed that the specifics of their medical conditions will not be disclosed. Clinician reports to management address only whether the worker's health status permits the worker to perform job tasks with or without restrictions. When restrictions apply to "nonessential" job tasks, current rules prohibit management from barring individuals from employment.

Drug Testing Evaluations

The exception to the confidential nature of an occupational health report is the evaluation of pre-employment drug testing results, usually involving measurement of metabolites in the urine from illicit recreational drugs. Here, an unexcused positive result requires a report to management that the candidate—not yet an employee—"does not meet the employer's standards for employment." Such a judgment does not involve a diagnosis of addiction, intoxication, or documented safety risk. It is simply an assessment of whether the urinary metabolites are present, based on confidential review of authorized prescriptions or reasonable dietary constituents.

The person who performs this evaluation is called a *medical review officer* (MRO). Becoming an MRO requires explicitly designated physician training and certification, especially for specific federal programs, such as those of the U.S. Department of Transportation (DOT). The evaluation requires forensic skills, including assessment of the documentation of the chain of custody of a urine sample, the worker's proof of authorized medications, and the confirmation that the specimen is from the worker.

Social policy establishing drug testing is also intended to create a deterrent against recreational drug abuse and to screen abusers from acquiring jobs in which they could endanger themselves or others. Although an MRO requires a clinical license, drug testing is quite distinct from protective assessments in OEH medicine. Drug testing is unusual in clinical practice, since the patient's history may be suspect and external documentation is required to confirm every assertion.

Other occasions for drug testing are similarly nonclinical, including (a) mandated randomly timed testing programs for safety-sensitive positions and (b) postinjury assessments. Workers' compensation regulations in some states allow employers' insurers to assume that metabolites of recreational drugs represent proof of worker impairment and permit them to remove workers' compensation coverage for these workers. No documentation of neurological, behavioral, or judgment impairment is required or sought.

Specific Work Approvals

Many work assignments require focused clinician assessment to permit the worker to engage in a single activity. The most common of these evaluations are respirator examinations and DOT certification examinations, both of which are covered by specific federal guidelines and evaluation criteria.

Required medical record management for OEH medical evaluations is unique and specific. The Occupational Safety and Health Administration (OSHA) specifies that medical records for employees receiving OSHA-mandated medical examinations be preserved and maintained for at least 30 years after a worker's employment ends. With rare exceptions, job-related evaluations are maintained by the employer (or designated clinical contractor) in permanently available files. Explicit arrangements are required to distinguish occupational health from other clinical documentation to establish permanent availability for written and radiological records.

Respirator evaluations are narrowly directed at whether or not the respiratory protection device would pose a health hazard to the worker. Employees with underlying pulmonary disease may be unable to cope with the supplemental inspiratory or expiratory demands of the respirator's filter. Some extremely claustrophobic employees are unable to withstand the perceived confinement of the face mask's opacity or compression. Clinicians should determine both the nature of the potential hazard for which respirators are needed and the type of respiratory protection required. Workers with highly reactive airways who are exposed to even low levels of an irritant may develop serious bronchospasm, resulting in their panicking and removing an otherwise protective device.

Spirometry is usually not required for approving a worker to use a respirator. Based on a worker's respiratory status and/or the respiratory hazards of potential exposures, a clinician may choose to perform pulmonary function tests to obtain objective data for approval of respirator use (Figure 10-1).

Facial hair or any facial deformities that prevent negative-pressure masks from forming adequate facial seals render negative-pressure respirators inadequate.[5] Clinical notes alert safety personnel to the need for individualized fit testing. Positive-pressure respirators may be required for these workers, even though they

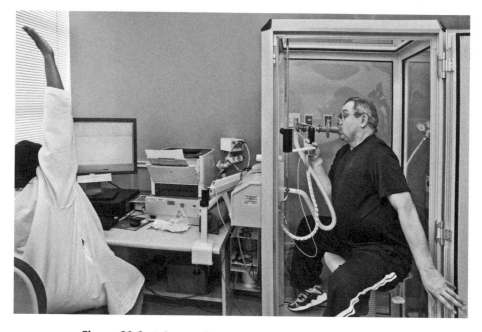

Figure 10-1. Pulmonary function testing. (Photograph by Earl Dotter.)

represent an increased cost to management over simple inspiratory filters.

Department of Transportation requirements for truck drivers of interstate or hazardous loads include a special set of considerations governed explicitly by regulatory language and by evolving agency guidelines. Special concerns include any medical condition associated with interrupted or reduced operator vigilance, such as coronary artery disease, sleep disorders, cardiac arrhythmias, diabetes, or seizures. Special training is available and published texts are helpful.

Exposure-specific assessments, based solely on workers' employment categories, may be the entire focus for clinical encounters in occupational health settings. These focused assessments include mandated evaluations for injury from specific situations.[6] A clinician's findings from a worksite walkthrough may suggest other circumstances, such as ergonomic stress, where medical monitoring can provide early recognition of potential harm. The following four examples represent a small fraction of the selective reasons for clinical monitoring for harm attributable to exposure. (Consult National Institute for Occupational Safety and Health [NIOSH] guidance documents at http://www.cdc.gov/niosh and specific OSHA regulations at http://

www.osha.gov for more comprehensive protocols on such monitoring.)

- Noise-exposed workers are monitored annually for personal compliance with hearing protection and for impaired hearing. An OSHA-defined standard threshold shift (change in hearing threshold, relative to a baseline audiogram, of an average of 10 decibels or more at 2000, 3000, and 4000 Hz in one or both ears) is a specific reportable degree of deterioration. Investigations regarding workplace policies and protections are often valuable for individual workers and the workforce as a whole. (See Chapter 12A.)

- Lead-exposed workers (those above the action level of 30 μg/m³ for more than 30 days each year) are required to be monitored for exposure (with blood lead levels) and for metabolic effects (with zinc protoporphyrin levels). Monitoring may detect proximal tubule involvement and kidney dysfunction, possibly due to lead exposure. Since significant exposure can result from accidental ingestion, worksite personal hygiene (lunchroom handwashing and cigarette contamination) should be considered. The OSHA lead standard offers specific regulatory requirements to remove workers from this exposure when findings show increased lead exposure. (See Chapters 7, 11, 23, 24, 26, and 28.)

- Asbestos-exposed workers are routinely provided personal protective equipment (PPE), such as clothing and respirators, and other protection, such as closed environments. The most immediate clinical challenge is to monitor these workers' ability to tolerate PPE, including monitoring for heat stress and respirator compliance. Regulatory requirements have not kept pace with recent evidence that supports screening of workers at high risk of lung cancer. In addition, regulatory requirements for clinical monitoring end when exposure ends, missing outcomes with long latency, such as mesothelioma. Nevertheless, chest X-rays and spirometry for restrictive disease are required. Since the risk of lung cancer due to asbestos exposure is greatly amplified by cigarette smoking, clinical encounters with these workers should routinely include counseling on tobacco cessation. (See Chapter 22.)

- Cadmium exposure (determined by environmental sampling exceeding a regulatory action level) requires biological monitoring for cadmium and for kidney dysfunction. Blood and urine cadmium levels and the urinary beta-2-microglobulin level (reported per gram of excreted creatinine) are indicators of potential disease. The clinician should also measure serum creatinine and ask about other risk factors for kidney disease. (See Chapters 11 and 28.)

Fitness-for-Duty and Return-to-Work Evaluations

Fitness for duty is defined as the ability of an individual to perform a job, based on the specific job requirements. A detailed understanding of the job duties is required, which may be problematic because job descriptions are often not informative or sufficiently oriented to behavioral aspects of the job. Ancillary information, such as interviews with workers in similar positions or with supervisors, may be needed to understand the essential requirements of the job.

When an employee has been out of work because of treatment of work-related or non-work-related illness or injury, or when a question arises about the employee's ability to function on the job, a fitness-for-duty evaluation may be requested. Fitness for duty can never be based solely on a diagnosis; rather, it must be based on an analysis of the employee's abilities. Past job performance is the best predictor of future job performance. In addition, a global assessment of functioning can be useful as a guide for the worker's current level of functioning and ability to perform daily tasks related to work. Overall, matching of an assessment of the employee's current behavioral and physical functioning with the essential functions required to perform a job as well as consideration of the employee's premorbid level of functioning on the job yields the best prediction of the employee's fitness for return to the job. Following such an evaluation, modified duty or work restriction may be recommended. In order to make this determination, the healthcare provider must know the physical and mental demands of the job in order to ensure rapid and safe return to work in the job the employee will be performing. Rehabilitative services and case management may be part of the return-to-work program so the employee remains fit for duty.

Reports to Workers and to Management

For all clinical evaluations, workers must be provided the results and interpretations of exposure and health outcome monitoring. Clinical management and follow-up are required in many circumstances, such as when blood pressure or liver function tests are abnormally increased.

In OSHA-mandated medical surveillance, employers must ensure regulatory compliance with screening or monitoring. The clinic needs to provide adequate documentation that these regulations are being followed. Individual clinical reports should reflect simply that each worker has been evaluated according to these requirements. Usually, individual results are suppressed unless a work-related health consequence has been found and therefore workers' compensation findings apply (see later discussion).

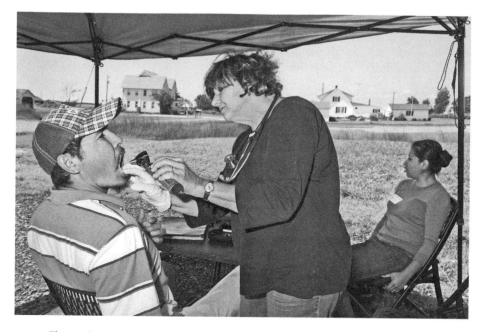

Figure 10-2. Nurse examining a crab picker in Maryland. (Photograph by Earl Dotter.)

An aggregate report should also be developed, combining results from similar workers to (a) demonstrate and document the number of screened workers (but not their names) and the proportion (or rate) of those with health findings of significance and (b) enumerate those evaluations that required either worker removal or exposure modification. Statistical reports regarding the distribution of numerical results (usually biological exposure indices), including comparison with previous years, and explanation of any changes contribute to improving the overall success of the occupational health and safety program. These aggregate reports are not confidential. They should be discussed with employers' health and safety professionals and also made available to workers and their representatives.

Work-Related Care and Workers' Compensation

Care for workers who have injuries and illnesses that are recognized as being related to work is influenced by state-specific workers' compensation laws and regulations. This care is affected by whether the worker or the employer selected the site of care. When workers are allowed to choose the site of care, it is usually in the same site as for their personal healthcare—usually because of comfort, confidence, and convenience. When employers choose the site of care, it is much more likely to be provided in a designated occupational medicine practice by health professionals known to management and familiar with the workplace and its activities and policies (Figure 10-2).

In workers' compensation care, HIPAA medical confidentiality rules do not apply. Once an employee files a claim, whether seeking lost wages or medical-care expenses, the employer or the workers' compensation insurer is permitted direct involvement in the review of decisions regarding clinical management, attribution, and specialty referrals. Release of personal health information, even for prior and unrelated illness, is permitted. Reports to management are not required to conceal diagnosis or medical details, and healthcare providers can choose to abandon the customary confidential "restricted-duty" reports in favor of simple photocopies of the clinical record. Where permitted by employers, reports that voluntarily respect the worker's privacy are preferred, but they are not required by regulation. (See Chapter 3.)

Often, even when the patient's care involves clinical specialists, employers will utilize the physicians and nurses with whom they have been working to monitor the care of employees with work-related conditions and the consequences of that care. Occupational health specialists review determinations of work absences and work restrictions, including those that enable workers to return to specially modified duty.

Setting Work Restrictions

Writing justifiable and protective health-motivated communications to supervisors, without disclosing medical diagnoses, can be challenging. The case examples of these communications that follow can be adapted to other clinical settings.

Case 1

A middle-aged worker in a manufacturing facility with hazardous machinery has type 1 diabetes, with poor control of blood glucose. Potential work restrictions and accommodations for this worker that need to be communicated to management might include:

- No unscheduled overtime
- No frequent work shift changes
- No skipped meal breaks
- Access to unscheduled snacks during work hours
- No work assignment above or adjacent to unprotected hazards, such as electrical, chemical, height, or mechanical dangers
- No operation of vehicles or hazardous powered equipment.

If neuropathy, retinopathy, cataracts, peripheral vascular disease, or coronary artery disease have developed, then other restrictions and accommodations may be necessary, including:

- No climbing ladders
- Practical vision testing for visually demanding assignments
- No exposure to extremes of temperature
- No strenuous physical activity
- Custom-fit, steel-toed shoes for all non-office work.

Case 2

A young worker entering a new work situation in a chemical packaging plant has mild persistent asthma. Even if this employee's physical exam is normal, work restrictions and accommodations may need to declare the following:

- No exposure to respiratory irritants, such as chlorine, ozone, cold, and smoke
- No work with diisocyanates or where these compounds have recently been used.

Case 3

A worker who developed a lumbar strain outside of work may be permitted to work in a modified assignment, with restrictions and accommodations for 5 days, possibly including the following:

- No lifting, carrying, pushing, or pulling of 25 pounds force (net weight)
- No sustained crouching, stooping, or kneeling
- Frequent position changes, including changes from sitting to standing, especially if computer work is involved that typically requires long periods of sitting
- Optional posture (employees' choice of sitting or standing) for half of any work hour.

Developing worker restrictions and accommodations includes consideration of risk assessment, pathophysiology, familiarity with job demands, and the culture of the employer's worksite.

ACCOMMODATION IN THE WORKPLACE

Since the ADA was passed in 1990, employers have been under increasing pressure to hire and accommodate workers with disabilities, including psychiatric illness. The number of discrimination claims against employers based on emotional or psychiatric impairment has also increased since the passage of the ADA. For example, in 1999, the Equal Employment Opportunity Commission reported that 15% of discrimination claims were related to emotional or psychiatric impairment—the largest category of claims in that year. The need to properly evaluate an individual's ability to perform a job and the ability to make reasonable accommodations is a growing concern among employers in the United States.

The ADA prohibits discrimination based on disability and provides that employers must make "reasonable accommodations" related to the disabilities of "qualified" applicants so long as this does not impose "undue hardship." "Qualified" means that the individual can perform the essential functions of the job, except for the disability. "Reasonable accommodations" refers to modifications or adjustments to a job or work environment that allows the qualified employee with the disability to perform the job functions. *Undue hardship* refers to "an action requiring significant difficulty or expense." Employers are not allowed to inquire about a disability before hiring, and a job applicant does not have to reveal a psychiatric history at the time of hire. Moreover, if a long-term employee who was previously performing the job develops a psychiatric disorder, the employer is obligated to make accommodations.

Individuals who are hospitalized for psychiatric diagnoses, such as schizophrenia, have low employment rates, often less than 20%. For those who are chronically mentally ill, the best predictors of future work performance seem to be ratings of work adjustment in a sheltered job site, ability to function socially with others, and previous employment history. Therefore, type of psychiatric diagnosis is not as predictive of work capacity as is assessment of objective behavioral performance. Although these findings apply specifically to psychoses, the same guideline seems to be applicable for all physical and psychiatric disorders.

Reasonable accommodations for persons with psychiatric disabilities include analysis of the individual employee's behavioral problems, such as anxiety or sensitivity to criticism, and development of accommodations based on individual needs. For example, when a sensitive employee returns from a hospitalization, the supervisor needs to be trained to offer positive feedback, along with critiques of performance.

A significant number of workers have diagnosable psychiatric conditions, especially depression, and some occupations have higher rates of such disorders that may significantly impact productivity. Some occupations appear to place workers at greater risk for traumas that result in psychiatric disorders, such as posttraumatic stress disorder. Whatever the causes, psychiatric illness will continue to affect workers and the workplace; therefore, they must be recognized, treated, and accommodated—rather than dismissed or ignored.

SENTINEL HEALTH EVENTS: RECOGNIZING THE PUBLIC HEALTH IMPACT OF INDIVIDUAL CASES

Sentinel health events are individual or multiple cases of occupational disease or injury that have significant public health importance. Clinicians need to report these to trigger investigations and intervention measures that are designed to protect a larger population. When a clinician diagnoses a worker with a disorder that is a sentinel health event, the clinician needs to report the problem to a government agency, usually a state health department, so that the employer can investigate it, assess affected workers and their work environment, and establish a plan to control the problem. (See Chapter 6.)

CASE MANAGEMENT AND SUPERVISED REHABILITATION

Occupational health clinicians often coordinate and monitor care provided by others, especially for patients receiving workers' compensation, to reduce miscommunication, delay, and even fraud. *Case management*, the coordination and use of healthcare resources to return employees to their optimal levels of health, includes planned activities to ensure appropriate use of medical facilities, early and appropriate referrals, and quality of care at controlled or reduced costs.[5] A written plan and protocols should be established to ensure quality of services and to evaluate results. The plan should also outline return-to-work procedures, including establishment of restricted- or modified-duty jobs.

The case manager, often an occupational health nurse (but sometimes an insurance company employee), works with the clinician to establish a proactive approach to case management, beginning with assessing worksite safety, identifying potential hazards, and working to control such hazards in collaboration with other health and safety professionals. The primary role of the case manager is to facilitate communication among the occupational health unit, management, the insurance carrier, the healthcare provider(s), and the employee. The case manager maintains frequent communication with the employee and all necessary persons but also advocates for the employee by facilitating open communication, rehabilitation, and the return-to-work process.

The case manager evaluates an employee's health needs and level of function, communicates essential information regarding work status and job requirements to the occupational healthcare provider, and keeps the employer apprised of employee progress or changes in the plan, such as return-to-work dates and work limitations. When determining readiness for work, the appropriateness of available modified job positions or accommodations that are needed should be considered in collaboration with the occupational healthcare provider.

Case monitoring is often achieved by telephone, email, or text messaging. Sometimes nurses accompany patients on visits to specialists to ensure that treatment and rehabilitation plans are received and acted upon. The employee should know that the nurse's role is observational and that the nurse is an advocate of the employee.

HEALTH PROMOTION AND HEALTH PROTECTION

The goals of health promotion and health protection are inextricably linked to prevention of illness and injury. The primary goal of health promotion is to maintain health and optimize an individual's health potential. Emphasis is placed on developing positive health behaviors, recognizing personal responsibility for health, and engaging families and communities in health promotion and disease prevention activities. However, a growing body of knowledge indicates that workers respond better to attempts at the workplace to improve nutrition, exercise, and smoking cessation when other workplace hazards

are also addressed. In addition, workers respond better when an ecologic approach that recognizes environmental impediments, such as improving stairwell lighting or lunch choices, is implemented.

Every 10 years, the Department of Health and Human Services provides national objectives for promoting health and preventing disease through its Healthy People project. Project publications have set and monitored national health objectives to meet a broad range of health needs, encourage collaboration across sectors, guide individuals toward making informed health decisions, and measure the impact of prevention activity. The framework of *Healthy People 2020*[7] provided 42 topic areas, each with targeted objectives. The overall goal for the occupational safety and health focus area was to "promote the health and safety of people at work through prevention and early intervention."[7] The Healthy People 2030 objectives will start to be developed soon. (See http://www.healthypeople.gov.)

NIOSH supports the integration of workplace health protection and efforts to promote worker health and well-being with the NIOSH Total Worker Health® (TWH) program.[8] TWH consists of policies, programs, and practices that integrate protection from occupational health and safety hazards with promotion of measures to prevent illnesses and injuries and to advance worker well-being. This holistic approach to address worker health, safety, and well-being aims to improve the quality of life of both individual workers and the workforce as a whole and to reduce organizational risk factors that can contribute to illness and injury. For example, understanding the connections among risk factors for occupational stress, cardiovascular disease, and sleep disorders can help to create better work environments and healthier workers.

REFERENCES

1. American Board of Occupational Health Nurses. Certification in occupational health nursing. Available at: https://www.abohn.org/certification. Accessed January 31, 2017.
2. National Institute for Occupational Safety and Health. Practical demonstrations of ergonomic principles (NIOSH Publication No. 2011-191, R1 9684). Cincinnati, OH: NIOSH, 2011. Available

at: https://www.cdc.gov/niosh/mining/userfiles/works/pdfs/2011-191.pdf. Accessed January 31, 2017.

3. Niu S. Ergonomics and occupational safety and health: An ILO perspective. Applied Ergonomics 2010; 41: 744–753.

4. Rogers B. Occupational health nursing: Concepts and practice. Beverly, MA: OEM Press, 2017.

5. Rogers B, Randolph SA, Mastroianni K. Occupational health nursing guidelines for primary clinical conditions (5th ed.). Beverly, MA: OEM Press, 2017.

6. Occupational Health and Safety Administration. Medical screening and surveillance. Available at: https://www.osha.gov/SLTC/medicalsurveillance/. Accessed January 31, 2017.

7. U.S. Department of Health and Human Services. Healthy People 2020. Available at: http://www.healthypeople.gov/2020/topics-objectives. Accessed August 19, 2017.

8. National Institute for Occupational Safety and Health. Total worker health. Available at: https://www.cdc.gov/niosh/twh/. Accessed January 31, 2017.

FURTHER READING

American College of Occupational and Environmental Medicine. Code of Ethics. Available at: http://www.acoem.org/codeofconduct.aspx. Accessed March 1, 2017. *Provides helpful guidelines on ethical issues.*

Boles M, Pelletier B, Lynch W. The relationship between health risks and work productivity. Journal of Occupational and Environmental Medicine 2004; 46: 737–745. *Provides evidence about health risks, such as from smoking and unhealthful diets, and work productivity. Occupational health professionals need to consider these risks in planning a comprehensive health program that will benefit the workforce and employer.*

Hartenbaum N. The DOT medical examination: A guide to commercial drivers' medical certification (6th ed.). Beverly, MA: OEM Press, 2017. *A helpful guide on DOT medical examinations.*

Occupational Safety and Health Administration. Recommended practices for safety and health programs. 2016. Available at: https://www.osha.gov/shpguidelines/docs/OSHA_SHP_Recommended_Practices.pdf. Accessed March 1, 2017. *A valuable resource.*

Rogers B, Randolph S, Mastroianni K. Occupational health nursing guidelines for primary clinical conditions (5th ed.). Beverly, MA: OEM Press, 2017. *A valuable resource guide that provides more than 135 guidelines for common clinical conditions typically seen in the occupational health setting and provides programmatic guides. Information on occupational health resources is also provided.*

SECTION III

HAZARDOUS EXPOSURES

11

Chemical Hazards

Michael Gochfeld and Robert Laumbach

There is a wide range of hazardous chemicals to which people may be exposed in the workplace or elsewhere. This chapter provides an overview and many illustrative examples of these chemicals and their adverse health effects, focusing mainly on metals, solvents, and pesticides. (See also Chapter 7.)

Chemicals are most broadly classified as being organic (containing one or more carbon atoms) or inorganic (Box 11-1). Chemicals can also be classified according to their structure, source, economic use, mechanism of action, environmental properties, and target organ. Sometimes, the only information available for a chemical is its class, such as pesticide or solvent. The classifications and examples presented in this chapter are intended to be illustrative, not comprehensive.

CLASSIFICATION BY STRUCTURE

Structure–activity relationships (SARs) are often useful in inferring the toxicity of an unfamiliar chemical from the known toxicity of familiar, or better-studied, chemicals of similar

chemical structure. Since only a few of the thousands of chemicals in commercial use have been adequately tested for toxicity, SARs may initially provide the only clues to likely toxicity, if any. For example, halogenated hydrocarbons with simple chain structure (alkanes) tend to share the target organ effect of central nervous system (CNS) depression, allowing some to be used as general anesthetics (Figure 11-1). Although their potency varies by the number of carbon atoms, presence or absence of double bonds, and the presence of chlorine, fluorine, or bromine atoms, their general effects on CNS depression are similar. In addition, many heavy metals are toxic to the proximal kidney tubule, and many hallucinogenic compounds share a common active group. SARs can also be predictive of carcinogenicity identified by long-term animal bioassays (Chapter 21). Yet one must be cautious since chemicals with similar structures do not always have similar properties. In some instances, SARs do not apply; for example, benzene causes leukemia, while compounds with similar chemical structure, such as phenol (hydroxybenzene) and toluene (methylbenzene), apparently do not.

Box 11-1. Chemicals Classified by Structure

Organic Chemicals

Aromatics, such as benzene and benzene derivatives (such as toluene and phenols)

Aliphatics, such as alkanes and alkenes

Chlorinated hydrocarbons, such as chlorinated alkanes and alkenes

Polycyclic aromatic hydrocarbons

Chlorinated polycyclic aromatics, such as dioxins, furans, and polychlorinated biphenyls

Amines

Organic acids, ethers, aldehydes, ketones, and alcohols

Inorganic Chemicals

Heavy metals, such as lead and mercury

Light metals, such as beryllium and lithium

Metalloids, such as arsenic and selenium

Acids and bases

Anions and cations, and salts

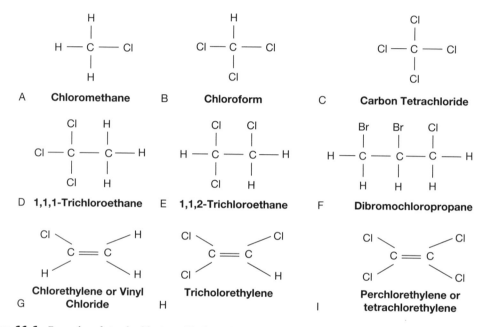

Figure 11-1. Examples of simple chlorinated hydrocarbons. Single carbon compounds are (A) chloromethane; (B) trichloromethane, or chloroform; and (C) tetrachloromethane, or carbon tetrachloride. Two-carbon compounds with a single bond (alkanes) include isomers (D) 1,1,1-trichloroethane and (E) 1,1,2-trichloroethane, as well as (F) dibromochloropropane (DBCP), or 1,2 dibromo,3-chloropropane. The bottom row shows the following chlorinated ethenes, each with a double bond: (G) chloroethene (vinyl chloride); (H) tricholoroethylene; and (I) tetrachlorethylene (better known as perchlorethylene or "perc").

CLASSIFICATION BY SOURCE

Chemicals can be classified by source (Box 11-2). The word *toxins* refers only to bioactive chemical substances produced naturally by plants and animals. Many plants and animals secrete chemicals designed to protect against being eaten. Monarch caterpillars may incorporate in their tissues alkaloids from the Milkweed leaves they eat, rendering themselves, and subsequently adult butterflies, toxic and unpalatable. Beetles may squirt hot cyanide compounds to deter predators. Plants that have been partially eaten by herbivores may load increased levels of distasteful tannin compounds in newly regenerated leaves. Similarly, many fungi secrete chemicals that inhibit bacterial growth, generating odors that we recognize as "spoilage," thereby protecting their own food source. Hymenoptera (such as bees and wasps), spiders, and some snakes have developed a variety of neurotoxic and hematotoxic venoms for immobilizing prey.

There is great diversity of toxins produced in the terrestrial and marine environment by

---

Box 11-2. Chemicals Classified by Source

Invertebrate
Vertebrate

Natural or Biologic Compounds (Toxins)

Plant
Bacterial
Fungal

Synthetic Compounds

Industrial reagent, by-product, or product
Pharmaceutical
Pesticide

Box 11-3. Chemicals Classified by Use

Glues
Pesticides

Solvents
Fuels
Paints, dyes, and coatings

Pharmaceutical agents and controlled substances
Detergents and cleansers
Acids and bases

---

organisms ranging from fungi and dinoflagellates to fish. The fungal toxin aflatoxin B1, which is produced by fungi that contaminate stored beans, peanuts, and other food items, is reputed to be the most toxic compound, by virtue of its very low LD_{50} (the dose that kills 50% of organisms tested). In humans, aflatoxin B1 can cause liver cancer. A wide variety of toxins have been adapted into some familiar pharmaceuticals, such as antibiotics. A compendium provides useful information on plant and animal toxins.[1]

CLASSIFICATION BY USE

Very often, the first aspect of a chemical that people recognize is its use—for example, as a solvent, a detergent, or a substance used for etching. For example, a worker may report having been overcome while "using a solvent." Or homeowners may report "some pesticide spray" having made them ill. Examples of common use classes of chemicals that may have toxic effects are shown in Box 11-3.

Pharmaceutical agents and controlled substances, including alcohol and tobacco, are grouped together, because very high concentrations of bioactive agents are deliberately introduced into the body. The most widespread toxic exposures involve the chronic inhalation of tobacco smoke by smokers and bystanders and chronic overconsumption of ethanol. Many substances of abuse that were originally developed as pharmaceuticals,

such as amphetamines, barbiturates, and narcotics, have profound toxic effects—quite apart from their addictive properties. By whatever route, and whether legal or illicit, these chemicals are used because of their high level of bioactivity. Toxicity may occur from excessive doses. Even when the dosage used is in the therapeutic range, there may be undesired side effects that are manifestations of toxicity. These effects may occur frequently, such as the soporific effects of the antihistamine diphenhydramine or, rarely, anaphylaxis due to penicillin.

CLASSIFICATION BY MECHANISM OF ACTION

Chemicals can be classified by biological mechanism of action (Box 11-4). For example, substances that block cellular respiration are categorized as asphyxiants. Methane and other gases are toxicologically inert, but they can function as *simple asphyxiants* by displacing oxygen from inhaled air, thereby decreasing the oxygen saturation of the blood and reducing its availability to cells. *Chemical asphyxiants*, which interfere with the transport or utilization of oxygen in the body, include carbon monoxide (CO), hydrogen sulfide (H_2S), and cyanide (HCN). Carbon monoxide has a strong affinity for hemoglobin, and the resultant carboxyhemoglobin is unable to transport oxygen from the lungs to cells elsewhere in the body (see below and Chapter 26).

Much exciting research in modern toxicology focuses on the mechanisms by which a bioactive

Box 11-4. Chemicals Classified by Mechanism of Action

Metabolic poisons and chemical asphyxiants
Hematotoxins, such as by methemoglobinemia (nitrites) and by hemolysis (arsine)
   Binders to macromolecules, such as DNA or protein
   Hydrogen ion effects, such as acids and bases
   Enzyme inducers

Genotoxins, including mutagens and carcinogens
   Cell membrane disrupters
   Competitive binders of active sites or receptors
   Formers of free radicals and active oxygen
   Chemicals causing redox reactions
   Chemicals interfering with signal transduction
   Chemicals interfering with hormone activity
Sensitizers
Irritants

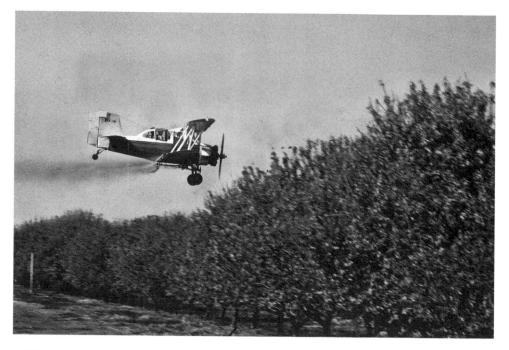

Figure 11-2. Aerial spraying of pesticides in an orchard in California. (Photograph by Earl Dotter.)

substance interacts with and alters its target organs to produce its adverse effects (toxicodynamics). Targets may include DNA, organelles, cell membranes, neurotransmitter receptors, hormone receptors, and metabolic enzymes and biochemical reactions.

CLASSIFICATION BY ENVIRONMENTAL PROPERTIES

The Environmental Protection Agency (EPA) has identified toxic chemicals that are persistent and bioaccumulative (PBTs) in the environment and the human body (Table 11-1). These are mainly chlorinated hydrocarbon pesticides and related compounds, which break down very slowly under ambient conditions (Figure 11-2).

Table 11-1. Persistent Bioaccumulative and Toxic Chemicals

Aldrin/dieldrin	Mercury
Benzo(a)pyrene	Mirex
Chlordane	Octachlorostyrene
DDT, DDD, and DDE	Polychlorinated biphenyls
Hexachlorobenzene	Dioxins and furans
Alkyl-lead	Toxaphene

Source: http://www.epa.gov/pbt/.

Some can be degraded by light, others by microorganisms. Most PBTs undergo some bioamplification through the food chain, so that organisms higher on the food chain, such as large predatory fish or birds, have higher tissue concentrations than organisms lower on the food chain.

Box 11-5. Chemicals Classified by Target Organ

Cardiotoxins
Pulmonary toxins
Neurotoxins   Metabolic toxins
Hematotoxins   Endocrine disruptors
Nephrotoxins   Dermatotoxins
Hepatotoxins   Reproductive agents and teratogens

CLASSIFICATION
BY TARGET ORGAN

Toxic chemicals can be classified by target organ (Box 11-5). Once absorbed into the bloodstream, chemicals are distributed to most organs but may have their major effects on a specific organ system. A chemical may have different target organ effects depending on the time course and intensity of exposure. For example, benzene is acutely neurotoxic (like many small organic molecules), but it is its chronic toxicity to the bone marrow that results in interference with normal production of red blood cells, white blood cells, and platelets, causing pancytopenia, leukemias, and other disorders. Once absorbed, lead is distributed to many organs, including bone, where it is stored in place of calcium; however, it is the neurotoxic effects of lead on both the developing brain and the mature nervous system that are the most important toxic effects of lead.

PROPERTIES OF CHEMICALS

Chemical Species

A chemical variant of an element, usually a metal element, is called a *species*. Different chemical species can have different chemical and toxicological properties. For example, trivalent chromium (Cr-III) and hexavalent chromium (Cr-VI), which differ in oxidation state, also differ in toxicity, carcinogenicity, and ability to pass through cell membranes. They represent different chromium species, yet they are interconvertible, depending on whether they are in an oxidizing or reducing environment. Cr-III is an essential nutrient, while Cr-VI is a lung and stomach carcinogen. Quantifying Cr-III and Cr-VI in environmental media or biological samples is complicated by the potential for redox reactions, which can occur in the environment, in the body, during transport to a laboratory, or

during analysis. Depending on how a soil sample is collected, transported, and analyzed, Cr-III can be oxidized and appear spuriously as Cr-VI when analyzed, or Cr-VI might be inadvertently reduced to Cr-III and reported as such.

The same chemical, such as mercury, may exist in several different chemical species. Slight modifications may have profound effects. Elemental mercury is a dense silvery liquid, with a specific gravity of 13.6. It is one of the few elements that are liquid at ambient temperature and also volatile, giving off an odorless, colorless but highly toxic vapor that is readily inhaled and absorbed into pulmonary capillaries. Mercury compounds used in industry are often inorganic salts, while many of the biocidal mercurial compounds, such as phenylmercuric acetate and thimerosal, are organic mercurials. The methylmercury produced in aquatic sediments by anaerobic bacteria from elemental or inorganic mercury biomagnifies in the food chain from plankton to small fish to large fish, potentially causing organic mercury poisoning in people who consume large amounts of fish.

In general, organic forms of metals have a different spectrum of toxicity than the inorganic forms of the same metals. Thus, organic mercury and organotin compounds are more highly toxic than the corresponding inorganic forms. Both have been used extensively as biocides, especially in antifouling paints used for ships to inhibit the growth of barnacles. As mercury and tin have leached out of paints into the sea, they have adversely impacted marine organisms and disrupted aquatic ecosystems. However, for some elements, such as arsenic, the inorganic compounds are more highly toxic than the organic compounds.

Isomers and Congeners

Two chemical compounds that have the same chemical formula but differ in structure are

```
        H   H   H   H
  H – C – C – C – C – H
        H   H   H   H
```
n-butane

```
        H   H   H
  H – C – C – C – H
        H   |   H
            |
        H – C – H
            H
```
isobutane (2-methylpropane)

Figure 11-3. N-butane and iso-butane (2-methyl pro-pane) are isomers of butane.

called *isomers*. Figure 11-3 shows two isomers of the common fuel, butane, which as a four-carbon chain can appear as either normal (linear) butane or branched isobutane. *Congeners* have the same basic structure but different numbers of atoms. For instance, dichlorophenol and trichlorophe-nol are congeners, while 2,4-dichlorophenol and 2,5-dichlorophenol are isomers. There are 209 different isomers and congeners of polychlori-nated biphenyls (PCBs), differing in the number and position of chlorine atoms on two attached benzene rings. Several of these compounds have four chlorines and therefore are isomers of tet-rachlorobiphenyl. Likewise, there are 209 con-geners of the polybrominated diphenyl ethers. The toxicity of isomers and congeners and their behavior in the human body may vary greatly.

Different chlorinated dibenzodioxins vary by orders of magnitude in their toxicity. The most toxic of these is 2,3,7,8-tetrachlorodibenzodioxin (TCDD or dioxin), which was a contami-nant in the production of the herbicide 2,4,5-trichlorophenoxyacetic acid (2,4,5-T). Each of the dioxin congeners can be assigned a *toxicity potency* (toxic equivalency factor[TEF]) relative to TCDD, which is given a value of 1. Some PCBs are considered dioxin-like in their biological effects and are assigned a TEF, while other PCBs, includ-ing the most common isomer (PCB-153), are not.

Polarity and Solubility

Polar compounds are readily soluble in water; *nonpolar compounds* are relatively insoluble in water but dissolve readily in a variety of organic solvents. Some compounds are insoluble in virtually all solvents, while a few dissolve readily in either water or organic solvents. The transition from polar to nonpolar is a continuum and is measured by the octanol:water partitioning coefficient. Nonpolar compounds have higher octanol solubility; polar compounds have higher water solubility.

Mixtures

Most toxicologic research is conducted with single chemicals. However, people are gener-ally exposed to mixtures of chemicals, present-ing a challenge for epidemiologists and others attempting to determine the adverse effects of individual chemicals and of the combined exposure to multiple chemicals (Figure 11-4). Chemicals may interact in the environmen-tal medium or in the lung, intestinal tract, or

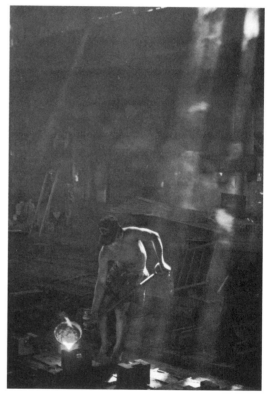

Figure 11-4. A barefoot worker pours molten iron into molds in a foundry in the Philippines as sunlight penetrates the emission-laden atmosphere containing carbon monoxide, crystalline silica, hydrocarbons, and carbon particles. The foundry was studied as part of an International Labor Organization–sponsored industrial hygiene course for government labor inspectors. (Photograph by Aaron Sussell.)

other organs. Interactions between chemicals may reduce or enhance their toxicities. There are a few examples of true synergy, in which the resulting toxicity is equal to the product of the effects of individual chemicals. Notable examples of synergy are the interactions between cigarette smoking and radon and between cigarette smoking and occupational exposure to asbestos.

There is now an abundance of reliable sources of information on toxic chemicals (see Further Reading at end of this chapter). The following section focuses on selected chemicals and groups of chemicals to illustrate some of the main themes in occupational and environmental health and toxicology. (See Chapter 7.) In addition, because many pharmaceuticals affect the same enzymes that metabolize occupational chemicals, it is important to evaluate the medication a person may be taking to assess whether there may be dangerous interactions with chemicals at work, in hobbies, or at home.

INORGANIC COMPOUNDS

Asphyxiants usually are grouped into two major categories: simple and chemical. Simple or inert asphyxiants, such as propane or hydrogen, act by displacing oxygen in the atmosphere. The most common scenario for this type of asphyxiation is work in a confined space, such as a manhole or a storage tank. The Occupational Safety and Health Administration (OSHA) requires special precautions for work in confined spaces, such as warning signs, air testing before entry, and the use of supplied-air respirators.

Chemical Asphyxiants

Chemical asphyxiants act by blocking the body's ability to use oxygen to support the basic life functions of cells. They can interfere with transport, delivery, or cellular utilization of oxygen in the body.

Carbon Monoxide

CASE 1

In December, a 50-year-old woman was brought to the emergency department of a

small rural hospital after collapsing at work at an onion farm. She reported no previous episodes of syncope or chest pain and had no significant past medical history other than treatment for mild hypertension. She was doing her ordinary work at the farm's packing shed, preparing onions for shipment, when she suddenly became dizzy and lost consciousness. Her electrocardiogram showed mild ischemic changes, and she was admitted to the intensive care unit for observation.

The next afternoon, two other workers from the same farm were brought to the emergency department complaining of headaches, dizziness, and nausea. Blood samples were drawn for determination of carboxyhemoglobin (COHb) concentration, and both workers had slightly increased levels (about 10%). Interpretation was complicated because more than 30 minutes had elapsed before they reached the hospital from the farm, and it was unclear whether they had been treated with oxygen during that time. The emergency department physician contacted the farm owner, who reported that he had called the gas company to check the propane heaters used in the barn. They had tested the barn with a "gas meter" and found no problem with carbon monoxide (CO) or other gases.

The two workers went back to work the next morning and again became ill. They returned to the emergency department. This time, their COHb levels were elevated (between 14% and 16%). A nurse from a local occupational health program was notified and visited the farm that afternoon. In discussing the situation with the farmer and other workers, she found several potential problems. Temperatures in the barn had been kept very cold. There was little ventilation. Several small propane heaters provided some heat. A propane-powered forklift was used intermittently in the barn. Because of weather conditions, the doors to the barn had been kept closed for the previous several days.

The nurse requested that an industrial hygienist visit the facility to conduct further air sampling. He arrived the next day. Long-term personal samples taken that day showed acceptable CO levels—up to 24 ppm, compared with the OSHA standard of 50 ppm. However, short-term samples showed levels up to 100 ppm at some locations, especially around the forklift. Doors in the facility were kept open during the day that sampling took place. Based on these findings, the farmer obtained an electric battery-powered forklift and improved ventilation in the facility.

Carbon monoxide is the most common chemical asphyxiant. It is produced by incomplete combustion of organic matter, such as occurs in gasoline and diesel engines, charcoal grills, or oil or gas stoves and heating systems. The presence of an unventilated source of CO indoors has usually been implicated in CO poisonings, as in Case 1. However, fatal CO poisoning has also occurred in outdoor settings where local conditions create the potential for high levels of gas to accumulate, such as near the exhaust of recreational boating craft. CO poisoning continues to be a very common cause of death in the workplace and elsewhere. Whereas the oxygen transport of hemoglobin relies on oxygen binding to hemoglobin in the lung and then being released in target tissues, CO binds 240 times more strongly than oxygen to hemoglobin (forming COHb), so that oxygen is not released in tissues. With continued CO exposure, the amount of COHb increases, leaving less and less unreacted hemoglobin to transport oxygen. Symptoms are nonspecific (Table 11-2). Onset is insidious. People become sleepy, without realizing that they are being poisoned. Drivers exposed to CO from faulty exhaust systems may fall asleep while driving. In acute exposure, the first symptom is usually headache, progressing to nausea, weakness, dizziness, and confusion.

Table 11-2. Symptoms and Signs Associated with Increasing Blood Levels of Carbon Monoxide

Percentage of Carbon Monoxide in Blood	Symptoms and Signs
10–20%	Headache and shortness of breath
20–30%	Nausea, dizziness, severe headache, and difficulty concentrating
30–40%	Lethargy, fainting, visual and auditory impairment, and chest pain
40–50%	Fainting, rapid heart rate, and seizures
>50%	Coma, convulsions, and death

Source: Sullivan JB Jr, Krieger GR (eds.). Clinical environmental health and toxic exposures (2nd ed.). Philadelphia: Lippincott, Williams & Wilkins, 2001, p. 725.

CO exposure should be considered in patients who collapse at work or report sudden headaches, lightheadedness, dizziness, or nausea. More severe poisoning can lead to unconsciousness and death.

The standard laboratory test for CO exposure is determination of the COHb concentration in the blood; this reveals the proportion of hemoglobin that is bound to CO. Normal COHb levels in nonsmokers range up to 4%, and smokers generally have levels as high as 10%. Serious medical problems usually do not develop unless levels exceed 20%. However, patients with ischemic heart disease are especially susceptible to the effects of CO. Interpretation of COHb levels is challenging because they return to normal within hours—even faster in patients who have been given oxygen. Therefore, if a patient collapses at work, is given oxygen, and is then brought to the emergency department, the COHb level measured in the emergency department may be well below the peak level the patient reached during the exposure. Hyperbaric oxygen therapy is used for severe CO poisoning, but even with such treatment permanent neurologic damage may occur.

Intermittent or episodic exposures to increased concentrations of CO can increase the risk of cardiovascular disease among groups such as tunnel workers and highway toll collectors. However, such exposures can be difficult to detect. In the case presented here, the original testing by the "gas meter" might have occurred when the ventilation was especially good (such as with a breeze blowing through the barn) (Figure 11-5), or the instruments might have been insensitive to slight CO elevations. Similarly, a worker's exposure from the forklift could vary with time and location in the facility. In this case, sampling with better instrumentation revealed the source of CO.

In chronic CO poisoning, effects may be direct or indirect from relative hypoxia. Carbon monoxide, including from cigarettes, is implicated in accelerating atherogenesis and promoting acute coronary hypoxia. Incomplete recovery from acute CO poisoning, especially after coma, may include residual neurobehavioral and cognitive impairment. Many residential building codes require installation of household CO monitors. Misuse of gasoline generators during power

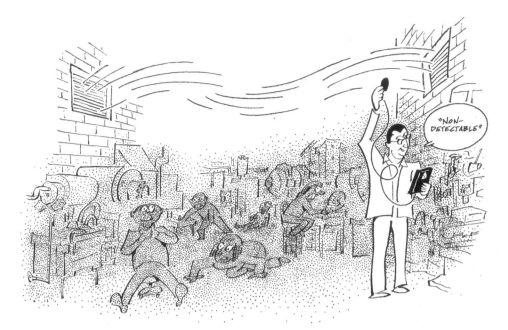

Figure 11-5. Location and timing of air sampling and use of appropriate measuring devices are all critically important. (Drawing by Nick Thorkelson.)

outages is a significant source of CO poisoning. (See Chapter 26 for further discussion of CO poisoning.)

Other Chemical Asphyxiants

In addition to CO, common examples include H_2S and HCN. Although these chemicals are sometimes used in a workplace, more frequently they are produced as a result of some other process, such as combustion or chemical mixing, and the asphyxiation occurs accidentally as a result of that process.

Hydrogen cyanide gas, a cellular asphyxiant, is acutely toxic and capable of causing death within seconds by poisoning cellular respiration. Workers with known potential for cyanide exposure must be trained to protect themselves against the known hazard of working with HCN gas under normal and upset operating conditions. However, they may be unaware of the potential of cyanide-containing salts to release HCN on contact with any acid and even with water. Cyanide compounds are used in the plating industry and in the commercial extraction of gold, silver, and mercury from metal ores. Alkaline cyanide solutions are used to reclaim metals from jewelry. Metals are extracted from the metal cyanide solutions by cathodic plating,

the basis for the application of metal cyanide in the plating industry. Cyanide compounds were formerly widely used as rodenticides and in the fumigation of ships. HCN is most commonly produced when acids come into contact with cyanide compounds. The burning of acrylonitrile plastics can also produce significant levels of HCN. Exposure to levels of about 100 ppm for 30 to 60 minutes can be fatal. HCN has a characteristic bitter almond taste, although not all people can identify it. In acute exposures, a person may absorb a lethal dose before the taste can be identified. The primary toxicity of HCN is its poisoning of the cytochrome electron transport system, blocking the oxidative phosphorylation formation of ATP, the energetic basis of cellular function. Initial symptoms include headache and palpitations, progressing to dyspnea and then convulsions.

Hydrogen sulfide, a colorless, chemical asphyxiant gas accounts for the rotten-egg odor associated with gas oozing out of marshes. It has been used in chemical analytic laboratories, metallurgy, and chemical synthesis and as a chemical disinfectant. At intermediate concentrations, H_2S acts as an irritant of the eyes and the respiratory tract. Although its odor is characteristic even at 1 ppm, exposure to a concentration above 150 ppm paralyzes the sense of smell before the odor is identified, so the worker is unaware of the exposure. Acute neurotoxic effects occur at 500 ppm. Delayed pulmonary edema has been reported. Acute H_2S poisoning may occur in a number of workplace settings, including leather tanning, sewage treatment, oil drilling, and other types of work. Hydrogen sulfide is a common cause of work-related fatalities in oil fields, where it occurs naturally as a contaminant of natural gas. Death may occur at 700 ppm. At higher levels, acute respiratory paralysis, or "knockdown," occurs. Serial fatalities may then take place as unprotected coworkers, attempting to rescue the fallen worker, also die.

A New Jersey community was exposed to high levels (above 100 ppb) of hydrogen sulfide when large quantities of wet wallboard (gypsum) were disposed of in a newly reopened landfill after Superstorm Sandy in 2012. Gypsum (calcium sulfate) breaks down with heat, acidity, and bacterial activity to release H_2S. Although the levels were below levels generally considered toxic (1 ppm or greater), residents reported headaches and symptoms and signs of stress from the storm's assault on their suburban environment. Perception and expectation are important modulators of toxicologic responses. Comparable air levels of H_2S at a mineral springs resort would be associated with health.

The outbreak of CO poisoning was described in Case 1 and consideration of other asphyxiants highlight several important principles:

1. Not every toxic exposure is exotic. Such familiar equipment as a forklift can cause fatal exposures.
2. Occupational medicine principles can be directly applicable to the general environment. For example, many cases of CO poisoning occur in the home and are caused by faulty heaters.
3. Workers, when exposed to an asphyxiant or intoxicant, become less alert and less able to react quickly and appropriately to hazards. This is a form of synergy, which increases the risk of injuries, further exposures, and other mishaps on and off the job.
4. In an environment with very high gas concentrations, every breath boosts the blood level of the gas, and toxicity can develop remarkably rapidly. Such acute toxicity is common in enclosed spaces, affecting not only the primary victims but also coworkers who rush in to provide assistance.
5. When a worker is found dead or unconscious after an unknown exposure, a blood sample should always be taken. COHb levels, thiosulfate levels, and other evidence suggesting acute asphyxiation should be obtained routinely.

The most important principle illustrated by asphyxiants is the primacy of prevention. Asphyxiation can almost always be anticipated. The hazards of confined spaces, forklifts, and other sources are well recognized. Abundant public messages warn about household generators. Once anticipated, exposures can be prevented by some combination of usual measures: (a) minimizing the formation of the asphyxiant, (b) proper ventilation, (c) proper work practices, (d) worker training, and (e) personal protective equipment.

METALS

Many elemental metals, such as cobalt, copper, chromium, iron, manganese, vanadium, iron, and zinc, have been identified as essential for human growth and physiology. Deficiency of any of these elements can lead to poor growth or abnormal function. However, all of them have also been implicated in toxicity, either through excessive ingestion or occupational exposures. Metalloids (nonmetallic elements that have some of the characteristics of metals) include selenium, which is essential for humans, and arsenic, which is not. For some trace elements that are micronutrients, such as cobalt, the daily dietary requirement is very low (measured in nanograms); for others that are macronutrients, such as iron, milligram amounts are required daily. Metals are often incorporated into biocides, such as lead arsenate insecticides, mancozeb (a manganese and zinc carbamate fungicide), mercurial fungicides, and copper algaecides. Arsenic compounds have been widely used to defoliate cotton prior to harvesting.

Lead

CASE 2

A 29-year-old laborer who worked intermittently for a construction firm that did bridge repair work complained to his family physician of intermittent stomach pains of several weeks' duration. The pain was not associated with meals. Onset had been gradual. He had no associated systemic or gastrointestinal symptoms. He had not experienced any unusual stress at home or at work. He reported drinking one or two cans of beer daily. Physical examination was normal. His physician treated him with antacids and his pain gradually resolved.

Approximately 2 months later, the patient returned complaining of more severe epigastric pain, associated with abdominal cramping, headaches, and fatigue. He recently started working at a new site, where he had used an oxyacetylene torch to remove paint from an old bridge. After consultation with an occupational medicine physician, the family physician obtained a blood lead level (BLL), which was 75 µg/dL. The patient stopped doing paint removal work, and his symptoms gradually improved. Within 4 weeks, his BLL decreased to 35 µg/dL. The contractor provided a ventilation system for use when paint was being removed from bridges. Subsequent quarterly monitoring of the patient's BLL showed a gradual further decline.

Although the use of lead pigment was discontinued in most paints in the United States by the 1970s, older lead-containing paints still cover many interior and exterior surfaces in older buildings and lead-based paints continue to be used on bridges and other steel structures. Blood lead levels in adults and children have declined over the past 40 years. However, indoor persistence of lead paint chips or lead dust still accounts for many cases of childhood lead poisoning. In addition, painters and other workers performing renovation work on bridges or buildings with lead paint can be significantly exposed to lead. Burning or torching of the surface to remove the paint produces a lead fume, which is readily absorbed through the respiratory tract.

Lead is a metal for which there is no known beneficial biological role. Lead poisoning among ship builders was described by Pliny the Elder (79 A.D.). Lead occurs in one oxidation state (+2). It is easy to analyze in biologic and environmental media because few things interfere with its measurement.

Childhood lead poisoning is caused primarily by ingestion and inhalation of paint dust and ingestion of paint chips by infants and toddlers. Many water distribution systems comprise lead pipes, which release lead into drinking water, thereby contributing significantly to lead exposure. Lead impairs cognitive development in children even at low doses.[2–4] and the adverse effects are detectable in adulthood.[5]

Occupational exposures to lead are mainly by inhalation of lead dust and fume, although ingestion can occur when workers smoke or eat on the job or where hygiene is poor. Lead exposure begins with mining and smelting, then continues into the industries that make lead products, including lead alloys and lead pigments, and those that fabricate products containing lead. A heavy, dense metal, lead is used in X-ray shields and weights, ranging from gram weights on fishing lines to multi-ton weights to stabilize construction cranes. Many lead-using factories have moved from high-income countries to low- and middle-income (LMICs) countries. Lead acid batteries continue to be manufactured in the United States but in decreasing numbers.

The combination of improved occupational and environmental hygiene and closure of lead factories greatly reduced the number of severe occupational lead poisoning cases in the United States. However, there remains an informal sector of backyard smelters, in which lead plates from vehicle batteries are melted to recover and recycle the lead. This source of urban lead exposure is difficult to detect and regulate. As environmental awareness led to removal of leaded paint from many structures in the 1980s, a new source of lead exposure emerged for workers performing or working near abrasive blasting, burning, welding, and cutting of steel structures, such as bridges that had been coated with anti-rust lead paint. To keep lead from contaminating the environment, lead-removal workers were enclosed in tents, which greatly increased

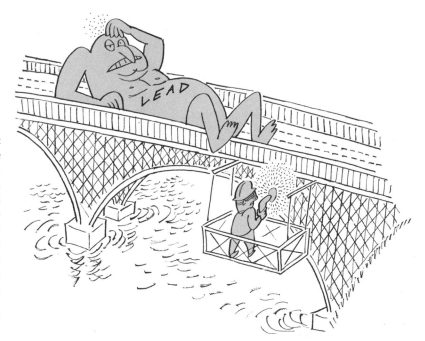

Figure 11-6. Lead paint on old structures can be released into the environment by maintenance work, such as the removal of leaded paint from bridges. To keep lead out of the ambient environment, EPA required this type of work to be enclosed, thereby greatly increasing the potential lead exposure to the workers—an unfortunate trade-off. (Drawing by Nick Thorkelson.)

their respiratory exposure to lead fume and dust (Figure 11-6).

Lead exposure is conveniently measured by analysis of lead in whole blood. During the period of use of leaded gasoline as an antiknock agent from the 1920s to the 1970s, BLLs in the United States averaged around 15 µg/dL. Since the removal of lead from gasoline, starting in the late 1970s, average BLLs have declined to below 2 µg/dL (Figure 11-7).

Lead is readily absorbed from the lungs and gastrointestinal tract. In adults, about 10% of ingested lead is absorbed; in children, whose bodies need calcium, about 50% of ingested lead is absorbed. Once absorbed, lead, some of it bound to protein, travels through the blood and gains access to all organs, including the brain.

Lead adversely affects many organ systems. Lead inhibits enzymes, such as delta-aminolevulinic acid dehydratase, which converts delta-aminolevulinic acid to porphobilinogen, and ferrochelatase, which inserts iron into the heme molecule. As a result, lead causes anemia and creates a build-up of protoporphyrin. Clinically apparent anemia may not occur until the BLL is above 50 µg/dL. Elevated blood pressure can occur when the BLL is approximately 20 µg/dL or higher. Peripheral nerve dysfunction starts to occur around 40 µg/dL. Moderate

hypertension is associated with elevated BLLs and may be partially related to toxic effects on the proximal renal tubule. Population increases in blood pressure have been associated with increases in lead exposure at very low levels.

The brain is a target organ for lead. Cognitive impairment and sleep disturbances are often

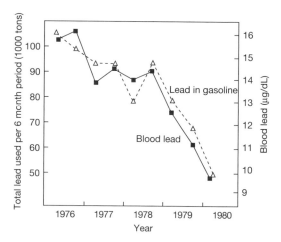

Figure 11-7. This graph tracks the dramatic decline in blood lead levels (BLLs) coincident with the reduction of leaded gasoline production in the United States (1976–1980). The decline reached 2.9 µg/dL by 1990 and has continued so that the mean BLL is below 2 µg/dL. (Source: U.S. Environmental Protection Agency.)

reported in adults with BLLs of 50 μg/dL or even lower. Encephalopathy may occur if the BLL reaches 100 μg/dL. Peripheral neuropathy may cause weakness and slowed reflexes. Motor neuron neuropathy predominates in lead poisoning, and "foot drop" is a classical symptom, often first detected by abnormal gait with circumduction of one foot. Classical lead poisoning, characterized by motor and sensory peripheral neuropathy leading to foot drop, gastrointestinal colic, weakness, and depression, is rarely encountered today in industrialized countries.

Blood lead level is a marker only for recent exposure to lead. Lead accumulates in organs, primarily bone, where K-wave X-ray fluorescence (K-XRF) can measure cumulative dose. Even in the presence of low current BLLs, a high bone lead, as measured by K-XRF, may be associated with chronic disease.[6] In lead-exposed workers, there is a close correlation between bone lead level and BLL.[7] The EDTA-mobilization test, in which administration of this chelating agent is followed by increased excretion of lead in the urine, can help assess body burden of lead and lead exposure in the distant past.

Lead was used as a pigment in oil-based paint. Approximately two-thirds of homes in the United States constructed before 1940 and one-half built between 1940 and 1960 contain heavily leaded paint. In 1978, the Consumer Product Safety Commission lowered the legal maximum lead content in most types of paint to 0.06%, a trace amount.[9] Residential and commercial painters encounter lead exposure when they prepare surfaces for painting by burning, scraping, sanding, or chiseling old paint. Buildings constructed before 1960 have a high likelihood of having leaded paint in them, which may have been covered by subsequent layers of paint.

From the 1920s to the 1980s, tetraethyl lead (TEL) was added to gasoline as an antiknock additive for automobile engines. The lead industry mounted an extensive campaign in the 1920s to gain acceptance of TEL, and its pervasive use in gasoline since then led to accumulation of lead in the environment and in people throughout the world. Acute organic lead poisoning was reported in the TEL workers as early as 1924. By the 1970s, the average BLL in the United States was 15 μg/dL, due largely to the lead contribution from gasoline. The decline in the use of leaded gasoline during the 1980s was accompanied by a decline in BLL (Figure 11-7). Although lead is no longer used as an additive in most gasoline, it is still used in certain fuels, such as aviation fuel. The story of lead in gasoline reflects major failures and successes of public health as well as corruption and integrity in science.[10,11] Cognitive impairment may occur in children even at BLLs below 5 μg/dL.[3] Two generations of children, from the 1930s to the 1980s, suffered at least subclinical effects from exposure to environmental lead.

In industrialized countries, concerns about lead focus mainly on (a) maternal exposure before and during pregnancy and (b) lead ingestion during infancy and young childhood, both of which interfere with the developing nervous system, causing cognitive impairment.[12] As the mean population BLL has fallen below 10 μg/dL, it has been recognized that there is no known threshold for this effect.[3,13] Because of lack of a threshold, lead is one of the very few environmental contaminants for which the EPA has declined to set a Reference Dose.

Lead dust from occupational exposure can be transported home on workers' clothes, skin, and hair, thus exposing children and other household members (Figure 11-8). Even in the 1990s, children of lead workers had elevated BLLs attributable to this type of paraoccupational exposure.[14]

Most states require clinical laboratories to report some or all BLL test results.[15] When funding allows, states investigate the source of reported elevated lead exposure. Such investigations are sometimes impeded by rules regarding privacy. Elevated BLLs in children are reportable to the Centers for Disease Control and Prevention (CDC) through state and local health departments. (See Chapter 6.)

The OSHA lead standard, promulgated in 1978, covers "general industry" (foundries and factories); a 1993 OSHA standard covers the construction industry (including exposures due to welding and lead abatement, like in Case 2). Both standards require employers to conduct air monitoring to determine whether workers are exposed to lead. Employers are required to keep airborne lead levels at or below the permissible exposure limit (PEL) level of 50 μg/m³ (8-hour time-weighted average [TWA]). Both standards require training and education as well as air sampling. If airborne lead exceeds 30 μg/m³, the

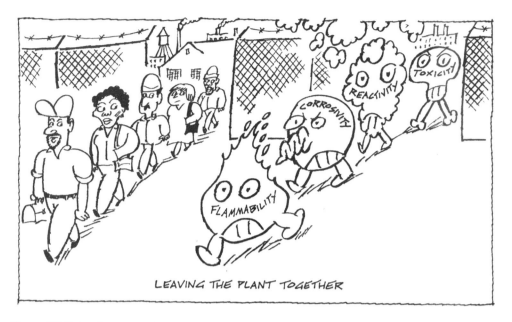

Figure 11-8. Workers can inadvertently bring toxic chemicals home with them. (Drawing by Nick Thorkelson.)

action level, medical surveillance is required. If airborne lead exceeds 50 μg/m³, employers must provide personal protective equipment, sanitation, and separation of work and street clothing.

The most important part of the OSHA lead standard for general industry is its medical removal clause with a rate retention provision. If a worker's BLL exceeds 60 μg/dL at any time or exceeds 50 μg/dL as the average of the last three tests (or of all tests within the past 6 months), the worker must be removed from exposure—with no loss of pay, seniority, or benefits. The worker may be returned to work when the BLL drops below 40 μg/dL. These standards, which have not been changed since first promulgated, are seriously out of date, allowing workers to maintain BLLs around 40 μg/dL, a level that is associated with adverse health effects.[16] With comparable exposure, workers who smoke at work and those who do not use gloves or wash hands before eating have more lead exposure than other workers.[17]

Lead-acid batteries are now the main use for lead, and recovery and reuse of lead from spent batteries is important economically and environmentally.[18] An undocumented industry in both high-income countries and LMICs is small-scale, often family-operated, battery recovery, which frequently results in household and neighborhood lead exposure.

Some drinking-water sources naturally contain high levels of lead (and other elements); others have been contaminated by lead from industrial or hazardous waste sites. More importantly, the continued reliance on leaded water pipe and the continued presence of lead solder in plumbing provides a direct exposure pathway. Depending on the water source, water may be leached out of older pipes, resulting in unacceptably high levels of lead in drinking water. This fact came to national attention in 2016, when high levels of lead in drinking water were reported in Flint, Michigan. (See Box 16-3 in Chapter 16.)

Some foods are high in lead because of environmental soil contamination, from past use of lead-containing pesticides and other sources (Figure 11-9). In the past, lead chromate dyes used in food packaging were identified as a potential source of lead exposure to children.[19] The EPA has developed the Integrated Exposure Uptake Biokinetic (IEUBK) Model for Lead in Children, which is available on its website; it enables the user to vary inputs from food, water, soil, and air to obtain a predicted distribution of BLLs for exposed children of varying ages.[20]

There are still other exposures of adults and children to lead. Whereas lead toys were once commonplace and identified as such, lead

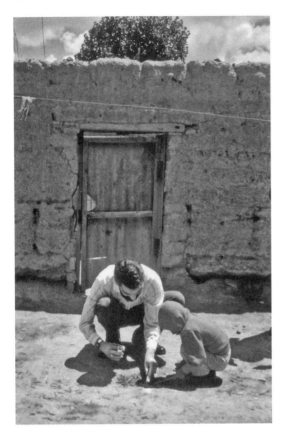

Figure 11-9. While a young resident looks on, a National Institute for Occupational Safety and Health physician and health scientist collects a residential soil sample as part of a study to assess heavy-metal contamination of a community near a large tin smelter in Bolivia. (Photograph by Aaron Sussell.)

contamination of toys imported from China emerged as a major public health issue in 2008. Scrap lead has also been melted into inexpensive jewelry. Lead has been identified in cosmetics, home remedies, and dietary supplements, especially from Latin American and Asian countries.

While it is beyond the scope of this book to address treatment recommendations, we note the following. Chelation treatment for lead poisoning relies on the use of sulfur-containing drugs that circulate through the body, binding lead and other metal atoms and extracting them from tissues so they can be excreted in the urine. Chelation is a controversial topic, because it has been recommended by alternative healers for many other conditions for which there is no evidence of benefit. Chelation is sometimes warranted and necessary for symptomatic patients with acute lead toxicity, especially if their clinical status is worsening. Chelation is of questionable benefit for chronic lead poisoning, because it may suddenly mobilize lead sequestered in bone and redistribute it to other organs, including the brain.[21] Chelation is potentially harmful if the source of exposure has not been identified and controlled. Dimercaptosuccinic acid (DMSA) has been approved by the Food and Drug Administration (FDA) for the treatment of childhood lead poisoning, although its efficacy has not been demonstrated for treating children with BLLs below 25 µg/dL.[22] and the CDC does not recommend it for children with BLLs below 45 µg/dL. It is unethical to treat lead-exposed workers with DMSA or other chelating drugs for prophylaxis while they are still being exposed to lead, and this practice is specifically prohibited in the OSHA lead standard. (See Chapters 23, 24, 26, 28, and 30 for further discussion of the adverse effects of lead.)

Mercury

Mercury, another element with no known essential function in the body, has many toxic effects.[23,24] It exists as elemental mercury (Hg^{o}), or quicksilver; as inorganic mercury, either as mercurous (Hg^{+}) or mercuric (Hg^{++}) salts; and in organic forms, mainly methylmercury (MeHg), dimethylmercury, ethylmercury, and phenylmercuric acetate. Elemental mercury, which is liquid at ambient temperatures, evaporates so that it can potentially saturate the air in closed rooms. Leaking or broken mercury-containing instruments, such as thermometers or sphygmomanometers, can be a source of mercury poisoning. Fine mercury droplets with greater surface-to-volume ratios release mercury more quickly than larger pooled droplets. Workers can be exposed to mercury during mining and distillation, production and use of mercury-containing products, and as bystanders when mercury-containing devices break.

Mercury is used in the manufacture of monitoring instruments and in certain industrial processes. It is important to distinguish the form of mercury (metallic [or elemental], inorganic, or organic) when evaluating toxic effects. Metallic and inorganic mercury affect the nervous system and the kidneys. At high doses, exposed persons may develop tremor. In addition, they may develop behavioral and personality changes, pathologic shyness, increased excitability, loss of memory, insomnia, and depression (a syndrome called erethism)—and in severe cases, delirium and hallucinations. Lower doses cause more subtle forms of these problems, such as visuomotor changes on neurobehavioral testing and slowed nerve conduction velocity. Kidney toxicity includes both glomerular and tubular dysfunction, with proteinuria and, in severe cases, impaired creatinine clearance. Exposure to metallic mercury is usually monitored through determinations of urine mercury levels, although blood levels may also be useful.

Organic mercury compounds (usually methylmercury) are sometimes encountered in workplace settings, but they are better known from outbreaks related to environmental contamination (usually human ingestion of contaminated fish). These exposures have been associated with severe disorders of the CNS and the peripheral nervous system and with birth defects in children of women exposed during pregnancy to high levels of methylmercury.

In the past, the felt-hat industry used mercuric nitrate to break down hairs to produce felt. Some hatters had very high mercury levels, and many showed symptoms of chronic mercurialism, including erethism and a tremor known as *hatters' shakes*. Community exposure to elemental mercury can also occur. Several volumes describe the history and status of mercury mining, exposure, and toxicity.[23,24] Bernardino Ramazzini (1713) wrote eloquently about the maladies of mercury-exposed gilders, mirror-makers, and even physicians. Of the mirror makers he wrote: "They learn by experience . . . how malignant is mercury. . . . Those who make the mirrors become palsied and asthmatic from handling mercury. At Venice, on the island called Murano, where huge mirrors are made, you may see these workmen . . . scowling at the reflection of their own suffering in their mirrors and cursing the trade they have chosen."

All forms of mercury are toxic and potentially lethal to humans and animals. Mercurial compounds have been widely used for their biocidal properties, such as in antiseptics, antibacterials, and fungicides. Phenylmercuric acetate has been used as a biocide in antifouling marine paints and indoor latex paint. In 1990, the EPA banned mercury for use in indoor paint. Increases in indoor mold and related symptoms since then may have been partially attributable to the removal of mercurial fungicides from indoor paint. Organomercurials have been used as seed dressings to prevent seed from becoming moldy in storage.

The dense liquid properties of elemental mercury, which has a specific gravity of 13.6 and a low coefficient of expansion, have made it valuable in instruments for measuring temperature and air pressure. Many thermometers and barometers have contained mercury. Many states, recognizing broken thermometers as a preventable source of household mercury exposure, have banned the sale of mercury thermometers. Hospitals have phased out many mercury-containing products; breakage of or a spill from one of these products may result in costly cleanups. Spillage during improper maintenance of gas meters that contain mercury can be a source of household mercury exposure.

The main route of exposure to elemental mercury is by inhalation of vapor. Contrary to popular opinion, elemental mercury is not absorbed through the skin and only negligibly in the gastrointestinal (GI) tract. Mercury has been used as a flexible weight in long tubes that are passed by gastroenterologists to dilate constrictions or obstructions in the GI tract; this use is being phased out. Physicians have been exposed to mercury when they have injected it into these tubes, which can rupture and release mercury into a patient's intestine or peritoneal cavity.[25]

Dental amalgams, popularly known as "silver amalgams" or "amalgam fillings," comprised of about 50% mercury, had been widely used in dentistry for a century. These amalgams, which are durable but not impervious to wear, release small amounts of mercury vapor, especially during chewing. Amalgams contribute up to about 1 µg of mercury daily in the urine of people who have them. Mercury has been rapidly replaced in dental practice by composite materials. Controversies arose during the 1990s, when many people were being urged to have their amalgams removed to alleviate nonspecific symptoms, usually not including the classic symptoms of elemental mercury poisoning. The

American Dental Association (ADA) stated that it was unethical for dentists to recommend amalgam removal for health reasons, although they could remove them at the request of patients. The ADA contends that, except for uncommon local allergic reactions, there is no evidence of systemic harm from amalgams.[26] In Europe, dental amalgams were phased out earlier as part of a more aggressive program to reduce all uses of mercury. The European Union has banned dental amalgams for children as well as women who are pregnant or breastfeeding.

During the late 1990s, many dentists began to develop mercury-free practices. Dental insurance companies reimbursed patients only for the cost of amalgams, not for the higher cost of composite fillings, thereby encouraging less affluent patients to settle for amalgam fillings. However, during removal of amalgams, patients have temporary increases in blood mercury levels, followed by decreases—with the biological half-life of mercury being about 2 months. Swallowing bits of amalgam is probably of negligible importance since elemental mercury is not well absorbed from the intestine.

Over many centuries, mercury has been used for many medicinal purposes, including treating syphilis. Mercury compounds, especially thimerosal (ethylmercury), was widely used as an antiseptic (in mercurochrome and merthiolate). Antiseptics now sold in pharmacies contain other ingredients. Thimerosal, used extensively as an antimicrobial to stabilize vaccines and other biologics, has been removed from vaccines for children and infants. Mercurial compounds are used by traditional healers in several cultures.[27] Calomel (mercurous chloride) was widely used for several disorders as a cathartic and purgative agent against parasites and for diphtheria by promoting the sloughing of mucosa in the throat.[28] Calomel, which was incorporated into teething powders used for infants, caused acrodynia (pink disease) with redness and pain in the hands and feet.

Minamata disease refers to severe methylmercury poisoning. In the mid-1950s, in fishing communities on Minamata Bay in southern Japan, people who regularly consumed fish from the Bay developed a serious progressive disorder that affected the cerebellum and peripheral nerves. Inorganic mercury had been released into Minamata Bay in effluent from a nearby factory and was subsequently transformed into organic mercury through the action of aquatic microorganisms and was then bioamplified through the food chain. Mild cases involved numbness and tingling and burning sensations around the mouth and in the fingers. More serious cases progressed to cognitive impairment, slurred speech, unsteady gait, deafness, tunnel vision, blindness, and death. There were hundreds of cases and at least 35 deaths. Infants born to affected mothers suffered congenital Minamata disease, characterized by motor impairment, mental retardation, and blindness. The syndrome was reproduced in cats that were fed fish from the bay. A similar epidemic occurred in Niigata, Japan, in the 1960s.[29]

Organomercurial fungicides, including those with methylmercury, were widely used as fungicides for protection of grain stored for seeding. In the 1970s, epidemics in Iraq and Guatemala occurred when people used mercury-treated grain for baking, rather than planting, and became severely poisoned. Mercury is no longer approved for seed treatment. The use of phenylmercuric acetate as an antibarnacle/antifouling additive to boat paints has also been banned, although its replacement (tributyltin) is equally harmful to aquatic life. Mercury was added to indoor latex paint as a preservative and to prevent mold growth and prolong shelf-life. All of the biocidal properties of mercury supported manufacturing industries in which workers were exposed to organic mercurial compounds. The formulation and application of mercury-containing fungicides exposed factory and agricultural workers.

Inorganic mercury, from both industrial and natural sources, can be converted to methylmercury in the sediment of bodies of water by anaerobic bacteria. Methylmercury absorbed by microorganisms bioaccumulates at every stage of the food chain, reaching $0.2 \ \mu g/g$ (0.2 ppm) in herbivorous fish and exceeding 1 ppm in many predatory fish, such as tuna, swordfish, and shark. Although the FDA has set an action level (the level at which commercial fish could be seized) of 1 ppm of methylmercury for commercially sold fish, mercury levels have been found as high as 4 ppm in fish being sold in supermarkets. (By comparison, in Minamata

Bay, mercury levels in fish exceeded 10 ppm.) People who consume fish frequently ingest significant quantities of mercury and, as a result, some develop symptoms. Susceptibility to mercury toxicity varies greatly, in part due to variants in metallothionein.

Elemental and inorganic mercury are excreted mainly in urine, but methylmercury is excreted mainly in feces. Therefore, urine is not a sensitive indicator of methylmercury ingestion. Some methylmercury deposits in hair, which grows at a rate of about 1 cm per month, and has been used to estimate the chronology of exposure. Most people have hair levels below 1 ppm, but hair levels above 8 ppm have been associated with symptoms of mercury poisoning. Hair levels above 50 ppm were seen in some people with Minamata disease.[29]

People who frequently eat large predatory fish, such as swordfish and tuna, are vulnerable to developing mercury poisoning. However, fish consumption has also been shown to benefit pregnancy outcome and reduce the risk of cardiovascular disease. These benefits have been attributed, in part, to omega-3 polyunsaturated fatty acids (PUFAs) and selenium present in fish. Benefits can also be achieved by consuming fish-oil supplements. Balancing the benefits of fish intake with contaminants, such as methylmercury and PCBs, has been challenging and controversial. It requires consideration of two separate dose–response curves, one for the benefits and one for the harms.[30,31] Most benefits may be realized at a consumption level below that causing toxic effects in most people. People who daily consume very large amounts of fish, including people who do subsistence fishing, often have elevated mercury levels, even if they eat fish that has low levels of mercury. Most predatory fish with high mercury levels are not high in PUFAs. However, salmon, herring, and some other fish are low in mercury and high in PUFAs.

Mercury exerts many of its toxic effects by its high affinity for sulfur, including binding to sulfhydrl groups of proteins and disrupting their tertiary configuration. Mercury has a high affinity for selenium as well; some manifestations of mercury toxicity may be due to its inhibition of selenoenzymes that are critical for antioxidant defense. Selenium in fish may offer some protection against mercury poisoning. Conversely, very high levels of selenium may cause symptoms, and mercury may confer some protection, making it difficult to sort out their combined effects.

Although minute amounts of dimethylmercury are present with methylmercury in aquatic environments or in hazardous waste, dimethylmercury is mainly a laboratory reagent used, for example, to calibrate nuclear magnetic resonance equipment. There are very few reports of poisoning due to dimethylmercury. However, a renowned chemist died from mercury poisoning 10 months after she spilled 3 to 5 drops of dimethylmercury on her latex-gloved hand. Dimethylmercury readily passes through latex and is absorbed by the skin. Her blood mercury levels exceeded 1,000 µg/L.[32]

When there has been chronic exposure to mercury, the source should be identified and eliminated. People who eat fish frequently (more than twice a week) should be especially attentive to choosing fish that are low in mercury. The 2013 Minamata Convention on Mercury "is a global treaty" that was designed to protect human health and the environment from the adverse effects of mercury.[33] The treaty aims to control anthropogenic releases of mercury, including shutting mercury mines, phasing out most uses of mercury, controlling emissions, and regulating mercury use in gold extraction.

In LMICs, mercury is widely used in small-scale gold mining, where riverbed gravel is washed with water and mixed with mercury to extract gold. The resulting gold amalgam is then heated to drive off the mercury. This is often done in homes, thereby exposing children and adults to the elemental mercury vapor. Many governments distribute mercury to miners free of charge to acquire gold for international trade. Where mercury is still in use, recycling of mercury, rather than mining of virgin mercury, should provide a sufficient amount. Surplus mercury could be inactivated, possibly by forming insoluble mercury sulfide.

Cadmium

Cadmium, another metal without known essential or beneficial biological functions, is nephrotoxic and carcinogenic. Because some cadmium is present in lead and zinc ores, cadmium pollution occurs near lead and zinc smelters. Cadmium has been used in alloys with other metals, in paint pigments, in nickel-cadmium batteries (now in very limited use), and in electroplating. It has also been used to stabilize plastic.

Cadmium fume can be absorbed through the lungs. Plants, especially rice, can absorb cadmium from soil, thereby making food a significant source of cadmium exposure, while conversely plants may be useful for bioremediation of cadmium-contaminated sites. Cadmium is present in tobacco and tobacco smoke, a major source of exposure. Once absorbed, cadmium is stored in soft tissues. Most of the body burden is in the kidney, where cadmium causes tubular damage. Cadmium has a long biological half-life (10 to 30 years). Cadmium exposure can be monitored by determining cadmium concentrations in urine or blood.

Cadmium induces the liver to synthesize metallothionein, a low-molecular-weight, sulfur-rich transport molecule, to which it binds avidly. The metallothionein-cadmium complex is transported in the blood to other organs. Metallothionein normally transports and regulates zinc, a cofactor for many enzymes.

Exposure to cadmium occurs during the smelting or refining of other metals or during torch cutting of steel that has been coated with cadmium. Acute cadmium poisoning is dramatic but not common. Cadmium has a relatively low boiling point (765°C), so that cadmium fume is generated at temperatures that do not release fumes from other metals. Cadmium fume is toxic to alveoli, resulting in cadmium-fume fever and pulmonary edema about 6 to 12 hours after exposure. It can be fatal.

Chronic lung and kidney disease developed in cadmium-exposed workers in Europe employed from the 1950s to 1970s, when exposures were higher than today. Chronic kidney disease begins with damage to proximal tubular cells, resulting in proteinuria, which can be monitored by increased urine levels of beta-2-microglobulin, retinol binding protein, or the brush border enzyme n-acetyl glucosaminidase. With low exposures, these changes are reversible. But with higher exposures, a tipping point is reached beyond which renal damage is progressive, even when exposure is terminated.

Tubular proteinuria is an early warning sign of possibly significant kidney damage. Cadmium also causes glomerular damage and proteinuria, especially in people with diabetes.[34]

Arsenic

Technically a metalloid rather than a true metal, arsenic is widely known as a classical poison. The organic forms that occur in seafood are much less toxic than the inorganic forms. Inorganic arsenic occurs in a trivalent state (arsenites) and a pentavalent state (arsenates). Soluble inorganic arsenicals are readily absorbed from the intestine. Pentavalent compounds are reduced to trivalent compounds, which undergo oxidative methylation to form monomethyl and dimethyl arsenous acids, which are water soluble and eliminated in the urine. (Methylation capability varies among individuals due to genetic polymorphisms in methyltransferase genes.) The main form of organic arsenic in seafood is arsenobetaine, which undergoes little metabolism and is quickly eliminated in the urine. Therefore, biomonitoring of persons for arsenic exposure must analyze urine for both inorganic and organic arsenic compounds.

Occupational exposures to arsenic occur in the smelting of metal ores (especially lead, zinc, and copper), the production and application of arsenical pesticides, the microelectronics industry (mainly in production of gallium arsenide), and the pharmaceutical industry (which produces some antihelminthic arsenical medications). However, most arsenic poisoning is due to nonoccupational exposure in drinking water from wells that tap aquifers with naturally occurring inorganic arsenic. This exposure to arsenic is widespread in South Asia. In the United States, where arsenical insecticides were widely used into the 1960s and arsenical defoliants were widely used more recently, high residues of arsenic in soil impede the conversion of contaminated land from agricultural to residential use.

Ongoing arsenic exposure can be evaluated with a 24-hour urine sample, which can provide an accurate indication of exposure. Urinary arsenic determinations usually include total arsenic and inorganic arsenic. The blood arsenic level may be informative, but the half-life of inorganic arsenic in blood is short (about

2 hours). Hair or nail samples are also used for biomonitoring of arsenic exposure.

Arsenic is released to the environment in some industrial and chemical processes, including smelting of some metal ores. It is readily absorbed from air, food, or water; distributes widely in the body; and is toxic to all organ systems. Acute occupational poisoning, which is rare, can be manifested with such symptoms as abdominal pain and cramping, difficulty swallowing, vomiting, watery diarrhea, and gastrointestinal bleeding. Shock and death can occur. Survivors may have liver and kidney damage and seizures.

Chronic arsenic poisoning can be manifested with hyperpigmentation of the skin and warty keratoses, especially on the soles of the feet and other parts of the body not exposed to the sun; ischemic heart disease; liver damage; anemia; lung irritation; diabetes; and a symmetrical distal polyneuropathy. People exposed to arsenic in drinking water are at increased risk of diabetes and hypertension. Arsenic can cause skin, liver, lung, and bladder cancer. Arsenic is unique among known human carcinogens in that there is no reliable animal model. Exposure to arsenic is usually monitored by measuring urinary arsenic levels.

Arsine (arsenic trihydride) is a colorless, odorless gas that is formed when acids leach arsenic ions out of metals. Occupational exposure occurs in metallurgical work, including etching and lead-acid battery manufacture. The use of acid cleaners to dislodge reaction residues from metal reactor vessels may generate arsine gas, and workers inside these vessels have been poisoned, sometimes fatally. Arsine gas is also used, in closed systems, in the doping process of microelectronic chips to form gallium arsenide. Arsine is a potent hemolytic agent. Following a prodrome of malaise, headache, trouble breathing, and vomiting, an exposed worker may experience severe abdominal pain and sudden onset of jaundice. Severe anemia may occur, with free hemoglobin in the serum and blood in the urine. In severe poisoning, fatal kidney failure may occur.

Manganese

Manganese is an essential trace element, but long-term inhalation of manganese dust or fumes can cause a parkinsonian syndrome by its toxic effect on the basal ganglia. Welders who use manganese-coated welding rods, workers in foundries, ceramics workers, workers who burn or grind ferromanganese alloy steel, and agricultural workers who spray manganese-containing fungicides are among those who may be exposed to manganese. The addition to gasoline of MMT (methylcyclopentadienyl manganese tricarbonyl), an organic manganese compound, as an anti-knock agent has been highly controversial, because of the potential health risks of this chemical and the widespread lead exposure that occurred when organic lead was added to gasoline.

Nickel

Nickel has important industrial uses in stainless steel, electroplating, batteries, coins, jewelry, and pigments. Nickel is absorbed from the lungs (about 20% to 35%) and the gastrointestinal tract (up to 40% from water), and it is excreted mainly in the urine. Nickel is an essential trace element, but it is toxic to the skin, respiratory tract, and the immune system. The most common adverse health effect is skin sensitization (in about 10% to 20% of the population), which results in contact dermatitis. At high occupational levels, nickel is toxic to both the upper and lower respiratory tract. Inhalation of some nickel compounds in the smelting and refining industries can cause lung and nasal cancer, and these compounds are considered human carcinogens by the International Agency for Research on Cancer (IARC) and the EPA. Nickel carbonyl, a highly reactive compound formed when nickel reacts with carbon monoxide, is rapidly absorbed and causes acute toxicity.

Beryllium

Beryllium, a lightweight metal with high tensile strength, is used as a modifier in nuclear reactors to capture neutrons. It is used in electronics and some other industries. Until beryllium was removed from fluorescent light bulbs, bulb manufacturing workers were at increased risk for beryllium poisoning. Machinists working with beryllium have potential exposure. Beryllium can cause acute or chronic poisoning as well as cancer. It is also immunotoxic, as demonstrated by a lymphocyte proliferation test, which can identify beryllium sensitization. Lymphocytes sensitized by beryllium undergo transformation and proliferate upon subsequent exposure to the antigen.

Chronic beryllium disease, resulting from inhalation of beryllium, is characterized by pulmonary granulomas that can reduce pulmonary function and cause dyspnea on exertion. Chest X-rays show diffuse infiltrates and enlarged lymph nodes. Lymphocyte transformation testing on blood or bronchial alveolar lavage fluid can assist with the early diagnosis of berylliosis. Sarcoidosis, a serious granulomatous disease of unknown etiology, can present with similar symptoms, and some cases initially diagnosed as sarcoidosis have proven to be beryllium disease. Harriet Hardy, a physician who was one of the founders of occupational medicine in the United States, established a registry of cases of beryllium disease that helped to increase recognition and understanding of this disease.

Thallium

Thallium was a commonly used household rodenticide until 1965, when it was banned for this purpose. Thallium is often implicated in fatal poisoning cases, with acute exposure due to ingestion resulting in severe gastrointestinal and neurologic symptoms. Whether accident, suicide, or homicide, death occurs within 3 weeks after acute exposure. Chronic exposure, which manifests mainly with neuropathy, is usually accompanied by hair loss.

Clerici solution is an especially toxic mixture of thallium formate and thallium malonate in water, used to establish gradients of very fine density for separation of precious metals. Synthesis of these organic compounds exposed workers to high levels of organic thallium, damaging the upper airway, discoloring the skin, and producing symptoms at thallium levels below those causing hair loss.

Chromium

Trivalent chromium (Cr-III) is an essential element, whereas hexavalent chromium (Cr-VI) is a human carcinogen in the respiratory and gastrointestinal tracts. These metal species are interconvertible through redox reactions in the environment and in the human body. Cr-VI compounds are more soluble and readily pass through cell membranes; however, once in the cell, Cr-VI is reduced to Cr-III. Metallic chromium is a very potent sensitizer. Industrial exposure to chromate and chromic acid result in skin and respiratory sensitization and upper-airway irritation. Inhalation of chromate may cause perforation of the nasal septum, which cannot be distinguished from perforation associated with cocaine.

INORGANIC ACIDS AND BASES

A wide variety of corrosive and caustic inorganic acids and bases are present in workplaces and homes. When acids dissolve in water, they release H+ ions; when bases dissolve in water, they release OH⁻ ions. At low concentrations, these compounds irritate the skin, eyes, and mucous membranes of the respiratory tract; at high concentrations, they produce chemical burns of these tissues.

The pH of a substance reflects its H+ concentration. The pH of pure water, which is completely neutral, is 7. Strong acids have a pH below 2; strong bases have a pH above 12. The pH of blood is maintained by homeostatic actions of the lung and kidney at about 7.4. The pH of stomach contents is generally below 2.

Hydrofluoric acid (HF), which is highly reactive and extremely corrosive, is used in chemical syntheses. In liquid and gaseous forms, it is used in manufacturing chemicals, etching glass and metals, pickling stainless steel, and etching computer chips. Even a few drops of HF on the skin can burn deeply—even down to bone. Small HF burns may require hospitalization. Exposure to higher concentrations or large volumes of HF may be fatal. Treatment requires removal from exposure and decontamination of the burned area and infiltration and intravenous treatment with calcium gluconate (which precipitates calcium fluoride).

ORGANIC COMPOUNDS

Due to its unique properties, carbon provides the backbone for many organic compounds with extremely diverse characteristics. Only a very small subset of organic compounds are described in this chapter to represent the main classes of these chemicals to which people are exposed in their workplaces, homes, and communities.

Some generalizations and broad classifications of organic compounds are useful. Many organic compounds are nonpolar and therefore soluble in organic solvents but not in water. Many are easily absorbed through the skin. Organic compounds of low molecular weight are volatile. Many polyaromatic organic compounds are considered to be semivolatile. (Organometallic compounds were described earlier in this chapter.)

Alkanes are compounds that range from methane, which has one carbon atom, to long-chain compounds of high molecular weight with many carbon atoms. They can be saturated (without double bonds) or unsaturated (with double bonds), and they may form straight-chain or branched-chain isomers. At ambient temperature, the alkanes with one to four carbon atoms (methane, ethane, propane, and butane) are gases, while pentane and alkanes with more carbon atoms are liquids. Gasoline is a mixture of mainly medium-chain alkanes (5 to 12 carbon atoms) that is produced from fractional distillation of crude oil.

Like other alkanes of low molecular weight, n-hexane is an acute depressant of the CNS. However, its unique metabolite, 2,5-hexanedione, causes an irreversible "dying-back" axonopathy, manifest by a peripheral neuropathy in a glove-and-stocking distribution. The effect is specific to the 2,5-dione structure, and neither n-pentane nor n-heptane has this metabolite or this toxicity. (See Chapter 23.)

A large variety of organic compounds are used in commerce, most of which have not been subject to extensive toxicologic testing or epidemiologic study. Some OSHA PELs that were established in 1970 are now outdated. In some instances, industries have established guidelines for occupational exposure limits for organic compounds in the absence of appropriate OSHA PELs.

Organic Solvents

CASE 3

During a routine medical examination, a 24-year-old man reported problems with concentration. He frequently lost his train of thought, forgot what he was saying in mid-sentence, and had been told by friends that he seemed to be forgetful. He also felt excessively tired after waking in the morning and at the end of his workday. He had occasional listlessness and frequent headaches. At work, he often felt drunk or dizzy. Several times, he had misunderstood simple instructions from his supervisor. All of these problems had developed insidiously during the previous 2 years. The patient thought that other employees in his area of the plant had complained of similar symptoms. He noted some relief during a week-long fishing vacation. He denied appetite or bowel changes, sweating, weight loss, fever, chills, palpitations, syncope, seizures, trembling hands, peripheral tingling sensations, and changes in strength or sensual acuity. He drank alcohol occasionally. He denied recreational drug use and cigarette smoking.

This man had worked for approximately 3 years as a car painter in a repair garage for railroad cars. At his physician's urging, he compiled a list of substances to which he had been exposed at work (Table 11-3).

When his plant had been inspected by OSHA 1 year before, only minor safety violations had been found. Physical examination, including a careful neurologic examination, was completely normal. Routine hematologic and biochemical tests, thyroid function studies, and a heterophile antibody assay were all negative. His erythrocyte sedimentation rate was 3 mm/hour (normal). He had slight elevations of serum gamma-glutamyl transpeptidase and alkaline phosphatase.

Table 11-3. List of Substances to Which Man in Case 3 Was Exposed

Paint Solvents	Paint Binders	Other Substances
Toluene	Acrylic resin	Organic dyes
Xylene	Urethane resin	Inorganic dyes
Ethanol	Bindex 284	Zinc chromates
Isopropanol	Solution Z-92	Titanium dioxide
Butanol		Catalysts
Ethyl acetate		
Ethyl glycol		
Acetone		
Methyl ethyl ketone		

This case illustrates many problems that confront clinicians. The patient reported vague, nonspecific symptoms that a busy clinician might easily dismiss. However, many toxicants (poisonous substances produced artificially by human activity) produce such nonspecific symptoms. In addition, the patient had multiple chemical exposures, making it difficult to identify one specific cause. This patient was unusual in that he was able to provide a list of his exposures, although this list had limitations. For example, it included two (fictional) trade names of chemicals whose identities were not known and might be difficult to determine. The absence of OSHA citations 1 year earlier may suggest—but not prove—that all exposures were then at permissible levels. However, the OSHA inspection might have been directed only at safety—not health—hazards, the plant may have been cleaned up just before the inspections, workplace conditions could have deteriorated in the year since the inspections, and new production processes could have been initiated or new materials introduced since then. In any event, all the symptoms that this man reported have been associated with exposure to concentrations of organic solvents below permissible exposure levels, so even substances in a well-maintained workplace could be the cause of his symptoms.

Organic solvents are used in many types of work, including oil refining and petrochemical production, plastics, chemical and pharmaceutical manufacturing, metal working, painting, and building maintenance. Often several different solvents are present in one product, and multiple products that contain solvents may be used in a workplace. Some products, such as paints, glues, and pesticides, are mixtures containing substantial proportions of solvents. The formulation of products containing solvents has changed over time because of economic factors and concern about the toxicity of specific solvents. These factors may make it difficult to reconstruct a worker's exposure over a long period of time.

As illustrated in Case 3, many organic solvents target the CNS, causing both acute effects (narcosis) and, in some persons, chronic neurobehavioral effects. In addition, several specific solvents, including carbon disulfide, n-hexane, and methyl n-butyl ketone, cause a peripheral neuropathy characterized by loss of distal sensation, progressing to include motor weakness and even paralysis. The disease may progress for several months after exposure has ceased, and permanent damage may occur. (See also Chapter 23.)

Benzene was commonly used as an industrial and commercial solvent in the past, but most uses have been eliminated because it is a carcinogen (see later discussion). Some other hydrocarbons, including ethylene oxide, the chloromethyl ethers, and epichlorohydrin, are also known carcinogens. Some chlorinated solvents, such as trichloroethylene and tetrachloroethylene, are human carcinogens. Many other solvents are suspected of being carcinogenic.

Many organic solvents are hepatotoxic. Carbon tetrachloride, chloroform, and tetrachloroethane can cause hepatic necrosis. Long-term exposure to carbon tetrachloride has been associated with the development of cirrhosis. Dimethylformamide and 2-nitropropane have caused outbreaks of chemically induced liver disease in exposed workers.

Some organic solvents, including the glycol ethers and ethylene oxide, adversely affect the reproductive system (Chapter 24). Solvents frequently cause skin irritation; these chemicals dry the skin by removing natural skin oils (Chapter 25). Many organic solvents are also acute respiratory tract irritants (Chapter 22).

The diagnosis of health problems related to solvent exposure relies on a thorough occupational and environmental history (Chapter 4). Biological monitoring may be helpful for ongoing exposures, but it is not useful for evaluating past exposures, because most solvents are metabolized and cleared from the body relatively quickly. Prevention of ongoing exposure through sound occupational and environmental hygiene is essential (Chapter 8).

Many of the low-molecular-weight aromatic and aliphatic compounds are widely used in a great variety of industrial processes as solvents or raw materials. They are volatile, and many are neurotoxic. These compounds have been used as anesthetics or abused for the "highs" they induce.

Benzene (C_6H_6), a colorless, pleasant-smelling volatile liquid, is the parent aromatic compound. It has been widely used as a solvent and as a raw material for building a wide variety of chemicals. Benzene is produced during the refining of petroleum. As a group, benzene, toluene, ethylbenzene, and xylene are referred to as BTEX compounds. Substitution has greatly reduced exposure to benzene; it is no longer used as a solvent and degreasing agent when other less toxic—but not innocuous compounds—can fulfill these functions. Benzene exposure still occurs in a variety of industries, including perfume manufacture, chemical research and development, and shoe manufacture. Benzene is present in unleaded gasoline (limited to the concentration of 1.3% in the United States by the EPA), resulting in some benzene exposure to gas-station attendants. It is also a constituent of cigarette smoke.

Like all organic solvents, benzene is a defatting agent that, with prolonged contact, dissolves lipids in the skin; therefore, it can cause dermatitis and can be absorbed through the skin. However, inhalation of benzene vapor is the main route of entry. About 50% of an inhaled dose is absorbed into the bloodstream. Benzene is very rapidly metabolized, in at least two pathways, to muconaldehyde and muconic acid or to quinones and phenol. Muconaldehyde and quinones are toxic to the bone marrow, causing anemias and leukemias. Measuring benzene in blood is not useful since it is cleared very quickly. Urinary phenol has been used as a nonspecific biomarker of benzene exposure.

Like other organic compounds of low molecular weight, benzene readily crosses the blood–brain barrier. Acute exposure to benzene causes CNS depression, ranging from lightheadedness and headache to coma, convulsions, and death. However, it is the chronic toxicity of benzene that is of greatest concern. Benzene depresses bone marrow production of red blood cells, white blood cells, and platelets, leading to pancytopenia and aplastic anemia, which is often irreversible and fatal. Benzene causes a wide variety of lymphohematopoietic diseases. The oldest, strongest epidemiologic evidence links benzene with acute myelogenous (myeloid) leukemia. However, multiple studies now show excesses of all other types of leukemia as well as multiple myeloma and non-Hodgkin lymphoma in benzene-exposed cohorts.

At its inception, OSHA adopted the ACGIH threshold limit value for benzene (10 ppm) as the OSHA PEL. But as epidemiologic evidence regarding leukemia increased, OSHA revised the (8-hour TWA) standard, in 1978, to 1 ppm. In 1980, in response to an industry challenge, the Supreme Court invalidated the standard because OSHA had failed to document "significant risk of material health impairment." Part of the controversy hinged on whether aplastic anemia was a necessary precursor of leukemia—if a 10 ppm standard were adequate to prevent aplastic anemia, it should also prevent leukemia. During the 1980s, studies by the IARC, EPA, and National Institute for Occupational Safety and Health provided convincing evidence of excess leukemia risk at exposures below 10 ppm, and, in 1987, OSHA promulgated and successfully defended a benzene standard of 1 ppm.

Toluene and xylene, both of which are methylated benzene compounds with many industrial applications, share the CNS depression properties of benzene, but they do not depress the bone marrow or cause leukemia.

Halogenated aliphatic solvents include a broad array of generally nonreactive, usually volatile liquids of low molecular weight, all of which depress the CNS and cause dermatitis. Most are hepatotoxic and nephrotoxic. Some are well-documented carcinogens. Long-term exposure can cause irreversible cognitive impairment. The most commonly encountered halogenated aliphatic solvents have one to four carbon atoms and up to one double bond. Among the best-known chemicals in this group are carbon tetrachloride (tetrachloromethane), chloroform (trichloromethane), methylene chloride (dichloromethane), trichloroethylene (trichloroethene), and perchlorethylene (tetrachloroethene). Dibromochloropropane (DBCP), an effective nematocide, was found to be a testicular poison (Chapter 24).

Bioactivity, toxic potency, and hazard of halogenated aliphatic solvents vary by structure and exposure. Many of these chemicals have been used as solvents in degreasing, cleaning, manufacturing, and laboratory work. Many workers have at least some potential for exposure to these chemicals. Dyes, paints, glues, pharmaceuticals, personal-care products, agrochemicals, and many other substances are either produced with these solvents or contain them as "inert ingredients."

In the past 50 years, use of specific chemicals as anesthetics and solvents has dramatically changed, in part because of concerns about their toxicity. Chloroform was replaced by other anesthetics because of toxicity and efficacy. Carbon tetrachloride was replaced as a solvent and spot remover because of its liver toxicity. Trichlorethylene has been largely replaced by the somewhat less toxic trichloroethane and, for dry-cleaning, by tetrachlorethylene (perchloroethylene, or "perc"), which is now being phased out because of its toxicity, in favor of "green" cleaning.

Occupations with regular use of solvents include chemical production; laboratory research; production and application of paints, dyes, and coatings; printing; metalworking and machine degreasing; development and production of pharmaceuticals; oil and chemical refining and production; and gas-station work. Solvents are found in many household products, including cleaning solutions, paints and stains, paint thinners, cosmetics, nail polish remover, and pesticides.

Solvents are often used as mixtures, such as gasoline, kerosene, and paint thinners, making it hard to evaluate the contribution of single compounds. *Mineral spirits* refers to mixtures of solvents containing both aromatic and aliphatic components. Volatility varies with the composition of low- and high-molecular-weight constituents and workplace temperature. Area air monitoring and personal breathing-zone air monitoring are useful in determining exposure potential. Personal breathing-zone monitoring is more reliable for individual exposure assessment since workers may move into and out of areas where air concentrations of solvents are high. Biological monitoring is useful in those few situations where there is a specific marker of exposure for a specific solvent.

Other Organic Chemicals

Vinyl chloride monomer (VCM), a gas, is the raw material for polyvinyl chloride (PVC), a ubiquitous plastic. Although PVC is inert, VCM is highly reactive. In the 1960s, VCM was found to cause acroosteolysis, a disorder characterized by osteoporosis, Raynaud phenomenon affecting the fingers, and skin thickening and nodule formation on the arms. In 1974, there was a report of three workers with angiosarcoma of the liver (an extremely rare disease) who had been exposed to VCM at a plant in Kentucky. Recognition of VCM as a carcinogen led to OSHA lowering the PEL from 500 to 1 ppm. Despite initial protests by industry, controlling occupational exposure to VCM below this PEL was feasible and even profitable due to reduced waste. Polyvinyl chloride continues to be widely produced and has many uses, including water pipes and construction material. Exposure to VCM has been effectively controlled by occupational and environmental hygiene, and cases of angiosarcoma are, again, very rare.[35]

Methyl-tert-butyl ether (MTBE) has been widely used as a gasoline additive (oxygenate) to improve its octane rating, promote more complete combustion, and reduce release of carbon monoxide, oxides of nitrogen, and other products of incomplete combustion. From about 1990 to 2006, MTBE was present in gasoline in concentrations higher than 10% (by volume). Many people who were exposed to MBTE reported symptoms of eye and respiratory tract irritation. In 2004, based partly on irritation and partly on carcinogenesis in several animals, several U.S. states banned MTBE. In 2006, gasoline companies stopped adding MTBE to gasoline, partly because of legal issues resulting from contamination of drinking-water supplies by MTBE spills and leaking underground gasoline storage tanks.

Bis(chloromethyl) ether (BCME) is a highly reactive chemical that is a known human carcinogen, which has been established as a cause of oat cell lung cancer among workers. This type of cancer, which is not associated with smoking, occurred in workers exposed to BCME alone and, to a lesser degree, in workers exposed to chloromethyl ether that had BCME as a low-level contaminant.[36]

Polybrominated diphenyl ethers (PBDEs) comprise a class of organobromines widely used as flame retardants in plastics, airplanes, motor vehicles, and textiles. They are structurally analogous to PCBs. These compounds are widespread in the home and community environment and show a broad range of toxicity, including endocrine disruption and reduced fertility in people. Polychlorinated diphenyl ethers have high toxicity and have been phased out of commerce. Like other chlorinated hydrocarbons, they show bioamplification in the food chain and are a threat to wildlife.

Formaldehyde, a highly reactive chemical that is used widely, has been recognized as a carcinogen for more than 30 years. A gas at ambient temperature, it has a characteristic odor. It irritates the eyes and, because it is highly soluble in water, it irritates the upper respiratory tract. It is also a potent sensitizer. Formaldehyde is used in producing plastics, resins, particle board, and paper. After the 1973 energy crisis, urea-formaldehyde foam was widely used as a retrofitting insulating material that was injected into the walls of homes. However, improper formulation resulted in off-gassing of formaldehyde and serious symptoms in residents of homes where it was used. Formaldehyde in solution (formalin) has been used as a preservative, exposing pathologists, laboratory technicians, and students in anatomy laboratories as well as museum workers and embalmers. Engineering controls can limit formaldehyde exposure. In anatomy and pathology laboratories, workers and students often use respiratory protection. Phenol has been substituted for formaldehyde as an anatomic preservative; however, workers who are sensitive to formaldehyde may eventually have to change occupations.

Formaldehyde is genotoxic, causing chromosomal breaks and forming cross-links in DNA and between DNA and proteins. Studies have found brain cancer, colon cancer, and leukemia among exposed pathologists and morticians and evidence for lung cancer in exposed industrial workers. In 2004, IARC finally determined that formaldehyde was a Group 1 carcinogen.[37]

Isocyanates are highly reactive compounds of low molecular weight that contain an -NCO group. They react with hydroxyl groups to form polyurethane polymers that are used in foams, thermoplastics, spandex fibers, and polyurethane coatings. Exposed workers include plastic manufacturers, foam makers, and producers of a wide range of polyurethane products. Incineration of polyurethane compounds releases isocyanates. Isocyanates are both strong irritants and sensitizers of the skin and respiratory tract. Isocyanates can cause or exacerbate asthma. Some isocyanates are animal carcinogens. Diisocyanates (with two –NCO groups) are the isocyanates that are most widely used,

especially methylene diphenyl diisocyanate and toluene diisocyanate.

Melamine, a cyclic cyanide-trimer, has been used, especially in China, as an adulterant to falsely elevate the apparent protein concentration of milk and pet foods, by increasing the nitrogen content. Melamine and its by-product cyanuric acid caused renal failure in dogs and cats fed pet food made in China, due to crystal formation in the kidneys. In 2008, over 300,000 babies became ill from melamine-contaminated milk formula, and several died of renal failure.

Perfluoroalkylated chemicals are a class of persistent anthropogenic chemicals that have been detected in human blood globally. Perfluorooctane sulfonate and perfluorooctanoic acid are eight-carbon-chain chemicals, sometimes called C8s, with complete fluorine substitutions. These chemicals have endocrine-disrupting, genotoxic, neurobehavioral, and reproductive effects in animals. A large population of people residing in the Ohio River Valley were exposed to C8 effluent and emissions from an industrial facility. As part of the legal settlement of a lawsuit, the C8 Science Panel was established to review serum C8 levels and epidemiologic data on health outcomes in this population. The panel concluded that there was a "probable link" between high C8 exposure and ulcerative colitis, thyroid disease, testicular cancer, kidney cancer, hypercholesterolemia, and pregnancy-induced hypertension.[38]

Endocrine-Disrupting Chemicals

Endocrine disruption refers to any mechanism that increases or decreases some function of the endocrine system. Chemicals may mimic some of the actions of hormones. For example, xenobiotics that mimic estrogen, known as *environmental estrogens*, may bind to estrogen receptors, either activating them or preventing estrogen from having its normal effects. Chemicals may stimulate the formation or release of estrogen or may induce enzymes that break it down. Endocrine disruptors may act on the hypothalamic-pituitary-adrenal axis, the thyroid, or sex hormone systems. For example, some PCBs and polybrominated biphenyls (PBBs) interfere with thyroid function, perhaps because of their structural resemblance to a thyroid hormone precursor.

Bisphenol A (BPA), a chemical used in plastics and epoxy resins has been considered acceptable by the FDA for use in plastic water bottles and the lining of food cans. Low levels of BPA have been widely detected in humans. This compound has been associated with endocrine disruption in animals.

DDT, an organochlorine insecticide, was the first endocrine disruptor identified. In the 1960s, researchers found that DDT interfered with reproduction in birds, causing them to lay thin-shelled eggs that broke during incubation. DDT and its metabolites are bioaccumulative compounds that are biomagnified in the food chain. As a result, fish-eating birds, such as bald eagles, brown pelicans, and ospreys and bird-eating hawks, such as peregrine falcons, suffered decades of reproductive failure due to DDT. The populations of these species have recovered slowly after organochlorine use has been greatly reduced since the 1970s. Among the multiple adverse effects on reproduction was induction of an enzyme that broke down both DDT and endogenous estrogens, thereby causing reproductive impairment.[39]

Endocrine disruptors have serious effects on aquatic wildlife, causing abnormal sexual development, sterility, and death of embryos.[40] In humans, endocrine disruptors adversely affect prenatal and infant development, especially of the urogenital system. Halogenated organic compounds, including polychlorinated dioxins and furans, disrupt male reproductive development, leading to undescended testes, hypospadias, and shortening of the penis. In the 1950s, diethylstilbestrol, which was prescribed to sustain pregnancy in women who showed signs of impending miscarriage, resulted in many cases of vaginal cancer in their daughters. In addition, grandsons of these women have had an increased rate of hypospadias.[41] Precocious puberty in girls, occurring as young as age 7, has been attributed to endocrine disrupting compounds, such as phthalates and PBBs.

Occupational exposure to endocrine disruptors also occurs. Men engaged in the manufacture of birth-control chemicals have experienced feminization, with loss of hair, increased pitch of voice, and gynecomastia. Maternal occupational exposure to phthalates or hair sprays has increased their likelihood of giving birth to boys with hypospadias, although this risk has been modified by folate supplements during pregnancy.[42]

Polycyclic Aromatic Hydrocarbons

Polycyclic aromatic hydrocarbons (PAHs) comprise a family of over 100 organic compounds built around two to six aromatic rings. They are formed by the incomplete combustion of petroleum compounds, coal, natural gas, wood, garbage, tobacco, and even food. PAHs are components of coal tar, creosote, and asphalt. They are ubiquitous in urban environments and detectable even in pristine environments due to atmospheric transport and deposition. PAHs with two to three rings are more volatile than those with four or more rings. They generally occur as mixtures. Benzo[a]pyrene (BaP), a carcinogenic PAH that typically comprises about 10% of PAH mixtures, is thought to be the primary carcinogen in tobacco smoke, charcoal-broiled meat, and chimney soot.

People are exposed to PAHs by inhalation of combustion products of tobacco, wood, or gasoline and by ingestion of food containing traces of them. PAHs are released from forest fires and volcanoes and from automobile exhaust, heating systems, and industrial plants. Soils near roadways have PAHs that may be a source of exposure to toddlers and gardeners. Occupational exposures occur in mines; refineries; metal works; factories producing coal tar, coke, and asphalt; smokehouses; and other smoky environments.

Seventeen PAHs are widespread in the environment.[43] Several are carcinogenic, with BaP being the most widespread and best-studied. PAHs irritate the skin. They vary in solubility in water (although most have low water solubility) and volatility. However, they adsorb readily to atmospheric particulates, enabling them to be transported long distances.

Coal-gas plants (manufactured gas plants) operated in many U.S. cities and towns from the late 1800s to about 1920. As they became obsolete, surface structures were removed and the land was leveled for residential development, covering over underground structures and pools of tar. PAHs, tar residues, and benzene and other volatile compounds eventually contaminated many homes that were built in those sites. Much remediation was performed in the 1980s and 1990s.

Polychlorinated Polyaromatic Compounds

Many isomers and congeners of PCBs were deliberately produced and formulated into compounds for commercial and industrial use. Depending on the number and location of chlorine atoms, PCB molecules can be flat (coplanar) or bent. PCBs demonstrate little acute toxicity, but, in animals, they produce a chronic syndrome with weight loss, chloracne, alopecia, skin edema, swelling around the eyes, shrinkage of the thymus and lymph glands, liver enlargement, bone marrow depression, and reproductive abnormalities. The syndrome is triggered through the aryl hydrocarbon (Ah) receptor. PCBs are well-documented animal carcinogens, causing liver cancer in several species, with the potency varying with degree of chlorination. PCBs are genotoxic. They can act as promoters of liver or lung cancer in animals. IARC has determined that PCBs are Group 1 carcinogens, based on evidence that they can cause malignant melanoma, breast cancer, and non-Hodgkin lymphoma.

PCBs and related compounds can cause *chloracne*, with lesions that are indistinguishable from adolescent acne but often dense and occurring on more parts of the body, including the face, ears, abdomen, and scrotum. Chloracne is a cutaneous manifestation of systemic exposure. PCBs can also cause hepatotoxicity, manifested by abnormal liver enzymes, but usually not by jaundice or clinically apparent liver disease. Women exposed prenatally to PCBs have had infants with lower birthweight, smaller head circumference, and impaired psychomotor and cognitive development.[44]

Although high blood levels of PCBs were widespread in the 1970s, the average concentration in blood has declined slowly since the imposition of restrictions on PCB production and use in the United States and Europe in the 1970s. In Yusho, Japan in 1968 and Yu-Cheng, Taiwan, in 1979, epidemics of furan poisoning occurred, from contamination of rice oil with dibenzofurans, which were derived from PCBs that had leaked from heating coils into the oil. Adults suffered chloracne and acute liver damage, which was fatal in some cases. Fetal exposure was associated with abnormal urogenital tract development and developmental neurotoxicity, including reduced psychomotor performance and spatial learning and impaired cognitive development.

Dioxins and furans are unwanted by-products of chemical synthesis or breakdown. *Dibenzodioxins* have two benzene rings connected through two oxygen atoms; *dibenzofurans* have two benzene rings connected by one oxygen atom. There are potentially 74 different dibenzodioxins and 134 different dibenzofurans. 2,3,7,8-tetrachlorodibenzo-p-dioxin (TCDD), or *dioxin*, is considered to be the most toxic synthetic chemical. It was present as a contaminant in the manufacture of the commonly used herbicide 2,4,5-trichlorophenoxy acetic acid (2,4,5-T), which comprised 50% of Agent Orange, a substance that was widely used to defoliate forests during the Vietnam War. Vietnam's forests have largely recovered, but TCDD is highly persistent and is still measurable in soils and aquatic sediments there. Human exposure, mainly through fish consumption, still occurs. There is a widespread belief in Vietnam that many currently occurring congenital defects or developmental abnormalities are due to persistent dioxin exposure.

Animal species vary widely in their susceptibility to TCDD toxicity. It affects many organ systems. Although it is not strongly genotoxic, it is a human carcinogen. Other dioxins and furans as well as some PCBs are given a toxic equivalency rating in comparison with TCDD. The natural combustion of wood yields dioxins and furans. Combustion of synthetic chlorinated compounds and application of chlorine bleaching compounds to wood yield chlorinated dioxins, such as TCDD, and chlorinated furans. The average background concentration of TCDD in body fat is about 4 parts per trillion (pg/g of lipid); in contrast, military personnel exposed to Agent Orange in Vietnam often had levels 10 times higher.[45]

Dioxins and furans can be ingested, inhaled, or absorbed through the skin; ingestion is generally the major route of entry. Dioxins can cause chloracne, induce liver enzymes, and exert anti-estrogenic activity.

Organophosphate Pesticides

CASE 4

A 38-year-old woman presented to the emergency department of a rural hospital complaining of a severe rash. The rash first appeared on her forearms several weeks before and during the previous 2 weeks had become more severe and spread to her face and neck. Itching kept her from sleeping for the previous 3 nights. She had no previous history of skin problems. She suspected that chemical exposures at work caused the rash. She worked at a greenhouse, where she had contact with pesticides, fungicides, fertilizers, and cleaning materials. Physical examination revealed a severe maculopapular rash on her hands, forearms, face, and neck. An emergency department physician treated her with topical steroids and an antihistamine and gave her free samples of each and prescriptions for more medication when these ran out. He referred her to a community clinic for follow-up, where she was seen 2 weeks later. The rash was then still severe. She had taken the free samples provided at the emergency department, but she could not afford to fill the prescriptions.

The physician at the community clinic asked her about chemicals she used at work, but she could not name any. She did not apply pesticides or fungicides, but she was exposed to them when the greenhouses were sprayed before she arrived at work each day and when she handled flowers. The physician provided her with medication for her rash, advised her to return in 2 weeks, and asked her to try to get the names of the pesticides and fungicides that were used at work.

Soon after, the physician at the community clinic saw two more workers from the greenhouse who presented with recent onset of headache and nausea. He reported the cluster of these patients from the same workplace to the state pesticide enforcement agency. Inspectors toured the greenhouse, where they found problems with labeling of pesticides and disposal practices but no serious violations of regulations. After the inspection, the owner of the greenhouse changed pesticide application procedures. All three patients recovered. When they returned to work, they were assigned to another area of the greenhouse, which did not have any hazardous exposures.

The worker in this case probably was acutely exposed to an organophosphate by inhalation (from pesticide fogging) and dermal absorption (from contact with pesticide-contaminated plants and surfaces). Once absorbed, organophosphates are metabolized by enzymes in the liver to form molecules that bind with acetylcholinesterase at cholinergic nerve endings, both centrally and peripherally. As a result, organophosphate poisoning causes a predictable constellation of muscarinic, nicotinic, and CNS symptoms. Typical symptoms include constricted pupils, salivation, sweating, and muscle fasciculation. At high exposures, diarrhea, incontinence, wheezing, bradycardia, and convulsions may occur. Severe cases can be fatal.

Cholinesterase inhibition can be measured by determining cholinesterase levels, but these measurements are difficult to interpret because the normal range is wide, accuracy of laboratories varies widely, and cholinesterase levels may quickly return to normal after exposure ceases. Cholinesterase levels are most useful for ongoing monitoring, if baseline levels are known, and in monitoring recovery from acute toxicity. Acute poisoning can be treated with atropine, with or without pralidoxime. A delayed neurotoxicity syndrome, with weakness, paresthesias, and paralysis of the lower legs, may occur in people after chronic exposure or severe acute exposure to organophosphate pesticides.

Biocides

Pesticides include insecticides, acaricides, molluscicides, nematocides, rodenticides, herbicides, fungicides, and other substances. They are designed to repel or kill living organisms ("pests"). Unlike most of the chemicals described previously, they are used specifically because of their toxicity. Although most pesticide use occurs in agricultural settings, people may also be occupationally exposed from pesticide use for structural pest control, especially in homes.

Compounds such as sulfur were used as pesticides more than 2,000 years ago. Many other pesticides also have a long history.[46] Pesticides, as a class of chemicals, affect almost every organ system, but individual pesticides usually have more specific toxicity. Because most pesticides have some human toxicity, new generations of pesticides are being designed to reduce human toxicity. Research and development have long aimed at developing pesticides that are target specific, with low toxicity for nontarget organisms, especially humans and aquatic life.

Workers are exposed to pesticides during production of active ingredients, formulation of commercial products, preparation and application (during mixing, loading, spraying, and cleaning equipment), and contact with treated crops (during inspection, weeding, and picking). Often agricultural field workers without special protection may be inadvertently exposed to nearby spray applications by wind drift. For many pesticides a *reentry time* (the time between application and when workers can, without protective equipment, enter a field to harvest the crops) of 1 to 7 days is specified. For many pesticides, efficacy requires achieving fine aerosols that can be easily inhaled. Exposure can occur by inhalation of vapors, dusts, or mists; dermal absorption; or ingestion—by eating food that has been sprayed or eating in the field without washing or changing clothes.

Fumigants

Fumigants are applied to buildings, warehouses, ship holds, and soil to eliminate rodent and invertebrate pests. They are highly toxic to people. For example, methyl bromide, the use of which has decreased because of high toxicity and its contribution to ozone depletion, can acutely affect the nervous and respiratory systems and the gastrointestinal tract. Metam sodium, a soil fumigant, is less toxic and is replacing methyl bromide. However, a huge spill of metam sodium into the Sacramento River in 1991 killed aquatic organisms for many miles and caused headache, nausea, and shortness of breath in people living along the river and in spill-response workers. Symptoms of irritant-induced asthma persisted.[47]

Ethylene dibromide (EDB), a strong alkylating agent, was widely used to fumigate stored grain. EDB is readily absorbed through the skin and by inhalation or ingestion. It is highly irritating to mucous membranes and is hepatotoxic. It is an animal carcinogen and is considered a probable human carcinogen (IARC Group 2A). Workers involved in fumigating and those who prematurely entered fumigated structures were

exposed. EDB was banned because of evidence of its carcinogenicity and the presence of significant residues in flour, cake mixes, and commercial baked goods.

Ethylene oxide (EtO), a highly reactive chemical, is used in chemical synthesis and in sterilizing reusable equipment and supplies in hospitals. Chemical operators and healthcare workers are exposed. It is considered a human carcinogen (IARC Group 1) and has been implicated in causing cancer of the blood and lymph systems.[48]

Carbon disulfide (CS_2) has been used to fumigate museum cases and agricultural products. Exposed workers in the rubber and rayon industries have developed acute psychoses at very high levels of exposure and cardiovascular disorders at intermediate levels. It causes a distal axonopathy.

Rodenticides

Rodenticides can have high specificity for mammals and can be incorporated into baits for rats and mice. Some kill quickly without exciting suspicion or aversion by the animals. They may also be used against other mammalian pests, including gophers, squirrels, and coyotes. Other rodenticides contain the anticoagulant warfarin, which leads to a deficiency of vitamin K (necessary for blood clotting) and causes poisoned animals to bleed to death but not before they have carried poisoned food back to their dens. These chemicals have a high potential to cause human poisoning, which may occur during production and formulation and in suicide attempts. Because they are highly toxic to people, rodenticides should only be used by trained personnel.

Insecticides

Insect pests are widespread in homes and on farms. A large variety of insecticides have been produced and formulated into hundreds of products. In organic farming, synthetic pesticides are not allowed, but naturally occurring compounds are permitted. *Integrated pest management* uses ecological approaches such as interspersing different crops, introducing biological controls, and selecting resistant strains, allowing crop production with little or no insecticide use.

Organochlorines (OCs) include (a) chlorinated ethanes, such as DDT; (b) cyclodiene chemicals, such as chlordane, aldrin, and dieldrin; and (c) saturated ring compounds, such as cyclohexanes (which include lindane). From the 1940s to the 1970s, OCs were widely used in agriculture and in programs to control human lice, structural termites, and malarial mosquitoes. As insects developed resistance, the effectiveness of the OCs declined. However, it was mainly their environmental and biological persistence that led to banning and replacement by less persistent insecticides. DDT use in the United States was banned in 1972. Acute toxicity of OCs is lower than for the organophosphates but higher than some pyrethroids. Some OCs have caused hepatotoxicity in formulation workers. They have been associated with Parkinson disease.[49] Chlordane was widely used as an agricultural insecticide until about 1978, after which its use became more restricted. From 1983 to 1988, it was frequently used around building foundations for termite control. Chlordane was banned in the United States for termite control in 1988 because of its carcinogenicity, environmental persistence, and bioaccumulation. Manufacture for export still continues.

DDT in talc was dusted on soldiers and others to kill lice, and lindane continues to be used for body lice control. DDT is still used in many LMICs for malaria control. DDT has low dermal absorption and low human toxicity when ingested. Acute exposure to high doses, as in suicide attempts, first manifests as a tingling sensation of the mouth and lips and progresses to muscle fasciculations and twitching, "jumpiness," involuntary movements, and tremors, which may progress to convulsions and death from respiratory failure. Chronic toxicity from DDT involves the liver. DDT is a potent inducer of liver enzymes, especially those in the CYP2B and CYP3A groups. DDT metabolites (DDD and DDE) cause liver and lung tumors in rodents, and DDT is considered a probable human carcinogen. DDT was probably the first widely recognized endocrine disrupting chemical. o,p-DDT activates the estrogen receptor and mimics estrogen, while its metabolite, p,p'-DDE, blocks the androgen receptor. However, in the long term, these effects are overridden by enzyme induction, which accelerates breakdown of estrogen.

Two other OCs are mirex and chlordecone. Mirex is an OC that has been used mainly to control fire ants in the southern United States. Chlordecone (Kepone) was used extensively to control cockroaches and other pests in homes, offices, and animal facilities. A chlordecone poisoning outbreak affected 148 workers in a Kepone factory in Virginia in the mid-1970s. Workers experienced a variety of effects, including reduced or absent sperm.[50]

Organophosphates (OPs) include some nerve gases, such as sarin and soman, that have high toxicity to humans, potentially causing rapid death after inhalation or dermal exposure to very low concentrations. Introduced into agriculture in the 1930s, OPs became widely used by the 1950s and are now almost universally used in agriculture. They include hundreds of compounds that have been synthesized to improve specificity and overcome resistance. OPs act by binding to the enzyme acetylcholinesterase, thereby inactivating it and preventing it from breaking down the neurotransmitter acetylcholine at every synapse and nerve–muscle junction. Once this enzyme is inactivated, nerve impulses are unable to cross the synapse or nerve–muscle junction, thereby causing paralysis.

Some OPs are directly toxic to mammals, whereas others are oxidized to a toxic metabolite. Metabolism of OP is very complex and involves several enzymes. For example, CYP2C19 activates diazinon, CYP3A4 activates parathion, and CYP2B6 activates chlorpyrifos. Chlorpyrifos and diazinon, OPs with relatively low acute toxicity to humans, have been widely used. Chlorpyrifos largely replaced chlordane in household treatment for termites. Both of these compounds have been restricted because of concerns over chronic toxicity. Exposure can be measured for some OPs by quantifying specific metabolites in urine, such as diethylphosphate, a metabolite of parathion, diazinon, and chlorpyrifos. Pyridostigmine, which also protects acetylcholinesterase from OPs, was taken prophylactically by U.S. troops in the Persian Gulf War in 1991.

Children are more susceptible to OP poisoning, probably due to their slower metabolism. Children who accompany parents into farm fields or work alongside them are therefore at especially high risk. The mnemonic SLUDGE is used to describe the symptoms of OP poisonin: *s*alivation, *l*acrimation, *u*rination, *d*efecation, *G*I distress, and *e*mesis.

Carbamates, such as carbaryl and aldicarb, are widely used insecticides that have variable human toxicity. Formulations containing solvents facilitate the dermal absorption of these compounds. Metabolism reduces the toxicity of carbaryl and increases the toxicity of aldicarb. Like OPs, these compounds are also anticholinesterases. However, unlike OPs, this effect is spontaneously reversible; recovery can occur within hours after an acute poisoning. The water-soluble aldicarb has high acute toxicity, but its anticholinergic effects are spontaneously reversible after a few hours. It is a systemic pesticide and has caused outbreaks of poisoning when used on hydroponic crops, such as cucumbers.

Pyrethrins, which are natural products produced by chrysanthenum-related plants, are used to deter insects. Pyrethroids, such as deltamethrin and resmethrin, are synthetic analogs. Both pyrethrins and pyrethroids are effective, do not promote insect resistance, have low mammalian toxicity, and break down relatively quickly in the environment. Therefore, they are widely used in homes and fields. Pyrethroids have been medically used to treat lice and mites. These chemicals disrupt sodium channels, which are necessary for transmission of nerve impulses along an axon. They are rapidly metabolized in the body. There are very few documented cases of human poisoning or death.

Nicotine, an alkaloid concentrated in tobacco plants, has been used in some pesticidal applications. It activates the nicotinic receptors, a subset of acetylcholine receptors, producing an initial polarization followed by receptor paralysis. Acute poisoning, characterized by nausea and vomiting, weakness, rapid heart rate, and even death, is very rare.

Rotenone, used to kill insects and mites, rarely causes acute poisoning. However, it causes selective nerve damage in experimental animals that is conducive to Parkinson disease. It has been linked to Parkinson disease in humans.[50]

N,N-diethyl-*m*-toluamide (DEET) is an insect repellent that is widely used for personal application. Its use increased greatly after recognition of widespread West Nile virus transmission in the late 1990s. Formulations vary from weak (5%) to very strong (higher than 90%), with most in the 20% to 40% range. DEET is used to repel insects, fleas, and ticks when applied to skin and clothing. Higher concentrations offer longer protection. DEET is absorbed through the skin. It has low acute toxicity, but it has been implicated as a neurotoxicant in children, leading to the recommendation that children under age 12 should not use repellants with more than 10% DEET.

Herbicides

Herbicides, which are toxic to plants, are not likely to have high human toxicity but can have both local and systemic toxic effects. By absorbing and incorporating chemicals, plants may convey toxic chemicals from water and soil to consumers. Some herbicides inhibit photosynthesis, such as triazines, including atrazine. Some inhibit plant respiration. Some act as growth regulators, such as the phenoxy acids. Some inhibit protein or lipid synthesis or block enzymes.

Chlorophenoxy compounds include 2,4-D (2,4-dichlorophenoxyacetic acid) and 2,4,5-T. These chemicals mimic growth hormone, producing lethal overgrowth in plants. They work in dicotyledenous plants but not in monocots, such as grasses; therefore, these chemicals suppress broad-leaved weeds in lawns without harming grass. Chlorophenoxy compounds have been associated with soft tissue sarcomas in exposed forestry workers. Agent Orange—a mixture of the butyl esters of 2,4-D and 2,4,5-T contaminated with up to 50 µg/g of TCDD—caused adverse effects, such as birth defects and cancer, among those exposed.[51]

Bipyridyl herbicides include paraquat, a nonselective, fast-acting contact herbicide used for weed control. It is highly acutely toxic to humans but not genotoxic or carcinogenic. Inhalation of paraquat, during spraying or by smoking tobacco or marijuana sprayed with paraquat, causes lung toxicity. Paraquat has been implicated in many cases of acute human poisoning. It is irritating to, but not well absorbed through, the skin. It also damages dopaminergic neurons and can cause or accelerate Parkinson disease, especially in combination with exposure to maneb, which contains manganese—another cause of parkinsonism.[52,53]

Triazines include atrazine, a widely used herbicide. Triazines have low dermal and oral toxicity. Atrazine is not genotoxic, but it causes mammary tumors in rats. Because of its adverse effects, including developmental defects in frogs, it has been banned in some European countries. (See Chapter 16.)

Glyphosphate kills plants, but it has very low toxicity for animals. However, the International Agency for Research on Cancer has classified it as a Group 2A probable human carcinogen. This herbicide is widely used by homeowners in their gardens. A surfactant in a common formulation probably accounts for its irritant effects. Genetic engineering of crops to be resistant to glyphosphate allows this broad-spectrum herbicide to be used for weed control on farms.

Fungicides

Plant pathogens, such as viruses and fungi, are extremely difficult to control. Chemical fungicides are most effective when used prophylactically on plants, prior to infection by the fungal spores; however, some achieve cures after infestation, either on contact or systemically. They generally have low mammalian toxicity; however, some fungicides are genotoxic and contribute significantly to estimates of cancer risk from food residues. Fungicides are also used to treat wood and seeds to prevent mold growth. Methylmercury is a very effective fungicide, but it was banned after an outbreak of mercury poisoning in Iraq that was caused by ingestion of treated seed.[54]

Antineoplastic Drugs

Hospital employees involved in preparing and administering chemotherapy can be exposed to highly toxic drugs.[55] Antineoplastic drugs, which are cytotoxic,[56] can cause adverse effects, including adverse reproductive outcomes, especially fetal loss during the first trimester of pregnancy, in nurses who mix these drugs. Use of fluorescent tracers has illustrated substantial opportunity for exposure during mixing. As a result, most hospitals require that mixing of these drugs be done in the pharmacy, not on the ward.

THE PRECAUTIONARY PRINCIPLE FOR NEW CHEMICALS

In 1998, a consensus statement described the *precautionary principle* as follows: "When an activity raises threats of harm to human health or the environment, precautionary measures should be taken even if some cause and effect relationships are not fully established scientifically."[57] The statement then listed four central components of this principle: (a) taking preventive action in the face of uncertainty, (b) shifting the burden of proof to the proponents of an activity, (c) exploring a wide range of alternatives to possibly harmful actions, and (d) increasing public participation in decision-making.[58] Regulatory policy is a sluggish and reactive way to reduce worker and public exposure to toxic chemicals and is fraught with delays over uncertainty.[9] Precautionary approaches provide an opportunity to identify potential hazards and limit exposure before widespread exposure and harm has occurred.[58] The statement "further research is needed" should never become a euphemism for failure to act.[59]

ACKNOWLEDGMENT

Cases 1 through 4 were adapted from cases developed by James Melius, MD.

REFERENCES

1. Barceloux DG. Medical toxicology of natural substances. Hoboken, NJ: John Wiley & Sons, 2008.
2. Agency for Toxic Substances and Disease Registry. Toxicological profile for lead. Atlanta: ATSDR, 2007.
3. Jusko TA, Henderson CR, Lanphear BP, et al. Blood lead concentrations <10 microg/dL and child intelligence at 6 years of age. Environmental Health Perspectives 2008; 116: 243–248.
4. Grandjean P, Landrigan PJ. Neurobehavioural effects of developmental toxicity. Lancet Neurol. 2014; 13: 330–338.
5. Mazumdar M1, Bellinger DC, Gregas M, et al. Low-level environmental lead exposure in childhood and adult intellectual function: A follow-up study. Environmental Health 2011; 10: 24. doi:10.1186/1476-069X-10-24.
6. Landrigan PJ. Strategies for epidemiologic studies of lead in bone in occupationally exposed populations. Environmental Health Perspectives 1991; 91: 81–86.

7. Morrow L, Needleman HL, McFarland C, et al. Past occupational exposure to lead: Association between current blood lead and bone lead. Archives of Environmental and Occupational Health 2007; 62: 183–186.

8. Specht AJ, Lin Y, Weisskopf M, et al. XRF-measured bone lead (Pb) as a biomarker for Pb exposure and toxicity among children diagnosed with Pb poisoning. Biomarkers 2016; 21: 347–352.

9. Consumer Product Safety Commission. What you should know about lead based paint in your home: Safety alert (CPSC Document #5054). Available at: https://www.deq.state.ms.us/MDEQ.nsf/pdf/Air_CPSCDocumentNo5054/$File/CPSC%20Document%20No_5054.pdf? Accessed October 10, 2016.

10. Kovarik W. Ethyl-leaded gasoline: How a classic occupational disease became an international public health disaster. International Journal of Occupational and Environmental Health 2005; 11: 384–397.

11. Michaels D. Doubt is their product: How industry's assault on science threatens your health. New York: Oxford University Press, 2008.

12. Needleman HL, Gunnoe C, Leviton A, et al. Deficits in psychologic and classroom performance of children with elevated dentine lead levels. New England Journal of Medicine 1979; 300: 689–695.

13. Needleman H. Low level lead exposure: History and discovery. Annals of Epidemiology 2009; 19: 235–238.

14. Czachur M, Stanbury M, Gerwel B, et al. A pilot study of take-home lead exposure in New Jersey. American Journal of Industrial Medicine 1995; 28: 289–293.

15. U.S. Department of Labor. States with adult blood lead level registries. Available at: http://www.osha.gov/SLTC/bloodlead/state.html. Accessed October 10, 2016.

16. Schwartz BS, Hu H. 2007. Mini-monograph: Adult lead exposure: Time for change. Environmental Health Perspectives 2007; 115: 451–454.

17. Karita K, Nakao M, Ohwaki K, et al. Blood lead and erythrocyte protoporphyrin levels in association with smoking and personal hygienic behaviour among lead exposed workers. Occupational and Environmental Medicine 2005; 62: 300–303.

18. Genaidy AM, Sequeira R, Tolaymat T, et al. An exploratory study of lead recovery in lead-acid battery lifecycle in U.S. market: An evidence-based approach. Science of the Total Environment 2008; 407: 7–22.

19. Weisel C, Demak M, Marcus S, Goldstein BD. Soft plastic bread packaging: Lead content and reuse by families. American Journal of Public Health 1991; 81: 756–758.

20. Environmental Protection Agency. Integrated exposure uptake biokinetic model for lead in children. Available at: https://www.epa.gov/superfund/lead-superfund-sites-frequent-questions-risk-assessors-integrated-exposure-uptake. Accessed October 10, 2016.

21. Cory-Slechta DA, Weiss B, Cox C. Mobilization and redistribution of lead over the course of calcium disodium ethylenediamine tetraacetate chelation therapy. Journal Pharmacology and Experimental Therapeutics 1987; 243: 804–813.

22. Liu X, Dietrich KN, Radcliffe J, et al. Do children with falling blood lead levels have improved cognition? Pediatrics 2002; 110: 787 791.

23. Goldwater L. Mercury: A history of quicksilver. Baltimore: York Press, 1972.

24. Hightower J. Diagnosis: Mercury: Money, politics, and poison (2nd ed.). Washington, DC: Island Press, 2008.

25. Haas NS, Shih R, Gochfeld M. A patient with postoperative mercury contamination of the peritoneum. Journal of Toxicology: Clinical Toxicology 2003; 41: 175–180.

26. American Dental Association. ADA positions & statements: ADA Statement on Dental Amalgam. Available at: http://www.ada.org/en/press-room/press-kits/dental-fillings-press-kit. Accessed October 10, 2016.

27. Riley DM, Newby CA, Leal-Almeraz TO. Incorporating ethnographic methods in multidisciplinary approaches to risk assessment and communication: Cultural and religious uses of mercury in Latino and Caribbean communities. Risk Analysis 2006; 26: 1205–1221.

28. Swiderski RM. Calomel: A drug in America. Boca Raton, FL: Universal Publishers, 2008.

29. Maruyama K, Yorifuji T, Tsuda T, et al. Methyl mercury exposure at Niigata, Japan: Results of neurological examinations of 103 adults. Journal of Biomedicine and Biotechnology 2012; 2012: 635075.

30. Gochfeld M, Burger J. Good fish/bad fish: A composite benefit-risk by dose curve. Neurotoxicology 2005; 26: 511–520.

31. Groth E 3rd. Fish consumption and blood mercury levels. Environmental Health Perspectives 2014; 122: A120.

32. Siegler RW, Nierenberg DW, Hickey WF. Fatal poisoning from liquid dimethylmercury: A neuropathologic study. Human Pathology 1999; 30:720–723.

33. United Nations Environmental Program. Minamata Convention on Mercury. 2013. Available at: http://www.mercuryconvention.org/ Convention. Accessed October 11, 2016.

34. Barregard L, Bergström G, Fagerberg B. Cadmium, type 2 diabetes, and kidney damage in a cohort of middle-aged women. Environmental Research 2014; 135: 311–316.

35. Collins JJ, Jammer B, Sladeczek FM, et al. Surveillance for angiosarcoma of the liver among vinyl chloride workers. Journal of Occupational and Environmental Medicine 2014; 56: 1207–1209.

36. Randall WS, Solomon SD. Building 6: The tragedy at Bridesburg. Boston: Little Brown, 1977.

37. International Agency for Research on Cancer. Formaldehyde, 2-butoxyethanol and 1-*tert*-butoxypropan-2-ol: Summary of data reported and evaluation. (Volume 88). Available at: http:// monographs.iarc.fr/ENG/Monographs/vol88/. Accessed October 10, 2016.

38. C8 Science Panel. The Science Panel website. Available at: http://www.c8sciencepanel.org. Accessed January 6, 2017.

39. Peakall DB. Pesticide-induced enzyme breakdown of steroids in birds. Nature 1967; 216: 505–506.

40. Colborn T, Myers JP. Our stolen future: Are we threatening our fertility, intelligence, and survival?—A scientific detective story. New York: Penguin Books, 1997.

41. Klip H, Verloop J, van Gool JD, et al. Hypospadias in sons of women exposed to diethylstilbestrol *in utero*: A cohort study. Lancet 2002; 359: 1102–1107.

42. Ormond G, Nieuwenhuijsen MJ, Nelson P, et al. Endocrine disruptors in the workplace, hair spray, folate supplementation, and risk of hypospadias: Case–control study. Environmental Health Perspectives 2009; 117: 303–307.

43. Agency for Toxic Substances and Disease Registry. Toxicological profile for polycyclic aromatic hydrocarbons. Atlanta: ATSDR, 2007.

44. Jacobson JL, Jacobson SW. Prenatal exposure to polychlorinated biphenyls and attention at school age. Journal of Pediatrics 2003; 143: 780–788.

45. Kahn PC, Gochfeld M, Nygren M, et al. Dioxins and dibenzofurans in blood and adipose tissue of Agent Orange-exposed Vietnam veterans and matched controls. Journal of the American Medical Association 1988; 259: 1661–1667.

46. Costa LG. Toxic effects of pesticides. In: Klaassen CD (ed.). Casarett & Doull's toxicology: The basic science of poisons (8th ed.). New York: McGraw Hill, 2013.

47. Cone JE, Wugofski L, Balmes JR, et al. Persistent respiratory health effects after a metam sodium pesticide spill. Chest 1994; 106: 500–508.

48. Hogstedt C, Aringer L, Gustavsson A. Epidemiologic support for ethylene oxide as a cancer-causing agent. Journal of the American Medical Association 1986; 255: 1575–1578.

49. Richardson J, Shalat S, Buckley B, et al. Elevated serum pesticide levels and the risk of Parkinson's disease. Archives of Neurology 2009; 66: 870–875.

50. Dhillon AS, Tarbutton GL, Levin JL, et al. Pesticide/environmental exposures and Parkinson's disease in East Texas. Journal of Agromedicine 2008; 13: 37–48.

51. Institute of Medicine. Veterans and Agent Orange: Update-2006. Washington, DC: IOM, 2006.

52. Rudyk C, Litteljohn D, Syed S, et al. Paraquat and psychological stressor interactions as pertains to Parkinsonian co-morbidity. Neurobiology of Stress 2015; 12: 85–93.

53. Costello S, Cockburn M, Bronstein J, et al. Parkinson's disease and residential exposure to maneb and paraquat from agricultural applications in the central valley of California. American Journal of Epidemiology 2009; 169: 919–926.

54. Bakir F, Damluji SF, Amin-Zaki L, et al. Methylmercury poisoning in Iraq. Science 1973; 181: 230–241.

55. McDevitt JJ, Lees PS, McDiarmid MA. Exposure of hospital pharmacists and nurses to antineoplastic agents. Journal of Occupational Medicine 1993; 35: 57–60.

56. Selevan SG, Lindbohm M-L, Hornung RW, Hemminki K. A study of occupational exposure to antineoplastic drugs and fetal loss in nurses. New England Journal of Medicine 1985; 313: 1173–1178.

57. Raffensperger C, Tickner J (eds.). Protecting public health and the environment: Implementing the precautionary principle. Washington, DC: Island Press, 1999.

58. Grandjean P, Bailar JC, Gee D, et al. Implications of the precautionary principle in research and policy-making. American Journal of Industrial Medicine 2004; 45: 382–385.

59. Gochfeld M. Why epidemiology of endocrine disruptors warrants the precautionary principle. Pure and Applied Chemistry 2003; 75: 2521–2529.

FURTHER READING

Brooks, S, Gochfeld M, Herzstein J, et al.
Environmental medicine. St. Louis,
MO: Mosby, 1995.
*A general textbook that has useful chapters on
chemical hazards.*

Bruckner JV, Anand SS, Warren DA. Toxic effects
of solvents and vapors. In: Klaasen CD (ed.).
Casarett & Doull's toxicology: The basic science
of poisons. New York: McGraw Hill Education,
2013, pp. 1031–1112.
*A summary of toxicity of solvents and other
volatile substances.*

Kendall RJ, Lacher Tem, Cobb GC, Cox SB. Wildlife
toxicology: Emerging contaminant and biodiversity
issues. Boca Raton, FL: CRC Press, 2010.
*Exposure, toxicology, and ecological effects of
chemicals on wildlife and ecosystems.*

Klaassen CD. Casarett & Doull's toxicology: The basic
science of poisons (8th ed.). New York: McGraw
Hill Education, 2013.
The best-known textbook of toxicology.

Nordberg GF, Fowler BA, Nordberg M, Friberg LT.
Handbook of the toxicology of metals (3rd ed.).
Amsterdam: Elsevier, 2007.
A valuable resource on the toxicology of metals.

Mendelsohn ML, Mohr LC, Peeters JP. Biomarkers:
medical and workplace applications.
Washington, DC: Joseph Henry Press, 1998.
*A useful book on biomarkers including
biomedical, epidemiologic, and ethical
principles.*

National Resource Council. Pesticides in the diets
of infants and children. Washington, DC:
National Academy Press, 1993. Available
at: http://books.nap.edu/openbook.php?record_
id=2126&page=13.
A valuable publication on childhood exposure.

Ramazzini B. [De Morbis Artificum Diatriba].
1713. Translated from the Latin by W.
C. Wright. New York: Hafner Publishing
Company, 1964.
*A book of historical significance written by the
founder of occupational medicine.*

12A

Noise Exposure and Hearing Disorders

David C. Byrne and Thais C. Morata

Exposure to unwanted sounds, or noise, is a common on-the-job occurrence. An unfortunate consequence is work-related hearing loss, a condition that has been one of the most prevalent occupational health concerns in the United States for many years.[1] Hearing loss can be a seriously disabling condition due to the integral role of hearing in human communication. Hearing-impaired individuals often avoid situations in which communication is difficult, rather than risking a misunderstanding and potentially embarrassing mistakes. This tendency leads to isolation, difficulties at work, and possibly adverse psychological consequences. The following scenarios illustrate difficulties associated with noise-induced hearing loss (NIHL):

- Going to restaurants, parties, or other social gatherings becomes a chore, since background noise or music makes conversation difficult, if not impossible.
- Watching television requires the volume to be set very loud, making it irritating or annoying for others to be in the same room.
- Working in noisy environments can make communication difficult and increase the risk of workplace injuries due to an inability

to hear environmental sounds and warning signals.
- Dealing with tinnitus (the perception of sound in the absence of external acoustic stimuli) becomes an unexpected consequence for some, who expected a hearing loss to result in silence, not an ever-present ringing in their ears.

Greater awareness and improved noise-control strategies are needed for the prevention of these hearing disorders.

PROPERTIES OF SOUND

Sound results from oscillations in pressure in any "elastic" medium. When transmitted through air, sound is usually described in terms of variations in pressure that alternate above and below the ambient atmospheric pressure. The characteristics of a particular sound depend on the rate at which the sound source vibrates, the amplitude of the vibration, and the properties of the conducting medium. Frequency is an objective description of the rate at which complete cycles of high- and low-pressure regions are produced by a sound source, and it is measured in hertz (Hz). Subjectively, frequency is often referred to as "pitch," although there is not an exact correlation between the two terms. Normal human ears respond to a very wide frequency range, from approximately 20 to 20,000 Hz.

A normal healthy human ear is also capable of detecting a remarkable range of sound levels. When the term *level* is used in acoustics, decibel notation is implied. By definition, the decibel (dB) is a dimensionless unit, related to the logarithm of the ratio of a measured quantity to a reference quantity. Decibel notation can cause confusion because it is often associated with different reference quantities. Acoustic intensity, acoustic power, hearing thresholds, electric voltage, electric current, electric power, and sound pressure level may all be expressed in decibels, each having a different reference. The decibel has no meaning unless a reference quantity is specified or the reference quantity is understood from the context in which it is being used. Sound pressure levels as high as those produced by jet engines (120 dB or greater) are found in some work areas, whereas sound levels approaching the threshold of hearing (approximately 0 dB) are used for audiometric testing.

ASSESSMENT OF NOISE EXPOSURE

The terms *noise* and *sound* are often used interchangeably; however, sound is normally used to describe useful communication or pleasant audible signals, whereas noise is typically considered as unpleasant or unwanted sound. Four major factors contribute to the occurrence of negative noise effects: (a) the overall noise level, (b) the frequency content, (c) the duration of exposure, and (d) the susceptibility of the individual.

There is a wide variety of measurement instrumentation for conducting noise-exposure assessments. A basic sound-level meter consists of a microphone that converts air pressure variations into an electrical signal, an amplifier/filter, an exponential time-averaging circuit, a device to determine the logarithm of the signal, and some type of output display. Some sound-level meters provide only the basic functions, while others are equipped with a very wide range of features, such as integration capability for determination of noise dose and measurement of impulse noise.

General-purpose sound-level meters are normally equipped with two filters or frequency-weighting networks, designated by the letters A and C. Other frequency-weighting networks, such as B and D, have been developed, but they are not used for industrial noise measurements. Most sound-level meters also will have a linear or flat response setting, which does not apply any correction values—that is, it weights all frequencies equally. The particular weighting network used must always be indicated when sound-level readings are obtained. The A, B, and C weighting curves approximate the human ear's perception of loudness at low, medium, and high sound levels, and, in the earliest sound-level meters, they could be easily produced with a few common electronic components. Empirically, the A-weighting has been found to give a good estimation of the risk potential for hearing damage from exposure to continuous noise. It is the weighting network used for measurements of occupational noise exposure, which are expressed as dBA.

A noise dosimeter consists of a miniature microphone connected to a small microprocessor-based sound-level meter, which stores the noise data. The microphone is positioned at the top of a worker's shoulder, and the sound-level meter hardware unit is clipped to the wearer's belt or placed in a pocket. Noise dosimeters continuously measure sound levels obtained near a worker's ear, then provide an average value for the exposure accumulated throughout an individual's workday. A dosimeter is essentially identical to any other sound-level meter, with the addition of an integrating function that keeps track of the noise level as well as the total exposure time. Dosimeters make it convenient to measure and assess a person's noise exposures by eliminating the need for the surveyor to follow a worker throughout the workday with a sound-level meter and a stopwatch to assess the worker's exact amount of exposure to different noise levels. Many instruments can continuously log or store noise exposure levels at 1-minute, 10-second, or 1-second intervals. This noise exposure history information can be saved and analyzed in many ways to help pinpoint periods of high noise levels or other significant occurrences during a work shift.

A worker's daily noise dose can be expressed as a percentage, with 100% constituting the limit of acceptable exposure. A noise dose is usually converted into an 8-hour time-weighted average (TWA). A TWA is a single value for noise level obtained by averaging all of the different sound levels that a worker is exposed to during the workday and normalizing that average to 8 hours. The TWA represents that constant noise level in dBA that has the same severity over 8 hours as the exposure to the actual noise in a workday.

Substantial interest and progress has been made in the development of smartphone apps to measure sound pressure level; some of these have been tested and shown to be quite accurate.[2,3] Apps for taking noise measurements in the work setting have been developed, and more will be available in the future.[4] This technology has the potential not only to raise the awareness of noise exposure but also to inform decisions concerning hearing protection.

NOISE-INDUCED HEARING LOSS

The Bureau of Labor Statistics has identified NIHL as one of the leading work-related conditions.[1] The reported prevalence of work-related hearing loss varies considerably among occupational groups.[5] With 10 or more years of noise exposure, it is estimated that 8% of the workers exposed to 85 dBA, 22% of the workers exposed to 90 dBA, 38% of the workers exposed to 95 dBA, and 44% of those exposed to 100 dBA will develop hearing impairment.[6] Noise-induced hearing loss is among the most common causes of acquired hearing loss. The National Institutes of Health estimates that approximately one-third of all hearing loss can be attributed, at least in part, to noise exposure.[7]

Noise-induced hearing loss is a specific condition with established symptoms and objective findings. The following features characterize cases of NIHL:

- Irreversible sensorineural (nerve-type) hearing loss that cannot be corrected by conventional medical or surgical procedures

- A history of long-term exposure to continuous noise levels greater than 85 dBA for 8 hours a day, or exposure to impact/impulse noise with peaks over 140 dB
- Hearing loss that has developed gradually over a period of years, most rapidly during the first 6 to 10 years of exposure—with the rate of loss decreasing as hearing thresholds increase
- Reduced hearing sensitivity in the high frequencies (difficulty hearing high-pitched sounds), with most affected persons showing a loss or "notch" in sensitivity at 4,000 Hz (If high-level noise exposures continue, the loss of hearing generally spreads to adjacent frequencies above and below 4,000 Hz.)
- An initial hearing loss that may be temporary, after which the original hearing sensitivity is usually restored within a matter of hours (However, in some cases temporary losses may last for days or weeks. Permanent losses result when these temporary losses do not recover completely.)
- Reduced ability to recognize words that is consistent with the degree of high-frequency hearing loss.

Hearing loss resulting from hazardous long-term exposure to noise progresses in a fairly well-established, recognizable pattern. Noise-induced hearing loss at the frequencies maximally affected (4,000 and 6,000 Hz) shows a rapid increase over the first 10 years of exposure; the development of the hearing loss then slows and tends to plateau. Hearing loss at frequencies below 4,000 Hz develops at a slower rate but gradually worsens if the exposure continues.

Noise-induced hearing loss has a gradual onset, and the affected individual might be unaware of any change until significant damage has occurred. Remedial behaviors, such as turning up the radio or television volume or blaming others for not speaking clearly, may conceal initial hearing difficulties. Affected people may be unaware of any hearing problem even when their hearing tests indicate decreased hearing ability. In some cases, damage may occur instantaneously, depending upon the noise characteristics and exposure circumstances. These cases are usually referred to as *acoustic trauma*. Generally, impulsive or impact noises are most likely to produce significant losses within short exposure periods, and steady-state continuous noises are responsible for impairments that develop over a long period of time.

Traditionally the mechanism underlying NIHL has been explained as physical trauma causing damage to the cochlea, which contains hair cells responsible for transforming the sound waves into neural signals that are transmitted to the auditory nerve and ultimately to the brain (Figure 12A-1). Hair cells are attached to the basilar membrane, and the stereocilia are in contact with the tectorial membrane (Figure 12A-2). Sound waves lead the basilar membrane to vibrate up and down. The vibration creates a shearing force between the basilar membrane and the tectorial membrane, causing the hair-cell stereocilia to bend back and forth. This leads to internal changes within the hair cells that create electrical signals. Auditory nerve fibers rest below the hair cells

and pass these signals on to the brain. Therefore, hair cells respond to sounds by bending of the stereocilia.[8,9]

The most common morphological finding in NIHL is degeneration of the hair cells (mainly the outer rows), which are thought to be the most vulnerable structures of the organ of Corti. The damage of inner hair cells and especially outer hair cells is described as a disarrangement of hairs, fusion of stereocilia, formation of giant hairs that exceed the normal stereocilia in length and thickness, and deformation of cuticular plates (Figure 12A-3). The loss of the outer hair cells induces retrograde degeneration of the efferent fibers, but it has little effect on the afferent cochlear neurons. Therefore, if there were damage to the outer hair cells alone, the lesion would be less obvious—because only rather extensive damage to the inner hair cells causes substantial degeneration of the afferent nerve fibers.

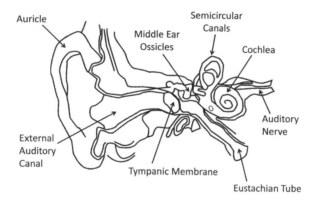

Figure 12A-1. Schematic drawing of the hearing mechanism.

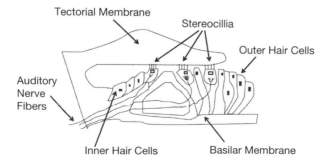

Figure 12A-2. Close-up drawing of the Organ of Corti in the cochlea.

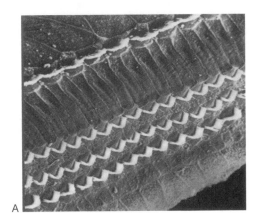 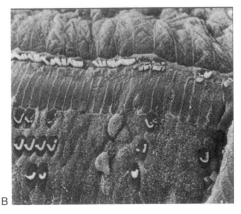

Figure 12A-3. Electron micrographs of (A) normal and (B) damaged inner ear hair cells.

Metabolic processes involving oxidative stress have been shown to contribute to NIHL. The generation of reactive oxygen species, or free radicals, has been associated with cellular injury in different organ systems. Free radicals produce cell damage by binding to macromolecules and producing lipid peroxidation—a basic mechanism of toxicity that is thought to be part of the mechanism of acquired hearing loss. Medical treatments, such as antioxidants, are being sought to prevent or minimize hair cell damage.

Hidden hearing loss, also known as *cochlear synaptopathy*, describes functional hearing impairment in individuals with normal behavioral audiometric thresholds. Normal results on routine testing of hearing acuity (on an audiogram) are possible, despite physical damage to connections between auditory nerve fibers and sensory cells. It is likely responsible for decreases in speech recognition ability, especially in noisy or difficult listening situations. Therefore, noise exposures that were traditionally considered to be safe (because they did not produce a permanent threshold shift) may not be safe at all.[10]

OTHER EFFECTS OF NOISE EXPOSURE

Exposure to excessive levels of noise is not restricted to the work environment, and the effects of noise exposure are not restricted solely to decreased hearing. Noise from power tools, powered lawn maintenance equipment, farm equipment, and shooting hobbies (such as skeet, targets, and hunting) or other recreational activities, such as attending music concerts, riding in motorboats, and watching automobile or motorcycle races, are examples of potentially hazardous nonoccupational sources of noise. In addition, excessive noise exposure is associated with hypertension, ischemic heart disease, respiratory disorders, annoyance, sleep disturbance, and decreased school performance. Noise can also disrupt communication. Some studies have suggested an association between accidents and both occupational noise exposure and hearing loss.[11,12]

THE IMPACT OF HEARING DISORDERS

Consequences of hearing disorders range from slight to seriously debilitating. At work, a hearing loss can increase difficulties associated with the use of hearing protectors, causing interference with verbal communication and detection of warning signals. In addition, the earnings of workers with severe hearing loss are estimated to be 50% to 70% of those than their peers without hearing impairment.[13]

One way to measure the impact or burden of health conditions is to calculate disability-adjusted life years (DALYs), the number of healthy years lost due to a disease or other health condition. For a condition like hearing loss, the DALYs calculation takes into account life limitations caused by hearing loss as a lost portion of a healthy year of life. It is an approach that can be used to quantify the impact of hearing loss on critical intangibles, such as communication and mental health. The National Institute for

Occupational Safety and Health (NIOSH) used DALYs to estimate the impact of hearing loss on quality of life by estimating the number of healthy years lost for every 1,000 workers each year by industrial sector.[5] It found that 2.5 healthy years were lost annually for every 1,000 noise-exposed U.S. workers due to hearing impairment (hearing loss that impacts daily activities). These lost years were shared among the 13% of workers with hearing impairment (130 out of every 1,000 workers). Workers in three industry sectors had the highest annual rate of healthy years lost (per 1,000 full-time workers): mining, 3.5; construction, 3.1; and manufacturing, 2.7.

However, hearing loss can have a severe impact on social interaction and family life that is difficult to quantify with precision. Hearing disabilities may have a negative effect on self-image, causing a perception of oneself as abnormal, prematurely old, or as a burden because affected individuals often ask others to repeat what they say. There are several barriers to seeking help and using hearing aids, including cost, pride, denial of a problem, and the stigma attached to deafness. People with hearing difficulties will often try to downplay or conceal its seriousness to minimize the risk of being marginalized, and they may avoid seeking help. People with untreated hearing loss are more likely to report depression and anxiety, and they are less likely to participate in social activities compared to those who wear hearing aids.[14] Unfortunately, less than 20% of the estimated 28 million U.S. residents who could benefit from hearing devices own them, and less than 20% of physicians include hearing testing in routine physical examinations.[15]

INFLUENCE OF OTHER FACTORS ON HEARING LOSS

The incidence and degree of hearing loss vary greatly among groups, partly due to endogenous factors or individual attributes that affect susceptibility, including age, gender, race, blood pressure, and use of certain medications. There is, however, limited knowledge about how noise impairment is influenced by, or interacts with, age-related hearing impairment. The effects of noise and age are challenging to differentiate, but they seem to be additive. Hearing acuity may decline with aging, but a healthy person who has not been exposed to ototraumatic or ototoxic agents may have normal hearing acuity even after age 65. The median hearing level (HL) across the frequencies of 1,000, 2,000, 3,000, and 4,000 Hz for 60-year-olds not exposed to noise is 17 dB HL for males and 12 dB HL for females.[16] Gender and race seem also to be associated with susceptibility to NIHL. White males have the highest rates of NIHL and African-American females the lowest.

Certain nonacoustic factors in the workplace, which may directly affect hearing or interact with noise, are considered possible contributors to variability in individual susceptibility to NIHL.[17] For example, workers with vibration-induced white finger syndrome have a higher rate of hearing loss than workers exposed to similar noise levels but not to vibration.[18] It is not known if whole-body vibration enhances risk for hearing loss. (See Chapter 12B.)

Some chemicals have ototoxic properties that can harm hearing and can also enhance the effects of noise. These include some metals, solvents, polychlorinated biphenyls (PCBs), pesticides, and asphyxiants (such as carbon monoxide).[19] This effect can be observed by the higher rates of hearing loss among groups exposed to chemicals or by the difference in the type of auditory function that is affected, such as a decreased ability to understand speech, especially in the presence of background noise. Some aromatic solvents reduce the protective role played by the middle-ear acoustic reflex.[20] A dysfunction of this reflex increases risks to hearing by allowing higher acoustic energy levels to penetrate the inner ear. The European Agency for Safety and Health at Work and the Nordic Expert Group have published comprehensive evaluations of ototoxic substances and have documented (a) disorders associated with workplace exposure to noise and ototoxic chemical substances, including qualitative information on noise–chemical interactions and (b) key policies from specific countries and multinational agencies.[21,22]

TINNITUS

Tinnitus is a condition often associated with many forms of hearing loss. It is usually described as "ringing in the ears," but other forms of sound have been reported, such as buzzing, pulsing, hissing, knocking, roaring, whooshing, chirping, whistling, and clicking. Tinnitus can be continuous or intermittent—lasting for minutes to a few hours at a time. It can be a minor annoyance or a serious and nearly intolerable condition. In severe cases, it may interfere with daily activities and sleep. Tinnitus is associated with noise exposure frequently and also with more than 200 medications as well as dietary, nutritional, hormonal, immunological, and stress factors.

Although the reported prevalence of work-related tinnitus ranges from 17% to 60% of cases among noise-exposed workers,[23,24] it has attracted relatively little interest. For example, only 13 U.S. states and a few countries (such as the United Kingdom, Canada, Australia, Germany, Denmark, and Sweden) provide workers' compensation for tinnitus.[24]

There are probably several mechanisms that cause tinnitus. It is often associated with an increase in the spontaneous neural activity in the auditory system. The first relay of the primary auditory pathway is in the cochlear nuclei in the brainstem, which tend to develop hyperactivity that might be relayed to higher levels in the brain. Alternatively, heightened activity of some descending pathway or other central mechanism might explain this hyperactivity.

GOVERNMENTAL REGULATIONS

Federal, state, and local governments set and enforce noise standards for aircraft, airports, interstate motor carriers, railroads, medium- and heavy-duty trucks, motorcycles, mopeds, and many commercial, industrial, and residential activities.

The Environmental Protection Agency (EPA) coordinated all federal noise-control activities until 1983. Most of the responsibility for regulating noise was then transferred to state and local governments. Although the EPA no longer plays a prominent role in regulating noise, its standards (regulations) are enforced by state and local governments, and federal agencies other than EPA continue to set and enforce noise standards for sources within their regulatory jurisdiction.

Workers in general industry who are exposed to noise levels above 85 dBA are required by the Occupational Safety and Health Administration (OSHA) to be in a hearing conservation program, which includes noise measurement, noise control, periodic audiometric testing, hearing protection, worker education, and recordkeeping.[25] Twenty-four states, Puerto Rico, and the U.S. Virgin Islands have OSHA-approved state plans and have adopted their own standards and enforcement policies. Most of these state standards are identical to those of federal OSHA. However, some states have adopted different standards or may have different enforcement policies. Most health and safety regulations are designed to keep damage risk within "acceptable limits"—that is, some people are likely to incur a hearing loss even when exposed to less than the maximum daily amount of noise specified in a regulation.

In the construction industry, noise exposures are required to be evaluated and controlled, and hearing protectors must be offered when exposures exceed 85 dBA. Apart from exposure limits, there is no mandatory hearing conservation program for construction workers. However, construction workers may choose to follow the criteria outlined in *Hearing Loss Prevention for Construction and Demolition Workers*, developed by the American National Standards Institute. These criteria, which help employers prevent occupational hearing loss among construction and demolition workers with potential exposures to continuous, intermittent, or impulse noise of 85 dBA and or higher, was approved by the American National Standards Institute and is available from the American Society of Safety Engineers.

The Federal Railroad Administration has issued a final rule, titled "Occupational Noise Exposure for Railroad Operating Employees," which requires railroads to conduct noise monitoring and implement a hearing conservation program for employees whose exposure to cab noise equals or exceeds an 8-hour TWA of 85 dBA. There is no hearing-loss prevention regulation for workers in agriculture, despite their high prevalence of hearing loss, or for workers in the service and public sectors.

Separate from the Occupational Noise Exposure Standard, OSHA's recordkeeping rule, when first implemented, significantly altered the criteria for documenting what constitutes a reportable hearing threshold shift. Work-related hearing loss in either ear is recordable when both of the following occur:

1. An average shift in hearing threshold of 10 dB or greater at 2,000, 3,000, and 4,000 Hz, relative to the audiometric baseline (called a *standard threshold shift*, or STS)
2. The average hearing level in the same ear is 25 dB or greater at 2,000, 3,000, and 4,000 Hz.

After the recording criteria were revised in 2004, it was anticipated that the number of recordable hearing loss cases would increase in most states,[26] possibly leading to improvements in hearing conservation and noise-control programs. From 2004 through 2010, rates of recordable hearing shifts reported to the Bureau of Labor Statistics declined in some industrial sectors but remained high (over 20 cases per 10,000) in subsectors such as primary metal manufacturing, air transportation, and food manufacturing.

NIOSH has established formal partnerships with audiometric service providers, occupational health clinics, hospitals, and others who conduct worker audiometric testing in order to collect audiometric data from a broad spectrum of sectors. These data have been analyzed to provide estimates of prevalence and describe trends for hearing loss by sector.[27] In general, the rates of hearing loss were found to range from about 11% to 25% of workers in various industries. The construction, mining, and manufacturing sectors have prevalence rates above 20%, suggesting that these sectors merit the attention given to them. Other industrial sectors, however, also have high rates; for example, the services sector has a prevalence of 20% and the public safety sector, which includes law enforcement, has unique exposures due to the need to maintain firearm skills. Law enforcement workers, more than 1 million of whom are at risk for hearing loss, are not covered by OSHA noise regulations, and their employers rarely intervene to protect their hearing.[28]

BEYOND COMPLIANCE: PREVENTING OCCUPATIONAL HEARING LOSS

Recommendations for measures to prevent hearing loss and the rationale for them can be found in two NIOSH publications: *Criteria for a Recommended Standard: Occupational Exposure to Noise (Revised Criteria)* and *Preventing Occupational Hearing Loss: A Practical Guide*.[29,30]

Initial steps of hearing-loss prevention programs are hazard assessment and control. Required noise measurements serve as the basis for assessing noise control alternatives. If employees' daily noise exposures are controlled to levels below a TWA of 85 dBA, a hearing conservation program is not legally required.

Exposure at the NIOSH recommended exposure limit (REL) for occupational noise (85 dBA TWA)[29] for 40 years increases the risk of NIHL by 8%—considerably lower than the 25% increased risk at the current permissible exposure limit (PEL) of OSHA and the Mine Safety and Health Administration (MSHA) (90 dBA TWA).

NIOSH previously recommended a 5 dB exchange rate for halving the exposure time when calculating TWAs—that is, starting at the 85 dBA REL for an 8-hour period, for each 5 dB increase in exposure, the permissible exposure time was to be halved. However, since 1998, NIOSH has recommended a 3 dB exchange rate, which is more firmly supported by scientific evidence.[29] The 5 dB exchange rate is still used by OSHA and MSHA.

Whenever there is hazardous noise in a workplace, measures should be taken to reduce noise levels as much as possible to protect exposed workers. The most effective way to prevent NIHL is to remove the noise source from the workplace, such as by engineering controls, or to remove the worker from exposure to hazardous noise.[31]

Noise Controls

When noise can be reduced or eliminated through engineering controls, the risk of hearing loss is also reduced or eliminated. Therefore, engineering controls should be the first priority for protecting workers from excessive noise exposure.[25] Any reduction in noise level—even if it is only a few decibels—serves to make the noise hazard more manageable, reduces the risk of hearing loss, improves communication, and lowers annoyance and related extra-auditory problems associated with high noise levels.[30]

The first step in a noise control program is to accurately define the problem and determine its extent, by answering questions such as "How many and which employees are affected?"

and "How much noise reduction is required?" After identifying a noise problem, its source(s) or "root cause" should be identified. Noise may be produced by mechanical impacts, vibrating surfaces, exhaust gases, rotating machinery, and other factors. There may be hundreds of potential noise-generating mechanisms within a relatively small space in a workplace. It may be difficult to determine all of the sources. The services of an acoustical consultant or noise control engineer may be helpful; however, many noise problems can be solved by individuals without extensive acoustical training by systematically tracking down the noise sources, such as by turning various pieces of equipment (or individual components) on and off, and/or by using temporary controls and observing their effects.

In controlling noise, one should prioritize engineering control measures. Installing a noise-control device on a specific piece of equipment simply because it is easy or relatively inexpensive may be ineffective because the device might not affect the overall noise level, depending on what else in the immediate area is also generating noise. One should consider the relative contribution of each noise source to the overall sound level.

Typical mechanisms for engineering control measures include reducing noise at the source, such as by installing a silencer or muffler; altering the noise path, such as by building an acoustic enclosure or barrier; reducing reverberation, such as by covering walls with sound-absorbing materials; and reducing equipment vibration, such as by installing vibration mounts or damping treatment. Trade journals and other publications, such as *Sound and Vibration*, periodically publish lists of manufacturers of available noise control materials.[32]

Successful noise control measures may not require purchasing and installing "acoustical" materials or products. A thorough equipment maintenance inspection should be done first to identify machinery needing adjustment, alignment, or repair. Restoring equipment to its optimal performance condition should be completed before investing in any noise control devices. It may be necessary to periodically inspect and/or replace existing noise control devices, because items such as pneumatic silencers will eventually become plugged and be rendered ineffective. Wherever possible, other maintenance-related controls should

be investigated. Even simple measures such as tightly closing access doors and panels will keep noise from "leaking out."

Engineering controls can be most effective when they are incorporated into the initial design of facilities and equipment. Similarly, the cost of including engineering controls during the design phase is generally much lower than retrofitting them later. Installing noisy equipment, such as motors, pumps, and fans, in unoccupied areas of a workplace, such as a rooftop or warehouse area, can greatly reduce workers' exposure to noise. Managers should adopt a "buy-quiet" policy for acquiring new equipment. An effective buy-quiet program includes selecting products or operations to be targeted for noise reduction through new purchases, setting criteria for new equipment noise levels, requesting noise-level specifications from manufacturers, and including these noise-level data in evaluation of bids. The ultimate goal is to encourage manufacturers to design quieter tools and equipment by creating a demand for quieter products.

When engineering control measures are inadequate, supplemental administrative controls may be used to help limit noise exposure. Administrative controls are defined as changes in the work schedule or operations that reduce worker noise exposures. For example, sometimes workers can be scheduled so that their time in a noisy environment is reduced. When extremely noisy operations are unavoidable, the number of workers permitted to work in such an environment should be minimized. In any situation, the application of administrative controls should not result in exposing more workers to noise. A quiet and conveniently located break area should be provided to give workers periodic relief from workplace noise.

Hearing Protection Devices

Hearing protection devices (HPDs) can be very effective against hazardous noise levels; however, in order to achieve the desired attenuation, workers must wear them consistently during exposure to noise levels greater than 85 dBA. Workers often find it difficult to do so because HPDs can be uncomfortable and interfere with communication. Consequently, use of HPDs is inconsistent and varies widely (Figure 12A-4). They are usually purchased

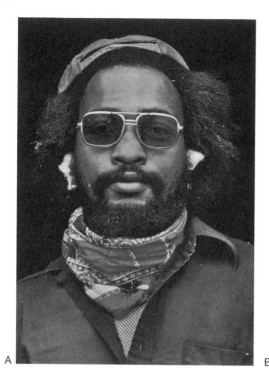
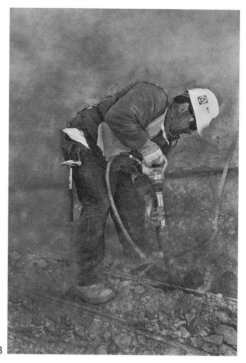

A   B

Figure 12A-4. Improper and proper hearing protection: (A) Cotton earplugs are ineffective in protecting a worker from loud noise. (B) This jackhammer operator is appropriately wearing earplugs. (Photographs by Earl Dotter.)

on the basis of minimum cost and maximum attenuation, often leading to use of uncomfortable devices that overprotect. New electronic HPDs are available that not only protect at appropriate levels but also facilitate communication. Recommendations to increase the use of HPDs include identifying devices that offer adequate attenuation and provide workers with better comfort.

The original rating system developed by the EPA to measure HPD attenuation is recognized as obsolete. Laboratory-derived attenuation values have been shown to fail to predict how HPDs function in the workplace. Therefore, OSHA has instructed its compliance officers to derate the labeled noise-reduction rating (NRR) of HPDs by 50% when enforcing the OSHA Occupational Noise Exposure Standard. NIOSH recommends derating by subtracting a percentage from the NRR: 25% for earmuffs, 50% for formable earplugs, and 70% for all other earplugs. This *variable* derating scheme, in contrast to OSHA's *fixed* derating scheme, distinguishes among the performance of different types of HPDs. Consensus standards have been developed with new strategies for a

more accurate determination of HPD attenuation provided in the field. The latest standards incorporate the variance of both (a) the fit of the protector among test subjects and (b) the variance of the HPD's performance over a wide range of noise spectra. These criteria have formed the basis of a proposed revision of EPA's Product Noise Labeling regulation.[33,34] The proposed regulation provides guidance for evaluating and labeling passive HPDs, active noise-reduction devices, and impulsive noise-reduction devices, such as sound restoration (or nonlinear) acoustic protectors.[35]

Regardless of how the NRR is calculated, a significant limitation of any labeling scheme is that the attenuation for an individual user cannot be predicted from the sample statistic derived from laboratory data. While the NRR may provide a good estimate of how much noise reduction a particular hearing protector is capable of providing, it is intended to inform the wearer about the potential performance of a protector and is not an indicator of the actual performance for any individual. Actual performance may only be determined by conducting individual fit-testing. Fit-testing measures how well an individual fits a specific hearing protector and is recommended as a "best practice" for hearing loss prevention programs.[36,37] Fit-testing generates a personal attenuation rating (PAR) that can be used to determine whether sufficient protection is being provided to individual workers in their work environments (Box 12A-1 and Figure 12A-5). Hearing protector fit-testing can improve the hearing loss prevention program and reduce cases of noise-induced hearing threshold shift by:

Box 12A-1. Example of Earplug Fit-Testing

At a site along the Gulf of Mexico, inspectors had to ride in a helicopter out to monitor oil rigs. Their main source of noise exposure was from the helicopter ride, which could be as high as 110 dBA and might last for up to 2 hours. Based on the high noise levels, it was decided that each worker should receive at least 25 dB of attenuation from their earplugs, which would bring their exposure level down to 85 dBA.

Initial fit-testing (with the earplugs they usually wore) showed that just over half of the workers received attenuation of 25 dB or more from their earplugs; they were adequately protected. On the other hand, the 33 people who did not get sufficient attenuation needed extra attention. First, an attempt was made for those people to refit their earplugs, and then they were tested again. If re-fitting the earplugs did not improve their results, then another type of earplug was chosen, until they found one that worked better. After refitting, retraining, and retesting, 92% of all workers were receiving at least a 25 dB PAR with the available earplug choices that were normally provided.

Results are depicted in Figure 12A-5. All 74 subjects are shown across from left to right, ordered from worst to best PAR. A line was drawn at 25 dB—the minimum level of desired attenuation for this situation. Workers on the left side of the graph (with less than the desired 25 dB attenuation) needed to be refitted and retested. A second data point (above the first) for each of these workers showed how much they improved after a little more instruction and practice time and/or by trying a different type of hearing protector. Most of the workers were able to obtain 25 dB or more just by reinserting their earplugs better; those few who still did not receive sufficient attenuation needed additional help—probably a different type or style of hearing protector.

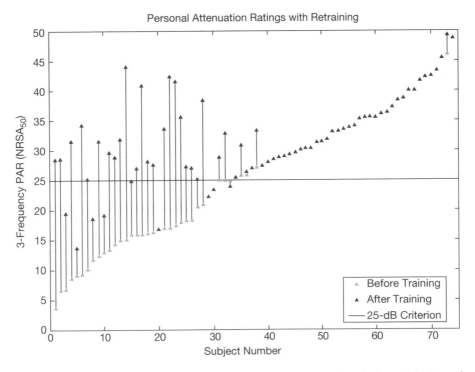

Figure 12A-5. This graph shows three-frequency personal attenuation ratings (PARs) obtained for 74 workers and compares them to the desired PAR of 25 (as indicated by the horizontal line). Before training, approximately half of the workers did not receive adequate protection from their earplugs. After these workers were given more individual instruction and practice time and/or a different type of earplug, most of them achieved the desired PAR or greater attenuation. (Source: Murphy WJ, Themann CL, Murata TK. Hearing protector fit-testing with off-shore oil-rig inspectors in Louisiana and Texas. International Journal of Audiology 2016; 55: 688–698.)

- Identifying workers who are at risk for NIHL
- Identifying hearing protection that is appropriate for a given noise exposure
- Training workers in the proper fitting technique and use of HPDs
- Increasing self-efficacy among workers who must wear hearing protection
- Improving the estimate of noise exposures for workers who wear hearing protection
- Implementing "best practices" for hearing loss prevention
- Reducing the potential liability for NIHL and workers' compensation.
- Reducing costs associated with maintaining an inventory of HPDs.

Audiometric Monitoring

Audiograms indicate a person's hearing threshold. Results are given in decibels, which indicate the intensity or loudness a sound has to be for the person to detect it. Thresholds below 25 dB HL are considered normal. NIOSH suggests that (a) monitoring audiometry be conducted on noise-exposed workers late in, or at the end of, their daily work shifts and (b) audiometry be repeated immediately after any monitoring audiogram indicates a significant threshold shift.[29] Before conducting retests, workers should be reinstructed and earphones refitted. Those who employ this retest strategy will find a significant reduction in the number of workers called back for a confirmation audiogram—because if the retest audiogram does not show the same shift as the initial audiogram, the retest audiogram becomes the test of record.

By testing workers during their work shifts, one may identify temporary threshold shifts (TTSs). Although the relationship between permanent threshold shifts and TTSs is not completely understood, workers with a TTS are being overexposed to noise. Discovering a TTS and taking action to prevent its recurrence will help protect workers from permanent hearing damage. If annual monitoring audiograms are performed before or at the beginning of work shifts, TTSs from noise exposure on the previous work shifts will have resolved so that any threshold shifts observed will represent permanent shifts in hearing.

Audiometry should be conducted again within 30 days of any monitoring or retest audiogram that continues to show a significant threshold shift. A minimum of 12 hours of quiet should precede the confirmation audiogram to determine whether the shift is a TTS or a permanent threshold shift. Hearing protectors should not be considered as a substitute for a quiet work environment.[29]

The OSHA criterion for the standard threshold shift (a change of 10 dB or more in the average of hearing thresholds at 2,000, 3,000, and 4,000 Hz) may not be the ideal method to identify and prevent permanent NIHL. NIOSH recommends a better criterion for the calculation of significant threshold shift: an increase of 15 dB in the hearing threshold level at any of the test frequencies in either ear (at 500, 1,000, 2,000, 3,000, 4,000, and 6,000 Hz), as determined by two consecutive audiometric tests.[29] This alternative criterion has both high sensitivity and high specificity.

Age Correction

Although many people experience a decrease in hearing acuity with age, others do not. It is not possible to predict who will and who will not develop hearing loss with aging. The median hearing loss attributable to aging for a given age group cannot be generalized to all individuals in that age group. Thus, when calculating significant threshold shifts, age-correcting hearing thresholds will overestimate the expected hearing loss for some people and underestimate it for others.

Unfortunately, the adjustment of audiometric thresholds for aging has become a common practice in workers' compensation litigation. Age corrections reduce the amount of hearing loss attributable to noise exposure, with a consequent reduction in the amount of compensation paid to workers for hearing loss.

Age-correcting audiograms obtained in an occupational hearing-loss prevention program are not recommended.[29] The purpose of the program is to prevent hearing loss. If an audiogram is age-corrected, regardless of the source of the correction values, the time required for a significant threshold shift to be identified will be prolonged. Delaying the identification of a worker with a significant threshold shift is counterproductive.

ACCOMMODATING WORKERS WITH HEARING LOSS

After a confirmation audiogram that indicates a permanent threshold shift, NIOSH recommends a written notification to the worker and a referral to the audiometric manager or professional supervisor for review and determination of probable etiology. This referral should explore all possible causes in addition to occupational noise, including ototoxic chemicals, age-related hearing loss, familial hearing loss, nonoccupational noise exposure, and medical conditions.[29]

Workers with a threshold shift due to causes other than noise should be counseled by audiometric managers and referred to their physicians for evaluation and possible treatment. Appropriate actions should be planned for workers showing a threshold shift that is determined by the audiometric manager to be due likely to occupational noise. At a minimum, these actions should include reinstruction and refitting of hearing protectors, additional training in worker responsibilities for effective hearing-loss prevention, and/or reassignment to a quieter work area. The professional supervisor should be responsible for identifying whatever changes may be necessary and for ensuring that they are implemented. According to OSHA's Hearing Conservation Amendment, the professional supervisor of the audiometric testing component of a hearing conservation program must be a licensed or certified audiologist or otolaryngologist or other physician.

The main factors that enable workers with hearing loss to continue working are ability to cope with the hearing loss, support from management and coworkers, adequate work conditions, psychological support from patient organizations and family members and friends, support from medical professionals and programs, and financial and other benefits.[38] A set of guidelines can be used by health professionals for managing the work-related conditions. Important to workers with hearing loss is knowledge about and availability of better hearing protectors and hearing aids, alternative means of obtaining and financing hearing aids, self-acceptance, a quiet work environment, determination and persistence to ask for needed accommodations at work, education of coworkers about hearing loss, and opportunities to communicate information and experiences with other affected workers.

ACCOMMODATING WORKERS WITH TINNITUS

Several standardized scales exist to evaluate in the interference of tinnitus on the quality of life. Most of them are short and easy to administer. Their use can offer valuable information on how to accommodate workers that suffer from tinnitus.[39] Most important in managing workers with tinnitus is to refer them to otolaryngologists or otologists (ear specialists), who will try to determine its cause by evaluating the auditory system, measuring blood pressure and kidney function, and assessing diet, allergies, and medications. Specialists determine treatment, which has included maskers (electronic devices the size of a hearing aids that use sound to make tinnitus less noticeable), support and counseling, surgery, drug therapy, diet, psychotherapy, electrical/magnetic stimulation, acupuncture, biofeedback, and hypnosis. They also should explain to patients the pathophysiology of their tinnitus, make recommendations for hearing aids when appropriate, and provide periodic monitoring.[40]

EFFECTIVENESS OF MEASURES TO PREVENT HEARING LOSS

While many workplaces comply with legal or other requirements to implement recommended interventions, few have evaluated the effectiveness of these interventions to prevent occupational NIHL.[41-44] Research, including broad systematic reviews, has been performed to evaluate the effectiveness of these interventions.[41-44] NIOSH has created an award program to identify and honor highly successful hearing loss prevention practices and innovations.[45] Since 2009, NIOSH has presented awards at the annual conference of the National Hearing Conservation Association.[46,47] Award competition has resulted in NIOSH acquiring high-quality field data on noise exposure monitoring and successful noise control programs.

ACKNOWLEDGMENT

This chapter is dedicated to the memory of Dr. Derek E. Dunn.

AUTHORS' NOTE

The findings and conclusions in this chapter are those of the authors and do not necessarily represent the views of the National Institute for Occupational Safety and Health.

REFERENCES

1. U.S. Department of Labor. Bureau of Labor Statistics. Injuries, illnesses, and fatalities. Available at: http://www.bls.gov/iif/oshsum.htm. Accessed December 22, 2016.
2. Kardous C, Shaw PB. Evaluation of smartphone sound measurement applications. Journal of the Acoustical Society of America 2014; 135: EL186–EL192.
3. Kardous C, Shaw PB. Evaluation of smartphone sound measurement applications (apps) using external microphones: A follow-up study. Journal of the Acoustical Society of America 2016; 140: EL327–EL333.
4. Williams W, Sukara Z. Simplified noise labelling for plant or equipment used in workplaces. Journal of Health and Safety, Research and Practice 2013; 5: 18–22.
5. Masterson EA, Bushnell PT, Themann CL, Morata TC. Hearing impairment among noise-exposed workers—United States, 2003–2012. Morbidity and Mortality Weekly Report 2016; 65: 389–394.
6. Prince MM, Stayner LT, Smith RJ, Gilbert SJ. A re-examination of risk estimates from the NIOSH Occupational Noise and Hearing Survey (ONHS). Journal of the Acoustical Society of America 1997; 101: 950–963.
7. National Institutes of Health. Noise and hearing loss. NIH Consensus Development Conference. Consensus Statement 1990, p. 8.
8. Lim DJ, Dunn DE. Anatomical correlates of noise induced hearing loss. Otolaryngologic Clinics of North America 1979; 12: 493–513.
9. Durrant JD, Lovrinic JH. Bases of hearing science (3rd ed.). Baltimore: Williams & Wilkins, 1995.
10. Liberman MC, Epstein MJ, Cleveland SS, et al. Toward a differential diagnosis of hidden hearing loss in humans. PLoS ONE 2016; 11: e0162726.
11. Picard M, Girard SA, Simard M, et al. Association of work-related accidents with noise exposure in the workplace and noise-induced hearing loss based on the experience of some 240,000 person-years of observation. Accident Analysis & Prevention 2008; 40: 1644–1652.
12. Dias A, Cordeiro R. Fraction of work-related accidents attributable to occupational noise in the city of Botucatu, São Paulo, Brazil. Noise Health 2008; 10: 69–73.
13. Mohr PE, Feldman JJ, Dunbar J, et al. The societal costs of severe to profound hearing loss in the United States. International Journal of Technology Assessment in Health Care 2000; 16: 1120–1135.
14. American Academy of Audiology. Untreated hearing loss linked to depression, social isolation in seniors. Available at: http://www.audiology.org/resources/documentlibrary/Pages/UntreatedHearingLoss.aspx. Accessed December 13, 2016.
15. Kochkin S, Rogin CM. Quantifying the obvious: The impact of hearing instruments on quality of life. The Hearing Review 2000; 7: 6–34.
16. American National Standards Institute. American national standard: Determination of occupational noise exposure and estimation of noise-induced hearing impairment. ANSI S3.44-1996. New York: American National Standards Institute, 1996.
17. Phaneuf R, Hetu R. An epidemiological perspective of the causes of hearing loss among industrial workers. Journal of Otolaryngology 1990; 19: 31–40.
18. Palmer KT, Griffin MJ, Syddall HE, et al. Raynaud's phenomenon, vibration induced white finger, and difficulties in hearing. Occupational and Environmental Medicine 2002; 59: 640–642.
19. Morata TC. Chemical exposure as a risk factor for hearing loss. Journal of Occupational and Environmental Medicine 2003; 45: 676–682.
20. Campo P, Venet T, Thomas A, et al. Neuropharmacological and cochleotoxic effects of styrene: Consequences on noise exposures. Neurotoxicology and Teratology 2014; 44: 113–120.
21. EU-OSHA—European Agency for Safety and Health at Work. Combined exposure to noise and ototoxic substances. Luxembourg Office for Official Publications of the European Communities, 2009. Available at: https://osha.europa.eu/en/tools-and-publications/

publications/literature_reviews/combined-exposure-to-noise-and-ototoxic-substances/view. Accessed December 13, 2016.

22. Johnson AC, Morata TC. Occupational exposure to chemicals and hearing impairment. The Nordic Expert Group for Criteria Documentation of Health Risks from Chemicals. Nordic Expert Group. Gothenburg. Arbete och Hälsa. 2010; 44: 1–177. Available at: https://gupea.ub.gu.se/bitstream/2077/23240/1/gupea_2077_23240_1.pdf. Accessed December 22, 2016.

23. Parving A, Hein HO, Suadicani P, et al. Epidemiology of hearing disorders: Some factors affecting hearing. The Copenhagen Male Study. Scandinavian Audiology 1993; 22: 101–107.

24. Axelsson A, Coles R. Compensation for tinnitus in noise-induced hearing loss. In: Axelsson A, Borchgrevink HM, Hamernik RP, et al (eds.). Scientific basis of noise-induced hearing loss. New York: Thieme, 1996, pp. 423–429.

25. Occupational Safety and Health Administration. Occupational noise exposure: Hearing conservation amendment; Final rule. Occupational Safety and Health Administration 1983, 29 CFR 1910.95, 48 Federal Register, 9738–9785.

26. Rabinowitz PM, Slade M, Dixon-Ernst C, et al. Impact of OSHA final rule—Recording hearing loss: An analysis of an industrial audiometric dataset. Journal of Occupational and Environmental Medicine 2003; 45: 1274–1280.

27. Masterson EA, Deddens JA, Themann CL, et al. Trends in worker hearing loss by industry sector 1981–2010. American Journal of Industrial Medicine 2015; 58: 392–401.

28. NIOSH Alert: Preventing occupational exposures to lead and noise at indoor firing ranges (DHHS [NIOSH] Publication No. 2009–136), April 2009. Available at: https://www.cdc.gov/niosh/docs/2009-136/pdfs/2009-136.pdf. Accessed December 22, 2016.

29. National Institute for Occupational Safety and Health. Criteria for a recommended standard: Occupational exposure to noise (revised criteria). NIOSH Publication No.98-126. Cincinnati, OH: NIOSH, 1998. Available at: https://www.cdc.gov/niosh/docs/98-126/pdfs/98-126.pdf. Accessed December 22, 2016.

30. Franks JR, Stephenson MR, Merry CJ. Preventing occupational hearing loss: A practical guide (Publication no. 96-110). Cincinnati, OH: National Institute for Occupational Safety and Health, 1996. Available at: https://www.cdc.gov/niosh/docs/96-110/pdfs/96-110.pdf. Accessed December 22, 2016.

31. Suter AH. The hearing conservation amendment: 25 years later. Noise Health 2009; 11: 2–7.

32. Sound & Vibration. Buyer's guide to products for noise and vibration control, July 2016. Available at: http://www.sandv.com/home.htm. Accessed January 17, 2017.

33. American National Standards Institute. Methods of estimating effective A-weighted sound pressure levels when hearing protectors are worn. ANSI S12.68-2007 (R2012). Melville, NY: Acoustical Society of America, 2012.

34. American National Standards Institute. Methods for measuring the real-ear attenuation of hearing protectors. ANSI S12.6-2016. Melville, NY: Acoustical Society of America, 2016.

35. Murphy WJ. How to assess hearing protection evaluation effectiveness: What is new in ANSI/ASA S12.68. Acoustics Today 2008; 4; 40–42.

36. Hager LD. Fit-testing hearing protectors: An idea whose time has come. Noise Health 2011; 13: 147–151.

37. Schulz TY. Individual fit-testing of hearing protectors: A review of uses. Noise Health 2011; 13: 152–162.

38. Detaille SI, Haafkens JA, van Dijk FJH. What employees with rheumatoid arthritis, diabetes mellitus and hearing loss need to cope at work. Scandinavian Journal of Work, Environment & Health 2003; 29: 134–142.

39. Steinmetz LG, Zeigelboim BS, Lacerda AB, et al. Evaluating tinnitus in industrial hearing loss prevention programs. International Tinnitus Journal 2008; 14: 152–158.

40. Dobie RA. A review of randomized clinical trials in tinnitus. Laryngoscope 1999; 109: 1202–1211.

41. Heyer N, Morata TC, Pinkerton L, et al. Use of historical data and a novel metric in the evaluation of the effectiveness of hearing conservation program components. Occupational and Environmental Medicine 2011; 68: 510–517.

42. Stephenson CM, Stephenson MR. Hearing loss prevention for carpenters: Part 1—Using health communication and health promotion models to develop training that works. Noise Health 2011; 13: 113–121.

43. Stephenson MR, Shaw PB, Stephenson CM, Graydon PS. Hearing loss prevention for carpenters: Part 2—Demonstration projects using individualized and group training. Noise Health 2011; 13: 122–131.

44. Verbeek JH, Kateman E, Morata TC, et al. Interventions to prevent occupational noise-induced hearing loss: A Cochrane systematic

review. International Journal of Audiology 2012; 53: S84–S96.

45. Safe in Sound: Excellence in Hearing Loss Prevention Award. Available at: www. safeinsound.us. Accessed December 22, 2016.

46. Meinke DK, Morata TC. Awarding and promoting excellence in hearing loss prevention. International Journal of Audiology 2012; 51: S63–S70.

47. Morata T, Meinke D. Uncovering effective strategies for hearing loss prevention. Acoustics Australia 2016; 44: 67–75.

FURTHER READING AND WEBSITES

American Tinnitus Association. Available at: http:// www.ata.org
The American Tinnitus Association promotes tinnitus awareness, prevention, and treatment. It offers information on prevention programs in schools, urges governmental and nongovernmental organizations to support hearing conservation, funds research, and facilitates self-help groups.

Cochlea.org. Available at: http://www.cochlea.org/en/
An educational website sponsored by several institutions and companies, it contains sections describing the anatomy, physiology, and pathophysiology of the auditory system.

National Institute for Occupational Safety and Health. Noise and hearing loss prevention. Available at: https://www.cdc.gov/niosh/topics/noise/
NIOSH's mission is to develop new knowledge in the field of occupational safety and health and to transfer that knowledge into practice. This web page includes facts, statistics, publications, and other information that is helpful for reducing occupational noise exposures and preventing hearing loss.

Occupational Safety and Health Administration. Occupational Noise Exposure Standard and Hearing Conservation Amendment, Code of Federal Regulations, Title 29, Chapter XVII, Part 1910, Subpart G. Available at: http://www. osha.gov/SLTC/noisehearingconservation/ standards.html
Noise and hearing conservation are addressed in this standard, which is applicable to general industry in the United States. It covers monitoring of noise exposure, audiometric testing, hearing protection, employee training, and recordkeeping.

Regarding guidance, OSHA's August 2013 OSHA technical manual (OTM), Section III: Chapter 5—Noise (Appendix G—Alternatives for evaluating benefits and costs of noise control). Available at: https://www.osha.gov/dts/ osta/otm/new_noise/appendixg.pdf
This chapter provides technical information and guidance to help compliance safety and health officers and others evaluate noise hazards and interventions in the workplace.

Suter A. Hearing conservation manual (5th ed.). Milwaukee, WI: Council for Accreditation in Occupational Hearing Conservation. Available at: http://www.caohc.org/
This manual covers all facets of developing a successful hearing-loss prevention program. This manual is designed as a reference text used during occupational hearing conservationist training courses. It is an excellent resource for practicing professionals.

U.S. Army Public Health Center Fact Sheet 51-002-0713: Occupational ototoxins (ear poisons) and hearing loss. Available at: https://phc.amedd. army.mil/PHC%20Resource%20Library/ Ototoxin_FS_51-002-0713.pdf
This is a fact sheet regarding ototoxic chemical exposures and guidelines for hearing conservation.

12B

Vibration

Peter W. Johnson and Martin G. Cherniack

Vibration has been traditionally divided into two categories: hand-arm (segmental) vibration (HAV) and whole-body vibration (WBV). Hand-arm vibration refers to tool-induced vibration, which affects the soft tissues (blood vessels, nerves, and tendons) in the fingers, hand, and arm. Whole-body vibration refers to predominantly vehicle-induced vibration, which affects the health and integrity of the spine as well as the gastrointestinal tract, kidney, and liver.

In order to characterize HAV and WBV, frequency and amplitude need to be objectively measured. The frequency of vibration, which is measured in oscillations per second or hertz (Hz), determines which bodily structures may resonate and may be potentially adversely affected—beyond damage caused by the direct transfer of energy. The amplitude of vibration, usually expressed as root-mean-squared acceleration—which is measured in g (a g is a unit of gravity) or more typically meters per second squared (m/s^2), determines the magnitude (intensity) of the vibration. Frequency and amplitude of vibration can be summarized by the average-weighted vibration, in which the frequency content of vibration is used to weight the amplitude over the period of exposure.

For HAV, the adverse health effects are related to both the frequency and the energy transfer to the upper extremities from either powered tools or stationary sources that produce oscillatory vibration, such as mounted drills and pedestal grinders. Both HAV and WBV are often measured with triaxial accelerometers (devices that measure acceleration in three orthogonal/perpendicular axes);[1,2] the time history of the accelerations is usually saved in a data-logging device. To assess HAV and WBV, vibration frequency-weighting curves have been developed to weight the vibration amplitude based on the frequency content in the vibration.

HAND-ARM VIBRATION

The international standard to assess HAV has been developed and published by the International Standards Organization (ISO), which uses a frequency weighting curve to quantify the vibration.[1] Based on this curve, the frequencies of interest from tool-transmitted HAV typically range between 6 and 1,250 Hz, with oscillations between 10 and 12 Hz given the greatest weighting for contributing to adverse health effects. Above 16 Hz, the importance of the vibration is progressively de-emphasized, with frequencies above 250 Hz adding very little to the exposure calculation. For HAV measurement and assessment, the accelerometer should be mounted to where the hand grips the tool,[3] then the three axes of vibration are added together and the vector sum measure is used to characterize the vibration exposure. The vibration exposure is then calculated based on what would be typical tool operation over an 8-hour work shift. In the United States, the same provisions are articulated in the ANSI standard (ANSI S2.70-2006) and the hand-arm vibration ACGIH threshold limit value (2016).

These frequency-weighting curves are based on physical principles of energy transfer across multiple frequencies, which were generally validated by epidemiologic studies of HAV. They can be a benefit or a detriment in assessing HAV and WBV exposures. The benefit is that this long-standing frequency-weighting methodology enables comparisons across all vibration studies. The disadvantage, especially in the realm of HAV, is that one generic frequency weighting-curve, as currently is employed by most standards and regulations, may not fit all tool applications. Evidence from newer biodynamic,[4] physiological,[5] and epidemiological[6] studies indicates that up to three frequency weighting curves may be needed to assess tool-induced vibration to the upper extremities—one for disorders of sensory nerves, one for disorders of blood vessels, and one for disorders of bones, tendons, muscle, and large nerves. The magnitude of the HAV that results from applying these alternative weighting curves can vary substantially; therefore, interpreting the HAV exposures, relative to the classical weighting curve in the current standards and regulations, is both complex and challenging. This is why consensus bodies, including the ISO, ACGIH, and ANSI have been reluctant to revise the existing weighting curve despite recognized limitations. There is both human and animal data suggesting injury from higher frequency exposures. For example, recent research using rat tails,[7] which are good anatomical analogs of the human finger (from a structural and tissue composition perspective), demonstrated that higher-frequency (60 to 250 Hz) vibration frequencies, which are heavily

discounted in the classical ISO 5439-1 vibration frequency-weighting curve, can damage the very small blood vessels in the rat tail. This type of high-frequency vascular damage may be analogous to what tool operators experience.

Adverse Effects of HAV

The deleterious effects from HAV induced by power tools on the peripheral nerves and small vessels of the upper extremity have been documented for more than a century.[8] Clinical recognition and control of HAV is based on reducing its most prominent manifestations: (a) tool- or cold-temperature-induced finger blanching and (b) signs and symptoms, such as numbness and tingling in the fingers, reduced sensitivity to touch, reduced circulation in the fingers, and decreased peripheral nerve function in the fingers. In 1918, Alice Hamilton, a pioneering occupational medicine physician, first described these manifestations of HAV in a group of quarry workers using air-powered tools.[9] Subsequent studies confirmed a strong association between duration and intensity of tool-induced vibration exposure and development of neurologic and vascular symptoms.[10]

Hand-arm vibration syndrome (HAVS) is more than just an incidental problem. In 1990, the National Institute for Occupational Safety and Health warned that up to 2 million U.S. workers were exposed to vibration at magnitudes and frequencies sufficient to provoke injury, with almost 40% of exposed workers experiencing symptoms.[10] The general decline in metalworking in many high-income countries, coupled with enhanced vibration-dampening in many tool designs, has substantially reduced symptom rates in specific industries, especially in forestry.

Many tools and exposures are associated with tool-induced, HAV-related disorders of the upper extremities.[11] The most recognized sources are air-powered rotary tools, such as grinders, sanders, and cutting wheels. However, gasoline-powered oscillating tools, such as chainsaws and brush cutters in the forestry industry, have also been associated with HAV-related upper-extremity disorders. The recent transition from air- and gas-powered tools to battery-powered tools, especially in construction, has not necessarily reduced the tool-related HAV exposures. In many instances, battery-powered tools may concentrate the vibration exposures over a narrower frequency range, which can have positive or negative effects, depending on the dampening properties and operating frequencies of the electric tool.[12]

Understanding HAV-related disorders of the upper extremity as measureable and quantifiable vascular and neurologic disorders, with controllable exposure-response features, began in the 1970s. In the past 30 years, characterization of the exposure–response relationship, identification of disorders, and addition of enhanced vibration-dampening in some tool designs have all helped to reduce exposure and occurrence of HAV-related upper-extremity disorders.

The causal relationship between HAV exposure and development of related disorders in the upper extremities has been well documented in the forestry industry. When lighter gas-powered chainsaws were widely introduced in the 1960s, forestry workers were exposed for longer durations to higher-frequency vibration. After a latency period of 5 to 10 years, many of these forestry workers started to develop vibration white finger (VWF), a disorder in which the vascular supply to the fingers is either temporarily or permanently disrupted, causing the fingers to turn white when exposed to vibration and/or cold.

From the 1970s to the 1990s, forestry industry studies demonstrated that reducing HAV exposure (by redesigning tool handles to isolate hands from tool vibration) was associated with a reduction in some important HAV-related disorders. In the longest established longitudinal study of vibratory disease, Finnish forest workers were surveyed multiple times from 1972 to 1995; [13,14] vibration exposures were reduced after the introduction of vibration-dampening chainsaws. During this period, the prevalence of VWF declined from 40% to 4% in exposed workers. From 1976 to 1995, VWF symptoms declined from 17% to 8% in the original group of workers. In addition, the prevalence of neurologically related hand and finger numbness fell from 78% in 1972 to 23% in 1976 but then increased to 40% in 1995—perhaps due to more proximally related neurological disorders, such as carpal tunnel syndrome (CTS) or rotator cuff syndrome.

In the mid-1980s, researchers determined that typical tool-induced vascular disorders could occur independently of sensory nerve impairment. In recognition of the differences between the signs and symptoms caused by vascular impairment and those caused by neurologic injury, the term *hand-arm vibration syndrome* was introduced to capture the multiple sites of injury. The accompanying Stockholm Workshop Scale[15,16] was designed to separately access vascular effects and neurologic effects. This scale, based on both objective and subjective components, provided a consensus rating system for both (a) vascular disorders, characterized by vasospasm and disturbances of digital circulation; and (b) sensory disorders, characterized by diffuse peripheral nerve trunk and mechanoreceptor injuries. However, the association of HAVS with other work-related upper-extremity disorders, such as reduced hand strength,[17] and bone and joint disorders (including traumatic osteoarthritis and diseases of the elbows, shoulders, and neck), is complicated and confounded by biomechanical and biodynamic factors, particularly because most segmental vibration does not extend beyond the wrist.[18] The development of CTS, the most frequently diagnosed concomitant disorder, has competing biomechanical and physiologic factors.[19] In addition, there appears to be interaction between HAV and biodynamic hand and arm loading.[20] Furthermore, the risk of CTS in vibration-exposed workers appears to be reduced by ergonomic redesign of jobs.[21]

Our understanding of the physiologic response in the upper extremities to tool-related vibratory stimuli continues to evolve. For example, a longitudinal study of shipyard workers reported that vascular abnormalities were diminished with reduced levels of exposure to tool-related vibration.[20] Another study demonstrated that workers who had reduced exposure to tool-induced vibration had very subtle, rather than gross, changes in quantitative sensory tests and lower morbidity than workers in the 1980s and 1990s who had used vibrating tools with less protection.[22] Other studies found that (a) tool-induced vibrations above 100 Hz may play an important role in tool-induced vibration disorders of the upper extremities[23,24] and (b) vibration-dampening gloves may help reduce worker exposures from higher-frequency (>150 Hz), tool-induced vibration.[25]

Anti-vibration (AV) gloves can provide some protection to workers from higher-frequency tool-induced vibration.[25,26] Selection of gloves for use with vibrating tools depends on several factors, which include the nature of the glove material, the oscillatory frequency of the tool source, and the trade-off between (a) mechanical isolation and (b) compensatory increased grip and transmission. A problem is that the fingers and palm of the hands are highly efficient shock absorbers, which effectively absorb all vibration with frequencies over 60 Hz; below this frequency, much of this vibration energy is transferred through the hand and into the arms, and, if the frequency is low enough, up to the shoulders. The fingers of tool operators appear to have resonant frequencies between 60 and 125 Hz. However, even if specific frequency signals could be isolated, the effect on tissue injury can be trivial, because of the greater impact from energy transfer directly to the fingers and palms. Vibrations at lower frequencies pass through the gloves and can excite (resonate with) the tool operator's forearms, elbows, and shoulders. However, evidence is modest for direct injury from these low-frequency vibrations, except for large inertial tools (heavy tools with large displacements), such as pavement breakers. In principle, gloves may attenuate frequencies higher than 125 Hz and provide some protection to the smaller anatomical structures within the fingers. For tools with frequencies 60 Hz and above, which includes many power tools, fingerless gloves should not be used—use of them leaves fingers unprotected and exposes them to the potentially harmful higher-frequency vibration. Anti-vibration gloves certified by the ISO are available, but the frequencies at which the gloves have been tested may not be the same frequencies to which the workers are exposed.

HAV Standards for Measurement and Regulation of Exposures

For measuring exposure to HAV, the ISO assumes that a relationship exists between the relative hazards presented by vibration at different frequencies.[1] To complement the ISO standard, the European Union (EU) adopted a vibration directive[27] by which companies in the EU were encouraged to implement either administrative or engineering controls based on the level of their employees' exposures to tool-related vibration. The EU regulations set a lower daily vibration exposure threshold (daily exposure action value = 2.5 m/sec^2), below which adverse health outcomes are expected to be less common. It also set an upper daily vibration exposure threshold (daily exposure limit value = 5.0 m/sec^2), at which adverse health effects are more likely.

Single-value vibration thresholds, as used in the ISO standard and the EU vibration directive, cannot substitute for a full array of preventive measures, which include warnings, health surveillance, instruction on proper use of tools, tool maintenance, restriction of daily maximum use, selection of appropriate gloves, and assessment of the total work environment.[28] In addition, measuring and characterizing tool-vibration frequency can lead to more appropriate selections of controls.

Factors Influencing HAV Exposures

Vibratory characteristics are highly specific to certain tools. For example, chainsaws and drills are primarily oscillatory and continuous-energy tools. Impact wrenches and rivet guns are highly impulsive, with vibration in both low and high frequencies.[29,30] Tools such as nut runners, which can be heavy, also can have major nonvibratory biomechanical consequences (lifting and holding these heavy tools); therefore, simple generic measurements may not capture the extent of a potential tool-specific hazard.

Tool-specific characteristics also influence the approach to exposure control. While personal protective equipment is not a first-line approach to control of vibration, some AV gloves can be effective if the tool has predominant frequencies above 125 Hz,[25,26] where the greatest risks are injuries to the smaller structures (smaller sensory nerves and mechanoreceptors) in the hands and fingers.

Frequency and direction of vibration as well as the position of the arm and hand all affect the transfer and absorption of, vibration energy. Push-and-pull forces as well as grip force affect the transmission of the vibration to the tool operator.[31] All tool vibration standards[1] and regulations[27] use frequency-weighting curves, which assume all vibrations are harmonic (cyclic or oscillatory), ignoring impact forces and instantaneous peak accelerations with percussing/impact tools, which may exceed 10^5 m/sec^2 (1,020 g). The dramatic reduction in vascular symptoms due to introduction of AV chainsaws in the 1970s has been best explained by the flattening of high-frequency, transient accelerations—rather than by a reduction in the lower-frequency average cyclic oscillatory vibrations.[29] In addition, in pedestal-grinder and stone-cutter operators, vascular symptoms were better accounted for when the unweighted or nondiscounted higher frequency content of peak impulsive tool exposures were accounted for and factored into the exposure assessment models. This is consistent with the high prevalence of VWF in platers and riveters, who use high-impulse tools for only a few minutes a day.[30]

A similar problem arises in working environments that use tools that oscillate at very high frequencies, such as small precision drills, saws, and tools used in medicine and dentistry.[32,33] The classical frequency-weighting curves used in standards and regulations exclude frequencies that exceed 1,250 Hz because (a) energy transfer is directly related to velocity and (b) there is no physiological evidence that the small blood vessels, sensory nerves, and mechanoreceptors in the fingers and hands respond to frequencies above 1,500 Hz. Nevertheless, neurologic and vascular symptoms have occurred in certain groups of workers, such as dentists, dental hygienists, and surgeons, who use these types of tools.[32,33]

Pathology, Diagnosis, and Treatment of Disorders Related to HAV

Sensorineural symptoms in the fingers and hands are the most common clinical presentation of workers with tool-related vibration disorders. In these workers, sensory nerve conduction velocity in the hands and fingers is slowed, especially distally.[34,35] These deficits in conduction velocity affect the small-diameter myelinated nerve fibers in the hands and fingers—distinct from the slowing in conduction velocity in the large diameter nerve fibers that pass through the shoulder, elbow, and wrist regions.

Temporal and chronic tool-induced changes in sensorineural symptoms in the fingers and hands can also be subjectively identified by assessing three mechanoreceptor populations in the fingertips: Meissner corpuscles, Merkel discs, and Pacinian corpuscles. Any temporal or chronic changes in sensory or tactile thresholds, often determined by vibrometry (subjecting the fingertips to oscillations of different magnitudes and frequencies), occur differentially among the three mechanoreceptor populations.[36] It appears that at least transient deficits in mechanoreceptor function occur at higher oscillatory frequencies (125 Hz or higher), and these frequencies are discounted by the classical frequency weightings used in the ISO standards[1] and EU regulations.[27] Damage to these mechanoreceptors can impair sensation and can eventually affect the larger motor nerves and muscle strength.

Primary HAV symptoms, digital vasospasm and progressive whitening of the fingertips (VWF), predominate in workers exposed to high magnitudes of vibration several hours a day. These symptoms often progress over time. However, companion vasoconstriction in the hands of individuals not exposed to vibration, such as people with diabetes, pregnant women, smokers, and older workers, results from central sympathetic mechanisms or other factors affecting peripheral blood vessels.[37] The characteristic objective finding of VWF and Raynaud's phenomenon is a local blanching of the fingers, often induced by exposure to cold.

Diagnosis of HAVS is based on a history of exposure, symptoms, physical examination findings, and, often, laboratory studies.[38] Finger blanching and small-fiber neuropathy are fairly specific to tool-induced vibratory disorders. However, disorders of large-diameter nerves and nerve compression disorders in the wrist, elbow, and shoulders as well as musculoskeletal pain and joint degeneration are nonspecific disorders that may not necessarily be associated with vibratory hand-tool use. To some extent, the diagnosis of HAVS is exclusionary, since both peripheral nerve dysfunction associated with vibrating tool use (VWF) and Raynaud's phenomenon can reflect serious underlying disorders that are unrelated to exposure to vibration, such as collagen vascular diseases, arterial occlusive diseases, pulmonary hypertension, neurologic disorders, blood dyscrasias, other forms of trauma, and adverse effects of medications.

The diagnosis of VWF can be difficult because of concurrent arterial or cutaneous disorders; however, these underlying disorders are not likely among workers who are intensely working with hand tools since it would limit or impair their ability to effectively operate their tools. Temperature sensitivity and hand weakness may reflect injury to small-diameter nerve fibers or may affect a more proximal, compression-related block of nerve conduction, such as CTS. In cases where CTS has been ruled out, mechanoreceptor injury may be the cause of (a) diffuse reduction of skin sensitivity and/or (b) paresthesia and an increased sensitivity to cold—a type of injury that can be acutely aggravated by exposure to vibratory tools. An association between HAV and upper-extremity osteoarthritis in a given patient is often not clear, in part because it may be difficult to rule out other factors.

As vibratory exposures are controlled and job tasks diversified, HAVS cases may present in atypical ways. Because affected nerves and blood vessels recover, low-grade exposure can produce a situation where onset of new symptoms is balanced by resolution of others.

When a worker has been highly exposed to HAV or when there are legal or administrative issues, a medical history focusing on HAVS symptoms and specific tests need to be done to determine if symptoms are vibration-related. HAVS is distinguished from other occupationally related disorders of the upper extremities with specific tests, such as (a) cold-challenge plethysmography or other cold-provocation tests for the diagnosis of Raynaud's phenomenon and (b) quantitative sensory tests for

detecting small-fiber neuropathies. However, these specific tests are not widely available and should not be done before a clinical evaluation is completed. If tests are eventually done, their extensiveness will depend on clinical findings, medical-legal criteria, and the availability of the patient for sequential follow-up. (Nerve conduction studies, which are used in the diagnosis of nerve entrapment syndromes, such as CTS, are less specific and therefore less useful in diagnosing HAVS.)

In a classic case of VWF, with damage of small nerve fibers, therapeutic options are limited and should be provided only by experienced clinicians. Rehabilitation should aim to transfer the affected worker to an alternative job, where hands are not exposed to HAV. Some affected workers who have mild symptoms (or whose symptoms have resolved) may be able to return to work using antivibration tools that may be complemented with the selection of the appropriate AV gloves.

WHOLE-BODY VIBRATION

Whole-body vibration, defined as vibration energy transmitted either through the buttocks when seated or through the feet and legs when standing, is transmitted up through the spine to organs and other anatomical structures. Common sources of WBV are listed in Table 12B-1.

The vibration frequencies relevant to WBV are lower than those for HAV, typically between 1 and 100 Hz. Fore-aft and side-to-side vibrations between 1 to 4 Hz and vertical vibrations between 6 to 12 Hz are most likely to cause adverse health effects. A vehicle operator's exposure to WBV is

Table 12B-1. Common Sources of Whole-Body Vibration

Activity	Source
Warehousing and material handling	Forklifts, tugs, and pallet trucks
Construction	Cranes, graders, scrapers, power shovels/excavators, bulldozers, off-road trucks, and wheel loaders
Farming	Tractors, all-terrain vehicles, and harvesters
Forestry	Forwarders, harvesters, and skid steer loaders
Mining	Haul trucks, power shovels/excavators, bulldozers, and wheel loaders
Transportation	Subways, buses, trains, helicopters, tractor-trailers, and watercraft
Work in buildings	Gross structural movement and ventilation systems

often associated with development of low back pain,[39-46] which is prevalent among truck drivers and heavy-equipment operators.[47,48,49] WBV exposure increases spinal load[50,51] and can contribute to muscle fatigue[52] and deterioration of intervertebral lumbar discs.[53] WBV can also adversely affect the cardiovascular, pulmonary, endocrine, and nervous systems and the gastrointestinal tract.[54,55]

Documenting the association between WBV exposure and its adverse effects on the spine is challenging because there may be no signs on physical examination and symptoms of neck or low back pain may be nonspecific.[56,57] Imaging studies of the spine can be helpful in some instances, but they often provide little or no useful diagnostic information.

Neck pain and low back pain are associated with WBV from various types of equipment and vehicles, ranging from relatively smooth-riding cars, to rougher-riding trucks and buses,[40,58,59] to the roughest-riding off-road machines and equipment in construction (Figure 12B-1),[60] farming,[41] forestry,[61] and mining.[62,63] These symptoms can also be experienced by (a)

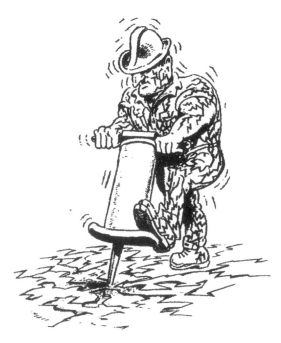

Figure 12B-1. Jackhammer operators are at high risk for disorders related to whole-body vibration, hand-arm vibration, and foot-transmitted vibration. (Drawing by Nick Thorkelson.)

operators of railway equipment[64] (trams, trains, and subways), watercraft, helicopters,[65] and fixed-wing aircraft,[66] and (b) workers standing on vibrating machines, platforms, or vehicles.[67]

Reducing WBV exposure can reduce low back pain and improve general health. The primary methods to reduce vehicle and heavy equipment operators' exposures to WBV is through the vehicle or equipment suspension and/or the seats. However, as the weight of a vehicle or equipment increases, the vehicle suspension becomes less effective and the role that the seat plays in protecting occupants from potentially harmful vibration becomes increasingly important.

Over time, design of vehicle and equipment seats has evolved. The first seats had no built-in suspension, and only the material of the seat cushion provided any protection from the vehicle and terrain-induced vibration. Then, in the mid-1960s, the supporting structure or pedestals of the seats were supplied with mechanical springs to assist the seat cushion and provide an additional means to absorb the vibration. Two decades later, air suspension seats were introduced as an enhancement to provide more protection from the vibration.

Despite the evolution of vehicle seats over more than 50 years and improvements being made in off-road vehicle seating, only modest improvements have been made in on-road vehicle seating.[68] In faster-moving on-road vehicles, the slow response of air suspension seats provides limited protection from WBV, typically only reducing vehicle and terrain-induced WBV by 5% to 15%.[58,59,68] In addition, many of these on-road, air-suspension seats amplify low-frequency (2 to 4 Hz) WBV exposures and do not adequately protect vehicle operators from the harmful intermediate frequencies (6 to 12 Hz), which may affect many of the structures in the torso (spine and internal organs).

In 2010, active suspension seats were commercially introduced for on-road vehicles. These seats monitor vibrations coming up through the seat base to the vehicle operator; an onboard computer controls a fast-acting linear electromagnetic motor in the seat base that cancels out much of the vibration induced by the vehicle and the terrain. In semi-trucks these seats can reduce WBV exposure by 50% relative to passive air-suspension seats.[69,70] A random-ized controlled trial that measured WBV expo-sures and health outcomes over a 1-year period demonstrated that truck drivers who received active suspension seats had substantially less WBV exposure and substantially less low back pain, compared to truck drivers who used new industry-standard air-suspension seats.[70]

WBV Standards for Measurement and Regulation of Exposure

The principle used to measure and assess WBV is analogous to those used to for HAV; the WBV exposure is typically expressed as root-mean-squared acceleration. Controlling WBV expo-sure depends on frequency, magnitude, and duration of exposure. Based on ISO standards,[2] measurements are performed in three orthogo-nal directions: up and down, fore and aft, and side to side. ISO standards provide numerical limits for exposure to vibrations transmitted to the human body between 1 and 100 Hz. The most critical frequencies (between 4 and 12 Hz) resonate the spine and several structures and organs in the torso.

Besides the continuous cyclic vibration, impulsive shock exposures are also thought to be of importance, and the ISO 2631-1 WBV standard[2] has a measurement parameter called *vibration dose value*, which is designed to mea-sure impulsive exposures that may be embedded within the cyclical vibration exposures. In addi-tion, there is a second ISO WBV standard, ISO 2631-5,[71] specifically for more accurately charac-terizing the impulsive exposures and the stresses on the spine.

To complement the ISO 2631-1 WBV stan-dard,[2] the European Union adopted a vibration directive,[27] in which companies in the European Union are encouraged to measure their employ-ees' WBV exposures, and, when vibration limits are exceeded, implement either administrative or engineering controls. The European Union regula-tions set a lower daily vibration exposure thresh-old (daily exposure action value = 0.5 m/sec²) and an upper daily vibration exposure threshold (daily exposure limit value = 1.15 m/sec²). When WBV exposures are above the daily exposure action value, employers are encouraged to implement administrative controls, and, when above the daily exposure limit value, engineering controls are preferred, due to the increased health risk associated with the higher exposures.

Health Effects of WBV

The main health effects associated with WBV occur at lower frequencies (2.5 to 30 Hz)—below the mainly higher-frequency vibrations that are associated with HAV-related disorders. Different parts of the human body have different resonant frequencies. Therefore, the response to WBV is complex since amplification or attenuation of WBV will vary in different parts of the body. The resonant frequencies of the structures and organs in the body are weight-dependant—the greater the weight of the structures or organs, the lower the resonant frequencies. The lower vibration frequencies that are characteristic of WBV will mainly resonate the structures and organs in the torso. The most harmful frequency for vertical WBV delivered through the feet (while stand-ing) or buttocks (while sitting) is between 4 and 8 Hz.[72,73] Vibratory frequencies between 6 and 12 Hz generate strong resonance in the vertebrae of the neck and lumbar region, with amplifica-tion of up to 240% above the vibration input at the vehicle operator's seat. These resonant vibra-tions may create chronic stresses and sometimes permanently damage organs or other structures in the torso.[54,55]

In addition to the concerns associated with lower-frequency vibrations, now higher-fre-quency vibrations (>60 Hz) may be of concern for some workers exposed to WBV while stand-ing. Workers exposed to higher-frequency vibra-tion for long periods of time while standing may develop skin blanching in the toes very similar to the finger changes with VWF.[74]

The greatest attention to the harmful effects of WBV in workers has been focused on low back disorders in vehicle operators. The daily action limit for WBV in the vibration directive of the European Union (0.50 m/s²)[27] is often exceeded for vehicle and equipment operators in con-struction, mining, agriculture, and forestry. In contrast, drivers of taxis, police cars, buses, and on-road trucks rarely have WBV exposures that exceed this action limit.

ISO standards on WBV also address comfort, fatigue-decreased proficiency, and acceptable exposure to vibration. The comfort standard applies to situations in which passenger comfort is important, such as on trains, subways, and buses. The fatigue-decreased proficiency standard applies to situations where maintaining a vehicle operator's efficiency is critically important, such as in reading gauges and screens, performing fine manipulation, and maintaining cognitive function. Limits to vibration exposure apply to situations where worker health and safety may be compromised by chronic injuries to the back, neck, and internal organs.

Databases on WBV exposure from industrial vehicles are available online;[75] however, WBV profiles based on relatively new equipment or vehicles can be misleading. The magnitude of WBV exposures in field settings is partially determined by vehicle age and maintenance, terrain, seat and cab design, and presence of other vibrating equipment on or in the vehicle.

Exposure to WBV is not the only factor adversely affecting equipment operators.[76] Awkward sitting postures, often required by drivers, can adversely affect the back. Drivers must also often adopt twisted postures when driving backward and looking to the side and/or behind. Depending on work shift and overtime schedules, drivers may have to work continuously for over 12 hours. Awkward postures, repetition of tasks, long duration of workshift, and forceful exertion are generally considered risk factors for the development of musculoskeletal disorders (see Chapter 20). In addition, poor ergonomic designs of cabs and seats as well as poorly located control gear, such as steering wheels and pedals, can adversely affect drivers. Cab and seat design modification most commonly addresses up-and-down WBV exposures to the spine; however, fore-and-aft and side-to-side WBV exposures also produce adverse health effects.

Finally, there are WBV standards for low-level and/or low-frequency vibration in buildings, trains, and large ships that address health effects that are presumed to be subtle and partly psychological. Vibration in buildings, which can be constant, intermittent, or impulsive, can occur as typical vertical WBV from the floor or, more commonly, as a combination of various gross building movements. Vibration in ships and trains typically consists of undulating rocking and/or rolling motion at very low frequency (less than 1 Hz); it can lead to motion sickness in susceptible individuals.

Prevention and Remediation of WBV

The control of WBV rests mainly on primary prevention and the selection of the appropriate equipment to reduce WBV exposure. For example, in the transportation sector, the evaluation and use of higher-quality, vibration-absorbent "air-ride" seats represents a focus on reducing vertical vibration. However, in off-road applications, more sophisticated seat designs that provide fore-and-aft and side-to-side attenuation, cab isolation, and improvements in vehicle suspension represent a more effective and integrated approach. In the industrial environment, antishock mounting of machinery, remote manipulation, and vibration-isolated cockpits are some examples of protection from vibration. Reducing exposures to WBV can help reduce or prevent back pain. In sum, reducing WBV exposure can reduce the occurrence of various disorders and contribute to workers' health and well-being.

REFERENCES

1. International Organization for Standardization. Mechanical vibration: Measurement and evaluation of human exposure to hand-transmitted vibration. Part 1: General requirements (ISO 5349-1), 2001.
2. International Organization for Standardization. Mechanical vibration and shock—Evaluation of human exposure to whole-body vibration. Part 1: General requirements (ISO 2631-1), 1997.
3. International Organization for Standardization. Mechanical vibration—Measurement and evaluation of human exposure to hand-transmitted vibration. Part 2: Practical guidance for measurement at the workplace (ISO 5349-2), 2001.
4. Griffin MJ. Frequency-dependence of psychophysical and physiological responses to hand-transmitted vibration. Industrial Health 2012; 50: 354–369.
5. Krajnak K, Miller GR, Waugh S, et al. Characterization of frequency-dependent responses of the vascular system to repetitive vibration. Journal of Occupational and Environmental Medicine 2010; 52: 584–594.

6. Bovenzi M. Epidemiological evidence for new frequency weightings of hand-transmitted vibration. Industrial Health 2012; 50: 377–387.

7. Krajnak K, Riley DA, Wu J, McDowell T, et al. Frequency-dependent effects of vibration on physiological systems: Experiments with animals and other human surrogates. Industrial Health 2012; 50: 343–353.

8. Loriga, G. Il lavoro coi martelli pneumatici. Boll. Ispett. Lavoro 1911; 2: 35.

9. Hamilton A. A study of spastic anemia in the hands of stone cutters. Washington, DC: U.S. Bureau of Labor Statistics. 236: Industrial Accidents and Hygiene Series 1918, No. 191, pp. 53–66.

10. National Institute for Occupational Safety and Health. Criteria for a recommended standard—Occupational exposure to hand-arm vibration. Washington, DC: Department of Health and Human Services, #89–106, 1989.

11. Health Safety Executive. Guide to good practice on hand-arm vibration. London: HSE, 2006.

12. Edwards DJ, Golt DG. Hand-arm vibration exposure from construction tools: Results of a field study. Construction Management and Economics 2006; 24: 209–217.

13. Pyykkö I, Korhonen O, Färkkilä M, et al. Vibration syndrome among Finnish forest workers: A follow-up from 1972 to 1983. Scandinavian Journal of Work, Environment & Health 1986; 12: 307–312.

14. Sutinen P, Toppila E, Starck J, et al. Hand-arm vibration syndrome with use of anti-vibration chain saws: 19-year follow-up study of forestry workers. International Archives of Occupational and Environmental Health 2006; 79: 65–71.

15. Gemne G, Pyykko I, Taylor W, Pelmear PL. The Stockholm Workshop scale for the classification of cold-induced Raynaud's phenomenon in the hand-arm vibration syndrome. Scandinavian Journal of Work, Environment and Health 1987; 13: 275–278.

16. Brammer AL, Taylor W, Lundborg G. Sensorineural stages of the hand-arm vibration syndrome. Scandinavian Journal of Work, Environment and Health 1987; 13: 279–283.

17. Koskimies K. Hand grip force among forest workers. Journal of Low Frequency Noise Vibration 1993; 12: 1–7.

18. Gemne G (ed.). Stockholm Workshop 1986. Symptomatology and diagnostic methods in the hand-arm vibration syndrome. Scandinavian Journal of Work, Environment and Health 1987; 13S: 265–388.

19. Koskimies K, Farkkila M, Pyykko I, et al. Carpal tunnel syndrome in vibration disease.

20. Cherniack M, Morse TF, Brammer AJ, et al. Vibration exposure, workplace modification, and disease in a shipyard: A 13-year revisit. American Journal of Industrial Medicine 2004; 45: 500–512.

21. Cherniack M, Brammer AJ, Lundstrom R, et al. The Hand-Arm Vibration International Consortium (HAVIC): Prospective studies on the relationship between power tool exposure and health effects. Journal of Occupational and Environmental Medicine 2007; 49: 289–301.

22. Hagberg M, Lundström R, Nilsson T, et al. Longitudinal epidemiological surveys in Sweden of workers exposed to hand-transmitted vibration. FP5 Project No. QLK4-2002-02650. European Commission Quality of Life and Management of Living Resources Programme. Annex 3 to Final Technical Report, January 7, 2007.

23. Burström L, Knutsson A. A descriptive study of women injured by hand-arm vibration. Annals of Occupational Hygiene 2002; 46: 299–307.

24. Bovenzi M. Longitudinal epidemiological surveys in Italy of workers exposed to hand-transmitted vibration. FP5 Project No. QLK4-2002-02650. European Commission Quality of Life and Management of Living Resources Programme. Annex 2 to Final Technical Report, December 13, 2006.

25. Welcome DE, Dong RG, Xu XS, et al. The effects of vibration-reducing gloves on finger vibration. International Journal of Industrial Ergonomics 2014; 44: 45–59.

26. Welcome DE, Dong RG, Xu XS, et al. Tool-specific performance of vibration-reducing gloves for attenuating fingers-transmitted vibration. Occupational Ergonomics 2016; 13: 23–44.

27. European Agency for Safety and Health at Work. Directive 2002/44/EC- vibration of 25 June 2002 on the minimum health and safety requirements regarding the exposure of workers to the risks arising from physical agents (vibration), June 7, 2002. Available at: https://osha.europa.eu/en/legislation/directives/19. Accessed February 24, 2017.

28. Griffin MJ. Negligent exposures to hand-transmitted vibration. International Archives of Occupational and Environmental Health 2008; 81: 645–659.

29. Starck J. High impulse acceleration levels in hand-held vibratory tools. Scandinavian Journal of Work, Environment & Health 1984; 10: 171–178.

British Journal of Industrial Medicine 1990; 47: 411–416.

30. Dandanell R, Engstrom K. Vibration from riveting tools in the frequency range 6 Hz to 10 MHz and Raynaud's phenomenon. Scandinavian Journal of Work, Environment & Health 1986; 12: 38–42.

31. Griffin M. Measurement, evaluation, and assessment of occupational exposures to hand-transmitted vibration. Occupational and Environmental Medicine 1997: 54: 73–89.

32. Cherniack MG, Mohr SM. Raynaud's phenomenon associated with the use of surgical pneumatic instruments. Journal of Hand Surgery 1994; 19A: 1008–1015.

33. Rytkönen E, Sorainen E, Leino-Arjas P, Solovieva S. Hand-arm vibration exposure of dentists. International Archives of Occupational and Environmental Health 2006; 79: 521–527.

34. Sakakibara H, Hirata M, Hashiguchi T, et al. Affected segments of the median nerve detected by fractionated nerve conduction measurement in vibration-induced neuropathy. Industrial Health 1998; 36: 155–159.

35. Cherniack M, Brammer AJ, Lundstrom R, et al. Segmental nerve conduction velocity in vibration exposed shipyard workers. International Archives of Occupational and Environmental Health 2004; 77: 159–176.

36. Brammer AJ, Piercy JE, Nohara S, et al. Vibrotactile thresholds in operators of vibrating hand-held tools. In: A Okada, W Taylor, H Dupuis (eds.). Hand-arm vibration. Kanazawa, Japan: Kyoei Press, 1990, pp. 221–223.

37. Hyvarinen J, Pyykko I, Sundberg S. Vibration frequencies and amplitudes in the aetiology of traumatic vasospastic diseases. Lancet 1973; 301: 791–794.

38. Olsen N, Hagberg M, Ekenvall L et al. In: Gemne G, Brammer AJ, Hagberg M, et al. (eds.). Proceedings of the Stockholm Workshop 94. Hand-arm vibration syndrome: Diagnostics and quantitative relationships to exposure. National Institute of Occupational Health, Solna, Sweden, May 25–28, 1994. Arb Hälsa 5: 181–186.

39. Boshuizen HC, Bongers PM, Hulshof, CT. Back disorders and occupational exposure to whole body vibration. International Journal of Industrial Ergonomics 1990; 6: 55–59.

40. Bovenzi M, Zadini A. Self-reported low back symptoms in urban bus drivers exposed to whole-body vibration. Spine 1992; 17: 1048–1059.

41. Bovenzi M, Betta A. Low-back disorders in agricultural tractor drivers exposed to whole-body vibration and postural stress. Applied Ergonomics 1994; 25: 231–241.

42. Bernard BP. Musculoskeletal disorders and workplace factors: A critical review of epidemiologic evidence for work-related musculoskeletal disorders of the neck, upper extremity, and low back. DHHS (NIOSH) 1997, Publication No. 97-141.

43. Schwarze S, Notbohm G, Dupuis H, Hartung E. Dose–response relationships between whole-body vibration and lumbar disk disease: A field study on 388 drivers of different vehicles. Journal of Sound Vibration 1998; 215: 613–628.

44. Bovenzi M, Hulshof CTJ. An updated review of epidemiologic studies on the relationship between exposure to whole-body vibration and low back pain (1986–1997). International Archives of Occupational and Environmental Health 1999; 72: 351–365.

45. Bovenzi M. Metrics of whole-body vibration and exposure-response relationship for low back pain in professional drivers: A prospective cohort study. International Archives of Occupational and Environmental Health 2009; 82: 893–917.

46. Burström L, Nilsson T, Wahlström J. Whole-body vibration and the risk of low back pain and sciatica: A systematic review and meta-analysis International Archives of Occupational and Environmental Health 2014; 88: 403–418.

47. Robb MJ, Mansfield NJ. Self-reported musculoskeletal problems amongst professional truck drivers. Ergonomics 2007; 50: 814–827.

48. Bovenzi M, Rui F, Negro C, et al. An epidemiological study of low back pain in professional drivers. Journal of Sound and Vibration 2006; 298: 514–539.

49. Waters T, Genaidy A, Viruet HB, Makola M. The impact of operating heavy equipment vehicles on lower back disorders. Ergonomics 2008; 51: 602–636.

50. Fritz M. Estimation of spine forces under whole-body vibration by means of a biomechanical model and transfer functions. Aviation, Space, and Environmental Medicine 1997; 68: 512–519.

51. Fritz M. Description of the relation between the forces acting in the lumbar spine and whole-body vibrations by means of transfer functions. Clinical Biomechanics 2000; 15: 234–240.

52. Wilder DG, Aleksiev AR, Magnusson ML, et al. Muscular response to sudden load: A tool to evaluate fatigue and rehabilitation. Spine 1996; 21: 2628–2639.

53. Palmer KT, Griffin M, Ntani G, et al Professional driving and prolapsed lumbar intervertebral disc diagnosed by magnetic resonance imaging: A case-control study. Scandinavian Journal of Work, Environment & Health 2012; 38: 577–581.

54. Thalheimer E. Practical approach to measurement and evaluation of exposure to whole-body vibration in the work-place. Seminars in Perinatology 1996; 20: 77–89.

55. Gruber GJ, Ziperman HH. Relationship between whole-body vibration and morbidity patterns among motor coach operators. (DHHS [NIOSH] Publication No 75-104), 1974.

56. Andersson GB. Epidemiological features of chronic low-back pain. Lancet 1999; 354: 581–585.

57. Airaksinen O, Brox JI, Cedraschi C, et al. European guidelines for the management of chronic nonspecific low back pain. European Spine 2006; 15: S192–S300.

58. Lewis CA, Johnson P. Whole-body vibration exposure in metropolitan bus drivers. Occupational Medicine 2012; 62: 519–524.

59. Kim JH, Zigman, M, Aulck LS, et al. Whole body vibration exposures and health status among professional truck drivers: A cross-sectional analysis. Annals of Occupational Hygiene 2016; 60: 936–948.

60. Miyashita K, Morioka I, Tanabe T, et al. Symptoms of construction workers exposed to whole body vibration and local vibration. International Archives of Occupational and Environmental Health 1992; 64: 347–351.

61. Rehn B, Lundstrom R, Nilsson L, et al. Variation in exposure to whole-body vibration for operators of forwarder vehicles—Aspects on measurement strategies and prevention. International Journal of Industrial Ergonomics 2005; 5: 831–842.

62. Smets MPH, Eger TR, Grenier SG. Whole-body vibration experienced by haulage truck operators in surface mining operations: A comparison of various analysis methods utilized in the prediction of health risks. Applied Ergonomics 2010, 41:763–770.

63. Burgess-Limerick R, Lynas D. Long duration measurements of whole-body vibration exposures associated with surface coal mining equipment compared to previous short-duration measurements. Journal of Occupational and Environmental Hygiene 2016; 13: 339–345.

64. Johanning E, Landsbergis P, Fischer S, et al. Whole-body vibration and ergonomic study of US railroad locomotives. Journal of Sound Vibration 2006; 298: 594–600.

65. Bongers PM, Hulshof CT, Dijkstra L, et al. Back pain and exposure to whole body vibration in helicopter pilots. Ergonomics 1990; 33: 1007–1026.

66. Simon-Arndt CM, Yuan H, Hourani LL. Aircraft type and diagnosed back disorders in US Navy pilots and aircrew. Aviation, Space, and Environmental Medicine 1997; 68: 1012–1018.

67. Chaudhary DK, Bhattacherjee A, Patra AK, Chau N. Whole-body vibration exposure of drill operators in iron ore mines and role of machine-related, individual, and rock-related factors. Safety and Health at Work 2015; 6: 268–278.

68. Jonsson PMG, Rynell PW, Hagberg M, Johnson PW. Comparison of whole-body vibration exposures in buses: Effects and interactions of bus and seat design. Ergonomics 2014; 58: 1133–1142.

69. Blood R, Dennerlein J, Lewis L, et al. Evaluating whole-body vibration reduction by comparison of active and passive suspension seats in semi-trucks. Proceedings of the Human Factors and Ergonomics Society's 55th Annual Meeting, 2011, pp. 1750–1754.

70. Johnson PW, Kim JH, Dennerlein J. A randomized controlled trial of new truck seats intended to reduce whole body vibration exposures and low back pain. Proceedings of the Sixth American Conference on Human Vibration, 2016.

71. International Organization for Standardization. Mechanical vibration and shock—Evaluation of human exposure to whole-body vibration—Part 5: Method for evaluation of vibration containing multiple shocks (ISO 2631-5). Geneva: International Organization for Standardization, 2004.

72. Rakhejaa S, Dong RG, Patra S, Boileau PE, Marcotte P, Warren C. Biodynamics of the human body under whole-body vibration: Synthesis of the reported data. International Journal of Industrial Ergonomics 2010; 40: 710–732.

73. Wilder DG. The biomechanics of vibration and low back pain. American Journal of Industrial Medicine 1993; 23: 577–588.

74. Eger T, Thompson A, Leduc M, et al. Vibration induced white-feet: Overview and field study of vibration exposure and reported symptoms in workers. Work 2014; 47: 101–110.

75. Centralized European whole-body vibration database. Available at: http://resource.isvr.soton.ac.uk/HRV/VINET/pdf_files/Appendix_W4B.pdf. Accessed February 24, 2017.

76. Salmon AW, Cann AP, Gillin EK, Eger TR. Case studies in whole-body vibration assessment in the transportation industry–Challenges in the field. International Journal of Industrial Ergonomics 2008; 38: 783–791.

12C

Extremes of Temperature

Ann M. Krake

This chapter describes extremes of temperature, their adverse health effects, evaluation and assessment, and strategies for prevention of heat- and cold-related illnesses and deaths. The appendix at the end of this chapter details physical hazards related to hyperbaric and hypobaric environments and their adverse effects.

HOT ENVIRONMENTS

Public Health and Extreme Heat

CASE 1

An 86-year-old woman was found unresponsive in her bedroom. She had no known medical history, but her grandson reported that she kept her bedroom windows closed for the previous 7 days during a heat wave. She had no fan or air conditioning. Her rectal temperature when she arrived at a hospital was 42.2°C (108°F). She had died of heat stroke.

Heat remains the leading cause of weather-related fatalities. Heat-related illnesses and deaths are expected to increase as hot summer temperatures and heat waves (defined in the northeastern United States as three consecutive days of air temperature 32.2°C [90°F] or greater) become more frequent, longer, and more intense and as the number of older people markedly increases.[1] (See Chapter 29.)

Between 1979 and 2013, more than 9,000 Americans died as a result of heat. The Centers for Disease Control and Prevention has reported an annual average of 658 heat-related deaths in the United States, most from work-related exposures, but also from exposure to excessive heat at home, in vehicles, and in community settings.[2] The actual number is likely much higher because of incomplete or incorrect information on death certificates, which, for example, may not indicate that heat was a contributing cause to a cardiac or respiratory death.[1]

Older people are highly vulnerable to extreme heat because they have a reduced ability to perspire and generally poorer cardiovascular responses (such as reduced skin blood flow and stiffer vessels)—and therefore less ability to release body heat through evaporation, the body's main mechanism for removing heat. Other factors that contribute to heat-related mortality include low socioeconomic status, substandard housing, lack of air conditioning, and inadequate access to healthcare and social services. People with chronic health problems, especially heart disease, or disabilities are more vulnerable to the adverse effects of heat. Also at increased risk are people who are not acclimatized to hot weather, those who overexert themselves, people who live in large cities, obese people, and those who consume alcohol or take certain medications including beta-blockers, anticholinergics (such as antihistamines and parkinsonism medications), sympathomimetics (such as amphetamines and pseudoephedrine), antihypertensives, and diuretics.

Before heat waves occur, public health and emergency response workers should develop preparedness and response plans that focus on identifying and limiting heat exposure of vulnerable populations. During heat waves, community residents should:

- Make daily checks on homebound neighbors, friends, and relatives, especially if they are elderly or disabled
- Encourage those without air-conditioned homes to go to cool places during the hottest parts of the day
- Encourage the drinking of nonalcoholic beverages
- Reduce or eliminate strenuous activities.

In addition, people should never leave children or pets alone in a car, even with the windows open and even on seemingly cool or cloudy days.

Infants and young children are also especially susceptible to heat. Children's bodies have a greater ratio of surface area to body mass, so they absorb more heat on a hot day (and lose heat more rapidly on a cold day). In addition, children have a considerably lower sweating capacity than adults and so are less able to dissipate body heat by evaporative sweating and cooling.

Heat stroke is the leading cause of non-crash vehicle deaths among children.[3] *Forgotten baby syndrome*, the failure to remember there is a child in one's car, is the leading cause of heat stroke in children under the age of 14. Since 1998, an average of 37 children have died annually in the United States as a result of being left, or becoming trapped, in hot vehicles.[4] The windows of a car act like a greenhouse, trapping

sunlight and heat. When the outside temperature is 15°C (59°F), car temperatures can rise well above 43.3°C (110°F). The darker the color of the vehicle interior, the faster and higher the temperature rises.[4]

Parents and policymakers need to be better educated about the dangers of leaving children unattended in vehicles. Most parents are unaware of the danger. Thirty states do not have laws that address leaving children unattended in vehicles; only 10 states have "Good Samaritan" laws that protect people who take action when they see a child in a car. However, there is evidence of progress. In 2015, a child vehicular heat-stroke law was passed in Texas, mandating hospitals to educate new parents on the dangers of hot cars; hospitals now distribute pamphlets and teddy-bear key chains to parents as a reminder that they are not riding alone in their cars.[5]

Occupational Health and Extreme Heat

CASE 2

A male worker, age 56, was harvesting ripe tobacco leaves by hand in North Carolina during his third day on the job. He had come from Mexico on a work visa. Coworkers reported that, during the mid-afternoon, he seemed confused. When they offered to carry him to the shade and have him drink water, he became combative. About 1½ hours after noticing his confusion, they took him to a hospital emergency department. His core body temperature (CBT) was 42.2°C (108°F). Despite treatment, he died. That day, the local high temperature was 34°C (93°F), with 44% relative humidity. Conditions had been similar for the previous 2 days. The man had been given health and safety training on pesticides but not on heat stress.[6]

An estimated 5 million to 10 million people in the United States work in industries where heat stress is a potential health and safety hazard.[7] (See Figures 12C-1 and 12C-2.) In all industries from 1992 to 2008, exposure to environmental heat was documented to have killed at least 488 workers and contact with hot objects or substances killed an additional 189.[8] Between

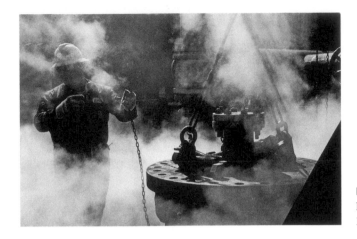

Figure 12C-1. Chemical worker exposed to heat while removing vessel lid. (Photograph by Earl Dotter.)

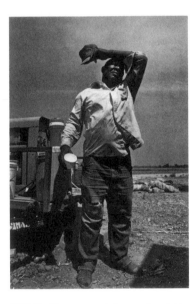

Figure 12C-2. Heat-stressed farmworker taking a water break as the ambient air temperature approached 105°F. (Photograph by Earl Dotter.)

1992 and 2006, the heat-related average annual death rate in the United States for crop workers, who work outdoors with exposure to heat and humidity, was 4 per 1 million workers, almost 20-fold higher than for non-agricultural workers (about 0.2 per 1 million workers).[6] And, partially because worksite conditions and job duties are usually not listed on hospital records or death certificates, occupational heat-related illnesses and fatalities are underestimated.[9]

Heat-related occupational illness and injury occur in situations where total heat load (environmental heat and heat generated by the body's metabolism) exceeds the capacity of the body to maintain normal bodily functions. Increased potential for heat strain comes from high ambient air temperatures, high humidity, strenuous physical activity, radiant heat sources (such as the sun, ovens, and foundry furnaces), and direct physical contact with hot objects. A hot, humid environment, which impedes evaporative cooling, combined with heavy work activity poses the highest risk for workers because the metabolic load placed on the body generates even more heat. However, work in cooler, less strenuous environments can also pose a risk, depending upon one's heat tolerance. Potential health risks of working in heat-stress conditions depend on one's physiology, level of heat acclimatization, and circumstances that allow effective heat exchange, rest, and hydration. In addition, professional expertise and judgment in evaluating heat stress and strain in a work environment provide essential information for preventing heat-related injuries and illnesses in workers.[10]

Heat stress is "the net heat load to which a worker is exposed from the combined contributions of metabolic heat [heat generated by the body], environmental factors, and clothing worn which results in an increase in heat storage in the body."[7] Air temperature and velocity, clothing, physical activity, humidity, and radiation are all contributors to the heat stress that workers experience.

Heat strain, which cannot be reliably predicted from heat stress, is defined as "the physiological response to the heat load (external or internal) experienced by a person, in which the body attempts to increase heat loss to the environment in order to maintain a stable body temperature."[7] Heat strain is unique to each person. Even in the same person with the same exposure, heat strain may be different, depending on the person's current physiological status.[10]

Many bodily responses to heat stress are desirable and beneficial because they help regulate internal temperature and, in situations of appropriate repeated exposure, help the body adapt, or acclimatize, to the work environment. However, at some individually determined stage of heat stress, compensatory measures of the body cannot maintain internal body temperature at a level required for normal functioning. As a result, risks of heat-induced disorders and "accidents" substantially increase.[7]

For normal body function deep-core body temperature must be maintained within the acceptable range of approximately 37°C (98.6°F) + 1°C (1.8°F), which requires a constant exchange of heat between the body and the environment. The amount of heat to be exchanged is a function of heat produced by the body (metabolic heat) and heat gained from the work environment. The rate of heat exchanged with both hot and cold environments is a function of air temperature, humidity, skin temperature, air velocity, evaporation of sweat, radiant temperature, and type, amount, and characteristics of clothing.[7] The basic heat balance equation, which can be used to evaluate both hot and cold situations, is as follows:

$$S = (M - W) \pm C \pm R \pm K - E$$

where S = change in body heat (either loss or gain by the body); (M − W) = heat produced by metabolism minus external work performed; C = convective heat exchange; R = radiative heat exchange; K = conductive heat exchange; and E = body heat lost by evaporation. To calculate the change in body heat (S), measurements of metabolic heat production, air temperature, water-vapor pressure, wind velocity, and mean radiant temperature are required.[7]

The major modes of heat exchange between people and their environments are convection, radiation, and evaporation. *Convection* refers to the rate of heat exchange between the individual's skin and the air immediately around the skin,

if the air is moving. Its value is a function of the difference between the skin and air temperatures and the rate of air movement over the skin. Skin temperature is normally assumed to be 35°C (95°F). Therefore, for a worker wearing a single layer of clothing (long-sleeved work shirt and trousers), an ambient air temperature of greater than 35°C will cause the body to gain heat from the air. In contrast, an ambient air temperature of less than 35°C will cause the body to lose heat into the air by convection.

Conduction, which is the transfer of heat to the skin from direct contact (touch) with hot equipment or floors or from hot liquids, plays a minor role in heat stress other than for brief periods of time when the body may come into contact with such objects. *Radiation*, or radiative heat exchange, also refers to heat that is transferred between the skin and solid surfaces or objects, cold or hot, but without direct skin contact. Working in direct sunlight and fighting fires are examples of radiative heat exposure.

Evaporation of water from the surface of the skin (sweating) is the primary method by which the body regulates internal temperature. Personal protective clothing and equipment can significantly affect regulation of body temperature. (See later discussion.)

Health Effects of Exposure to Hot Environments

CASE 3

A 43-year-old male, who was a new, seasonal park employee on a day off from work, hiked down a trail in Grand Canyon National Park during the hottest part of the day. Although he was carrying water, he had brought nothing to eat. Park rangers found him that evening wandering around a campground "in a state of shock." His pulse was 100 and his oral temperature was 39.2°C (102.6°F). He was treated for hyponatremia (decreased serum sodium) with intravenous fluids, kept under observation overnight, and medically evacuated the following morning. He later reported that when he was told by hikers coming up the trail that there was no water or shade along the 7-mile route, he decided to continue even more quickly to his destination—the campground at Phantom Ranch at the bottom of the canyon on the Colorado River. He noticed that although he was drinking and urinating frequently, his urine became clearer the farther he hiked. When asked why he did not try to cool off by getting into the creek running alongside the campground, he told the rangers he did not think to do that and hardly noticed it was there.

The level of heat stress at which excessive heat strain will result depends upon the heat tolerance capabilities of each individual. A person's sensitivity to heat is affected by age, weight, degree of physical fitness, degree of acclimatization, metabolism, level of hydration, use of alcohol or drugs, and medical conditions such as hypertension and diabetes. At greatest risk are:

- Unacclimatized people
- People performing physically strenuous work
- Those with previous heat illness
- Older people
- People with cardiovascular or circulatory disorders
- Those taking medications that impair cooling mechanisms of the body
- People who abuse alcohol or are recovering from recent use
- People in poor cardiovascular fitness
- Those recovering from illness
- Dehydrated individuals.

Heat disorders and adverse health effects of people exposed to hot work environments include, in increasing order of severity, irritability, lack of judgment and loss of critical thinking skills, skin disorders (such as heat rashes and hives), heat syncope (fainting), heat cramps, heat exhaustion, and heat stroke. Heat syncope happens when blood flow is directed to the skin for cooling, resulting in decreased supply to the brain, and most often strikes workers who stand in place for extended periods in hot environments. Heat cramps, caused by sodium depletion due to sweating, typically occur in the muscles employed in strenuous work. Heat cramps and syncope often accompany (a) heat exhaustion, or (b) weakness, fatigue, confusion, nausea, and

other symptoms that generally prevent a return to work for at least 24 hours to give the individual time to replenish lost electrolytes and body water. A CBT increase of only 1°C (1.8°F) above normal can adversely affect brain function. As heat-stress levels rise, so do the risks of "accidents" and injuries.[11] The dehydration, sodium loss, and CBT above 38°C (100.4°F) due to heat exhaustion usually result from performing strenuous work in hot conditions with inadequate water and electrolyte intake. Heat exhaustion may lead to heat stroke if the affected person is not quickly cooled and rehydrated.

While *heat exhaustion* victims continue to sweat as their bodies struggle to stay cool, *heat stroke* victims usually stop sweating as their bodies fail to maintain an appropriate core temperature. Heat stroke is defined as either *classic* or *exertional*, depending upon the characteristics of the individual (age and health status), type of activity (strenuous or sedentary), and whether the affected person has dry skin or is sweating. Exertional heat stroke is more common in work environments and occurs when hard work, hot environment, and dehydration overload the capacity of the body to cool itself. This thermoregulatory failure is a life-threatening emergency that requires immediate medical attention. Signs and symptoms include irritability, confusion, nausea, convulsions or unconsciousness, hot wet or dry skin, and a CBT above 40.6°C (105°F). Death can result from damage to the brain, heart, liver, or kidneys.[10] Because many workers have been incorrectly taught they are not in danger of heat stroke if they are still sweating, they need to be re-educated about symptoms.[7]

Prolonged increase in CBT and chronic exposures to high levels of heat stress are associated with disorders, such as temporary infertility in both men and women,[7] increased heart rate, sleep disorders, fatigue, irritability, kidney stones, and serious gastrointestinal disease. *Rhabdomyolysis* (the breakdown of muscle tissue), which can be caused by a very high body temperature, often results in permanent disability. Muscle tissue can be damaged or die when overheated or overexerted and then circulate in the blood, causing potentially fatal heart or kidney disorders. The case-fatality rate may be as high as 8%.[7] During the first trimester of pregnancy, a sustained CBT greater than 39°C (102.2°F) may endanger the fetus. In addition, one or more occurrences of heat-induced illness predisposes a person to subsequent heat-related injuries and can result in temporary or permanent loss of ability to tolerate heat stress.[7,12]

Acclimatization

Acclimatization is a low-cost, effective way to improve the safety, comfort, and productivity of employees in heat-stress situations.[10] It allows workers to withstand heat stress with a reduction in heat strain by a series of physiological adaptations. Acclimatized individuals perspire more abundantly and more uniformly over their body surface and start to sweat earlier than unacclimatized individuals, resulting in lower CBT and less cardiovascular strain. In addition, plasma volume is increased in acclimatized individuals, and they can therefore withstand greater water loss from sweating.[13]

Acclimatizing to a job with heat stress by working at even a moderate rate brings about physiological changes that lead to improved safety and comfort for healthy workers. Exposure to heat only, however, will not bring about sufficient acclimatization needed for the combination of heat and physically demanding work; an elevated metabolic rate, such as occurs during work activities, is also required. The ability of a worker to tolerate heat stress requires adequate cardiac, pulmonary, and renal function. It also requires adequate function of the heat-loss thermoregulatory mechanism (modulation of skin blood flow and sweat) and the body's ability to balance fluids and electrolytes. Impairment or reduction of any of these functions may interfere with a worker's capacity to acclimatize to heat or, once acclimatized, to perform strenuous work in the heat.[7] Acclimatization at a certain temperature and work load is effective only for those conditions; a person exposed to higher levels of heat stress will not be fully acclimatized at that level—only to the lower level.[10] About 5% of workers may not be able to acclimatize to heat stress adequately to work under extreme heat exposure.[7]

The effects of acclimatization can begin with as little as 30 minutes of daily physical activity for 1 week. Rapid changes within the first few days provide most of the benefits of lower CBT, skin temperature, and heart rate; a faster onset of sweating; and increased sweat production. Further improvements in water and electrolyte management in the body occur during the second and third weeks. Figure 12C-3 shows a typical acclimatization schedule for workers during a 10-hour shift.

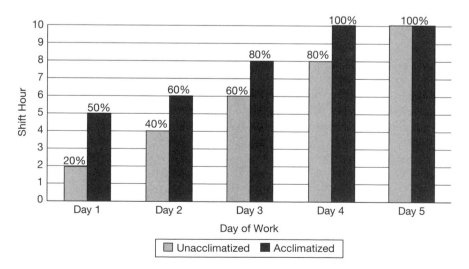

Figure 12C-3. Work schedule for heat acclimatized and unacclimatized employees. (Based on a 10-hour shift.) (Source: Adapted from National Institute for Occupational Safety and Health. Criteria for a recommended standard: Occupational exposure to heat and hot environments (DHHS [NIOSH] Publication No. 2016-106). Cincinnati, OH: NIOSH, 2016.)

Although heat acclimatization for most individuals begins early during work in the heat, it is also quickly lost if the exposure is discontinued. The loss of acclimatization begins when the activity under heat-stress conditions is discontinued, with a noticeable loss occurring after only 4 days. This loss is usually rapidly made up, so that by Tuesday, workers who were not working on the previous weekend are as well acclimatized as they were on the preceding Friday. However, if there is no exposure to heat stress for 1 to 2 weeks, full acclimatization can require up to an additional 3 weeks of continued physical activity under heat-stress conditions similar to those anticipated for the work.[10] A worker's capacity to acclimatize may be reduced by chronic illness, the use or misuse of pharmacologic agents, a sleep deficit, a suboptimal nutritional state, or a disturbed water and electrolyte balance. In addition, an acute episode of mild illness, especially if it includes fever, vomiting, respiratory impairment, or diarrhea, may cause abrupt, transient loss of acclimatization.[7]

Acclimatization alone, however, should never be relied on to manage working in a heat-stress environment. Adequate rest and rehydration are always necessary (Table 12C-1).

Evaluating and Assessing Heat Stress

In an attempt to understand a worker's level of heat-stress exposure, one must evaluate how the *combination* of environmental conditions, work demands, and clothing requirements affect an individual's ability to maintain thermal equilibrium.[10] Assessing heat stress in workers involves measuring the environmental contributions to heat stress at the work location, assessing metabolic work rates for each task, and adjusting for clothing factors.

The wet-bulb globe temperature (WBGT) index, most commonly used to assess the environmental contribution to heat stress, is a simple approximation of the combined effects of air movement, temperature, humidity, and radiative heat.[7] It gives an indication of how a worker feels or perceives the work environment. The WBGT is a function of dry bulb (ambient air) temperature, natural wet bulb temperature (which simulates the effect of evaporative cooling), and black globe temperature (which estimates radiant, or infrared, heat load). Individual and task metabolic rates can be estimated using the table on "Comparison of WBGT Exposure Limits for Acclimatized Workers" in *Occupational Exposure to Heat and Hot Environments*,[7] a NIOSH criteria document,

Table 12C-1. Screening Criteria for TLV® and Action Limit for Heat-Stress Exposure

Allocation of Work in a Cycle of Work and Recovery	TLV® (WBGT Values in °C)				Action Limit (WBGT Values in °C)			
	Light	Moderate	Heavy	Very Heavy	Light	Moderate	Heavy	Very Heavy
75 to 100%	31.0	28.0	–	–	28.0	25.0	–	–
50 to 75%	31.0	29.0	27.5	–	28.5	26.0	24.0	–
25 to 50%	32.0	30.0	29.0	28.0	29.5	27.0	25.5	24.5
0 to 25%	32.5	31.5	30.5	30.0	30.0	29.0	28.0	27.0

Notes. Wet-bulb globe temperature (WBGT) values are expressed to the nearest 0.5°C.

The thresholds are computed as a time-weighted average (TWA)-metabolic rate, where the metabolic rate for rest is taken as 115 W and work is a representative mid-range value. The time base is taken as the proportion of work at the upper limit of the percent work range (such as 50% for the range of 25% to 50%).

If work and rest environments are different, hourly TWAs should be calculated and used. TWAs for work rates should also be used when the work demands vary within the hour, but note that the metabolic rate for rest is already factored into the screening limit.

Values in this table are applied by reference to the "Work-Rest Regimen" section of the Documentation and assume 8-hour workdays in a 5-day workweek with conventional breaks, as discussed in the Documentation (reference 10). When workdays are extended, consult the "Application of the TLV®" section of the Documentation.

Because of the physiological strain associated with heavy and very heavy work among less fit workers, regardless of WBGT, criteria values are not provided for continuous work and not provided for up to 25% rest in an hour for very heavy work. The screening criteria are not recommended, and a detailed analysis and/or physiological monitoring should be used.

This table is intended as an initial screening tool to evaluate whether a heat stress situation may exist and, thus, the table is more protective than the TLV® or Action Limit. Because the values are more protective, they are not intended to prescribe work and recovery periods.

Source: From ACGIH®, 2017 TLVs® and BEIs® Book. Copyright 2017, p. 238. Reprinted with permission.

or by using the metabolic rate categories table of ACGIH.[14] In addition, the ACGIH publication *Heat Stress and Strain: Documentation of the TLV (2009 Supplement)* is an excellent resource on the proper use, limitations, and accuracy of the WBGT monitor.[10]

Many heat-stress guidelines have been developed to protect people from heat-related illnesses. The objective of any heat-stress index is to prevent the CBT from rising excessively. Core body temperature should not exceed 38°C (100.4°F), and oral temperature should not exceed 37.5°C (99.5°F) in prolonged daily exposure to heavy work and/or heat.[11] A CBT of 39°C (102.2°F) should lead to termination of exposure, even when CBT is being monitored. This does not mean that a worker with a CBT exceeding these levels will necessarily experience adverse health effects; however, above these levels, the rate of unsafe acts committed by workers increases as does the risk of illness from heat stress.

The Occupational Safety and Health Administration (OSHA) does not have a specific heat-stress standard; however, exposure to heat stress is enforced by the Secretary of Labor under the General Duty Clause of the OSH Act. The OSHA technical manual[12] provides investigation guidelines that approximate those found in the 2017 ACGIH publication *Threshold Limit Values (TLVs) for Chemical Substances and Physical Agents and Biological Exposure Indices.*[14]

NIOSH recommends that total heat exposure be controlled so that unprotected healthy workers, who are medically and physically fit for their required level of activity and are wearing, at most, long-sleeved work shirts and trousers or equivalent, are not exposed to conditions exceeding the applicable NIOSH criteria. Almost all healthy employees, working in hot environments and exposed to combinations of environmental and metabolic heat less than the NIOSH recommended action limits for unacclimatized workers or the NIOSH recommended exposure limits for acclimatized workers, should be able to tolerate total heat stress without substantially increasing their risk of incurring acute adverse health effects.[7]

ACGIH guidelines require the use of a decision-making process that provides step-by-step situation-dependent instructions that

factor in clothing insulation values and physiological evaluation of heat strain (Figure 12C-4). ACGIH WBGT screening criteria (Table 12C-1) factor in the ability of the body to cool itself (considering clothing insulation value, humidity, and air movement), and, like the NIOSH criteria, can be used to develop work/rest regimens for acclimatized and unacclimatized employees. The ACGIH WBGT-based heat exposure assessment was developed for a traditional work uniform of long-sleeved shirt and pants. It represents conditions under which nearly all adequately hydrated, unmedicated, healthy workers can be repeatedly exposed without adverse health effects. Clothing insulation values and the appropriate WBGT adjustments, as well as descriptors of the other decision-making process components, can be found in *Threshold Limit Values for Chemical Substances and Physical Agents and Biological Exposure Indices* by ACGIH.[14] The ACGIH TLV for heat stress attempts to provide a framework for the control only of heat-related disorders. Although the rates of "accidents" and injuries can increase with increasing levels of heat stress, the TLVs are not directed toward controlling them.

NIOSH and ACGIH criteria can only be used when WBGT data for the immediate work area are available, and they must not be used when encapsulating suits or garments that are impermeable or highly resistant to water vapor or air movement are worn. Further assumptions regarding work demands include an 8-hour workday, 5-day workweek, two 15-minute breaks, and a 30-minute lunch break, with rest area temperatures the same as, or less than, those in work areas and "at least some air movement." NIOSH and ACGIH guidelines do not establish a fine line between safe and dangerous levels but, to ensure protection in each situation, require professional judgment and a heat-stress management program.

Evaluating and Assessing Heat Strain

It is impossible to predict in any given environment who will suffer heat strain from excessive heat stress. However, knowing what to look for and how to intercede can prevent injuries and save lives. Supervisors and workers must be educated on (a) risk factors for, and early warning

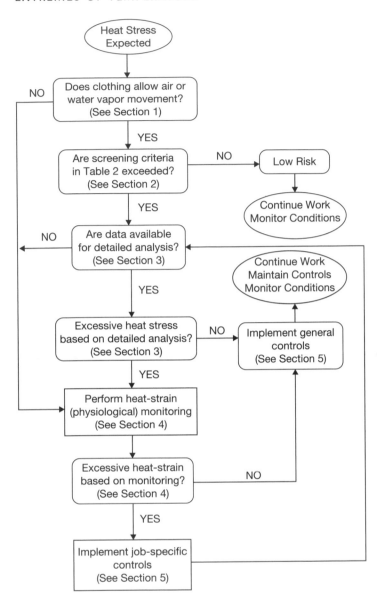

Figure **12C-4.** Algorithm for evaluating heat stress and strain. (Source: ACGIH®, 2017 TLVs® and BEIs® [Copyright 2017], p. 235. Reprinted with permission.)

signs and symptoms of, heat strain and (b) how to monitor themselves and coworkers. Knowing the signs and symptoms of heat strain is the best way to prevent heat-related illnesses. The presence of one symptom deserves attention; the presence of two or more symptoms requires intervention.

Physiological monitoring for heat strain is necessary when impermeable clothing is worn or when heat-stress screening criteria are exceeded. Sustained peak heart rate, an indicator of physiological strain, is considered by ACGIH to be the best sign of acute, high-level exposure

to heat stress. Sustained peak heart rate, defined by ACGIH as 180 beats per minute (bpm) minus an individual's age, is a leading indicator that thermal regulatory control may not be adequate and that an increase in core temperature has occurred, or will soon, occur. Sustained peak heart rate represents an equivalent cardiovascular demand of about 75% of maximum aerobic capacity. During an 8-hour work shift, even if sustained peak demands do not occur, there may still be excessive demand placed on the cardiovascular system. These "chronic" demands can be measured by calculating the average heart rate over the shift. Decreases in physical job performance have been observed when the average heart rate exceeds 115 bpm over the entire shift. This level is equivalent to working at approximately 35% of maximum aerobic capacity, a level sustainable for 8 hours.

An individual's heat-stress exposure should be discontinued when any of the following excessive heat strain indicators occur: (a) for those with normal cardiac performance, heart rate is sustained for several minutes over 180 bpm minus the individual's age in years; (b) CBT is greater than 38.0°C (100.4°F) for unselected, unacclimatized workers and greater than 38.5°C (101.3°F) for medically fit, heat-acclimatized workers; (c) recovery heart rate 1 minute after a peak work effort exceeds 110 bpm; or (d) there are symptoms of sudden and severe fatigue, confusion, nausea, dizziness, lightheadedness, or the sensation of a pounding pulse within the body. An individual may be at greater risk of heat strain if (a) profuse sweating is sustained over several hours, (b) weight loss over a shift is greater than 1.5% of body weight, or (c) 24-hour urinary sodium excretion is less than 55 millimoles.

A variety of equipment is available for monitoring heat strain in an individual. One of the simplest devices is a standard body-weight scale. Employees should weigh themselves fully clothed, without equipment belts, just before starting a shift and again, wearing the same clothing, just before ending a shift; however, one should recognize that sweat-loaded clothing will adversely affect the validity of this measurement. Weight loss over the shift (hydration status) can then be calculated by subtracting postshift weight from preshift weight and dividing that total by preshift weight. Multiplying by 100 gives percentage body weight lost or gained. Weight loss should not exceed 1.5% of total body weight in a workday. If it does, fluid and food intake should be increased until a return to baseline is achieved.

A simple and inexpensive method for monitoring heat strain is to use a heart-rate monitor. Measurements should be taken at appropriate intervals (that is, 15 to 30 minutes) covering at least a full 2-hour period during the hottest parts of the day and again at the end of the day to ensure a return to baseline.[7]

There are also currently two methods of monitoring internal (core) body temperature—but they are practical only for research purposes. Both involve swallowing a disposable sensor that sends a signal to a direct-readout data logger that is worn by the worker. One sensor incorporates a crystal that vibrates in direct proportion to the worker's CBT, while the other is a thermistor-based system. Both offer radio-frequency capabilities and can monitor CBT and heart rate in multiple workers within a direct line of sight. Both systems are fairly costly, and users should be familiar with the limitations of the equipment prior to use with employees. In addition, when considering use of this equipment, one should remember that most heat-related illnesses may result with little or no increase in CBT and that problems can arise sooner than an increase in CBT is recognized. Most heat strain occurs because, at some point during heat exposure, the body is limited in its ability to distribute and store heat. Heat strain can occur without the body experiencing hyperthermia -- when the body is not able to maintain thermal equilibrium.

Preventing Heat Stress and Heat Strain

Preventing heat stress and heat strain is the best method of keeping workers safe. Keeping workers fully hydrated is critically important. Where sweat production may reach 6 to 8 liters in a workday, voluntary replacement of water lost in the sweat is usually incomplete unless water is readily available and accessible. The thirst mechanism is generally sensitive enough to drive an individual to drink enough to prevent dehydration. However, thirst should not be exclusively relied upon for adequate water replacement, so workers in hot work environments are encouraged to regularly drink water or other fluids that ideally are less than 15°C (59°F). Work requiring higher levels of activity in hot environments for longer than 2 hours can lead to a loss of electrolytes (from sweating) and hyponatremia from excessive consumption of plain water without eating. Sports drinks containing carbohydrates and electrolytes should be provided.[7]

Prevention always requires professional judgment that considers both environmental conditions and personal risk factors. Administratively, employers can (a) evaluate ways to reduce the physical demands of the work, (b) ensure that new workers and those returning from an absence of 4 or more days begin with only 20% of the workload on the first day and increase incrementally by no more than 20% each subsequent day, and (c) limit work for hot jobs to morning and evening hours and/or institute work/rest regimens in accordance with NIOSH, OSHA, or ACGIH guidelines. Employers should require workers to use a buddy system, ensure all supervisors and workers are trained in recognizing symptoms of heat strain, and institute preplacement and periodic medical surveillance exams that include testing of aerobic capacity and assessing mental and physical qualifications. Those with low heat tolerance or poor physical fitness should be excluded from hot jobs. Continuing education programs can provide workers with information on the hazards of heat stress, awareness of its symptoms, and the dangers of using energy drinks, drugs, and alcohol while working in hot and physically demanding environments. Workers should be allowed to acclimatize to a hot work environment, which may require additional staffing for the same job until all workers are acclimatized. Note that in especially harsh job and environmental climates, such as those in construction and agriculture in the southern and western U.S. states, where long hours in extreme WBGT conditions prevail, the capacity to protect workers is a serious challenge. For example, temperatures and working conditions may require alternating work and rest periods, with the duration of the rest period being as long as three times the duration of the work period—which realistically will not be tolerated by most employers. It is therefore vital that other mitigation measures discussed here are taught, implemented, and enforced, including use of a buddy system, pre- and postshift weighing, and heart-rate monitoring. In addition to regularly scheduled breaks, employers and supervisors must allow employees to take breaks when they feel they need to, thereby self-limiting their exposure.

Employees can help themselves by ensuring that they are well-hydrated, well-nourished, and not sleep-deprived. Those working in hot, dry environments will also benefit from soaking their

clothing with water before and during their shift to aid in evaporative cooling. Equipment such as an ice vest or a capillary cooling system, which can be worn either under air- and vapor-impermeable protective suits or with regular workclothes, will help keep workers cooler during specific short-term, high-intensity tasks; however, use of this equipment may only be practical in some industrial environments, but generally not in agricultural work environments. A comprehensive heat-stress management program that includes an emergency action plan for severe heat illness can prevent heat strain in all work environments.

COLD ENVIRONMENTS

CASE 3

One January day, the frozen body of a 93-year-old man was found by neighbors who became concerned when they saw the windows of his house icing over. Four days before, the local utility company had installed on his electric meter a "limiter," which restricts the amount of electricity a house can use, because he had not paid his electric bills. After the limiter was installed, a cold front settled over the area, dropping temperatures to −24°C (−11.2°F).

Hypothermia (abnormally low body temperature) causes approximately 700 deaths a year in the United States, half of which occur in people age 65 and older.[15] Like hyperthermia, hypothermia is always preventable. Yet dozens of people freeze to death every winter, especially during exceptionally cold periods. Those most at risk include older people who live in inadequately heated structures and homeless people. In the United States between 2003 and 2014, approximately 13,500 people died as a result of exposure to excessive natural cold. Of those who died of hypothermia, 67% were men. Death rates were highest among older people. Of all the deaths, 10% were attributed to alcohol or drug intoxication. A study conducted in Wisconsin, where 27 hypothermia deaths occurred in early 2014, found that 67% of those who died were found outdoors. Of those found indoors, 15% resided in homes with unused or nonfunctional furnaces. Among those who died,

56% lived alone and 7% were homeless. In addition, 19% had a history of mental illness.[16]

Occupational Cold Stress

CASE 4

During construction of the Alaskan pipeline, a man was killed because of the cold-weather clothing he was wearing. The worker had tunnel vision and impaired hearing because of his wool cap and fur-lined hood. As a result, he failed to see a pickup truck that backed over him. Had he not been wearing a bulky parka, he may have escaped with only minor injuries, but his clothing got entangled in the truck's drive shaft, and he was quickly crushed. One of the lessons of this incident is that failing to manage and properly use personal protective equipment can do more harm than good; ideally *every* hazard is considered and mitigated on the job.[17]

Occupational illness, injury, and reduced productivity related to cold stress result from (a) net body heat loss (decrease in CBT) or (b) heat loss from limbs, feet, hands, or head. Workers in agriculture, transportation, oil and gas extraction, construction, warehousing, food production, and utilities, and especially those who work outdoors, as open-water divers, and in cold storage, are at increased risk of the adverse effects of cold stress.

Workers' compensation claims for cold injury reflect the expected association between environmental factors and cold injuries. The highest rates of cold injury occur in the oil and gas industry; trucking and warehousing; protective services; interurban and local transportation; electric, gas, and sanitation; auto sales, service, and repair; food and related products industries; and heavy construction. Most workers with cold injury are men under age 35 who do "routine outdoor work."[18] Cold injuries correlate with periods of extreme cold. As wind speed increases, the rate of cold injury increases.

Heat loss occurs in the following ways: (a) radiation (up to 65%), (b) conduction (up to 15% but greater in cold water where body heat is lost up to 25 times faster), (c) convection (as the wind increases), (d) respiration, and (e) evaporation. Rates of heat loss by respiration and evaporation

depend on the ambient temperature and relative humidity.[19] Working conditions of low temperatures, high winds, wet clothes, or wet body pose the highest risk of causing cold-stress injuries and illnesses. However, hypothermia can result even when air temperatures are above freezing or whenever water temperature is below normal body temperature: 37°C (98.6°F).

The CBT of a worker must remain within 1% to 4% of normal body temperature—no lower than 36°C (96.8°F)—the temperature at which the metabolic rate increases in an attempt to compensate for heat loss and a temperature slightly above the point at which maximal shivering begins. For single occupational exposures, a drop in CBT to no lower than 35°C (95°F) is permissible under ACGIH guidelines.[19] However, CBT is maintained at the expense of other parts of the body, as peripheral blood flow decreases to reduce heat lost from the skin's surface. Therefore, extra care must be taken to protect arms and legs from discomfort and damage.

Health Effects of Exposure to Cold Environments

As with hyperthermia, workers exposed to cold environments often are slow to recognize they are in danger. Hypothermia can lead to carelessness and disorientation especially in those who are not regularly exposed to cold weather and are distracted by other job hazards.[17] Workers beginning to experience hypothermia may shiver and stomp their feet. They may lose coordination, have slurred speech, and fumble hand-held items. As body temperature continues to fall, these symptoms will worsen and shivering will stop. Workers may become unable to walk or stand.

Exposure to a cold environment causes intense stimulation of the sympathetic nervous system, which results in reduced heat loss through the skin (vasoconstriction) and often pain and numbness of fingers and toes. The most common nonfreezing cold injuries are chilblains (pernio) and immersion (trench) foot. With chilblains, repetitive exposure to drier temperatures just above freezing to as high as 16°C (60°F) causes damage to the capillary beds in the skin. This damage is permanent and the redness and itching, which typically occur on cheeks, ears, fingers, and toes, will return with additional exposure. Trench foot, which can progress to gangrene, is caused from repetitive exposure to a cold, wet environment above the freezing point, conditions common to commercial fishing, for example. Symptoms include tingling or itching, burning, swelling, and, in more extreme cases, blisters.[20] *Frostbite*, which occurs when the skin tissue falls below 0°C (32°F), can occur when workers touch cold metal or chemicals or wear constrictive clothing or shoes. Frostbite, which can be superficial or deep, is classified in degrees, ranging from redness and numbness (first degree) to frostbite affecting bone and muscle (fourth degree).[15] Freezing in deeper layers of tissue causes the affected area to look waxy and pale and feel hard to the touch.

If exposure to cold continues and CBT falls to around 36°C (96.8°F), metabolic rate, the respiratory rate, pulse, and blood pressure increase in an attempt to maintain homeostasis. At a CBT of 35°C (95°F), maximal shivering occurs and physical work and mental processes are impaired. Workers should be removed from the environment when shivering, the most inefficient way of producing heat, becomes evident.[19] Severe hypothermia results if CBT falls below 33°C (91.4°F). Consciousness becomes clouded and progressively lost, respiration and pulse decrease, and blood pressure falls and becomes difficult to measure. The skin becomes cold and may turn bluish. When CBT reaches 28°C (82.4°F), loss of consciousness, little or no breathing, and ventricular fibrillation may occur. Worker fatalities from exposure to cold have almost always resulted from failure to escape from environments with low temperature of air or water.[19]

Workers at greatest risk of cold stress are older workers, those with cardiovascular disorders, and those taking medications that interfere with body temperature regulation or reduce tolerance to working in the cold. The danger of hypothermia is also increased in people who use alcohol and other depressants of the central nervous system. Workers routinely exposed to temperatures below −25°C (−13°F) at wind speeds greater than 2 m/sec (5 mph) or air temperatures below −18°C (0.4°F) at wind speeds less than 2 m/sec (5 mph) should be medically qualified for work in such environments. Employees suffering from diseases or taking medication that interferes with body temperature regulation or reduces the

tolerance for cold work should be excluded from working at or below −1°C (30.2°F).[19]

Assessing the Cold Work Environment

Whenever environmental temperatures are expected to go below 16°C (60.8°F), the air temperature should be monitored, and workers performing barehanded tasks for more than 20 minutes should be provided with ways to warm their hands. These may include radiant heaters or warm air jets. When they fall below −1°C (30.2°F), air temperatures should be monitored at least every 4 hours and metal tool handles and control bars should be wrapped in insulating material. Wind speed should also be monitored when it exceeds 2 m/sec (5 mph) or whenever air temperatures drop below −1°C. Workers should be provided with anticontact gloves, such as those made of silk, to prevent contact frostbite from surfaces that are less than −7°C (19.4°F).

Workers in an environment that is continually at or below −7°C (19.4°F) should be provided a work-warming regimen. Table 12C-2 is an example of a work/warm-up schedule for a 4-hour work shift. Heated shelters stocked with warm, noncaffeinated drinks and food should be readily available. Workers should remove their outer layers of clothing while in the shelter. (The work rate should not be so high that heavy sweating results; however, dry clothing should be available if necessary to prevent a return to the work environment in wet clothing.)

Preventing Cold-Related Injuries

Cold-related injuries can be prevented by developing and using a cold-weather management plan. Plans may include scheduling maintenance and repair jobs during warmer weather or warmer parts of the day; reducing physical demands; using relief workers or assigning extra workers for long, demanding jobs; monitoring workers who are at risk of cold stress; and providing cold-weather training that includes information about risks, prevention, symptoms, monitoring, and personal protective equipment.[21]

Protective clothing is the most important way to avoid cold stress. The following

Table 12C-2. Threshold Limit Values (TLVs) Work/Warm-up Schedule for a 4-Hour Shift

Air Temperature, Sunny Sky		No Noticeable Wind		5 mph Wind		10 mph Wind		15 mph Wind		20 mph Wind	
°C (approx.)	°F (approx.)	Max. Work Period	No. of Breaks	Max. Work Period	No. of Breaks	Max. Work Period	No. of Breaks	Max. Work Period	No. of Breaks	Max. Work Period	No. of Breaks
−26° to −28°	−15° to −19°	(Norm. breaks)	1	(Norm. breaks)	1	75 min	2	55 min	3	40 min	4
−29° to −31°	−20° to −24°	(Norm. breaks)	1	75 min	2	55 min	3	40 min	4	30 min	5
−32° to −34°	−25° to −29°	75 min	2	55 min	3	40 min	4	30 min	5	Non-emergency Work should cease	
−35° to −37°	−30° to −34°	55 min	3	40 min	4	30 min	5	Non-emergency Work should cease			
−38° to −39°	−35° to −39°	40 min	4	30 min	5	Non-emergency Work should cease					
−40° to −42°	−40° to −44°	30 min	5	Non-emergency Work should cease							
−43° and below	−45° and below	Non-emergency Work should cease									

Notes.
- Schedule applies to any 4-hour work period with moderate to heavy work activity, with warm-up periods of 10 minutes in a warm location. For light to moderate work (limited physical movement), apply the schedule one step lower. For example, at −35°C (−30°F) with no noticeable wind (Step 4), a worker at a job with little physical movement should have a maximum work period of 40 minutes with 4 breaks in a 4-hour period (Step 5).
- The following is suggested as a guide for estimating wind velocity if accurate information is not available: 5 mph—light flag moves; 10 mph—light flag fully extended; 15 mph—raises newspaper sheet; 20 mph—blowing and drifting snow.
- If only the wind-chill cooling rate is available, a general rule of thumb for applying it rather than the temperature and wind velocity factors given above are (a) special warm-up breaks should be initiated at a wind-chill cooling rate of about 1,750 W/m² and (b) all non-emergency work should have ceased at or before a wind chill of 2,250 W/m². In general, the warm-up schedule provided above slightly undercompensates for the wind at the warmer temperatures, assuming acclimatization and clothing appropriate for winter work. On the other hand, the chart slightly overcompensates for the actual temperatures in the colder ranges, because windy conditions rarely prevail at extremely low temperatures.
- Threshold limit values apply only for workers in dry clothing.

Source: From ACGIH®, 2016 TLVs® and BEIs® Book. Copyright 2016, p. 210. Reprinted with permission.

are recommendations for working in cold environments:

- Wear at least three layers of clothing:
  1. An outer layer, like Gortex or nylon, to break the wind and allow some ventilation
  2. A middle layer of down or wool to absorb sweat and provide insulation even when wet
  3. An inner layer of cotton or synthetic weave to allow ventilation
- Wear a hat. Up to 40% of body heat can be lost when the head is left exposed
- Wear insulated boots or other footwear
- Keep a change of dry clothing available in case workclothes become wet
- Do not wear tight clothing; loose clothing allows better ventilation.

The thirst mechanism is usually not strong enough to drive an individual to drink enough to replace the water lost in sweat, especially when the temperature is cold, so workers should take care not to become dehydrated. As in hot weather, workers should drink plenty of liquids and avoid energy drinks, drugs, and alcohol. Workers should also take frequent breaks out of the cold, avoid fatigue, and consume warm, high-calorie food to maintain energy reserves. As with heat stress, supervisors should enforce appropriate work schedules and allow workers to interrupt their work if they express extreme discomfort.

When temperatures in the work environment are at or below −12°C (10.4°F), workers should pair up or be under constant protective observation. Workers new to the environment should be allowed to acclimatize. They should not be required to work full time in the cold during the first few days of work while they adjust to the conditions and protective clothing.[19]

Workers should also be educated about symptoms of cold-related illnesses and should be encouraged to seek shelter and medical attention if they or fellow workers experience pain, numbness or tingling, severe shivering, or drowsiness. In general, workers who are provided with insulated protective clothing, assigned to work in areas where drafts and wet conditions are minimized, and given adequate breaks with access to a warm shelter and food are far less likely to suffer adverse health effects from exposure to cold.

REFERENCES

1. Environmental Protection Agency. Climate change indicators in the United States: Heat-related deaths. Updated June 2015. Available at: www.epa.gov/climatechange/indicators. Accessed September 28, 2016.
2. Centers for Disease Control and Prevention. Heat-related deaths after an extreme heat event—four states, 2012, and United States, 1999–2009. Morbidity and Mortality Weekly Report 2013; 62: 433–436.
3. National Highway Transportation Safety Administration. Consumer advisory: Parents and caregivers reminded that summer heat makes it especially dangerous to leave children in cars. June 2010. Available at: http://www.nhtsa.gov/About+NHTSA/Press+Releases/2010/Consumer+Advisory:+Parents+and+Caregivers+Reminded+Never+to+Leave+Children+in+Cars. Accessed September 28, 2016.
4. Null J. Heatstroke deaths of children in vehicles. Updated October 31, 2016. Department of Meteorology and Climate Science, San Jose State University. Available at: http://noheatstroke.org/. Accessed September 28, 2016.
5. Pelletierre N. "Forgotten baby syndrome": A parent's nightmare of hot car death. July 14, 2016. Available at: https://gma.yahoo.com/forgotten-baby-syndrome-why-parents-forget-kids-hot-113304573--abc-news-parenting.html#. Accessed July 15, 2016.
6. Centers for Disease Control and Prevention. Heat-related deaths among crop workers—United States, 1992–2006. Morbidity and Mortality Weekly Report 2008; 57: 649–653.
7. National Institute for Occupational Safety and Health. Criteria for a recommended standard: Occupational exposure to heat and hot environments (Publication No. 2016-106). Cincinnati, OH: National Institute for Occupational Safety and Health, DHHS (NIOSH), 2016.
8. U.S. Bureau of Labor Statistics. Tabular data, 1992–2002: Census of fatal occupational injuries (1992–2002). Fatalities by detailed event or exposure, all industries, exposure to environmental heat and contact with hot objects or substances. Available at: http://www.bls.gov/iif/oshwc/cfoi/cftb0186.pdf. Accessed October 16, 2016.

9. Centers for Disease Control and Prevention. Fatalities from occupational heat exposure. Morbidity and Mortality Weekly Report 1984; 33: 410–412.

10. ACGIH. Heat stress and strain: Documentation of the TLV, 7th edition (2009 Supplement). Cincinnati, OH: ACGIH, 2009.

11. World Health Organization. Health factors involved in working under conditions of heat stress. Technical Report Series No. 412. Geneva: World Health Organization, 1969.

12. Occupational Safety and Health Administration. Technical manual, section III: Chapter 4, Heat stress, 1999. Available at: http://www.osha.gov/dts/osta/otm/otm_iii/otm_iii_4.html. Accessed September 28, 2016.

13. Malchaire J, Kampmann B, Havenith G, et al. Criteria for estimating acceptable exposure times in hot working environments: A review. International Archives of Occupational and Environmental Health 2000; 73: 215–220.

14. ACGIH. 2017 TLVs and BEIs: Threshold limit values for chemical substances and physical agents & biological exposure indices. Cincinnati, OH: ACGIH, 2017.

15. Danzel DF. Hypothermia and frostbite. In: Kasper DL, Fauci AS, Hauser SL et al. (eds.). Harrison's principles of internal medicine (19th ed.). New York: McGraw-Hill Company, 2015, p. 478e-1–478e-5.

16. Centers for Disease Control and Prevention. Hypothermia-related deaths—Wisconsin, 2014, and United States, 2003–2014. Morbidity and Mortality Weekly Report 2015; 64: 141–143.

17. Occupational Hazards Editorial Staff. Protecting workers in cold conditions. EHS Today. November 1999. Available at: http://ehstoday.com/news/ehs_imp_33546/. Accessed November 26, 2016.

18. Sinks T. A joint NIOSH/Division of Safety and Hygiene study identified workers at greatest risk of frostbite and hypothermia. Ohio Monitor 1987; Jan: 12–15.

19. ACGIH. Cold stress: Documentation of the TLVs and BEIs with other worldwide occupational exposure values CD-ROM-2009. Cincinnati, OH: ACGIH (2001 suppl.), 2009.

20. Occupational Safety and Health Administration. Cold stress can be prevented. Available at: https://www.osha.gov/dts/weather/winter_weather/windchill.html. Accessed November 27, 2016.

21. National Institute for Occupational Safety and Health. Safety and health topic: Cold stress. Available at: http://www.cdc.gov/niosh/topics/coldstress/. Accessed November 27, 2016.

FURTHER READING

ACGIH. Heat stress and strain: Documentation of the TLVs and BEIs with other worldwide occupational exposure values CD-ROM 2009. Cincinnati, OH: American Conference of Governmental Industrial Hygienists (2009 suppl.), 2009.

National Institute for Occupational Safety and Health. Criteria for a recommended standard: Occupational exposure to heat and hot environments—Revised criteria. Cincinnati, OH: U.S. Public Health Service, Centers for Disease Control and Prevention, National Institute for Occupational Safety and Health, DHHS (NIOSH) Publication No. 2016-106, 2016. *These two publications are the best technical guides for keeping workers safe from the effects of heat stress and strain. The NIOSH document also covers international standards and recommendations.*

Crippen E, Davis K (eds.). Staying alive in the Arctic: A cold weather survival manual. Washington, DC: American Petroleum Institute, 1978. *While most workers do not ordinarily face the harsh conditions that builders of the Alaska pipeline did, lessons learned there are still helping safety professionals protect workers from the cold. This publication should be required reading for cold-weather workers.*

APPENDIX TO CHAPTER

PHYSICAL HAZARDS RELATED TO HYPERBARIC AND HYPOBARIC ENVIRONMENTS AND THEIR ADVERSE HEALTH EFFECTS

Juan C. Dapena

The human body has evolved to function at a surface pressure of 760 mm Hg (1 Atmosphere Absolute, or 1 ATA). At this pressure, air-filled cavities (such as the inner ear, sinuses, and lungs) and the gases dissolved in tissues and fluids (mostly oxygen and nitrogen) are at equilibrium. Relatively healthy individuals can easily manage the physiological changes associated with exposure to hyperbaric (increased-pressure) or hypobaric (decreased-pressure) environments.

Boyle's law states that, at a constant temperature, the volume (V) of a given mass of gas is inversely proportional to the absolute pressure (P) exerted—described by the formula $P_1V_1 = P_2V_2$. By using the standard conversion of 1 ATA for every 10 meters of seawater, one can predict volumetric changes according to a rise or fall in pressure. A closed bottle with a volume of 1 liter at 1 ATA (sea level) will shrink to 0.5 liter at a depth of 10 meters of sea water, where the absolute ambient pressure is 2 ATA (1 ATA at surface + 1 ATA at depth). At 3 ATA, the volume will be one-third of the original, and so forth.

The bottle in this example could maintain the original volume if it is connected to a source of air capable of providing enough pressure to equal that of the external environment.

The density of the medium in which a subject travels determines the rate of pressure changes exerted on the subject. An additional 1 ATA is reached for every 33 feet of seawater in which one descends. In contrast, 0.5 ATA is reached at 18,000 feet (5,500 meters) of altitude. This difference is important when planning dives on lakes at high altitudes, which require specialized training and specific dive tables.

Injuries caused by pressure changes affecting air-filled cavities are known as *barotrauma*. Ear barotrauma (*ear squeeze*) is the most common disorder in divers while descending, resulting from inability to equalize pressure between the middle ear and the external environment through the Eustachian tube, which connects the middle ear with the throat. An inward bulging of the tympanic membrane results from the relative negative pressure in the middle ear, potentially causing hearing loss, pain, and/or accumulation of blood or serous fluid. Failure to act with remedial measures to equalize the pressure can lead to rupture of the tympanic membrane, which may be suspected when ear pain is suddenly relieved. Unilateral tympanic membrane rupture can result in nausea, vertigo, and disorientation. *Reverse squeeze*, which can occur during a diver's ascent, is caused by increased middle ear pressure, leading to the outward bulging of the tympanic membrane. (This rarely results in tympanic membrane rupture.) "Squeeze" and "reverse squeeze" are commonly experienced, to a lesser degree and severity during flight (even in commercial aircraft), sky diving, and mountain climbing.

Sinus barotrauma, which occurs with descent, is commonly manifested as sinus pressure, headache, and nosebleed. Allergies, infections, and anatomical abnormalities can lead to mechanical obstruction of openings between the sinuses and the nasal cavity. The frontal sinus is the sinus most commonly obstructed due its anatomical tortuosity.

Pulmonary overinflation syndrome (POIS), a more serious form of barotrauma, is caused by a diver's failure to exhale during ascent to the surface, resulting in lung and blood vessel damage. Air that has accumulated in the pleural space (between the lungs and the chest wall) can create a pneumothorax. Accumulation of air in the pericardial cavity can compress the heart, creating mediastinal emphysema. Rupture of alveolar capillaries can introduce air into the blood, creating an arterial gas embolism with neurologic manifestations that may resemble a stroke and causing loss of consciousness. Any of these POIS-related conditions should be considered a medical emergency that requires immediate evaluation and treatment.

Henry's law describes the direct relationship between the amount of a gas that will dissolve in a liquid and the partial pressure of the gas over the liquid. The rate at which the gas dissolves depends on the nature of the gas dissolved and the duration of the pressure. When exposed to hyperbaric conditions, tissues and body fluids readily absorb nitrogen, which readily dissolves in blood. Upon a diver's ascent to the surface, ambient pressure may be rapidly reduced, causing the formation of nitrogen bubbles in the blood, as it comes out of solution. *Decompression sickness* (DCS), which is caused by air bubbles in blood vessels or other fluid-filled spaces, can lead to injury. A mild form of DCS (Type I) is manifested by joint and muscle pain, with onset about 4 to 6 hours after ascent from depth. A more serious form (Type II), which is manifested by neurologic and cardiopulmonary symptoms, can be fatal.

Dalton's law, which is related to two other disorders related to the effects of gases at depth, states that the total pressure exerted by a mixture of gases is the sum of the partial pressures that would be exerted by each of the gases if it alone occupied the total volume. Since air consists of

80% nitrogen and 20% oxygen, the partial pressure of each gas at 1 ATA is 0.8 ATA nitrogen and 0.2 ATA oxygen. At increased partial pressure, nitrogen can cause narcosis, with symptoms similar to the effects of alcohol intoxication, which increase as depth increases. At increased partial pressure, oxygen can become neurotoxic, with paresthesias, visual changes, tinnitus, nausea, vertigo, confusion, and seizures. Preventive measures include managing time spent at depth and carefully controlling the rate of descent and ascent. More specific recommendations can be found by referring to dive tables and instructions at the Divers Alert Network (http://www.diversalertnetwork.org) and National Association of Underwater Instructors (http://www.naui.org).

Hypobaric environments are encountered by hikers and climbers at high-altitude mountain settings as well as pilots and passengers in unpressurized aircraft. At altitudes greater than 2,500 meters (about 8,200 feet), the partial pressure of oxygen becomes markedly reduced, so that altitude-related illness can occur, especially in those who have not acclimatized because they ascended too rapidly. Acute mountain sickness, the most common form of altitude-related illness, is manifested by headache, nausea, vomiting, fatigue, and loss of appetite. It may be due to an imbalance between hypoxia-induced vasodilation and hypocarbia-induced vasoconstriction of blood vessels in the brain.

High-altitude pulmonary edema, a more serious form of altitude-related illness, affects the lungs. It may be due to hypoxia-induced vasoconstriction and resultant leakage of fluid from pulmonary capillaries. Onset, usually insidious, occurs within 24 to 60 hours of arriving at high altitude. Initial symptoms, which include headache, shortness of breath, cough, and weakness, may progress to cough productive of bloody sputum, low-grade fever, and pulmonary congestion. If untreated, severe headache, confusion, ataxia, hallucinations, and coma may occur due to high-altitude cerebral edema. Preventive measures for illness due to hypobaric environments include proper acclimatization and early recognition of symptoms that indicate that descent is warranted. More specific recommendations can be obtained from the International Society for Mountain Medicine (http://www.ismmed.org).

AUTHORS' NOTE

The findings and conclusions in this chapter and the appendix to this chapter are those of the authors and do not necessarily represent the views of the United States Army and the United States Navy. The author of this chapter is not responsible for the content of the appendix to the chapter, and the author of the appendix is not responsible for the content of the chapter.

FURTHER READING

Edmonds C, Bennet M, Lippmann J, Mitchell S. Diving and subaquatic medicine (5th ed.). Boca Raton, FL: CRC Press, 2015.
An excellent source for understanding diving-related physiology and injury.

Lesham E, Pandey P, Shlim DR, et al. Clinical features of patients with severe altitude illness in Nepal. Journal of Travel Medicine 2008; 15: 315–322.
A good description of the demographic characteristics and clinical course of patients with altitude-related illness who were evacuated for medical treatment from mountainous regions in Nepal.

Tetzlaff K, Thorsen E. Breathing at depth: Physiologic and clinical aspects of diving while breathing compressed gas. Clinics in Chest Medicine 2005; 26: 355–380.
An excellent review of the physics, pathophysiology, and clinical features of breathing in a hyperbaric environment

U.S. Navy Diving Manual, Revision 6, April 15, 2008. Washington, DC: U.S. Government Printing Office, 2008. Available at: http://www.usu.edu/scuba/navy_manual6.pdf.
A global standard for diving.

12D

Ionizing and Non-ionizing Radiation

John Cardarelli II

T he term *radiation* initiates certain feelings and responses in people based on their past experiences and knowledge of the subject. Although humans evolved in an environment consisting of ionizing and non-ionizing background radiation for millions of years, it was not until 1895 that the discovery of X-rays (ionizing radiation) was made—by Wilhelm Conrad Roentgen. The following year, Antoine Henri Becquerel discovered that uranium emits another form of invisible energy, later termed *radioactivity* by Marie Curie, another pioneer in ionizing radiation.

Since these discoveries, ionizing and non-ionizing radiation has successfully been used for beneficial purposes in the nearly all industries, employing millions of workers (Table 12D-1). Despite its enormous benefits, ionizing radiation suffers from a negative societal perception, which has been influenced by the nuclear weapons industry and the reported adverse health effects of workers in this industry. In addition, society often judges ionizing radiation on the basis of highly publicized negative events: the use of atomic bombs in Hiroshima and Nagasaki (1945); nuclear power plant accidents at Three Mile Island (1979), Chernobyl (1986), and Fukushima (2011); criticality at a nuclear fuels

fabrication facility in Tokaimura, Japan (1999); the dispersion of cesium-137 from a teletherapy machine in Goiania, Brazil (1987), where four people died and more than 100,000 requested screening for potential contamination; and the concern over the potential use of radioactive "dirty bombs." In contrast, non-ionizing radiation has a positive image in society because of its tangible benefits, such as wireless communications, and lack of negative events or strong evidence of adverse health effects.

IONIZING RADIATION

Terminology

Ionizing radiation is caused when an electron is ejected from its atomic structure. *Non-ionizing radiation* does not eject electrons but causes molecules to vibrate. *Exposure* represents the amount of ionizing-radiation energy that is absorbed in air. *Dose* refers to the amount of energy absorbed in a specified material other than air, usually tissue. *Half-life* is the amount of time that it takes for half of an amount of radioactive material to decay. *Activity* represents the decay rate or how quickly that radioactivity

289

Table 12D-1. Types of Workers, by Sector, Who May Be Exposed Occupationally to Ionizing and Non-ionizing Radiation

Accelerator Personnel	Medical and Dental
Department of	Dental workers
Defense (DOD)	Medical clinic workers
Department of	Nuclear medicine
Energy (DOE)	(fluoroscopy) workers
Contractor employees	Radiologists and
Visitors	Radiology Technicians
Reactor facility	Veterinarians
employees	Chiropractors
Weapons fabrication	Podiatrists
personnel	Nuclear Power Plant workers
Office workers	Commercial plants
Uranium fuel cycle	Naval fleet and shipyard
Miners	workers
Millers	Transportation
Fuel fabricators	Airline crews
Fuel processors	Screening personnel
Uranium enrichment	Trucking and other
workers	shipping workers
Educational Institutions	Regulatory
Industry	Inspectors
Radiographic workers	Research
(in non-destructive	Other
testing)	
Manufacturing workers	
Distribution workers	
Well logging workers	

Adapted from National Council on Radiation Protection and Measurements. NCRP Report No. 101: Exposure of the U.S. Population from Occupational Radiation, NCRP, Washington, DC, 1989; and National Council on Radiation Protection and Measurements. NCRP Report No. 160: Ionizing Radiation Exposure of the Population of the United States, NCRP, Washington, DC, 2009.

Table 12D-2. Radiation Units

Unit	Conventional Units	SI Units
Exposure	**Roentgen (R)** 87.6 ergs per gram (air) 2.58×10^{-4} Coulomb/kg (air)	**Coulombs/kg**
Dose	**rad** 100 ergs per gram (tissue) 1 rad = 0.01 Gy	**Gray (Gy)** 1 Gy = 100 rad
Dose Equivalent	**rem** 1 rad $\times w_r$,* 1 rem = 0.01 Sv	**Sievert (Sv)** 1 Sv = 100 rem
Activity	**Curie (Ci)** 3.7×10^{10} decays per second	**Becquerel (Bq)** 1 decay per second

* w_r = Radiation weighting factor is a dimensionless number that depends on the way in which the energy of the radiation is distributed along its path through the tissue. In general, it is 20 for exposures to alpha particles, 1 for exposures to beta particles and gamma and X-rays, and 5 to 20 for exposures to neutrons.

keep abreast of changing developments. With use of terms and units, those outside the field will begin to better understand ionizing radiation.

The Basics of Ionizing Radiation

The various types of radiation and how they interact with matter can be described by our understanding of the atom. *Alpha* (α) *radiation*, which is a helium nucleus (two protons and two neutrons), is typically associated with heavy elements, such as radon, radium, uranium, and plutonium. It is a large positively-charged particle and easily interacts with other atoms to quickly deposit its energy. Depending on its energy, which is measured in million electron-volts (MeV), an alpha particle can travel up to 10 cm in air. However, most only penetrate 1 to 3 cm (less than 5 MeV) before dissipating all their energy. Alpha particles with at least 7.5 MeV can penetrate the nominal protective layer of the skin (0.07 mm), but only 14% of all alpha emissions occur above this level of energy, and most of these 14% are human-made with very short half-lives. Therefore, alpha radiation does not pose an external hazard to people, who are easily shielded (such as by air, skin, or paper), but can be hazardous if the emitting radionuclide is inhaled, ingested, or injected into the body.

material decays. *Risk* is the increment of some adverse health affect associated with a known amount of cumulative radiation dose.

The multiple units and scientific terms used to define and describe ionizing radiation do little to bring understanding to those outside the field. These problems have existed for decades and will continue to exist until scientific organizations, industries, and national governments achieve harmonization. Scientific organizations are providing leadership by publishing internationally recognized standards through the International Commission on Radiation Protection (ICRP) and the International Atomic Energy Agency. In contrast, industry continues to produce instrumentation that provides results in conventional units (Table 12D-2), and governments, with their complex legislative processes, struggle to

Beta (β) radiation consists of electrons emitted by atoms. The mass of a proton is 1,836 times larger than that of a beta particle, which can penetrate further into materials or tissue.[1] Due to their small size and charge, beta particles can travel about 12 feet per MeV in air and need only 0.07 MeV to penetrate the skin. Most beta particles do not normally penetrate beyond the top layer of skin, but exposure to higher-energy beta particles (>0.07 MeV) can cause skin burns. Beta radiation is easily shielded with plastic, glass, or metals, but layers of plastic or glass are preferred in the workplace because X-rays can be produced from beta interactions with metal shielding. These characteristics make beta radiation both an external and internal hazard to people.

Photon (gamma or X-ray) radiation is a form of electromagnetic radiation, such as light, with energies high enough to cause ionization. There are several differences between gamma rays and X-rays, most importantly their points of origin. Gamma rays originate from within nuclei of atoms, whereas X-rays originate from surrounding orbital electrons. Gamma ray emissions are very specific and are often used to identify radionuclides with special instruments. X-ray emissions are generally not specific because they are produced artificially by the rapid slowing down of an electron beam (*bremsstrahlung radiation*). Since the rate of slowing is not specific, various X-ray energies exist within a continuum of energies that peak at the maximum energy of the incident electron beam or beta particle on the target surface. *Characteristic X-rays* are one exception where X-rays with specific energies are emitted due to the specific energy levels between electron shells. An electron shifting from a higher energy shell to a lower energy shell will emit an X-ray of fixed energy that is equal to the energy difference between shells. Gamma rays commonly encountered in medical and industrial workplaces are generally higher in energy (0.2 MeV to 1.5 MeV) than X-rays (typically less than 0.5 MeV). Finally, photon-emitting radionuclides found in natural background generally have higher energies (such as postassium-40, with 1.46 MeV) than artificial radionuclides (such as cobalt-60, with 1.125 MeV and 1.33 MeV, and cesium-137, which is commonly associated with its initial decay product Ba-137, which emits 0.662 MeV).

Neutron radiation is essentially zero for background radiation levels at ground level. It is an occupational concern only at commercial nuclear power plants and research facilities and for airplanes or spacecraft. Neutrons have no charge. Therefore, they are not influenced by other charged particles and can easily penetrate materials. Water or concrete are effective shielding materials because they contain many similar-sized atoms close to that of a neutron (hydrogenous materials). As the neutrons penetrate these materials, they interact with the atomic nuclei of the material—like billiard balls. Neutron radiation is also capable of creating radioactive materials through a process called *activation*. When a neutron is absorbed by an atomic nucleus, the atom becomes "excited" and often releases the excess energy in the form of other types of radiation, especially protons. Protons originate from the nucleus and hold an electric charge of +1 elementary charge. Since the number of protons in the nucleus identifies an element, any change in this number will change the element and its chemical properties. The most common activation product encountered in various industries is cobalt-60.

Measuring External and Internal Doses

Alpha, beta, gamma, and X-radiation do not cause the body to become radioactive. However, most materials in their natural state, including body tissues, contain measurable amounts of naturally occurring radioactive material, especially potassium-40, uranium, and thorium decay products. *External doses* occur when the body is irradiated by a radioactive source outside the body. This dose can be measured by using a dosimeter. A qualified individual should select the most appropriate dosimeter for a given application, based on its advantages and limitations. All of these technologies can be built to detect the types of radiation (beta, gamma, or neutron) and their respective energies, but they cannot identify the specific radionuclide emitting the energy. Other types of detectors and electronics are needed to identify radionuclides. Additional considerations when selecting a dosimeter include the type of radiation encountered, the monitoring frequency (immediate, hourly, weekly, monthly, or quarterly), the required sensitivity, processing time, and cost.

Internal doses occur when a radioactive material enters the body via inhalation, ingestion, injection, or absorption through the skin and deposits its energy in the tissues. Typical external and internal radioactive sources and their industrial uses are listed in Table 12D-3. Doses from internal exposures are more difficult to assess than external exposures because individual characteristics, such as diet, health status, and age, vary greatly within a population. In an attempt to standardize the dosimetry methodology, ICRP has developed human reference models to estimate internal doses.[2,3] These models are used to derive airborne radiation concentration limits (called *derived air concentrations*) for workplaces. Internal dose estimates are determined by direct measurements and/or biological samples. Direct measurements, such as of thyroid, bone, or the entire body, employ very sensitive instruments that measure photon radiation (gamma or characteristic X-rays) emitted from within the body. Specific gamma energies identify radionuclides, while measurements estimate the amounts internally deposited. These data are then used, together with knowledge of the initial time of exposure and the ICRP standardized models, to estimate dose. Biological samples, such as urine, feces, exhaled breath, sweat, and hair, are used when the type of exposure, chemical properties (such as solubility), and radionuclide are known. The amount of radioactive material measured in these samples can estimate internal dose by using the ICRP models. In the workplace, both methods are used to refine internal dose estimates, as more information is obtained on the individual's elimination rate of the radioactive materials.

Background Radiation and the Environment

The National Council on Radiation Protection and Measurements published a complete review of all radiation exposures to U.S. residents for 2006, such as terrestrial, cosmic, medical, consumer-products, security, research, and occupational exposures.[4] The average annual dose was 6.2 mSv (620 mrem), which represented a 170% increase over the average annual dose to U.S. residents from the late 1980s (3.6 mSv or 360 mrem).[5]

Radon and thoron exposure, which is responsible for about 36% of background dose (about 2.28 mSv), is highest where naturally occurring radioactive material (uranium and thorium) is found. Cosmic radiation, which accounts for about 5% (0.33 mSv) of background levels, increases at higher altitudes and at longitude positions closer to the poles. Terrestrial radiation (rocks and soil) accounts for about 3%

Table 12D-3. Occupational Dose Limits or Recommendations (Annual unless otherwise specified)

Dose Limits	DOE	NRC	OSHA	NCRP (1993)	ICRP* (1991)
Occupational	50 mSv (external plus internal doses)	50 mSv (external plus internal doses)	12.5 mSv per quarter for the whole body (head and trunk; active blood-forming organs or gonads)	50 mSv	20 mSv averaged over 5 years (100 mSv in 5 years), with a further provision that the effective dose should not exceed 50 mSv in any single year
Lens of eye	150 mSv	150 mSv	12.5 mSv per quarter	150 mSv	20 mSv
Hand and forearms, feet and ankles	500 mSv	500 mSv	187.5 mSv per quarter	500 mSv	500 mSv
Skin	500 mSv	500 mSv	75 mSv per quarter	500 mSv	500 mSv
Cumulative	None	None	50(N − 18) mSv N = age (years)	10 mSv × age (years)	100 mSv in 5 years

Note. DOE = Department of Energy; NRC = Nuclear Regulatory Commission; OSHA = Occupational Safety and Health Administration; NCRP = National Council on Radiation Protection and Measurements; ICRP = International Commission on Radiological Protection.

* The 2005 ICRP recommendations continue to endorse these limits, except for the dose limit to lens of the eye, which was lowered from 150 mSv to 20 mSv in 2011 (in ICRP Publication 118).

(0.21 mSv). Internal exposures (radioactive substances inside the body, especially potassium-40) account for about 5% (0.29 mSv). Occupational and manmade radiation sources (radiation from consumer products, industrial and security uses, and education and research) account for about 2% (0.14 mSv). Medical exposures, which account for 49% (3 mSv) of the total annual dose, have increased 700% since the 1980s—due mainly to increases in medical imaging and the growth of the U.S. population.

Health Effects

Health effects from radiation exposures vary with the type, amount, and duration of exposure. When radiation exposes a cell, it may (a) pass through without doing any damage, (b) interact and damage the cell but with later repair by the cell, (c) interact and damage the cell in such a way that it continues to reproduce itself in a damaged state, or (d) kill the cell. The death of a single cell may not be harmful, but if many cells are killed within an organ then that organ may not function properly. The likelihood of damage is also related to the mitotic cycle of the cell. In 1906, the Law of Bergonie and Tribondeau concluded that the most radiosensitive cells have a high division rate and a long dividing future and are not specialized. In general, tissues that are young and rapidly growing are most likely to be radiosensitive. Therefore, mature lymphocytes are more radiosensitive than (in order) intestinal crypt cells, mature spermatocytes, erythorcyes, and nerve cells.

The acute health effects of ionizing radiation are nonstochastic, in that the severity of the effect varies with the dose. They occur within a range of minutes to days after exposure. If the dose is kept below a given threshold, usually about 0.10 Gy (10 rad), no effect has been observed. Above this value, especially above 1 Gy (100 rad), acute radiation sickness begins to develop, which includes the hematopoietic syndrome, gastrointestinal syndrome, central nervous system syndrome, and cutaneous radiation syndrome, the last of which often complicates the recovery process of the affected individual due to an increased potential for infection.

The hemopoietic syndrome, which results from penetrating gamma or X-ray doses ranging between 2 to 10 Gy (200 to 1,000 rad), is characterized by deficiencies of white blood cells overall, lymphocytes, and platelets. It consists of four phases: prodromal (with nausea, vomiting, and anorexia lasting up to 48 hours), latent (without symptoms but with changes in blood elements lasting up to 3 weeks), bone marrow depression, and recovery.

The gastrointestinal syndrome, which results from penetrating gamma or X-ray doses greater than 10 Gy (1,000 rad), is characterized by an immediate onset of nausea, vomiting, and diarrhea, followed by a short latent period. Severe dehydration is caused by the massive denuding of the gastrointestinal tract. Most patients do not survive.

The central nervous syndrome, which results from penetrating gamma or X-ray doses above 100 Gy (10,000 rad), is characterized by vomiting and diarrhea (within minutes of exposure), confusion, disorientation, hypotension, and fever, resulting in death within a short time.

The severity of the cutaneous syndrome is determined by the dose of *beta radiation*, energy of the radiation, and type of exposure (skin contamination, contact with contaminated clothing, or distant exposure). Effects depend on uniformity of exposures and location of contamination on the body. Most radiosensitive are moist areas (axilla, groin, and skin folds), followed by the inner aspect of the neck, the antecubital and popliteal spaces, the flexor surfaces of the extremities, and the chest, abdomen, face, and back. Least sensitive are the nape of the neck, scalp, palms, and soles. The larger the area irradiated, the lower the dose needed for adverse reactions. Conversely, the smaller the area irradiated, the higher the dose needed for a similar reaction. A temporal scheme classifies the effects as acute effects (within the first 6 months), subacute effects (within the second 6 months), in the chronic clinical period (2 to 5 years), and in the late clinical period (after 5 years). The skin response depends on the dose. Skin responses include erythema (3 to 10 Gy; 14 to 21 days), hair loss (> 3 Gy; 14 to 18 days), dry desquamation (8 to 12 Gy; 25 to 30 days), moist desquamation (15 to 20 Gy; 20 to 28 days), blister formation (15 to 25 Gy; 15 to 25 days), ulceration (>20 Gy, 14 to 21 days), and necrosis (>25 Gy; >21 days). Workers in the commercial nuclear power industry can face a unique skin hazard of highly localized, radioactive material (usually cobalt-60 or cesium-137) called *hot particles, fleas,* or *specks.* These particles range from 1 to 100 μm in diameter, deliver very high doses to a local area, and are difficult to remove. In the event of a terrorist attack involving nuclear material (involving fission) or radioactive (nonfissile) material, these particles may become a primary radiological concern, but they are not likely to result in whole-body doses causing significant adverse health effects.

Chronic effects (stochastic effects) are those in which the probability of the effect may increase with increasing dose. The Bradford Hill perspectives (see Chapter 4) can be used to determine the cause-and-effect relationship between exposures to varying degrees of ionizing radiation and adverse or beneficial health effects.[6] The scientific community has adopted a linear, no-threshold, dose–response model to set occupational dose limits, based primarily on atomic bomb survivors and patients undergoing radiation therapy who have received very large exposures in a very short period of time. There is little controversy about the linear response between high cumulative doses (>1 Gy; 100 rad) and adverse health effects. However, controversy continues as to whether the linear no-threshold model is appropriate for lower cumulative doses (measured in Sv or rem) and dose rate (measured in Sv/hour or mrem/hour) as found in the workplace.[7-11] Over the past several decades, several response models have been studied and proposed in the scientific literature, including the linear quadratic model (cancer risk increases exponentially with dose), the threshold model (cancer risk does not exists until dose reaches a particular level), the supra-linear model (cancer risk is substantially increased at lower dose and dose-rate levels), and the hormesis model (a health benefit is recognized at low levels and cancer risk only becomes a concern at a particular dose level). (Figure 12D-1).[12]

Pregnancy Issues

Thousands of pregnant workers are exposed to ionizing radiation each year. Inadequate knowledge about ionizing radiation contributes to much anxiety and unnecessary consideration of pregnancy termination. Fears and concerns can often be alleviated by an understanding that the radiation risks during pregnancy are related to radiation dose and stage of pregnancy. Preconception irradiation of either parent's gonads does not result in increased risk of cancer or congenital malformations. Radiation risks are most significant during organogenesis in the early fetal period and lower in the second and third trimesters. Congenital malformations, which have a threshold ranging between 0.1 and 0.2 Gy (10 to 20 rad), typically involve the central nervous system. Fetal doses of 0.1 Gy are not reached even with three pelvic CT scans or 20 conventional diagnostic X-ray examinations. Ionizing radiation increases the risk of leukemia and other malignancies in adults

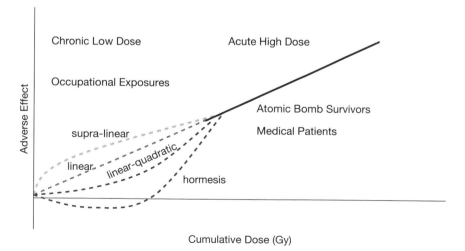

Figure 12D-1. Health effects associated with dose of ionizing radiation.

and children under 18 years of age. The embryo/fetus is assumed to be at about the same risk for carcinogenic effects as children. After exposure in utero to 0.01 Gy, the absolute risk of a fatal cancer from birth to age 15 is about 1 per 1,700. This suggests that the probability of bearing a healthy child is very high, even if the pregnant worker receives a radiation dose that exceeds the occupational dose limit for nonpregnant workers. These risks must be considered in the context of the occurrence of abnormal pregnancy outcomes of pregnant women who are not exposed to radiation: spontaneous abortion, more than 15%; genetic abnormalities, 4% to 10%; intrauterine growth retardation, 4%; and major malformations, 2% to 4%.

Exposures of more than 0.1 Gy (10 rad) are extremely rare in the workplace, especially if a woman informs her employer of her pregnancy. The dose to a declared pregnant worker is limited in the United States to 0.005 Gy (0.5 rad) per gestation period (one-tenth of the occupational dose limit for nonpregnant workers). The ICRP states that pregnant workers may work where there is a potential for exposure to ionizing radiation as long as there is reasonable assurance that the fetal dose can be kept below 0.001 Gy (0.1 rad) above background throughout the pregnancy. This dose is about the same as that which all people receive annually from penetrating natural background radiation, excluding radon, and 1/50th of the nonpregnant occupational dose limit of 0.05 Gy (5 rad).

Termination of pregnancy is rarely contemplated due to of an occupational exposure, but it may become a dominant concern after an attack with a nuclear weapon or "dirty bomb." High fetal doses (0.1 to 1.0 Gy; 10 to 100 rad) during late pregnancy are *not* likely to result in congenital malformations since all the organs have been formed by then. There is less than a 1% chance that childhood cancer or leukemia will result from a fetal dose of about 0.1 Gy (10 rad). Therefore, termination of pregnancy at fetal doses less than 0.1 Gy (10 rad) is not justified on the basis of radiation risk. As the fetal dose increases to above 0.5 Gy (50 rad), there can be significant fetal damage, depending on the stage of the pregnancy. At fetal doses between 0.1 and 0.5 Gy (10 and 50 rad) decisions should be based upon individual circumstances.[13]

Radiation Protection

Radiation protection standards have evolved since the discovery of X-rays in 1895 and continue to undergo changes, additions, and revisions. International and national organizations recommend scientifically based protection standards, and national governments promulgate regulations with occupational dose limits (Table 12D-3). The latest recommendations differ from regulatory standards since these are based on recent findings from the Radiation Effects Research Foundation and the United Nations Scientific Committee on the Effects of Atomic Radiation. The most recent dose-limit recommendations were reduced in order to be commensurate with the basic philosophy that radiation workers ought to have at least the same level of protection as those in safe industries (about 1 death per 10,000 workers per year).[14]

Radon

Occupational exposure limits for radon and radon progeny (radon daughters) were derived to protect the health of underground miners over a working lifetime of 30 years.[15] When radon gas and radon progeny are inhaled, the radiation dose is primarily caused by the (short-lived) radon progeny. Because it was not feasible to routinely measure individual radon progeny, the concept of the working level (WL) was introduced and defined as 1.3×10^5 MeV of alpha radiation emitted from the short-lived radon progeny in 1 liter of air. An exposure of 1 WL for a working period of 1 month (170 hours) results in a cumulative exposure of 1 working level month (WLM). A WLM, which is the common unit of measurement for human exposure to radon progeny, is the basis for the occupational exposure limits.

Radiation Protection Programs

Radiation protection programs, which reflect application of management's responsibilities for radiation protection and safety, implement policies, procedures, and organizational structures commensurate with the nature and extent of radiation risks (Figure 12D-2). Three principles

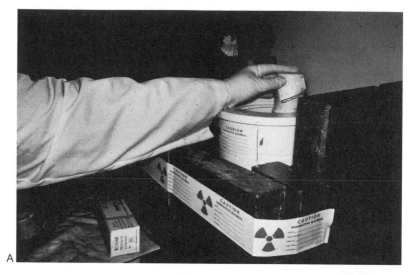

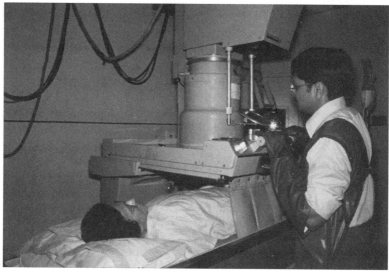

Figure 12D-2. Examples of protection of healthcare workers from ionizing radiation. (A) Worker wearing leather glove in nuclear medicine supply storage area. (B) X-ray technician wearing protective apron. (Photographs by Earl Dotter.)

of radiation protection and safety include justifying, limiting, and optimizing exposures. Radiation exposures may be justified if an activity produces sufficient benefit—considering social, economic, and other relevant factors—to offset the harm it might cause exposed workers. Dose limitation is necessary to limit the risk of stochastic effects from exposures considered to be unacceptable. Protection and safety should be optimized to ensure that the magnitude of worker doses, the number of workers exposed, and the likelihood of incurring exposure are all kept as low as reasonably achievable, after accounting for social and economic factors (cost and cost-effectiveness of engineering controls, emergency response activities, and the potential impact to the public). A "safety culture," which contributes to a successful radiation protection program, depends on management's commitment to encouraging a questioning and learning attitude toward protection and safety and discouraging complacency. A neutral or negative attitude by management toward radiological protection can cause unnecessary or excessive radiation exposure in the workplace, as can inaccurate or incomplete radiation surveys, inadequately prepared radiological work permits, failure of radiological technicians to react to changing or unusual conditions, failure of workers to follow procedures, and inadequate involvement of supervisors.

The basic structure of a radiation protection program should include:

1. Assignment of responsibilities to various levels of management
2. Designation of controlled or supervised areas
3. Local rules for workers to follow and the supervision of work (site-specific considerations and accountability procedures)
4. Arrangement for monitoring workers and the workplace with appropriate dosimeters and instrumentation
5. A system to record and report all relevant information to appropriate decision-makers
6. Education and training programs on the nature of the hazards, protection, and safety
7. Methods to periodically review and audit performance of the program
8. Emergency response plans
9. A health surveillance program
10. A quality assurance and quality control program.

Emergency Response and Recovery

Terrorist attacks have focused attention on preparedness to address large-scale radiological and nuclear threats as well as threats of small-scale industrial radiation releases. Since 9/11, response capabilities of federal and state governments in the United States have been improved by creating the Department of Homeland Security, consolidating many federal emergency-response plans into a national response framework, and providing funding to state and local governments. Emergency-response workers may be highly exposed to radiation at levels requiring additional precautions and medical intervention. (See Chapter 31.) Most important for health professionals responding to emergencies is to always treat life-threatening injuries first before addressing radioactive contamination or radiation exposure. Even if people have been heavily irradiated or contaminated with radioactive material, they should be first evaluated for other forms of injury, such as mechanical

trauma, burns, and smoke inhalation.[16] One should be especially cautious of wounds containing metallic objects since these can be a major source of radiation. Decisions during an initial response to a large-scale radiological incident are based on protecting life and critical infrastructure. Decisions during the recovery phase that follow include consideration of law enforcement, mass casualties, damage to infrastructure, psychosocial impacts, and environmental concerns.[17] *Protective action guides* support actions to protect the public and emergency workers responding to or recovering from a radiological or nuclear incident.[18] (See Chapter 31 and the list of Websites for Further Information at the end of the chapter.)

NON-IONIZING RADIATION

Everyone is exposed daily to non-ionizing radiation, which is both naturally occurring and manmade. It can be beneficial or detrimental to those exposed. Like ionizing radiation, one cannot see it except for visible light (wavelength = 400 to 760 nm), taste it, or smell it. But unlike ionizing radiation, one may be able to feel it by sensing heat or through electrostimulation. The phenomenon of hearing certain radiofrequencies is also a well-established biological effect with no known adverse health consequences. *Non-ionizing radiation* is the energy absorbed by any material without causing ionization (ejection of electrons surrounding the atoms within the material). It takes many forms, including television and radio signals, radar, mobile phone signals, microwaves, visible light, infrared and ultraviolet light, and lasers. The presence of non-ionizing radiation is growing, fueling anxiety and speculation about its possible adverse health effects. Levels of exposure will continue to grow as technology advances and as society increasingly demands the conveniences it brings.

The electromagnetic spectrum includes ionizing and non-ionizing radiation. All non-ionizing radiation presents in *electromagnetic fields* (EMFs), which can be described by frequency or corresponding wavelength by the equation

$$\lambda = c / f$$

where λ = wavelength in meters (m), c = velocity of light (about 300 million meters per second), and f = frequency in cycles per second (hertz, or Hz). Most of the non-ionizing radiation spectrum is partitioned into specified radiofrequency bands. Hazards potentially associated with exposure to EMFs in various bands may result in (a) currents produced in the body by contact with energized sources or without such contact (electrostimulation), (b) increased core-body temperature, or (c) increased body surface temperature (Table 12D-4). How efficient these fields interact with the body depends on several factors. For example, materials with high water content (muscles) absorb EMF energy at higher rates than dry materials. The absorption rate is higher

when (a) the incident electric field is parallel to the body and (b) the incident magnetic field is perpendicular to a larger cross-sectional area. Sharp corners, edges, and points concentrate electric fields. Depth of penetration of EMF energy decreases as conductivity or frequency increases and as wavelengths decrease.

Electric fields (E-fields) exist when electric charges exert forces on one another, whether in motion or not. Electric field strength describes the strength of forces on charges (in volts per meter [V/m]). Electric fields can be visualized as lines of force that emanate from a positively charged object to a negatively charged object.

The strength of *magnetic fields* (M-fields), measured in amperes per meter (A/m), is associated with the strength of these additional forces

Table 12D-4. Frequency Bands and Their Associated Biological Impacts

Band	Frequency Range (Hz)	Wavelength Range (m)	Biological Impact
SELF Sub-extremely low frequency	0–30	$0–10^7$	$0–10^5$ Hz 0–3,000 m
ELF Extremely low frequency	30–300	$10^7–10^6$	
VF Voice frequency	300–3,000	$10^6–10^5$	Electro Stimulation (primary dosimetric parameter is internal current density)
VLF Very low frequency	$3,000–3 \times 10^4$	$10^5–10^4$	
LF Low frequency	$3 \times 10^4–3 \times 10^5$	$10^4–10^3$	
MF Medium frequency	$3 \times 10^5–3 \times 10^6$	$10^3–10^2$	$10^5 – 6 \times 10^9$ Hz 3,000 – 0.05 m Specific Absorption Rates (Heating effects)
HF High frequency	$3 \times 10^6–3 \times 10^7$	$10^2–10$	
VHF Very high frequency	$3 \times 10^7–3 \times 10^8$	10–1	
UHF Ultra-high frequency	$3 \times 10^8–3 \times 10^9$	1–0.1	
SHF Super-high frequency	$3 \times 10^9–3 \times 10^{10}$	$0.1–10^{-2}$	Above 6×10^9 Hz, below 0.05 m:
EHF Extremely high frequency	$3 \times 10^{10}–3 \times 10^{11}$	$10^{-2}–10^{-3}$	
SEHF Supra-extremely high frequency	$3 \times 10^{11}–3 \times 10^{12}$	$10^{-3}–10^{-4}$	Surface Heating (Radiant)
Infrared Radiation	IR-C	0.3 μm–1 mm	Corneal burns, thermal skin burns
	IR-B	0.14 μm–0.3 μm	
	IR-A	760 nm–1,400 nm	Retinal burns, cataracts of lens, thermal skin burns
Visible Light		400–760 nm	Retinal burns, thermal skin burns
Ultraviolet Radiation	UV-A	400–320 nm	Cataract of lens, thermal skin burns
	UV-B	320–280 nm	Corneal injuries, cataracts of lens, photokeratitis, photoconjunctivitis, erythema
	UV-C	280–200 nm	

on moving charges. An ampere is the SI unit for electric current. Magnetic fields exist in a direction perpendicular to the direction of the electrical current, and their intensity is proportional to amount of current present. Magnetic fields are related to another quantity called the *magnetic flux density* (B) by B = μH, where μ is the permeability of the medium. B is the sum of the components of magnetic fields passing through a given area and is the quantity used for hazard evaluation. Its SI unit is the telsa (T), and the cgs unit is the gauss (G) (1 T = 10,000 G). A useful factor to convert B and H is 1 G = 80 A/m.

The relationship between the E and H fields is described by the *power density*, which is the power incident on a surface per unit surface area. Abbreviated as *S*, it can be calculated from E- or H-field measurements by the following equation:

$$S = E^2 / 377 \text{ or } 377H^2$$

where S = power density in watts per square meter (W/m^2 or VA/m^2), E = electric field strength measurement (V/m), and H = magnetic field strength measurement (A/m), and 377 = the constant = the impedance of free space (in ohms, Ω or V/A). Impedance describes the resistance experienced by electromagnetic radiation travelling through space. The quantitative nature of an electromagnetic field changes with increasing distance from the source. In the near field, a distance from the source to about one-sixth of the associated wavelength, E and H fields are not perpendicular because the radiator is not an ideal source. These differences prevent the use of the power density equation, cited previously, and require the measurement of individual components of the E- and H-field strengths. At distances greater than about one-half of the wavelength to about three times the wavelength from the source, called the *far field*, the E and H fields are perpendicular, allowing the use of the power density equation. In this region, the E- and H-field strengths decrease linearly with distance from the source and the power density decreases as the square of the distance from the source. The distance between the near and far fields, the *intermediate field*, is a transitional region where the power density equation still does not apply. The E- and H-field strengths decrease linearly

with distance following a 1/r relationship (where r is the radius from the source).

Exposure Limits

The transfer of energy from electric and magnetic fields in any material is described by the *specific absorption rate* (SAR). "Specific" refers to the normalization to mass of the material exposed, "absorption" refers to the absorption of the energy in a specific medium (tissue), and "rate" refers to the time rate of change of the energy absorption. SAR is the most reliable indicator or predictor of the potential for biological effects in test animals and a measure of what is happening inside the human body. It is expressed in units of watts per kilogram (W/kg) or milliwatts per gram (mW/g). Since SAR is difficult to evaluate or measure outside the laboratory, the measurable quantities of magnetic or electric field strengths and power density as well as induced and contact currents are used to define the radiofrequency (RF) environment. They have been correlated with SAR to determine the maximum permissible exposure (MPE) levels (Table 12D-5). In the far field, measuring field strengths or power density provides reliable exposure assessments. Measuring field strengths or power density is unreliable near or in contact with RF sources or other metallic objects. The MPE values provided are those from the Institute of Electrical and Electronics Engineers standard, which incorporates the latest scientific findings and recommendations for occupational exposures.[19,20] Guidelines for limiting RF exposure have also been developed by several other scientific organizations and government agencies, but the differences are minor and work is underway to harmonize the various exposure limits.[21,22] In the case of exposure of the whole body, a human adult (height = 175 cm) absorbs RF energy most efficiently when the wavelength is 40% of the long axis of the body and parallel to the incident E-field vector. This occurs at a frequency of about 70 megahertz (MHz). The RF exposure limits, which are called basic restrictions, reflect this dependency on frequency and were derived from a SAR of 4 W/kg for those frequencies associated with heating affects (100 kilohertz to 3 Gigahertz). In terms of human metabolic

Table 12D-5. Maximum Permissible Exposure for the Occupational Environments[*]

Frequency Range (MHz)			RMS E-Field[†] Strength (V/m)	RMS H-Field[†] Strength (A/m)	Power Density (S) E Field, H Field (W/m²)	Averaging Time |E|², |H|², or S (min)
0.1	–	1.0	1842	$16.3/f_M$	$(9000/f_M^2, 100,000/f_M^2)^{‡}$	6
1.0	–	30	$1842/f_M$	$16.3/f_M$	$(9000/f_M^2, 100,000/f_M^2)$	6
30	–	100	61.4	$16.3/f_M$	$(10,100,000/f_M^2)$	6
100	–	300	61.4	0.163	10	6
300	–	3,000			$f_M/30$	6
3,000	–	30,000			100	$19.63/f_G^{1.079}$
30,000	–	300,000			100	$2.524/f_G^{0.476}$

Note. Data from IEEE (2005). f_M = frequency in MHz; f_G = frequency in GHz.

[*] An occupational environment is also called a controlled environment—an area where the occupancy and activity of those within it are subject to control and accountability, as established by an RF safety program for the purpose of protection from RF exposure hazards.

[†] For exposures that are uniform over the dimension of the body, such as certain far-field exposures, the exposure field strengths and power densities are compared with the MPEs in this table. For nonuniform exposures, the mean values of the exposure fields, as obtained by spatially averaging the squares of the field strengths or averaging the power densities over an area equivalent to the vertical cross-section of the human body, or a smaller area depending on the frequency, are compared with the MPEs in this table.

[‡] These power density values are commonly used as a convenient comparison with MPEs at higher frequencies and are displayed on some instruments.

heat production, 4 W/kg represents a moderate activity level, such as with housecleaning. A safety factor of 10 was applied resulting in a RF exposure limit of 0.4 W/kg, virtually an indistinguishable heating affect from normal temperature variation, exercise, or exposure to the sun. For localized exposures in an occupational environment where the field strength is more than 20 times the spatial average, the SAR should not exceed 10 W/kg. For the extremities and the pinnae (the cartilaginous projection portion of the outer ear consisting of the helix, lobule, and anti-helix), the SAR should not exceed 20 W/kg. RF exposures below this level are intended to prevent adverse health effects. Exposures in excess of the limits are not necessarily harmful. However, without intended life-saving or medical benefits, these situations are not recommended.

Interpreting RF Measurement Data

Occupational limits (sometimes referred to as a controlled environment) apply to persons exposed at work, provided they are fully aware of the potential for their exposure and can exercise control over it. There are three fundamental concepts when interpreting measurement data: (a) the difference between exposure and emission limits, (b) spatial averaging, and (c) time averaging.

Emission limits are the maximum power output authorized by government authorities for companies or individuals. However, these transmitting signals are often not emitted at the maximum power output. This is especially true for cell-phone base stations or towers, since the amount of power used is proportional to the number of calls handled. For this reason, it is important to note that the emission limit (maximum power output) may not be directly related to exposure potentials. Unlike emission limits, exposure guidelines apply to *exposure limits*, and they are relevant only to locations that are accessible by workers.

Spatial Averaging

The exposure limits are based on the concept that the exposures are applied to a whole-body averaged SAR. This means that spot measurements exceeding the stated exposure limits do not imply noncompliance or harmful exposure scenarios if the spatial average of RF fields over the body does not exceed limits. A spatial average measurement may consist of three or more measurements averaged together that span a length of an adult.

Time Averaging

Another feature of the exposure guidelines is that EMF exposures should be averaged over a 6-minute period for workplaces (controlled environments). The MPE standard uses 0.1 hour (6-minute) averaging time since the whole-body thermal time constant is known to be 1 hour or more. Therefore, 6 minutes, which corresponds to a time constant for partial body heating, is scientifically conservative for short periods of time (less than 6 minutes)—and extremely conservative for both the whole-body and localized exposures in the main (resonance) frequency range (100 kHz to 3 GHz).

To properly apply field measurements to exposure limits, one must consider the length of time individuals are exposed. For example, during any given 6-minute period, workers could be exposed to twice the applicable limit for 3 minutes as long as they are not exposed for the preceding or following 3 minutes. Similarly, a worker could be exposed at 3 times the limit for 2 minutes as long as no exposure occurs during the preceding or subsequent 4 minutes.

Protective Measures

Engineering Controls

Protection of workers from unnecessary or excessive exposure to RF radiation is accomplished through engineering and administrative controls. Engineering controls are preferred since they eliminate or reduce the potential exposures at the source, but they require a sophisticated level of knowledge to install. Improperly installed controls may enhance worker exposures. Interlocks, shielding, bonding, grounding, and filtering are some of the more common controls employed. The Occupational Safety and Health Administration (OSHA) requires a lockout/tag-out program for working with sources of hazardous energies, which may include installing many of the RF controls described previously.

The effectiveness of shielding materials varies with the material, geometry, frequency, and where the field reduction is measured. Some properties are more effective for reducing electric fields while others are more suitable for reducing magnetic fields. One of the most recognizable types of shielding is that used on microwave ovens. The perforated screen is designed to allow penetration of visible light (wavelength about 0.7×10^{-6} to 0.4×10^{-6} meters, or 430 million to 750 million Hz) but prevents leakage of microwave radiation (wavelength about 12 cm,

or 2,450 MHz). Perforated or continuous shielding materials reduce exposures by reflection, absorption (attenuation), and internal reflection. The proper selection of material is complex and should be done by qualified individuals.

Techniques that may supplement the use of engineering controls include prudent placement of RF sources, resonant frequency shift, and personal protective equipment (shoes, clothing, and special suits). Consideration should be given to building-construction materials and layout when installing RF equipment to reduce or prevent unnecessary enhancement of reflected energy at the worker's location. If the operating frequencies are around 10 to 40 MHz, the whole-body SAR may be reduced by *resonant frequency shift*, separating the body from the ground plane by a small distance with electrically insulating materials. This measure reduces the worker's absorption characteristics by reducing the flow of current from the body to a grounded surface. Resonant frequency shift may be especially useful for dielectric-heater (plastic-sealer) operators by having them stand on nonconductive platforms made of wood or rubber. For factory worksites, metal-reinforced concrete floors act as ground planes. Footwear that reduces the grounding effect also achieves the same effect as a resonant frequency shift. The level of RF exposure reduction is dependent on the RF frequency and the types of shoes and socks worn by the worker. Wool socks and rubber-soled shoes provide the greatest reduction for frequencies below 100 MHz (wavelengths above 3 meters). RF protective suits may be helpful when work must be done in "hot" areas, such as continual-radar, onboard naval vessels, and some communication and broadcast environments. Suit material is typically wool, polyester, or nylon impregnated with a highly conductive threaded metal. Some are more effective than others, depending on frequency, orientation of the worker in the environment relative to the incident electric fields, and construction of openings for feet, hands, and head. Washing these suits may reduce their protective capabilities. Some experts recommend against use of RF-protective suits because they may be hazardous to individuals near the wearer and may increase the hazard to the wearer by allowing closer proximity to open circuits that may act as secondary sources.

Administrative Controls

Administrative controls include increasing the distance between the source and workers (often used and easy to bypass), controlling the duration of exposure, restricting access, placing warning signs, providing training commensurate with the level of potential hazard, and real-time monitoring via dosimetry. Horizontal and vertical distance should be considered when determining the appropriate distance, which is often the distance that results in a radiation level equal to the limit (the *hazard distance*). There is no simple way to calculate the reduction of field strength with distance since the calculation depends on so many factors; however, some researchers measured magnetic field strengths that showed a reduction by $1/r^5$ for induction heaters.[23] Controlling the duration of exposure is achieved by applying the time-averaging technique discussed previously. Finally, real-time monitoring devices (dosimeters) are especially useful in identifying potentially harmful exposures, allowing the recipient to take protective actions and reduce risk of injury. Dosimeters provide an audible and visual alarm when exposures exceed a predetermined level (usually 50% of the maximum permissible exposure) and allow the wearer to quickly identify if changes occur during work activities.

Health Effects Associated with EMF Below 100 kHz

Exposures to electric and magnetic fields emanating from the generation, transmission, and use of electricity have been studied extensively. Recommendations of various scientific organizations and regulatory agencies acknowledge controversy regarding the potential health effects of chronic low-level EMF exposures. However, there is no convincing evidence of a health risk.[24-27] One of the most comprehensive reviews of health effects associated with extremely low frequency (ELF) exposures was published by IARC,[28] which found that there is:

1. Limited evidence in humans for the carcinogenicity of ELF magnetic fields in relation to childhood leukemia
2. Inadequate evidence in humans for the carcinogenicity of ELF magnetic fields in relation to all other cancers
3. Inadequate evidence in humans for the carcinogenicity of static electric or magnetic fields and ELF electric fields
4. Inadequate evidence in experimental animals for the carcinogenicity of ELF magnetic fields
5. No available data for the carcinogenicity of static electric or magnetic fields and ELF electric fields in experimental animals.

IARC concluded that ELF magnetic fields are possibly carcinogenic to humans and that static electric and magnetic fields and ELF electric fields are not classifiable as to their carcinogenicity to humans.

Health Effects Associated with EMF Above 100 kHz

More than 100 million U.S. residents use wireless communication devices, with 50,000 new users daily; cell phones are now being used by 91% of U.S. adults.[29,30] If the use of wireless communication devices is ever associated with even the slightest increase in risk of adverse health effects, it could become a significant public health problem. At frequencies above 100 kHz, studies support the basic restrictions and MPE recommendation described earlier. These recommendations were made on the basis of a comprehensive review of the scientific data to protect against established adverse health effects from RF exposures. An adverse health effect is defined as a harmful change in health that is supported by the consistent findings in the peer-reviewed literature, demonstrated by independent laboratories, with consensus in the scientific community. The established adverse health effects associated with RF exposure above the basic restrictions and MPEs are (a) aversive or painful electrostimulation due to excessive RF internal electric fields, (b) RF shock or burns due to contact with excessively high RF voltages, (c) heating pain or tissue burns due to excessive localized RF exposures, and (d) behavioral disruption, heat exhaustion, or heat stroke due to excessive whole-body RF exposures.[22] Adverse effects do not include things like biological effects (sensations) without a harmful health effect, indirect effects caused by electromagnetic interference with electronic devices, or changes in subjective feelings of well-being that are a result of anxiety about RF effects or impact.

Debate continues on the level of protection necessary to prevent long-term health effects from RF exposures. The World Health Organization (WHO) and many European countries promote a precautionary approach by discouraging the widespread use of mobile phones by children for nonessential calls; children may be more likely to develop adverse effects because their nervous system is still developing and they could face a lifetime of various hazardous exposures.[31] The Russian National Committee on Non-Ionizing Radiation Protection extends the WHO recommendations for children to pregnant women and to those suffering from specific diseases and recommends that duration of cellular phone calls be limited to 3 minutes each with at least 15 minutes between calls. The United States does not necessarily endorse the precautionary approach because without clear, convincing epidemiologic evidence that a health hazard exists from RF exposures, this approach could negatively impact industry growth and development.

Cancer-related studies on animals have not provided consistent evidence of physiological, pathological, or disease-specific effects of long-term RF exposures. One study found a slightly increased incidence of brain and heart tumors in male, but not female, rats who had RF exposures from the major radio systems used in cell phones.[32] Epidemiological studies show no clear or consistent evidence to indicate a causal role of RF exposures in human cancer or other disease endpoints at exposures below the basic restrictions and MPEs. However, it is scientifically impossible to prove absolute safety (the null hypothesis) of any physical agent. Many of the original studies lack adequate exposure-assessment information and biological measures and include confounding factors, recall bias, and participation bias. More recent studies have benefitted from improved dosimetry and modeling techniques and better clinical testing protocols.

Infrared and Ultraviolet Radiation

Infrared radiation (IR) lies at frequencies higher than those of radar waves and microwaves (Table 12D-4). Nearly half of the sun's radiant energy is emitted as IR. IR is highly absorbed by water and the earth's atmosphere and invisible to the eye. However, its warmth can be detected by the skin. All objects with temperatures above absolute zero emit infrared radiation. In industry, significant levels of IR are produced directly by lamps and indirectly by heat sources, such as heating and drying devices. The primary biological effect of IR is thermal due to absorption in the water within body tissues. For this reason, IR cannot penetrate the skin but leaves a sensation of heat, which often serves as an adequate warning sign to take protective action or risk skin burns. The lens of the eye is particularly vulnerable to IR because the lens has no heat sensors and a poor heat-dissipating mechanism. Cataracts may be produced by chronic IR exposure at levels far below those that cause skin burns. Occupations typically at risk of IR exposure include glass blowers, furnace workers, foundry workers, blacksmiths, solderers, oven operators, those who work near baking and drying heat lamps, and movie projectionists. Like RF radiation, IR exposure limits are frequency-based; however, they represent conditions under which it is believed that nearly all healthy workers may be repeatedly exposed without acute adverse effects. The limits for IR most recognized in the scientific community are published by ACGIH.[32] Control of IR hazards require (a) shielding of the IR source and eye protection with appropriate IR filters, (b) maximizing the distance between workers and the IR source, and (c) reducing the time spent in areas with high levels of IR exposure.

Ultraviolet radiation (UVR) is produced by the sun and artificially by incandescent, fluorescent, and discharge types of light sources. It is characterized by three distinct energy bands known as UV-A (400 to 320 nm), UV-B (320 to 280 nm), and UV-C (280 to 200 nm). The first two bands are principal UV components in sunlight. Nearly all UV-A reaches the earth's surface, but most UV-B is absorbed by the stratospheric ozone layer. UV-C is completely absorbed by the ozone layer and oxygen in the air, but it can be artificially produced. Industrial sources of UVR include welding arcs, plasma torches, electric arc furnaces (full spectrum of UVR), germicidal and black-light lamps (mostly UV-C), and certain types of lasers (full spectrum of UVR). Because wavelengths of UVR are so short, UVR presents a surface heating hazard.

The most common adverse health effect from overexposure to UVR is sunburn (erythema). Chronic low-level UVR exposure to the sun is also associated with various skin effects, including skin cancer (basal cell carcinoma, squamous cell carcinoma, and malignant melanoma), premature aging of the skin, solar elastosis (wrinkling), and solar keratoses (premalignant lesions). Basal cell carcinoma and malignant melanoma are more strongly associated with a history of multiple episodes of sunburn, whereas squamous cell carcinoma is associated with total exposure. UVR exposure has also been associated with suppressing the immune system and developing cortical cataracts (UV-B exposure). Photosensitizing agents, such as coal tar, plants (including figs, lemon and lime rinds containing furmocoumarins and psoralens, celery, and parsnips), and pharmaceutical drugs (including chlorpromazine, chlorpropamide, and tolbutamide) can increase susceptibility to UVR. All of these effects vary with individual susceptibilities (lighter skin is more susceptible than darker skin and people on medicine for diabetes are more susceptible) and geographic location (UVR levels are highest near the equator, at higher altitudes, when the sun is directly overhead, when there is no cloud cover or ozone coverage, during the summer, and in highly reflective environments). Acute high-level UVR exposures, especially from UV-B, result in eye injuries, which are often only recognized several hours after the exposure. Photokeratitis (inflammation of the cornea) and photoconjunctivitis (inflammation of the thin transparent mucous membrane lining the inner surface of the eyelids) are usually reversible within several days. Intense UVR exposure also has an indirect impact on health through its ability to cause photochemical reactions. Small amounts of oxygen and nitrogen can be converted into ozone and oxides of nitrogen, which are respiratory irritants. Halogenated hydrocarbon solvent vapors can decompose into toxic gases, such as perchloroethylene decomposing to hydrogen chloride and trichloroethylene decomposing to phosgene. Chronic low-level

UVR exposures can be controlled by use of protective clothing, eyewear, and sunscreen lotions and by reduction of duration of exposure. Controlling UVR from acute high-level photochemical exposures may require local exhaust ventilation and isolation of UVR sources from industrial processes that involve solvents. Only qualified personnel should determine the effectiveness of any particular form of personal protection. (See Chapter 25.)

Laser Radiation

Laser is an acronym for *light amplification by the stimulated emission of radiation*. Uses in industry include heat treatment, glazing, alloying, cladding (providing or encasing with a covering or coating), cleaning, brazing, soldering, conduction welding, penetration welding, cutting, hole drilling, marking, trimming, and photolithography.[33] Health and safety decisions are based on the class of laser and the wavelength of the laser source. The hazard classification system places lasers into four categories depending on their potential to cause harm from direct beam exposures (Table 12D-6). These exposures may result in at least four types of injury to the eyes and skin, each requiring a special consideration for selecting the appropriate personal protective equipment:

1. An injury caused by ultraviolet photochemical exposure, which could require eye protection whenever a blueish-white light is visible
2. Blue-light photochemical injury, which can cause retinal burn (solar eclipse blindness)
3. Thermal injury, which is the most common injury from laser radiation exposures, especially from carbon dioxide and Nd:YAG laser
4. Near-infrared thermal injury, which results from molten metal or large, heated surfaces during treatment—a hazard that is only of concern for repeated, chronic exposures.

Nonbeam laser hazards constitute the greatest source of noncompliance with federal safety codes. Sources of nonbeam hazards include (a) improper electrical design or improper use of grounding, component, or shielding; (b) lack of

Table 12D-6. Laser Classification

Class of Laser*	Hazard Potential
1	Pose no potential for injury. No safety measures required to either the eye or skin.
2, 2a	Visible beam posing no significant potential for injury. Blinking response limits exposure.
3, 3a, 3b	Modest potential for injury. Normal aversion response is not sufficient to limit eye exposure to a safe level. Skin hazards normally do not exist. May require safety precautions and personal protective equipment. Class 3b lasers require more safety precautions than Class 3a.
4	Serious potential for injury of the eye and skin. Requires safety precautions and personal protective equipment. Diffuse reflection viewing hazard. Potential fire hazard. Most laser systems for cutting, heat treating, and welding are Class 4.

* When Class 3 and 4 lasers are fully enclosed to prevent potentially hazardous laser radiation exposures, the system may be classified as a Class 1 system.

knowledge for production of laser-generated air contaminants; (c) unwanted plasma radiation; (d) excessive noise levels; (e) inadequate ventilation controls; (f) fire hazards; (g) explosive hazards from high-pressure tubes; (h) exposure to toxic chemicals and laser dyes; and (i) fire hazards. Most of these hazards are associated with Class 3b and 4 lasers. In practice, it is always desirable to totally enclose the laser and beam path to prevent both direct-beam and nonbeam exposures.

Unlike most other workplace hazards, there is generally no need to perform workplace measurements for lasers because of highly confined beam dimensions, minimal likelihood of changing beam paths, and the difficulty and expense of using laser radiometers. However, measurements must be performed by manufacturers to ensure proper laser classification. Laser safety standards are published by government agencies and by independent and industrial standards organizations. In the United States, the American National Standards Institute has developed the *Standard for the Safe Use of Lasers* (Z136.1) and publishes general safety requirements for users. Although this standard is not a law, it forms the basis for OSHA and many states' regulations. There are other laser safety standards and state-specific regulations, but they apply primarily to Class 3b and 4 installations and maintenance activities.

The International Organization for Standardization (ISO) and International Electrotechnical Commission have published standards similar to those in the United States. Two requirements in the ISO documents that affect manufacturers are that (a) all systems must be Class 1 during operation and (b) manufacturers must specify which are the materials that equipment is designed to process. A Class 1 laser rating can be achieved by installing appropriate engineering controls.

Controlling all aspects of potential laser exposures is complex and requires a qualified individual to assess direct and nonbeam hazards. Control measures include process isolation, local-exhaust and building ventilation, training and education, restricted access, proper housekeeping, preventive maintenance, and use of appropriate personal protective equipment.

AUTHOR'S NOTE

The findings and conclusions in this chapter are those of the author and do not necessarily represent the views of the United States Environmental Protection Agency.

REFERENCES

1. Turner JE. Atoms, radiation, and radiation protection. New York: Pergamon Press, 1986.
2. International Commission on Radiological Protection. Publication 68: Dose coefficients for intakes of radionuclides by workers. Philadelphia: Elsevier Health Publishing, 1995.
3. International Commission on Radiological Protection. Publication 66: Human respiratory tract model for radiological protection. Philadelphia: Elsevier Health Publishing, 1995.
4. National Council on Radiological Protection and Measurements. Ionizing radiation exposure of the population of the United States (Report number 160). Bethesda, MD: NCRP, 2009.

5. National Council on Radiological Protection and Measurements. Exposure of the U.S. populations from occupational radiation (Report number 101). Bethesda, MD: NCRP, 1989.

6. Hill AB. The environment and disease: Association or causation? Proceedings of the Royal Society of Medicine 1965; 58: 295–300.

7. Preston, RJ. Update on linear non-threshold dose-response model and implications for diagnostic radiology procedures. Health Physics 2008; 95: 541–546.

8. Sack B, Meyerson G, Siegel J. Epidemiology without biology: False paradigms, unfounded assumptions, and specious statistics in radiation science. Biological Theory 2016; 11: 69–101.

9. Health Physics Society. Radiation risk in perspective. Position statement of the Health Physics Society, 2016. Available at: https://hps.org/documents/radiationrisk.pdf. Accessed December 27, 2016.

10. National Council on Radiological Protection and Measurements. Uncertainties in the estimation of radiation risks and probability of disease causation. (Report No. 171). Bethesda, MD: NCRP, 2012.

11. National Council on Radiological Protection and Measurements. Health effects of low doses of radiation: Perspectives on integrating radiation biology and epidemiology (NCRP Commentary No. 24). Bethesda, MD: NCRP, 2015.

12. BEIR VII. Health risks of exposure to low levels of ionizing radiation. Report of the Advisory Committee on the Biological Effects of Ionizing Radiation. Washington, DC: National Academy Press, 2005.

13. International Commission on Radiological Protection. Publication 84: Pregnancy and medical radiation. Philadelphia: Elsevier Health Publishing, 2001.

14. Meinhold CB, Lauriston S. Taylor Lecture: The evolution of radiation protection—from erythema to genetic risks to risks of cancer to . . .? Health Physics 2004; 87: 240–248.

15. National Institute for Occupational Safety and Health. A recommended standard for occupational exposure to radon progeny in underground mines (DHHS Publication No. 88-11). Washington, DC: NIOSH, 1987.

16. Christodouleas JP, Forrest RD, Ainsley CG, et al. Short-term and long-term health risks of nuclear-power-plant accidents. New England Journal of Medicine 2011; 364: 2334–2341.

17. National Council on Radiation Protection and Measurement. Management of terrorist events involving radioactive material (Report 138). Bethesda, MD: NCRP, 2001.

18. U.S. Environmental Protection Agency. PAG Manual: Protective action guides and planning guidance for radiological incidents. EPA-400/R-16/001, November 2016. Available at: https://www.epa.gov/sites/production/files/2016-12/documents/cpa-pag-manual-2016-prepublication.pdf. Accessed December 27, 2016.

19. Institute for Electrical and Electronics Engineers. IEEE standard for safety levels with respect to human exposure to radio frequency electromagnetic fields, 3 kHz to 300 GHz. New York: IEEE, 2005

20. Institute for Electrical and Electronics Engineers. IEEE standard for safety levels with respect to human exposure to radio frequency electromagnetic fields, 3 kHz to 300 GHz. Amendment 1: Specifies ceiling limits for induced and contact current, clarifies distinctions between localized exposure and spatial peak power density. New York: IEEE, 2010.

21. National Council on Radiation Protection and Measurements. Biological effects and exposure criteria for radio frequency electromagnetic fields (Report 86). Bethesda, MD: NCRP, 1986, pp. 1–382.

22. World Health Organization. Framework for developing EMF standards. International EMF project. Geneva: WHO, 2003.

23. Conover DL, Murray WE, Lary JM, Johnson PH. Magnetic field measurements near RF induction heaters. Bioelectromagnetics 1986; 7: 83–90.

24. Institute of Electrical and Electronics Engineers. Possible health hazards from exposure to power-frequency electric and magnetic fields—a COMAR technical information statement. IEEE Engineering in Medicine and Biology Magazine 2000; 19: 131–137.

25. McColl N, Auvinen A, Kesminiene A, et al. European Code against Cancer 4th Edition: Ionising and non-ionising radiation and cancer. Cancer Epidemiology 2015; 39: S93–S100.

26. Scientific Committee on Emerging and Newly Identified Health Risks. Potential health effects of exposure to electromagnetic fields (EMP). 2015. Available at: https://ec.europa.eu/health/scientific_committees/emerging/docs/scenihr_o_041.pdf. Accessed December 27, 2016.

27. Taki M. Bioelectromagnetics researches in Japan for human protection from electromagnetic field exposures. IEEJ Transactions of Electrical and Electronic Engineering 2016; 11: 683–695.
28. International Agency for Research on Cancer. IARC monographs on the evaluation of carcinogenic risks to humans. Volume 80, Non-ionizing radiation, part 1: Static and extremely low-frequency (ELF) electric and magnetic fields. Lyon, France: IARC, 2002.
29. National Toxicology Program. Fact sheet: Studies on radiofrequency radiation emitted by cellular phones, 2005. Available at: http://pulse.pharmacy.arizona.edu/resources/toxicology/cellphones.pdf. Accessed December 22, 2016.
30. National Toxicology Program. Cell phone radiofrequency radiation studies, 2016. Available at: https://www.niehs.nih.gov/health/assets/docs_a_e/cell_phone_radiofrequency_radiation_studies_508.pdf. Accessed December 22, 2016.
31. Maisch D. Children and mobile phones . . . is there a health risk? Journal of Australasian College of Nutritional & Environmental Medicine 2003; 22: 3–8.
32. ACGIH. Threshold limit values for chemical substances and physical agents & biological exposure indices. Cincinnati, OH: ACGIH, 2016.
33. Ready JF, Farson DF (eds.). LIA handbook of laser materials processing. Orlando, FL: Manolia Publishing, 2001.

WEBSITES FOR FURTHER INFORMATION

Government Agencies

Centers for Disease Control and Prevention, http://www.cdc.gov/nceh/radiation/default.htm
EPA Radiation Protection Program, http://www.epa.gov/radiation/
FDA Center for Devices and Radiological Health, http://www.fda.gov/Radiation-EmittingProducts/default.htm
Federal Emergency Management Agency, http://www.fema.gov/
International Atomic Energy Agency, http://www.iaea.org/
National Library of Medicine, http://www.remm.nlm.gov/
Occupational Safety and Health Administration, http://www.osha.gov/SLTC/radiation/index.html

Scientific Organizations

American Association of Physicists in Medicine, http://www.aapm.org/
American Association of Radon Scientists and Technologists, http://www.aarst.org/
Conference on Radiation Control Program Directors, http://www.crcpd.org/
Health Physics Society, http://www.hps.org/
International Commission on Radiological Protection, http://www.icrp.org/
International Radiation Protection Association, http://www.irpa.net/

13

Biological Hazards

Mark Russi

Occupationally and environmentally related infectious diseases continue to cause morbidity and mortality, facilitated by many factors, including poverty, climate change, stress migration, human encroachment in remote environments, and an increasingly contiguous global society.

In order to identify occupational infectious diseases, one needs to understand situations likely to enhance contact between workers and infectious agents or those in which the usual microbial environment is altered. Examples include (a) workplaces where patients are treated (Figure 13-1); (b) settings where people have contact with animals and zoonotic agents; (c) activities that provide increased opportunities for exposure to soil or other media in which infectious agents, such as fungal or other spores, persist; (d) environments with enhanced contact with mosquitoes or other arthropod vectors that carry infectious agents; (e) research or clinical laboratories (Figure 13-2); and (f) circumstances where exposure to an altered range of diseases in the general environment exists, such as in tropical countries or settings where many people live or train in close proximity.

In healthcare settings, workers are exposed to pathogens spread by direct contact, droplet, airborne, fecal-oral, and bloodborne transmission. Infectious diseases spread by airborne or droplet transmission include tuberculosis (TB), influenza, pertussis, varicella, parvovirus B19 infection, measles, and rubella. Principal bloodborne pathogens of concern are the human immunodeficiency virus (HIV), hepatitis B virus (HBV), and hepatitis C virus (HCV). Fecal-oral transmission of Salmonella and Shigella bacteria, enteroviruses, and hepatitis A virus may occur in hospitals and other work settings. In recent years, healthcare institutions have had to prepare for emerging and re-emerging organisms, such as those that cause severe acute respiratory syndrome (SARS), novel H1N1 influenza, Middle Eastern respiratory syndrome (MERS), Ebola virus disease (EVD), and Zika virus disease.

Beyond healthcare, other infectious diseases pose increased risks to a wide spectrum of workers. Zoonoses may occur by direct contact with animals or their respiratory secretions or excreta. Veterinarians, farmers, cat and dog breeders, and animal handlers are at heightened

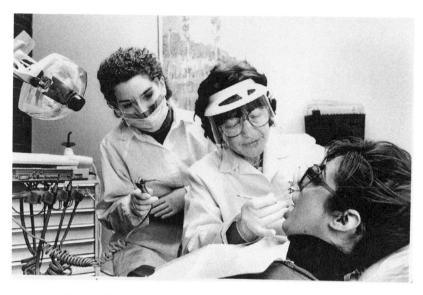

Figure 13-1. Dentists and dental technicians are at increased risk of exposure to HIV, hepatitis B and hepatitis C viruses, and other pathogens. They require protection of the eyes, nose, and mouth from splashes of blood and saliva. The worker closest to the patient has eye protection, but no surgical mask whereas the other worker has a mask, but lacks eye protection. Both workers should have masks and eye protection. (Photograph by Marvin Lewiton.)

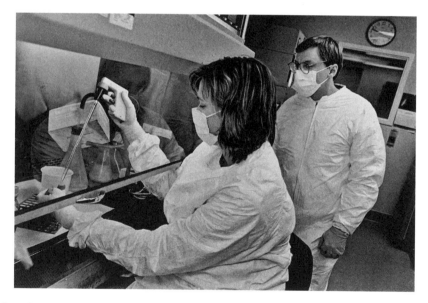

Figure 13-2. Laboratory workers who may be risk for acquiring specific infections may need to use personal protective equipment and work under a hood with exhaust ventilation. (Photograph by Earl Dotter.)

risk. Outdoor work settings increase the risks of arthropod-borne diseases and fungal infections for forestry, farm, construction, landscape, and other workers because of (a) increased contact with mosquitoes and ticks and (b) increased exposure to *Coccidioides immitis, Histoplasma capsulatum,* or other pathogens in soil and dust. Workers who move within or between countries may be exposed to unfamiliar agents that cause endemic infectious diseases, such as Lyme disease, malaria, and other parasitic diseases; nematode infestations; and viral and bacterial illnesses. The risk of contracting disease is greater in low- and middle-income countries (LMICs); however, foodborne illnesses and other infectious diseases are also common in high-income countries.

BIOLOGICAL HAZARDS IN HEALTHCARE AND LABORATORY SETTINGS

Bloodborne Pathogens

Prevention

More than 500,000 needlesticks occur annually in the United States, of which at least 5,000 involve HIV-contaminated blood. Unfortunately, underreporting of blood and body fluid exposures is common. Studies of percutaneous exposures with hollow-bore needles have demonstrated significant differences between the number of needlesticks reported and the number estimated retrospectively by questionnaires. In the operating room, where injuries may occur during as many as 15% of all procedures and blood contact may occur in as many as 50%,[1,2] underreporting is substantial—one study found that only approximately 2% to 11% of blood exposures were reported.[3] Because early prophylactic therapy is indicated for certain exposures, underreporting places healthcare workers at unnecessary risk of infection.

Guidelines and regulations have been designed to reduce bloodborne exposures among healthcare workers. Universal Precautions, developed by the Centers for Disease Control and Prevention (CDC) in 1987, were incorporated into the Occupational Safety and Health Administration (OSHA) Bloodborne Pathogen Standard of 1991, along with a requirement for annual training, planning for exposure reduction, implementing engineering controls, and providing the HBV vaccine to potentially exposed healthcare workers. In 1995, Standard Precautions were introduced, combining Universal Precautions with isolation of body substances, to establish a single set of procedures for patient care and handling of blood and other potentially infectious body fluids.

Needlestick injuries can be reduced by educational programs and replacement of standard instruments with safer devices (Figure 13-3). Use of phlebotomy devices with engineered safety features and needleless intravenous delivery systems have reduced needlestick injuries. Use of blunt needles for certain procedures has the potential to reduce percutaneous injuries among operating room personnel, but acceptance among surgeons of blunt needles has been limited. Interventions in operating room settings that may reduce needlesticks include use of stapling or adhesives for wound closures, use of electrocautery for some incisions, and robotics. The Needlestick Safety and Prevention Act of 2000, which recognized the potential for safer devices to reduce bloodborne pathogen exposures among healthcare workers, mandated OSHA to amend the Bloodborne Pathogens Standard so that employers would be required to document consideration and use of effective safer medical devices to eliminate or minimize occupational exposure to blood.[4]

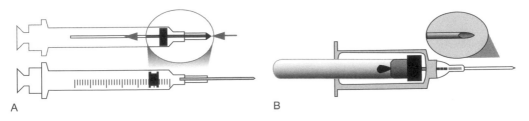

Figure 13-3. Shown here are two devices that help prevent accidental needlesticks (sharp sticks). (A) Syringe with retractable needle: After the needle is used an extra push on the plunger retracts the needle into the syringe, thus removing the hazard of needle exposure. (B) Blunt-tipped blood-drawing needle: After blood is drawn, a push on the collection tube moves the blunt-tip needle forward through the needle and past the sharp needle point. The blunt point tip of this needle can be activated before it is removed from the vein or artery. (Source: Occupational Safety and Health Administration.)

Although a broad range of infections can be transmitted percutaneously or mucocutaneously, the bloodborne pathogens of greatest significance for healthcare workers are HIV, HBV, and HCV.

Human Immunodeficiency Virus

As of 2015, the CDC has documented 58 healthcare workers in the United States who had become HIV-positive following occupational exposure: 24 nurses, 20 laboratory workers, 6 physicians, 2 surgical technicians, 2 housekeepers or maintenance workers, 1 dialysis technician, 1 respiratory therapist, 1 health aide, and 1 morgue technician. Of these 58 healthcare workers, 49 had percutaneous exposure to HIV, 5 mucocutaneous exposure, 2 both cutaneous and mucocutaneous exposure, and 2 exposure from an unknown route. It is noteworthy that only a single confirmed case of occupational HIV transmission to a healthcare worker has taken place since 1999.[5] This may be due to widespread use of antiretroviral therapy resulting in lower viral loads among HIV-positive patients, as well as the institution of antiretroviral prophylactic therapy following healthcare worker exposure to HIV-contaminated blood and body fluids.

A 0.3% risk of HIV seroconversion following needlestick exposure has been commonly quoted.[6] A higher risk of seroconversion is associated with deep injury, visible contamination of a device with blood, needle placement directly into an artery or vein, and exposure to a person with a high titer of HIV. Risk of seroconversion following mucous membrane exposure has been estimated to be 0.09%.[7] The risk of seroconversion following isolated skin exposure has not been quantified but is likely to be extremely low.

The U.S. Public Health Service recommendation for antiretroviral prophylaxis is supported by several lines of evidence, including a case-control study of healthcare workers who became HIV-positive following bloodborne occupational exposure to HIV[8] and a study of HIV-positive pregnant women administered zidovudine during pregnancy.[9] Drug efficacy is decreased if it is not begun soon after exposure or prematurely discontinued.

Drug resistance is a major challenge to the efficacy of antiretroviral therapy. Seroconversions have occasionally occurred after bloodborne HIV exposure despite prophylaxis with one or more antiretrovirals, possibly due to viral resistance, late initiation of therapy, inadequate duration of therapy, or an overwhelming inoculum of virus. In prescribing combination anti-retroviral therapy to exposed healthcare workers, probable patterns of viral resistance should be considered, based on the medication history of the source patient. Drug toxicities also should be monitored closely in healthcare workers receiving prophylaxis. A broad range of mild and serious side effects has been reported.[10]

Many people who are potentially exposed to HIV at work are concerned that they may place sexual partners or other family members at risk. Many worry about future pregnancies and career options. Clinicians treating HIV-exposed workers should counsel them on barrier protection to prevent pregnancy and disease transmission, and the clinicians may also counsel sexual partners and family members, if necessary.

Healthcare workers exposed to HIV-infected blood or body fluids should receive prophylaxis as soon as possible following exposure. Healthcare workers working in HIV-endemic countries where antiretrovirals may not be readily available should be provided access to prophylaxis.[11]

Hepatitis B Virus

Due to the implementation of Standard Precautions in medical centers and widespread hepatitis B vaccination, the estimated incidence of HBV infections among healthcare workers is approximately one-fifth that of the general population. Among unvaccinated healthcare workers, percutaneous exposure to HBV-infected blood confers a seroconversion risk of 1% to 6% if the source patient is e-antigen negative and 22% to 31% if the source patient is e-antigen positive.[12] Viral titers may be as high as 1 billion virions per millilter of blood or serous fluid; however, they are usually several orders of magnitude lower in saliva, semen, and vaginal secretions. Hepatitis B virus is resistant to drying, ambient temperatures, simple detergents, and alcohol. It may survive on environmental surfaces for up to 1 week.[8] An HBV-contaminated sharp object may pose a threat to healthcare workers for several days after last contact with a source patient.

Less than half of people who become infected with HBV manifest acute symptoms. Acute illness generally consists of several weeks of malaise, jaundice, and anorexia. Fulminant hepatitis may develop in approximately 1% of patients. Chronic HBV infection develops in approximately 5% of those infected and is usually accompanied by persistent presence of hepatitis B surface antigen (HBsAg) in the blood for more than 6 months. In those whose infections do not become chronic, hepatitis B surface antibody (anti-HBs) develops as HBsAg levels fall. IgM antibodies to hepatitis B core antigen (HBcAg) indicate current infection, while IgG core antibodies indicate past infection. The e antigen, which is separated from HBcAg during intracellular processing, is a marker of HBcAg production and viral replication. Cirrhosis develops in approximately 20% to 35% of people with chronic HBV infection, 20% of whom will develop hepatocellular carcinoma.

Administration of the hepatitis B vaccine generates immunity in more than 90% of people who receive three vaccine doses. Once established, immunity appears to persist even as anti-HBs titers fall or become undetectable, although the number of years during which immunity is sustained is not known. Periodic booster doses are not recommended. Individuals who do not produce anti-HBs following vaccination should receive three additional doses of vaccine. Those who do not mount an anti-HBs response to the vaccine following three additional doses should be counseled regarding their susceptibility to HBV and receive hepatitis B immune globulin (HBIG) and possibly additional vaccine if exposed percutaneously or mucocutaneously to HBV-contaminated blood or body fluids. HBIG, which should be administered as soon as possible following exposure, is approximately 75% effective in preventing HBV infection in those without vaccine-induced protection.

Hepatitis C Virus

Among healthcare workers, the prevalence of HCV infection is about the same as that of the general population: 1.5%. Following percutaneous exposure of healthcare workers to infected blood, the risk of hepatitis C seroconversion ranges from 0% to 10%, with an average of 1.8%.[13] Infection following mucocutaneous exposure appears to be much less common. The incubation period for hepatitis C varies from 2 to 24 weeks, with an average of 6 to 7 weeks. Antibodies to HCV (anti-HCV) may be detected within 5 to 6 weeks of infection, and they may persist regardless of whether virus is actively replicating. Most people who become infected with HCV have no acute symptoms. Chronic hepatitis develops in approximately 85% of those infected.

No hepatitis C vaccine is available. Administration of immune serum globulin is ineffective. A number of medication regimens are effective in treating chronic HCV infection. Treatment during acute HCV infection or early in the course of chronic HCV infection may be associated with higher cure rates, but there is limited experience with newer hepatitis C medications, such as ledipasvir/sofosbuvir, in treatment of acute disease.[14,15] Symptomatic patients with acute hepatitis C are more likely to spontaneously clear the virus than are patients with asymptomatic infection.[16]

For those who are acutely infected and symptomatic, delaying therapy until 12-24 weeks after onset of symptoms may reduce unnecessary therapy in those destined to clear HCV spontaneously. Given the lower apparent likelihood of spontaneous clearance among those with asymptomatic acute infections, initiation of therapy after infection is documented by seroconversion and polymerase chain reaction (PCR) assay may be prudent. Currently there is no role for prophylaxis in individuals exposed percutaneously or mucocutaneously to HCV-infected blood or other body fluids. Testing with PCR may be used to detect early infection or to confirm presence of virus.

Other Infections

Tuberculosis

Following a resurgence of TB in the United States during the 1980s and early 1990s, disease incidence has fallen in recent years. However, TB remains the single most important infectious cause of death worldwide. It is important to distinguish between *infection* with the organism (*Mycobacterium tuberculosis*) that causes TB and *active disease.* Approximately 95% of people who become infected will contain the organism with a healthy immune response and never develop active disease. Such people have latent infections, which are not contagious. Risk for developing active disease is highest within the first 2 years of infection. It also is increased when the infected person's immune response is compromised, which may occur with HIV infection, malnutrition, cancer chemotherapy, diabetes mellitus, or other diseases. In 2014 in the United States, 9,421 cases of active TB were reported. The incidence rate of 2.96 cases per 100,000 population represented a decrease of approximately 60% since 1992, when cases most recently peaked. More than 65% of active TB cases in the United States occur among those born in other countries; their rate is 13 times that of those born in the United States. Among cases where susceptibility testing was performed, the proportion of active TB patients in the United States with multidrug-resistant tuberculosis was 1.3%.[17]

Without careful adherence to engineering, administrative, and personal protective controls, healthcare workers remain at increased risk for active TB. In response to increasing TB rates in the late 1980s and early 1990s and occupational transmission in several medical centers, the CDC issued guidelines recommending that healthcare facilities at high risk for TB transmission develop and implement programs to prevent occupational exposure.[18] CDC guidelines, most recently updated in 2005, address early identification of potentially contagious patients, engineering controls to minimize spread within a medical center, use of personal protective equipment, and medical surveillance among healthcare workers. For the potentially contagious patient placed in negative-pressure isolation, work-practice controls include respiratory isolation signage, use of N95 respirators by all persons entering the isolation room, and restriction of diagnostic and therapeutic procedures to negative-pressure isolation settings.

Tuberculin skin testing (TST) for TB, which is based on a healthy immune response to the presence of *Mycobacterium tuberculosis*, may be positive in persons with latent infection and those with active disease. A decreasing incidence of TST conversion among healthcare workers is testament to the success of administrative,

engineering, and personal protective controls in healthcare facilities.[19] Administrative controls (early isolation of suspected TB patients) and engineering controls (adequate ventilation rates) have been strongly associated with reduced rates of TST conversion among healthcare workers.[20,21] In the past, outbreaks in healthcare facilities caused substantial morbidity among healthcare workers. In 11 outbreaks from 1928 to 1991, TST conversion rates ranged from 15% to 100%, and active TB occurred in 11% to 61% of skin-test converters. However, healthcare workers who were TST-positive at time of exposure did not develop elevated risk of active TB.[22]

Tuberculin skin testing is the most widely used method for TB surveillance among healthcare workers. Healthcare workers with previously negative tuberculin tests must be tested at time of hire. Because skin-test positivity can wane over time and can be "boosted" by repeated skin testing, those in whom testing has not been performed within the preceding year should receive a two-step test (TST test repeated several weeks following an initial test) to ensure adequate TST sensitivity. In addition to prior infection, vaccination with Bacillus Calmette-Guerin (BCG)—a live, attenuated form of *Mycobacterium bovis* used in many LMICs to reduce TB infections among children—may produce a positive skin test either initially or on two-step testing, especially if BCG vaccination has been recent. A new infection requires an intensive public health search for a source patient and carries with it specific recommendations for chemoprophylaxis. Therefore, one should establish accurate baseline skin-testing results to avoid mistakenly identifying a "boosted" response as a new infection.

The recommended frequency of ongoing testing is based on community TB prevalence and frequency of inpatient TB admissions. People with documented positive TSTs should not be retested. They should be monitored for symptoms suggestive of active TB. After TST conversion and a negative chest X-ray, additional screening chest X-rays should not be done. Tuberculin skin testing reactions may be suppressed by illnesses or medications that alter the normal immune response, and they may be difficult to interpret in areas where non-TB mycobacterial infections are common.

An alternative or supplemental screening method involves assays that measure the release of interferon gamma (IFN-g) in whole blood incubated with TB-like synthetic peptides, such as QuantiFERON-TB Gold, QuantiFERON-TB Gold In-Tube, and T-SPOT.TB. There is much variability in sensitivity for both TST and IFN-g release assays and no clear advantage of either test. In non-BCG vaccinated populations, specificity for both types of tests is 96% or higher.[23] The principal advantage of QFT-g is its greater specificity among people who have been vaccinated with BCG, probably because peptides used in QFT-g assays are not found in BCG vaccine. Therefore, for people who have received BCG vaccine, QFT-g assays are often used after a positive TST. A negative QFT-g result in people who have received BCG vaccine indicates a lower likelihood of latent TB; a positive result is presumptive evidence of latent or active disease.

OSHA requires employers to meet the general duty clause of the OSH Act—to provide a workplace free of recognized hazards. This requirement includes identifying potential respiratory hazards and providing a respiratory protection program specific to the hazard.

Re-emergent or Newly Emergent Diseases: Novel H1N1 Influenza, Middle Eastern Respiratory Syndrome, Ebola Virus Disease

In 1997, of transmission of avian influenza (H5N1) to a human was first documented. As of 2016, more than 800 cases had been documented, occurring principally in children, in adults under the age of 40, and in areas of the world where people and animals live in close proximity or where people live near slaughtered poultry. The case-fatality rate has been approximately 60%. Human-to-human transmission is very rare. Increased viral transmission among humans would represent a global public health emergency.

In the spring of 2009, a novel H1N1 influenza virus, derived from swine, avian, and human strains, emerged from rural Mexico. Novel H1N1 spread rapidly, primarily via droplet spread, and the World Health Organization declared a Phase 6 pandemic within months. The case-fatality rate of H1N1 influenza was estimated at 0.4%. In contrast to seasonal influenza, novel H1N1

disproportionately affected children as well as adults below the age of 60. In New York City, for example, a relatively small percentage of those hospitalized with novel H1N1 influenza were older than 60. More severe disease and higher case fatality occurred among pregnant women and people with chronic medical problems, including asthma, other chronic lung disease, diabetes, immunosuppression, and obesity.

The absence of an effective vaccine at the start of the epidemic, the difficulty in distinguishing between early influenza and other common wintertime viral syndromes, and the poor sensitivity of clinic-based testing for H1N1 created challenges for healthcare workers, as did conflicting recommendations about and availability of personal protective equipment.[24] In order to reduce the likelihood of transmission via short-range aerosol transmission, N95 respirators were recommended for healthcare workers treating patients with novel H1N1 influenza.

Middle Eastern respiratory syndrome was first reported in Saudi Arabia in 2012, and, as of late 2016, had infected more than 1,800 people globally with a mortality rate of approximately 35%. Like SARS, it is caused by a coronavirus. The disease predominantly affects the respiratory tract, and most deaths have occurred among those with comorbid illnesses. The virus has been detected in camels, and spread from camels to humans may occur. As of June 2017 there had been only two cases in the United States. It is likely spread via respiratory droplets; however, the precise way the virus spreads is not fully characterized. Current guidance calls for the imposition of airborne and contact precautions in caring for patients suspected or confirmed to have MERS.

During 2014, an outbreak of EVD of unprecedented magnitude took place in the West African countries of Sierra Leone, Guinea, and Liberia. More than 28,000 people were infected, and more than 11,000 died. Case tallies outside of West Africa were limited; only four cases occurred in the United States, one of which was fatal. Although multiple studies have demonstrated that close contact with an infected individual is required for disease transmission, there is limited evidence (from two animal studies and one human study) that transmission may occur in the absence of documented close contact.[25-27] Based on the high hazard level of EVD and disease transmission to healthcare workers, the CDC enhanced its guidance for the protection of healthcare workers to include use of respirators, face shields, contact precautions, and enhanced precautions where exposure to effluent was possible. Considerable attention was devoted to donning and doffing procedures, including the use of an assistant and a trained observer to detect procedural lapses that could result in contamination. Although there were EVD cases reported in the Democratic Republic of the Congo in May 2017, as of June 2017, there had been no additional cases in West Africa. A vaccine, currently in Phase 2 and 3 clinical trials, appears to be effective based on early studies.[28]

BIOLOGICAL HAZARDS IN SCHOOLS, HEALTHCARE SETTINGS, AND OTHER WORKPLACES

Measles

Despite control of measles in the general population, healthcare facilities should continue to maintain measles vaccination programs for their personnel because several past measles epidemics have been linked to healthcare facilities. Since measles may be spread by large droplets and airborne transmission, precautions must be used when caring for patients with confirmed or suspected measles. Hospitals, schools, and day-care centers should be vigilant for imported measles cases, especially from Europe and Asia.

Rubella

The principal hazard of rubella is its potential to adversely affect fetal development. In a 1980 outbreak, 47 (13%) of healthcare workers at a Boston hospital developed rubella; one healthcare worker terminated her pregnancy. In another outbreak, 56 hospital employees developed rubella; three women terminated their pregnancies. More recently, outbreaks have tended to occur in nonhospital workplaces that employ a large proportion of foreign-born workers.[29] Rubella, which is spread by droplet transmission, is most contagious at the time the rash is erupting, although virus may be shed from 1 week before to 5 to 7 days after the onset of rash. Infants with congenital rubella may excrete virus for years. Droplet Precautions must be used when caring for patients with rubella, and healthcare workers should be vaccinated if they do not have evidence of rubella immunity.

Mumps

Mumps is an acute viral syndrome, which may cause parotitis and less frequently deafness, orchitis, oophoritis, and mastitis. Transmission occurs from direct contact or via respiratory droplets. Incubation is usually 16 to 18 days. Infected people may be contagious prior to manifesting symptoms. One dose of measles-mumps-rubella (MMR) vaccine protects 80% of vaccinees from mumps; two doses protect 90%.

An outbreak, which occurred in Iowa and surrounding states in 2005 and 2006, primarily involved people age 18 to 25, most of whom had been vaccinated. The viral genotype was identical to one associated with a large mumps outbreak in the United Kingdom, which also occurred principally among unvaccinated individuals. Due to their increased risk of acquiring and transmitting mumps, healthcare workers should receive two doses of MMR vaccine. Persons suspected of having mumps should remain isolated for 9 days following onset of symptoms.

Varicella (Chickenpox)

Varicella may be spread by contact with infected lesions or by airborne transmission. The incubation period ranges from 10 to 21 days. People at risk for severe disease include immunocompromised individuals, pregnant women, and premature infants. Adults generally have more severe disease than children. Outbreaks may occur in hospitals when personnel without immunity care for patients with unrecognized disease. A varicella vaccine was licensed in 1994 and is recommended for nonimmune healthcare workers, teachers of young children, day-care workers, military personnel, those who work in institutions and prisons, and international travelers. It is contraindicated for pregnant women. Exposed hospital personnel who do not have varicella immunity should be furloughed from patient contact from days 10 to 21 after contact with an infected patient.

Parvovirus B19 Infection

Episodes of parvovirus B19 transmission to healthcare workers occur infrequently. Risk of infection among school and day-care teachers generally exceeds that of healthcare workers. Parvovirus is spread via large droplets, direct contact, or fomites. Patients with erythema infectiosum rash (fifth disease) are contagious before the appearance of the rash. Infected adults generally suffer a self-limited viral arthropathy. Those with parvovirus-associated aplastic crisis are contagious for up to 1 week following onset of illness. Infected immunocompromised persons may be contagious for years. Patients hospitalized during a phase of disease when transmission may occur should be treated using Droplet Precautions. When women become infected during the first half of pregnancy, there is a small risk of fetal death due to hydrops or spontaneous abortion.

Pertussis

Pertussis, which is easily spread by droplets or direct contact, has an attack rate of 80% in unvaccinated individuals. Estimates of annual incidence in the United States range from 800,000 to 3.3 million cases.[30] Several pertussis outbreaks have occurred in hospitals and involved healthcare workers.[31] Infants are at highest risk of death.

An acellular pertussis vaccine (Tdap) is recommended to the general population—with an accelerated schedule of vaccination to healthcare workers. Vaccine efficacy is approximately 92%. Antibiotic prophylaxis continues to be recommended following acute unprotected exposure to a pertussis patient, regardless of whether the exposed individual has received Tdap.

Seasonal Influenza

More than 100,000 U.S. residents are hospitalized annually due to influenza or its complications, and between 3,000 and 49,000 die each year. Hospitals have a high risk of influenza transmission, which generally occurs by large droplets.

Patients hospitalized with influenza should be treated using Droplet Precautions. In adults, virus may be shed from 1 day prior to illness to 7 days after onset. Children may excrete virus for longer periods. The most effective means of prevention is annual vaccination, which is specifically recommended for healthcare workers. Vaccine consists of killed virus or recombinantly produced antigen from three (trivalent) or four (quadrivalent) strains designed to closely match circulating strains. Average efficacy of influenza vaccination, based upon several decades of data is 59%.[32] Antivirals may be administered during outbreaks to prevent influenza in nonimmunized adults.

Hepatitis A

Although outbreaks of hepatitis A have occurred in healthcare facilities, hepatitis A prevalence among healthcare workers is similar to that in the general population. The CDC does not specifically recommend hepatitis A vaccination for healthcare workers. Transmission has occurred in hospitals (a) during care of patients with diarrhea who were later discovered to be acutely infected with HAV and (b) through contamination of food due to improper handwashing after patient care. Outbreaks may occur in day-care centers, especially if there is community transmission, but day-care center workers do not have increased prevalence of infection.[33]

Bioterrorism

Following the 9/11 attack on the World Trade Center and the dissemination of anthrax spores through the U.S. mail during 2001, there has been increased attention on preparedness for terrorist attacks. Bioterrorism agents are viewed as credible threats due to their capacity for widespread dissemination and potential to affect or kill many people. The CDC classifies such agents into three categories. Category A agents can be easily disseminated or transmitted from person to person, can result in high case-fatality rates, can have major public health impact, might cause public panic and social disruption, and require special action for public health preparedness. Category B agents are moderately easy to disseminate, result in moderate morbidity rates and low case-fatality rates, and require specific enhancements of diagnostic capacity and disease surveillance. Category C agents could be engineered for mass dissemination in the future due to their availability, ease of production and dissemination, and potential for high morbidity and case-fatality rates. (See Chapter 31.)

Agents of bioterrorism vary widely in their propensity for transmission from person to person. Standard precautions are all that is required to prevent transmission to healthcare workers caring for those affected by anthrax, tularemia, Q fever, and biological toxins. However, patients who have not been adequately decontaminated may harbor disease agents on their skin or clothing that could cause disease in healthcare providers. For some agents, such as smallpox virus and Lassa fever virus, the primary means of transmission is close contact, but isolated examples of airborne spread dictate use of respiratory protection when providing patient care.[34,35] Healthcare workers should use Droplet Precautions when caring for patients with pneumonic plague and viral encephalitis viruses and Standard Precautions when caring for patients with brucellosis.

As a result of the 2001 dissemination of anthrax spores, 23 people contracted inhalational or cutaneous disease, 17 of whom survived. They had symptoms that included fever, flu-like symptoms, cough, dyspnea, pleuritic chest pain, nausea, vomiting, headache, and chest discomfort. Presence of shortness of breath, nausea, and vomiting and lack of rhinorrhea helped to distinguish the initial clinical presentation of anthrax from influenza or influenza-like illness. For affected postal workers, the most important factor in survival was physicians' clinical suspicion of anthrax, based on occupational history, which led them to initially obtain blood cultures.

Considerable attention has been directed to smallpox virus as a potential biological weapon, although the only known remaining stocks of the virus are safeguarded in the United States and Russia. A major campaign was undertaken by the U.S. government to vaccinate military personnel stationed in areas considered to be at risk and healthcare workers who might need to care for smallpox victims in a bioterrorist attack. Many military personnel were vaccinated. Due to widespread concern about adverse effects of smallpox vaccine, a smaller than anticipated proportion of healthcare workers chose to be vaccinated. Common adverse effects of vaccination include fever, lymph node swelling, and injection site pain. Less common, potentially serious adverse effects include erythema multiforme, generalized vaccinia, myocarditis, transmission to contacts, and inadvertent inoculation (such as people inoculating their eyes with virus shed from the vaccine site or inoculating vulnerable family members). The marginal acceptance by healthcare workers of the smallpox vaccination campaign and the absence of a documented threat resulted in a policy shift to rapidly vaccinate healthcare workers only if smallpox cases were to occur.

Measures to enhance preparedness for bioterrorist attacks have included the following:

- Upgrading of epidemiological detection systems to recognize unusual disease clusters that may indicate exposure to bioterrorist agents
- Building capacity of laboratories to detect bioterrorism-related agents
- Improving communication systems among first responders, law enforcement personnel, and staff medical centers
- Increasing awareness of bioterrorism-related disease among physicians.
- Stockpiling vaccines and drugs
- Improving supply lines for rapid delivery of vaccines and drugs
- Performing research on relevant diagnostic tests, vaccines, and therapies.

BIOLOGICAL HAZARDS ASSOCIATED WITH ANIMAL CONTACT

Many bacterial, fungal, parasitic, viral, and rickettsial diseases can be transmitted from animals to humans (Table 13-1). Workers who have frequent contact with wild animals, farm animals, or domestic pets are at increased risk.

Workers including park rangers, hunters, ranchers, forestry workers, trappers, fur traders, geologists, other scientific field workers, butchers, rendering workers, expedition leaders, and zoo workers have contact with wild animals. These include rats, mice, bats, rabbits, raccoons,

Table 13-1. Illustrative Zoonoses and Transmitting Animals

Zoonoses	Transmitting Animals
Bacterial Diseases	
Brucellosis (Brucella species [spp.])	Farm animals and dogs, bison, and deer
Campylobacteriosis (Campylobacter spp.)	Cats, dogs, farm animals, and improper food preparation
Cat scratch disease or cat scratch fever (*Bartonella henselae*)	Cat scratches and bites
Escherichia coli O157:H7	Cattle and improper food preparation
Fish tuberculosis (Mycobacterium spp.)	Fish and aquarium water
Leptospirosis (Leptospira spp.)	Livestock, dogs, rodents, wildlife, and contaminated water
Lyme disease (*Borrelia burgdorferi* infection)	Ticks on deer, mice, dogs, and other animals
Plague (*Yersinia pestis*)	Wild rodents, cats, and fleas
Psittacosis (*Chlamydia psittaci*)	Pet birds, including parrots and parakeets
Q fever (*Coxiella burnetti*)	Cattle, sheep, goats, dogs, and cats
Salmonellosis (Salmonella spp.)	Reptiles, birds, dogs, cats, horses, farm animals, and improper food preparation
Tuberculosis (*Mycobacterium tuberculosis*)	Deer, elk, bison, and cattle
Tularemia (*Francisella tularensis*)	Sheep and wildlife, especially rodents and rabbits
Yersiniosis (*Yersinia enterocolitica*)	Dogs, cats, and farm animals
Fungal Diseases	
Cryptococcosis (Cryptococcus spp.)	Wild birds, especially pigeon droppings
Histoplasmosis (Histoplasma spp.)	Bat guano (stool)
Ringworm (Microsporum spp. and Trichophyton spp.)	Mammals, including dogs, cats, horses, and farm animals
Parasitic Diseases	
Cryptosporidiosis (Cryptosporidium spp.)	Cats, dogs, and farm animals
Giardiasis (*Giardia lamblia*)	Various animals and water contaminated by animal excrement
Hookworm (*Ancylostoma caninum, Ancylostoma braziliense, Uncinaria stenocephals*)	Dogs and their environment
Leishmaniasis (Leishmania spp.)	Dogs and sandflies
Raccoon roundworm infection (*Baylisascaris procyonis*)	Raccoons
Roundworm (*Toxocara canis, T. cati,* and *Toxocaris leonina*)	Cats, dogs, and their environment
Tapeworm infection (*Dipylidium caninum*)	Flea infections in cats and dogs
Toxoplasmosis (*Toxoplasma gondii*)	Cats and their environment
Viral Diseases	
Hantavirus (hantavirus pulmonary syndrome)	Wild mice
Herpes B virus	Macaque monkeys
Lymphocytic choriomeningitis	Rodents, such as rats, guinea pigs, and house mice
Monkeypox	Recently suspected to be associated with prairie dogs, Gambian rats, and rabbits
Rabies	Mammals, including bats, skunks, raccoons, dogs, cats, and others
West Nile virus	Spread by mosquitoes; can affect birds, horses, and other mammals
Rickettsial Diseases	
Rocky Mountain spotted fever (*Rickettsia rickettsii*)	Dogs and ticks

skunks, deer, and bison. For some diseases, relatively close animal contact is required for transmission; for giardiasis, illness may occur after ingesting small amounts of water or food contaminated by animal waste, and for histoplasmosis, illness may occur after breathing dusts contaminated with animal excrement. Workers are at increased risk for brucellosis (if they have contact with, for example, bison or deer), raccoon roundworm (raccoons), giardiasis (water contaminated by animal excrement), hantavirus infection (wild mice), histoplasmosis (bat guano), lymphocytic choriomeningitis (rodents, including house mice), TB (deer, elk, or bison), plague (wild rodents), rabies (raccoons, skunks, or bats), and tularemia (rodents, rabbits, or hares). Chronic wasting disease of deer and elk, which is endemic in Colorado, Wyoming, and Nebraska, may be caused by a prion; it is not clear if this represents a threat to humans.

Contact with macaque monkeys, which may occur in an animal laboratory setting, a monkey cell culture facility, or among veterinarians, is associated with transmission of herpes B simiae, which can cause fatal encephalomyelitis in humans. Infection is caused by animal bites, scratches, or exposure to the tissues or secretions of macaques. Immediate and thorough wound cleansing is indicated following a macaque bite. Prophylactic treatment with acyclovir or valacyclovir is indicated for percutaneous or mucocutaneous exposures to potentially infected animals.

Farmworkers and those who process farm products, such as meatpackers, butchers, and slaughterhouse workers, may be exposed to cattle, sheep, pigs, goats, domestic fowl, horses, and other animals. Farm workers have much contact with livestock and livestock waste. Agents that may be transmitted in the farm environment include Brucella, Campylobacter, Cryptosporidium, *Escherichia coli* 0157:H7, *Coxiella burnetti*, rabies virus, ringworm, Salmonella, and *Yersinia enterocolitica*. Bovine spongiform encephalopathy (BSE, or "mad cow disease"), a neurological degenerative disease of cattle, is likely caused by a prion; eating contaminated meat has been associated with variant Creuzfeldt-Jakob disease in humans, but farmworkers are not at increased risk.

Enhanced contact with pet animals may occur among breeders, delivery personnel, veterinarians, pet shop workers, and others. Illnesses associated with dogs include brucellosis (rare), Campylobacter infection, cryptosporidiosis, giardiasis, leptospirosis, Lyme disease, Q fever, rabies, Rocky Mountain spotted fever, salmonellosis, and infestations with tapeworm, hookworm, ringworm, and roundworm. Many of these same illnesses are associated with cats. Cat scratch disease, caused by *Bartonella henselae*, and plague (rarely) can also be transmitted from cats. Bird-associated illnesses may occur among veterinarians, pet shop workers, poultry workers, and bird breeders, including psittacosis (parrots and parakeets), Q fever (ducks and geese), cryptococcosis (wild bird and pigeon droppings), and salmonellosis (chickens, baby chicks, and ducklings). Human monkeypox cases have been reported in association with pet prairie dogs. Smallpox virus is closely related to monkeypox virus. Smallpox vaccine, which may be 85% protective against monkeypox, is recommended for workers investigating monkeypox outbreaks or involved in caring for infected people or animals.

BIOLOGICAL HAZARDS ASSOCIATED WITH ARTHROPOD VECTORS

Contact with arthropod vectors, especially mosquitoes and ticks, may occur frequently among park rangers, landscapers, nursery workers, farmers, ranchers, trappers, construction workers, soldiers, and others who work outside.

Zika Virus

The Zika virus, named after the Zika Forest in Uganda where it was first discovered in 1947, is spreading rapidly via mosquito vectors in tropical and subtropical areas of the Americas. In most individuals, the virus causes only mild symptoms, most commonly fever, rash, joint pain, and conjunctivitis, typically lasting from several days to a week. Those who become infected are likely protected from future infections. In a very few affected people, the virus has been linked to the Guillain-Barre syndrome, which may or may not resolve completely. Zika virus has also been associated with microcephaly and other severe birth defects in infants of women infected during pregnancy. In June 2017, CDC reported that, among 2,549 completed pregnancies with laboratory evidence of recent possible Zika virus infection, 5% of the fetuses or infants resulting from these pregnancies had birth defects potentially associated with the Zika virus infection, including brain abnormalities, microcephaly, neural tube defects and other early brain malformations, eye abnormalities, and consequences of central nervous system dysfunction, such as congenital and sensorineural deafness.[36]

As of June 2017 the vast majority of U.S. cases had occurred in individuals returning from countries where the Zika virus is spread by mosquitoes. In the United States, there also has been sexual and laboratory transmission.

The principal vector of Zika virus disease is the *Aedes aegypti* mosquito whose range in the United States is generally in the South, although it may extend further northward. It may also spread less efficiently via the *Aedes albopictus* mosquito, a species more likely to be present in the northern United States. Because there is no vaccine against the Zika virus, the best prevention is mosquito control and avoidance of mosquito contact when visiting areas where there has been local spread. General recommendations include use of insect repellents, wearing long-sleeved shirts and long pants, and avoiding being out around the time of dawn and dusk, when mosquitoes are more likely to bite.

In healthcare settings, person-to-person spread is thought to be extremely unlikely unless there is contact with blood via a needlestick or splash onto mucous membranes. The CDC has published guidance addressing the diagnostic work-up of pregnant women with known exposure to the virus, as well as fetal growth monitoring. Much is unknown regarding the likelihood of (a) infection among exposed persons, (b) transmission to the developing fetus, and (c) fetal abnormalities in infants of infected pregnant women.

Viruses That Cause Encephalitis

Several types of encephalitis are transmitted in the United States by mosquito vectors. Eastern equine encephalititis, transmitted primarily from birds to humans by mosquitoes, accounts for an average of five reported cases a year in the United States; it has a 35% case-fatality rate. Coastal areas and freshwater swamps have the highest transmission risk. Western equine encephalitis, also rare, has a lower case-fatality rate. LaCrosse encephalitis, which is reported in the United States approximately 70 times a year, is typically transmitted from chipmunks or squirrels to humans by the treehole mosquito (*Aedes triseriatus*). Workers in woodland areas are at increased risk. St. Louis encephalitis is transmitted from birds to humans primarily by Culex mosquitoes.

West Nile virus, a flavivirus common in Africa, West Asia, and the Middle East, is closely related to St. Louis encephalitis virus. It appears to have been introduced to the eastern United States during 1999 or earlier. It is transmitted primarily from birds to humans by mosquitoes, with outbreaks in temperate regions predominating in late summer and early fall. Year-round transmission takes place in milder climates.

Agents Spread by Ticks

Tick bites represent another occupational hazard for those who work in outdoor settings. The most important illnesses associated with tick vectors are Lyme disease, Rocky Mountain spotted fever, babesiosis, and ehrlichiosis. Lyme disease is caused by *Borrelia burgdorferi* and transmitted to humans by black-legged ticks (*Ixodes scapularis* in north central and northeastern United States, and *Ixodes pacificus* on the Pacific coast). Infection is most likely to be transmitted if the tick has fed for at least 2 days. Workers in woodland areas of the northeastern and north central United States, as well as a limited region of the northwestern Pacific coast, are at highest risk. If recognized early, Lyme disease can be effectively treated with oral antibiotics. Rocky Mountain spotted fever is caused by *Rickettsia rickettsii* and spread by the American dog tick and the Rocky Mountain wood tick.

Babesiosis is caused by Babesia protozoan parasites (primarily *Babesia divergens* and *Babesia microti*). Disease, which is spread from mice to humans primarily by the *Ixodes scapularis* tick, is characterized by fevers, chills, myalgias, hepatosplenomegaly, and hemolytic anemia. Ehrlichiosis is caused primarily by three distinct bacterial species of the genus Ehrlichia. In the United States, ehrlichiosis due to *Ehrlichia chaffeensis* occurs primarily in the southeastern and south central states and is transmitted by the lone star tick, *Amblyomma americanum*. Ehrlichia ewingii has caused a few human cases of ehrlichiosis in Missouri, Oklahoma, and Tennessee. Human granulocytic ehrlichiosis is caused by a third Ehrlichia species, and it is transmitted by black-legged ticks (*Ixodes scapularis* and *Ixodes pacificus*).

Prevention

Preventive measures that should be implemented by outdoor workers to prevent transmission of mosquito-borne or tickborne illnesses include wearing lightly colored, long-sleeved shirts tucked into pants and lightly colored, long pants tucked into socks; using DEET-containing insect repellents; using mosquito netting if sleeping outdoors; avoiding outdoor work at dawn and dusk; and checking of skin and hair for ticks daily. Permethrin-containing repellents may be used on clothing, shoes, bed nets, and camping gear.

TRAVELERS' HEALTH

Detailed discussion of diseases typically encountered in tropical countries and LMICs, as well as their prevention and treatment can be found at http://www.cdc.gov/travel. The most common cause of illness in travelers is contamination of food or water. Travelers' diarrhea can be due to bacteria, including *E. coli*, Salmonella, and *Vibrio cholerae*; viruses; or parasites. Many illnesses are transmitted to travelers via arthropod vectors, including malaria, yellow fever, dengue, filariasis, leishmaniasis, trypanosomiasis, and onchocerciasis. Schistosomiasis can be transmitted through the skin during swimming in fresh water.

Vaccination and prophylaxis vary by destination country. General recommendations for travelers include frequent handwashing, drinking only bottled or boiled water or canned drinks, eating only thoroughly cooked food or self-peeled fruits and vegetables, complying with any recommended malaria prophylaxis, and protecting oneself from mosquitoes. One should not eat food purchased from street vendors, drink beverages with ice, eat unpasteurized dairy products, handle animals, or swim in fresh water. Prior to departure, workers assigned to tropical countries or LMICs should consult with a travel medicine specialist.

REFERENCES

1. Centers for Disease Control and Prevention. Evaluation of blunt suture needles in preventing percutaneous injuries among health-care workers during gynecologic surgical procedures–New York City, March 1993–June 1994. Morbidity and Mortality Weekly Report 1997; 46: 25–29.
2. Quebbeman EJ, Telford GL, Hubbard S, et al. Risk of blood contamination and injury to operating room personnel. Annals of Surgery 1991; 214: 614–620.
3. Lynch P, White MC. Perioperative blood contact and exposures: A comparison of incident reports and focused studies. American Journal of Infection Control 1993; 21: 357–363.
4. Occupational Safety and Health Administration. Occupational exposure to bloodborne pathogens; needlestick and other sharps injuries. Federal Register January 18, 2001; 66: 5317–5325.
5. Joyce MP, Kuhar D, Brooks JT. Notes from the field: Occupationally acquired HIV infection among health care workers—United States, 1985–2013. Morbidity and Mortality Weekly Report 2015; 63: 1245–1246.
6. Beltrami E, Williams I, Shapiro C, Chamberland M. Risk and management of blood-borne infections in health care workers. Clinical Microbiology Reviews 2000; 13: 385–407.
7. Cardo DM, Culver DH, Ciesielski CA, et al. A case-control study of HIV seroconversion in health care workers after percutaneous exposure. New England Journal of Medicine 1997; 337: 1485–1490.
8. Beltrami EM, Williams IT, Shapiro CN, Chamberland ME. Risk and management of blood-borne infections in health care workers. Clinical Microbiology Reviews 2000; 13: 385–407
9. Sperling RS, Shapiro RE, Coombs RW, et al. Maternal viral load, zidovudine treatment, and the risk of transmission of human immunodeficiency virus type 1 from mother to infant. New England Journal of Medicine 1996; 335: 1621–1629.
10. Centers for Disease Control and Prevention. Serious adverse events attributed to nevirapine regimens for postexposure prophylaxis after HIV exposures–Worldwide, 1997–2000. Morbidity and Mortality Weekly Report 2001; 49: 1153–1156.
11. Russi M, Hajdun M, Barry M. A program to provide antiretroviral prophylaxis to health care personnel working overseas. Journal of the American Medical Association 2000; 283: 1292–1293.
12. Centers for Disease Control and Prevention. Updated U.S. Public Health Service Guidelines for the management of occupational exposures to HBV, HCV, and HIV and recommendations for postexposure prophylaxis. Morbidity and Mortality Weekly Report 2001; 50: 1–52.
13. Centers for Disease Control and Prevention. Recommendations for follow-up of health-care workers after occupational exposure to hepatitis C virus. Morbidity and Mortality Weekly Report 1998; 47: 603–606.
14. Jaeckel E, Cornberg M, Wedemeyer H, et al. Treatment of acute hepatitis C with interferon alfa-2b. New England Journal of Medicine 2001; 345: 1452–1457.

15. Wiegand J, Buggisch P, Boecher W, et al. Early monotherapy with pegylated interferon alpha-2b for acute hepatitis C infection: the HEP-NET Acute HCV-II study. Hepatology 2006; 43: 250–256.

16. Gerlach JT, Diepolder HM, Zachoval R, et al. Acute hepatitis C: high rate of both spontaneous and treatment-induced viral clearance. Gastroenterology 2003; 125: 80–88.

17. Scott C, Kirking HL, Jeffries C, Price SF, Pratt R. Tuberculosis trends, United States, 2014. Morbidity and Mortality Weekly Report 2015; 64: 265–269.

18. Centers for Disease Control and Prevention. Guidelines for preventing the transmission of mycobacterium tuberculosis in health care facilities, 1994. Morbidity and Mortality Weekly Report 1994; 43: 1–132.

19. Tokars JI, McKinley GF, Otten J, et al. Use and efficacy of tuberculosis infection control practices at hospital with previous outbreaks of multidrug-resistant tuberculosis. Infection Control and Hospital Epidemiology 2001; 22: 449–455.

20. Blumberg HM, Watkins DL, Berschling JD, et al. Preventing the nosocomial transmission of tuberculosis. Annals of Internal Medicine 1995; 122: 658–663.

21. Menzies D, Fanning A, Yuan L, Fitzgerald JM. Hospital ventilation and risk for tuberculous infection in Canadian health care workers. Canadian Collaborative Group in Nosocomial Transmission of TB. Annals of Internal Medicine 2000; 133: 779–789.

22. Stead WW. Management of health care workers after inadvertent exposure to tuberculosis: a guide for the use of preventive therapy. Annals of Internal Medicine 1995; 122: 906–912.

23. Madhukar P, Zwerling A, Menzies D. Systematic review: T-cell-based assays for the diagnosis of latent tuberculosis infection: an update. Annals of Internal Medicine 2008; 149: 177–184.

24. Centers for Disease Control and Prevention. Novel influenza A (H1N1) virus infections among health-care personnel–United States, April-May, 2009. Morbidity and Mortality Weekly Report 2009; 58: 641–645.

25. Dalgard DW, Hardy RJ, Pearson SL, et al. Combined simian hemorrhagic fever and Ebola virus infection in cynomolgus monkeys. Labatory Animal Science 1992; 42: 152–157.

26. Jaax N, Jahrling P, Geisbert T, et al. Transmission of Ebola virus (Zaire strain) to uninfected control monkeys in a biocontainment laboratory. Lancet 1995; 346: 1669–1671.

27. Roels TH, Bloom AS, Buffington J, et al. Ebola hemorrhagic fever, Kikwit, Democratic Republic of the Congo, 1995: Risk factors for patients without a reported exposure. Journal of Infectious Diseases 1999; 179: S92–S97.

28. Henao-Restrepo AM, Longini IM, Egger M, et al. Efficacy and effectiveness of an rVSV-vectored vaccine expressing Ebola surface glycoprotein: Interim results from the Guinea ring vaccination cluster-randomised trial. Lancet 2015; 386: 857–866.

29. Centers for Disease Control and Prevention. Control and prevention of rubella: Evaluation and management of suspected outbreaks, rubella in pregnant women, and surveillance for congenital rubella syndrome. Morbidity and Mortality Weekly Report 2001; 50: 1–23.

30. Cherry JD. The epidemiology of pertussis: a comparison of the epidemiology of the disease pertussis with the epidemiology of Bordetalla pertussis infection. Pediatrics 2005; 115: 1422–1427.

31. Weber DJ, Rutala WA. Management of healthcare workers exposed to pertussis. Infection Control and Hospital Epidemiology 1994; 15: 411–415.

32. Osterholm MT, Kelley NS, Sommer A, Belongia EA. Efficacy and effectiveness of influenza vaccines: A systematic review and meta-analysis. Lancet Infectious Diseases 2012; 12: 36–44.

33. Centers for Disease Control and Prevention. Prevention of hepatitis A through active or passive immunization: Recommendations of the Advisory Committee on Immunization Practices (ACIP). Morbidity and Mortality Weekly Report 1999; 48: 1–37.

34. Carey DE, Kemp GE, White HA, et al. Lassa fever. Epidemiological aspects of the 1970 epidemic, Jos, Nigeria. Transaction of the Royal Society of Tropical Medicine and Hygiene 1972; 66: 402–408.

35. Gelfand HM, Posch J. The recent outbreak of smallpox in Meschede, West Germany. American Journal of Epidemiology 1971; 93: 234–237.

36. Shapiro-Mendoza CK, Rice ME, Galang RR, et al. Pregnancy outcomes after maternal Zika virus infection during pregnancy – U.S. territories, January 1, 2016-April 25, 2017. Morbidity and Mortality Weekly Report 2017; 66: 615–621.

FURTHER READING

Heymann DL (ed.). Control of communicable diseases manual (20th ed.). Washington, DC: American Public Health Association, 2015.

An extremely useful guide on the identification, prevention, and control of a wide range of infectious diseases.

Wright WE (ed.). Coutrier's occupational and environmental infectious diseases (2nd ed.). Beverly Farms, MA: OEM Press, 2008.

A comprehensive overview of the recognition, management, and prevention of infectious diseases in the workplace.

14

Occupational Stress

Paul A. Landsbergis, Marnie Dobson, Anthony D. LaMontagne, BongKyoo Choi, Peter Schnall, and Dean B. Baker

Occupational stress contributes to a wide range of health problems, including acute traumatic injuries, psychological disorders, musculoskeletal disorders, gastrointestinal illnesses, and cardiovascular disease (CVD).[1-7] As a group, these disorders are responsible for much morbidity, mortality, and disability, as well as healthcare utilization.

The following are some examples:

- A 49-year-old bus driver, who commutes 1 hour for a 12-hour split shift, driving through the congested streets of a large city, is trying to keep his hypertension under control. He does not smoke cigarettes or drink alcohol.
- A 56-year-old hotel housekeeper, who works without rest breaks to complete the many rooms she has to clean daily, is experiencing back and shoulder pain.
- A 39-year-old temporary worker for a major software company, who works long hours yet gets fewer holidays, vacation days, and pay raises than his salaried coworkers, is experiencing headaches, irritability, and difficulty sleeping.
- A 52-year-old nurse, who cares for seven high-needs patients, does not eat lunch, and

often works extra hours, feels emotionally drained, experiences palpitations, and was recently diagnosed with hypertension.

Workers have been active in reducing sources of stress at work. For example, nurses, through their labor unions, have lobbied for legislation and bargained for union contracts that mandate minimum staffing levels in hospitals and make overtime work voluntary. Hotel room cleaners, through their union, have bargained for reductions in the number of rooms that they have to clean daily.

DEFINITIONS

The *occupational stress process* refers to the ways in which sources of stress in the work environment (*stressors*) can lead to psychological, behavioral, or physiologic manifestations of stress (*strain*), and to longer-term health effects. The National Institute for Occupational Safety and Health (NIOSH) and the International Labour Office have defined *occupational stress* as the harmful physical and emotional responses that occur when job requirements do not match or exceed a worker's capabilities, resources, or needs. As NIOSH has stated,

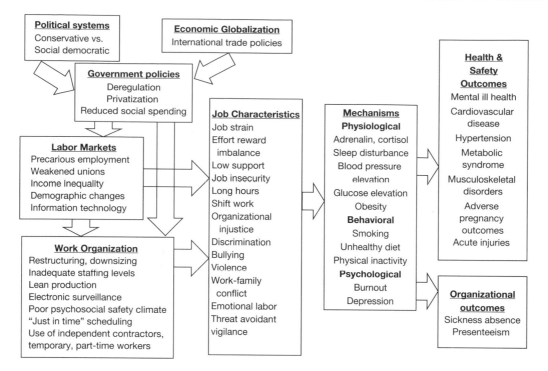

Figure 14-1. A perspective on occupational stress in the context of political systems and economic globalization. (Source: Adapted from Schnall P, Dobson M, Landsbergis P. Globalization, work and cardiovascular disease. International Journal of Health Services 2016; 46: 656–692).

stressful working conditions (stressors) "play a primary role in causing job stress," but *modifiers* "can intervene to strengthen or weaken this influence."[8] These modifiers include individual factors, such as coping style, and other work environment factors, such as social support.

Occupational stressors are often considered in the context of the *organization of work*, which NIOSH defines as "the work process (the way jobs are designed and performed)" and "the organizational practices (management and production methods and accompanying human resource policies) that influence job design."[3] According to NIOSH, work organization also includes external factors, such as the social, economic, and legal environment, as well as technological factors that encourage or enable new organizational practices.[3] The NIOSH conception of work organization can be expanded to explicitly include the following factors that influence organizational practices:

- The impact of political systems
- Economic globalization

- Policies of privatization
- Deregulation
- Reduced societal spending on education, healthcare, and social services, all of which are often features of international trade policies or conservative political policies
- Growing social inequality
- The changing labor market. (See Figure 14-1.)

OCCUPATIONAL STRESSORS AND THE CHANGING WORK ENVIRONMENT

Over the past 40 years, economic globalization policies, which have influenced labor markets and work organization, have increased work stressors. John Howard, Director of NIOSH, has stated: "Fierce competition in the globalized world of commerce pressures employers to structure work in the most efficient or leanest way possible. . . . As the employment relationship continues to undergo change, stress related to work organization, scheduling, and staffing may heighten risks for worker injury or illness."[9]

Other contributors to increasing job stress have included use of new information technologies that reduce the number of workers needed to produce goods or services, thereby increasing job insecurity, as well as declines in both union membership and labor protection.[2] Employers in manufacturing, healthcare, social services, and government are implementing new systems of work organization, known as *lean production, lean sigma, total quality management,* or *new public management* and all of which are modern versions of *scientific management* or *Taylorism,* which can increase occupational stress.[10] Deregulation and privatization policies have made labor markets more precarious, increased job insecurity and time pressure, and limited job control and support in the workplace. Global slowing in economic growth since the 2008 global economic crisis and implementation of austerity policies in some countries have worsened working conditions for many people.[11]

OCCUPATIONAL STRESS MODELS

Current understanding of the occupational stress process evolved from early research on the physiology and cognitive psychological component of the stress response.

Physiologic Stress Models

Early physiologic stress response models focused on two main mechanisms: (a) the adrenal medullary response, involving epinephrine (adrenalin) and norepinephrine, and (b) the hypothalamic–pituitary–adrenal (HPA) axis, involving cortisol. Walter Cannon's *fight-or-flight response* is most associated with stimulation of the adrenal medulla and epinephrine secretion. This pattern, occurring in conjunction with sympathetic arousal of the cardiovascular system, is an active response mode in which an organism is able to use metabolic energy to support both mental and physical exertion. Although this response mechanism is a basic element in the behavior of all animals, it can be taxing in the short term. In the long term, arousal of psychoendocrine mechanisms

can lead to difficulties with relaxation and a state of chronic overarousal. Adrenal medullary mechanisms reflect the importance of sustained arousal conditions: threats to security, time pressures for increased performance, and a range of workplace social situations, including challenges to one's authority. In contrast, the HPA axis is often activated in situations in which people face threats over which they have little control. In such situations, the HPA axis mediates a behavioral response of defeat, withdrawal, and conservation of resources.[2]

Allostasis, or *allostatic load,* describes the "wear and tear" on the body of sustained physiological arousal due to chronic exposure to stress, including heightened and fluctuating neural mechanisms and neuroendocrine responses that contribute to the development of hypertension and atherosclerosis.[12] However, in contrast to research on the HPA axis and the sympathetic nervous system, research on allostasis has not focused on control over one's environment.[2]

Contributions from Cognitive Psychology

A central tenet of cognitive stress models is that processes of perception and interpretation of the external world help determine the development of psychological states and ensuing risk for chronic disease. This tenet led to the development in the 1980s of the *person-environment (PE) fit model,* which assumes that strain develops when there is a discrepancy (a) between the demands of the job and the abilities of the person to meet those demands or (b) between the motives of the person, such as obtaining income, and the "supplies" of the environment to satisfy the person's motives. The PE fit model assumes that strain arises because of poor fit between individuals' motives and abilities and their perceptions of the environment. Because the PE fit model has limited ability to predict what objective work conditions are likely to result in stress, it is no longer widely used. While currently used models of occupational stress still recognize subjective perceptions in the stress process, the focus of these models is identifying work factors that could potentially harm workers and should therefore be the targets of interventions.

INTEGRATED OCCUPATIONAL STRESSOR MODELS

Newer, more integrated models of the occupational stress process focus on human behavior in complex environments, rather than solely on psychological processes or physiologic brain functions. These models, which typically are multidimensional in order to capture requisite complexity, offer more complete ways of understanding stressful job conditions. Since the stress process may involve some subjective perceptions and cannot be easily measured objectively—as chemical or physical hazards can—occupational stress research has been advanced mainly through development of theoretical models of the stress process. These models have then been used to develop and test theories of occupational stress. This testing has involved using surveys containing standardized questionnaires based on these models in epidemiological studies to assess stressors and stress in the workplace. The fields of sociology and labor relations have contributed important insights to these integrated models.

The Job Demand–Control Model

The *job demand–control (JDC) model*, also known as the *job strain model*, views stress and subsequent strain as arising primarily due to characteristics of work, rather than subjective perceptions of workers. This model assumes that strain arises from an imbalance between demands and decision latitude (control) in the workplace, where lack of control is seen as an environmental constraint on response capabilities.[12] Decision control consists of two components, which are highly correlated in job situations: (a) personal control over decision-making (autonomy) and (b) opportunities to develop skills.

The JDC model characterizes jobs by their combination of demands and control. Jobs with high demands and low control, such as those of waiters, data-entry operators, and machine-paced assembly-line workers, result in strain. High demand-low control work is typically found in, but not limited to, occupations with a high division of labor and deskilling of tasks. The model assumes that jobs in which psychological demands are accompanied by high control result in active learning and high motivation, which promote mental health and social participation.

Examples of high-demand task characteristics are work overload and time pressure (or work with tight deadlines). Low decision latitude arises in tasks that are too narrow in content, lack stimulus variation, have rigid and unmodifiable information formats, and/or do not allow creativity, problem-solving, the opportunity to learn new skills, participation in decision-making, or worker control over work pace, work methods, or work schedules, such as assembly-line or fast-food work.

The JDC model parsimoniously captures the two primary physiologic mechanisms described previously: (a) the adrenal medullary response, which has been shown to correspond to increased job demands, and (b) increased adrenal cortical output (part of the HPA axis), which is associated with decreased decision latitude or control. This model also integrates insights from (a) research on stressful life events (demands) and (b) industrial/organizational psychology (job autonomy and skills).

The JDC model can also be conceptually expanded to include consideration of demands versus control over a range of physical and organizational factors at work. The lack of control over all aspects of the job is recognized as a key factor in the development of occupational stress.

Recent epidemiologic research on occupational stress and disease risk has usually been performed with the *job demand-control-support (JDCS) model*, which includes social support as an additional dimension.[13] Lack of social support can include social isolation from coworkers, few opportunities for collaboration and therefore a lack of new learning, competition among workers, and bullying and harassment.

The Effort–Reward Imbalance Model

The *effort-reward imbalance (ERI) model*, also widely used, shares some elements with the JDCS model, while emphasizing social reciprocity and the imbalance between the effort required on a job and the rewards provided by the job.[6] In the ERI model, "effort" can be due to extrinsic factors, such as high workload, or intrinsic characteristics, such as the worker's "overcommitment". "Reward" includes *esteem reward*, such as respect and support, income, and *status control*, such as job security, job stability, and prospects for promotion or demotion. In the ERI model, the work role is considered a basic tool to link a person's important emotional and motivational needs, such as self-esteem and self-efficacy, with the opportunity structure. Therefore, occupational stress arises from both (a) the immediate conditions of work and (b) the broader context of career and the role of work in a person's life. The ERI model is especially relevant to the evolving U.S. labor market, in which an increasing proportion of jobs are becoming insecure, and thus providing less *reward*, as corporations frequently restructure to compete in a global marketplace. (See Chapter 2.)

The Job Demands-Resources Model

Building upon the JDCS and ERI models as well as early industrial/organizational psychology research, the *job demands-resources (JDR) model* assumes that job *resources*, such as performance feedback, rewards, job control, participation in decision-making, job security, and supervisory coaching, can buffer the effects of various physical, psychological, and organizational demands. Demands are often predictors of exhaustion or burnout, while resources are often predictors of work motivation and work engagement. In a sense, the JDR model mirrors two main pathways of the JDCS model: (a) demands plus low resources lead to ill health (burnout) and (b) demands plus high resources lead to motivation (work engagement).

The JDR model includes more types of demands and resources than the JDCS model. The flexibility of this model is both an advantage and limitation, because it may be unclear which of the many possible resources and demands are most important for worker health and how demands and resources are interrelated. In addition, it may be difficult to differentiate job demands from job resources; for example, should a job characteristic, such as a high level of responsibility at work, be considered a job demand or a job resource?[14] Another limitation is that the JDR model has been tested only with mental health outcomes, not physical health outcomes.

OCCUPATIONAL STRESSORS

Epidemiologic studies have also demonstrated associations among more specific stressors, short-term and long-term stress responses, and enduring health outcomes. The following section describes the most commonly studied specific stressors, some of which are embedded in the more comprehensive models described previously.

Long Work Hours

Duration of work can be very long in low- and middle-income countries that have inadequate protections; it continues to be long in some high-income countries, such as the United States. In contrast to many other high-income countries, where work hours have declined, average annual work hours in the United States have not changed substantially over the past several decades. The United States ranks first in annual work hours among high-income countries (1,787 in 2011), about 1 workweek longer than Japan, 3 workweeks longer than the United Kingdom, and 10 workweeks longer than Germany. In 2014, full-time employees in the United States reported working 47 hours weekly, with salaried employees working 5 hours longer than hourly employees. Among salaried employees, 50% reported working 50 or more hours weekly, and 25% reported working 60 hours weekly.[15] There is no federal legislation guaranteeing U.S. workers paid vacations, as is present in other high-income nations. U.S. workers frequently choose not to take all available paid vacation time because of high workloads and fear of job loss.

With the growth of women's participation in the U.S. workforce, the proportion of married couples in which both spouses work has increased from 42% in 1970 to 74% in 2009. From 1979 to 2007, combined annual hours worked by married men and women, age 25 to 54, with children increased between 6.3 and 19%, depending on income level.[16] Over the same period, the percentage of families that were "single-parent" increased from about 10% to about 20%. Long workweeks can cause adverse health and social effects on workers, their partners, and their children. One-third of parents in the United States complain that they have insufficient time with their children; and 37% of working parents say they always "feel rushed."[17]

Shift Work

Shift work refers to work activity scheduled outside standard daytime work hours (between 7 A.M. and 7 P.M.), and where there may be a handover of duty from one individual or work group to another on the same job within a 24-hour period. Examples of shift work include: (a) work during the afternoon, night, or weekend outside standard daytime work hours; (b) extended work periods of 12 hours or more; (c) rotating hours of work (usually alternation among two or three shifts); (d) *split shifts*, in which a person's workday is divided into two distinct periods, with several hours of break between these periods (Figure 14-2). In 2010, 29% of workers in the United States reported working other than a regular day shift.[18]

In one-third of dual-earner families with children, a parent works either a rotating shift or a nonstandard work shift.[19] Nonstandard work shifts can have adverse effects on sleep, physical health, leisure time, and family activities, especially activities requiring involvement of parents at their children's schools or associated with standard schedules.

Precarious Work and Job Insecurity

Job insecurity among workers in high-income countries, which has increased as a result of economic globalization and other changes in the labor market, is associated with work intensification and lower job control.[2] In 2010, 19% of workers in the United States reported nonstandard work arrangements, which include being an independent contractor or consultant, a freelance worker, an on-call worker, or a worker paid by a temporary agency. Job insecurity ("I am worried about becoming unemployed") was reported by 32%.[20]

Threat-Avoidant Vigilant Work

Threat-avoidant vigilant (TAV) work involves a worker continuously maintaining a high level of vigilance in order to avoid disaster, such as loss

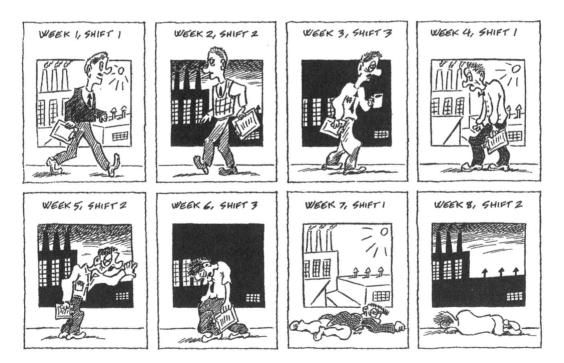

Figure 14-2. Shift work is stressful and causes a number of adverse effects on health and well-being. (Drawing by Nick Thorkelson.)

of human life. Many workers in TAV work, such as operators of urban mass transit, truck drivers, and air traffic controllers, are at high risk for cardiovascular disease, particularly hypertension.[2,21]

Organizational Justice

Organizational justice is defined as the extent to which a workplace is considered fair and just by its employees. It includes (a) *procedural justice*, whether or not decision-making and procedures in the workplace are applied consistently and ethically, with affected workers having input, and (b) *relational justice*, with workers being treated fairly and with dignity and respect by their supervisors.[2]

Workplace Injustice: Discrimination, Harassment, and Bullying

Workplace injustice includes both institutional (or structural) forms of discrimination, such as labor stratification, with placement of women and people of color into more hazardous jobs, and interpersonal forms of abuse and aggression, such as harassment and bullying.[22] The U.S. Equal Employment Opportunity Commission is "responsible for enforcing federal laws that make it illegal to discriminate against a job applicant or an employee because of the person's race, color, religion, sex (including pregnancy, gender identity, and sexual orientation), national origin, age (40 or older), disability or genetic information. It is also illegal to discriminate against a person because the person complained about discrimination, filed a charge of discrimination, or participated in an employee discrimination investigation or lawsuit."[23]

Workplace discrimination refers to actions taken by organizations or individuals that intentionally or unintentionally impair a member of a protected group's ability to work. *Workplace harassment* includes negative actions taken against a worker due to attributes, such as race or gender, which create a hostile environment. The experience of harassment and discrimination is highest among those who live below the poverty line and among African-American and Latino workers.[22] *Bullying* is a type of interpersonal aggression in the workplace associated with a persistent and repeated targeting of one or more individuals, using verbal abuse, humiliation, and other behaviors, all of which create a power imbalance and a hostile work environment. The prevalence of workplace bullying is higher in the United States than in European countries.[24] In the United States, the prevalence of reporting being bullied at work during the previous year ranges from 7.8%[20] to 9.4%.[24] However, a much higher percentage of workers (28%) report "at least two negative acts (of bullying), weekly or more often," for at least 6 months, suggesting that negativity at work may be normalized as part of the work culture in the United States or that reporting it as "bullying" is seen as a sign of weakness.[24]

Workplace Violence

Workplace violence (WPV) can include physical assaults, and nonphysical WPV events, such as threats, sexual harassment, verbal abuse, and bullying. Occupational groups at increased risk of physical violence include taxi drivers, bus drivers, retail workers, and public employees, such as police and corrections officers, healthcare providers, social workers, and special-education teachers.[25]

Other Specific Stressors

Machine-paced work means that the pace of the operation and work output are controlled, to some extent, by a source other than the operator. Such work typically presents a harmful combination of short-interval demands with lack of control. It requires vigilance yet is monotonous and repetitive. Machine-paced assembly-line work is highly stressful, as documented by research using the JDC model (Figure 14-3).[13]

In *piecework*, the worker's income is based on the quantity of products produced. This system has been shown to induce stress responses similar to those of machine-pacing (Figure 14-4). Piecework workers may increase their work pace even to the point of discomfort; for example, a study found that when invoicing clerks were paid based on piecework, in contrast to their usual hourly pay rate, they doubled their work pace, also increased their urinary epinephrine and norepinephrine levels by about one-third.

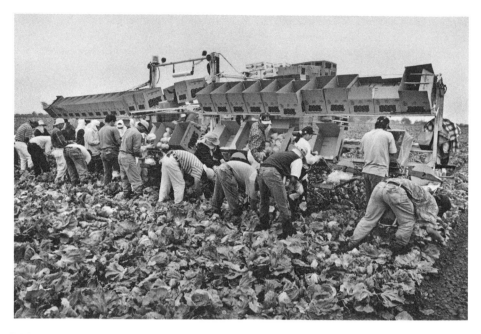

Figure 14-3. California farmworkers stoop to harvest, wrap, and box iceberg lettuce for shipment direct from the farm field. The speed of the mechanical equipment sets the work pace. (Photograph by Earl Dotter.)

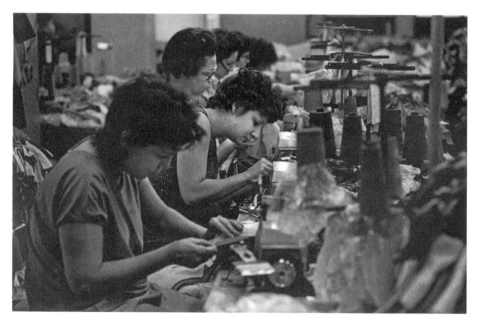

Figure 14-4. Garment workers, who often work on a piecework basis, are often under much stress at work. (Photograph by Earl Dotter.)

Electronic surveillance (performance monitoring) is performed by listening to calls and providing time quotas for customer-service operators, such as in "call centers"; conducting camera surveillance; monitoring computer usage; and tracking of mobile workers, such as package-delivery drivers or utility workers, by GPS-enabled vehicles, hand-held computers, or mobile phones. The result is often less worker control over schedules and how work is done (similar to machine-pacing), an emphasis on quantity and speed over quality, deadline pressure, and a climate of threat and fear.[4] *Role ambiguity* results from lack of clarity concerning job requirements so that workers do not know the objectives, scope, and responsibilities of their jobs. *Role conflict* occurs when conflicting demands are made on a worker by different groups in a worker's organization or when workers are required to perform work that they dislike or believe to be beyond job requirements (Figure 14-5).

Work–family conflict is a type of role conflict in which the demands of work and family are incompatible, making participation in both more difficult. It can be due to the number of work hours or inflexibility of work schedules, or lack of supervisor or spousal support.[26] The proportion of U.S. workers reporting work-family conflicts has ranged from 16% to 50%.[20,27]

Emotional labor describes the management of emotion, typically part of human service work. Emotional labor can include both the suppression of negative emotions, such as anger that a nurse may feel when dealing with a patient's hostile family members, and the requirement for displaying positive emotions, such as "service with a smile" in the retail sector. Strategies to perform the appropriate emotional expression can include *surface acting* ("putting on a mask")— that is, faking the required emotion—and *deep acting*, a change in internal feeling state to match the externally required emotional display.[28]

Psychosocial safety climate (PSC) is a measure of organizational policies, practices, and procedures that are designed to protect worker psychological health and safety. The 12-question version of the PSC survey consists of four subscales: Management Commitment, Management Priority, Organizational Communication, and Organizational Participation.[29]

Low income can be conceptualized as a component of socioeconomic position, along with education and occupation, or contributing to exposure to stressors. Low-wage workers are more likely to experience job insecurity, less likely to receive paid sick days, and are more likely to be female, black, or Hispanic.[30]

Unsafe and unpleasant working conditions can be psychosocial or physical stressors. These stressors include improper lighting, excessive noise, inadequate work space, unsafe machines, tools, buildings, depressing surroundings,

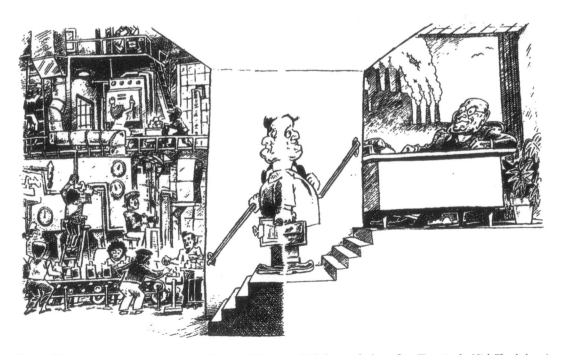

Figure 14-5. A supervisor's job may be highly stressful due to its high degree of role conflict. (Drawing by Nick Thorkelson.)

unsanitary conditions, and toxic chemical exposures—all of which can contribute to mental health problems. For example, investigations of complaints among office workers have found that stress responses are associated with uncomfortable workstations, crowding, and inadequate ventilation and temperature control.

ADVERSE HEALTH OUTCOMES

The pathophysiologic effects of chronic stress (strain), resulting from work-related stressors, contribute to a wide range of unhealthy behaviors and illnesses, including mental disorders, CVD and its risk factors (hypertension, obesity, diabetes, and the metabolic syndrome), and musculoskeletal disorders (Figures 14-1 and 14-6). Some evidence also exists that work stressors contribute to gastrointestinal disorders, some cancers, adverse pregnancy outcomes, and acute traumatic injuries.

Mental Disorders

Occupational stressors are risk factors for a wide range of mental disorders, including psychological distress, anxiety, depression, "burnout," and suicidal ideation and behavior.[5,31-34] Occupational stressors associated with mental disorders include job strain (in jobs with high demands and low control),[5] effort-reward imbalance,[6] job with demands and low resources,[14] job insecurity,[2] organizational injustice,[32] bullying,[31] harassment (especially sexual harassment of women workers),[22] mandatory overtime,[2] emotional labor (surface acting but not deep acting),[28] and work–family conflict.[26] Unemployment also increases risk of mental disorders.[35] Workers who are targets of bullying often feel isolated, demoralized, and unable to escape or prevent the situation. As a result, they may suffer from chronic mental (and somatic) disorders, including depression and post-traumatic stress disorder (PTSD). Bullying also reduces work performance and increases worker turnover, therefore reducing productivity.[22] Poor psychosocial safety climate predicts job strain, bullying, and harassment and related mental disorders.[29] Job autonomy can buffer the effects of emotional labor and protect against burnout.[28] Certain acute stressors faced by workers, such

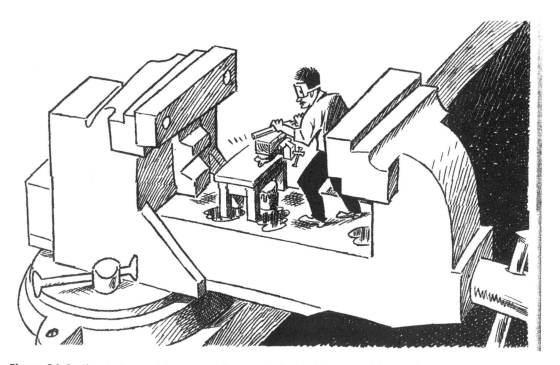

Figure 14-6. Chronic stress contributes to a wide range of unhealthy behaviors and illnesses. (Drawing by Nick Thorkelson.)

as emergency responders' exposure to traumatic events, can lead to PTSD.

Burnout, which consists of emotional exhaustion, depersonalization or cynicism, and experiencing a lack of personal accomplishment, can affect any worker, but human service workers are at especially increased risk. Burnout may be a prelude to depression.[1]

Reducing exposure to occupational stressors can lead to substantial benefits to workers' mental health. For example, a study estimated that reducing or eliminating exposure to occupational stressors could prevent up to 13% of prevalent depression in working men and up to 17% of depression in working women.[36]

Health Behaviors

In some studies, associations have been found between occupational stressors and a variety of health-related behaviors, such as smoking, alcohol consumption, physical inactivity, and unhealthy eating habits and resulting weight gain;[26,37,38] however, in some other studies these associations have not been found.

In addition, many studies show positive relationships between occupational stressors and sickness absence from work, which can be considered a health *outcome* or, alternatively, a *behavior*.[39] Attending work when ill (*presenteeism*) is a consequence of exposure to occupational stressors. Reducing exposure to occupational stressors could lead to multiple benefits to the health behavior of workers, which could also benefit employers through improved employee health, and reduced sickness absence, presenteeism, and associated costs.

Physiologic Reactions

Occupational stressors induce a variety of short-term physiologic reactions.[12,21] Substantial advances in understanding these effects have resulted from the development and use of ambulatory (portable) monitoring and biochemical measurement techniques. Bioelectric measures of stress reactions include heart rate and rhythm, electromyography, and galvanic skin response. Stress can affect the immune system and increase inflammation,[12] and increase platelet coagulation,[12] which contribute to atherosclerosis and other forms of cardiovascular disease (CVD).[19]

When employees are exposed to occupational stressors over an extended period of time, leading to chronic overarousal, disorders develop. For example, chronic stress can reduce heart-rate variability, thereby increasing the risk of heart disease.[2] The cumulative physiological toll on biological systems (*allostatic load*) is often measured by blood pressure; serum levels of glucose, high-density lipoproteins, total cholesterol, and triglycerides; and waist circumference—all of which are associated with increased risk of CVD. Some research demonstrates that increased secretion of both adrenalin and cortisol in demanding, low-control jobs increases both blood pressure and serum levels of lipids, thereby increasing the risks of the metabolic syndrome and heart disease.[21] Cortisol can also stimulate glucose production in the liver and promote insulin resistance in peripheral tissues, both of which increase the risk of diabetes.[2]

Shift work can produce a variety of adverse physiological effects by disrupting circadian rhythm, disturbing sleep, altering dietary patterns, and promoting unhealthy behaviors. These effects include increased sympathetic activity, impaired glucose metabolism, increased blood pressure, abnormal blood coagulation, endothelial dysfunction, inflammation, and altered immune system function.[40] Long work hours and work–family conflict have also been linked to insufficient sleep, a risk factor for many adverse health effects.[26] Work stressors may also lead to weight gain by disturbing circadian rhythm or chronically activating the HPA axis.[11]

Work stressors, specifically lack or loss of job control, can inhibit anabolism (regeneration or growth of tissues). Whereas release of energy occurs through the HPA axis, recovery is facilitated by the hypothalamic-pituitary-gonadal axis. The regeneration of cells is governed largely by the same hormones that stimulate reproduction. Psychosocial stressors at work appear to inhibit anabolic hormones, such as dehydroepiandrosterone sulfate, testosterone, and estradiol, therefore not only inhibiting tissue regeneration but also potentially affecting the reproductive system.[41]

Chronic Diseases

Cardiovascular Disease

About 10% to 20% of all deaths due to CVD among working age populations are related to work,[42] and many of them are associated with occupational stressors. Job strain, effort-reward imbalance (ERI), job insecurity, long work hours (more than 50 hours a week or more than 10 hours a day), and shift work increase the risk of CVD.[1,2,6,21] Some studies show that lack of control over work hours exacerbates the effects of long hours; for example, mandatory over-time has been associated with coronary heart disease. A few studies link unfairness, bullying, and lower levels of "organizational justice" to CVD.[22] Some studies have found that return-ing to a job with job strain or ERI after myo-cardial infarction leads to an increased risk of a recurrence.[2,11]

Hypertension

Blood pressure and risk of hypertension can be increased by work stressors, especially job strain (defined here as a specific type of stressor (low job control plus high job demands), but sometimes also used (mostly in psychology) to describe an outcome, which can lead to confu-sion in interpretation of this term), long work hours, effort–reward imbalance, and TAV work (mainly professional driving).[2,6] More consis-tent evidence is found when blood pressure is measured with a portable monitor that mea-sures blood pressure over 24 hours (ambulatory blood pressure).[2] Essential hypertension (and other CVDs) are primarily diseases of modern industrial society; they are mostly absent among small-scale agricultural communities and soci-eties of hunter-gathers.[11]

Diabetes and the Metabolic Syndrome

Evidence exists for a slightly increased risk of type 2 diabetes and the metabolic syndrome in workers with job strain, long work hours,[2] and/or shift work.[40]

Work-Related Musculoskeletal Disorders

Occupational stressors increase the risk of work-related musculoskeletal disorders (WMSDs), even with controlling for the physical demands of the job.[43] There are at least two mechanisms that may explain this association. First, work organi-zation shapes exposure to WMSD risk factors, including overtime, lack of breaks, machine-paced work, repetitive tasks, excessive standing, and increased work demands, which contribute to inadequate recovery time. Second, the body's response to stress, including stress-related ten-sion causing increased static loading of the muscles, reduced pain tolerance, increased sleep disturbance, and reduction in both immune function and the capability to heal microtrauma, may explain this association. Workers under stress may alter their work behavior in a way that increases the risk of WMSDs. For example, workers may strike a keyboard with greater force or increase their work pace, leading to greater muscle strain.[4] Physically demanding work, such as agricultural work, or fast-paced and repeti-tive tasks, such meat cutting, can increase risk of WMSDs.

Cancer

Shift work involving night work and circadian rhythm disruption is a probable human carcino-gen, especially the association of long exposure (more than 20 years) to night work and breast cancer.[44] No consistent evidence has been found linking other occupational stressors to cancer.

Gastrointestinal Illnesses

Work stressors have been associated with the development of gastric ulcer and irritable bowel syndrome.[7]

Adverse Pregnancy Outcomes

Some research indicates that irregular work hours are associated with a small increase in the risk of miscarriage and reduced fertility.[45] Some evidence also suggests that job strain is a risk factor for preterm delivery and preeclampsia.[45]

Acute Traumatic Injuries

Risk of accidents and injuries are higher on the night shift.[40] These risks are greater for work shifts longer than 8 hours, for successive shifts (especially night shifts), and for shifts without sufficient rest breaks. Some studies have shown associations between injuries and various work stressors, including downsizing, long hours, work intensification, understaffing, and jobs with low job control.[4]

MODIFIERS

The association between stressors and stress responses may be modified by characteristics of the person and the environment, an idea intrinsic to all models of stress. Positive emotional, informational, and instrumental support can ameliorate the stress response. Another potential modifier is socioeconomic status; occupational stressors have a greater adverse impact on health in workers with lower levels of occupational status, education, or income.[2,4]

Individual personality or psychological characteristics, such as hardiness, limited locus of control (the extent to which people believe they have control over events in their lives), poor self-esteem, ineffective coping style, Type A behavior, and hostility, may also increase workers' vulnerability to stressors. However, such characteristics may also be shaped by psychosocial stressors at work.[1,12] Thus, reducing work stressors, especially by increasing job control, may also help enhance workers' ability to develop more effective coping strategies.

PREVENTION OF OCCUPATIONAL STRESS

Preventing or reducing occupational stressors and occupational stress is challenging, given the economic, political, and labor-market factors that are increasing stressors at work (Figure 14-1). Therefore, developing and implementing multiple types of preventive measures is necessary (Table 14-1).

The first step in developing preventive measures is identifying work stressors. Employers, managers, employees, labor union representatives, and occupational health specialists can assess occupational stressors and the risk of occupational stress at their workplaces. This can be done using qualitative methods, such as

focus groups, other discussions, and individual interviews, and by quantitative methods, such as by performing surveys and analyzing existing organizational data. For example, managers and workers can perform the NIOSH surveys on work stressors and health at their workplaces, obtaining information on disorders such as depression, hypertension, and sleep problems. (Survey questions specific to the issues in a given workplace can be added to the NIOSH survey.) If the workplace, or specific jobs in the workplace, have high levels of stressors or stress-related health problems compared to national averages, preventive measures need to be developed and implemented. (See list of widely used occupational stressor and symptom surveys at the end of this chapter.)

Additional sources of data can provide helpful information on the relationship between work stressors and injuries and illnesses. More data can be collected from company records on sick leave and turnover, OSHA–recordable injuries and illnesses, workers' compensation, and health insurance. In addition, inexpensive portable monitors can be used to measure blood pressure at and outside of work to obtain a better estimate of a worker's cardiovascular risk.[2] Time trends of data on stressors and stress-related disorders can identify persistent problems and can help evaluate the effectiveness of preventive measures.[4]

Stress Prevention and Reduction through Work Reorganization

Occupational stress can be prevented and controlled most effectively using a comprehensive, or systems, approach that integrates primary, secondary, and tertiary prevention and integrates multiple levels of intervention (Table 14-1).[1,4,46,47] Primary prevention interventions, which proactively aim to prevent illness and injury among healthy workers, address occupational stressors by improving laws and regulations, workplace policies, and design of jobs and tasks.[1] Examples include:

- State laws that ban mandatory overtime or require safe staffing levels for nurses
- Employer-initiated child care or flexible work schedule (work–family) programs

Table 14-1. Strategies and Programs to Prevent and Reduce Occupational Stressors and Stress[1,4,46,47]

Type of Intervention	Level of Prevention			Typical Intervention Methods
	Primary	Secondary	Tertiary	
	Prevent disease in healthy workers **Eliminate or reduce job stressors**	**Detect stressors and symptoms, and intervene early** **Improve workers' ability to cope with stressors**	**Treat, rehabilitate, and compensate workers with job stress-related illness or injury**	
Legislative/ Policy	U.S.: Federal, state, and local laws, such as bans on mandatory overtime, safe staffing for nurses, work-hour limits for medical residents and transportation workers, and paid family leave Canada: 2013 National Standard for Psychological Health and Safety in the Workplace Scandinavian countries: Job stressors included in national health and safety laws	National surveillance systems Paid sick leave	Workers' compensation Social Security Disability Health insurance	Legislation Regulation Voluntary standards
Employer/ Organization	Worksite surveillance programs Worksite health & safety programs Work-family programs Participatory ergonomics programs Healthier shift work scheduling Eliminate on-call scheduling	Worksite screening and surveillance programs Expanded health promotion programs to address job stressors	Health insurance Rehabilitation and return-to-work programs (with reduced job stressors)	Collective bargaining Employer-initiated programs/ policies Worker cooperatives
Job/Task	Job/task redesign, such as elimination of machine-pacing and piecework, increased job control, and skill development Adequate rest breaks Job rotation Supervisor training Opportunities for social interaction Clear promotion pathways		Provide light-duty jobs and accommodations	Labor-management committees and initiatives Participatory action research Worker participation in planning, decision-making Employer-initiated job redesign
Individual	Stress resilience training for emergency responders	Health promotion Stress management Employee assistance programs Disease management programs	Medical care	Employer-initiated programs Labor-management initiatives

- Elimination of "on-call" scheduling in retail businesses as a result of pressure from worker advocates and regulators
- Quotas for the number of rooms hotel housekeepers are required to clean daily as a result of labor-management collective bargaining
- Elimination of machine-paced work in call centers as a result of the work of a labor-management committee[1,4]

- Training supervisors to improve work–life balance.[26]

Raising the minimum wage is a primary prevention measure that can improve mental health.[48]

Secondary prevention interventions aim to detect stressors and symptoms at an early stage and to intervene to improve workers' ability to cope. Examples include surveillance and screening programs to identify workers and groups at high risk of occupational stress-related disorders, and stress management classes, which provide training in relaxation or meditation skills or help employees adopt strategies on how to handle stressful situations.

Tertiary prevention interventions are reactive, aiming to minimize the effects of stress-related conditions once they have occurred, through treatment or management of symptoms, illnesses, or injuries. Examples include counseling (such as through employee assistance programs), medical or psychological treatment, compensation for occupational stress-related conditions, and return-to-work programs.

The development, implementation, and evaluation of occupational stress prevention programs should include the meaningful participation of groups targeted by interventions – a fundamental concept in public health.[1,46,47] Where labor unions or worker centers are present, they too are important participants in assessment of needs as well as development, implementation, and evaluation of interventions. Worker participation, a form of job control, demonstrates organizational fairness and justice and it builds mutual support among workers and between workers and managers.

The European Psychosocial Risk Management-Excellence Framework provides a comprehensive "best-practice" framework for psychosocial risk management in the workplace for policymakers, employers, trade unions, occupational safety and health professionals, and employees in the European Union.[49] It has identified seven key features of successful workplace intervention projects to reduce occupational stress:[49]

1. Workplace interventions need to be developed with a full understanding of theory and evidence-based practice.
2. A systematic and stepwise approach needs to be utilized with development of clear aims, goals, tasks, and intervention plans.
3. A proper risk assessment needs to be carried out to identify risk factors and groups of workers with potentially high exposure.
4. Interventions need to be tailored for an industrial sector, occupation, or workplace size, while remaining flexible and adaptable for implementation in a specific workplace.
5. The most effective interventions are those that are accessible and user-friendly in their format, process, and content to individuals at all levels of an organization.
6. A systematic approach is the most effective, with components of the intervention aimed at both the individual and the organization.
7. Intervention programs that facilitate competency building and skill development are important because, at the organizational level, they build leadership and management skills that facilitate and support the continuous improvement cycle and organizational change and, at the individual level, they enable workers to identify and manage work-related stress.[49]

Prevention and control of occupational stress can be integrated with other approaches to protect and promote worker health and well-being. NIOSH recommends the "Total Worker Health"® (TWH) approach, which integrates (a) health promotion and stress management aimed at individuals with (b) "health protection" (occupational health), with the goal of reducing both physical and psychosocial hazards in the workplace. The TWH approach has the potential to identify and change barriers to healthier behaviors, such as inflexible schedules, shift work, and long duration of work, and to reduce risks of chronic disease caused by stressful work. However, few employers have adopted the TWH approach.[2] Other integrated approaches have also been articulated, including the 2013 National Standard of Canada for Psychological Health & Safety in the Workplace, and an Australia integrated approach to workplace mental health, which targets the prevention and control of work-related risks to mental health, the promotion of the positive aspects of work, and addressing mental health problems as they manifest at work, whether or not they are work-related.[50]

REFERENCES

1. Schnall P, Rosskam E, Dobson M, et al. (eds.). Unhealthy work: Causes, consequences and cures. Amityville, NY: Baywood Publishing, 2009.

2. Schnall P, Dobson M, Landsbergis P. Work, stress and cardiovascular disease. In: Cooper CL, Quick JC. Handbook of stress and health: A Guide to research and practice. Chichester: Wiley, 2017, pp. 99–124.

3. Sauter SL, Brightwell WS, Colligan MJ, et al. The changing organization of work and the safety and health of working people: Knowledge gaps and research directions. Cincinnati, OH: NIOSH, 2002. Available at: https://www.cdc.gov/niosh/docs/2002-116/pdfs/2002-116.pdf. Accessed December 27, 2016.

4. Landsbergis P, Sinclair R, Dobson M, et al. Occupational health psychology. In: Anna D (ed.). The occupational environment: Its evaluation, control, and management. Fairfax, VA: American Industrial Hygiene Association, 2011, pp. 1086–1130.

5. Theorell T, Hammarstrom A, Aronsson G, et al. A systematic review including meta-analysis of work environment and depressive symptoms. BMC Public Health 2015; 15: 738.

6. Siegrist J, Wahrendorf ME. Work stress and health in a globalized economy: The model of effort-reward imbalance. Switzerland: Springer, 2016.

7. Huerta-Franco MR, Vargas-Luna M, Tienda P, et al. Effects of occupational stress on the gastrointestinal tract. World Journal of Gastrointestinal Pathophysiology 2013; 4: 108–118.

8. National Institute for Occupational Safety and Health. Stress . . . at work (DHHS Publication Number 99-101). Cincinnati, OH: NIOSH, 1999. Available at: (https://www.cdc.gov/niosh/docs/99-101/). Accessed December 27, 2016.

9. Howard J. The changing employment relationship and its impact on worker well-being. NIOSH E-news 2015; 12. Available at: http://www.cdc.gov/niosh/enews/enewsV12N12.html. Accessed December 27, 2016.

10. Landsbergis P, Cahill J, Schnall P. The impact of lean production and related new systems of work organization on worker health. Journal of Occupational Health Psychology 1999; 4: 108–130.

11. Schnall P, Dobson M, Landsbergis P. Globalization, work and cardiovascular disease. International Journal of Health Services 2016; 46: 656–692.

12. McEwen BS. Protective and damaging effects of stress mediators: Central role of the brain. Dialogues in Clinical Neuroscience 2006; 8: 367–381.

13. Karasek RA, Theorell T. Healthy work: Stress, productivity, and the reconstruction of working life. New York: Basic Books, 1990.

14. Bakker AB, Demerouti E. Job Demands-Resources Theory: Taking stock and looking forward. Journal of Occupational Health Psychology 2017; 22: 273–285.

15. Saad L. The "40-hour" workweek is actually longer—by seven hours. August 29, 2014. Available at: http://www.gallup.com/poll/175286/hour-workweek-actually-longer-seven-hours.aspx. Accessed December 27, 2016.

16. The state of working America. Annual hours worked by married men and women age 25–54 with children, by income group, selected years, 1979–2010, May 22, 2012. Available at: http://www.stateofworkingamerica.org/chart/swa-income-table-2-17-annual-hours-work-married. Accessed December 27, 2016.

17. Parker K, Wang W. Modern parenthood: Roles of moms and dads converge as they balance work and family. Pew Research Center, 2013. Available at: http://www.pewsocialtrends.org/2013/03/14/modern-parenthood-roles-of-moms-and-dads-converge as they balance work-and-family/. Accessed December 27, 2016.

18. Alterman T, Luckhaupt SE, Dahlhamer JM, et al. Prevalence rates of work organization characteristics among workers in the U.S.: Data from the 2010 National Health Interview Survey. American Journal of Industrial Medicine 2013; 56: 647–659.

19. Presser HB, Ward BW. Nonstandard work schedules over the life course: A first look. Monthly Labor Review 2011; 3–16.

20. Alterman T, Luckhaupt SE, Dahlhamer JM, et al. Job insecurity, work-family imbalance, and hostile work environment: Prevalence data from the 2010 National Health Interview Survey. American Journal of Industrial Medicine 2013; 56: 660–669.

21. Schnall PL, Belkić K, Landsbergis P, Baker D. Why the workplace and cardiovascular disease? Occupational Medicine 2000; 15: 1–6.

22. Okechukwu CA, Souza K, Davis KD, de Castro AB. Discrimination, harassment, abuse, and bullying in the workplace: contribution of workplace injustice to occupational health disparities. American Journal of Industrial Medicine 2014; 57: 573–586.

23. U.S. Equal Employment Opportunity Commission. Overview. Available at: https://www.eeoc.gov/eeoc/index.cfm. Accessed December 28, 2016.

24. Lutgen-Sandvik P, Tracy S, Alberts J. Burned by bullying in the American workplace: Prevalence, perception, degree and impact. Journal of Management Studies 2007; 44: 837–862.

25. Lippel K. Addressing occupational violence: An overview of conceptual and policy considerations viewed through a gender lens. Geneva: International Labour Office, 2016.

26. Hammer L, Demsky C. Work-life balance. In: Day A, Kelloway K, Hurrell J Jr (eds.). Workplace well-being: Building positive and psychologically healthy workplaces. New York: Wiley, 2014, 90–111.

27. Schieman S, Milkie MA, Glavin P. When work interferes with life: Work-nonwork interference and the influence of work-related demands and resources. American Sociological Review 2009; 74: 966–988.

28. Grandey AA. Emotion regulation in the workplace: A new way to conceptualize emotional labor. Journal of Occupational Health Psychology 2000; 5: 95–110.

29. Bailey T, Dollard M, Richards P. A national standard for psychosocial safety climate (PSC): PSC 41 as the benchmark for low risk of job strain and depressive symptoms. Journal of Occupational Health Psychology 2015; 20: 15–26.

30. Oxfam. Millions of low-wage workers in the US are struggling to survive. June 21, 2016. Available at: https://www.oxfamamerica.org/explore/stories/millions-of-low-wage-workers-in-the-us-are-struggling-to-survive/. Accessed December 27, 2016.

31. Verkuil B, Atasayi S, Molendijk M. Workplace bullying and mental health: A meta-analysis on cross-sectional and longitudinal data. PLoS One 2015; 10: e0135225.

32. Ndjaboué R, Brisson C, Vézina M. Organisational justice and mental health: A systematic review of prospective studies. Occupational and Environmental Medicine 2012; 69: 694–700.

33. LaMontagne A, Keegel T, Louie A, Ostry A. Job stress as a preventable upstream determinant of common mental disorders: A review for practitioners and policy-makers. Advances in Mental Health 2010; 9: 17–35.

34. LaMontagne A, Milner A. Working conditions as modifiable risk factors for suicidal thoughts and behaviours. Occupational and Environmental Medicine 2017; 74: 4–5 doi:10.1136/oemed-2016-104036.

35. Milner A, Page A, LaMontagne A. Cause and effect in studies of unemployment, mental health, and suicide: A meta-analytic and conceptual review. Psychological Medicine 2013; 44: 909–919.

36. LaMontagne A, Keegel T, Vallance D, et al. Job strain-attributable depression in a sample of working Australians: Assessing the contribution to health inequalities. BMC Public Health 2008; 8: 181. doi:10.1186/1471-2458-8-181.

37. Siegrist J, Rodel A. Work stress and health risk behavior. Scandinavian Journal of Work, Environment & Health 2006; 32: 473–481.

38. LaMontagne A. Job strain and health behaviours-developing a bigger picture. American Journal of Epidemiology 2012; 176: 1090–1094.

39. Milner A, Butterworth P, Bentley R, et al. Sickness absence and psychosocial job quality: An analysis from a longitudinal survey of working Australians, 2005–2012. American Journal of Epidemiology 2015; 181: 781–788.

40. Kecklund G, Axelsson J. Health consequences of shift work and insufficient sleep. British Medical Journal 2016; 355: i5210.

41. Theorell T. Anabolism and catabolism— Antagonistic partners in stress and strain. Scandinavian Journal of Work, Environment & Health Suppl 2008; 136–143.

42. International Commission on Occupational Health. The Tokyo Declaration on Prevention and Management of Work-Related Cardiovascular Disorders. International Commission on Occupational Health Newsletter 2013; 11: 4–6.

43. Lang J, Ochsmann E, Kraus T, Lang J. Psychosocial work stressors as antecedents of musculoskeletal problems: A systematic review and meta-analysis of stability-adjusted longitudinal studies. Social Science & Medicine 2012; 75: 1163–1174.

44. IARC Working Group on the Evaluation of Carcinogenic Risks to Humans. Painting, firefighting, and shiftwork. IARC Monographs on the Evaluation of Carcinogenic Risks to Humans 2010; 98: 9–764.

45. Figa-Talamanca I. Occupational risk factors and reproductive health of women. Occupational Medicine (London) 2006; 56: 521–531.

46. LaMontagne AD, Keegel T, Louie AM, et al. A systematic review of the job stress intervention evaluation literature: 1990–2005. International Journal of Occupational and Environmental Health 2007; 13: 268–280.

47. LaMontagne AD, Keegel T, Vallance DA. Protecting and promoting mental health in the workplace: Developing a systems approach to job stress. Health Promotion Journal of Australia 2007; 18: 221–228.

48. Reeves A, McKee M, Mackenbach J, et al. Introduction of a national minimum wage reduced depressive symptoms in low-wage workers: A quasi-natural experiment in the UK. Health Economics 2017; 26: 639–655. doi: 10.1002/hec.3336.

49. Leka S, Vartia M, Hassard J, et al. Best practice in interventions for the prevention and management of work-related stress and workplace violence and bullying. In: Leka S, Cox T (eds.). The European Framework for Psychosocial Risk Management: PRIMA-EF. Nottingham, UK: Institute of Work, Health and Organisations, 2008, pp. 136–173.

50. LaMontagne AD, Martin A, Page KM, et al. Workplace mental health: Developing an integrated intervention approach. BMC Psychiatry 2014; 131: 1–11.

FURTHER READING

Karasek R, Theorell T. Healthy work: Stress, productivity, and the reconstruction of working life. New York: Basic Books, 1990.
The first major book on the processes by which occupational stress leads to ill health, focusing on the demand-control-support model, and proposals to reduce occupational stress and promote healthy work.

Siegrist J, Wahrendorf ME. Work stress and health in a globalized economy: The model of effort-reward imbalance. Geneva: Springer, 2016.
A comprehensive, updated summary of research on the effects of stressful working and employment conditions on workers' health, focusing on the effort–reward imbalance model.

Schnall P, Belkic K, Landsbergis PA, Baker D. The workplace and cardiovascular disease. In: Occupational medicine: State-of-the-art reviews. Philadelphia, PA: Hanley and Belfus, 2000.
An in-depth book on the association between working conditions, including occupational stress, and CVD, as well as strategies to prevent work-related CVD.

Schnall P, Rosskam E, Dobson M, et al (eds.). Unhealthy work: Causes, consequences and cures. Amityville, NY: Baywood Publishing, 2009.

This textbook reviews the major changes occurring in the workplace in the context of the global economy, scientific findings on the effects of work stressors on workers' health, and in-depth case studies of measures to improve working conditions, prevent disease, and improve health.

WEB RESOURCES

Copenhagen Psychosocial Questionnaire
http://www.arbejdsmiljoforskning.dk/en/publikationer/spoergeskemaer/psykisk-arbejdsmiljoe
Widely used questionnaire that measures occupational stress and health.

Effort-Reward Imbalance Questionnaire
http://www.uniklinik-duesseldorf.de/unternehmen/institute/institut-fuer-medizinische soziologie/forschung/the-eri-model-stress-and-health/eri-questionnaires/questionnaires-download/
Widely used questionnaire that measures job efforts and job rewards.

European Psychosocial Risk Management-Excellence Framework (PRIMA-EF)
http://www.prima-ef.org/
Provides policymakers, employers, trade unions, experts, and employees with a comprehensive best-practice framework for psychosocial risk management at the workplace.

Job Content Questionnaire
http://www.jcqcenter.org/
A widely used questionnaire, focused on measuring job demands, job control, and workplace social support. Newly expanded to measure additional job characteristics.

The following NIOSH websites provide a comprehensive source of information on occupational stress and related topics and links to additional resources:

http://www.cdc.gov/niosh/topics/stress/
Information about occupational stress and worker health.

http://www.cdc.gov/niosh/programs/workorg/
Information about the organization of work and worker health.

http://www.cdc.gov/niosh/topics/workschedules/
Information about work schedules and worker health.

https://www.cdc.gov/niosh/docs/99-101/
A thorough booklet on occupational stress and worker health.

http://www.cdc.gov/niosh/topics/stress/qwlquest.html
The NIOSH Quality of Worklife questionnaire, including questions on occupational stress and

health, which has been used in national surveys and in workplaces.

https://www.cdc.gov/niosh/topics/nhis/
    The NIOSH Occupational Health Supplement to the national Health Interview Survey, which contains questions on occupational stress and health.

https://www.cdc.gov/niosh/twh/
    The NIOSH Total Worker Health program, designed to integrate occupational health and safety with health promotion.

National Standard of Canada for Psychological Health and Safety in the Workplace
http://www.mentalhealthcommission.ca/English/national-standard
    A voluntary set of guidelines, tools, and resources for promoting workers' psychological health and preventing psychological harm due to workplace factors.

UK Health and Safety Executive Management Standards for Work-Related Stress
http://www.hse.gov.uk/stress/standards/before.htm
    Guidelines for reducing occupational stress.

Unhealthy Work (Center for Social Epidemiology)
http://unhealthywork.org/
    A comprehensive website on occupational stress and health with a focus on CVD.

"Working on Empty" (film)
http://workingonempty.org/
    A documentary film on occupational stress.

VicHealth's Creating Healthy Workplaces Program
https://www.vichealth.vic.gov.au/media-and-resources/publications/creating-healthy-workplaces-publications
    This Australian website focuses on preventing chronic disease in the workplace by identifying best practices for addressing alcohol-related harm, prolonged sitting, stress, race-based discrimination, and violence against women.

Work and Family Researchers Network
http://workfamily.sas.upenn.edu/content/about
    An international membership organization of work and family researchers, policymakers, and practitioners.

15

Air Pollution

Horacio Riojas-Rodríguez, Isabelle Romieu,
and Mauricio Hernández-Ávila

In the mid-20th century, dramatic episodes of outdoor (ambient) air pollution in high-income countries demonstrated that air pollution could cause many deaths. For example, in the London Fog of 1952, during which there were high concentrations of smoke from coal-burning household stoves, an estimated 12,000 excess deaths occurred. The proportion of deaths due to respiratory causes was increased. Infants, young children, and older people were at especially increased risk.[1] Ambient air pollution is now an established risk factor for respiratory and cardiovascular morbidity.[2–5] Although levels of air pollutants have been markedly decreased in high-income countries, adverse health effects still occur frequently in many urban areas at levels that were previously considered to be safe.[6,7]

Exposure to air pollutants at the global level has increased due to the increased number of people who live in urban environments, especially in low- and middle-income countries (LMICs). Over 80% of people in these countries live in cities where the air does not meet international health-based guidelines.[8] By 2050, an estimated 66% of the world's population will live in urban areas, with heavy traffic, pollution, poor housing, limited access to water and sanitation services, and other health risks.[9]

In most healthy adults, the lung can store about 5 L of air (6 L in many athletes). We inhale and exhale about 500 mL per breath, an average of about 15 times per minute, for a total of 7.5 mL per minute, 450 L an hour, 10,800 L a day, and 3.9 million L a year. We, therefore, can inhale a large dose of chemicals if the air we breathe is contaminated with chemicals.

The World Health Organization (WHO) estimated that, in 2012, approximately 7 million people died—about half prematurely—due to exposure to indoor and/or outdoor air pollution—about 12% of all deaths. In addition, air pollution caused much morbidity—almost 8% of disability-adjusted life years.[10]

Ambient air pollutants arise mainly from combustion of fossil fuels (Figure 15-1). They include (a) primary pollutants, such as sulfur dioxide (SO_2), oxides of nitrogen (NOx), and particulate matter (PM); (b) secondary acidic aerosols and other particles; and (c) oxidant pollutants, primarily ozone (O_3), that are produced by photochemical reactions involving hydrocarbons and NOx. High emission of oxidant pollutants is often associated with heavy motor-vehicle traffic, especially in large cities of LMICs.[3,7,9] In cities and some rural areas of these countries, home cooking and heating as well as cooking with solid fuel (biomass

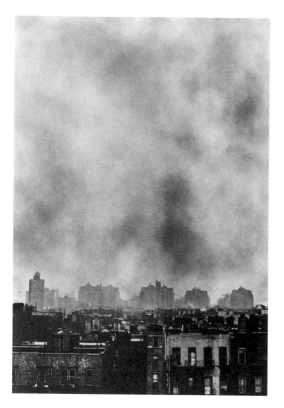

Figure 15-1. Air pollution in New York City in 1968. (Photograph by Earl Dotter.)

or coal) can significantly contribute to ambient air pollution—and indoor air pollution. Industrial processes contribute to ambient air pollution by emitting volatile organic compounds (VOCs), black carbon (BC), and other pollutants that may adversely affect health. Increasingly, air pollution is also both a contributing cause and an adverse consequence of climate change (Chapter 29).

To understand related health effects, one should understand the sources and properties of major ambient air pollutants, as described next.

MAJOR AMBIENT AIR POLLUTANTS

Particulates

Particulate air pollution consists of mixtures of solid and liquid particles that form aerosols. Airborne particles vary in shape, size, composition, and origin. They can be classified as (a) primary, those emitted directly into the atmosphere from mobile or fixed anthropogenic fuel sources, road dust, fires, and other sources; or (b) secondary, those formed in the atmosphere by chemical reactions involving gases, such as SO_2, NOx, VOCs, and ammonia (NH_3).[11,12]

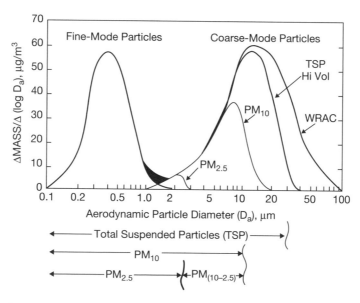

Figure 15-2. Example of a mass distribution of ambient particulate matter as a function of aerodynamic particle diameter. The y axis represents an estimate of the concentration. (Source: Environmental Protection Agency. Air quality criteria for particulate matter. National Center for Environmental Assessment, 1996.)

Typically particles are classified according to their size (Figure 15-2).[10] Particle size affects deposition in the respiratory tract and, consequently, the potential to cause adverse health effects. Particles less an 10 μm in diameter (PM_{10}) comprise the *inhalable fraction* of airborne particles.[13] Particles between 2.5 and 10 μm, the *coarse fraction*, include mainly soil material, such as suspended road dust and windblown dust, and particles generated by handling, crushing, and grinding operations. Particles less than 2.5 μm ($PM_{2.5}$), the *inhalable fraction* or *fine fraction*, comprise all particles capable of entering the alveoli. They are produced by fuel and biomass combustion and by the atmospheric reaction of gases. A subset of $PM_{2.5}$, *ultrafine particles* smaller than 0.1 μm, are formed by combustion exhaust.[10]

During the past 15 years, the highest levels of PM_{10} (300 μg/m³) occurred in large cities in the Eastern Mediterranean region. In megacities of more than 14 million residents (Dehli, Cairo, and Dhaka), the highest levels of PM_{10} ranged from 160 to 240 μg/m³.[14]

Black Carbon

Black carbon is formed by the incomplete combustion of fossil fuels, biofuels, and biomass. Its half-life in the atmosphere is from days to weeks. Black carbon, which also contains organic carbon, is a major component of soot, which is directly emitted into the air in the form of $PM_{2.5}$.[15]

By absorbing light, BC influences climate. It can absorb 1 million times more energy than carbon dioxide. It deposits on snow and ice, thereby reducing their reflectivity ("albedo"), leading to increased temperature and accelerating melting.[16]

Most BC emissions come from mobile sources (diesel-powered engines and vehicles) and biomass (including forest fires); some come from residential heating and cooking as well as industry. In the year 2000, there were about 8.4 million tons of BC emitted.[15] In 2005, the United States emitted almost 640,000 tons of BC. Globally, BC represents 8% of all emissions (0.64 million tons).[15]

Ozone

Ozone is a colorless gas that occurs naturally in the stratosphere, where it filters out ultraviolet (UV) radiation. At ground level in cities and many rural areas, O_3 is the prime oxidant ingredient of smog, along with other oxidant species and $PM_{2.5}$. Ozone is a secondary pollutant formed as the product of the atmospheric photochemical reaction of primary emissions, such as NOx and VOCs, in the presence of sunlight and accelerated at high temperature.[2] This photochemical pollution is especially prevalent in the many large cities with heavy vehicle traffic, as more than half of the ingredients necessary to produce O_3 come from car exhaust pipes, especially those located in sunny regions and/or at high altitude, such as Mexico City.[7,11]

Sulfur Dioxide

Sulfur dioxide is a water-soluble gas formed from the oxidation of sulfur, which contaminates coal and petroleum fuels. Consequently, SO_2 is emitted by coal- and oil-fired power plants and by industrial processes involving fossil-fuel combustion.[3] In the air, SO_2 can be transformed into sulfuric acid and sulfates. Exposure to 100 ppm of SO_2 is an immediate threat to health and life.[17] Sulfur dioxide and PM pollution, which are typically emitted together by combustion sources, exist as components of a complex mixture.[3] However, depending on the source, the proportion of PM to SO_2 varies greatly. For example, in areas where low-sulfur fuel is used, the ambient level of SO_2 is low. In contrast, in areas where high-sulfur fuel is used or where much coal is burned, the ambient level of SO_2 is high.

From 2000 to 2005, global emissions of SO_2 were approximately 5.6 million metric tons. From 2005 to 2010, SO_2 emissions likely increased in China, Eastern Europe, India, the Caucasus Region, and Central Asia, as well as in international sea transportation. However, total global SO_2 emissions decreased by 9.9 million metric tons, compared to 2000–2005, because of reduced emissions in the United States, Canada, and Western Europe.[18,19]

Oxides of Nitrogen

Like SO_2, nitrogen dioxide (NO_2) and other NOx are produced by high-temperature combustion processes and contribute to the formation of acid aerosols (from exhaust combustion of motor vehicles and from the combustion of charcoal, petroleum, or natural gas).[20] Outdoors, NOx are nearly always present together with other combustion pollutants. Initially, almost all NOx emissions are in the form of nitric oxide (NO), which is then oxidized in air to form NO_2, a more toxic compound and a major precursor of photochemical smog. In addition, the reaction of NO_2 to chemicals produced by sunlight contributes to the formation of nitric acid, the main constituent of acid rain.[20] In 2008, the countries with the highest NOx emissions were China, the United States, India, and Russia.[21]

Polycyclic Aromatic Hydrocarbons

Polycyclic aromatic hydrocarbons (PAHs) comprise several hundred organic compounds, each of which consists of carbon and hydrogen atoms grouped in two or more condensed aromatic rings. Since PAHs are formed during the incomplete combustion of coal, petroleum, and gasoline, the airborne concentrations of these chemicals are associated with urbanization, industrialization, and vehicular traffic. Polycyclic aromatic hydrocarbons of low molecular weight (with less than 4 rings) remain in a gaseous state until they are eliminated by precipitation; PAHs of high molecular weight (with 4 or more rings), tend to attach to particles.[22]

Lead

Lead, mainly in the form of lead oxide, polluted the air in most urban areas, when it was used as an antiknock agent in gasoline from the mid-1920s to the late 1970s. In the United States, removal of lead from gasoline lowered the average blood lead level (BLL) from 13 to 3 µg/dL.[12] In Mexico City, removal of lead from gasoline lowered the annual average ambient lead level from 1.2 to 0.2 µg/m³ and the average BLL in children in Mexico City by about 7.6 µg/dL.[6] (See Chapters 11, 23, 24, 28, and 30). By 2016, only Algeria, Yemen, and Iraq continued to sell leaded gasoline (along with lead-free gasoline).

Volatile Organic Compounds

Volatile organic compounds, which are present in ambient air, mainly as gases, include alkenes, aldehydes, and aromatic hydrocarbons (such as benzene and toluene). VOCs are involved in the formation of secondary pollutants, like O_3.[23,24] Some VOCs, such as trichloroethylene and tetrachloroethylene, are chlorinated compounds. Sources of VOCs include evaporation and combustion of fossil fuels, use of solvents, and industrial processes.

Carbon Monoxide

Carbon monoxide (CO) is produced by incomplete combustion of fossil fuels (mainly derived from mobile sources), deforestation, and the burning of waste. Most of the carbon in automotive fuel is oxidized to carbon dioxide, with only a small fraction incompletely oxidized to CO.[25,26]

AMBIENT AIR QUALITY STANDARDS AND GUIDELINES

In the past half-century, much progress has been made in many countries to control ambient air pollution and thereby reduce adverse health and environmental consequences. In the United States, the Clean Air Act of 1970 mandated that the federal government develop and promulgate national ambient air quality standards (NAAQS), specifying uniform nationwide limits for certain major air pollutants ("criteria air pollutants"): CO, lead, NO_2, O_3, PM, and SO_2. The act has been amended several times, most recently in 1990.[14] (See Chapter 3.)

Under the act, the Environmental Protection Agency must identify pollutants that "may reasonably be anticipated to endanger public health or welfare" and issue air quality criteria for them—"primary" and "secondary" NAAQSs for these pollutants. Primary standards set limits to protect public health, including the health of sensitive populations, such as people with asthma, children, and older people. Secondary standards protect against other effects, such as decreased visibility and damage to animals, crops, vegetation, and buildings. Standards are

Table 15-1. National Ambient Air Quality Standards, United States*

Pollutants	NAAQS Concentrations		Standard Type
	In ppm	In μg/m^3	
Particulate matter < 10 μm (PM$_{10}$)			
24-hour average not to be exceeded more than once per year, on average, over 3 years		150	Primary and secondary
Particulate matter <2.5 μm (PM$_{2.5}$)			
Annual mean, averaged over 3 years		12	Primary
Annual mean, averaged over 3 years		15	Secondary
24-hour average, 98th percentile, averaged over 3 years		35	Primary and secondary
Ozone (O$_3$)			
Annual fourth-highest daily maximum 8-hour concentration, averaged over 3 years	0.070		Primary and secondary
Sulfur dioxide (SO$_2$)			
99th percentile of 1-hour daily maximum concentrations, averaged over 3 years	0.075		Primary
3-hour average not to be exceeded more than once per year	0.5		Secondary
Nitrogen dioxide (NO$_2$)			
98th percentile of 1-hour daily maximum concentrations, averaged over 3 years	0.100		Primary
Annual mean	0.053		Primary and secondary
Carbon monoxide (CO)			
1-hour average not to be exceeded more than once per year	35		Primary
8-hour average not to be exceeded more than once per year	9		Primary
Lead (Pb)			
Rolling 3-month average not to be exceeded		0.15	Primary and secondary

* For detailed information on scientific bases and policy considerations underlying decisions establishing the NAAQS listed here, see the air quality criteria, staff papers, and NAAQS promulgation notices.

Source: U.S. Environmental Protection Agency. NAAQS Table. Available at: https://www.epa.gov/criteria-air-pollutants/naaqs-table. Accessed August 18, 2017.

set for two types of averaging-time periods: long term (such as annual average) and short term (such as 24 hours or less) (Table 15-1). The act requires that NAAQSs be reviewed periodically and, if appropriate, revised. In 1997, the NAAQS for PM$_{2.5}$ was added. The NAAQS for O$_3$ was last revised in 2014. Air quality guidelines have been established in 109 (56%) out of 193 countries, and 73 countries (38%) have a specific air quality policy, act, or regulation.[15,27]

The World Health Organization has developed air quality guidelines for international use.[13,28] These guidelines, which consist of concentration limits of air pollutants for certain averaging times, are used by national governments promulgating air quality standards.[14]

EXPOSURE ASSESSMENT

Assessment of the exposure consists in quantitatively and qualitatively estimating the contact of an individual or a population with a specific toxicant and its entry into the body.[29] Exposure assessment considers exposure route and pathways, dose and duration, and frequency and intensity.[30]

Exposure assessment, which is one of the four steps in risk assessment, is used to estimate the increased risk of health impacts in individuals as a result of exposure to a toxic air pollutant. This step is used to determine the amount of pollutants to which individuals are exposed and the number of people exposed. It consists of four steps:

1. Identifying the pollutants that are likely to be present in air
2. Estimating the amount of pollutants emitted by various sources
3. Estimating the concentrations of pollutants for the geographical areas of interest
4. Estimating the number of individuals who breathe different levels (or a selected level) of polluted air.[31]

Individuals within a population differ considerably in their personal exposure to air pollutants. However, nearly all routine monitoring and regulation of air pollution are based upon environmental, rather than personal, measurements performed at fixed locations. Assessment of individual and population exposure to air pollution should consider variations of sources of exposure among individuals.[32] Personal exposure assessments include identifying (a) key sources of selected pollutants, (b) their emission rates, (c) their concentration in outdoor and indoor air, and (d) the duration of personal contact with the pollutants.[32] Knowing where people are and what they do is essential for determining personal exposure.

People living in high-income countries or in urban areas of LMICs spend most of their time indoors, where they are exposed to both outdoor air pollutants that penetrate indoors and pollutants that are generated indoors. For particles as small as 1 μm, the correlation between outdoor and indoor air concentrations is very high. Penetration of outdoor air pollutants to indoor air is a function of the air exchange rate, which is determined by type of construction, air conditioning, and other factors. Carbon dioxide, SO_2, and NO_2 penetrate from outdoor to indoor air with great efficiency. Ozone exposure is directly related to the amount of time spent outdoors.[10] In the absence of air conditioning, an estimated 70% of $PM_{2.5}$ from outdoors penetrates the indoor environment.

Three factors govern the risk of tissue injury from pollutants and their metabolites: (a) their chemical and physical properties, (b) the dose that reaches critical tissues (target site), and (c) how these tissues respond to the pollutants and their metabolites. The physical form and properties, such as the solubility of airborne contaminants, influences distribution in the atmosphere and body tissues—and, therefore, the dose delivered to these critical tissues. Since dose is very difficult to determine, surrogate measures are used, ranging from atmospheric concentration of pollutants to concentrations of biomarkers. For some pollutants, mathematical models of the relationship between exposure and dose can be used to develop surrogate measures. The interaction of pollutants with biological receptors can trigger mechanisms of toxic response, by direct stimulation or by initiating a cascade of molecular and cellular events that ultimately lead to tissue damage.[3,17] Pathways of pollutant sources—from exposure to inhalation to toxic effects—are shown in Figure 15-3.

PATTERNS OF AMBIENT AIR POLLUTION

During the past 25 years in high-income countries, urban air quality has tended to improve. However, 56% of these countries still fail to comply with WHO's air quality guidelines.[9,33]

In contrast, in many LMICs, air quality has tended to worsen due to urbanization, industrialization, intensification of traffic, use of diesel and other highly polluting fuels, burning of waste, energy inefficiency, and inadequate control measures. In addition, in these countries, many households burn biomass for heating and cooking, thereby generating air pollutants.[34] Among cities in LMICs with more than 100,000 residents, 98% exceed WHO air pollution guidelines.[7,18,19] WHO's Air Management Information System provides air-pollution data for cities in more than 60 countries.[18,35] In addition, WHO's Global Urban Ambient Air Pollution Database provides information on air pollution and its health impacts for more than 100 countries.[19,36,37]

ADVERSE HEALTH EFFECTS OF AMBIENT AIR POLLUTANTS

Exposure to ambient air pollution is associated with cardiorespiratory mortality, exacerbations of asthma, increased respiratory disorders and associated symptoms, decreased pulmonary function, increased airways reactivity, increased

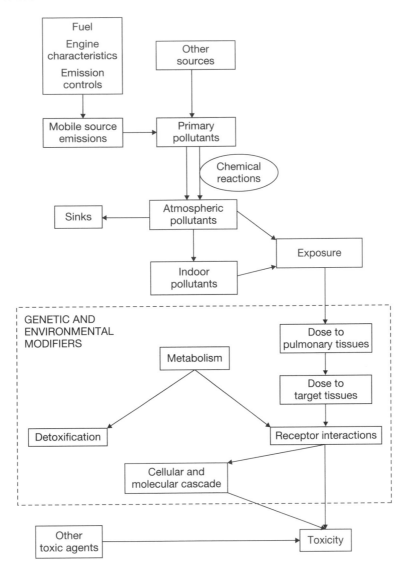

Figure 15-3. Pathway from motor vehicle pollutant sources to toxic effects in humans by exposure through inhalation. (Source: Watson AY, Bates RR, Kennedy D [eds.]. Air pollution, the automobile, and public health. Sponsored by the Health Effects Institute. Washington, DC: National Academy Press, 1988, p. 21.)

lung inflammation and systemic inflammatory markers, decreased heart-rate variability, increased plasma viscosity, reduced immunological defense, and increased healthcare utilization.[2] These associations are based on toxicology and epidemiology studies and exposure assessments.

Levels of ambient air pollutants usually correlate with one another, because either (a) emission sources often emit multiple pollutants or (b) pollutants in the air interact with one another. Although the health effects of specific pollutants have usually been studied separately

and are regulated separately, exposure to mixtures of pollutants, which commonly occur, may be responsible for adverse health effects.[2] It is often difficult to interpret data in epidemiological studies of people exposed to such mixtures. Correct interpretation may depend on (a) comparing results from different locations and (b) considering data from acute human exposures and experimental animal exposures to the primary pollutant.[10]

The next section considers adverse health effects of the *criteria air pollutants* regulated by the NAAQS, except for lead. (See Table 15-2.)

Table 15-2. Health Effects of Air Pollutants and Populations at Greatest Risk

Agent	Susceptible Population	Clinical Consequences	
Particles (PM$_{10}$ and PM$_{2.5}$)	Children	Increased acute cardiovascular and respiratory mortality	Effects seen alone or in combination with sulfur dioxide
	People with chronic heart and lung disease, including asthma	Increased cardiovascular mortality with chronic exposure	Probable effects:
		Increased hospital admissions for respiratory and cardiac conditions	• Acute respiratory infections in children
		Increased respiratory symptoms	• Decreased rate in lung function growth
		Decreased lung function	• Low birth rate
		Increased asthma exacerbations	• Postneonatal mortality
		Increased prevalence of chronic bronchitis	
		Increased risk of lung cancer	
		Increased blood fibrinogen	
		Increased inflammatory markers	
		Reduced heart-rate variability	
Sulfur dioxide	Healthy adults and COPD patients	Increased respiratory symptoms	Highly soluble gas with little penetration to distal airways
		Increased respiratory mortality and increased hospital visits for respiratory disease	
	People with asthma	Acute bronchoconstriction in people with asthma	Observations related to short-term exposures
Acid aerosols	Healthy adults	Increased respiratory illness	Currently not a criteria pollutant; no NAAQS established
	Children	Decreased lung function	
	People with asthma	Increased hospitalizations	Effects seen in combination with ozone and particles
	Others		
Ozone	Athletes	Increased hospital admissions for acute respiratory illnesses	Effects found at or below current NAAQS; effects increased with exercise
	Outdoor workers	Aggravation of asthma	Effects seen in combination with acid aerosols and particles
	People with asthma and other respiratory illnesses	Increased bronchial responsiveness	Probable increased mortality
	Children	Decreased lung function	Possible effects:
		Lung inflammation	• Aggravation of acute respiratory infections
		Increased respiratory symptoms	• Chronic bronchiolitis with repetitive exposure
		Decreased exercise capacity	
		Increased hospitalizations	
Nitrogen dioxide	Children with asthma	Increased respiratory morbidity	Effects occur at levels found indoors with unvented sources of combustion
	Young children	Increased airway reactivity	
		Decreased lung function	
		Increased respiratory symptoms	
		Increased respiratory illnesses	
Carbon monoxide	Healthy adults	Increased cardiac ischemia	Effects increase with anemia or chronic lung disease
	Patients with ischemic heart disease	Decreased exercise capacity	Possible effects:
			• Low birthweight
			• Preterm birth

Note. COPD = chronic obstructive pulmonary disease; NAAQS = national ambient air quality standards.

Particulate Matter and Sulfur Dioxide

The health effects of PM and SO$_2$ are presented together because they are both products of fossil-fuel combustion and are often present together in complex mixtures. Epidemiological studies suggest that (a) increased morbidity and mortality are associated with levels of airborne particles below the current standards and (b) PM$_{2.5}$, which contains more-reactive substances, is more closely associated with adverse health effects.[4,38] Globally, PM$_{2.5}$ pollution causes over 3.2 million premature deaths annually and a loss of 76 million disability-adjusted life years.[39]

Experimental Studies

Sulfur dioxide may cause bronchitis-like pathology in animals exposed to levels far above ambient air concentrations. In asthmatics, exposure to airborne concentrations from 0.25 to 0.5 ppm elicits acute bronchoconstriction, with increased airway resistance and decreased air flow. Sulfur dioxide can also reduce pulmonary defenses.[40]

Fine particulates, especially ultrafine particles (<100 nm), are toxic to the lungs due to their small size, particle surface area, number, particle surface chemistry, and potential for becoming internalized from the airway lumen into the interstitial space.[41] In addition, transition metals (those with the capacity of generating free radicals, such as manganese and vanadium) contained in particles may cause oxidative stress, augmented by the release of reactive oxygen species from the influx of inflammatory cells that results from the primary interaction between the lung and particles. Short-term exposure to high levels of concentrated ambient particles (200 µg/m³

of PM$_{2.5}$) can induce a transient, mild pulmonary inflammatory reaction[41] and changes in blood indices and heart-rate variability.[22] Figure 15-4 summarizes the pathways by which deposition of particles in the airways can induce adverse health effects in the airways and systematically.[42] In addition, combustion products may (a) modulate the immune system, impairing inflammatory and host-defense functions of the lung, and (b) act in synergy with allergens to enhance allergen-specific IgE production, initiate a TH$_2$ cytokine environment, and promote primary allergic sensitization.[43]

Population-Based Studies of Mortality

Acute exposure to airborne PM increases mortality. Occurrence of deaths is related to daily changes in air pollution levels.[3,4] A study in 20 U.S. cities found increases in total mortality (0.51%) and cardiovascular mortality (0.68%) for each 10 µg/m³ increase in PM$_{10}$.[8,44] The relationship appears to be linear, even at the lowest levels, without any

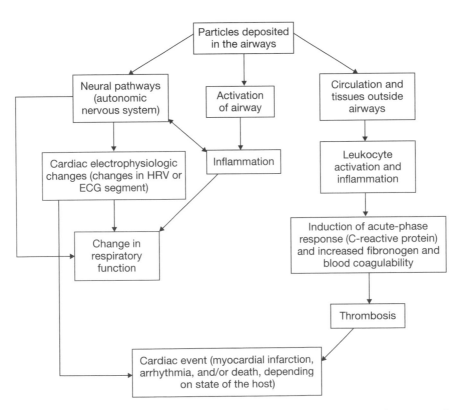

Figure 15-4. Adverse effects of particles on airways and the cardiovascular system: Possible pathways. ECG, electrocardiogram; HRV, heart-rate variability. (Source: Adapted from Health Effects Institute. Understanding the health effects of components of the particulate matter mix: progress and next steps. Boston: Health Effects Institute, 2002.)

threshold. People who otherwise might have survived for a long time are among those who died. Daily mortality appears to be more strongly associated with concentrations of $PM_{2.5}$ than with concentrations of larger particles[40]—an important finding for urban areas of LMICs, where vehicular traffic with poorly maintained engines and extensive use of diesel fuel is a major source of PM pollution. Increased infant mortality in these countries has been partially linked to exposure to airborne PM.[7,45] Each 10 µg/m³ increase in PM_{10} causes an estimated 1% increase in nonaccidental deaths in young children.[23]

Chronic exposure to $PM_{2.5}$ also increases mortality.[24] Fine particulate pollution appears to be associated with mortality from all causes combined, cardiopulmonary diseases, and lung cancer. Each 10 µg/m³ elevation in $PM_{2.5}$ air pollution has been associated with a 4% increase in all-cause mortality, a 6% increase in cardiopulmonary mortality, and an 8% increase in lung cancer mortality.[38] Cardiopulmonary mortality has also been associated with residing near major roads.[46]

Population-Based Studies of Morbidity

Acute exposure to high concentrations of SO_2 can cause bronchoconstriction, chemical bronchitis, and tracheitis. Asthmatics appear to be more sensitive. There is a linear exposure–response relationship between SO_2 and each of these three outcomes.[3]

Acute exposure to PM has been associated with morbidity in children and older people. Among children, PM has been associated with emergency-department visits and hospital admissions, increased upper respiratory infection and pneumonia, respiratory symptoms, and decrease in lung function.[3,47] Among older people, ambient levels of PM_{10} have been associated with increased hospital admissions for respiratory illnesses (including chronic obstructive pulmonary disease [COPD] and pneumonia) and cardiovascular disorders (including ischemic heart disease).[48] Ambient levels of PM has also been associated with (a) increases in systemic inflammatory markers, such as fibrinogen, C-reactive protein, and plasma viscosity, and (b) decreases in neural control of heart function, manifested by decreases in heart rate and heart-rate variability.[42] People with asthma appear to be more susceptible to the impact of PM_{10}, with increases in respiratory symptoms and decreases in lung function.[2,49] Diesel particles increase allergic response and can lead to the development of allergy and asthma.[5,6] Long-term exposure to SO_2 has been related to chronic bronchitis, especially in cigarette smokers.[3]

Long-term exposure to PM air pollution has been associated with chronic cough, bronchitis, and chest illness. A 10 µg/m³ increase in PM_{10} seems to be associated with a 5% to 25% increase in bronchitis or chronic cough and a 1% to 3% decrease in lung function.[49] Exposure to PM may lead to a reduction in maximum attained lung function, which occurs early in adult life and, ultimately, to an increased risk of chronic respiratory illness.[43,48]

Black Carbon

Population-Based Studies of Morbidity

Scientific evidence, although limited, suggests that short- and long-term exposure to BC can be associated with respiratory disorders (including childhood asthma), cardiovascular disorders (including increased blood pressure), and premature death.[16,29,50]

Population-Based Studies of Mortality

Black carbon has been found to be associated with cardiovascular mortality[51] and reduced pulmonary function.[52] Increased prior BC concentrations have been found in patients with major cardiovascular adverse effects.[53] An estimated 14,000 deaths due to BC occurred globally in 2010. Control of BC emissions could yield substantial public health benefits.[54]

Ozone

Ozone is a powerful oxidant that can react with a wide range of cellular components and biological material. Its biological effects are likely caused by intermediates, such as free radicals, lipid hydroperoxides, aldehydes, and hydrogen peroxide. The primary target organ for O_3 is the lung, where exposure produces cellular and structural changes that reduce lung function. Exposure to low concentrations of O_3, even for 10 to 30 minutes, causes irritation of the eyes, nose, throat, and lungs. Exposure to high concentrations of O_3 cause cough, chest pain, pneumonitis, and other respiratory problems. People with COPD and asthma are especially sensitive to O_3.[32]

Experimental Studies

Ozone causes oxidation or peroxidation of biomolecules via free radical reaction. Ozone reacts rapidly with substrates in the lung lining fluid, preferentially with antioxidants; however, low content of lung lining fluid (antioxidant defense) or high O_3 exposure leads to the oxidation product responsible for adverse health effects. Lipoperoxidation of polyunsaturated fatty acids of lung cells can release arachidonic acid, which is subsequently converted into prostaglandin E_2 and prostaglandin F_{2alpha}, both of which act on neuroreceptors in airways and induce an inflammatory response.[30]

Ozone damages the respiratory tract, increasing permeability and inflammation, which causes morphological, biochemical, and functional changes and decreases host defenses. Ozone exposure causes a major lesion in the centriacinar area, affecting the efficiency of gas exchange. In animals, it causes fibrotic changes,[31] which are believed to cause airflow obstruction.

In humans, O_3 induces an increase in the constituents of the bronchoalveolar lavage fluid. Levels of O_3 frequently measured in urban areas in the United States reduce lung function. Decrement in lung function and physical performance, aggravation of respiratory tract symptoms, increased airway reactivity, and acute inflammation have been observed at exposure levels as low as 0.08 ppm. Acute reversible reductions in lung function have been observed in exercising children exposed to 0.12 ppm.[3,30] After repeated exposure to O_3, decrement in lung function observed after single exposures attenuated, suggesting adaptation, but airway inflammation persisted despite attenuation of some markers of inflammation.

These studies, taken together, show wide but reproducible variability among individuals' sensitivity to O_3, and they suggest that adults and children who engage in prolonged exercise or work outdoors may be at risk of adverse health effects of O_3 concentrations near the ambient standard.[55]

Population-Based Studies of Mortality

Significant associations have been found between O_3 exposure and COPD, other respiratory disorders, cardiac disorders, and cerebrovascular disease.[56] When the airborne concentration of O_3 is high, O_3 levels are associated with daily mortality. A pooling of 15 time-series studies found that an increase of 200 µg/m³ (100 ppb) in O_3 concentration was associated with a 3.6% increase in mortality.[57]

Population-Based Studies of Morbidity

Exposure of healthy individuals, including children, to relatively low concentrations of O_3 can cause lung inflammation, acutely decreased lung function, and respiratory impairment, as well as increases in emergency department visits and hospital admissions due to respiratory diseases, respiratory symptoms (such as cough, throat dryness, and chest discomfort and pain), headache, eye discomfort, and temporary lung function decrement. The combined relative risk estimate for respiratory-disease hospital admission from major time-series studies for all ages has been estimated at 1.18 per 100 ppb increase in daily 1-hour maximum O_3 concentrations.[55] People with asthma appear to be more sensitive to O_3 exposure; increases in respiratory-related emergency department visits and symptoms and decreases in lung function have been reported.[3,6] In clinical studies, O_3 potentiates the effect of allergen exposure in sensitive people with asthma, perhaps as a consequence of increased penetrability of the respiratory epithelium from O_3 exposure.[30]

Because of the acute health effects associated with short-term O_3 exposure and the available studies on long-term animal exposure to O_3, there is concern that long-term exposure may have a cumulative adverse impact on human health. Studies of long-term exposure to O_3 suggest both a decrease in baseline pulmonary function and induction of asthma.[55] In communities with high O_3 concentration, O_3 exposure has been linked to the incidence of asthma in children participating in heavy exercise.[58]

In children under age 15, the incidence of upper respiratory infections has been found to be associated with airborne O_3 concentration. In children under age 5, a 20 ppb increase in O_3 level was found to be associated with a 13% increase in consultations for respiratory infections.[59] Studies have found that O_3 levels are associated with cough, use of bronchodilator medications, and increases in biomarkers of respiratory tract inflammation.[39,60] In asthmatic children, decreases in pulmonary function have been associated to O_3 exposure.[54] There is evidence that O_3 may be associated with abnormal pregnancy outcomes. A significant relationship has been found between O_3 exposure of pregnant women and low birthweight of their infants.[61]

Nitrogen Dioxide

Nitrogen dioxide is highly reactive. It causes bronchitis and pneumonitis and increases susceptibility to respiratory infections. Much exposure to NO_2 takes place indoors, where sources include cooking stoves and space heaters. Brief exposure to concentrations as high as 0.5 ppm may be experienced while cooking with gas stoves or driving in traffic.[57] In ambient air, NO_2 does not generally occur alone but as part of a complex mixture of pollutants. Consequently, characterizing the effects of NO_2 in ambient air has proven to be challenging. The contribution of NO_2 to secondary particles (those that form the atmosphere from other gaseous pollutants) and the role of NO_2 in the formation of O_3 may be more relevant to public health than any of its direct effects.

Exposure to *low concentrations* of NO_2 in the air may cause irritation in the eyes, nose, throat, and lungs as well as cough and shortness of breath, fatigue, and nausea. It can cause fluid accumulation in the lungs 1 or 2 days after exposure. Exposure to *high concentrations* of NO_2 can cause irritation, inflammation, and spasms in the throat and the upper airways.[20]

Experimental Studies

Animal experiments show that exposure to NO_2 concentrations at levels about 10 times those generally found in outdoor air in cities can impair both cellular and humoral immunological mechanisms of the lung.[62]

Population-Based Studies of Mortality

There is a significant association between exposure to NO_2 and daily mortality. An increase of 50 µg/m³ in NO_2 has been associated with a 1.3% increase in daily deaths. Nitrogen dioxide has also been associated with daily mortality in children under age 5 and fetal death.[6] Studies

have also found that NO_2 is associated with respiratory mortality,[39] cardiovascular mortality,[63] and all-cause mortality.[51]

Population-Based Studies of Morbidity

Results of studies of short-term effects among children and adults exposed to O_3 outdoors have been inconsistent. One study indicated an increase in asthma admissions related to ambient levels of NO_2.[64] Pathological effects in the lung resulting from occupational exposure to NOx range from mild inflammatory response in the tracheobronchial mucosa at low concentrations to bronchitis, bronchopneumonia, and acute pulmonary edema at high concentrations.[3]

Long-term exposure to outdoor NO_2 has been associated with increased chronic respiratory symptoms and infections among children and possibly to a decrease in lung function. A meta-analysis of 11 epidemiological studies reported an increase in respiratory illness in children under age 12 associated with long-term exposure to high concentrations of NO_2 from gas stoves.[65] A study demonstrated (a) a significant deficit in lung growth related to exposure to NO_2 and $PM_{2.5}$ and (b) in communities with relatively high exposure to NO_2, more frequent chronic cough and phlegm among children with asthma.[58]

Among adults, chronic NO_2 exposure has been associated with increased respiratory symptoms and reduced lung function. A cohort study of over 800,000 patients age 40 to 89 found that NO_2 exposure was associated with hospital admissions for exacerbation of COPD.[27] Another study found an inverse association between NO_2 and forced expiratory volume (FEV_1).[54]

Polycyclic Aromatic Hydrocarbons

Several polycyclic aromatic hydrocarbons (PAHs) have the potential to cause cancer. The International Agency for Research on Cancer has determined that benzo[a]pyrene (BaP) and several other PAHs are potential human carcinogens.[66]

Experimental Studies

Studies in laboratory animals have shown that benzo[k]fluoranthene, benzo[a]anthracene, chrysene, BaP, dibenzo[a,h]anthracene, benzo[j] fluoranthene, indeno[1,2,3-c,d]pyrene, and benzo[b]fluoranthene can cause tumors.[52] Other animal studies have observed that certain PAHs, when inhaled, can cause lung cancer; some PAHs, when ingested, can cause stomach cancer; and, some PAHs, when applied to the skin, can cause skin cancer.[66] Other studies have shown that the offspring of female mice, after being fed high levels of BaP during pregnancy, had higher rates of birth defects and lower birthweight.[66]

Population-Based Studies

Studies in humans have shown that chronic dermal or respiratory exposure to PAHs may cause cancer. Other studies suggest that exposure of pregnant women to high levels of BaP may cause birth defects and a low birthweight in their infants.[52] Another study found that elementary-school students with heavy indoor exposure to PAHs (due to outdoor traffic) substantially increased their risk of cancer.[67]

Volatile Organic Compounds

The adverse health effects of VOCs may vary according to the compound, its toxicity, and the duration of exposure. Long-term exposure can cause liver, kidney, and central nervous system injuries. Even short-term exposure can cause irritation of the eyes and the respiratory tract as well as fatigue, headaches, nausea, dizziness, and allergic skin disorders.[68]

Carbon Monoxide

High exposure to CO has occurred mainly in firefighting and certain other occupations (Table 15-3), in suicide attempts, and in unintended poisoning, such as due to defective or improperly used combustion devices. High exposure can cause acute poisoning, resulting in coma and death. Most fatal CO poisoning occurs in confined spaces, such as inside garages, automobiles, weather-sealed houses, and ice skating rinks.

Carbon monoxide is produced by the incomplete combustion of fossil fuels, mainly derived from mobile sources. Most of the carbon in automotive fuel is oxidized to carbon dioxide, with only a small fraction incompletely oxidized to CO.[25]

The health impacts of CO exposure are weakness, dizziness, nausea, vomiting, headaches, chest pain, and confusion. People with chronic respiratory or cardiac disorders, such as those with coronary artery disease or peripheral vascular disease, are highly vulnerable. Workers in small, poorly ventilated workplaces are at increased risk of CO poisoning.

Fatal CO poisoning has also occurred outdoors, such as on recreational houseboats near generators and the exhaust of other gasoline-powered motors, which led to hazard warnings and boat redesign.

Although outdoor CO exposures in urban environments are generally much lower than those associated with CO poisoning, some urban CO exposures may adversely affect the heart and the brain, the most oxygen-sensitive organs.[3] (See Chapters 7, 11, 23, and 26.)

Experimental Studies

Carbon monoxide decreases capacity for oxygen uptake, leading to decreased work capacity under maximum exercise conditions. A blood carboxyhemoglobin (COHb) concentration of about 5% is required to decrease oxygen-uptake

Table 15-3. Predicted Carboxyhemoglobin (COHb) Levels for People Engaged in Different Types of Work in Different Concentrations of Carbon Monoxide

CO Concentration in ppm	in mg/m³	Exposure Time	Predicted COHb Level for Those Engaged in Sedentary Work	Light Work	Heavy Work
100	115	15 minutes	1.2	2.0	2.8
50	57	30 minutes	1.1	1.9	2.6
25	29	1 hour	1.1	1.7	2.2
10	11.5	8 hours	1.5	1.7	1.7

capacity. Reduced cognitive abilities have been observed at COHb levels as low as 3.2%. Headaches can occur at a COHb level of 15% and dizziness at 20%. Above 30%, severe headaches and cardiovascular symptoms can occur. Above COHb levels of about 40%, there is considerable risk of coma and death.[3]

Population-Based Studies

Daily increases in CO exposure have been associated with increases in premature mortality and hospitalizations from congestive heart failure.[3] However, epidemiologic studies on the health effects of CO need to be interpreted with caution because measurements of CO in air by fixed monitors correlate poorly with personal CO measurements. Therefore, CO may be a proxy for other pollutants, such as $PM_{2.5}$.[3]

Carbon monoxide exposure may also adversely affect the developing fetus directly by creating an oxygen deficit—without elevating the COHb level in fetal blood. During high CO exposure, a pregnant woman's hemoglobin gives up oxygen less readily (than a woman who is not pregnant), with resultant lowering of the oxygen pressure in the placenta and in fetal blood.

In animals, CO causes low birthweight and developmental effects.[2] In humans, CO exposure during pregnancy has been associated with adverse pregnancy outcomes, including intrauterine fetal death and low birthweight.[6]

SUSCEPTIBILITY FACTORS

Susceptibility of individuals to air pollutants varies widely. Susceptibility is a function of both (a) intrinsic factors, such as age, gender, race, pre-existing health impairment, and genetic factors, and (b) extrinsic factors, such as the nature, magnitude, and frequency of exposures to pollutants as well as concomitant hazardous exposures, environmental conditions, nutritional status, and lifestyle factors.[69]

Intrinsic Factors

Certain subgroups are more susceptible to the health effects of air pollution, including children, older people, people with respiratory and cardiovascular disorders, and those with certain genetic factors. Several factors are responsible for the high susceptibility of children to ambient air pollutants. Children spend more time outdoors than do most adults, and they often engage in vigorous play. Since they also have higher respiratory rates than adults, they may receive higher doses of pollutants in proportion to body weight. Intensive growth and development processes in children create windows of great vulnerability to environmental toxicants. Older people are more likely to suffer from respiratory and cardiovascular disorders and impairment of immune response, all of which increase their susceptibility to air pollutants, especially to $PM_{2.5}$. People with asthma are generally more adversely affected by short-term exposure to inhaled agents, especially PM and O_3.

Genetic factors can play a major role in responsiveness to air pollutants, especially to PM and O_3.[2,70] Certain genetic polymorphisms affect synthesis of enzymes involved in the response to oxidative stress, such as glutathione-S-transferase, which could increase one's susceptibility to O_3 and enhance one's allergic response to diesel exhaust. These genetic factors might explain some of the large variability among individuals in response to O_3 exposure.

Extrinsic Factors

Most air pollution exposures involve a complex mixture of chemicals. In studies of the health effects of vehicular exhaust emissions, it is difficult to assess the effect of individual pollutants, especially $PM_{2.5}$ and NO_2. Some studies have reported a synergistic effect of O_3 and PM, or of O_3 and diesel exhaust, in increasing an individual's susceptibility to allergens.

Dietary antioxidants modulate the response to photo-oxidant exposure in animals and humans. Water-soluble antioxidants, such as ascorbate, urate, and reduced glutathione, are abundantly present in lung fluid and provide protection against damaging oxidation reactions in the extracellular components of lung fluid. Within the cell, alpha-tocopherol and glutathione peroxidase may act to prevent the propagation of lipid peroxidation reactions. Vitamin E may prevent O_3-induced peroxidation, especially in vitamin E–deficient animals. Vitamin E, vitamin C, and betacarotene may protect against the adverse health effects of O_3 on lung function.[71,72] Other micronutrients, such as omega-3 fatty acids, may decrease the adverse cardiovascular response to PM exposure. Deficiency of these micronutrients could increase susceptibility to PM and photo-oxidants, especially where populations are chronically exposed to high ambient air levels of pollutants.

Low socioeconomic status increases the association between air pollution and adverse health effects. Several factors, such as poor living conditions, poor nutrition, concomitant exposure, and limited access to healthcare, likely interact to increase the vulnerability to air pollutants.[73]

Although outdoor air pollutants have been linked to several adverse respiratory and cardiovascular disorders, this risk is not uniformly distributed and may vary in relation to the proximity to emission sources. Therefore, people who reside or work close to major roads or highways may have a greater risk of suffering health effects compared to similar people who reside or work further away.[74] This new area of environmental research relies heavily on exposure metrics, such as distance to major roads (as determined by geographic information systems) and measures of traffic density.[75] Geographic information systems may incorporate variables on terrain, population density, and pollutant levels and help to construct a model to predict the spread of pollution in an area.[76] This technique may be useful in identifying "hot spots" of higher concentration for ecological studies or in evaluating rates of chronic disorders in relation to exposures.

Traffic-related emissions have been associated with severity and frequency of respiratory symptoms, asthma exacerbations, increased airway inflammation, and reduced lung volumes[29]—as well as cardiovascular and cerebrovascular morbidity and mortality. Living near a major road increases the risk of deep venous thrombosis, a risk factor for pulmonary embolism.[77]

The physical and chemical properties of the mixture of air pollutants near vehicular traffic may explain why this type of exposure causes serious health problems. Near vehicular emissions there is a much higher burden of $PM_{2.5}$ and ultrafine particles, with greater content of organic and elemental carbon.[78] These highly toxic particles are more likely to enter the distal airways and the systemic circulation. High CO levels may also play a role in increasing risk for cardiovascular disease.

There are inconsistencies among studies, with some reporting no association between traffic emission and health effects.[79-81] Given that populations with lower socioeconomic status are more likely to reside close to major roads or highways, factors other than environmental exposures could be biasing the results.[61]

Many unanswered questions remain, including:

- What constitutes proximity to a road?
- Is there a threshold, either based on distance to the exposure or traffic density that could offer some degree of protection to an exposed population?
- Should people with severe asthma or congestive heart failure minimize their exposure to traffic, such as by residing and working further from traffic?

With more studies standardizing their approach and controlling for bias, more information will be available to translate results into effective health policies and public health interventions that may reduce morbidity and mortality due to traffic emissions.

AUTHORS' NOTE

The findings and conclusions in this chapter are those of the authors and do not necessarily represent the views of the Instituto Nacional de Salud Pública of Mexico or the Ministry of Health of Mexico.

REFERENCES

1. Logan WP. Mortality in the London fog incident, 1952. Lancet 1953; 336–338.
2. Bascom R, Bromberg PA Costa D. Health effects of outdoor air pollution. Part I & Part II. American Journal of Respiratory and Critical Care Medicine 1996; 153: 3–50 and 447–498.
3. Romieu I. Epidemiological studies of health effects arising from motor vehicle air pollution. In: Schwela D, Zali O (eds.). Urban traffic pollution. London E&FN Spon. 1999; pp. 9–69.
4. Pope CA III. Epidemiology of fine particulate air pollution and human health: biologic

mechanisms and who's at risk? Environmental Health Perspectives 2000; 108: 713–723.

5. Brunekreef B, Holgate ST. Air pollution and health. Lancet 2002; 360: 1233–1242.

6. Romieu I, Hernandez M. Air pollution and health in developing countries: A review of epidemiological evidence. In: McGranahan G, Murray F (eds.) Air pollution and health in rapidly developing countries. London: Earthscan, 2003, pp. 49–67.

7. Romieu I, Korc M. Contaminación del aire exterior. In: Romieu I, Lopez S (eds.). Contaminación ambiental y salud de los niños en América Latina y el Caribe. Cuernavaca, Mor, Mexico: Instituto Nacional de Salud Publica, 2003, pp. 109–129.

8. Romieu I, Samet JM, Smith KR, Bruce N. Outdoor air pollution and acute respiratory infections among children in developing countries. Journal of Occupational and Environmental Medicine 2002; 44: 640–649.

9. Prüss-Ustün A, Wolf J, Corvalán C, et al. Preventing disease through healthy environments: A global assessment of the burden of disease from environmental risks. 2016. Available at: http://apps.who.int/iris/bitstream/10665/204585/1/9789241565196_eng.pdf?ua=1. Accessed January 12, 2017.

10. Brauer M. Sources, emissions, concentrations, exposures, and doses. In: Bates DV (ed.). A citizen's guide to air pollution (2nd ed.). Vancouver, Canada: Cambridge University Press, 2002, pp. 11–47.

11. Agency for Toxic Substances and Disease Registry. Introduction—Survey of toxic substances: Outdoor air pollutants. Available at: https://www.atsdr.cdc.gov/training/toxmanual/modules/4/lecturenotes.html. Accessed January 18, 2017.

12. Annest JL, Pirkle JL, Makuc D, et al. Chronological trend in blood lead levels between 1976 and 1980. New England Journal of Medicine 1983; 308: 1373–1377.

13. Organización Mundial de la Salud. Guías de calidad del aire de la OMS relativas al material particulado, el ozono, el dióxido de nitrógeno y el dióxido de azufre, 2005, p. 25.

14. Grant LD, Shoaf CR, Davis M. United States and international approaches to establishing air standards and guidelines. In: Holgate ST, Koren HS, Samet JM, Maynard RL (eds.). Air pollution and health. London: Academic Press, 1999, pp. 947–982.

15. Environmental Protection Agency. Criteria air pollutants. NAAQS table. Available at: https://www.epa.gov/criteria-air-pollutants/naaqs-table. Accessed January 12, 2017.

16. World Health Organization. Ambient (outdoor) air quality and health. Fact sheet, updated September 2016. Available at: http://www.who.int/mediacentre/factsheets/fs313/en/. Accessed January 12, 2017.

17. Health Effects Institute. Diesel Workshop: Building a research strategy to improve risk assessment. 1999. Available at: https://www.healtheffects.org/publication/diesel-workshop-building-research-strategy-improve-risk-assessment. Accessed January 12, 2017.

18. Krzyzanowski M, Schwela D. Patterns of air pollution in developing countries. In: Holgate ST, Koren HS, Samet JM, Maynard RL (eds.). Air pollution and health. London: Academic Press, 1999, pp. 105–113.

19. World Health Organization. Public health, environmental and social determinants of health (PHE). WHO global urban ambient air pollution database (update 2016). Available at: http://www.who.int/phe/health_topics/outdoorair/databases/cities/en/. Accessed January 12, 2017.

20. Holdren JP, Smith KR. Energy, the environment and health. In: Goldenburg J (ed.). Energy assessment: Energy and the challenge of sustainability. New York: United Nations Development Programme, 2000, pp. 61–110.

21. European Commission. EDGAR Emissions of Greenhouse Gases. Main air pollutant emissions in most polluting countries. Available at: http://edgar.jrc.ec.europa.eu/background.php. Accessed January 9, 2017.

22. Ghio AJ, Huang YC. Exposure to concentrated ambient particles (CAPs): A review. Inhalation Toxicology 2004; 16: 53–59.

23. Cohen AJ, Anderson HR, Ostro Bea. Urban air pollution. In: Ezzati M, Lopez AD, Rodgers A, Murray CJL (eds.). Quantification of health risks. Global and regional burden of diseases attributable to selected major risk factors. Geneva: World Health Organization, 2004, pp. 1353–1433.

24. Dockery DW, Pope III CA, Xu X. et al. An association between air pollution and mortality in six U.S. cities. New England Journal of Medicine 1993; 329: 1753–1759.

25. Holman C. Sources of air pollution. In: Holgate ST, Koren H, Maynard R (eds.). Air pollution and health. London: Academic Press, 1999, pp. 115–148.

26. Intergovernmental Panel on Climate Change, Working Group I: The Scientific Basis. Reactive gases: Carbon monoxide (CO) and hydrogen (H2).

Available at: https://www.ipcc.ch/ipccreports/tar/wg1/139.htm. Accessed January 12, 2017.

27. Atkinson RW, Carey IM, Kent AJ, et al. Long-term exposure to outdoor air pollution and the incidence of chronic obstructive pulmonary disease in a national English cohort. Occupational and Environmental Medicine 2015; 72: 42–48.

28. World Health Organization. Air quality guidelines—global update 2005. Available at: http://www.who.int/phe/health_topics/outdoorair/outdoorair_aqg/es/. Accessed January 13, 2017.

29. Louwies T, Nawrot T, Cox B, et al. Blood pressure changes in association with black carbon exposure in a panel of healthy adults are independent of retinal microcirculation. Environment International 2015; 75: 81–86.

30. Mudway IS, Kelly FJ. Ozone and the lung: A sensitive issue. Molecular Aspects of Medicine 2000; 21: 1–48.

31. Paige RC, Plopper CG. Acute and chornic effects of ozone in animal models. In: Holgate ST, Koren HS, Samet JM, Maynard RL (eds.) Air pollution and health. London: Academic Press, 1999, pp. 531–557.

32. Ozkaynak H. Exposure assessment. In: Holgate ST, Koren HS, Samet JM, Maynard RL (eds.). Air pollution and health. London: Academic Press 1999, pp. 149–162.

33. World Health Organization. Air pollution levels rising in many of the world's poorest cities. May 12, 2016. Available at: http://www.who.int/mediacentre/news/releases/2016/air-pollution-rising/en/. Accessed January 13, 2017.

34. Ng CFS, Ueda K, Nitta H, Takeuchi A. Seasonal variation in the acute effects of ozone on premature mortality among elderly Japanese. Environmental Monitoring and Assessment 2013; 185: 8767–8776.

35. Biblioteca Virtual de Desarrollo Sostenible y Salud Ambiental-Organización Panamericana de la Salud. The Air Management Information System (AMIS) and a Global Air Quality Partnership. Available at: http://www.bvsde.paho.org/bvsci/i/fulltext/amis/amis.html. Accessed January 13, 2017.

36. World Health Organization. WHO's urban ambient air pollution database—Update 2016. Data summary. Available at: http://www.who.int/phe/health_topics/outdoorair/databases/AAP_database_summary_results_2016_v02.pdf?ua=1. Accessed January 13, 2017.

37. World Health Organization. Public health, environmental and social determinants of health (PHE). WHO Global Urban Ambient Air Pollution Database (update 2016). Available at: http://www.who.int/phe/health_topics/outdoorair/databases/cities/en/. Accessed January 13, 2017.

38. Klemm RJ, Mason RMJ, Heilig CM, et al. Is daily mortality associated specifically with fine particles? Data reconstruction and replication of analyses. Journal of the Air Waste Management Association 2000; 50: 1215–1222.

39. Beelen R, Hoek G, van den Brandt PA, et al. Long-term effects of traffic-related air pollution on mortality in a Dutch cohort (NLCS-AIR study). Environmental Health Perspectives 2008; 116: 196–202.

40. Schlesinger RB. Toxicology of sulphur oxides. In: Holgate ST, Koren HS, Samet JM, Maynard RL (eds.). Air pollution and health. London: Academic Press 1999, pp. 583–611.

41. MacNee W, Donaldson K. Particulate air pollution: Injurious and protective mecahnisms in the lungs. In: Holgate ST, Koren HS, Samet JM, Maynard RL (eds.). Air pollution and Health. London: Academic Press, 1999, pp. 653–672.

42. Health Effects Institute. Understanding the health effects of components of the particulate matter mix: Progress and next steps. Boston: Health Effects Institute, 2002.

43. Thomas PT, Zelikoff JT. Air pollutants: Modulators of pulmonary host resistance against infection. In: Holgate ST, Koren HS, Samet JM, Maynard RL (eds.). Air pollution and health. London: Academic Press, 1999, pp. 357–379.

44. Aga E, Samoli E, Touloumi G, et al. Short-term effects of ambient particles on mortality in the elderly: Results from 28 cities in the APHEA2 project. European Respiratory Journal Supplement 2003; 40: S28–S33.

45. Romieu I, Samet JM, Smith KR, Bruce N. Outdoor air pollution and acute respiratory infections among children in developing countries. Journal of Occupational and Environmental Medicine 2002; 44: 640–649.

46. Hoek G, Brunekreef B, Goldbohm S, et al. Association between mortality and indicators of traffic-related air pollution in the Netherlands: A cohort study. Lancet. 2002; 360: 1203–1209.

47. Schwartz J. Air pollution and children's health. Pediatrics 2004; 113: 1037–1043.

48. Samet JM, Zeger SL, Dominici F, et al. The National Morbidity, Mortality, and Air Pollution Study. Part II: Morbidity and mortality from air pollution in the United States. Research Report (Health Effects Institute) 2000; 94: 5–79.

49. Pope CA III, Dockery D. Epidemiology of particle effects. In: Holgate ST, Koren HS, Samet JM, Maynard RL (eds.) Air pollution and health. London: Academic Press, 1999, pp. 671–705.

50. Cheng Y, Kan H. Effect of the interaction between outdoor air pollution and extreme temperature on daily mortality in Shanghai, China. Journal of Epidemiology 2012; 22: 28–36.

51. Deguen S, Petit C, Delbarre A, et al. Neighbourhood characteristics and long-term air pollution levels modify the association between the short-term nitrogen dioxide concentrations and all-cause mortality in Paris. PLoS One 2015; 10: 1–14.

52. Agencia para Sustancias Tóxicas y el Registro de Enfermedades. Resúmenes de Salud Pública— Hidrocarburos aromáticos policíclicos (HAP) [Polycyclic Aromatic Hydrocarbons (PHA)]. Available at: http://www.atsdr.cdc.gov/es/toxfaqs/es_tfacts69.html. Accessed September 7, 2016.

53. Crouse DL, Peters PA, Villeneuve PJ, et al. Within- and between-city contrasts in nitrogen dioxide and mortality in 10 Canadian cities: A subset of the Canadian Census Health and Environment Cohort (CanCHEC). Journal of Exposure Science & Environmental Epidemiology 2015; 25: 1–8.

54. Barone-Adesi F, Dent JE, Dajnak D, et al. Long-term exposure to primary traffic pollutants and lung function in children: Cross-sectional study and meta-analysis. PLoS One 2015; 10: 1–16.

55. Thurston GD, Ito K. Epidemiological studies of ozone exposure effects. In: Holgate ST, Koren HS, Samet JM, Maynard RL (eds.). Air pollution and health, London: Academic Press, 1999, pp. 486–510.

56. Peters A, von Klot S, Heier M, et al. Exposure to traffic and the onset of myocardial infarction. New England Journal of Medicine 2004; 351: 1721–1730.

57. Bernard SM, Samet JM, Grambsch A, et al. The potential impacts of climate variability and change on air pollution-related health effects in the United States. Environmental Health Perspectives 2001; 109: 199–209.

58. Kunzli N, McConnell R, Bates DV, et al. Breathless in Los Angeles: The exhausting search for clean air. American Journal of Public Health 2003; 93: 1494–1499.

59. Sweeney LM, Sommerville DR, Goodwin MR, et al. Acute toxicity when concentration varies with time: A case study with carbon monoxide inhalation by rats. Regulatory Toxicology and Pharmacology 2016; 80: 102–115.

60. Snow SJ, Gordon CJ, Bass VL, et al. Age-related differences in pulmonary effects of acute and subchronic episodic ozone exposures in Brown Norway rats. Inhalation Toxicology 2016; 28: 313–323.

61. O'Neill MS, Jerrett M, Kawachi I, et al. Health, wealth, and air pollution: Advancing theory and methods. Environmental Health Perspectives 2003; 111: 1861–1870.

62. Morrow PE. Toxicological data on NOx: An overview. Journal of Toxicology and Environmental Health 1984; 13: 205–227.

63. Chen R, Pan G, Kan H, et al. Ambient air pollution and daily mortality in Anshan, China: A time-stratified case-crossover analysis. Science of the Total Environment 2010; 408: 6086–6091.

64. Ackermann-Liebrich U, Rapp R. Epidemiological effects of oxides of nitrogen, especially NO2. In: Schwela D, Zali O, (eds.). Urban traffic pollution. London: E & FN Spon, 1999, pp. 561–584.

65. Hasselblad V, Eddy DM, Kotchmar DJ. Synthesis of environmental evidence: nitrogen dioxide epidemiology studies. Journal of the Air and Waste Management Association 1992; 42: 662–671.

66. Agencia para Sustancias Tóxicas y el Registro de Enfermedades. Hidrocarburos aromáticos policíclicos (HAPs). 1996. Available at: http://www.cvs.saude.sp.gov.br/pdf/toxfaq120.pdf

67. Oliveira M, Slezakova K, Madureira J, et al. Polycyclic aromatic hydrocarbons in primary school environments: Levels and potential risks. Science of the Total Environment 2017; 575: 1156–1167.

68. Tox Town. Volatile organic compounds (VOCs). Available at: https://toxtown.nlm.nih.gov/espanol/chemicals.php?id=41. Accessed September 2, 2016.

69. American Thoracic Society. What constitutes an adverse health effect of air pollution? American Journal of Respiratory and Critical Care Medicine 2000; 161: 665–673.

70. Kleeberger SR. Genetic aspects of susceptibility to air pollution. European Respiratory Journal Supplement 2003; 21: S52–56.

71. Grievink L, Smit HA, Brunekreef B. Anti-oxidants and air pollution in relation to indicators of asthma and COPD: A review of the current evidence. Clinical & Experimental Allergy 2000; 30: 1344–1354.

72. Romieu I, Trenga, C. Diet and obstructive lung disease. Epidemiology Reviews 2001; 23: 268–287.

73. O'Neill M, Ramirez-Aguilar M, Meneses-Gonzalez F, et al. Ozone exposure among Mexico City outdoor workers. Journal of the Air & Waste Management Association 2003; 53: 339–346.

74. Holguin F. Traffic, outdoor air pollution, and asthma. Immunology and Allergy Clinics of North America 2008; 28: 577–588, viii–ix.

75. Briggs D. The role of GIS: Coping with space (and time) in air pollution exposure assessment. Journal of Toxicology and Environment Health: Part A 2005; 68: 1243–1261.

76. Mukerjee S, Smith LA, Johnson MM, et al. Spatial analysis and land use regression of VOCs and NO(2) from school-based urban air monitoring in Detroit/Dearborn, USA. Science of the Total Environment 2009; 407: 4642–4651.

77. Baccarelli A, Martinelli I, Pegoraro V, et al. Living near major traffic roads and risk of deep vein thrombosis. Circulation 2009; 119: 3118–3124.

78. Brunekreef B, Beelen R, Hoek G, et al. Effects of long-term exposure to traffic-related air pollution on respiratory and cardiovascular mortality in the Netherlands: The NLCS-AIR study. Research Reports 2009; 5–71; discussion 73–89.

79. Venn A, Lewis S, Cooper M, et al. Local road traffic activity and the prevalence, severity, and persistence of wheeze in school children: Combined cross sectional and longitudinal study. Occupational and Environmental Medicine 2000; 57: 152–158.

80. Wilkinson P, Elliott P, Grundy C, et al. Case-control study of hospital admission with asthma in children aged 5–14 years: Relation with road traffic in north west London. Thorax 1999; 54: 1070–1074.

81. Lewis SA, Antoniak M, Venn AJ, et al. Secondhand smoke, dietary fruit intake, road traffic exposures, and the prevalence of asthma: A cross-sectional study in young children. American Journal of Epidemiology 2005; 161: 406–411.

FURTHER READING

Phalen RF, Introduction to air pollution science: A public health perspective. Burlington, MA: Jones and Bartlett Learning, 2013.

Vallero D. Fundamentals of air pollution (5th ed.). Waltham, MA: Academic Press, 2014.

Cooper CD, Alley FC. Air pollution control: A design approach (4th ed.). Long Grove, IL: Waveland Press, Inc., 2010.

Major books on air pollution, its adverse health effects, and its control.

Correia AW, Pope CA 3rd, Dockery DW, et al. Effect of air pollution control on life expectancy in the United States: An analysis of 545 U.S. counties for the period from 2000 to 2007. Epidemiology 2013; 24: 23–31.

Chafe ZA, Brauer M, Klimont Z, et al. Household cooking with solid fuels contributes to ambient PM2.5 air pollution and the burden of disease. Environmental Health Perspectives 2014; 122: 1314–1320.

Riojas-Rodríguez H, da Silva AS, Texcalac-Sangrador JL, Moreno-Banda GL. Air pollution management and control in Latin America and the Caribbean: Implications for climate change. Revista Panamericana de Salud Pública 2016; 40: 150–159.

Journal articles that focus on specific issues concerning air pollution.

16

Water Contamination

Jeffery A. Foran and Amaryl Griggs

Although there are more than 3.5×10^{20} gallons of water on earth, only a very small percentage is freshwater and even less is available for human use. Effectively, about 0.01% of all of this water is usable, and this amount is unevenly distributed. Almost 800,000 people in low- and middle-income countries (LMICs) lack access to safe water for drinking, personal hygiene, and domestic use, and an estimated 2.4 billion people lack access to adequate sanitation facilities. Lack of access to clean drinking water contributes to hundreds of millions of cases of water-related disease and about 1.5 million deaths annually.

Access to adequate amounts of clean water is not a significant problem in the United States; however, water shortages impacting ecological and human health do occur, for example, during prolonged droughts and exceptional contamination events, such as hurricanes and major floods. But even in these cases, advanced technology and infrastructure, including bottling and movement of water through pipes and aqueducts, facilitates transport over great distances from areas of abundance to areas of need.

The average person needs to consume a minimum of 5 liters (1.3 gallons) of water a day to survive in a moderate climate at an average activity level. The minimum amount of water needed for drinking, cooking, bathing, and sanitation is between 50 and 100 liters (13 to 26 gallons) a day. However, rates of water use among people in different countries are markedly different. For example, the average person in Somalia uses about 10 liters (2.6 gallons) of water a day, while the average person in the United States uses approximately 500 liters (132 gallons) of water a day for drinking, cooking, bathing, and watering domestic property. Similarly, each individual in North America has, on average, access to over 6,000 cubic meters of stored water (in reservoirs), while each individual in the poorest countries in Africa has, on average, access to less than 700 cubic meters and each person in Ethiopia has, on average, access to less than 50 cubic meters of stored water.[1,2]

Seven hundred million people in 43 countries face *water scarcity* (less than 1,000 cubic meters of water available per person annually). By 2025, an estimated 1.8 billion people will live in countries that face *absolute water scarcity* (less than 500 cubic meters of water per person annually), while two-thirds of the world's population will

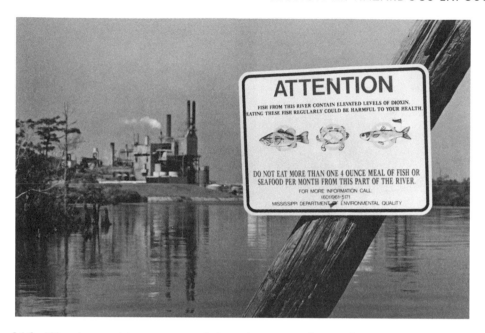

Figure 16-1. Although non-point sources account for increasing amounts of water pollution in the United States, stationary point sources still account for a substantial amount of water pollution, such as with dioxin, a by-product of the manufacture of bleached white paper at this Mississippi plant. (Photograph by Earl Dotter.)

live in countries experiencing *water stress* (less than 1,700 cubic meters of water per person annually).[2]

Water scarcity will not affect all countries and regions in the same way. For example, population increases and growing demands are projected to push many countries into water scarcity. By 2030, up to 700 million people will be displaced by water scarcity, and up to 250 million Africans will live in water-stressed countries, mainly in North Africa and sub-Saharan Africa.

The greatest drinking-water hazard globally is microbial contamination. Access to safe (uncontaminated) water—treated or untreated—is unevenly distributed throughout the world. Over 600 million people lack access to improved water sources, and more than 2 billion lack sanitation facilities. As a result, 1.7 billion people suffer from diarrheal disease each year, resulting in about 750,000 deaths of children under age 5. The vast majority of these people live in LMICs.

Adequate water treatment in many countries has reduced pathogen concentrations to levels that pose little threat to public health. However, pathogen contamination of water supplies has not been eliminated, in part because of pathogens that are resistant to conventional treatment, such as Cryptosporidium species. Chemical contaminants in surface water and groundwater, from natural sources and human activities, also pose a threat to human health (Figure 16-1). The nature and sources of chemical contamination may be similar or differ greatly among high-income countries and LMICs.

The global disparities in access to clean freshwater are readily apparent. The adverse effects of these disparities on individual and community health as well as on ecosystems are becoming better understood. This chapter, which addresses water quality and its effects on health, provides overviews of (a) pathogen and chemical contamination of surface water and groundwater, (b) contaminant sources, (c) effects of exposure to contaminants on human health, (d) approaches to treatment of sanitary waste and drinking water (Boxes 16-1 and 16-2), and (e) regulatory and nonregulatory approaches to address contamination of surface water, groundwater, and drinking water.

Box 16-1. Generalized Steps in the Treatment of Sanitary Waste Prior to Its Discharge to Surface Waters

Screening

Screening involves removal of items, such as wood, rocks, and dead animals, prior to wastewater entering the treatment plant. Most of these materials are sent to a landfill.

Pumping

Gravity moves sewage from homes and businesses to the treatment plant. If the plant is built above the ground level, wastewater must be pumped up to the aeration tanks, where gravity moves wastewater through the treatment process.

Aeration

Aeration causes some dissolved gases that cause taste and odor problems, such as hydrogen sulfide, to be released from the water. Wastewater then enters a series of long, parallel concrete tanks. Each tank is divided into two sections. In the first section, air is pumped through the water. As organic matter decays, it uses up oxygen. Aeration replenishes oxygen. Bubbling oxygen through the water also keeps the organic material suspended while it forces grit (coffee grounds, sand, and other small dense particles) to settle out. Grit is pumped out of the tanks and taken to landfills.

Sludge Removal

Wastewater then enters the second section or sedimentation tanks. The sludge, the organic portion of the sewage, settles out of the wastewater and is pumped out of the tanks.

Some of the water is removed in a step called thickening. The sludge is processed in large tanks called digesters.

Scum Removal

As sludge is settling to the bottom of the sedimentation tanks, lighter materials, termed scum, float to the surface. This scum includes grease, oils, plastics, and soap. Slow-moving rakes skim the scum off the surface of the wastewater. Scum is thickened and pumped to the digesters along with the sludge. After solids are removed, the liquid sewage is filtered through a substance, usually sand, by the action of gravity. This method removes almost all bacteria, reduces turbidity and color as well as odors, reduces the amount of iron, and removes most other solid particles from the water. Water is sometimes filtered through carbon particles to remove organic particles.

Disinfection

Finally, the wastewater flows into a tank where chlorine is added to kill bacteria. The chlorine is mostly eliminated as the bacteria are destroyed, but sometimes it is neutralized by adding other chemicals. This protects fish and other aquatic organisms as the treated waste is discharged to surface waters. The treated water, called effluent, is then discharged to a local river, lake, or the ocean.

Residuals

Treating wastewater includes dealing with the solid-waste material. Solids are kept for 20 to 30 days in large, heated enclosed tanks, called digesters, where bacteria break down (digest) the material, reducing its volume and odors, and remove organisms that can cause disease. The finished product is sent to landfills or is sometimes used as fertilizer.

Source: http://ga.water.usgs.gov/edu/wwvisit.html.

Box 16-2. General Steps in the Treatment of Drinking Water

Aeration

Water is mixed to liberate dissolved gases and to suspend particles in the water column.

Flocculation

Materials and particles present in drinking water (clay, organic material, metals, and microorganisms) are often quite small and will not settle out from the water column without assistance. To help the settling process, "coagulating" compounds are added to the water. Suspended particles stick to these compounds and create large and heavy clumps of material.

Sedimentation

Water is left undisturbed to allow the heavy clumps of particles and coagulants to settle out.

Filtration

Water is run through a series of filters that trap and remove particles still remaining in the water column. Typically, beds of sand or charcoal are used to accomplish this task.

Disinfection

Water, now largely free of particles and microorganisms, is treated to destroy any remaining disease-causing pathogens, commonly done with chlorination (the same process used to eliminate pathogens in swimming pools), ozone, or ultraviolet radiation. Water is now safe to drink and is sent to pumping stations for distribution.

CONTAMINANTS OF SURFACE WATER AND GROUNDWATER

Contaminants of surface water and groundwater include discharges of pathogens and chemicals from industrial and wastewater-treatment plants; runoff of pesticides, fertilizers, and pathogens from farms; household use of cleaners, pharmaceuticals, and pesticides; leaking septic systems; and stormwater runoff. Human exposure to water contaminants occurs from (a) direct exposure through ingestion of water, dermal absorption, and inhalation, and (b) ingestion of aquatic organisms that have accumulated contaminants.

Pathogens

There is a long history of human morbidity and mortality due to pathogens in drinking water. In 1854, John Snow identified contaminated drinking water as the source of a cholera epidemic that killed more than 600 people in London. Subsequently, water treatment, primarily with chlorine, became widespread and reduced pathogen-associated diseases. However, many LMICs continue to have inadequate water treatment and significant waterborne illness as a result.

Pathogen-associated disease has re-emerged as an important public health threat in many countries with advanced water treatment, partially due to runoff from agricultural areas, the inadequacy of water treatment to kill chlorine-resistant pathogens, and increased frequency of downpours associated with climate change that can lead to sewage contamination of drinking water. (See Chapter 29.) At least half of waterborne disease outbreaks in the United States between 1948 and 1994 coincided with extreme precipitation.[3] For example, in Milwaukee in 1993, a waterborne disease outbreak, attributed to heavy rainfall, washed pathogens and other contaminants into Lake Michigan. More than 400,000 cases of the gastrointestinal illness and 54 deaths resulted from contamination of drinking water by Cryptosporidium that was resistant to water chlorination. As a result, water treatment facilities in Milwaukee and other cities have now added specialized filtration systems to reduce risks from Cryptosporidium and similar pathogens.

Bioterrorism

Bioterrorists could contaminate drinking water with pathogens or biotoxins, although the likelihood appears to be extremely low.[4] Concern has focused on (a) *Clostridium perfringens* (which causes acute gastroenteritis), *Bacillus anthracis* (which causes anthrax), *and Yersinia pestis* (which causes plague) and (b) biotoxins, such as botulinum, aflatoxin, and ricin. These pathogens are potentially resistant to disinfection by chlorination, and these biotoxins are stable for relatively long periods in water.[5] Because of the risk of bioterrorist contamination of water supplies, security at water treatment plants and sources of potable water has been increased. Rapid detection methods, such as with DNA microchip arrays, immunologic techniques, micro-robots, optical technologies, flow cytometry, and molecular probes, are also under development.

Contamination at Swimming Beaches

Ingestion of pathogen-contaminated water while swimming has also become a public health concern. Swimming beaches in the United States are visited by more than one-third of U.S. residents. Approximately 3.5 million people are sickened each year because of contact with water polluted by sewage at swimming beaches.[7] Contamination of water at swimming beaches can cause ear, nose, and throat infections (such as swimmer's ear, or otitis externa), respiratory infections, and diarrheal diseases. Some of these disorders may be life-threatening to young children, older people, and individuals with compromised immune systems.

During 2012, U.S. beaches had more than 20,000 closing and advisory days, more than 80% because testing found bacteria levels above public health standards; the primary known cause was massive stormwater runoff and sewage.[6] In 2013, 10% of all monitoring samples from coastal U.S. beaches exceeded Environmental Protection Agency (EPA) Beach Action Values, which are considered to be precautionary benchmarks for making swimming safety decisions.[7] Public health or natural resources agencies monitor water quality at swimming beaches. Monitoring focuses on *Escherichia coli* or fecal coliforms and also includes pH, nutrients, and temperature. Although the strain of *E. coli* commonly found in fecal-contaminated water and fecal coliforms do not cause human disease, they are used as indicators of human pathogens, such as Giardia and Cryptosporidium species.

Chemical Contaminants

Lead

Lead occurs naturally in the earth's crust and is used in a variety of industrial applications. In the past, airborne lead from its use in gasoline contaminated surface waters, although at very low levels that have not likely resulted in significant human exposure. (However, airborne lead from its use in gasoline caused soil contamination, which continues to be a public health concern.)

Because of its malleability and corrosion resistance, elemental lead has been used in water supply pipes since Roman times. (The word *plumbing* comes from the Latin for "lead.") In older cities, public water supply pipes may still contain lead, although more than 99% of all public drinking water systems have lead concentrations of less than 0.005 ppm. However, lead concentrations in the water of homes and other buildings may be significantly higher and may pose a threat to human health. Homes built before 1986 are more likely to have lead pipes, joints, and solder, although new homes are also at risk. Even pipes that are considered "lead-free" may contain up to 8% lead and can leave significant amounts of lead in the water for the first several months after their installation.

The acidity of drinking water plays an important role in the availability of lead, with higher concentrations occurring in waters that are acidic. Acidic water (water with pH below 6.0) corrodes leaded pipes and solder and results in leaching of lead into the water distribution system. When water is acidic and remains in contact with the pipe for hours, the lead concentration in the first draw may be considerable. Changes in water supply or treatment have resulted in widespread contamination leading to increased blood lead levels in children in Flint, Michigan, and in Washington, DC, impacting low-income and minority residents the most. (See Box 16-3.) Since the situation in Flint was discovered, there has been increased testing of lead concentrations in drinking water throughout the United States,

with a focus on measuring lead concentrations in drinking water consumed by children.

The EPA's maximum contaminant level goal for lead in drinking water is zero. However, the EPA has not developed a reference dose or maximum contaminant level (MCL) for lead in water because health effects occur at very low levels and likely lack a threshold. The EPA requires drinking water systems to install or improve corrosion control to minimize lead levels at the tap, install treatment to reduce lead in source water entering the distribution system, and replace lead service lines when more than 10% of targeted tap samples exceed lead concentrations of 15 µg/L. Drinking water systems are also required to conduct public education programs if levels remain above 15 µg/L after reduction actions are taken. Where lead contamination occurs as a result of plumbing, removal of the existing plumbing and installation of lead-free plumbing and fixtures should prevent further exposure. When this is not practical, running water for 30 seconds before drinking or cooking may reduce the lead concentration, especially when water has not been used for a prolonged period. (See Chapters 11, 23, 24, 26, 28, and 30 for further discussion of lead.)

Arsenic

Arsenic, an element that occurs naturally in soil and rock, is released to the environment via leaching to water and from anthropogenic sources, including ore-smelting operations. The average concentration of arsenic in surface water and groundwater is about 1 ppb, although much higher concentrations can occur locally.

Arsenic in water can be lethal at concentrations of 50 to 60 ppm. At concentrations as low as 300 ppb, arsenic can cause nausea, vomiting, and diarrhea. Chronic exposure to lower levels of arsenic can cause skin changes, including darkening and small corns or warts. The International Agency for Research on Cancer, the EPA, and the National Toxicology Program have classified arsenic as a known human carcinogen. The EPA has set an MCL for arsenic in drinking water (10 ppb, or 10 µg/L).

Arsenic has been found in groundwater throughout the United States (Figure 16-2), in some cases at concentrations greater than the

Box 16-3. Lead in Drinking Water

Two incidents have highlighted the continuing challenges of ensuring safe drinking water for everyone in the United States. Lead contamination of drinking water in Washington, DC, and in Flint, Michigan, suggests that initiatives to improve water treatment and protect human health may have unintended consequences.

In 2002, elevated lead levels were discovered in water supplied to more than 6,000 homes in Washington, DC. Chlorination of the city's water to kill pathogens, as required by the Safe Drinking Water Act (SDWA), created carcinogenic disinfection by-products. To reduce disinfection by-products as required under the SDWA, corrosive chloramines were added to the city's water, mobilizing lead in its aging pipes and resulting in lead concentrations in the drinking water of some homes 20 times greater than the EPA-recommended level. The District of Columbia replaced approximately 11,000 public service pipes and encouraged homeowners to replace private portions of water pipes containing lead. However, replacement of public feeder or service lines has slowed recently because the process appeared to disturb lead in pipes on private land. The city government has informed the public about the lead hazard, provided recommendations to reduce lead exposure, and continues to provide lead testing kits to individuals. In addition, the city has optimized corrosion control by adding orthophosphate, a corrosion inhibitor, during water treatment. These measures have helped reduce lead levels in tap water. The District of Columbia Water and Sewer Authority claims that its water is safe to drink; as of 2015, the lead concentration of water leaving the treatment plant was less than 4 µg/L. However, lead-based pipes and solder continue to be problems in private residences and buildings.

In April 2014, the city of Flint, Michigan, temporarily switched its water supply from Lake Huron to the Flint River in an attempt to save money while a new pipeline to Lake Huron was built. The water from this new source, which was treated at Flint water facilities, was significantly more corrosive than the previously used water from Lake Huron, which had been treated by the Detroit Water and Sewage Department. Along with other factors, including high chloride levels, Flint's water was not treated with corrosion inhibitors, which increased the deterioration and leaching of lead from the old network of lead-containing pipes. In September 2014, Virginia Tech University sampled water from 252 homes in Flint. It found that 101 homes had first-draw lead levels of 5 ppb (5 µg/L) or higher; the 90th percentile lead concentration was 25 ppb, well above the EPA action level of 15 ppb. Some levels exceeded 100 ppb, and one exceeded 1,000 ppb, even after flushing.

A study conducted by Mona Hanna-Attisha, a pediatrician, found that the number of Flint children under age 5 with elevated blood lead levels increased from 2.4% to 4.9% after the change of water source.[1] The number of children with elevated blood lead levels in the areas with the highest lead concentrations in water had increased from 4.0% to 10.6%. In October 2015, Flint switched its water source back to Lake Huron;. however, many children may have suffered irreversible brain damage from lead exposure.

Reference

1. Hanna-Attisha M, LaChance J, Sadler RC, Schnepp AC. Elevated blood lead levels in children associated with the flint drinking water crisis: A spatial analysis of risk and public health response. American Journal of Public Health 2016; 106: 283–290.

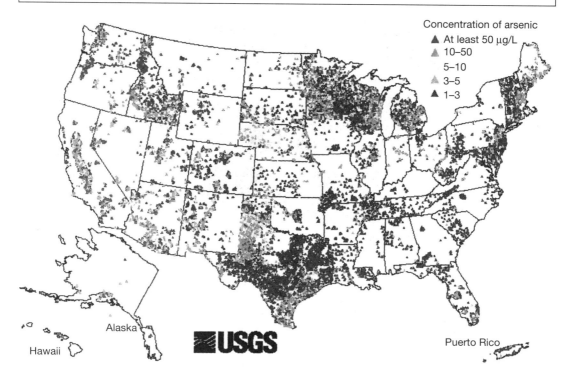

Concentration of arsenic
▲ At least 50 µg/L
▲ 10–50
  5–10
▲ 3–5
▲ 1–3

Alaska
Hawaii
Puerto Rico

Figure 16-2. Arsenic concentrations in groundwater in the United States. (Source: Ryker SJ. Mapping arsenic in groundwater. Geotimes 2001; 46: 34–36. © 2001 American Geological Institute and reprinted with their permission.)

MCL. Rice grown in the United States has also been contaminated with arsenic, resulting in elevated concentrations of arsenic in baby food. As a result, the Food and Drug Administration (FDA) has proposed a tolerance level for arsenic in baby food of 100 μg/L (100 ppb). While there is some concern about the health risks of exposure to arsenic in the United States, the health risks associated with these concentrations pales in comparison to the disaster that has occurred in Bangladesh and in West Bengal, India, where millions of people drank groundwater heavily contaminated with arsenic.

Bangladesh and West Bengal have had some of the highest global rates of waterborne infectious disease, including shigellosis, typhoid, cholera, and hepatitis A. To address this problem, well water has been heavily promoted and developed as a safe alternative to untreated surface water, and the public has been instructed to rely on groundwater as its primary source of drinking water. As a result, the incidence of waterborne infectious disease has declined dramatically. However, in the 1980s, arsenic contamination was found in groundwater, and, during the mid-1990s, the public became well aware of this problem. More than 30 million people in Bangladesh and West Bengal may be exposed to arsenic concentrations in drinking water greater than 50 μg/L (Figure 16-3).

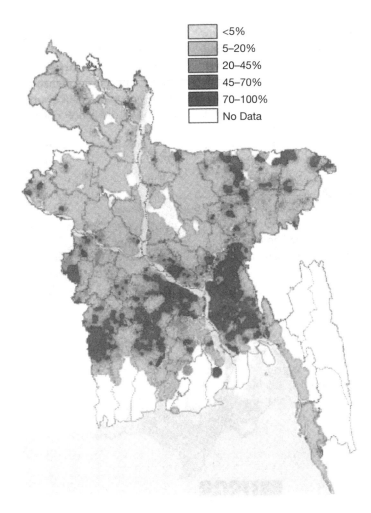

Figure 16-3. Probability of groundwater concentration in Bangladesh exceeding 50 ppb (50 μg/L). (Source: McArthur JM, Ravenscroft P, Safiullah S, Thirlwall F. Arsenic in groundwater: Testing pollution mechanisms for sedimentary aquifers in Bangladesh. Water Resources Research 2001; 37: 109–117. Reprinted with permission.)

Drinking arsenic-contaminated water in Bangladesh has likely caused more than 100,000 cases of skin disorders. Skin and internal cancers caused by arsenic exposure have become major health issues in the region with considerable associated social and economic hardship. Preventive measures have been implemented, including extensive water-quality testing and on-site mitigation, through use of deep arsenic-free wells, rainwater harvesting, installation of treatment plants, home treatment, and extensive training and education. However, these programs have been relatively ineffective in reducing arsenic exposure and the risk of associated disease.[8] As of 2013, 12% of people were still drinking and cooking with arsenic-contaminated water (arsenic concentrations greater than 50 μg/L), and 25% of people were drinking water that did not meet the WHO arsenic guideline (10 μg/L).[8,9]

Atrazine

Atrazine, a triazine pesticide, has been used for over 35 years and is applied in the United States to corn, sorghum, sugar cane, macadamia nuts, and conifer trees. In the United States, approximately 71 million pounds of this restricted-use pesticide are applied annually to 70 million acres, with 88% of atrazine use occurring on corn.

The use of atrazine results in runoff, leaching, and volatilization from agricultural soils and transport to surface water, groundwater, and the atmosphere. The EPA estimates that atrazine is present in over 1,500 community water supplies and over 70,000 rural domestic wells nationwide. Atrazine has been detected in drinking water in over 40% of municipal wells tested in Midwestern states and in over 31% of drinking water wells tested in Maine. Atrazine concentrations in finished drinking water monitored from 2005 to 2008 ranged from 0.1 to 6.7 ug/L. Atrazine has also been found in more than 98% of samples collected from Midwestern streams, rivers, and lakes after it was used on crops. Surface water concentrations of atrazine ranged from 0.3 to 9.1 ug/L in monitoring conducted in 2007 and 2008, while maximum concentrations of atrazine in Great Lakes tributaries monitored between 2010 and 2013 were 1.1 ug/L in urban areas and 0.5 ug/L in nonurban areas.[10] Atrazine has also been the most commonly detected pesticide in southern Florida canals.

As would be expected of a broad-spectrum herbicide, atrazine is toxic to primary producers (plants and algae) in surface waters. Chronic, lower-level atrazine exposure causes changes in species composition of aquatic plant and algal communities and the productivity of these systems. In turn, the feeding behavior and efficiency of organisms that consume plants and algae are affected, resulting in changes in species composition and abundance at higher levels in the food chain.

Atrazine has relatively low mammalian acute toxicity (its median lethal dose in rats is greater than 1,000 ppm). However, because of its widespread use and its occurrence in surface water and groundwater, concern has arisen over adverse effects in humans and on aquatic or semiaquatic organisms associated with chronic, low-level exposures. Atrazine may cause cancer in humans and affect human reproduction and development via disruption of the endocrine system. Atrazine also causes developmental and reproductive toxicity in laboratory animals and in naturally occurring amphibians.

Because of the widespread use of atrazine, its occurrence in groundwater and surface water systems, and concern with its potential to cause cancer, endocrine disruption, and reproductive and developmental effects in human and nonhuman organisms as well as significant ecological effects, the European Union banned its use in 2003. While there have been efforts to further restrict or ban the use of atrazine in the United States, it continues to be applied as a restricted-use pesticide. However, in 2016, the EPA completed a reassessment of the ecological risks of atrazine and concluded that the substance poses significant health risks to birds, mammals, fish, amphibians, and terrestrial and aquatic plants. As a result, the EPA may further restrict or discontinue some uses of atrazine. Also in 2016, the state of California listed atrazine as a reproductive toxicant under its Proposition 65 program.

Mercury

Mercury is an important contaminant of many surface water systems; it accumulates in fish and other aquatic organisms that feed high in the food chain. People consuming mercury-contaminated aquatic organisms (primarily fish)—the most important, nonoccupational

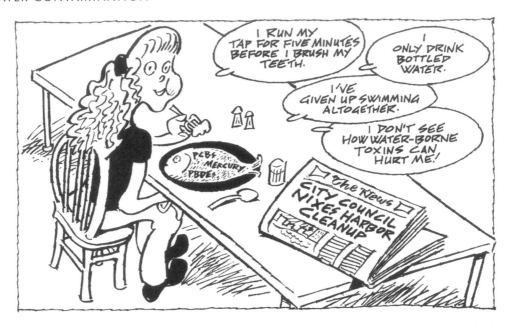

Figure 16-4. Contamination of fish with mercury or other hazardous substances is a concern. (Drawing by Nick Thorkelson.)

source of human exposure to mercury—may be exposed to concentrations that pose threats to health (Figure 16-4).

Mercury is a naturally occurring element that is found in the earth's crust. It occurs in surface waters as a result of direct solubilization and from direct and indirect industrial discharges. Discharges from chloralkali plants, leaking landfills, incineration of mercury-containing products, and combustion of coal are important sources of mercury contamination of surface water. While some of these discharges are direct and result in local contamination, incineration of mercury-containing products, such as in medical waste, and combustion of coal used for electrical generation discharge mercury to the atmosphere, where it is transported long distances and deposited in lakes. Nearly 80% of anthropogenic emissions of mercury to the air come from fossil-fuel combustion, mining and smelting, and incineration of waste.

Inorganic mercury that enters lakes is relatively insoluble; however, it is readily transformed by bacteria to its organic form (methylmercury), which accumulates in the tissues of aquatic organisms, including fish. Because biomagnification (accumulation and concentration up the food chain) is the predominant mechanism of accumulation in aquatic ecosystems, mercury concentrations are highest

in fish that feed at the top of the food chain, such as pike, shark, tuna, and swordfish. Mercury concentrations in these fish may be biomagnified as much as 100,000 times over concentrations in surface water. The concentration of mercury in aquatic food chains is influenced by pH, with more accumulation occurring in water with lower pH. Acid precipitation, which results from the discharge of sulfates and nitrates from combustion of fossil fuels, may therefore play an important role in mercury accumulation in organisms in acidified lakes.

At high concentrations, mercury can damage the brain, kidneys, and other organs. Chronic prenatal exposure to lower concentrations of methylmercury and exposure of infants via breast milk cause developmental disorders, such as delayed onset of walking, and abnormalities of language, attention, and memory.

While a contaminant of many foods, most adult intake of mercury is from seafood. Concentrations of mercury in shark, swordfish, tile fish, mackerel, and albacore tuna occur at levels that have triggered warnings to women of childbearing age, pregnant women, nursing mothers, and young children to avoid consumption of these fish.[11] Similarly, 30 state natural resource and health agencies in the United States have advised these same individuals to reduce or avoid consumption of fish, including perch, northern and walleye pike, muskie, and other species caught recreationally.[12]

Polychlorinated Biphenyls

Polychlorinated biphenyls (PCBs) are representative of a class of nonpolar, chlorinated organic compounds that include DDT, chlorinated dioxins, toxaphene, and many others. Polychlorinated biphenyls and other compounds in this class are relatively insoluble in water, persistent in some environmental compartments (such as sediments), and accumulate to a high degree in animals and plants. While they are present in water at extremely low concentrations, they occur at very high concentrations in aquatic organisms, such as fish, posing health risks to people who consume them.

Polychlorinated biphenyls were manufactured and sold in the United States from 1929 to 1977, when the EPA banned their manufacture. During this period, over 1 billion pounds were produced. Despite a ban on their manufacture, PCBs continue to be encountered in various products and applications, including transformers and capacitors, heat-transfer fluids, flame retardants, and pigmented products, printed papers, plastics, and paints as well as in wastewater from recycling these products.[13] They have also been found in over 500 hazardous waste sites in the United States.

Polychlorinated biphenyls concentrate in the fatty tissues of aquatic organisms, including fish. Bioconcentration and biomagnification of PCBs in upper levels of the food chain can lead to concentrations in the tissues of predatory fish that are over 1 million times greater than concentrations in surrounding water. As a result, fish are the most significant source of PCB exposure to humans and other fish-eating animals.

Polychlorinated biphenyls are classified by the International Agency for Research on Cancer as *Carcinogenic to Humans* (Group 1) and as probable human carcinogens by EPA. The hepatotoxic effects of PCBs include induction of microsomal enzymes, liver enlargement, increased serum levels of liver-related enzymes and lipids, altered porphyrin and vitamin A metabolism, and histopathologic alterations that progress to noncancerous lesions and tumors. Polychlorinated biphenyls also cause adverse dermal effects (chloracne), ocular effects (Meibomian gland hypersecretion and abnormal conjunctival pigmentation), and immunological effects (including increased susceptibility to respiratory tract infections, increased prevalence of ear infections in infants, decreased antibody levels, and changes in T lymphocytes). Exposure to PCBs has also been associated with adverse effects on sperm morphology and production as well as menstrual disorders. Anthropometric effects, including reductions in head circumference and birthweight, and neurobehavioral abnormalities, including decreased neuromuscular maturity, abnormal reflexes, reduced psychomotor scores, impairment of short-term memory, decreases in visual recognition, and reduced activity levels, have been observed in children exposed to PCBs in utero. Some of these effects have persisted into later childhood.

As a result of high PCB concentrations in the tissues of many fish species, warnings have been issued to reduce consumption of the most contaminated species, including salmon, trout, and walleye caught by recreational anglers in the Great Lakes and from other inland water bodies. Concern has also been raised regarding PCB contamination in farm-raised Atlantic salmon.[14]

Polybrominated Diphenyl Ethers

Polybrominated diphenyl ethers (PBDEs) comprise a relatively new class of compounds used as flame retardants in many commercial and household products. The use of PBDEs has increased dramatically in recent years, with annual sales reaching more than 70,000 metric tons.[15] PBDEs are released to, and accumulate in, soils, surface waters, and aquatic organisms from manufacturing, widespread use, disposal in and leaching from landfills, and incineration.

Polybrominated diphenyl ethers are relatively insoluble in water but highly lipophilic; thus, they bioaccumulate in fish and other aquatic organisms as well as terrestrial species, including humans, that consume aquatic organisms. Concentrations of PBDEs in fish are highly variable depending on the type of fish and its location. For instance, PBDE concentrations in fish from Europe are about one-tenth those in fish from North America, likely due to the proximity of fish feeding areas to PBDE sources.[15] Regional distribution of PBDEs may also be associated with Europe's more aggressive approach of banning PBDE manufacture and use.

Polybrominated diphenyl ethers are present in human blood, milk, and fatty tissues. Concentrations in people have increased 100-fold over the past 30 years, with a doubling time of about 5 years, and concentrations in North Americans are significantly higher than concentrations in Europeans.[15]

Some PBDE congeners are metabolically active and induce hepatic cytochrome P450 IIB1 and IA1. They also have weak or moderate binding affinity to the Ah receptor; PBDEs disrupt spontaneous behavior, impair learning and memory, and induce other neurotoxic effects in adult mice exposed neonatally. Polybrominated diphenyl ethers are endocrine disruptors, altering thyroid hormone homeostasis and causing a dose-dependent depletion of thyroxine. They are agonists of estrogen receptors (both ERα and ERβ), an effect that may be enhanced by in vivo metabolism. Polybrominated diphenyl ethers have not been demonstrated to be carcinogenic in rodent bioassays, although some concern for PBDE carcinogenesis continues to be raised. If humans are as sensitive as experimental animals to the adverse effects of PBDEs, current concentrations in humans may leave little or no margin of safety—arguing for close evaluation of the management of PBDEs and potentially aggressive regulation.

Disinfection By-products

Disinfection by-products (DBPs) are created by the interaction of organic matter in source waters with chlorine and other water disinfectants. Disinfection by-products include trihalomethanes, such as chloroform; haloacetic acids, such as trichloroacetic acid; bromate, which is formed when ozone is used for water disinfection; and chlorite, formed when chlorine dioxide is used for disinfection. The health effects of exposure to these substances include carcinogenicity (primarily bladder, colon, and rectal cancer) and reproductive and developmental effects, including spontaneous abortions, stillbirths, neural tube defects, preterm births, intrauterine growth retardation, and low birthweight.

Disinfection by-products are formed by treatment of drinking water. Without treatment, the occurrence of pathogens that cause cholera,

typhoid, cryptosporidiosis, and other diseases would increase with commensurate threats to public health. To address the DBP problem, the EPA issued the Stage 1 Disinfectants and Disinfection Byproducts Rule in 1998, which requires drinking-water treatment plants to attain certain levels of disinfection and, at the same time, reduce DBPs to specified levels prior to distributing water. The rule also sets goals for the complete removal of some DBPs, although deadlines to achieve these goals were not specified. Treatment plants that use surface waters with high concentrations of organic materials were also required to reduce the concentrations of these materials to specified levels prior to treatment to decrease or avoid the formation of DBPs. The EPA issued the Stage 2 Disinfectants and Disinfection Byproducts rule in 2006. The Stage 2 rule refines the Stage 1 rule and attempts to strengthen health protection for customers of systems that deliver disinfected water. The rule focuses specifically on two important DBPs: trihalomethanes and haloacetic acids.

The EPA estimates that the nationwide cost of complying with the Stage 1 rule is about $700 million, with an additional cost of about $80 million annually for compliance with the Stage 2 rule. However, the agency also indicates that the benefits of implementation of the rules, which include the prevention of cancer as well as reproductive and developmental disorders, far outweigh the costs. For example, the EPA estimates that nearly 300 cases of bladder cancer will be prevented by implementation of the Stage 2 rule, providing an annual benefit of $1.5 billion. Additional benefits, including prevention of reproductive and developmental effects, will also accrue from implementation of the Stage 2 rule, with a similar annualized cost/benefit ratio.

Pharmaceuticals and Personal Care Products

Pharmaceuticals and personal care products (PPCPs) include thousands of chemicals that are used daily in cosmetics, personal medicines, and agricultural products. Over 4,000 pharmaceutical products are currently in use, and many of these substances enter surface water and groundwater from human waste disposal (discharged from wastewater treatment plants and septic systems), improper disposal of pharmaceuticals and other personal products, and agricultural runoff. PPCPs can have a variety of adverse effects on aquatic ecosystems and on human health although the full extent of exposure to, and adverse effects of, PPCPs are unknown. Exposure to PPCPs in the environment has raised concern for endocrine disruption (disruption of compounds that alter the normal function of hormones), reproductive toxicity, developmental toxicity (some effects that may be delayed until adulthood), and other effects. Of particular concern is the buildup of antibiotic resistance of microorganisms because animals and humans are exposed unintentionally to antibiotics in food, water, and other sources.

Removal of PPCPs from wastewater is difficult and highly variable; various treatment processes have removal rates ranging from 20% to over 90%. Most conventional wastewater treatment plants utilize activated sludge as a means to break down organic compounds. The sludge is concentrated with microorganisms that use organic pollutants in wastewater for energy, thereby removing contaminants from water. Because chemical and physical properties of individual PPCPs vary greatly, each treatment process relying on activated sludge may be more or less efficient at removing individual compounds.[16]

Ozonation has been found to be more effective in removal of pharmaceuticals compared with activated sludge. However, the effectiveness of ozonation in the treatment of pharmaceuticals is also highly variable, ranging from 1% to 100%, with greater removal efficacy occurring for analgesics and anti-inflammatories such as diclofenac, naproxen, ketoprofen, mefenamic acid, and aspirin. Despite its comparative efficiency at removing some pharmaceuticals, ozonation is one of the least used treatment methods in the United States, likely due to the high costs of equipment and maintenance, which render it uncompetitive with other treatment options.[17]

The EPA has begun to consider development of numeric water quality criteria for PPCPs, which will be especially important for wastewater treatment plants that receive and discharge these compounds. Numeric water quality criteria are used to establish permit limits for wastewater treatment plants and other point source discharges, and these limits typically force the development and use of technology that removes pollutants to levels that protect water quality. Numeric criteria for PPCPs will also enhance identification and management PPCPs, especially antibiotics that derive from nonpoint sources, such as animal feedlots.

REGULATING AND MANAGING WATER QUALITY

Water quality and the adverse health effects associated with water pollution can be managed by (a) preventing pollution before it occurs, (b) treating water after pollution has occurred, and (c) implementing public health practices that reduce or eliminate human exposure when pollution prevention and treatment have not occurred or are ineffective.

Treatment-Based Approaches

The primary statutes governing the management of water quality in the United States are the Clean Water Act (CWA) and the Safe Drinking Water Act (SDWA). The Clean Water Act, adopted in 1972, emphasizes treatment of wastes before they are discharged to surface water. Treatment thresholds are guided by chemical-specific water quality criteria, which are risk-based contaminant concentrations that, if not exceeded, should prevent adverse impacts of pollutants on human health and the environment. Treatment thresholds are also based on technology guidelines that require industrial sectors to install the best available, economically achievable levels of water treatment to remove pollutants prior to their discharge to surface waters. The Clean Water Act has been remarkably successful in reducing toxic chemicals, such as PCBs, and pathogens, such as bacteria and viruses, discharged from point sources—waste pipes of industrial facilities and wastewater treatment plants. As a result, surface waters are cleaner now than before the adoption of the CWA. However, the focus of the CWA on point sources has addressed only a portion of surface water quality problems in the United States.

Non-point-source pollution, also called polluted runoff, enters lakes and streams from farms and animal feeding operations, leaking hazardous waste and sanitary landfills, septic systems, stormwater runoff that carries pollutants from city streets and sidewalks to surface waters and the atmosphere. Non-point contaminants, such as PCBs (from contaminated sediments), mercury (from atmospheric deposition), atrazine (from agricultural runoff), and many pathogens (from animal feeding operations, leaking septic systems, and runoff from urban areas) enter surface waters relatively uncontrolled by the Clean Water Act.

Before 1972, discharges of pollutants, such as PCBs from paper mills, occurred with little control and accumulated to very high concentrations in the sediments of lakes and rivers. They have persisted in sediments and are resuspended in surface waters during floods and other disturbances—an especially challenging nonpoint pollutant source. In the Great Lakes region, dozens of hotspots (areas of concern) have been identified, where sediments are highly contaminated with persistent, bioaccumulative toxicants, such as PCBs. In only a few cases are measures being implemented to cap or remove contaminated sediments, often at very significant expense. However, without cleanup, these contaminants will continue to accumulate in fish and other organisms that will be consumed by humans and wildlife.

The Safe Drinking Water Act, passed in 1974, is a treatment-based statute designed to control and reduce toxic and pathogenic compounds in drinking water, which in the United States is provided by over 155,000 public water treatment systems. The SDWA gives the EPA authority to set national, health-based standards for both naturally occurring drinking-water contaminants, such as bacteria and viruses, and contaminants of anthropogenic origin, such as lead and atrazine. Implementation of the standards occurs typically at the treatment plant, with enforcement provided either by states or the EPA. While much of the SDWA focuses on treatment to reduce contaminant concentrations at the tap, revisions in 1996 gave the EPA and the states greater authority to protect groundwater and surface water that serves as a source of drinking water. The SDWA also requires water suppliers to notify the public when there is a contamination problem in a drinking water system and treatment plants to provide annual reports to their users on the quality of their tap water.

Exposure Reduction

The Clean Water Act has been relatively effective in regulating the discharge of contaminants from point sources, and the Safe Drinking Water Act has accomplished much of its goal of ensuring that contaminants do not occur in drinking water. However, these statutes have not addressed the vast quantities of in-place pollutants (in sediments) and other non-point sources of pollutants, such as leaking hazardous waste landfills or the atmosphere. As a result, PCBs, mercury, and other bioaccumulative contaminants have become concentrated in the tissues of fish and other aquatic organisms, posing threats to human health and the environment. Regulation of contaminants in fish sold commercially, such as PCBs and mercury, occurs under the Federal Food Drug and Cosmetic Act. The FDA sets regulatory thresholds, called tolerance levels, for PCBs, mercury, and other compounds in fish. When the concentration of a contaminant in fish or other foods exceeds a tolerance level, the FDA can remove the food from commercial markets or it can issue a consumption warning as it has, in conjunction with the EPA, for mercury in shark, swordfish, tilefish, and mackerel.[18] However, many fish are caught and consumed by sport or recreational anglers, and contaminants in these fish are not regulated by the FDA.

The EPA has developed methods to manage the health risks of toxicant exposure through consumption of contaminated fish caught by sport or recreational anglers. Its risk-based method is used to develop fish consumption advisories for compounds, such as PCBs and mercury, that are commonly found in sport-caught fish. Consumption advisories are typically issued by states and warn anglers and their families to restrict or eliminate consumption of specific species and size classes, based on tissue concentrations of individual contaminants and combinations of contaminants.

The risk-based approach to consumption advisories developed by the EPA conflicts, in many cases, with the tolerance levels set by the FDA for commercially sold fish. (One important exception is mercury, for which the FDA and EPA have developed a consensus approach.) For example, a PCB concentration of 1 mg/kg (ppm) will trigger stringent "do-not-eat" consumption advice for a recreationally caught salmon in the Great Lakes, while the same salmon may be sold in commercial markets without restriction since this concentration is below the FDA tolerance level for PCBs (2 mg/kg). This issue gained significant attention in 2004 when some types of commercially sold salmon were found to have concentrations of PCBs, toxaphene, dieldrin, and other contaminants at levels that would trigger stringent EPA-based consumption advice but no action by the FDA.[10] The difference in the two approaches is attributable to the reliance of the EPA on a public health protective, risk-based approach to the development of fish consumption advisories, while the FDA incorporates considerations not based on health, such as economic benefit and analytical detection capabilities in the development of tolerance levels. FDA confirmed the 2 mg/kg tolerance level for PCBs in fish in 2016.

Source Control and Prevention

Water quality managers have recognized the limitations of end-of-pipe, treatment-based controls as a water quality management tool. This approach is not useful for many of the nonpoint sources that plague surface waters. It also becomes cost prohibitive as toxicant concentrations have been reduced to very low yet still harmful levels. As a result, prevention-based approaches for the management of water quality are being pursued that (a) address all phases of the water cycle in structuring management approaches; (b) recognize water as one part of a total environmental management plan to avoid transferring problems from one environmental medium to another; (c) acknowledge the link between land use and water quality; and (d) promote source reduction, waste minimization, water conservation, and reuse.

Source reduction and waste minimization are being promoted in industry and agriculture and in many communities. Recycling and reuse of industrial waste has reduced point sources of pollutants and, concurrently, saved money by decreasing the need to purchase raw or unused

resources. Similarly, measures in agriculture are being implemented to change crop rotation and tillage practices to reduce the need for large quantities of pesticides. Organic farming practices and produce from organic farms are increasing in popularity, with the concurrent benefit of reducing both leaching of pesticides to groundwater and runoff to surface water.

THE FUTURE OF WATER QUALITY MANAGEMENT

Hundreds of millions of people live without access to safe, clean water. Targeted approaches to point and nonpoint source controls of contaminants in the United States and other high-income countries either are not available or are irrelevant to address the water needs of people in LMICs experiencing water stress. In 2000, the United Nations set millennium development goals (MDGs) to address the needs of the world's poorest people. The goals, which were to have been met by 2015, focused on child and maternal mortality, hunger, malnutrition, education, and, pertinent to this chapter, water and sanitation. By 2015, 2.1 billion people had gained access to improved water sanitation, 147 countries met the MDG for drinking water, 95 countries met the MDG for sanitation, and 77 countries met both. However, some regions, including South Asia, Oceania, and sub-Saharan Africa, did not meet the sanitation or drinking-water MDGs. The United Nations predicts that, by 2050, 25% of all people will be affected by recurring water shortages. It is therefore likely that the new Sustainable Development Goal of ensuring, by 2030, universal access to safe and affordable drinking water for all, will not be met.

Water management is challenged by a convergence of water quality and water quantity issues. Technologies are available that can conserve enough water to reduce stress on threatened natural resources while accommodating agricultural, industrial, and residential uses.[2] By 2020, enough water could be saved by conservation during indoor residential use to meet the needs of over 5 million people, and sustainable irrigation practices could save 450,000 acre-feet of water per year, enough to satisfy the needs of another 3.6 million people. In some cases, water that is conserved is also water that does not have to be treated and discharged, eliminating the costs and adverse effects of treatment and discharge processes. However, water distribution and water quality issues will continue to impose constraints on addressing the world's water needs.

While conservation will play an important role in addressing both water quantity and quality, global management of water will be challenged by existing and new stressors. The world's growing population, which relies on the 0.01% of water globally that is usable, poses formidable challenges for water quality managers, health professionals, and government officials. The global effects of climate change also pose daunting challenges. The United Nations Intergovernmental Panel on Climate Change predicts that increases in global mean temperature due to continued accumulation of greenhouse gases may account for up to 20% of the global increase in water scarcity. Climate change–induced disruption of traditional weather and runoff patterns will increase the frequency and severity of droughts and floods, with resultant impacts on the structure and function of riparian ecosystems as well as on human health and human-made structures. Climate change also will impact stratification and mixing patterns in surface waters, altering nutrient and contaminant cycles with potentially profound effects on aquatic communities and on organisms—including humans—that rely on aquatic systems for sustenance. Potential climate change–induced emergence of new or modified pathogens may pose additional challenges to water treatment systems designed to protect people and marine and freshwater ecosystems. (See Chapter 29.)

REFERENCES

1. Gleick, PH, Ajami, N, Christian-Smith, J, et al. The world's water (Vol. 8): The biennial report on freshwater resources. Washington, DC: Island Press, 2014.

2. United Nations Department of Economic and Social Affairs. International Decade for Action "Water for Life" 2005–2015. Available at: www.un.org/waterforlifedecade/scarcity.shtml. Accessed October 20, 2016.

3. Curriero FC, Patz JA, Rose JB, Lele S. The association between extreme precipitation and waterborne disease outbreaks in the United States, 1948–1994. American Journal of Public Health 2011; 91: 1194–1199.

4. Foran JA, Brosnan T. Early warning systems for hazardous biological agents in potable water. Environmental Health Perspectives 2000; 108: 993–995.

5. Burrows WD, Renner SE. Biological warfare agents as threats to potable water. Environmental Health Perspectives 1999; 107: 975–984.

6. Wei J. NRDC annual beach report: Water pollution ruins over 20,000 days at the beach for third straight year, June 26, 2013. Available at: https://www.nrdc.org/media/2013/130626. Accessed October 19, 2016.

7. National Resources Defense Council. Testing the waters: A guide to water quality at vacation beaches (24th ed.), June 2014. Available at: https://www.nrdc.org/sites/default/files/ttw2014.pdf. Accessed October 19, 2016.

8. Smith AH, Lingas EO, Rahman M. Contamination of drinking water by arsenic in Bangladesh: A public health emergency. Bulletin of the World Health Organization 2000; 78: 1093–1103.

9. BBS/UNICEF 2015. Progotir Pathey: Bangladesh Multiple Indicator Cluster Survey 2012–2013. Dahka, Bangladesh: Bangladesh Bureau of Statistics and UNICEF.

10. Baldwin, AK, Corsi SR, DeCicco LA, et al. Organic contaminants in Great Lakes tributaries: Prevalence and potential aquatic toxicity. Science of the Total Environment 2016; 554–555: 42–52.

11. U.S. Food and Drug Administration. What you need to know about mercury in fish and shellfish, March 2004. Available at: http://www.fda.gov/food/resourcesforyou/consumers/ucm110591.htm. Accessed October 20, 2016.

12. U. S. Environmental Protection Agency. Fish advisories and health. 2016 Available at: http://www.epa.gov/waterscience/fish. Accessed October 20, 2016.

13. Gorsman E. Nonlegacy PCBs: Pigment manufacturing by-products get a second look. Environmental Health Perspectives 2013; 121: A87–A93.

14. Hites RA, Foran JA, Carpenter DO, et al. Global assessment of organic contaminants in farmed salmon. Science 2004; 303: 226–229.

15. Hites RA. Polybrominated diphenyl ethers in the environment and in people: a meta-analysis of concentrations. Environmental Science and Technology 2004; 38: 945–956.

16. Radjenović J, Petrović M, Barceló D. Fate and distribution of pharmaceuticals in wastewater and sewage sludge of the conventional activated sludge (CAS) and advanced membrane bioreactor (MBR) treatment. Water Research 2009; 43: 831–841.

17. Ziylan A, Ince NH. The occurrence and fate of anti-inflammatory and analgesic pharmaceuticals in sewage and fresh water: Treatability by conventional and non-conventional processes. Journal of Hazardous Materials 2011; 187: 24–36.

18. U.S. Environmental Protection Agency. EPA-FDA advisory on mercury in fish and shellfish, 2014. Available at: www.epa.gov/fish-tech/ epa-fda-advisory-mercury-fish-and-shellfish. Accessed October 20, 2016.

FURTHER READING

Adler RW, Landman JC, Cameron DM. The Clean Water Act, 20 years later. Washington, DC: Island Press, 1993.
A review of the Clean Water Act: its successes and failures.

Agency for Toxic Substances and Disease Registry. Toxicological profiles. U.S. Dept. of Health and Human Services, Public Health Service. Available at: http://www.atsdr.cdc.gov/toxfaq.html.
These profiles provide comprehensive reviews of the toxicology and health effects of contaminants discussed in this chapter and many others.

Foran, JA. Regulating toxic substances in surface water. Boca Raton, FL: Lewis Publishers/CRC Press, 1993.
An overview of approaches and mechanisms for management of toxic substances in surface waters.

National Resources Defense Council. Testing the waters: A guide to water quality at vacation beaches (24th ed.), June 2014. Available at: https:// www.nrdc.org/sites/default/files/ttw2014.pdf.
A report on the extent, frequency, and causes of beach closings in the United States.

Water Quality 2000. A national water agenda for the 21st century. Phase III report. Washington, DC: Water Environment Federation, 1992.
A forward-looking document intended to guide water management decisions in the 21st century.

West Bengal and Bangladesh Arsenic Crisis Information Center. Available at: http://bicn. com/acic/
Provides information on arsenic contamination in drinking water.

World Bank Arsenic Mitigation Project. Available at: http://web.worldbank.org/external/projects/ main?pagePK=104231&piPK=73230&theSitePK =40941&menuPK−228424&Projectid=P050745
A summary of World Bank efforts to address arsenic contamination of drinking water in Bangladesh.

World Health Organization: Water, sanitation, and health. Available at: http://www.who.int/water_ sanitation_health/en/
A general overview of global water, sanitation, and health issues.

17

Food Safety

Craig W. Hedberg

Foodborne illnesses occur as the result of dynamic interactions among agents, hosts, and the environments in which these interactions occur (Figure 17-1). This is a fundamental concept that can help us understand the nature of threats to food safety and to develop strategies to prevent the transmission of foodborne illness.

For example, *Escherichia coli* O157:H7 are enteric bacteria that are carried by cattle. During slaughter, the surfaces of carcasses may be contaminated. Carcass trimmings may be ground, which spreads contamination throughout large batches of ground beef. Because *E. coli* O157:H7 can cause bloody diarrhea in people of all ages and a life-threatening complication of the kidneys in young children and older people, the presence of *E. coli* O157:H7 in ground beef is an important public health problem. However, if a hamburger made from contaminated ground beef is thoroughly cooked, the bacteria will be destroyed, and no transmission will occur.

Similarly, a salad maker in a restaurant who is infected with hepatitis A virus (HAV) and has poor personal hygiene and handwashing practices may contaminate salads served to the restaurant's patrons. However, if the restaurant's patrons have been vaccinated against HAV, they would no longer be susceptible to infection, and no transmission of illness would occur.

These two examples highlight the interactions among agents, hosts, and environment that lead to disease transmission or, alternatively, can be altered to prevent transmission. For each of these diseases, a much broader range of environmental, technical, and policy interventions are used, and could be used, to prevent transmission, as described later in this chapter.

Food safety can be viewed in terms of a specific food product or an entire food system. For a specific food product, this requires a systematic approach that accomplishes the following:[1]

- Describes the food and its production, distribution, and intended use
- Identifies hazards that can cause illnesses associated with the food and evaluates the need for measures to prevent or minimize the likelihood of foodborne illness
- Establishes preventive measures, as appropriate, to ensure the safety of the food
- Monitors the implementation of the preventive measures
- Initiates corrective actions, when appropriate.

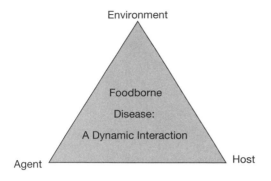

Figure 17-1. This triangle demonstrates the dynamic interactions between agent, host, and environment that result in the occurrence of foodborne disease.

All of these functions have corresponding functions that can be described for an entire food system. Food safety represents the combined use of all of these tools to detect, prevent, and abate foodborne illness hazards in the food supply. Because these hazards are the result of dynamic interactions, food safety is a constantly moving target that depends on a strong system of public health surveillance to (a) detect new and emerging food safety hazards and (b) provide feedback on the efficacy of control strategies.

PUBLIC HEALTH SURVEILLANCE FOR FOODBORNE DISEASES: THE KEY TO HAZARD IDENTIFICATION

Public health surveillance is the ongoing, systematic collection, analysis, interpretation, and dissemination of data regarding a health event for use in public health action to reduce morbidity and mortality and to improve health (Chapter 6).[2] Historically, foodborne disease surveillance has been conducted to accomplish the following:[3]

- Control and prevent outbreaks
- Determine the causes of foodborne disease
- Monitor trends in occurrence of foodborne disease.

Accomplishing these tasks requires the coordination of three separate but related activities: (a) case surveillance for specific foodborne pathogens, such as Salmonella and *E. coli*

O157:H7; (b) collection and evaluation of complaints of foodborne illness from consumers; and (c) investigation of foodborne illness outbreaks identified from pathogen-specific surveillance or consumer complaints.

The role of surveillance in driving the cycle of public health prevention related to foodborne disease outbreaks has been depicted by the Centers for Disease Control and Prevention (CDC) (Figure 17-2). Surveillance identifies outbreaks, which are then investigated using a combination of epidemiological, laboratory, and environmental methods. Results of investigations that identify the source of contamination and factors contributing to its occurrence can (a) lead to direct public health interventions or (b) stimulate applied targeted research to improve existing interventions or develop new ones. As new interventions are implemented, surveillance monitors their effectiveness, based on the occurrence of new outbreaks. (See Chapter 6.)

Although data on foodborne illness surveillance are frequently compiled at a national level, responsibility for foodborne disease surveillance in the United States resides at the state or local level, as authorized by state laws and regulations governing the reporting of communicable diseases. These laws vary widely by state; there is therefore no consistent organization of foodborne disease surveillance in the United States.[4] A state legal analysis project of the Council to Improve Foodborne Outbreak Response

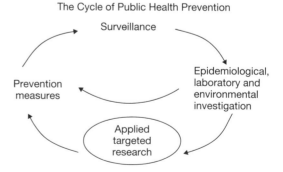

Figure 17-2. This drawing demonstrates how surveillance for foodborne disease outbreaks leads to preventive measures to improve food safety. (Adapted from Tauxe RV. Molecular subtyping and the transformation of public health. Foodborne Pathogens and Disease 2006; 3: 4–8.)

examined legal authorities for foodborne disease surveillance and outbreak response in 12 states. In three states, foodborne disease surveillance was performed by a central state office, in four states surveillance responsibilities were shared between state and local health agencies, and in five states it was performed primarily by local health agencies.[4] In addition to differing legal structures, resources to conduct surveillance activities vary widely by state and contribute to observed disparities in the distribution of reported foodborne outbreaks.[5]

In the United States, the CDC compiles reports of nationally notifiable diseases.[6] Unfortunately, only a few important foodborne diseases are nationally notifiable, and reported case counts do not provide any information about the source of the illnesses. In order to provide better data to determine trends in the occurrence of foodborne disease and to evaluate the causes of sporadic infections, the CDC established in 1996 the Active Surveillance Network for Foodborne Diseases (FoodNet). FoodNet has conducted, since 1996, active, population-based surveillance for seven major bacterial causes of foodborne disease at five sites and, since 2007, at 10 sites (with 49 million people, 15% of the U.S. population).[7] FoodNet data provided the framework for the CDC's estimate that the annual burden of foodborne illness in the United States is 48 million cases, 128,000 hospital admissions, and 3,000 deaths.[8]

Trend data for the occurrence of *E. coli* O157:H7 and Salmonella infections have been very useful for evaluating the effectiveness of the regulatory efforts of the Food Safety Inspection Service of the U.S. Department of Agriculture to reduce foodborne illnesses associated with meat and poultry products. For example, reduction in contamination of ground beef with *E. coli* O157:H7 and improved cooking practices for ground beef in fast-food restaurants helped to reduce the incidence of these infections from 2.1 to 1.0 cases per million, successfully attaining the Healthy People 2010 goal for *E. coli* O157:H7 incidence in the United States.[9] In contrast, rates of Salmonella infection have remained largely unchanged despite government and industry measures to reduce Salmonella contamination of meat and poultry products. FoodNet case-control studies, which have shown an increased

risk of Salmonella infections associated with eating foods prepared outside the home, have helped explain Salmonella trend data and have confirmed the importance of restaurants as sources for foodborne disease outbreaks.[10]

Although FoodNet has provided valuable information regarding the incidence and cause of sporadic infections, it was not established to detect or investigate outbreaks of foodborne disease. To enhance the usefulness of pathogen-specific surveillance, the CDC established the national molecular subtyping network for foodborne disease surveillance (PulseNet) in 1998. PulseNet is a national network of public health and food regulatory agency laboratories that perform standardized molecular subtyping of *E. coli* O157:H7, Salmonella, and Listeria by pulsed-field gel electrophoresis. Patterns from cases are submitted electronically to the CDC, stored in a database, and periodically reviewed to detect unusual, large, or multistate clusters that may represent a foodborne outbreak. More rapid identification of outbreaks by PulseNet has annually resulted in prevention of 270,000 cases of Salmonella, *E. coli* O157:H7, and Listeria illness along with an annual reduction of $507 million in costs.[11] The development and implementation of whole-genome sequencing in PulseNet will further improve outbreak detection.

The CDC collects data on foodborne disease outbreaks from all states and territories through the National Outbreak Reporting System.[5] The overall goal of a foodborne outbreak investigation is to rapidly obtain sufficient information to implement specific interventions to abate the outbreak. Secondary goals of outbreak investigations include identifying the agent, vehicle, source of contamination, and factors contributing to the occurrence of the outbreak. Identifying these factors is critical for identifying new hazards, evaluating the effectiveness of existing control measures, and developing new prevention methods.

Results from 2014 illustrate the potential benefits and limitations of foodborne outbreak surveillance.[3] A total of 864 outbreaks were reported, resulting in 13,246 cases and 21 deaths. An etiology could be identified for 677 (78%) outbreaks. Norovirus accounted for 42% of outbreaks with a known etiology and 33% of all foodborne outbreaks reported. The next most common cause was Salmonella, which accounted for 22% of outbreaks with a known etiology and 17% of all foodborne outbreaks reported. However, among 25 multistate outbreaks detected, 11 were attributed to Salmonella, 10 were attributed to Shiga-toxin-producing *E. coli* (STEC), and 3 were attributed to *Listeria monocytogenes*. Etiologic agents isolated from implicated foods in 13 multistate outbreaks included Salmonella in nut butters, chia seed powder, cucumbers, and mung bean sprouts. STEC was isolated from ground beef, clover sprouts, prepackaged salads, cabbage, and leaf lettuce.[3] *L. monocytogenes* was isolated from stone fruits, apples, and mung bean sprouts.[3] Assessment of pathogen-commodity pairs identified Salmonella as causing the most outbreak-associated cases of illness—in seeded vegetables (357 cases), in chicken (227 cases), and in sprouts (115 cases).[3]

The CDC's National Outbreak Reporting System collects available information on etiology, number of cases and hospitalizations, and implicated vehicle for each outbreak reported. States also report information on the outbreak setting and factors identified as contributing to the occurrence of the outbreak. Therefore, these data provide a rich framework for analyzing the relative contributions of raw material source contamination, cross-contamination, and ill food workers as the likely causes of foodborne outbreaks in restaurants or other settings. Unfortunately, concerns over the quality and completeness of these data have limited the willingness of the CDC or other investigators to analyze these data and present the findings, contributing to a self-perpetuating problem. Because the data are not being actively used and reported, states see little benefit in making a greater effort to improve the quality or completeness of the data on contributing factors.

Based on the results of surveillance of sporadic infections and outbreaks of foodborne illness, three major foodborne disease problems can be identified:

- Pathogen contamination of raw ingredients
- Scales of production and distribution that turn minor errors into large outbreaks
- Contamination by food handlers of ready-to-eat foods.

ABATING HAZARDS IN THE FOOD SYSTEM: PREVENTING CONTAMINATION, CONTROLLING AMPLIFICATION OR SPREAD, AND REDUCING OR ELIMINATING THE HAZARD

Preventing Contamination

As a general principle of environmental microbiology, it is always better to prevent contamination from occurring rather than to manage the contamination or try to eliminate it during the processing of a food product. However, some contamination of these raw ingredients is inevitable, given the process of growing fresh fruits and vegetables in an open field or of converting living animals into meat and poultry products in an abattoir. For foods processed with a heat treatment or other control measure capable of killing pathogens, the primary concern is to prevent contamination from environmental sources in the postprocessing environment. In a restaurant setting, persistent concerns are cross-contamination from raw to ready-to-eat foods and contamination of ready-to-eat foods from infected food workers.

When dealing with issues of chemical contamination, preventing contamination is paramount, since most toxic chemicals are resistant to inactivation by heat or chemical sanitizers. The series of outbreaks and recalls due to contamination of wheat gluten and milk with melamine in China was especially disturbing.[12] These events occurred because of the intentional addition of melamine to these products to increase their apparent protein content. This type of economic fraud has far-reaching implications for food safety and defense that go beyond normal considerations of food safety from a microbiological standpoint. Food processors need to know their suppliers and have some system for ensuring the integrity of their supply chain to prevent future recurrence of this type of problem. Supply chain integrity, supported by a strong regulatory structure that can respond to cross-border contamination issues, is a prerequisite for food safety in a global economy.

Several outbreaks highlight the importance and challenges of preventing microbial contamination. During the summer of 2006, there were 238 cases of *E. coli* O157:H7 infection, including

31 cases of hemolytic uremic syndrome (HUS) and five deaths, caused by spinach that was produced on a single U.S. farm and harvested on a single day.[13] Extensive environmental evaluations were conducted to identify the source of contamination in this outbreak. Multiple strains of *E. coli* O157:H7 were isolated from feces of cattle on a nearby ranch, soil in the cattle pasture, feces of feral swine, surface water, and river sediment samples. The outbreak-associated strain was isolated only from cattle and feral swine feces.[14] Because the environmental evaluations were conducted 2 to 3 months following the contamination event, it is possible that transient contamination of water used in irrigation or processing of the spinach may have caused the outbreak. However, several lines of evidence suggest that the feral swine may have been the critical vector of *E. coli* O157:H7 from the cattle ranch to the spinach field.

First, at the time of the environmental evaluations, the outbreak-associated strains were only isolated from feces of cattle and feral swine. Although the cattle were restricted to their pasture land and had no direct access to the spinach fields, feral swine were observed in both cattle pastures and spinach fields.[14] There was no evidence that cattle manure had been directly applied to the spinach field or that the spinach field could have been contaminated from flooding events or runoff from the cattle pasture.

In addition, following this outbreak, a company committed $2 million for a novel academic research program to fast-track studies of *E. coli* O157:H7 in leafy greens.[15] Results of these studies established that spinach and leaf lettuce plants do not take up *E. coli* O157:H7 through their roots under field conditions and that application of bacteria on leaves is unlikely to lead to internalization and distribution of the bacteria throughout the plants' vegetative tissues. In contrast, *E. coli* O157:H7 applied to cut surfaces were readily taken up and transported through vascular tissue. In addition, blades used to harvest and core head lettuce were shown to be capable of contaminating multiple heads of lettuce following the initial contamination of the blade.[16] These findings support the suggestion that feral swine feces in the spinach field may have contaminated harvesting equipment and may have been transferred to the freshly harvested spinach. Uptake of *E. coli* O157:H7 at the cut end of the spinach would have likely led to internalization of the contamination and reduced the effectiveness of subsequent efforts to wash and sanitize spinach leaves.[17]

For food items such as fresh produce that will be consumed without an effective treatment measure, preventing contamination at the time of harvest is critical. The investigation of factors associated with outbreaks, such as this one, were used to help develop good agricultural practices for the production of fresh produce items.[18] These practices are the core of the Produce Safety Rule under the Food Safety Modernization Act.

Controlling Amplification or Spread

Hazard analysis and critical control point (HACCP) systems were originally established as process-control systems to protect the safety of foods served to astronauts in space. They have evolved to become a major framework for food safety, which form the basis for preventive measures under the Food Safety Modernization Act (Table 17-1).[1,19] A notable success of the application of HACCP to fresh produce has been the implementation of regulations requiring the development of HACCP plans for the production of fruit juices. During the 1990s, a series of *E. coli* O157:H7 and Cryptosporidium outbreaks were associated with consumption of unpasteurized apple juice and cider.[20] Several outbreaks of Salmonella infection were associated with unpasteurized orange juice. In response to these outbreaks, the Food and Drug Administration (FDA) implemented process control measures to regulate the production of fruit juices. These rules were phased in over a 3-year period to accommodate the needs of small producers. In particular, the rules specified the implementation of treatments that could accomplish a 5-log reduction in the presence of *E. coli* O157:H7 as a critical control point in the HACCP plan.[21] Surveillance by the CDC has demonstrated that fewer juice-associated outbreaks have been reported since implementation of these rules. However, outbreaks continue to be associated with processors who are exempt from the rule or who are not in compliance.[20]

Since 1999, the CDC and FDA have recommended that persons at high risk for

Table 17-1. The Principles of Hazard Analysis and Critical Control Point (HACCP) Systems Compared to Preventive Control Systems

HAACP Systems	Preventive Control Systems
Identify hazards that are reasonably likely to occur in the food item	Identify known or reasonably foreseeable hazards for which illness or injury will likely occur in the absence of preventive controls
Determine the critical control points (CCPs) at which the hazard can be prevented, minimized, or eliminated	Establish risk-based procedures, practices, and processes to significantly minimize or prevent identified hazards
Establish critical limits to assure the effective control of the hazard at CCPs	Establish parameters and minimum/maximum values for process controls
Establish monitoring procedures to detect violations of the critical limits	Monitor parameters to ensure that minimum/maximum values are met and ensure that control activities are conducted following defined procedures
Establish corrective actions to prevent the distribution of potentially contaminated foods and to regain control over the process	Establish and implement corrective action procedures that would apply if preventive controls are not properly implemented
Establish verification procedures to ensure that corrective actions are taken when critical limits are exceeded	Establish verification procedures as appropriate for all preventive controls, including validation for process controls and supplier verification when a supplier controls a hazard
Establish recordkeeping and documentation procedures to assure that monitoring procedures and corrective actions are being properly performed	Establish recordkeeping and documentation procedures to assure that monitoring procedures and corrective actions are being properly performed
	Establish a recall plan for hazards requiring a preventive control.

complications of infection with Salmonella and *E. coli* O157:H7, such as older people, young children, and those with compromised immune systems, not eat raw sprouts. At the same time, the FDA issued *Guidance for Industry for Reducing Microbial Food Safety Hazards for Sprouted Seeds*, which emphasizes the importance of good agricultural practices for the production of seeds and good manufacturing practices for manufacturing, packaging, and holding human food. Two specific interventions are recommended: antimicrobial treatment of seeds to reduce pathogens and testing of spent irrigation water for the presence of pathogens before products are distributed.[17] This second intervention is recommended because available antimicrobial treatments cannot eliminate all pathogens from seeds and because the conditions required to germinate the seeds and grow the sprouts are also ideal conditions to grow Salmonella and *E. coli* O157:H7. Therefore, any contaminants that survive the treatment would be likely to replicate to dangerous levels prior to distribution.

In contrast to the implementation of the juice HACCP regulation, the FDA's sprout guidance has not been effective at reducing the occurrence of sprout-associated outbreaks.[22] Twenty-eight Salmonella and four *E. coli* O157:H7 outbreaks that were reported to the CDC from 1998 through 2010 were linked to sprouts.[23] Inadequate disinfection, sampling, and testing procedures as well as incorrect interpretation of test results were identified in most of these investigations.[23] The continuing occurrence of similar outbreaks has led to the inclusion of specific recommendations for sprout production under the Produce Safety Rule of the Food Safety Modernization Act.[24] Requirements specific to sprouts include treating seeds or beans that will be used for sprouting and pathogen testing of spent sprout irrigation water from each production batch for pathogens. In addition, sprouts cannot be allowed to enter commerce until pathogen testing is negative.[24]

A large outbreak of HUS caused by STEC O104:H4, which occurred in Europe in 2011, highlights the interactions between global-sourcing and local-production practices that defines the risks of sprout production and consumption.[25] In May 2011, a large increase in HUS cases, primarily among adult women, was recognized in Germany. A series of case-control studies, a recipe-based study of an implicated restaurant, and trace-back investigations of sprouts from the distributor that supplied the restaurant identified a specific source of fenugreek sprouts that had been imported from Egypt as the cause of the outbreak.[25] In June 2011, a smaller cluster of HUS cases was reported in France.[26] All of those affected had attended the same event. A retrospective cohort study among adults who attended the event implicated fenugreek as the source of illness. Both the French and German STEC O104:H4 outbreak investigations identified a common source of fenugreek sprouts and resulted in implementation of Europe-wide control measures in 2011.[26]

Contamination of alfalfa and other seeds represents a special concern because the raw seed is not a desirable food item, and sprouting the seeds necessarily amplifies the initial contamination. For many raw food items, contamination may be a sporadic occurrence, and the levels of contamination may be low. For example, raw shell eggs emerged as a public health problem during the 1980s due to trans-ovarial transmission of *Salmonella enteritidis* from infected hens. However, only 1 in 1,000 to 10,000 shell eggs was contaminated with *S. enteritidis*, and, typically, only a few cells of *S. enteritidis* were deposited in each egg. Egg-associated outbreaks were caused by practices such as pooling multiple eggs together, letting the pooled egg mix sit on a kitchen counter out of refrigeration for several hours, and using the pooled egg mix to make lightly cooked food items. Therefore, the low numbers present in a few eggs were amplified sufficiently to provide an infectious dose to many patrons.[27] The same patterns of amplification have been demonstrated in outbreaks of Salmonella associated with tomatoes and in a series of Shigella outbreaks traced to contaminated parsley imported from Mexico, in which the parsley was chopped, held in a large bowl in the kitchen, and sprinkled as a garnish on dishes ready to be served.[28] In many of these restaurants, food workers and servers became infected as a result of handling and eating contaminated foods. These ill food workers served as additional sources for amplifying transmission during the outbreaks. Therefore, maintaining temperature

control and preventing cross-contamination can effectively reduce the risk of an outbreak associated with contaminated food items or ingredients.

The role of infected food workers in transmitting foodborne illness in restaurants is most notable in outbreaks due to norovirus.[5] The CDC's environmental health specialists network has evaluated food workers' experiences and beliefs about working while ill.[29] Among food workers studied, 20% reported that they had worked while ill (with vomiting and diarrhea) during the previous year. A variety of reasons, including the lack of paid sick leave and understaffing at the restaurant, were cited as reasons.[29] Most restaurant managers let ill food workers decide whether or not to work, and most of these managers work while ill.[30] These findings suggest that a lack of effective monitoring of employee illness or a lack of commitment to enforcing policies regarding ill food workers is an antecedent condition that fosters the transmission of norovirus in restaurants. These same antecedent conditions may also contribute to the role of infected food workers in transmitting Salmonella in restaurants.[31] Whether they are actively contributing to transmission to restaurant patrons or merely serving as indicators of transmission within the restaurant, illnesses among food workers are important health events that should be actively monitored by restaurant managers.

Reducing or Eliminating the Hazard

The ultimate control for abating food safety hazards is to reduce or eliminate the hazard. Cooking is an effective way to destroy foodborne pathogens such as *E. coli* O157:H7 and Salmonella that are associated with raw meat and poultry products. Cooking times and temperatures required to ensure the microbial safety of these foods are well characterized and have been widely publicized and incorporated into food safety regulations. For example, poultry should be cooked to an internal temperature of 165°F to kill Campylobacter and Salmonella, while a hamburger should be cooked to 160°F to ensure destruction of *E. coli* O157:H7. Unfortunately, most households do not have thermometers that are suitable for measuring the internal temperature of a hamburger.[32]

Pasteurization is another highly successful public health intervention that has virtually eliminated transmission of foodborne pathogens through milk.[33] The success of pasteurization is demonstrated by the occurrence of outbreaks among persons who seek out raw milk. For example, outbreaks in the United States caused by nonpasteurized milk increased from 30 in the 2007-2009 period to 51 in the 2010-2012 period. Most outbreaks (77%) were caused by Campylobacter species and by non-pasteurized milk purchased from states in which nonpasteurized milk sale was legal (81%).[33] The absence of outbreaks associated with pasteurized milk confirms the effectiveness of the intervention. The success of milk pasteurization has led to the development of pasteurization conditions that have been validated to achieve a 5-log reduction of *Salmonella enteritidis* in shell eggs, without coagulating egg proteins and destroying the physical characteristics or culinary uses of the raw egg.[34]

The success of pasteurization has also provided a model for the use of irradiation as a public health intervention to reduce food safety hazards associated with contamination of raw ingredients.[35] The FDA approved the use of irradiation to control microbes in spices and dried herbs in 1983.[36] Following nationwide concern regarding the emergence of *E. coli* O157:H7 in ground beef during the 1990s, the FDA approved in 1997 the use of irradiation to control pathogenic bacteria in red meat. Two years later, the U.S. Department of Agriculture (USDA) amended its regulations to allow irradiation of refrigerated and frozen uncooked meat, and commercially irradiated ground beef became available in 2000.[37] In 2008, the FDA approved the use of irradiation to control pathogens in fresh spinach and head lettuce.

Although low-dose irradiation has been shown to be effective at reducing levels of pathogen contamination in these products without materially affecting the nutritional content or sensory appeal of these products, it has not yet gained widespread acceptance in the marketplace.[37] Consumers continue to shun the technology despite consistent reassurances from public health professionals that there is no risk associated with the consumption of food that has received low-dose irradiation and that these food products are inherently safer microbiologically.[38]

REGULATORY POLICIES AND EDUCATION: PROHIBITING BAD PRACTICES AND INSTITUTIONALIZING GOOD PRACTICES

Regulation of food production historically developed as a tool to prohibit bad practices that jeopardized the safety of food. Both the Food and Drugs Act and the Meat Inspection Act were passed in 1906 in response to unsanitary conditions in meatpacking plants and the use of poisonous preservatives and dyes in foods.[39] These first federal food safety laws—which are still in force in the United States— established the jurisdictions of the USDA for meat and poultry products and the FDA for the rest of the food system. The occurrence of high-profile, multistate foodborne disease outbreaks since 2000 and the lack of progress demonstrated by FoodNet toward meeting *Healthy People 2010* targets for reduction of foodborne pathogens drove Congress to pass the Food Safety Modernization Act, which was signed into law in 2011 to translate the principles of HACCP into a system of preventive controls.[40]

The act represents a considerable enhancement of HACCP and its regulatory use, with the food industry being charged with identifying problems and developing solutions under the scrutiny of regulatory oversight. This shift represents an important distinction, which is needed to deal with the growing complexity of food production and distribution systems that are not easily governed by a simple and consistent set of specific rules.

In the restaurant setting, this shift has been accompanied by inspections systems that have moved away from basic observations of the cleanliness of floors, walls, and ceilings to risk-based inspections that focus on managers demonstrating knowledge of food safety.[41] Promoting "active managerial control" in restaurant operations and using inspections as opportunities to consult with managers to help them solve food safety problems have been shown to improve restaurant operations.[42,43] However, institutionalizing good practices still requires regulatory oversight with strong enforcement capabilities.

Although most food producers strive to produce safe and wholesome food in a profitable manner, there are some who are willing to jeopardize safety in order to make more money. The most egregious example of this irresponsibility caused an outbreak involving at least 714 cases of Salmonella in 46 states and Canada with at least 166 hospitalizations and 9 deaths from September 2008 to April 2009.[44] Following the recognition of unusual multistate *Salmonella typhimurium* clusters by PulseNet, investigations by state and local health departments led to the identification of peanut butter and peanut-containing products as the source of the outbreak. The outbreak strains were confirmed in unopened peanut butter containers produced at a single facility in Georgia. During investigations of this facility, it was disclosed that the company had been testing its peanut butter for Salmonella so that it could provide a "Salmonella-free" certificate of analysis to its customers. In fact, several samples from the company during the outbreak period were positive. However, when confronted with a positive sample, the company retested the product. If the follow-up sample was negative, the product was shipped with the "Salmonella-free" certificate of analysis. Neither the company nor the laboratories that performed these tests for the company were required to report the results to regulatory authorities. As a result, an ongoing problem within the plant was ignored until the size of the outbreak finally allowed investigators to identify its source.

Education of managers and food workers is critical to food safety. Education of consumers is also important to help them reduce their risk for foodborne illness by following safe food-handling and food-preparation recommendations and by avoiding consumption of potentially hazardous foods. In particular, the importance of handwashing should be emphasized in general education programs, beginning in preschool. Because the food industry is one of the major sources of employment in the economy, all consumer education activities should help to prepare food industry workers for safe food-handling practices at work. (Detailed information on food safety practices is available at http://www.foodsafety.gov and http://www.fightbac.org.)

CONCLUSION

Although methods to abate specific hazards, such as *E. coli* O157:H7 contamination of ground beef, can be developed solely based on knowledge of the agent and the characteristics of the food system, public health surveillance is needed to monitor the effectiveness of control measures on a population basis. Monitoring systems at a plant level may not be sufficiently sensitive to prevent the release of large quantities of contaminated products. People represent the ultimate bioassay for this type of contamination, and epidemiology is the tool needed to detect it.

The unique ability of public health surveillance to identify new hazards and provide population-based evaluation of the effectiveness of control measures make it a prerequisite for effective food control programs and a primary tool for food control research. Improving public health surveillance for foodborne diseases will require considerable investments at multiple levels. However, such investments are critical to the improvement of our food safety systems.

REFERENCES

1. U.S. Food and Drug Administration. Current good manufacturing practice and hazard analysis and risk-based preventive controls for human food. Federal Register 2015; 80: 55907–56168.
2. Centers for Disease Control and Prevention. Updated guidelines for evaluating public health surveillance systems. Morbidity and Mortality Weekly Report 2001; 50; 1–35.
3. Centers for Disease Control and Prevention. Surveillance for foodborne-disease outbreaks, United States, 2014, Annual report. Atlanta: U.S. Department of Health and Human Services, CDC, 2016.
4. Elliot P, Morse D. Analysis of state legal authorities for foodborne illness detection and outbreak response. In: Council to Improve Foodborne Outbreak Response. Guidelines for Foodborne Disease Outbreak Response (2nd ed.). Atlanta: Council of State and Territorial Epidemiologists, 2014.

5. Centers for Disease Control and Prevention. Vital signs: Multistate foodborne outbreaks—United States, 2010–2014. Morbidity and Mortality Weekly Report 2015; 64: 1221–1225.

6. Centers for Disease Control and Prevention. Summary of notifiable infectious diseases and conditions—United States, 2013. Morbidity and Mortality Weekly Report 2015; 26: 1–119.

7. Huang JY, Henao OL, Griffin PM, et al. Infection with pathogens transmitted commonly through food and the effect of increasing use of culture-independent diagnostic tests on surveillance—Foodborne Diseases Active Surveillance Network, 10 U.S. sites, 2012–2015 Morbidity and Mortality Weekly Report 2016; 65: 368–371.

8. Scallan E, Hoekstra RM, Angulo FJ, et al. Foodborne illness acquired in the United States—Major pathogens. Emerging Infectious Diseases 2011; 17: 7–15.

9. Henao OL, Jones TF, Vugia DJ, et al. Foodborne Diseases Active Surveillance Network—2 decades of achievements, 1996–2015. Emerging Infectious Diseases 2015; 21: 1529–1536.

10. Jones TF, Angulo FJ. Eating in restaurants: A risk factor for foodborne disease? Clinical Infectious Diseases 2006; 43: 1324–1328.

11. Scharff RL, Besser J, Sharp DJ, et al. An economic evaluation of PulseNet: A betwork for foodborne disease surveillance. American Journal of Preventive Medicine 2016; 50: S66–S73.

12. Coulombier D, Heppner C, Fabiansson S, et al. Melamine contamination of dairy products in China—Public health impact on citizens of the European Union. Eurosurveillance 2008; 13: 1–2.

13. Centers for Disease Control and Prevention. Ongoing multistate outbreak of *Escherichia coli* serotype O157:H7. Infections associated with consumption of fresh spinach—United States, September 2006. Morbidity and Mortality Weekly Report 2006; 55: 1045–1046.

14. Jay MT, Cooley M, Carychao D, et al. *Escherichia coli* O157:H7 in feral swine near spinach fields and cattle, central California coast. Emerging Infectious Diseases 2007; 13: 1908–1911.

15. Osterholm MT, Ostrowsky J, Farrar JA, et al. A novel approach to enhance food safety: Industry-academia-government partnership for applied research. Journal of Food Protection 2009; 72: 1509–1512.

16. Taormina PJ, Beuchat LR, Erickson MC, et al. Transfer of Escherichia coli O157:H7 to iceberg lettuce via simulated field coring. Journal of Food Protection 2009; 72: 465–472.

17. Zhang G, Ma L, Beuchat LR, et al. Evaluation of treatments for elimination of foodborne pathogens on the surface of leaves and roots of lettuce (*Lactuca sativa L.*). Journal of Food Protection 2009; 72: 228–234.

18. Lynch MF, Tauxe RV, Hedberg CW. The growing burden of foodborne outbreaks due to contaminated fresh produce: Risks and opportunities. Epidemiology and Infection 2009; 137: 307–315.

19. Food and Drug Administration. Standards for the growing, harvesting, packing, and holding of produce for human consumption. Federal Register 2016; 80: 74353–74568.

20. Vojdani JD, Beuchat LR, Tauxe RV. Juice-associated outbreaks of human illness in the United States, 1995 through 2005. Journal of Food Protection 2008; 71: 356–364.

21. Food and Drug Administration. Hazard analysis and critical control point (HAACP): Procedures for the safe and sanitary processing and importing of juice: Final rule. Federal Register 2001; 66: 6137–6202.

22. Food and Drug Administration. Guidance for industry: Reducing microbial food safety hazards for sprouted seeds. Available at: http://www.fda.gov/Food/GuidanceRegulation/GuidanceDocumentsRegulatoryInformation/ProducePlantProducts/ucm120244.htm Accessed November 11, 2016.

23. Dechet AM1, Herman KM, Chen Parker C, et al. Outbreaks caused by sprouts, United States, 1998–2010: Lessons learned and solutions needed. Foodborne Pathogens and Disease 2014; 11: 635–644.

24. U.S. Food and Drug Administration. Standards for the growing, harvesting, packing, and holding of produce for human consumption. Federal Register 2015; 80: 74353–74568.

25. Buchholz U, Bernard H, Werber D, et al. German outbreak of *Escherichia coli* O104:H4 associated with sprouts. New England Journal of Medicine 2011 365: 1763–1770.

26. King LA, Nogareda F, Weill FX, et al. Outbreak of Shiga toxin-producing *Escherichia coli* O104:H4 associated with organic fenugreek sprouts, France, June 2011. Clinical Infectious Diseases 2012; 54: 1588–1594.

27. Schroeder CM, Latimer HK, Schlosser WD, et al. Overview and summary of the Food Safety and Inspection Service risk assessment for *Salmonella* enteritidis in shell eggs, October 2005. Foodborne Pathogens and Disease 2006; 3: 403–412.

28. Naimi TS, Wicklund JH, Olsen SJ, et al. Concurrent outbreaks of Shigella sonnei and enterotoxigenic Escherichia coli infections associated with parsley: implications for

surveillance and control of foodborne illness. Journal of Food Protection 2003; 66: 535–541.

29. Carpenter LR, Green AL, Norton DM, et al. Food worker experiences with and beliefs about working while ill. Journal of Food Protection 2013; 76: 2146–2154.

30. Norton DM, Brown LG, Frick R, et al. Managerial practices regarding workers while ill. Journal of Food Protection 2015; 78: 187–195.

31. Medus C, Smith KE, Bender JB, et al. Salmonella outbreaks in restaurants in Minnesota, 1995 through 2003: Evaluation of the role of infected foodworkers. Journal of Food Protection 2006; 69: 1870–1878.

32. Takeuchi MT, Edlefsen M, McCurdy SM, Hillers VN. Educational intervention enhances consumers' readiness to adopt food thermometer use when cooking small cuts of meat: an application of the transtheoretical model. Journal of Food Protection 2005; 68: 1874–1883.

33. Mungai EA, Behravesh CB, Gould LH Increased outbreaks associated with nonpasteurized milk, United States, 2007–2012. Emerging Infectious Disease 2015; 21: 119–122.

34. Hank CR, Kunkel ME, Dawson PL, et al. The effect of shell egg pasteurization on the protein quality of albumen. Poultry Science 2001; 80: 821–824.

35. Osterholm MT, Norgan AP. The role of irradiation in food safety. New England Journal of Medicine 2004; 350: 1898–1901.

36. Food and Drug Administration, U.S. Department of Health and Human Services. Irradiation in the production, processing and handling of food. Final rule. Federal Registry 2008; 73: 49593–49603.

37. Neal JA, Cabrera-Diaz E, Márquez-González M, et al. Reduction of Escherichia coli O157:H7 and Salmonella on baby spinach, using electron beam radiation. Journal of Food Protection 2008; 71: 2415–2420.

38. Fan X, Sokorai KJ. Retention of quality and nutritional value of 13 fresh-cut vegetables treated with low-dose radiation. Journal of Food Science 2008; 73: S367–S372.

39. Bruhn CM. Consumer perceptions and concerns about food contaminants. Advances in Experimental Medicine and Biology 1999; 459: 1–7.

40. U.S. Food and Drug Administration. Significant dates in U.S. food and drug law history. Available at: http://www.fda.gov/AboutFDA/WhatWeDo/History/Milestones/ucm128305.htm. Accessed November 11, 2016.

41. U.S. Government Publishing Office. Public Law 111–353. January 4, 2011. Available at: https://www.gpo.gov/fdsys/pkg/PLAW-111publ353/pdf/PLAW-111publ353.pdf. Accessed November 11, 2016.

42. Buchholz U, Run G, Kool JL, Fielding J, et al. A risk-based restaurant inspection system in Los Angeles County. Journal of Food Protection 2002; 65: 367–372.

43. Reske KA, Jenkins T, Fernandez C, et al. Beneficial effects of implementing an announced restaurant inspection program. Journal of Environmental Health 2007; 69: 27–34, 76.

44. Cavallaro E, Date K, Medus C, et al. Salmonella typhimurium infections associated with peanut products. New England Journal of Medicine 2011; 365: 601–610.

FURTHER READING

Council to Improve Foodborne Outbreak Response. Guidelines for foodborne disease outbreak response (2nd ed.). Available at: http://www.cifor.us/documents/CIFOR%20Industry%20Guidelines/CIFOR-Industry-Guideline.pdf. Accessed August 25, 2017.
This book provides descriptions of model practices for surveillance and outbreak response, and rationale for their development.

U.S. Food and Drug Administration. Bad bug book: Handbook of foodborne pathogenic microorganisms and natural toxins. Available at: http://www.fda.gov/downloads/Food/FoodSafety/FoodborneIllness/FoodborneIllnessFoodbornePathogensNaturalToxins/BadBugBook/UCM297627.pdf. Accessed on August 25, 2017.
This book describes basic characteristics of foodborne pathogens and associated diseases.

18

Hazardous Waste

Ken Silver, Gary A. Davis, and Denny Dobbin

With the growth of cities during the Industrial Revolution in the 19th century, waste became a significant societal problem—dumped onto grounds, released into water, and dispersed into the air. Unmanaged urban garbage supported proliferation of pathogen-transmitting vectors, such as rodents and insects. Waste was increasingly recognized for its impacts on public health, the environment, and land use. Local governments in the United States accepted responsibility for managing municipal solid waste.[1]

In the 20th century, advances in chemical technology, especially synthesis of organic chemicals, exponentially increased the volume of toxic material produced and resultant waste generated, outpacing methods for managing it. National limits on air and water discharges led to greater reliance by industry on land disposal.[2] Nuclear power generation, begun in the 1950s, continues to produce much radioactive and highly toxic waste that will persist for many years and is difficult to manage.

As we, as a society, produce, use, and discard products, we may generate waste at each stage— "cradle to grave." We process raw materials, creating waste. We produce and package goods,

creating waste. We consume or otherwise use products, creating waste. And we discard products at the end of their useful life, creating waste. All this waste needs to be treated and disposed.

Hazardous waste can adversely affect workers and community residents. Workers are potentially at risk of harm at each of the cradle-to-grave stages. They are engaged in production, where hazardous waste is generated. They are engaged in treatment, storage, and disposal of waste. (See Figure 18-1.) They are engaged in remediation of uncontrolled hazardous waste sites. In addition, they respond to emergencies, including spills of hazardous materials. Emergency responders may be at the greatest risk because of the urgent and chaotic nature of their work.

Community exposure to hazardous waste disproportionately affects poor people and minorities. They have historically been less able to control the location of abandoned waste sites and actively polluting industries. They are often exposed to multiple environmental stressors and suffer a variety of adverse impacts, ranging from chronic disease to loss of property value.[3] Hazardous exposures faced by community residents tend to be at lower concentrations, but of longer duration, than those of workers.

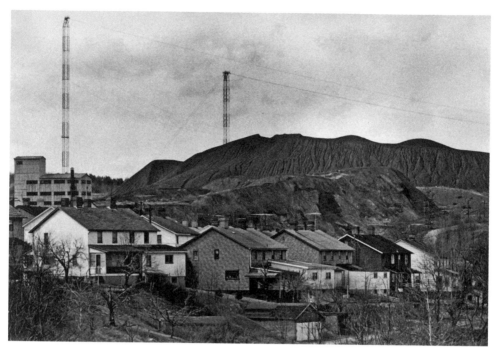

Figure 18-1. "Company town" in Pennsylvania with coal slag heaps. (Photograph by Earl Dotter.)

DEFINITION OF HAZARDOUS WASTE

Hazardous waste is defined as discarded solid or liquid material that may, directly or indirectly, cause adverse health effects, unless properly treated, stored, or disposed in a manner that meets specific governmental regulatory definitions. For example, *radioactive waste*, comprised of discarded materials and products that emit harmful radiation, can include spent nuclear fuel rods, high-level radioactive material left over from producing nuclear weapons, mill tailings (radioactive sands left over after uranium metal is separated from its ore), and low-level radioactive waste. *Industrial waste* includes manufacturing waste, waste from mining and other mineral extraction, coal combustion, and gas and oil production. *Municipal solid waste* includes household garbage, food waste, and trash from public and commercial buildings in communities. *Medical waste* includes waste from clinics, hospitals, and biomedical research laboratories.

The Environmental Protection Agency (EPA) estimates that, by volume, 94% of waste is industrial waste, 5% hazardous waste, and 1% municipal solid waste. Radioactive and medical waste represent, by volume, less than 0.1% of total waste. Typical per-capita daily generation of waste in the United States includes about 4 pounds of municipal waste, about 10 pounds of hazardous waste, as much as 300 pounds of industrial waste, and as little as 1 ounce of medical waste.

Each year in the United States, as much as 2.5 billion tons of solid, industrial, and hazardous waste is produced. There are as many as 550,000 generators of hazardous waste.[4] Chemical manufacturers generate approximately 80% of the total. More than 90% of hazardous waste is discharged as wastewater from industrial production streams. The remaining 10% includes inorganic solids, including contaminated soil and metals, organic solvents in liquid form, and sludge and other residues from water-pollution and air-pollution control systems.

All chemical wastes are potentially toxic, but only those that are specifically designated by regulation are legally considered hazardous. Hazardous waste has a precise legal meaning in laws and regulations adopted to control threats to the environment and human health. Designating a material as hazardous waste sets in motion a series of controls and actions to contain the material. However, just because a chemical is *defined* as "not hazardous" does not mean that it *is* not hazardous. Lobbying by special-interest trade associations, which cite economic hardship and market conditions, has led to the exclusion of some chemicals from hazard regulation.[5]

Under the federal Resource Conservation and Recovery Act (RCRA), a waste may be classified as "hazardous" if it meets one of the following four characteristics:

- *Ignitability*: The relative likelihood that a chemical will burst into flame in the presence of an ignition source (has a flashpoint at or less than 140°F)
- *Corrosivity*: The potential of strong acids (with a pH of 2 or less) and strong bases (with a pH of 12.5 or more) to eat through steel or chemically burn living organisms
- *Reactivity*: The potential for a chemical waste to explode or emit toxic gases
- *Toxicity*: The capability of a chemical to poison living organisms.

ADVERSE HEALTH EFFECTS

When evaluating adverse health effects of industrial chemicals discharged or dumped as waste into the environment, extrapolation from occupational data may be helpful. However, standard assumptions and methods that apply to workplaces must be adapted. In the community, as compared with the workplace, people are generally exposed to much lower levels of chemicals and to more complex mixtures of chemicals. Occupational exposure standards for chemicals, designed primarily to protect healthy, working men for 8-hour work shifts, are not sufficient to protect community residents exposed to chemicals—including children, pregnant women (and their fetuses), older people, and people with chronic illnesses or disabilities.

In environmental epidemiology, nondifferential misclassification of exposure can obscure exposure–disease relationships (Chapter 5). Patterns of exposure to chemicals in the environment can be difficult to characterize in time and space, due to (a) variations in daily activities of people and (b) episodic and seasonal fluctuations in highly complex physical processes, such as flow of groundwater and change in atmospheric conditions.

Compared to historic industrywide studies that enrolled thousands of workers who worked in the same location for many years with high levels of exposure, epidemiologic studies of people living around hazardous waste sites tend to be based on relatively small (neighborhood-sized) populations and often face challenges in exposure assessment, leading to misclassification bias, as described previously. Additional difficulties include loss of follow-up due to changes in residence, wide interindividual variability in the population, and potential exposure to the dozens of chemicals that can migrate from a waste site, typically at much lower levels than in workplaces. These challenges make it difficult to obtain findings that are statistically significant. The long latency period for most cancers to develop presents additional difficulties. Government agencies and clean-up consultants often construct computerized risk-assessment models that are based on relatively few exposure measurements. Clean-up priorities are strongly influenced by predictions based on these models, typically in the form of a risk of cancer in the range of 1 in 10,000 (10^{-4}) to 1 in 1,000,000 (10^{-6}). Seldom do epidemiologic studies or personal health data provide relevant information to assist with clean-up decisions. Obtaining persuasive scientific evidence of adverse health outcomes may require several years of costly research, during which time contaminants will continue to migrate offsite via groundwater and other pathways. (See Box 18-1.) Risk modeling, however imperfect, allows clean-up projects to be prioritized and implemented without waiting for epidemiologic evidence of a "body count."

Investigations of possible health effects from hazardous waste sites are performed in the most public of settings. Residents of a community often want scientists to confirm that their health effects are causally associated with exposure to hazardous waste.[6] Ideally, cluster investigations, which may be necessary initially, lead to communication among scientists and community residents on the desirability and feasibility of population-based epidemiologic studies. Early stages of this communication can be marked by conflict between community residents who are experiencing real-life tragedies and scientists

Box 18-1. Use of Analytical Epidemiology for Assessing In-Utero Exposures at Hazardous Waste Sites

Rarely have community cluster investigations near toxic waste sites led to positive findings in analytical epidemiologic studies utilizing quantitative estimates of residents' past exposure to chemicals. Two such studies of childhood cancer at federal Superfund sites, conducted in the glare of media attention and with extensive involvement by public stakeholders, have replicated important findings. Each of these two studies demonstrated that in-utero exposure to chemicals in hazardous waste may be significantly associated with risk of childhood cancer.

Woburn

A cluster of leukemia cases in Woburn, Massachusetts, a suburb of Boston, was discovered in the 1970s.* Affected families, brought together by a local clergyman, plotted cases on a street map to illustrate apparent clustering. Local residents used advocacy and popular epidemiology to attract the attention of government officials, scientists, and the general public. They pointed to a nearby tannery, chemical plant, and industrial laundry as likely sources of contamination of municipal Wells G and H.

Harvard researchers, operating with limited resources, collaborated with the local citizens' group to conduct a telephone survey. They found associations between past exposure to water from Wells G and H and rates of perinatal deaths, two of five categories of congenital anomalies, childhood disorders of the urinary and respiratory tracts, and childhood leukemia.[1] The study's findings were debated.

To obtain more-precise estimates of individuals' past exposures, the Massachusetts Department of Public Health (MDPH) contracted with a civil engineer to refine its water distribution model, which had been used in the Harvard study. Fifty hydraulically distinct zones of exposure within Woburn were defined by integrating well pumping records, dimensions of water pipes, and historical modifications to the municipal system.[2] This modeling project yielded quantitative estimates of the industrial solvent trichloroethylene (TCE) in the tap water of homes during the 1960s.

In a case-control study, MDPH researchers assessed the risk of childhood leukemia in relation to past tap water exposure to TCE, based on mothers' residential and pregnancy histories. Random misclassification of exposure, which routinely biases epidemiologic findings toward "the null" (no effect), was thereby minimized. The study found that risk of childhood leukemia in Woburn increased with maternal consumption of contaminated drinking water during pregnancy; a statistical test for trend across exposure categories was significant for the period of pregnancy, suggesting a dose-response relationship between drinking water exposure during pregnancy and childhood leukemia.[3]

---

* Featured in the PBS Nova documentary *Toxic Trials* (1986) and the book *A Civil Action* by Jonathan Harr (1995), followed by a fictionalized film (1998).

Toms River

Another cluster of childhood cancer was discovered in the 1980s, providing conditions similar to Woburn for epidemiologists and public stakeholders to move beyond cluster investigations to analytical epidemiology utilizing individual-level estimates of exposure.[4]

A chemical factory, operating since the 1950s in Toms River, a suburban community in Ocean County, New Jersey, came under intense public scrutiny for its disposal practices. As early as the 1960s, chemicals from the plant's dyestuffs and resin manufacturing processes that had been discharged into the Toms River were drawn into a public drinking water well through the area's sandy soil. After shifting to land disposal, the company incurred in the 1980s state criminal sanctions and clean-up costs for its unlined waste lagoons and chemical landfill. At an old egg farm located 1 mile from the plant, another company's toxic waste leached from an illicit disposal trench into a second public drinking water source, the "Parkway" wells.

Initially unconnected to the toxic waste issue, a support network of families dealing with childhood cancer formed in Ocean County in the early 1980s. Protest actions by environmental activists opposed to the chemical company's 7-mile pipeline discharging waste into the Atlantic Ocean thrust the community into the national spotlight. Local leaders emerged to demand accountability of government agencies and companies.

An apparent cluster of childhood brain cancer and leukemia cases in Toms River led to an investigation by ATSDR and state agencies, in cooperation with local government agencies, community groups, and academic researchers. Incidence data from the state cancer registry from 1979 to 1995 for girls under age 5 in the Toms River area revealed a significant 9-fold elevation in acute lymphocytic leukemia and a significant 11-fold elevation in brain and other central nervous cancers.[5]

A case-control study found a significant association between prenatal exposure to water from the Parkway wellfield over a 15-year period and incidence of leukemia in girls. It also found an exposure-response relationship between prenatal air exposures, modeled from historical production records of the chemical plant, and leukemia risk in girls under 5 years of age.

References

1. Lagakos SW, Wessen BJ, Zelen M. An analysis of contaminated well water and health effects in Woburn, Massachusetts. Journal of the American Statistical Association 1986; 81: 583–596.
2. Bureau of Environmental Assessment. Appendix XI: Murphy Water Distribution Model, in Woburn Childhood Leukemia Follow-up Study, Volume II Appendices. Boston, MA: Massachusetts Department of Public Health, 1997, p. 131.
3. Costas K, Knorr RS, Condon SK. A case-control study of childhood leukemia in Woburn, Massachusetts: The relationship between leukemia incidence and exposure to public drinking water. Science of the Total Environment 2002; 300: 23–35.
4. Fagin D. Toms River: A story of science and salvation. New York: Bantam Books, 2013, p. 538.
5. Maslia ML, Reyes JJ, Gillig RE, et al. Public health partnerships addressing childhood cancer investigations: Case study of Toms River, Dover Township, New Jersey, USA. International Journal of Hygiene and Environmental Health 2005; 208: 45–54.

with cool rationality.[7] To respond effectively to communities, public health professionals need to be able to educate the public and health professionals, actively listen, and respectfully support the detective work of community residents (popular, or participatory, epidemiology).[8,9] Health officials accustomed to doing "just science" often discover they must share power with citizens' groups.[10-12]

The term *hazardous waste* is a social construct: its meaning changes with societal perceptions and concerns. Originally, it denoted industrial liquid chemicals leaking from corroded barrels at disposal sites that migrated into the drinking water, backyards, basements, and sumps of nearby residences. Love Canal, a community built on a hazardous waste site in Upstate New York, was the site of an historic event in the 1970s, when residents noted a wide range of adverse health effects that seemed to be related to wastes at the site.[13] Over time, however, it was recognized that Love Canal was not that unusual; any garbage dump that was active before about 1985 might, in fact, be a hazardous waste site.

The term *hazardous waste* also applies to problems as disparate as (a) one-time environmental releases of chemicals, such as by spills, leaks, fires, and explosions; (b) medium-duration exposure of military personnel near burn-pits on bases in Iraq and Afghanistan;[14] and (c) long-term problems, such as the presence of radioactive and chemical wastes from the Cold War era at facilities of the military and the U.S. Department of Energy.[15] The wide variety of contaminants, settings, and populations available for study has challenged scientists, required innovation, and generated a social movement that has challenged traditional modes of scientific inquiry and governmental decision-making, while stimulating cooperative projects among communities and public health scientists.[16,17]

With the enactment of federal community right-to-know legislation in 1986, which required industrial facilities emitting toxic substances to file public reports, the term *hazardous waste* expanded to include air and water pathways of factory pollution. Increasingly, stringent disposal regulations spurred the expansion of a "treatment, storage, and disposal" industry for chemical wastes. This industry generally took

the path of least resistance and expanded into minority and working-class communities—in both urban and rural areas.[18,19] And the Environmental Justice Movement was born.

Environmental justice advocates refer to racial and class-based disparities in the siting of polluting industries. Evidence of disparate levels of exposure and increased occurrence of illness form the basis for grassroots campaigns and lawsuits, based on both civil-rights and environmental laws, to hasten clean-up projects and implement other interventions.

To overcome the limited statistical power of neighborhood-sized populations, environmental epidemiologists seek ways to increase the size of study groups and/or the numbers of countable events. National and state-level registries of adverse birth outcomes have revealed ecologic associations between (a) proximity to hazardous waste sites and (b) low birthweight and certain congenital anomalies.[20-24] A crude exposure surrogate of proximity to hazardous waste sites enables epidemiologists to include geographic areas large enough to capture many rare outcomes. Knowledge of each waste site's principal contaminants, such as solvents, metals, and pesticides, allows for the testing of more specific hypotheses.[25,26] While ecologic studies suffer from various biases due to a lack of individual-level data, some analytical (cohort and case-control) studies have also found elevated rates of congenital anomalies, including neural-tube and cardiac defects, that are associated with hazardous waste contamination.[27,28]

Enhanced statistical power, facilitated by the availability of large health-agency datasets with tens of millions of person-years of observation, has revealed ecological associations between proximity to hazardous waste sites and chronic diseases, including chronic obstructive pulmonary disease, hematologic malignancies, and breast cancer.[29-31] These findings are often consistent with the results of analytical studies.[32-36] Innovations in geographic methods have enhanced exploratory studies of possible associations between environmental exposures and adverse health outcomes.[37]

An alternative approach to investigating the possible health effects of hazardous waste is by studying the prevalence of symptoms in neighborhoods near hazardous waste sites.[38,39] Recall bias and confounding are major potential limitations of these studies. However, some increases in the prevalence of symptoms among exposed residents persist after controlling for recall bias and confounding and can be used as a basis for further research.[40]

Biological markers show promise as refined measures of exposures to synthetic organic chemicals. For example, the impact of public health advisories recommending that pregnant women reduce their fish intake has been assessed by concentration of polychlorinated biphenyls (PCBs) in breast milk, which has decreased.[41] However, use of biological markers as precursors of disease still presents major interpretative challenges.

Among genetic markers, chromosomal abnormalities are generally recognized as steps in—or very near to—causal pathways to cancer and certain congenital anomalies. However, the clinical significance of sister chromatid exchanges and point mutations in specific genes is less clear. Micronuclei, small chromosomal fragments arising from errors in or interruption of DNA synthesis, are measurable in both exfoliated cells (such as in buccal smears) and lymphocytes. An increased frequency of micronuclei may be an index of accumulated DNA damage as well as future risk of cancer.[42]

Application of a battery of immune markers may reveal associations with exposure (or residential proximity) to a waste site, but the clinical significance of this association may remain unknown.[43,44] Correlations observed between specific biomarkers and exposures in groups of study participants may not be interpretable at the level of individuals.

HAZARDOUS WASTE MANAGEMENT

Hazardous waste management includes treatment, storage, and disposal. It may also include reclamation and incineration—depending on technology, cost, regulation, and physical and chemical properties. Treatment, such as diluting or neutralizing a strong acid or base, can alter the chemical and physical composition of waste, making it less likely to cause harm. Treatment also includes filtering, solidifying,

or evaporating waste. Waste treatment is often done in surface impoundments, such as diked lagoons or ponds, where hazardous waste is temporarily contained. These sites, which are open surface facilities that can hold liquid or partially solidified hazardous waste, vary widely in size. To prevent leakage, barriers of clay or other impermeable material are used to line these holding areas, and groundwater is monitored for possible contamination. Hazardous waste may also be stored before treatment or disposal; for example, a treatment operator may hold a volume of waste targeted for reclamation until markets are favorable to sell the reclaimed product.

Disposal is defined as burial of hazardous waste. Land disposal, which is regulated, includes injection into deep wells, landfilling, and land farming. Injection, used for disposing most hazardous waste, requires wells with depths greater than drinking-water aquifers. Abandoned oil and gas wells in Texas and other oil-producing states are often used for this purpose.

Landfills are holes below ground level where hazardous waste may be stored permanently. Landfills must be lined with impermeable material, such as clay. Liquids that leach out must be collected and treated. Groundwater must be periodically tested by monitoring wells surrounding the site. Some hazardous wastes are banned from landfills, and generators must treat certain wastes to lessen their toxicity before they are sent to landfills.

In *land farming*, which relies on bacterial decomposition of hazardous waste, waste from petroleum refineries or elsewhere, is sprayed onto land that is then tilled to mix waste, soil, and oxygen from the air with nutrients and bacteria. The resultant mixture enhances breakdown of waste into safer substances.

Incineration (thermal decomposition of material) is a method used for hazardous waste comprised of organic compounds that can be broken down to simpler chemical components in kilns containing a flame at 1,600°F or higher. While waste volume is greatly reduced, ashes may contain high concentrations of heavy metals, and the stack emissions contaminate the air. Toxicants of concern include particulate matter, heavy metals (such as mercury and lead), irritant gases (such as nitrogen oxides and sulfur dioxide), volatile organic compounds, and dioxins and furans.[45] Since incineration is relatively expensive, less than 3% of hazardous waste in the United States is treated in this manner. Incinerators come in a variety of forms that are appropriate to the waste being treated. For example, rotary kilns are used for solids, injection incinerators for liquids, and specially designed furnaces for explosives. Properly operating incineration—with accurately controlled temperature, turbulence, and oxygen concentrations—breaks down organic waste into carbon dioxide, water, and ash. If combustion is incomplete, carbon monoxide may form. Measurement of carbon monoxide in flue gas is used to determine the effectiveness of incinerator performance. Although in reduced volume, inorganic hazardous waste may still be hazardous after incineration.

Hazardous waste may be reclaimed as a commercially useful product. Heavy metals, such as lead, can be reclaimed or recycled from discarded lead-acid batteries, silver can be reclaimed from certain types of photographic processes, and spent degreasing solvents can be cleaned and reclaimed. Some hazardous wastes can be reclaimed in other than their original forms. One popular means of reclamation is use of combustible hazardous waste as fuel in kilns to produce cement. Further attempts at source reduction, cradle-to-grave stewardship, recycling, and reclamation can reduce hazardous waste volumes and increase efficiency of production.

RCRA enacted in 1976 and administered by the EPA, is the primary federal legislation for managing solid waste, including hazardous waste. The RCRA is structured around controlling hazardous waste from cradle to grave, including generation, treatment, storage, and disposal.[46] RCRA covers waste from mines, municipalities, and oil and gas production, manufacturing, and coal production facilities. Although the EPA's authority to directly regulate medical wastes under RCRA lapsed in 1991, federal regulations on air emissions from incinerators at healthcare facilities have spurred the development alternative treatment methods, with stakeholder participation by environmentally concerned health professionals.[47]

POLLUTION PREVENTION AND TOXICS USE REDUCTION

The phrase "Pollution prevention pays" was coined by the 3M Company in the 1970s to describe practices that focused on process and material changes rather than end-of-the pipe treatment. Shortly after federal RCRA landfill regulations went into effect, California produced, in 1981, a report on alternatives to land disposal, such as incineration, physical treatment, and pollution prevention.[48] Next, the state implemented a land disposal ban of certain priority chemicals, which was adopted by Congress in the 1984 amendments to RCRA.

With the Pollution Prevention Act of 1990, Congress mandated the hierarchy of managing waste:

- Pollution should be prevented or reduced at the source whenever feasible.
- Pollution that cannot be prevented should be recycled in an environmentally safe manner.
- Pollution that cannot be prevented or recycled should be treated in an environmentally safe manner.
- Disposal or other releases into the environment should be employed only as a last resort.

In two states, legislative strategies emerged. In California, a 1986 referendum (Proposition 65) led to a law that required public notification of carcinogens and reproductive toxins in products sold to consumers or released into sources of drinking water; the law has resulted in many products being reformulated to eliminate reportable chemicals. In Massachusetts, a state Toxics Use Reduction Act was enacted in 1989, requiring companies to submit annual plans for reducing their use of toxic chemicals and to demonstrate reductions over time. The act also established the Toxics Use Reduction Institute at the University of Massachusetts Lowell to assist industry.[49] As a result of the act, from 1990 to 2005, facilities using the most-toxic chemicals reduced their use by 40%, toxic by-products by 71%, toxics shipped in product by 41%, on-site releases of toxics to the environment by 91%, and transfers of toxics offsite for further waste management by 60%.[50]

Tools for Pollution Prevention

The hazardous waste problem is first and foremost a toxic chemical use problem. Proposals have been made, mainly by the European Union, to "sunset" (phase out) the use of high-priority chemicals. Policymakers in the United States have focused on tools to evaluate and encourage the use of alternatives.[51] These tools can be voluntarily adopted by businesses; their use is also encouraged by incentives, such as environmental labeling programs, and government-business partnerships.

The EPA, in cooperation with industry and academia, has developed chemical ranking and scoring tools. Less toxic alternatives have been referred to as "safe substitutes" and "safer chemical substitutes." Methodologies utilized have been termed *cleaner technology substitute assessments, chemicals alternative analysis,* and *alternatives assessment.*[52-55] These methodologies evaluate comparative risk, performance, cost, and resource conservation alternatives by industry sector. Businesses can use these methodologies. In addition, the EPA Design for the Environment Program performs voluntary cooperative assessments with chemical manufacturers and other entities, including consumers, over the entire lifecycle of a product—from cradle to grave, including raw material acquisition, production, transportation, use, and end-of-life disposition.[56] Life-cycle assessment (LCA) was developed to ensure that the safer substitutes do not create worse environmental impacts, such as introduction of other more-toxic raw materials, increased energy use, or waste disposal problems. LCA provides for a well-informed comparison of alternatives.

Emerging Pollution Prevention Policies

A centerpiece of U.S. toxic chemicals regulation, the Toxic Substances Control Act of 1976, was found to be inadequate to address new and existing toxic chemicals. In 2016, a political consensus was forged to reform the law. New amendments to the law direct the EPA to prioritize chemicals for assessment; create a fast-track process for addressing certain persistent, bioaccumulative, and toxic chemicals; permit the EPA to ban chemicals when unreasonable risks are identified; and require the EPA to make an affirmative finding on the safety of a new chemical (or significant new use of an existing one) before the chemical is permitted to enter the marketplace. These amendments will preempt certain state regulations.

An even more fundamental approach has evolved to target how industry chooses materials. The concept of *green chemistry* is the design of products and processes that reduce or eliminate the generation of hazardous substances. It has evolved from a set of principles to an EPA-sponsored research program and an annual awards program, the Presidential Green Chemistry Challenge.[57] Prominent academics have advocated for rethinking of the materials that we, as a society, use and for developing a policy framework that includes methods for characterizing, classifying, and prioritizing chemicals; generating and using new chemical information; and promoting transitions to safer chemicals.[58,59] California's Green Chemistry Initiative, two parts of which became law in 2008, contains elements of this approach.[60]

Environmental labeling is a voluntary, incentive-based approach to award an environmental seal of approval to consumer products with reduced environmental impacts, as compared to other products that perform the same function. Green Seal, Inc., a nonprofit organization founded in 1989, operates the oldest environmental labeling program in the United States. The program has several standards that focus on reducing the use of toxic chemicals, including standards for paints and household cleaners. Products that are evaluated and comply with the standards can display the Green Seal on their label. Recently, the EPA has begun a similar initiative, its Safer Choice labeling program.

Extended producer responsibility (EPR) is a policy to promote environmental improvements of product systems by extending the responsibilities of the manufacturer to the entire lifecycle of the product, especially to take-back, recycling, and final disposal.[61,62] EPR evolved from a requirement in Germany for producers to take back the packaging of products and bear the expense of recycling it. *Take-back policies,* in general, require producers to arrange or take financial responsibility for managing products or packaging them after their use. There are similar policies, sometimes called *extended product responsibility (product stewardship)*, the purpose of which is to require or encourage cooperation for environmental improvements through the lifecycle of the product, including reduction in toxic chemical use and hazardous waste generation. For example, producer responsibility for handling products at the end of their lifecycle has resulted in reduction in the use of mercury in batteries and use of lead in electronics products. However, EPR programs requiring take-back of products have not always resulted in reduction in exposure to toxic chemicals; certain programs have simply exported the end-of-life products to low- and middle-income countries where recycling is performed without regard to exposure of workers and the general public.[63]

REMEDIATING ABANDONED AND ILLEGAL HAZARDOUS WASTE SITES

Public awareness of hazardous waste was heightened in the second half of the 20th century with reports of abandoned and uncontrolled hazardous waste sites and spilled, or illegally dumped, hazardous waste that posed a threat to public health or the environment.[13] Too often, extensive sites were abandoned, with no one to hold responsible for cleaning them up.[2] A series of legislative acts to address the problem became known as the *Superfund Law*. To support remediation of abandoned sites, the U.S. federal government established Superfund from taxes on chemical manufacturers.

Superfund

Superfund began in 1980 with enactment of the Comprehensive Environmental Response, Compensation and Liability Act (CERCLA). It was updated and improved by the Superfund Amendments and Reauthorization Act (SARA) in 1986. Administered by the EPA, Superfund established (a) liability, in the event of releases or spills for generators, transporters, and managers of hazardous waste, and (b) an almost $9 billion fund, which has been used for remediation of hazardous waste sites when those responsible

for them cannot be identified or lack resources to conduct clean-up. (Superfund excludes petroleum products and radioactive material waste.)

Superfund clean-up is based on a multistep approach beginning with site discovery, preliminary assessment, and a site inspection to determine whether emergency action is required. In the first step of long-term remediation, which can last 10 or more years, site data are entered into the EPA's *Hazard Ranking System* to determine if the degree of public health hazard merits a site's inclusion on the National Priorities List (NPL). A remedial investigation/feasibility study is performed on each NPL site to (a) detail the nature and extent of its health and safety risks and (b) develop recommendations for clean-up. Remedy selection follows analysis of recommended alternatives. In the next phase, remedial design, engineering plans are developed for the remediation. Ultimately, remedial action is implemented through construction work. After remedial action has been completed, project close-out is done and the site is removed from the NPL (delisted).

The EPA provides technical assistance grants for community groups to hire independent experts to review technical documents and facilitate public engagement in Superfund remediation projects. Reconceiving an NPL site as a primarily public works project—with environmental benefits—may be helpful in overcoming technocratic inertia and in building support for remedial action among the Superfund program's key constituencies: community groups, private-sector firms, and construction-worker unions.[64]

As of May 2017, the EPA reported to have conducted or overseen 1,184 clean-up construction projects under the Superfund program. There were then 1,336 hazardous waste sites on the NPL; 393 sites had been delisted and 53 new sites had been proposed to be added. (An updated list of NPL sites may be found at https://www.epa.gov/superfund/national-priorities-list-npl-sites-state.) The many complexities of the Superfund clean-up program relate to inadequate information for subsurface geologic investigations, costly engineering remedies, involvement of multiple stakeholders with differing interests, and ongoing proposals for fundamental reforms in program administration.[65-67]

In 1998, the EPA developed the concept of a *brownfields* site, defined as "real property, the expansion, redevelopment, or reuse of which may be complicated by the presence or potential presence of a hazardous substance, pollutant, or contaminant."[68] Other locally unwanted land uses, such as actively polluting factories, typically fall outside the definition of brownfields.[3] Decision-makers involved with preparing brownfields sites for productive reuse often require technical and legal assistance to fully understand the complexities of investigating and cleaning up contaminated sites. (Additional information about brownfields programs may be found at http://www.brownfieldstsc.org/.)

ROLES OF OTHER FEDERAL GOVERNMENT ENTITIES

As it enacted various laws, Congress recognized the significance of the public health impact of unregulated hazardous waste and releases. Superfund has helped address public health issues related to hazardous wastes by establishing federal programs to respond to documented needs. For example, a program was established at the National Institute of Environmental Health Sciences to conduct research on preventing adverse health effects related to hazardous waste.[69] Prodded by labor unions working in coalition with environmentalists, Congress has recognized the need to protect workers in hazardous waste operations and emergency responses, has directed the Occupational Safety and Health Administration to promulgate relevant protective workplace standards and has provided funding for occupational safety and health training (Figure 18-2).[64]

CERCLA was designed to address past hazardous waste disposal activities, even if disposal or the substance was not previously considered hazardous. The EPA was mandated to investigate sites, develop clean-up plans, and negotiate payment by responsible parties. Congress recognized the need to address the health concerns of communities and, as part of CERCLA, established the Agency for Toxic Substances and Disease Registry (ATSDR) to work with the EPA by assessing the adverse public health impacts of these sites.[70]

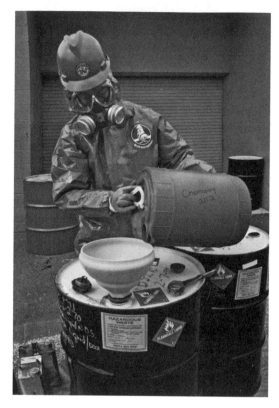

Figure 18-2. Hazardous waste worker. (Photograph by Earl Dotter.)

Consolidated administratively with the National Center for Environmental Health at the Centers for Disease Control and Prevention, ATSDR has a multidisciplinary staff of epidemiologists, toxicologists, physicians, public health educators, and others. Clinicians, community members, and others can request assistance from ATSDR to address concerns about potential health effects from hazardous waste sites by submitting a written petition that should include available relevant environmental data and the facility name, location, description of hazardous waste release, and relevant health data. ATSDR performs health consultations, which are written evaluations about hazardous substances released at a site and the likelihood that human exposure can occur or has occurred, and if the level of exposure could result in harm. ATSDR also performs public health assessments, which are more comprehensive evaluations that examine multiple exposure pathways. In addition, ATSDR makes public health recommendations to the EPA and other government agencies concerning hazardous waste sites.

Federal Plans for Emergency Response

Unplanned spills and releases of hazardous waste present special problems for public health protection, depending on the toxicity and physical characteristics of the chemicals involved. Congress anticipated these emergency situations as it enacted hazardous waste–related legislation and provided means to address these situations through governmental agencies.

For multimedia accidental chemical releases, oil spills, and other smaller scale events, fire and police personnel are universally recognized as first responders. Specific large-scale events—such as train derailments, chemical plant explosions, aerospace accidents, and natural disasters—may require other professionals, not generally recognized as first responders, to participate with first responders. (See Chapter 31.)

The National Oil and Hazardous Substance Pollution Contingency Plan (NCP), the first comprehensive system of accident reporting, spill containment, and clean-up requirements, was promulgated in the 1968 Clean Water Act and has since been refined. It established the requirements for response headquarters and national and regional reaction teams, which were the precursors to the current National Response Team and Regional Response Teams. The NCP identifies the responsibilities of 15 participating federal agencies during an emergency. The National Response Team is responsible for the administration and implementation of the NCP, as well as the planning and coordination of all national response activities.

When releases are serious enough to be considered "nationally significant incidents," the National Response Framework (NRF) is activated and works in conjunction with the NCP. The NRF is the federal government's comprehensive, all-hazard approach to crisis management and provides a mechanism for coordinating federal assistance to state governments and localities.[71] The development of an NRF was mandated by the Homeland Security Act (2002) and the Homeland Security Presidential Directive-5 (2003). The plan was completed in 2005 and has been revised periodically.[72] The NRF integrates the NCP and other national-level contingency plans addressing terrorism, radiological incidents, and natural disasters. A National Incident Management System delineates the Incident Command System for coordination across agencies and jurisdictions. (See Box 31-1 in Chapter 31.)

Hazardous releases are most likely to occur in industrial disasters such as chemical plant fires and explosions. But natural disasters, such as floods, hurricanes, and earthquakes, can also cause oil and chemical tanks to be displaced and their contents released. Facilities that store large quantities of acutely toxic materials may also be vulnerable to terrorist attacks. Progress has been slow in reducing these "vulnerable targets" through legally enforceable limits and mandates for the use of less toxic materials.[73]

CONCLUSION

Uncontrolled hazardous waste can cause acute or chronic disease and threaten the environment. Contaminated land can be a barrier to economic revitalization of a community. Since clean-up of contaminated communities costs more than prevention and control of hazardous waste, more emphasis needs to be placed on prevention and control measures. Through regulation and other systematic approaches, governmental agencies can encourage waste managers to reduce waste at its source, ensure that hazardous and solid wastes are managed safely at industrial facilities, recycle waste to conserve materials or energy, manage waste to prevent spills and releases of toxic materials, and clean up contaminated sites. Federal research and monitoring programs can help identify adverse health effects of hazardous waste, and they can help develop better ways to manage streams of hazardous waste and to clean up uncontrolled sites.

REFERENCES

1. Melosi MV. The sanitary city: Urban infrastructure in America from colonial times to the present. Baltimore & London: Johns Hopkins University Press, 2000.

2. Colten CE, Skinner PN. The road to Love Canal: Managing industrial waste before EPA. Austin: University of Texas Press, 1996, p. 217.

3. Lerner S. Sacrifice zones: The front lines of toxic chemical exposure in the United States. Cambridge, MA: MIT Press, 2010, p. 346.

4. U.S. Environmental Protection Agency. RCRA's critical mission and the path forward (EPA 530-R-14-002). Washington, DC: EPA, 2014, p. 24. Available at: https://www.epa.gov/sites/production/files/2015-09/documents/rcras_critical_mission_and_the_path_forward.pdf. Accessed October 25, 2016.

5. Princen T. The cultural: The magic, the vision, the power. In T Princen, JP Mano, PL Martin (eds.). Ending the fossil fuel era. Cambridge, MA: MIT Press, 2015, pp. 53–95.

6. Ozonoff D, Boden LI. Truth and consequences: Health agency responses to environmental health problems. Science, Technology and Human Values 1987; 12: 70–77.

7. Fagin D. Toms River: A story of science and Salvation. New York: Bantam Books, 2013, p. 538.

8. Brown P. Popular epidemiology and toxic waste contamination: Lay and professional ways of knowing. In S Kroll-Smith, P Brown, VJ Gunter (eds.). Illness and the environment: A reader in contested medicine. New York: NYU Press, 2000, pp. 364–383.

9. Clapp R. Popular epidemiology in three contaminated communities. Annals of the American Academy of Political and Social Sciences 2002; 584: 35–46.

10. Till JE. Building credibility in public studies. American Scientist 1995; 83: 468–473.

11. Maslia ML, Reyes JJ, Gillig RE, et al. Public health partnerships addressing childhood cancer investigations: Case study of Toms River, Dover Township, New Jersey, USA. International Journal of Hygiene and Environmental Health 2005; 208: 45–54.

12. Allen BL. Uneasy alchemy: Citizens and experts in Louisiana's Chemical Corridor disputes. In R Gottlieb (ed.). Urban and industrial environments. Cambridge, MA: MIT Press, 2003; p. 211.

13. Adeola FO. Hazardous wastes, industrial disasters, and environmental health risks. New York: Palgrave Macmillan, 2011, p. 235.

14. Institute of Medicine. Long-term health consequences of exposure to burn pits in Iraq and Afghanistan. Washington, DC: National Academies Press, 2011, p. 180.

15. Rahm D. (ed.). Toxic waste and environmental policy in the 21st century United States.

16. Jefferson, NC: McFarland & Company, 2002, p. 184.

16. Brown P, Morello-Frosch R, Zavestoski S (eds.). Contested illnesses: Citizens, science, and health social movements. Berkeley: University of California Press, 2012, p. 324.

17. Quigley D, Lowman A, Wing S (eds.). Tortured science: Health studies, ethics, and nuclear weapons in the United States. In RH Elling (ed.). Critical approaches in the health social sciences series. Amityville, NY: Baywood Publishing, 2012, p. 265.

18. Bullard RD. Dumping in Dixie: Race, class, and environmental quality. Boulder, CO: Westview Press, 1990, p. 165.

19. Murdock SH, Krannich RS, Leistritz FL, et al (eds.). Hazardous wastes in rural America: Impacts, implications, and options for rural communities. Lanham, MD: Rowman & Littlefield, 1999, p. 231.

20. Croen LA, Shaw GM, Sanbonmatsu L. Maternal residential proximity to hazardous waste sites and risk for selected congenital malformation. Epidemiology 1997; 8: 347–354.

21. Vrijhedi M, Dolk M, Armstrong B. Chromosomal anomalies and residence near hazardous waste landfill sites. Lancet 2002; 359: 320–322.

22. Orr M, Bove F, Kaye W, Stone M. Elevated birth defects in racial or ethnic minority children of women living near hazardous waste sites. International Journal of Hygiene and Environmental Health 2002; 205: 19–27.

23. Dolk M, Vrijhedi M, Armstrong B. Risk of congenital anomalies near hazardous-waste landfill sites in Europe: EUROHAZCON study. Lancet 1998; 352: 423–427.

24. Baibergenova A, Kudyakov R, Zdeb M, Carpenter DO. Low birth weight and residential proximity to PCB-contaminated waste sites. Environmental Health Perspectives 2003; 111: 1352–1357.

25. Kuehn CM, Mueller BA, Checkoway H, Williams M. Risk of malformations associated with residential proximity to hazardous waste sites in Washington State. Environmental Research 2007; 103: 405–412.

26. Mueller BA, Kuehn CM, Shapiro-Mendoza CK, Tomashek KM. Fetal deaths and proximity to hazardous waste sites in Washington state. Environmental Health Perspectives 2007; 115: 776–780.

27. Malik S, Schechter A, Caughy M, Fixler DE. Effect of proximity to hazardous waste sites on the development of congenital heart disease.

Archives of Environmental Health 2004; 59: 177–181.

28. Ruckart PZ, Bove FJ, Maslia M. Evaluation of exposure to contaminated drinking water and specific birth defects and childhood cancers at Marine Corps Base Camp Lejeune, North Carolina: a case-control study. Environmental Health 2013; 12: 104.

29. Carpenter DO, Ma J, Lessner L. Asthma and infectious respiratory disease in relation to residence near hazardous waste sites. Annals of the New York Academy of Sciences 2008; 1140: 201–208.

30. Boberg E, Lessner L, Carpenter DO. The role of residence near hazardous waste sites containing benzene in the development of hematologic cancers in upstate New York. International Journal of Occupational and Environmental Health 2011; 24: 327–338.

31. Lu X, Lessner L, Carpenter DO. Association between hospital discharge rate for female breast cancer and residence in a zip code containing hazardous waste sites. Environmental Research 2014; 134: 375–381.

32. Rennix CP, Quinn MM, Amoroso PJ, et al. Risk of breast cancer among enlisted Army women occupationally exposed to volatile organic compounds. American Journal of Industrial Medicine 2005; 48: 157–167.

33. Talbott EO, Xu X, Youk AO, et al. Risk of leukemia as a result of community exposure to gasoline vapors: a follow-up study. Environmental Research 2011; 111: 597–602.

34. Nirel R, Maimon N, Fireman E, et al. Respiratory hospitalizations of children living near a hazardous industrial site adjusted for prevalent dust: A case-control study. International Journal of Hygiene and Environmental Health 2015; 218: 273–279.

35. Ruckart PZ, Bove FJ, Shanley E 3rd, Maslia M. Evaluation of contaminated drinking water and male breast cancer at Marine Corps Base Camp Lejeune, North Carolina: A case control study. Environmental Health 2015: 14: 74.

36. Aschengrau A, Rogers S, Ozonoff D. Perchloroethylene-contaminated drinking water and the risk of breast cancer: Additional results from Cape Cod, Massachusetts, USA. Environmental Health Perspectives 2003; 111: 167–173.

37. Shaddick G, Zidek JV. Spatio-temporal methods in environmental epidemiology. Boca Raton, FL: CRC Press, 2016, p. 365.

38. Dayal H, Gupta S, Trieff N. Symptom clusters in a community chronic exposure to chemicals in

two Superfund sites. Archives of Environmental Health 1995; 50: 108–111.

39. Baker DB, Greenland S, Mendlein J, Harmon P. A health study of two communities near the Stringfellow Waste Disposal site. Archives of Environmental Health 1988; 43: 325–334.

40. Ozonoff D, Colten ME, Cupples A. Health problems reported by residents of a neighborhood contaminated by a hazardous waste facility. American Journal of Industrial Medicine 1987; 11: 581–597.

41. Fitzgerald EF, Hwang S-A, Langguth K, et al. Fish consumption and other environmental exposures and their associations with serum PCB concentrations among Mohawk women at Akwesasne. Environmental Research 2004; 94: 160–170.

42. Mateuca RA, Decordier I, Kirsch-Volders M. Cytogenetic methods in human biomonitoring: Principles and uses. Methods in Molecular Biology 2012; 817: 305–334.

43. Vine MF, Stein L, Weigle K. Effects on the immune system associated with living near a pesticide dump. Environmental Health Perspectives 2000; 108: 1113–1124.

44. Williamson DM, White MC, Poole C, et al. Evaluation of serum immunoglobulins among individuals living near six Superfund sites. Environmental Health Perspectives 2006; 114: 1065–1071.

45. Committee on Health Effects of Waste Incineration, Board on Environmental Studies and Toxicology, National Research Council. Waste incineration and public health. Washington, DC: National Academies Press, 2000, p. 334.

46. U.S. Environmental Protection Agency. The National Biennial RCRA Hazardous Waste Report (based on 2011 data). Washington, DC: National Analysis, 2012, p. 62.

47. Gerwig K. Greening health care: How hospitals can heal the planet. Oxford: Oxford University Press, 2014, p. 280.

48. Stoddard SK, Davis GA, Freeman H. Alternatives to the land disposal of hazardous wastes: An assessment for California. Sacramento: California Governor's Office of Appropriate Technology, Toxic Waste Assessment Group, 1981.

49. Ellenbecker M, Geiser K. At the source: The origins of the Massachusetts toxics use reduction program and an overview of this special issue. Journal of Cleaner Production 2011; 19: 389–396.

50. Executive Office of Energy and Environmental Affairs. Toxics Use Reduction Act (TURA)

Program Overview. Available at: http://www.mass.gov/eea/agencies/massdep/toxics/tur/toxics-use-reduction-act-tura-program-overview.html. Accessed September 28, 2016.

51. Davis GA. The sun also rises: Evaluating the potential for safe substitutes for priority chemicals. In: K Geiser, F Irwin (eds.). Rethinking the materials we use: A new focus for pollution policy. Washington, DC: World Wildlife Fund, 1993.

52. Geiser K, Tickner J, Edward S, Rossi M. The architecture of chemical alternatives analysis. Risk Analysis 2015; 35: 2152–2161.

53. Davis GA, Kincaid L, Swanson M. Chemical hazard evaluation for management systems: A method for ranking and scoring chemicals by potential human health and environmental impacts. Cincinnati, OH: Risk Reduction Engineering Laboratory, Office of Research and Development, 1993.

54. Davis GA, Kincaid L, Menke D. The product side of pollution prevention: Evaluating the potential for safe substitutes. Cincinnati, OH: Risk Reduction Engineering Laboratory, Office of Research and Development, 1994.

55. U.S. Environmental Protection Agency, Office of Pollution Prevention & Toxics. Design for the Environment Program Alternatives Assessment Criteria for Hazard Evaluation Version, 2011. Available at: https://www.epa.gov/sites/production/files/2014-01/documents/aa_criteria_v2.pdf. Accessed October 26, 2016.

56. U.S. Environmental Protection Agency. Design for the Environment Alternatives Assessments. Available at: https://www.epa.gov/saferchoice/design-environment-alternatives-assessments. Accessed September 28, 2016.

57. Anastas PT, Warner JC. Green chemistry: Theory and practice. Oxford: Oxford University Press, 1998.

58. Geiser K. Chemicals without harm: Policies for a sustainable world. Cambridge, MA: MIT Press, 2016.

59. Geiser K. Materials matter: Toward a sustainable materials policy. Cambridge, MA: MIT Press, 2001.

60. California Department of Toxic Substances Control. Green chemistry resources. Available at: http://www.dtsc.ca.gov/PollutionPrevention/GreenChemistryResources/index.cfm. Accessed August 20, 2017.

61. Davis GA, Wilt CA, Barkenbus JN. Extended product responsibility: A tool for a sustainable economy. Environment 1997; 39: 10–15, 36–38.

62. Lindhqvist T. Extended producer responsibility in cleaner production: Policy principle to promote environmental improvements of product systems, 2000. Available at: http://portal.research.lu.se/portal/files/4433708/1002025.pdf. Accessed October 26, 2016.

63. Grossman E. High tech trash: Digital devices, hidden toxics, and human health. Washington, DC: Island Press, 2016.

64. Slatin C. Environmental unions: Labor and the Superfund. In: C Levenstein, R Forrant, J Wooding (eds.). Work, health, and environment series. Amityville, NY: Baywood Publishing, 2009, p. 246.

65. Macey GP, Cannon JZ (eds.). Reclaiming the land: Rethinking Superfund institutions, methods and practices. New York: Springer, 2007, p. 305.

66. Sara MN. Site assessment and remediation handbook (2nd ed.) Boca Raton, FL: Lewis Publishers, 2003, p. 944.

67. Lehr J, Hyman M, Gass T, Seevers WJ (eds.). Handbook of complex environmental remediation problems. New York: McGraw-Hill, 2001.

68. Greenberg M. Measuring the success of the federal government's Brownfields program. Remediation 2005; 15: 83–94.

69. National Institute for Environmental Health Sciences. Superfund basic research program: Balancing scientific excellence with research relevance, October 2008, p. 27. Available at: https://www.niehs.nih.gov/research/supported/assets/docs/r_s/superfund_basic_research_program_balancing_scientific_excellence_with_research_relevance_508.pdf. Accessed October 26, 2016.

70. Johnson BL. Impact of hazardous waste on human health: Hazard, health effects, equity, and communications issues. Boca Raton, FL: CRC Press, 1999, p. 389.

71. Department of Homeland Security. National Response Framework, 2016, p. 52. Available at: https://www.fema.gov/media-library-data/1466014682982-9bcf8245ba4c60c120aa915abe74e15d/National_Response_Framework3rd.pdf. Accessed October 26, 2016.

72. Lindsay BR. The National Response Framework: Overview and possible issues for Congress, 2008, p. 18. Available at: https://www.fas.org/sgp/crs/homesec/RL34758.pdf. Accessed October 26, 2016.

73. Perrow C. The next catastrophe: Reducing our vulnerabilities to natural, industrial, and terrorist disasters. Princeton: Princeton University Press, 2007, p. 377.

WEBSITES FOR ADDITIONAL INFORMATION

Agency for Toxic Substances and Disease Registry. Available at: http://www.atsdr.cdc.gov/Asbestos/sites/libby_montana/
This website describes findings of the public health assessment for the Libby, Montana, asbestos site and related activities.

Brownfields and Land Revitalization Technology Support Center. Available at: http://www.brownfieldstsc.org/
This website describes the Brownfields and Land Revitalization Initiative of the EPA and the U.S. Army Corps of Engineers.

National Oil and Hazardous Substance Pollution Contingency Plan. Title 40 Code of Federal Regulations Subchapter J Superfund, Emergency Planning, and Community Right-to-Know Programs (Part 300 et seq). GPO fdsys.gov. Available at: https://www.gpo.gov/fdsys/pkg/CFR-2015-title40-vol28/pdf/CFR-2015-title40-vol28-chapI-subchapJ.pdf
These are the federal regulations for responding to both oil spills and releases of hazardous substances.

U.S. Environmental Protection Agency. NPL Site Status Information. Available at: https://www.epa.gov/superfund/current-npl-updates-new-proposed-npl-sites-and-new-npl-sites
This website organizes current and proposed Superfund sites by state, date, remediation status, milestones, and other criteria.

U.S. Environmental Protection Agency. Office of Emergency Management. https://www.epa.gov/emergency-response
This website provides an overview of EPA activities in emergency management, including downloadable computer models, links to laboratories, and pending revisions to the National Contingency Plan, the U.S. government blueprint for responding to oil spills and releases of hazardous substances.

U.S. Federal Emergency Management Agency. National Response Framework, 3d edition. 2016. Available at: http://www.fema.gov/media-library/assets/documents/117791
This website describes the National Response Framework, which provides a comprehensive approach to domestic incident management to prevent, prepare for, respond to, and recover from major disasters and other emergencies.

Worker Training Program, National Institute of Environmental Health Sciences https://tools.niehs.nih.gov/wetp/
This website compiles lesson plans from worker training curricula developed by grantees and provides links to related resources.

SECTION IV

ADVERSE HEALTH EFFECTS

19

Injuries and Occupational Safety

Dawn N. Castillo, Timothy J. Pizatella, and Nancy A. Stout

Occupational injuries are caused by acute exposure in the workplace to safety hazards, such as mechanical energy, electricity, chemicals, and ionizing radiation, or from the sudden lack of essential agents, such as oxygen or heat. Examples of events that can lead to worker injury include motor-vehicle crashes, assaults, falls, being caught in parts of machinery, being struck by tools or objects, and contact with electrical energy. Resultant injuries include fractures, lacerations, abrasions, burns, amputations, poisonings, and damage to internal organs.

Occupational and nonoccupational injuries represent a serious public health problem (Box 19-1). More than 4,830 workers died from occupational injuries in the United States in 2015.[1] Another 3.5 million workers sustained nonfatal injuries in 2015;[2] this estimate is conservative because it relies on employer reporting, excludes important groups of workers (such as workers who are self-employed and workers on small farms), and may miss counting many cases.[3] An estimated 2.5 million workers were treated in emergency departments for work-related injuries and illnesses in 2014, with approximately 4% of them being hospitalized immediately or transferred to another hospital, such as a trauma

or burn center.[4] The direct cost of serious occupational injuries in the United States in 2014 was estimated at $59.9 billion,[5] an amount that includes only wages and medical payments to workers whose injuries resulted in more than 6 days away from work.

CAUSES OF INJURY

Although the immediate cause of injury is exposure to energy or deprivation from essential agents (such as oxygen deficiency), injury events arise from a complex interaction of factors associated with materials and equipment used in work processes, the work environment, and the worker. These factors include safety hazards in workplaces or work settings; hazards and safety features of machinery and tools; the development and implementation of safe work practices; the organization of work; the design of workplaces; the safety culture of the employer and workplace safety climate; availability and use of personal protective equipment (PPE); demographic characteristics of workers; training, experience, and knowledge of workers; and economic and social factors.

Box 19-1. Injuries Are a Major Public Health Problem

In addition to the workplace, injuries occur at home and school, while traveling, and during recreation. In the United States, injuries are the leading cause of death for persons aged 1 to 44 years, surpassing deaths from cancer, heart disease, and infectious diseases. In 2015 in the United States, 214,008 injury deaths occurred (age-adjusted rate of 64 per 100,000 persons). Injuries contributed to more than 3.5 million years of potential life lost before age 65. In 2015, an estimated 32 million nonfatal injuries required treatment in an emergency department (age-adjusted rate of 9,948 per 100,000 persons).[1]

Many injury causes are common in multiple environments, such as the workplace and home; others are more common in the workplace. Transportation events, violence, falls, and being struck by objects are examples of injury causes that are common in multiple settings; machinery, electrocutions, explosions, and overexertion injuries are more common in the workplace. Strategies for reducing and preventing injuries in multiple settings include changes to the environment (such as changes in roadway design), regulatory policy (such as specifying product safety parameters), and educational approaches. Broad injury prevention measures, such as those focused on improving roadway safety, improve workplace safety. Injury prevention measures in the workplace complement those occurring in other settings.

Reference

1. National Center for Injury Prevention and Control. Injury Prevention & Control: Data & Statistics (WISQARSTM). Available at: http://www.cdc.gov/injury/wisqars/index.html. Accessed June 20, 2017.

Further Reading

Chen G, Jenkins EL, Marsh SM, Johnston JJ. Work-related and non-work-related injury deaths in the U.S.: A comparative study. Human and Ecologic Risk Assessment 2001; 7: 1859–1868.

Smith GS, Sorock GS, Wellman H, et al. Blurring the distinctions between on and off the job injuries: similarities and differences in circumstances. Injury Prevention 2006; 12: 236–241.

CASE 1

A 28-year-old male temporary worker was fatally injured while cleaning and sanitizing a machine at a company that manufactured food products. Although the incident was not witnessed, the victim was reportedly cleaning the augers inside the bottom of the machine's tub while they were rotating. Both of the victim's arms became caught in the augers. A coworker heard the victim yell and noticed him being pulled into the machine. The coworker then stopped the machine via an emergency stop button while another coworker called emergency medical services. The victim was transported to a local hospital where he was pronounced dead. Subsequent investigation found several inches of water mixed with food product on the floor, which made it slippery, and floor drains clogged with food product, which prevented the water from draining. It is likely the slippery floor caused the worker to fall into the machine's rotating augers.[6]

This case illustrates how occupational injuries can be caused by a variety of factors and circumstances, some of which are clearly established while others are presumed:

- The victim was employed through a temporary staffing agency, which apparently did not provide him with training on safety hazards associated with his work tasks or on safe work practices and did not require the company to provide such training. (See Chapter 2.)

- The company provided new workers with orientation and in-house on-the-job training that focused on good manufacturing practices but did not provide comprehensive safety training on hazards in the workplace or on safe work practices. (See Chapter 4.)

- The company did not have a comprehensive written health and safety program. It provided lockout/tagout training only to permanent maintenance workers, not to temporary employees.

- The company had a manager responsible for health and safety, but he spent only 2 hours weekly on health and safety. The company's health and safety committee was defunct and therefore had not been meeting.

- The process for cleaning and sanitizing the machine included removing the tub cover and spraying water into the equipment after turning it on, creating the possibility of workers coming into contact with moving parts.

- The floor, with several inches of water due to clogged floor drains, was slippery, which increased the likelihood of workers falling into the machine.

- The equipment did not have engineering controls that could help prevent injuries to workers cleaning it, such as an interlock into the auger power control circuit to shut down or prevent start-up of the auger motors when the tub cover was removed.

This case demonstrates how injury events can arise from a complex array of factors, not all of which contribute equally. In addition, the responsibilities for a safe work environment and safe work practices are not borne equally by all involved parties. Employers bear the greatest responsibilities, as they are responsible for providing a safe work environment, including the identification of potential safety hazards and the implementation of hazard controls and safe work practices and procedures. Workers are responsible for following established procedures, although they should be empowered by supervisors to report problems with established procedures and provided with the training and support to identify and report safety hazards to employers. This case also highlights how multiple employer arrangements can endanger worker safety when workers are hired by a temporary staffing agency but work in an environment controlled by another employer. (The Occupational Safety and Health Administration has issued a series of guidance documents to clarify the responsibilities that employers have in this type of situation.[7])

THE EPIDEMIOLOGY OF INJURIES

Occupational injuries are not random events. They cluster or are associated with specific types of workplaces and jobs, workplace exposures, and worker characteristics. Because occupational injuries are not random, they can be anticipated and steps can be taken to prevent them.

Epidemiologic data allow those involved in injury prevention efforts to target groups and settings with high numbers or rates of occupational injuries and to anticipate and take steps to prevent injuries in specific workplaces or work settings. Epidemiologic data on fatal and nonfatal occupational injuries differ and thus are addressed separately. Both categories of injuries require attention—fatal injuries, because they represent the most severe consequence of occupational injury and are devastating to families, communities, and workplaces, and nonfatal injuries, because of the sheer volume and aggregate costs to workers, families, employers, and society as a whole.

Fatal Injuries

In the United States, data on fatal occupational injuries are considered to be very complete. Beginning in 1992, the U.S. Bureau of Labor Statistics (BLS) began collecting data through the Census of Fatal Occupational Injuries (CFOI), which uses multiple sources of data and involves verification of the work-relatedness of deaths.[1] A less complete system based only on death certificates, the National Traumatic Occupational Fatalities (NTOF) system, provides additional data for the years 1980 through 1995.[8] Both CFOI and NTOF provide data for each state and for the United States as a whole. Data, such as medical-examiner records, also exist at the state level. (See Chapter 6.)

In 2015 there were 4,836 fatal occupational injuries in the United States—3.4 fatal occupational injuries for every 100,000 U.S. full-time equivalent workers.[1] The distribution and risks for fatal occupational injury differ by demographic characteristics of workers. Men account for more than 90% of occupational fatalities and have occupational fatality rates approximately 10 times higher than those for women.[8-9] In 2015, of all occupational fatal injuries, 67% were among white non-Hispanic workers, 19% among Hispanic workers, 10% among black non-Hispanic workers, and 2% among non-Hispanic Asian workers.[9] Of all fatal occupational injuries, 19% occurred among workers born in other countries, with the largest proportion born in Mexico.[1] An analysis of fatal occupational injuries from 2005 through 2009 found that high rates, by race, ethnicity, and foreign birth, were largely associated with work in high-risk industries, such as agriculture, mining, transportation, and construction.[10] Of all fatal occupational injuries in 2015, 57% occurred to workers between 25 and 54 years of age, 8% to workers younger than 25, and 35% to workers 55 and older.[11] Rates of fatal occupational injury generally increase with age, with the highest rates among workers 65 and older.[1,8-9] The youngest and oldest workers present both challenges and opportunities for occupational injury prevention (Box 19-2).

In 2015, of all fatal occupational injuries, 78% were among wage and salary workers; the remainder were among self-employed workers, whose fatality rate is more than four times greater than that of wage and salary employees.[9] In 2015, 17% of the deaths occurred among workers identified as contractors.[1] From 2011 to

---

Box 19-2. The Youngest and Oldest Workers Present Challenges and Opportunities for Prevention

The U.S. workforce is characterized by involvement of workers from early adolescence to beyond traditional retirement ages. The United States is somewhat unique among industrialized nations in the high participation of youth less than 18 years of age in the workforce. As the U.S. population has aged and people have lived longer than in the past, the number of older workers has increased—and this number is expected to continue to grow. The number of workers 55 years and older increased 47% between 2004 and 2014, and it is expected to increase an additional 20% by 2024 to more than 40 million.[1] In 2016, there were nearly 5 million workers 16 to 19 years of age and 1.6 million workers 75 years and older in the United States.[2]

Because of their biologic, social, and economic characteristics, the youngest and oldest workers have unique patterns and risks for work-related injuries. While younger workers have lower rates than older workers for fatal injuries, their rates for nonfatal occupational injury are higher. The higher rates of nonfatal injury are frequently attributed to less experience and training on safety hazards in the workplace. In contrast, the oldest workers have the highest rates of fatal occupational injury, lower rates of nonfatal injury, and longer recovery times once injured. Decreased physical ability to tolerate and recover from injuries may account for the longer recovery times and increased fatality rates. While normal decrements in health associated with aging, such as reductions in visual acuity and slower reaction times, would theoretically lead to increased injuries among older workers, it would appear that work and life experiences contribute to the lower rates of nonfatal occupational injury among older workers. Furthermore, older workers may be assigned to less physically demanding tasks.

It is important to ensure that employers provide new workers with training on the specific safety hazards in their work environment and guidance on how to safely perform their jobs. In addition, there is potential value in providing youth with basic training on occupational safety before they enter the workforce, as a means of helping to keep them safe in their first jobs, and potentially contributing to a more safety conscious generation of new workers. Along these lines, NIOSH and its partners

have designed curricula that can be integrated into high-school programming or be used in other group settings, such as in apprentice training.[3] Several government and private-sector entities have also developed educational materials to increase the safety of young workers up to 24 years of age.

At the other end of the age spectrum, older workers bring a wealth of experience and perspective to the workplace. As the workforce continues to age, it is important to understand workplace programs and policies that reduce the risk for injury among an older population facing the realities of the aging process and to make reasonable accommodations to increase the safety of older workers. Modifying work tasks to account for age-related decrements in functioning may have the added benefit of increasing safety for workers of all ages.

References

1. Bureau of Labor Statistics. Employment projections: 2014–2024 summary. Washington, DC: Bureau of Labor Statistics, News Release, USDL 15-2327, December 8, 2015. Available at: http://www.bls.gov/news.release/pdf/ecopro.pdf. Accessed September 10, 2016.
2. Bureau of Labor Statistics. Employment status of the civilian noninstitutional population by age, sex, and race. Washington, DC: BLS, 2017. Available at: http://www.bls.gov/opub/ee/2017/cps/annavg3_2015.pdf. Accessed June 20,2017.
3. National Institute for Occupational Safety and Health. Youth@Work: Talking safety. Cincinnati, OH: NIOSH, 2015. Available at: http://www.cdc.gov/niosh/talkingsafety/. Accessed: September 10, 2016.

Further Reading

National Institute for Occupational Safety and Health. Productive aging and work. Available at: http://www.cdc.gov/niosh/topics/productiveaging/default.html. Accessed September 10, 2016.
National Institute for Occupational Safety and Health. Young worker safety and health. Available at: www.cdc.gov/niosh/topics/youth/. Accessed September 10, 2016.
National Research Council and the Institute of Medicine. Protecting youth at work: Health, safety and development of working children and adolescents in the United States. Committee on the Health and Safety Implications of Child Labor. Washington, DC: National Academies Press, 1998.
National Research Council and the Institute of Medicine. Health and safety needs of older workers. In: Wegman DH, McGee JP (eds.). Division of behavioral and social sciences and education. Washington, DC: National Academies Press, 2004.

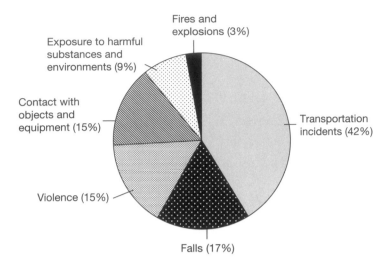

Figure 19-1. Events or exposures leading to occupational injury deaths, United States, 2015. (Source: Bureau of Labor Statistics, U.S. Department of Labor.)

2015, most fatally injured contractors were male and identified as wage and salary workers (as opposed to self-employed workers), and many worked in construction.[12] (See Chapter 32B.)

Transportation-related events accounted for 42% of the 4,836 occupational injury deaths in the United States in 2015 (Figure 19-1).[1] These events involved motor vehicles and mobile equipment, such as tractors and forklifts; occurred on and off the highway; and included pedestrians and bystanders as well as operators and drivers. Work-related motor-vehicle crashes provide unique challenges and opportunities for prevention (Box 19-3). Falls, mostly to a lower

---

Box 19-3. Unique Challenges for Prevention of Work-Related Motor Vehicle Deaths and Injuries

Motor vehicle crashes are the leading cause of occupational injury deaths in the United States. Between 2003 and 2015, crashes killed 16,005 workers who were drivers or passengers in motor vehicles, averaging more than three deaths daily[1]. Truck drivers account for more crash fatalities than any other occupation (46% in 2015[2]), and they have the highest rates of occupational deaths due to motor vehicle crashes. However, crash risk affects workers in all industries and occupations, whether they drive heavy or light vehicles on the job and whether driving is a main or incidental job duty.

Preventing work-related motor vehicle crashes is a responsibility shared by employers and workers and requires a multipronged approach to reduce risks related to the driver, the vehicle, and the work environment. Although employers cannot exert full control over the conditions their workers face while on the road, they can take a number of steps to help keep their workers safe when driving, such as:

- Promoting road safety by the highest levels of company leadership
- Conducting a thorough assessment of road risks drivers face
- Considering if work can be accomplished without traveling by motor vehicle or use safer modes of travel, such as air or rail

- Implementing and enforcing policies for mandatory use of seat belts
- Ensuring that workers assigned to drive on the job have valid driver's licenses appropriate for the types of vehicles they drive
- Conducting motor vehicle record checks for prospective employees and periodic rechecks after hiring
- Providing driver training at the time of hiring and periodic refresher driving training
- Providing fleet vehicles with high safety ratings based on crash testing
- Selecting vehicles with advanced safety features, such as forward-collision and lane-departure warning systems, automated emergency braking, and adaptive cruise control
- Maintaining complete and accurate records of workers' driving performance
- Reviewing motor vehicle crashes to determine if changes in policies and practices are needed
- Incorporating fatigue management into motor vehicle safety programs
- Avoiding requiring workers to drive irregular hours or to extend their workday far beyond their normal working hours as a result of driving responsibilities
- Establishing schedules that allow drivers to obey speed limits and follow applicable hours-of-service regulations
- Preventing distracted driving by banning text messaging and the use of hand-held phones while driving

(continued)

Box 19-3. (Continued)

- Setting safety policy in accordance with state graduated-driver licensing laws so that company operations do not place younger workers in violation of these laws
- Offering periodic vision screening and assessment of physical health for all workers for whom driving is a primary job duty.

Many of these recommendations are included in the American National Standards Institute/American Society of Safety Engineers (ANSI/ASSE) Z15.1–2017 standard, *Safe Practices for Motor Vehicle Operations.*[3] This voluntary consensus standard provides minimum guidelines for employers to develop a motor vehicle safety program. These guidelines are meant for use by employers with vehicle fleets of all sizes and vehicle types.

Workers can also take steps to increase their safety while driving in the performance of their work, including:

- Following employer policies and traffic laws
- Using seat belts at all times and insisting that passengers do the same
- Not texting or using a hand-held phone while driving
- Avoiding placing or taking cell phone calls while operating a motor vehicle
- Ensuring they are well-rested before operating a motor vehicle at work

- Talking to their healthcare provider about whether medical conditions or medications may affect their ability to drive safely
- Maintaining work vehicles in good operating condition.

Source: Preventing work-related motor vehicle crashes. DHHS (NIOSH) Publication No. 2015-111, Cincinnati, OH: NIOSH 2015. Available at: http://www.cdc.gov/niosh/docs/2015-111/pdfs/2015-111.pdf. Accessed September 14, 2016.

References

1. Bureau of Labor Statistics. Table A-2: Fatal occupational injuries due to transportation incidents and homicide, all United States [2003–2015]. Available at: http://www.bls.gov/iif/oshcfoi1.htm. Accessed June 20, 2017.
2. Bureau of Labor Statistics. Table A-6: Fatal occupational injuries due to transportation incidents and homicide by occupation, all United States, 2015. Available at: http://www.bls.gov/iif/oshwc/cfoi. Accessed June 20, 2017.
3. ANSI/ASSE Z15.1 Safe practices for motor vehicle operations. Des Plaines, IL: American Society of Safety Engineers, 2017.

Further Reading

National Institute for Occupational Safety and Health. Fact sheet: Older drivers in the workplace: How employers and workers can prevent crashes. Cincinnati, OH: NIOSH, 2016, DHHS (NIOSH) Publication No. 2016-116. Available at: http://www.cdc.gov/niosh/docs/2016-116/pdfs/2016-116.pdf. Accessed September 10, 2016.
National Institute for Occupational Safety and Health. Motor vehicle safety at work. NIOSH Center for Motor Vehicle Safety webpage. Available at: http://www.cdc.gov/niosh/motorvehicle. Accessed September 10, 2016.

level, accounted for 17% of the fatalities in 2015.[1] Violence accounted for 15% of the fatalities, with most involving homicides and many involving suicides. Assaults against workers occur in a variety of work situations, and consequently prevention strategies vary (Box 19-4). Contact with objects or equipment accounted for 15% of the fatalities, including being struck by falling objects, being caught in running equipment or machinery, and being caught in or crushed by collapsing materials, such as in trench cave-ins or collapsing buildings. Rapid technological advances in robotic machinery require vigilant attention to safety implications for workers (Box 19-5). Exposure to harmful substances or environments, such as electric current, temperature extremes, hazardous substances, and oxygen deficiency, accounted for 9% of fatalities. Fires and explosions accounted for 3% of the fatalities.[1] Demographic characteristics vary; for example, homicide accounts for a higher proportion of deaths among women than in men.[1,8]

The incidence of occupational injury deaths varies by industry sector (Table 19-1), with the most deaths in 2015 occurring in the construction sector and the highest fatality rates in agriculture, forestry, fishing and hunting; transportation and warehousing; and mining, quarrying, and oil and gas extraction.[19] Numerous specific industries and occupations have injury rates far above the average for all industries and occupations. For example, occupations with fatality rates (deaths per 100,000 full-time equivalent workers) more than 10 times higher than the national average in 2015 include logging workers (133), fishers and related fishing workers (55), aircraft pilots and flight engineers (40), roofers (40), and refuse and recyclable materials collectors (39).[1,9]

Nonfatal Injuries

There is no single data system in the United States that collects data on all nonfatal occupational injuries. The two primary national sources

(continued)

Box 19-5. (Continued)

workers. However, increased interaction between robots and workers presents safety risks for workers and others. Job safety analysis and site hazard assessments are necessary to ensure that risks to workers and the public are identified, that engineering controls are implemented to prevent injuries, and that administrative controls, such as worker training, are used to ensure that workers and others understand the operation of robots, associated risks, and safety measures. Robot safety standards are being developed and updated. It is critical that these standards keep pace with rapidly advancing robot technologies so that the potential of robots is realized while the safety of workers is protected.

References

1. National Institute for Occupational Safety and Health. Preventing the injury of workers by robots. Cincinnati, OH: NIOSH, 1984,

DHHS (NIOSH) Publication No. 85-103. Available at: http://www.cdc.gov/niosh/docs/85-103/default.html. Accessed September 10, 2016.
2. National Institute for Occupational Safety and Health. Safe maintenance guidelines for robotic workstations. Cincinnati, OH: NIOSH, 1988, DHHS (NIOSH) Publication No. 88-108. Available at: https://www.cdc.gov/niosh/docs/88-108/88-108.pdf. Accessed September 10, 2016.
3. ANSI/RIA 15.06. National Standard for Industrial Robots and Robot Systems—Safety Requirements Ann Arbor, MI: Robotics Industry Association, 2012.

Further Reading

Murashov V, Hearl, F, Howard J. Working safely with robot workers: Recommendations for the new workplace. Journal of Occupational and Environmental Hygiene 2016; 13: D61–D71.

Sheridan T. Human-robot interaction: Status and challenges. Human Factors, 2016; 58: 525–532.

Table 19-1. Number and Rate of Fatal Occupational Injuries, by Industry Sector, United States, 2015

Industry Sector	Number of Fatalities	Fatality Rate*
Construction	937	10.1
Transportation and warehousing	765	13.8
Agriculture, forestry, fishing and hunting	570	22.8
Professional and business services	477	3.0
Government	457	1.9
Manufacturing	353	2.3
Retail trade	269	1.8
Leisure and hospitality	225	2.0
Other services, except public administration	202	3.0
Wholesale trade	175	4.7
Educational and health services	139	0.7
Mining, quarrying, and oil and gas extraction	120	11.4
Financial activities	83	0.9
Information	42	1.5
Utilities	22	2.2
Total	**4836**	**3.4**

* Rate per 100,000 full-time equivalent workers.
Source: Bureau of Labor Statistics. Census of Fatal Occupational Injuries Charts, 1992-2015 (revised data). Washington, DC. Available at: http://www.bls.gov/iif/oshwc/cfoi/cfch0014.pdf.

of data on nonfatal work-related injuries are data from the BLS annual survey of employers[3] and from emergency departments.[4] Neither system is designed to capture all work-related injuries and both have limitations. The BLS survey is based

on employer reports of injuries documented in records required by the Occupational Safety and Health Administration (OSHA). Based on the BLS survey, there were an estimated 3.5 million occupational injuries in 2015.[2] The BLS survey excludes the self-employed, farms with fewer than 11 employees, and federal government employees, and it may miss many cases that should be counted.[3] Data on worker demographics and the circumstances of injuries are available only for lost workday cases in the BLS survey.[13] The emergency department system collects data on injuries treated in a nationally representative sample of emergency departments, with an estimate of 2.8 million (± 397,000) occupational injuries and illnesses in 2014.[4] The identification of these cases requires documentation in the emergency department record that the injury was work-related. Research on the completeness of the emergency department data has not been conducted, and information on industry and occupation are not regularly available in the emergency department data. Data collected in both systems overlap and are not mutually exclusive. Illnesses, such as dermatitis, are included in both the emergency department data and lost workday data from the BLS employer survey, but they represent less than 15% of cases in both systems.[4] Although the data from the BLS survey and emergency departments have limitations and undoubtedly underrepresent the true burden of occupational injuries, they are likely to represent the majority of the more-serious injuries, and they provide useful information on epidemiologic patterns of injury.

Although not as dramatic as for fatal injuries, differences are seen across demographic categories for nonfatal injuries. Men accounted for approximately 64% of nonfatal work-related injuries treated in emergency departments in 2014 and approximately 75% of the hospitalizations.[4] In 2015, men accounted for 61% of employer-reported injuries requiring days away from work (lost worktime injuries), had a rate about 24% higher than women, and had injuries that, on average, required more time away from work.[13] In 2014, most injuries treated in emergency departments (51%) were among white, non-Hispanic workers, with fewer among Hispanic workers (10%) and black, non-Hispanic workers (11%).[4] About 66% to 68% of nonfatal injuries occur among workers 25 to 54 years of age.[4,13] Those younger than 25 account for about 18% of injuries treated in emergency departments[4] and 10% of lost work-time injuries.[13] Workers older than 54 account for 15% of injuries treated in emergency departments[4] and 22% of lost work-time injuries reported by employers.[13] Age-group-specific rates of nonfatal occupational injuries follow patterns that vary according to data source. In the emergency department data for 1998 to 2007, workers 16 to 24 years of age were found to have rates about double those of older groups.[14] In contrast, in employer-reported data, rates are similar by age group and do not follow a clear pattern.[13] The median number of days away from work, based on employer-reported data, was 8 in 2015, with the median days increasing steadily from a low of 4 days for workers 14 to 15 years of age to a high of 14 days for workers 65 and older.[13]

In 2015, of employer-reported cases, 10% occurred among employees who had worked for less than 3 months for the employer, 17% among employees with 3 to 11 months of service, 31% with 1 to 5 years of service, and 40% with more than 5 years of service.[13] Most employer-reported injuries requiring time away from work in 2015 occurred Monday through Friday (85%),[15] and when reported, 62% occurred between 8:00 A.M. and 4:00 P.M.[16] Of all employer-reported injuries, 64% occurred between 2 and 8 hours into the work shift, with the largest proportion (26%) occurring 2 to 4 hours into the shift.[17]

The types of events leading to nonfatal occupational injuries follow a different pattern than fatal occupational injuries. The most common events resulting in nonfatal occupational injuries include contact with objects and equipment, bodily reaction and exertion, and falls.[4,13] Figure 19-2 shows the distribution of nonfatal occupational injuries treated in emergency departments in 2014. Demographic characteristics vary; for example, bodily reaction and exertion, as well as falls, account for a higher proportion of injuries among women than in men.[4]

The number and rate of nonfatal injuries by industry division vary greatly from the number

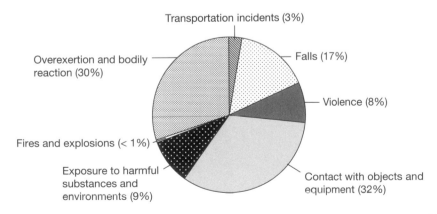

Figure 19-2. Events or exposures leading to occupational injuries treated in emergency departments, United States, 2014. (Source: NIOSH. Work-related injury statistics query system, http://wwwn.cdc.gov/wisards/workrisqs/. Unpublished queries by John Myers on June 19, 2017.)

Table 19-2. Number and Rate of Nonfatal Occupational Injuries Reported by Employers, by State and Local Government and Private Industry Sector, United States, 2015

Industry Division	Number of Injuries	Injury Rate*
State and local government	705,200	4.8
Education and health services	599,600	3.8
Manufacturing	425,700	3.4
Retail trade	399,600	3.4
Leisure and hospitality	322,300	3.3
Professional and business services	201,800	1.3
Transportation and warehousing	194,200	4.4
Construction	199,600	3.4
Wholesale trade	170,200	3.0
Financial activities	75,400	1.0
Other services, except public administration	70,000	2.3
Agriculture, forestry, fishing and hunting	53,000	5.4
Information	30,900	1.2
Mining, quarrying and oil and gas extraction	12,100	1.4
Utilities	11,000	2.0
Total	**3,470,600**	**3.1**

* Rate per 100 full-time equivalent workers.
Source: Bureau of Labor Statistics. Employer-reported workplace injuries and illnesses—2015. News Release USDL 16-2056. Washington, DC: BLS. Available at: http://www.bls.gov/news.release/osh.nr0.htm.

and rate for injury deaths (Table 19-2).[2] Most injuries in the private sector in 2015 occurred in the education and health services sector, and the highest injury rates were in the agriculture, forestry, fishing, and hunting sector.[2] The injury rate for workers in state and local governments exceeded that in all private-industry sectors combined. The occupational injury rate in 2015, averaged across all industries and state and local governments, was 3.1 per 100 full-time equivalent workers. Because the BLS annual survey of employers excludes farms with fewer than 11 employees, the numbers and rates of nonfatal occupational injuries reported for the agriculture, forestry, fishing, and hunting sector should be considered as conservative estimates.

Clinical Presentation and Course of Injuries

In 2014, the most common diagnoses of workers treated for occupational injuries in emergency departments were as follows: sprains and strains (22%); lacerations, punctures, amputations, and avulsions (19%); contusions, abrasions, and hematomas (14%); dislocations and fractures (7%); and burns (3%).[4] Most sprains and strains (54%) were to the trunk area (shoulder, back, chest, or abdomen), followed by the lower extremities (legs, feet, and toes, 25%). About 77% of the lacerations, punctures, amputations, and avulsions were to the upper extremities (arms, hands, or fingers). An estimated 4% of occupational injuries resulted in hospital admission.[4] The most common event resulting in hospitalization was a fall (21%), and the most common diagnosis was fracture (27%).[4]

Of the estimated 1.2 million injuries and illnesses with lost workdays in 2015, the median time away from work was 8 days. Median time away from work was highest for fractures (31 days), carpal tunnel syndrome (28 days), and multiple traumatic injuries with fractures (31 days).[13]

PREVENTION OF INJURIES

Prevention through Design

One of the best ways to prevent occupational injuries is to "design out" hazards and risks early in the design or redesign process, commonly referred to as *prevention through design*. This approach seeks to eliminate or reduce occupational hazards and risks in work facilities, equipment, machinery, tools, and work processes. While prevention through design is not a new concept, in 2007, the National Institute for Occupational Safety and Health (NIOSH) initiated a national prevention through design initiative "to foster designing out occupational hazards in equipment, structures, materials, and processes that effect workers."[18] Through partnerships with external stakeholders, the national NIOSH plan includes specific goals in research, education, practice, policy, and small business "to more effectively protect workers from injury and disease."[18] In 2011, the consensus standard Z590-3, *Prevention through Design: Guidelines for Addressing Hazards and Risks in Design and Redesign Processes,* was released.[19] This standard complements several provisions of ANSI Z10

Occupational Health and Safety Management Systems[20] aimed at preventing workplace serious injuries and fatalities. Case 2 illustrates a situation in which an engulfment hazard could have been reduced or eliminated by application of prevention through design.

CASE 2

A 36-year-old male Hispanic laborer died after becoming engulfed in sawdust inside a sawmill storage silo. The flat-bottomed silo used a three-armed rotating sweep auger mechanism to funnel stored sawdust through an opening in the silo floor to a transfer auger, which transported the sawdust to another part of the sawmill for use in generating electricity for the mill. Due to the flat-bottom design of the silo, the sweep auger was prone to frequent clogs, requiring workers to manually unclog the system with rakes and poles. The worker had entered the silo to manually clear a clog; soon afterward, sawdust that had accumulated on the sides of the silo collapsed, completely engulfing him.

Although several factors contributed to this worker's death, NIOSH investigators recommended retrofitting the silo with a mechanical leveling/raking device that would improve the flow of loose materials, such as sawdust, to minimize or eliminate the need for workers to enter into this confined space.[21]

The Hierarchical Approach to Occupational Injury Control

In addition to the concept of prevention through design, several models for occupational injury control have evolved over the years. Some of these models categorize worker protection strategies based on a hierarchy of controls: (a) hazard elimination, (b) hazard substitution, (c) engineering controls, (d) warning systems, (e) administrative controls, and (f) PPE (Table 19-3).[22]

William Haddon Jr. proposed 10 basic strategies for injury prevention that have several similarities to the hierarchical approach, such as hazard elimination, hazard reduction, and use of barriers for protection.[23] He also introduced

Table 19-3. Hierarchy of Controls

A	Elimination—Eliminate or reduce hazards through system design and redesign
B	Substitution—Substitute less hazardous methods, materials, or processes for more hazardous ones
C	Engineering Controls—Prevent access to hazards
D	Warnings—Alert workers to hazards (Warnings are often considered an administrative control because they require an active response from workers in order to be effective.)
E	Administrative Controls—Change the way people work
F	PPE—Protect workers from hazards with personal protective equipment

Source: Manuele FA. Advanced safety management: Focusing on Z10 and serious injury prevention (2nd ed.). Hoboken, NJ: John Wiley & Sons, 2014.

the concept that injuries were caused by a chain of multifactorial events, each of which provided opportunities for intervention. Epidemiology, safety engineering, biomechanics, ergonomics, psychology, safety management, and other types of expertise comprise a multidisciplinary approach that is useful for identifying injury risk factors and developing control strategies.

Elimination and Substitution

The most effective approach is to eliminate a hazard completely—the top tier of the hierarchy of controls and a tenet of prevention through design. One example is locating pumps, agitators, and gauges outside of confined spaces so that worker entry is not required for maintenance, repair, or monitoring. Substitution replaces hazardous materials, processes, or equipment with those that are less hazardous, such as using materials handling equipment in place of manual materials handling.

Engineering Controls

If a hazard cannot be eliminated completely through design or an appropriate substitution, then the next strategy should be to implement engineering controls that prevent or reduce hazards through the application of safeguards. For example, many types of industrial equipment require power transmission units that include belts, pulleys, gears, shafts, and other mechanisms necessary for the equipment to function. Workers can be exposed to serious, or even fatal, injury hazards if they contact these rotating or moving components. A fixed barrier guard that completely encloses the power transmission unit is an engineering control that protects workers from being caught in or struck by hazards by preventing worker contact with any moving parts. As long as the guard remains in place, the worker is protected from injury. Another engineering control is an optical sensor, also called a light curtain, used to protect the worker from injury when operating a mechanical power press (Figure 19-3). The optical sensor is integrated into the press control mechanism so that if any part of the worker's body breaks the plane of light in front of the hazardous point of operation, the downward motion of the press ram cannot be initiated or, if motion has begun, the press ram is automatically disengaged.

Many engineering controls are interlocked to ensure that they cannot be removed without disabling the machine or equipment. An interlock is a device that is integrated into the control mechanism of a machine or work process to prevent the work cycle from being initiated until the interlock is closed, signaling the equipment that the work cycle can be initiated. One example is a skid-steer loader with interlocked driver controls

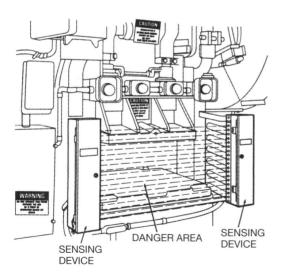

Figure 19-3. Photoelectric (optical) sensor installed on a mechanical power press to protect the point of operation. (Source: Occupational Safety and Health Administration. Concepts and techniques of machine safeguarding. Washington, DC: OSHA, 1980.)

that require the operator be properly positioned inside the equipment, with the seat belt fastened, before the equipment can be started and the bucket raised. Interlocks, which are usually electrical or mechanical controls, need to be designed so that they are not easily bypassed or disabled.

Elimination, substitution, and engineering controls are often referred to as *passive controls* since they typically do not require worker involvement to be protective. However, passive controls should be designed so that they do not adversely interfere with work processes or introduce additional hazards. Although passive controls are generally more effective prevention strategies than those that require worker involvement, it is not possible to implement them for all potentially hazardous work situations.

Warnings and Other Administrative Controls

Administrative controls are management-directed work practices or procedures that, when implemented, will reduce exposure to hazards and the risk of injury. They are sometimes referred to as *active controls* because they require worker involvement to be effective. Warning systems, safe work practices and procedures, and worker training are examples of administrative controls. Workers must react to warnings, such as back-up alarms and smoke detectors, follow prescribed safe work practices and procedures and apply the training they have received in order to prevent injuries. Other examples of administrative controls include housekeeping procedures requiring that spills or debris be cleaned up quickly to reduce the potential for a slip, trip, or fall injury (Figure 19-4) and implementation of hazardous energy-control policies, such as for lockout/tagout procedures, for workers performing maintenance on machines. (Figure 19-5). These procedures should be written and consistently implemented, and workers should be trained in their use.[24]

Personal Protective Equipment

If hazardous injury exposures cannot be prevented through elimination, substitution, engineering, or administrative controls, then PPE provides the last line of defense for worker protection. Personal protective equipment consists of devices worn by workers to reduce (a) the risk

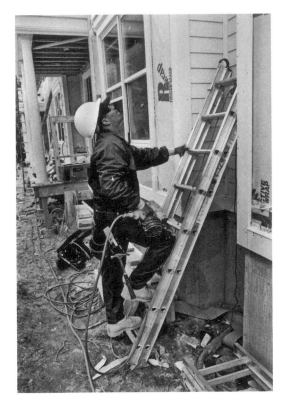

Figure 19-4. Example of poor housekeeping on a construction site. Loose bricks, lumber, and other debris create a potential tripping hazard for workers. (Photograph by Earl Dotter.)

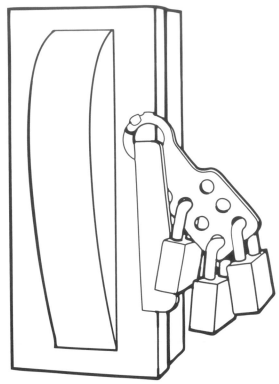

Figure 19-5. Lockout hasp on an electrical control panel that provides a method for applying a lock (lockout) to the panel during maintenance or repair to ensure that the equipment is not energized until the work has been completed. The control panel should also be tagged (tagout) with a label indicating that work is being performed. Workers should be provided with individually keyed locks, and only the worker who applied the lock should remove it. (Source: Occupational Safety and Health Administration. Concepts and techniques of machine safeguarding. Washington, DC: OSHA, 1980.)

that exposure to a hazard will injure the worker or (b) the severity of an injury if one does occur. Although the hazard still exists, the potential for worker injury is mitigated by using PPE. The use of PPE in many work environments is essential for worker protection. However, PPE is usually viewed as the least effective approach for injury prevention and is the lowest tier on the hierarchy of controls. Active decision-making by management to identify required PPE, worker consultation to identify the most comfortable or user-friendly PPE, policies that encourage appropriate use, and follow-up evaluation to determine effectiveness are necessary to achieve the intended protection for which the PPE is designed. Examples of PPE for reducing worker injuries include protective hard hats, eyewear and face shields, steel-toed safety shoes, fall restraint devices, and personal flotation devices (Figure 19-6). When worn properly and as necessary, PPE can prevent, or at least reduce the severity of, traumatic injuries.

Fall-restraint devices, such as lanyards and body harnesses, do not prevent workers from falling, but protect them from suffering more serious injuries or fatalities due to falls from elevations (Figures 19-7A and 19-7B).

Combined Application of Controls

A comprehensive approach to worker injury prevention inevitably includes all tiers of the control hierarchy to achieve maximal worker protection. In most work environments, a combination of elimination, substitution, engineering controls, warning systems, administrative controls, and PPE will often be required to have a complete and effective injury prevention program. The following examples illustrate how the combined

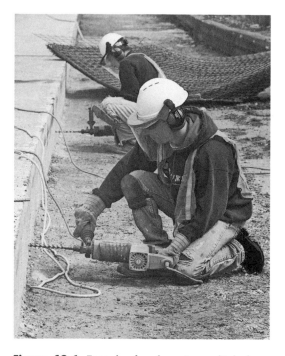

Figure 19-6. Example of worker using multiple forms of personal protective equipment, including hard hat, face shield, hearing protection, work gloves, knee pads, and work boots. (Photo Courtesy of Mine Safety Appliance Company.)

application of controls can be used to achieve an optimal level of worker protection.

Tractors equipped with a rollover protective structure (ROPS), an engineering control, significantly reduce the risk that the operator will be injured in a rollover event (Figure 19-8). However, more effective protection can be achieved if a seat belt, an administrative control, is worn to keep the operator within the protective envelope of the rollover protective structure. Another example is the increased protection afforded by the combined use of seat belts, mandated in company safety policies and programs, in motor vehicles that are also equipped with air bags and advanced safety features, such as traction-stability control systems and forward-collision avoidance systems with automatic braking.

Training

Training refers to methods that help individuals acquire knowledge (safety information on potential workplace hazards), change attitudes (perceptions and beliefs regarding safety), and practice safe work behaviors (organizational,

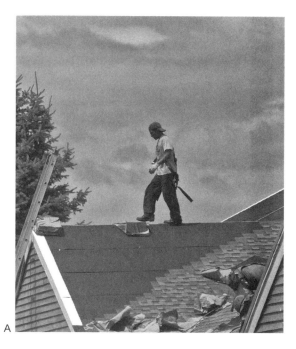

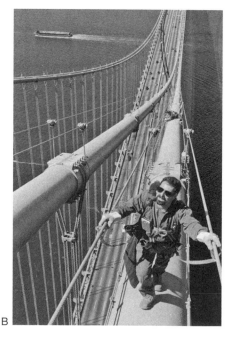

A   B

Figure 19-7. (A) Roof worker without fall protection. (Photograph by Marvin Lewiton.) (B) Bridge inspector with ropes that provide fall protection. (Photograph by Earl Dotter.)

management, or worker performance). Despite inadequate data on the direct relationship between training and injury, evidence suggests a positive impact of training on establishing safe working conditions.[25] Training is one of the key factors accounting for differences between companies with low and high injury rates. It is often critically important for developing and implementing effective hazard control measures.[25,26] Training increases hazard awareness and knowledge, facilitates adoption of safe work practices, and leads to other workplace safety improvements. Training is an administrative control, as workers must properly use training they have received on a consistent basis for it to be effective in preventing injuries.

Effective training programs (a) assess training needs specific to the work task, (b) develop training to address these specific needs, (c) set clear training goals, and (d) evaluate the post-training knowledge and skills and provide feedback to the workers.[25] Another important characteristic of a successful program is management commitment to safety and training that is initiated as soon as a worker is hired and continued through periodic retraining and reinforcement.[25,26]

Unique characteristics of the specific workforce must be considered when developing or implementing safety training programs. Language, literacy, cognition, and cultural issues may diminish the effectiveness of training when programs are not tailored to account for unique or diverse characteristics of the workforce. Workplace safety training appears to be most effective when it includes active learning experiences that stress worksite application and when it is developed and implemented in the context of a broader workplace-based prevention approach.[25]

Standards

Many standards aim to protect workers from traumatic injury. These standards cover a multitude of hazards and address the work environment, work practices, equipment, PPE, and worker training. The two primary types of worker protection standards consist of (a) mandatory standards, such as those promulgated by OSHA or other regulatory agencies, and (b)

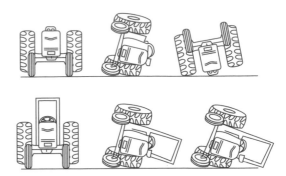

Figure 19-8. The tractors on the lower of the two rows shown above each have a two-post roll-over protective structure (ROPS) frame installed. The ROPS is designed to reduce the risk of injury or death by preventing the tractor from rolling onto and crushing the operator. A properly fastened seat belt greatly improves the chances that the operator will stay within the protective envelope of the ROPS. (Source: National Institute for Occupational Safety and Health. Safe grain and silage handling (DHHS [NIOSH] Publication No. 95-109). Washington, DC: NIOSH, 1995.)

voluntary standards, such as those developed through independent organizations, like the American National Standards Institute, through a consensus process involving various stakeholders in an industry—typically including representatives from labor, management, government, academia, and manufacturers. Numerous specifications, codes, and guidelines for machinery, equipment, tools, and other materials can also assist engineers and designers in developing safer products and systems, many of which have application in the workplace. Examples include the National Electric Code published by the National Fire Protection Association as well as numerous consensus standards from the American Society of Mechanical Engineers and the American Society for Testing and Materials.

Injury Control: Roles and Responsibilities

Occupational injury prevention is not the sole responsibility of a single person or group. Employers, workers, public health and safety practitioners, researchers, regulators, and policymakers each share in the responsibility for prevention. A multidisciplinary approach involving interaction among diverse groups is crucial to developing and implementing effective occupational injury prevention strategies.

Within an organization, active participation by both management and workers is essential to an effective safety program. Employers are responsible for establishing written safety policy, developing a comprehensive safety program, and effectively implementing that program at the workplace. A competent person or committee should be designated with responsibility for overall planning and implementation of company safety policy. This person or committee should have sufficient knowledge concerning safety policy, standards, regulations, and hazard abatement and should actively participate with managers and workers in coordinating and overseeing the safety program.

An effective safety program will strive to identify hazards through job safety analysis or other methods of systems safety analysis and will eliminate or control identified hazards through the various approaches previously described. Workers, managers, and safety specialists should work together to analyze the job and potential hazards and to recommend changes or controls to abate them to avoid an injury event. Table 19-4 includes injury hazards with examples from each of the three main categories of hazard control strategies: passive (elimination/substitution/engineering controls), active (warning systems and administrative controls), and PPE. The most comprehensive safety programs will typically require strategies from all six tiers from the hierarchy of controls. In industries or jobs where the work environment is not constant, site hazard assessments should be performed prior to beginning work in any new or changing environment. Occupations such as farming, logging, construction, oil and gas extraction, and mining are characterized by frequently changing work sites and require a site hazard assessment prior to commencing work in any new or changed environment. This requirement is particularly important in industries such as construction and utility maintenance, where worksites change not only from job to job but also from day to day—even hour to hour—with constant potential for new hazards.

Employers are also responsible for ensuring proper maintenance of vehicles, equipment, and machinery and their safety features, such as machine guarding, interlocks, warning systems, and barriers. Where job hazards cannot be eliminated or controlled, employers are responsible for providing appropriate PPE, such as fall arrest systems, respirators, hearing protectors, hard hats, or protective eyewear.

Employers must also ensure that workers receive appropriate training in minimizing their risk—including training on safety policy and practice, hazard recognition and control technologies, and the appropriate use of PPE. Enforcement of safety policies is also a critical employer responsibility. The demonstrated commitment of management to safety is a major factor in successful workplace safety programs.[27-29] Employers are more likely to have successful safety programs when they demonstrate concern by having top managers personally involved in safety activities and routinely involve workers in decision-making about safety matters. As part of a comprehensive safety program, employers should require systematic reporting and tracking of occupational injuries and "near-miss" events as well as assessment of this information for corrective action to prevent similar occurrences.

In the case of multiple employers, such as temporary staffing agencies providing workers to other employers, it is critically important that responsibilities for worker safety be clearly delineated in contracts. Both the temporary staffing agency and the worksite employer should play an active role in worker safety.[30] This may include the temporary staffing agency conducting site visits and reviewing safety records before entering into contractual arrangements with other employers and ensuring that the tasks, job safety analyses, and training and supervision that will be provided to employees are documented. Worksite employers will have responsibility for task-specific safety training, supervision, and the provision of a safe work environment.

Workers also play a vital role in workplace safety. Their participation is essential. Workers share in the responsibility for complying with safe work practices and policies, maintaining a safe work area, and using appropriate PPE when required by their employer. Workers should also participate in company-sponsored training. They should report injuries, near-miss events, and unsafe conditions for corrective action. As the experts in their jobs, workers should be involved in systems safety analysis and development of safe solutions. Workers' input into recommended design or modification of safety

Table 19-4. Injury Hazards and Illustrative Control Strategies by Category

Injury Hazard	Passive Controls: Elimination/Substitution/ Engineering Controls	Warnings and Other Administrative Controls	Personal Protective Equipment
Motor vehicle crashes	Ensure all vehicles are equipped with air bags and advanced safety features, such as forward collision avoidance systems with automatic braking and traction stability control	Implement a mandatory seat belt policy; purchase vehicles with blind-spot monitoring and lane-departure warning systems	Provide helmets and eye protection for workers whose jobs require operating motorcycles or bicycles
Assaults	Install bullet-resistant barriers or enclosures in retail settings	Train workers in nonviolent response when confronted with volatile situations	Provide body armor for public safety workers
Falls from elevation	Install grids or screens over skylight fixtures that meet OSHA standards for protection from falls through skylights	Train workers to set up extension ladders at the optimal inclination angle of 75° using the NIOSH ladder safety smart phone app*	Provide personal fall-arrest systems during work at elevations
Falls to same level	Redirect downspouts away from walkways with high pedestrian traffic	Implement a policy encouraging workers to clean up or report floor spills promptly	Provide or require workers to wear shoes with slip-resistant soles
Caught in	Ensure that controls on skid-steer loaders are interlocked and require operators to be properly positioned with seat belts fastened before the vehicle can be started and the bucket raised	Develop standard procedures for safely clearing material jams on machinery and equipment	Ensure long hair is tied back or covered when working around machinery with rotating or moving components
Struck by	Install fencing or other physical barriers around robots or other moving equipment, with access through interlocked gates	Minimize forklift traffic during shift changes to reduce exposure to moving forklifts during times when large numbers of worker pass through an area during a short time period	Provide protective hard hats, eyewear, and shoes
Contact with electrical energy	Install ground fault circuit interrupters in damp or wet locations	Develop and implement a hazardous energy control policy for all maintenance and repair activities	Provide electricians with properly rated dielectric gloves when procedures require work on energized components, such as troubleshooting an electrical panel
Overexertion	Use mechanical lifting devices, such as ceiling mounted cranes, to lift heavy and bulky items	Use job rotation schedules with different physical demands to reduce the frequency of lifting and repetitive motion tasks	Provide workers with nonslip safety gloves during manual materials handling tasks
Confined spaces	Where possible, locate serviceable components, such as pumps, agitators, and gauges outside of confined spaces so that entry is not required for maintenance, repair, or monitoring	Ensure workers test any confined space for flammable, toxic, or oxygen-deficient atmospheres prior to entry; identify and post warning signs outside of all confined spaces	Provide self-contained breathing apparatus or other appropriate air-supplied respirators if entry is required into spaces with flammable, toxic or oxygen-deficient atmospheres

Note. OSHA = Occupational Safety and Health Administration; NIOSH = National Institute for Occupational Safety and Health.
* NIOSH Ladder Safety Mobile Application. Available at: http://www.cdc.gov/niosh/topics/falls/mobileapp.html.

controls, processes, or technology and into the development of safe work practices increases the acceptance of positive changes and, thus, the success of safety programs.

An effective workplace safety program that minimizes injuries results from a multidisciplinary effort that actively involves every level of the workforce, from the employer and upper-level managers to employee representatives and workers. Each must assume some responsibility for safety and must work together interactively to achieve the common goal of preventing injuries.

Researchers provide science-based approaches to workplace injury prevention. The development of injury prevention strategies and technologies, through laboratory studies and field evaluations, yields evidence-based strategies and solutions to existing and emerging hazards. It is important for researchers and industry to work together in partnership throughout the research process to ensure that prevention strategies are relevant and applicable to the workplace, to demonstrate and evaluate prevention effectiveness in actual work settings, and to facilitate the transfer of research results to implementation and practice in the workplace. Injury prevention research results will only be effective in reducing injuries if they are directly communicated and transferred to employers, trainers, safety practitioners, regulators, and policymakers who can implement research results for prevention action. This research-to-practice process, developing and applying science-based prevention strategies in the workplace, is also a shared responsibility of the multiple entities with vested interest in workplace injury prevention.

Government agencies also play a role in preventing occupational injuries. Federal and state labor agencies are involved in data collection on occupational deaths and injuries through the BLS, and they serve a regulatory function by establishing standards for safe work practices and enforcing those regulations. Federal OSHA and 28 states and territories authorized by OSHA promulgate and enforce mandatory minimum standards for occupational safety and health in most industry sectors. The Mine Safety and Health Administration collects data and has regulatory responsibilities for miners. Other governmental agencies have prevention responsibilities for segments of the workforce, including agencies within the U.S. Department of Transportation for workers in trucking, transit, railroads, and aviation. Federal and state labor agencies also provide consultative services to employers and education to raise awareness about their standards and injury prevention practices. State health departments are involved in occupational safety at varying levels, including the collection, analysis, and interpretation of unique data not collected by BLS; disseminating occupational injury prevention recommendations using state networks; and ensuring that occupational injury prevention is encompassed within state injury prevention plans. Increasing state health department involvement in occupational safety holds considerable potential for improving worker safety (Box 19-6). (See Chapters 3 and 6.)

Box 19-6. Unique Role for Public Health Agencies in Occupational Safety

In 2008, NIOSH, in conjunction with the Council of State and Territorial Epidemiologists (CSTE), updated the publication *Guidelines for Minimum and Comprehensive State-Based Public Health Activities in Occupational Safety and Health*.[1] This publication highlights the important role of state public health agencies in fostering occupational safety and health, based on the three core functions of public health identified by the Institute of Medicine in 1988: assessment, policy development, and assurance.

Assessment: Assessment involves the regular and systematic collection, analysis, and communication of the public's health, including statistics on health status. There are numerous state-level data sources for assessing occupational injuries that include injuries not captured in the national occupational injury systems overseen by the BLS. These unique state-level data include hospital discharge data, emergency department data, workers' compensation records, burn center data, and poison control centers' data. CSTE has identified key occupational injury indicators that use existing state-level data to assess and track trends in occupational injuries at the state level, and these have been reported by 27 states to date. In-depth analyses of state-based occupational injury surveillance data have been conducted in several states, leading to state-specific injury prevention efforts, including prevention of burns and injuries among teen workers.

Policy development: Policy development involves the responsibility to develop public health policies based on scientific knowledge. Examples of how state health departments can contribute to sound policy development to improve worker safety include collaborating with stakeholders in establishing statewide

(continued)

Box 19-6. (Continued)

occupational safety objectives, such as the Healthy People 2020 objectives for the nation[2] to reduce occupational injuries; collaborating with public health partners to encompass the prevention of occupational injuries in broad statewide injury prevention programs and plans (such as those focused on reducing transportation injuries and injuries to adolescents); developing programs and working relationships with partners, such as state labor departments and OSHA, to collectively work toward preventing occupational injuries; and developing program capacity to identify and respond to emerging occupational safety hazards or unique prevention opportunities.

Assurance: Assurance involves making sure that services are available at the state level to achieve agreed-upon goals, such as injury prevention generally, or occupational injury specific goals. State health departments should have sufficient occupational safety expertise and resources to meet their populations' information needs and be able to provide appropriate referrals for technical assistance.

Public health agencies have statutory, regulatory, and philosophical commitments to protect the health of the public, including vulnerable groups who may fall outside the jurisdiction of federal or state regulatory agencies. The NIOSH/CSTE publication noted here provides guidelines on developing state-based public health programs in occupational safety and health, ranging from minimum activities that can be performed with existing state health department staff and data to more comprehensive approaches that require additional resources. It is intended that these guidelines will be used by state health agencies to develop the capacity for minimum activities in every state and to enhance existing programs. Numerous examples of state-based public health activities in occupational safety and health suggest that state public health agencies have a critical and complementary role to state labor agencies in preventing occupational injuries.

References

1. Stanbury M, Anderson H, Rogers P, et al. Guidelines for minimum and comprehensive state-based public health activities in occupational safety and health. DHHS (NIOSH) publication no. 2008-148. Cincinnati, OH: National Institute for Occupational Safety and Health, 2008. Available at: http://www.cdc.gov/niosh/docs/2008-148/pdfs/2008-148.pdf. Accessed September 14, 2016.
2. Healthy People.gov: Healthy People 2020, www.healthypeople.gov. Accessed September 14, 2016.

Further Reading

Council of State and Territorial Epidemiologists. Occupational health: Overview. Available at: http://www.cste.org/members/group.aspx?id=106606. Accessed September 11, 2016.

Davis L, Souza K. Integrating occupational health with mainstream public health in Massachusetts: An approach to intervention. Public Health Reports, 2009; 124: 5–14.

CONCLUSION

Occupational injuries continue to exert too large a toll on the workforce. While the rate of fatal injuries in the United States has decreased markedly over time, the rate of nonfatal injuries has not been reduced as much. The prevention of workplace injuries requires concerted and consistent efforts from multiple parties using multiple strategies. In addition to the primary stakeholders in the workplace, additional groups can help reduce occupational injuries. These groups include researchers who provide the evidence base for effective prevention strategies and technologies, manufacturers and distributors of industrial equipment and tools that design and promote safety features of equipment, insurers who provide monetary incentives for good safety records and practices, and healthcare providers and public health practitioners who provide their patients and constituents with information on preventing workplace injuries.

AUTHORS' NOTE

The findings and conclusions in this chapter are those of the authors and do not necessarily represent the views of the National Institute for Occupational Safety and Health (NIOSH). Mention of company names or products does not constitute endorsement by NIOSH. In addition, citations to websites external to NIOSH do not constitute NIOSH endorsement of the sponsoring organizations or their programs or products. Furthermore, NIOSH is not responsible for the content of these websites. All web addresses referenced in this document were accessible as of the publication date.

ACKNOWLEDGMENT

The authors acknowledge Dr. Stephanie Pratt, Director of the NIOSH Center for Motor Vehicle Safety, for her assistance in updating Box 19-3 and John Myers, Chief of the NIOSH

Surveillance and Field Investigations Branch, for his assistance in updating the CFOI, BLS, and NEISS data, Tables 19-1 through 19-3, and Figures 19-1 and 19-2.

REFERENCES

1. Bureau of Labor Statistics. Census of fatal occupational injuries charts, 1992–2015 (revised data). Available at: http://www.bls.gov/iif/oshwc/cfoi/cfch0014.pdf. Accessed June 19, 2017.

2. Bureau of Labor Statistics. Table SNR05: Incidence rate and number of nonfatal occupational injuries by industry and ownership, 2015. Available at: https://www.bls.gov/iif/oshwc/osh/os/ostb4740.pdf. Accessed June 19, 2017.

3. Committee on Education and Labor, U.S. House of Representatives. Hidden tragedy: Underreporting of injuries and illnesses. A majority staff report by the Committee on Education and Labor, U.S. House of Representatives, The Honorable George Miller, Chairman. Washington, DC: U.S. Government, June 2008.

4. National Institute for Occupational Safety and Health. Work-related Injury Statistics Query System, http://wwwn.cdc.gov/wisards/workrisqs/. Unpublished queries by Dawn Castillo on June 19, 2017.

5. Liberty Mutual Insurance. The most serious workplace injuries cost U.S. companies 59.9 billion per year, according to 2017 Liberty Mutual Workplace Safety Index. Boston, MA: Liberty Mutual Insurance. Available at: https://www.libertymutualgroup.com/about-lm/news/news-release-archive/articles/2017-lm-wsi. Accessed June 20, 2017.

6. Massachusetts Department of Public Health. Temporary worker died while cleaning a double auger screw conveyor machine-Massachusetts. Massachusetts Fatality Assessment and Control Evaluation Report 11-MA-050-01. Boston: Massachusetts Department of Public Health, Occupational Health Surveillance Program, 2014. Available at: https://www.cdc.gov/niosh/face/pdfs/11MA050.pdf. Accessed September 5, 2016.

7. Occupational Safety and Health Administration. Protecting temporary workers. Washington, DC: U.S. Department of Labor. Available at: https://www.osha.gov/temp_workers/ Accessed June 21, 2017.

8. Marsh SM, Layne LA. Fatal injuries to civilian workers in the United States, 1980–1995: National and state profiles. DHHS (NIOSH) Publication No. 2001-129S. Cincinnati, OH: U.S. Department of Health and Human Services, Centers for Disease Control and Prevention, National Institute for Occupational Safety and Health, 2001. Available at: http://www.cdc.gov/niosh/docs/2001-129/pdfs/01-129S.pdf. Accessed September 14, 2016.

9. Bureau of Labor Statistics. Fatal occupational injuries, total hours worked, and rates of fatal occupational injuries by selected worker characteristics, occupations, and industries, civilian workers, 2015. Washington, DC: U.S. Department of Labor, Bureau of Labor Statistics. Available at: http://www.bls.gov/iif/oshcfoi1.htm. Accessed June 19, 2017.

10. Steege AL, Baron SL, Marsh SM, Menendez CC, Myers JR. Examining occupational safety and health disparities using national data: A cause for continuing concern. American Journal of Industrial Medicine 2014, 57: 527–538.

11. Bureau of Labor Statistics. Table A-8. Fatal occupational injuries by event or exposure and age, all United States, 2015. Available at: http://www.bls.gov/iif/oshcfoi1.htm. Accessed June 21, 2017.

12. Bureau of Labor Statistics. Fatal occupational injuries incurred by contracted workers, 2011–2014. Available at: http://www.bls.gov/iif/oshcfoi1.htm/contractor.xlsx. Accessed June 20, 2017.

13. Bureau of Labor Statistics. Nonfatal occupational injuries and illnesses requiring days away from work, 2015. Washington, DC: BLS, 2016, News Release USDL 16-2130. Available at: http://www.bls.gov/news.release/osh2.nr0.htm. Accessed June 20, 2017.

14. Estes CR, Jackson LL, Castillo DN. Occupational injuries and deaths among young workers, United States, 1998–2007. Morbidity and Mortality Weekly Report, 2010; 59: 449–455. Available at: http://www.cdc.gov/mmwr/preview/mmwrhtml/mm5915a2.htm. Accessed September 11, 2016.

15. Bureau of Labor Statistics. Table R89: Number of occupational injuries and illnesses involving days away from work by selected worker characteristics and day of the week event occurred, private sector, 2015. Available at: https://www.bls.gov/iif/oshwc/osh/case/ostb4841.pdf. Accessed June 21, 2017.

16. Bureau of Labor Statistics. Table R96: Number of nonfatal occupational injuries and illnesses involving days away from work by selected worker characteristics and time of day event occurred, private industry, 2015. Available

at: https://stats.bls.gov/iif/oshwc/osh/case/ostb4848.pdf. Accessed June 21, 2017.

17. Bureau of Labor Statistics. Table R82: Number of nonfatal occupational injuries and illnesses involving days away from work by selected worker characteristics and hours on the job before event occurred, private industry, 2015. Available at: https://www.bls.gov/iif/oshwc/osh/case/ostb3284.pdf. Accessed June 21, 2017.

18. National Institute for Occupational Safety and Health. Prevention through design: Plan for a national initiative. Cincinnati, OH: NIOSH, 2010. DHHS (NIOSH) Publication No. 2011-121. Available at: http://www.cdc.gov/niosh/docs/2011-121/pdfs/2011-121.pdf. Accessed September 11, 2016.

19. ANSI/ASSE Z590-3-2011 (R2016). Prevention through design: Guidelines for addressing occupational hazards and risks in design and redesign processes. Des Plaines, IL: American Society of Safety Engineers, 2016.

20. ANSI/AIHA Z10-2012. Occupational health and safety management systems. Fairfax, VA: American Industrial Hygiene Association. Note: ASSE is now the secretariat for this standard.

21. deGuzman G, Higgins DN. Hispanic sawmill worker dies inside storage silo after being engulfed in sawdust—North Carolina. Morgantown, WV: NIOSH Division of Safety Research, 2005, Fatality Assessment and Control Evaluation Report 2004-09. Available at: http://www.cdc.gov/niosh/face/In-house/full200409.html. Accessed September 14, 2016.

22. Manuele, Fred A. Advanced safety management: Focusing on Z10 and serious injury prevention (2nd ed.). Hoboken, NJ. John Wiley & Sons, 2014.

23. Baker SP, O'Neill BO, Ginsburg MJ, Li G. The injury fact book (2nd ed.). New York: Oxford University Press, 1992.

24. Moore P, Pizatella T. Request for preventing worker injuries and fatalities due to the release of hazardous energy. DHHS (NIOSH) publication no. 99-110. Cincinnati, OH: U.S. Department of Health and Human Services, Centers for Disease Control and Prevention, National Institute for Occupational Safety and Health, 1999. Available at: https://www.cdc.gov/niosh/docs/99-110/. Accessed September 14, 2016.

25. Cohen A, Colligan MJ. Assessing occupational safety and health training. Cincinnati, OH: National Institute for Occupational Safety and Health, 1998, DHHS (NIOSH) publication no. 98-145. Available at: https://www.cdc.gov/niosh/docs/98-145/. Accessed September 14, 2016.

26. Johnston JJ, Cattledge GH, Collins JW. The efficacy of training for occupational injury control. Occupational Medicine: State of the Art Reviews 1994; 9: 147–158.

27. Hofmann DA, Jacobs R, Landry F. High reliability process industries: Individual, micro and macro organizational influences on safety performance. Journal of Safety Research 1995; 26: 131–149.

28. Shannon HS, Mayr J, Haines T. Overview of the relationship between organizational and workplace factors and injury rates. Safety Sciences 1997; 26: 201–217.

29. Zohar D. A group level model of safety climate: testing the effect of group climate on microaccidents in manufacturing jobs. Journal of Applied Psychology 2000; 85: 587–596.

30. OSHA-NIOSH. Recommended practices. Protecting temporary workers. Washington, DC: OSHA, 2014, DHHS (NIOSH) publication no. 2014-139. Available at: http://www.cdc.gov/niosh/docs/2014-139/pdfs/2014-139.pdf Accessed September 11, 2016.

FURTHER READING

American National Standards Institute. Safety of Machinery; General Requirements and Risk Assessment Electronic Standard. B11.0-2015. Park Ridge, IL: American Society of Safety Engineers, 2015.
This standard specifies basic terminology, principles, and a methodology for achieving safety in the design and the use of machinery. It specifies principles of risk assessment and risk reduction to help designers, integrators, and users of machinery in achieving this objective. These principles are based on knowledge and experience of the design, use, incidents, accidents, and risks associated with machinery. Procedures are described for identifying hazards and estimating and evaluating risks during relevant phases of the machine life cycle and for the elimination of hazards or the provision of sufficient risk reduction. Guidance is given regarding the documentation and verification of the risk assessment and risk reduction process.

Baron S, Cone J, Souza K (Eds). Special issue: Occupational health disparities. American Journal of Industrial Medicine, May 2014.
This special journal issue includes papers presented at Eliminating Health and Safety Disparities at Work, a 2014 multidisciplinary

national conference. *The issue includes commentaries and research papers addressing disparities by demographics, such as race and ethnicity; employment arrangements, such as temporary workers and day laborers; and illustrative industries, such as the hotel industry.*

Haight JM (Ed.). Safety professionals handbook, Vol. 1: Management applications and Vol. 2: Technical applications (2nd ed.). Park Ridge, IL: American Society of Safety Engineers, 2012. *This handbook serves as a reference for managers to improve safety, occupational health, or environmental programs addressing safety engineering management, hazard communication and right-to-know, environmental management, safety and health training, workers' compensation, and fleet safety. It also explains regulatory issues, applied science and engineering principles, cost analysis and budgeting, benchmarking and performance criteria, and best practices.*

Manuele FA. On the practice of safety (4th ed.) Hoboken, NJ: John Wiley & Sons, 2013. *This textbook addresses a broad range of topics on the practice of safety useful to managers, safety professionals, educators, and students. It includes chapters ranging from defining the practice of safety, the costs of worker injuries and illnesses, incident investigation, system safety, prevention through design, risk management, and measuring safety performance.*

Myers ML. Occupational safety and health policy. Washington, DC: American Public Health Association Press, 2015.

This comprehensive book provides information on occupational safety and health policy. It includes information on worker safety and health legislation, such as the Occupational Safety and Health Act and the Mine Safety and Health Act; how these laws have been implemented; and how they are enforced. Information is provided on other legislation and policy that impacts worker safety and health, including workers' compensation and right-to-know and privacy laws.

Occupational Safety and Health Administration. Concepts and techniques of machine safeguarding. OSHA 3067. Washington, DC: U.S. Department of Labor, Occupational Safety and Health Administration, 1992 (revised). Available at: https://www.osha. gov/Publications/Mach SafeGuard/toc.html. Accessed September 14, 2016. *An excellent reference for identifying potential hazards when working with industrial machinery. The publication also provides general principles of machine safeguarding to protect workers from injury.*

Wallerstein N, Rubenstein H. Teaching about job hazards: A guide for workers and their health providers. Washington, DC: American Public Health Association, 1993. *This comprehensive manual provides guidance for health and safety education to workers, including guidance specific to healthcare providers, as well as information for occupational safety and health training resources.*

20

Musculoskeletal Disorders

Carisa Harris-Adamson, Stephen S. Bao, and Bradley Evanoff

Work-related musculoskeletal disorders (WMSDs) commonly result from excessive physical and psychosocial demands of work. These disorders, which arise from nontraumatic injury of soft-tissue structures, such as muscles, tendons, ligaments, and nerves, are caused and/or exacerbated by workers' physical interactions with their work environments.

In the early 1700s, Bernardino Ramazzini first noted the harmful effects of unnatural postures and repetitive movements, such as numbness in the arms of scribes due to continual hand movements and sciatica among potters due to continual turning of the potter's wheel. People used a variety of terms to describe these common disorders, including *repetitive strain injury, washerwoman's sprain, telegrapher's cramp, carpet layer's knee*, and, more recently, *mouse hand* (or *mouse shoulder*) and *cellphone thumb*.

The most commonly affected body areas are the neck, arms, hands, and the low back. However, some WMSDs affect the hips and the knees.

Tendonitis and tenosynovitis, the most common types of WMSDs, are inflammatory disorders of the tendon and tendon sheath. These disorders include rotator cuff tendonitis, elbow epicondylitis, wrist extensor and flexor tendonitis, peripatellar knee tendonitis, peripheral entrapment neuropathies (such as carpal tunnel syndrome [CTS]), and mechanical or nonspecific disorders of the low back or neck.

WMSDs can cause pain, weakness, burning, and/or numbness and tingling, resulting in days away from work and reduced productivity. Symptoms can initially be intermittent and mild, but, without treatment and/or work continuation of exposure, they may become more frequent and severe.

Figure 20-1 presents a conceptual model of the contributors to WMSDs, including workplace factors (both physical and psychosocial), individual factors (gender, age, and other disorders), and their interaction. Causal attribution of specific cases of musculoskeletal disorders (MSDs) to work can be difficult and controversial (Box 20-1).

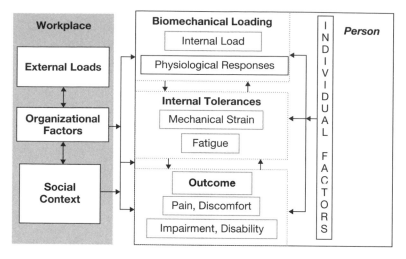

Figure 20-1. Conceptual model of contributors to musculoskeletal disorders. (Adapted from Institute of Medicine. Musculoskeletal disorders and workplace: Low back and upper extremities. Washington, DC: National Academies Press, 2001.)

Box 20-1. Plumber's Knee

A plumber was forced to retire at age 50. He was a plumber for 32 years. He spent 65% of his work time kneeling and squatting. This was frequently combined with heavy lifting. This led to numerous knee surgeries.

- First sought treatment for pain and swelling in 1980
- Arthroscopic surgery to repair torn meniscus in the knees in 1985
- Filed initial workers' compensation claim in 1983–1985
- Filed another claim in 1998 because first surgery not fully successful
- In 2003, the Vermont Supreme Court ruled that knee deterioration after 1995 was wholly attributable to the earlier injuries.

Comment: There are at least three features of WMSDs that contribute to controversy over attribution: (a) gradual onset (days to years), (b) none are uniquely caused by work, and (c) ubiquity of risk factors.

The basic mechanism for these disorders appears to be overloading tissue tolerance with insufficient recovery time. A variety of individual (gender and age) and lifestyle (obesity, smoking, and exercise), biomechanical, organizational, and social factors may contribute to the tension between overload and recovery.

Source: Workplace Ergonomics News 2003; 5: 6.

INCIDENCE AND SEVERITY

For 2015, the Bureau of Labor Statistics (BLS) reported 356,910 WMSDs[1] in private industry in the United States, for an annual incidence rate of 29.8 per 10,000 full-time workers.[1]

---

[1] BLS includes the following disorders and circumstances in its definition of MSDs: a pinched nerve; herniated disc; meniscus tear; sprain, strain, or tear; hernia; pain, swelling, and numbness; carpal tunnel syndrome and tarsal tunnel syndrome; Raynaud's syndrome and Raynaud's phenomenon; musculoskeletal system and connective tissue diseases and disorders, and when the event or exposure leading to the injury or illness is overexertion and bodily reaction, unspecified; overexertion involving outside sources; repetitive motion involving microtasks; other and multiple exertions or bodily reactions; and rubbed, abraded, or jarred by vibration.

Work-related musculoskeletal disorders, which resulted in a median of 12 days away from work, accounted for 32% of all injuries and illnesses reported to BLS. The service and manufacturing sectors together accounted for about 50% of cases. Incident cases and rates, by occupation, are shown in Table 20-1.

Workers' compensation for WMSDs in the United States accounts for about $16 billion in direct costs annually—almost 25% of all workers' compensation costs.[2] Incidence and direct costs for workers' compensation cases of WMSDs, by body area and specific conditions, have been reported by Washington State (Table 20-2). Indirect costs range from two to five times direct costs. WMSD cases are underreported in BLS surveys and workers' compensation data;[3] time

Table 20-1. Incidence of Work-Related Musculoskeletal Disorders in Private Industry, United States, 2015

Occupation	Number of Incident Cases	Incidence Rate per 10,000 Workers
Laborers and freight handlers	21,990	111.0
Nursing aides and orderlies	19,360	180.5
Janitors and cleaners	15,810	102.6
Heavy and tractor-trailer truck drivers	15,320	95.6
Emergency medical technicians/paramedics	3,980	187.4
Firefighters	5,630	168.5
Telecommunication line installers/repairers	2,190	224.6

Table 20-2. WMSDs of the Neck, Back, Upper Extremity, and Knee, Washington State Workers' Compensation Compensable* Claims, State Fund and Self-Insured, 2002–2010

Type	Incidence per 10,000 FTEs	Median Lost Workdays[†]	Median Cost[‡]
All	90.0	56	$11,183
Back	40.8	35	$6,032
Sciatica[§]	2.3	303	$46,872
Shoulder	14.8	129	$28,228
Rotator cuff syndrome[§]	6.2	192	$37,835
Elbow/forearm	5.3	116	$18,083
Epicondylitis[§]	1.6	129	$19,484
Hand/wrist	15.3	79	$14,166
Carpal tunnel syndrome[§]	6.4	100	$17,536
Tendonitis[§]	3.4	95	$15,721
Knee	10.1	56	$14,245
Bursitis[§]	0.2	60	$12,424

Note. WMSD = work-related musculoskeletal disorders; FTE = full-time equivalent employees.

* Claims involving 4 or more lost workdays.

[†] Lost workdays data are only available for State Fund claims.

[‡] Cost data are only available for State Fund claims and are adjusted to 2010 dollars.

[§] Data on incidence, lost workdays, and costs for specific WMSD diagnoses are only available for State Fund claims.

Source: Anderson N, Adams D, Bonauto D, et al. Work-related musculoskeletal disorders of the back, upper extremity, and knee in Washington State, 2002–2010. Technical Report 40-12-2015 SHARP Program. Tumwater: Washington State. Department of Labor and Industries, 2007.

away from work and reduced productivity are also underreported in official statistics.[4]

Changes in BLS case definitions over time have likely led to more underreporting. The Occupational Safety and Health Administration (OSHA) 200–300 logs underestimate the occurrence of WMSDs because they may be included in the "injuries" or the "all other illnesses" categories—or not at all.

Effectively addressing WMSDs involves early recognition, appropriate treatment, and exposure reduction. Early recognition depends on surveillance of worker symptoms and on worker education. Once a WMSD does occur, prompt appropriate medical treatment is essential. In addition, the workers' exposures should be assessed and task-specific interventions should be implemented. It may also be necessary to limit or modify the workers' duties. Comprehensive programs that integrate ergonomic improvements and medical treatment are effective in reducing the incidence and severity of WMSDs.[5]

Early recognition and treatment of WMSDs prevent progression to more severe and more costly conditions. (See Box 20-2.) Workers who are treated in the early stages of WMSDs have better prognoses and are less likely to have prolonged disability than workers treated only after prolonged duration of symptoms and development of functional deficits. Conservative management is most effective when begun in the early stages of these disorders.[6] With some disorders, such as CTS, workers can often be successfully treated with conservative measures in the early stages; however, if significant nerve conduction abnormalities develop, surgery may be necessary.[7]

Both healthy and injured workers benefit from workplace evaluations that identify physical stressors, many of which can be reduced or eliminated. Simple modifications can often maintain work productivity with less effort, thereby reducing risk of injury among healthy workers and enabling injured workers to safely return to their usual jobs more quickly.[8] Early and safe return to work is facilitated when clinicians have more information about workers' tasks and exposures and when worksite modifications reduce physical exposures.[9]

Comprehensive ergonomic programs incorporate primary and secondary prevention of WMSDs. Important components of prevention programs include job surveillance, symptom surveillance, and timely access to clinical evaluation. Job surveillance uses checklists or other tools to identify high-risk tasks needing

---

Box 20-2. The Choice of a Healthcare Provider for Injured Workers Is Important

Ideally, healthcare providers should have training or experience in ergonomics and the role of work modifications in the treatment of WMSDs. Effective diagnosis and treatment require knowledge of specific job duties. The best way for a healthcare provider to obtain knowledge of job duties is through a worksite visit. Since this is impractical in some clinical settings, information about exposures and job duties can also be obtained through a written work description or a videotape of the job task. Employers should have a contact person with knowledge of job activities and the ability to coordinate appropriate job placement during a recovery period. Working knowledge of the industry and the specific workplace is also needed to make appropriate recommendations regarding temporary or permanent job modifications. Many employers will provide detailed information about job duties and physical exposures to the treating physician. It is difficult to provide optimal care for employees when this information is not available.

---

ergonomic modifications. Symptom surveillance includes analyzing medical reports, monitoring OSHA 300 logs and/or administering symptom surveys. If workers and managers are trained to recognize symptoms early and clinical evaluation is accessible, many problems can be avoided. Secondary prevention can reduce the severity of WMSDs that are identified. Recommendations for diagnosing and treating WMSDs and for modifying jobs to reduce physical exposures (ergonomic hazards) and facilitate early and safe return to work have been published.[8]

Goals for medical management include:

- Eliminating or reducing pain and inflammation, with the goal of striving to break the pain/spasm cycle, which often occurs with MSDs (There are numerous medical treatments and therapeutic modalities, which are beyond the scope of this book; patients' self-management of pain is important.)
- Preventing progression of WMSDs
- Maximizing function to prevent disability
- Reducing risk of reinjury.

The vast majority of injured or symptomatic workers are able to return to productive work quickly, as long as their jobs are modified to reduce ergonomic hazards. Job modifications, which are frequently simple and inexpensive, can help employees safely return to work sooner and reduce risk of future injury. Examples of job modifications include:

- Training or retraining in work procedures that reduce physical exposure
- Implementing simple job changes, such as with a step stool or tilted work surface, to prevent awkward postures

- Changing tool design to reduce awkward postures and high hand forces
- Reducing force in use of equipment and tools
- Changing procedures, such as implementing job rotation
- Using conveyors, hoists, slides, and carts to reduce heavy lifting, pushing, pulling, and carrying. (See Chapter 9.)

When there is no simple fix to reduce or eliminate physical exposures that are causing or exacerbating WMSDs, temporary job transfer or restrictions can enable workers to recover. It is helpful to understand job requirements by reading about the physical demands of a job or observing workers performing job tasks, either in person or on video. Examples of temporary restrictions include:

- Reducing pace or quantity of work
- Restricting certain tasks
- Limiting work hours
- Setting functional restrictions for activities at work and at home, such as not lifting more than 5 pounds or not elevating shoulders beyond 90°.

If a worker needs to be transferred to a different job, the employer and a clinician should assess the new job to ensure that the worker will not be exposed to physical risk factors similar to those on the job that first caused or aggravated the condition. When this cannot be accomplished, temporary removal from work, to allow for healing, may the best option. In most cases, keeping an injured or symptomatic person working in an appropriate modified-duty position is preferable to lost worktime. Nonspecific low back pain will resolve relatively quickly among 90% of those injured; however, those who miss work for more than 12 weeks have a 40% probability of missing work for the remainder of the year and those who miss work for 2 years will likely never return.[10] With exposure reduction, modified duty, and supervised therapy as needed, injured workers can regain their physical capacity and confidence to return to work.[11]

Successful prevention programs have decreased the occurrence, duration, and severity of disability by improved early recognition and management of WMSDs and integration of ergonomic interventions with medical treatment of injured workers.[12] For example, an integrated program designed for sheet-metal workers at an aircraft manufacturer combined preplacement evaluations of workers with ongoing surveillance for symptoms and signs of upper-extremity WMSDs. Jobs were modified for those with signs of early disorders by restricting work hours and restricting use of vibrating hand tools. After implementation of this program for screening, surveillance, early medical evaluation, and job modification, there were decreases in workers' compensation costs, time away from work, and severity of injuries.[13]

Most major corporations have ergonomics programs that reduce the occurrence and severity of WMSDs. Successful approaches have most often combined ergonomic principles for prevention and improved recognition and management of WMSDs.

NECK AND UPPER-EXTREMITY DISORDERS

Five workplace physical exposures cause WMSDs of the upper extremity and neck:

- Forceful exertions
- Repetitive or prolonged duration of exertions
- Static or awkward postures
- Hand-arm vibration
- Mechanical or contact stresses.

Combinations of physical exposures within the same task increase risk.[14,15] The effects of these exposures can be exacerbated by workplace psychosocial factors, such as the perception of intense workload, monotonous work, and low levels of social support at work.[14] The way in which work is organized largely determines the physical and psychosocial dimensions of the work. Duration, frequency, and intensity of individual and combined occupational risk factors should be considered.

Physical Load Factors

Force, Repetition, and Sustained Exertion

Three types of muscle activity may contribute to the development of WMSDs:

- Sustained low force muscle contractions, such as moderate neck flexion while working at a computer for several hours without rest breaks (Note that the weight of the head in flexion is equivalent to that of a bowling ball.)
- Occasional high-force muscle contractions, such as intermittent use of heavy tools in overhead work
- Repetitive forceful exertions with inadequate work/rest cycles, which lead to fatigue.

Sustained static contractions or lack of adequate rest during repetitive forceful exertions can lead to increases in intramuscular pressure, potentially impairing blood flow to muscle cells and leading to fatigue and muscle soreness. Peak force exertions may cause small tears of tendons or muscle fibers, leading to inflammation and pain. High levels of exposure to repetitive and forceful movements, especially those of long duration or with awkward posture, are strongly associated with several WMSDs of the upper extremity.[14–17] Repetitive motions, such as by a data-entry operator performing thousands of keystrokes an hour (often in an awkward posture, with forearms pronated and wrists in ulnar deviation) or by a worker in a meat-processing plant who performs thousands of knife cuts a day, may eventually exceed ability of muscles, tendons, and nerves to recover from stress, especially if motions involve forceful contractions or prolonged static contractions of muscles.

Failure to recover usually implies some type of tissue damage or dysfunction, which may represent acute inflammation that is totally reversible. In WMSDs, the sites of likely tissue damage are most commonly tendons, tendon sheaths, and tendon attachments to bones, bursae, and joints.

Too many forceful contractions of muscles increase tension on tendons, compressing microstructures of the tendons and leading to ischemia, microscopic tendon tears, progressive lengthening, and sliding of tendon fibers through the ground substance matrix. Three primary pathophysiological pathways for the development of WMSDs have been hypothesized, including central nervous system reorganization, tissue injury or compression, and tissue reorganization.[18] All of these events can cause systemic inflammation, acutely or chronically, leading to fibrosis and eventual pain, discomfort, and/or loss of function.[18]

Posture, Mechanical Stress, and Vibration

In addition to repetitive and sustained forceful exertions, three other physical exposures that influence the development of WMSDs are external mechanical stress, work performed in awkward postures, and segmental (localized) vibration.

Posture is relevant because some postures (a) increase tension of tendons around bony prominences, increasing their susceptibility to injury; (b) lengthen muscles under tension, increasing their susceptibility to injury; (c) shorten or lengthen muscles, increasing the need to produce more muscle force on an object, due to the length-tension relationship of muscles; and (d) change the geometry of nerves and tendons, resulting in increased internal pressure and possible inflammation. For example, pinching while the wrist is flexed causes more stress on muscles and tendons than pinching while the wrist is in a neutral posture; when combined with high force, the stress would be even greater.[14]

Another source of mechanical stress results from a work surface or a hand-held tool with hard, sharp edges or the ends of a short handle that press on soft tissues. The tool exerts just as much force on the hand as the hand does on the tool. These stresses can lead to (a) neuritis due to forceful contact between one's thumb or fingers and the edge of scissors handles or (b) cubital tunnel syndrome in workers, such as microscopists, who must position their elbows on a hard surface for long periods. Short-handled tools, such as needle-nosed pliers, can dig into the base

of the palm and compress superficial branches of the median nerve.

Work with an arm elevated more than 60° from the trunk is more stressful for rotator cuff tendons than work performed with the arm at one's side. Rotator cuff tendonitis has been associated with a combination of increasing duration of shoulder extension/flexion and high hand forces.[14,19] Work performed in static postures that require prolonged, low-level muscle contractions of the arm or trapezius muscle may also trigger chronic localized pain even in jobs without high-force demands.

Segmental vibration is transmitted to the arm from impact tools, power tools, and bench-mounted buffers and grinders. Raynaud phenomenon and other disorders, including CTS, have been associated with several types of power tools, including chain saws, rock drillers, chipping hammers, and grinding tools. (See Chapter 12B.)

Changes in Work Load

Abrupt increases in workload that increase any of the physical risk factors of a job can cause various WMSDs. These abrupt increases can affect new workers, performing unaccustomed forceful or repetitive work,[2] and veteran workers who have an abrupt change in their type of duration of work or the way it is performed. For example, increases in the number of repetitive motions performed or the force with which they are performed can lead to tendonitis. Workers should be allowed to gradually adjust to increases in workload.

Nonoccupational Factors

Personal risk factors may influence the risk of developing WMSDs, including age and obesity,[14,20] as well as coexisting medical conditions, such as rheumatoid arthritis, diabetes, pregnancy, and acute trauma. Women seem to be at increased risk for some WMSDs. Few personal factors strongly predict susceptibility to WMSDs of the arm.

Psychosocial Factors

Psychosocial factors may be important in the risk of developing an WMSD and, subsequently, the risk of developing long-term disability.[21] (See

Chapter 14.) Multiple pathophysiological processes, such as sympathetic arousal, peripheral vasoconstriction, increased muscle tension, and immunosuppression, may explain the association between psychosocial factors and WMSDs.[22] The effects of psychosocial stress may operate by increasing muscle tension and decreasing micropauses in muscle activity or by interacting with increased catecholamine and cortisol secretion, thereby increasing pain perception and prolonging recovery.[22] Psychological factors may be especially important in determining whether specific WMSDs evolve into chronic pain syndromes due to responses of the central nervous system to high job stress.

Psychosocial factors predict MSD severity better than MSD incidence. The risk of arm disorders is increased by high structural constraints and perception of low decision latitude, and by high strain and low levels of social support at work.[14,23-25] Several measures have been used to define intense or stressful workloads, such as lack of control over how work is done, perceived time pressure, deadlines, work pressure, or lack of workload variability.[26] (See Chapter 14.)

Diagnosis

Evaluation of patients for suspected WMSDs of the neck or arm has three major components: (a) a history, (b) a physical examination of the neck and arm; and (c) assessment of the worksite and work tasks.[27,28]

The history should characterize symptoms by determining their location, radiation, duration, evolution, time patterns, and exacerbating and relieving factors. The worker's description of work activities is useful. The worker should be asked to describe the nature of specific work tasks and their risk factors (forceful exertions, repetitive activities, and other adverse exposures). Physical demands of job tasks should be reviewed or viewed, in person or on video. The history should include chronic stable exposures as well as acute changes in work tasks, tools, materials, and work pace or duration, such as more overtime, longer workdays, or fewer days off, with less time for recovery from fatigue and occult injury.

Determining whether an affected worker has a predisposing medical condition, such

as previous injury to the symptomatic area, is important. However, since causation of MSDs is frequently multifactorial, the presence of non-occupational risk factors does not negate the importance of coexisting occupational factors.

Awareness of industries and occupations associated with increased risk upper-extremity disorders can alert clinicians (Table 20-3). Since there are also high-risk jobs in low-risk industries, assessment of a worker's physical exposures is important.

Table 20-3. Most Frequent Occupations in High-Risk Industries for Compensable Work-Related Musculoskeletal Disorder Claims in Washington State

Industries	Occupations
Forest nurseries and forest-product gathering	Nursery workers
	Laborers/farmworkers
	Production inspecting/packing
	Floral design
Masonry, stonework, tile, plastering	Drywall installers
	Insulation installers
	Brick masons
Roofing	Roofers
	Carpenters
	Laborers
Meat products	Butchers and meatcutters
	Laborers and freight stocking/handling
	Hand packers
Dairy products	Laborers and freight handlers/stockers
	Truck drivers
	Hand packers
Sawmills	Lumber handlers
Millwork	Laborers
	Woodworking machine operators
	Assemblers
	Cabinetmakers
Iron and steel foundries	Mold and core
	Furnace/oven
	Grind/polish machine operators
	Laborers
	Machine operators
Heating, ventilation, and air conditioning	Welder/cutter
	Assembler/fabricator
	Laborer
	Grinding/polishing machine operators
Nursing and personal care facilities	Nursing aides and orderlies
	Health aides
	Nurses
	Maids/housekeeping

(continued)

Table 20-3. (Continued)

Industries	Occupations
Local and suburban passenger transport	Emergency medical technicians Bus drivers Physician assistants/nurses Mechanics Taxi/drivers
Trucking and courier services	Truck drivers Freight handlers/stockers Refuse and recyclable collectors Grader/sorters
Air transportation scheduled and air courier services	Freight/stock handlers Flight attendants Couriers/messengers Transport/ticket/reservations Mechanics
Examples of high-risk occupations that cross over most industries	Housekeeping/janitorial Data-entry operators Stockers/receivers Assembly, packaging
Dairy product manufacturing	Laborers and freight stockers Production workers Truck drivers (heavy and light) Packagers and package handlers
Waste collection	Refuse and recycled materials collectors Truck drivers (heavy and light) Laborers Bus and truck mechanics Welders and cutters
Nursing care facilities	Nursing aides and orderlies

Source: Silverstein B, Kalat J, Fan ZJ. Work-related musculoskeletal disorders of the neck, back, and upper extremity in Washington State, state fund and self insured workers' compensation claims 1993–2001. Tumwater: Washington State Department of Labor and Industries, 2003.

Physical examination of the upper extremity involves inspection, assessment of the range of motion, strength, palpation, and evaluation of peripheral nerve function. Numbness and paresthesia can result from peripheral nerve compression as well as diabetes, alcohol abuse, exposure to organic solvents, and many other causes. Increased pain on resisted maneuvers often results from lesions in a tendon or at its insertion to bone. In some cases, it is not possible to determine the precise source of pain in the upper extremity; in others, it is possible to determine the specific disorder that is present. The severity of these disorders varies widely. Published guidelines provide standardized methods for diagnosis, for use in epidemiological studies and clinical practice.[27–30]

Workers in certain occupations, such as keyboard operators, musicians, and newspaper reporters, often have an increased rate of pain in the upper extremity or neck.

Diagnosis of a WMSD of the upper extremity involves three steps:

1. Determining, usually by history and physical exam, whether the individual has a specific disorder, such as flexor tendonitis of the forearm.
2. Obtaining evidence from a detailed occupational history, direct observation of work tasks (in person or on video), and/or review of detailed job descriptions and job safety analyses. Table 20-4 lists illustrative exposures of concern.[31]
3. Considering nonoccupational causes, based on the history and physical exam. Review and analysis of surveillance and epidemiologic data of similar work may provide information on the relative contributions of occupational and nonoccupational factors in causing a specific WMSD in the worker's occupation and industry. Except for tests of nerve conduction, sophisticated diagnostic or laboratory studies are often not necessary, unless the worker (a) has a history of trauma, (b) has symptoms suggestive of underlying systemic disease, or (c) fails to improve with conservative treatment.

Determining the relative contributions of occupational factors in causing WMSDs is often challenging. The critical question is: Were the physical exposures at work of sufficient magnitude, frequency, and duration to have caused or aggravated the WMSD in a worker? Intense periods of high exposure for even just a few days can cause many WMSDs. Commonly, a worker is simultaneously exposed to multiple risk factors, such as repetitive and forceful hand exertion, shoulder abduction, and vibration from hand tools.

Neck Disorders

Nonradiating neck pain is often called *tension neck syndrome*, suggesting muscular origin. Nonradicular radiating neck pain is often reported by patients with neck-shoulder pain. Arm pain

Table 20-4. Caution Zone Risk Factors, Washington State Ergonomics Rule/Guideline, 2000

Movements or postures that are a regular and foreseeable part of the job, occurring more than 1 day per week and more frequently than 1 week per year

Awkward postures	Working with the hand(s) above the head, or the elbow(s) above the shoulders, more than 2 hours total per day
	Working with the neck or back bent more than 30° (without support and without the ability to vary posture) more than 2 hours total per day
	Squatting more than 2 hours total per day
	Kneeling more than 2 hours total per day
High hand forces	Pinching an unsupported object(s) weighing 2 or more pounds per hand, or pinching with a force of 4 or more pounds per hand, more than 2 hours per day (comparable to pinching half a ream of paper)
	Gripping an unsupported objects(s) weighing 10 or more pounds per hand, or gripping with a force of 10 or more pounds per hand, more than 2 hours total per day (comparable to clamping light duty automotive jumper cables onto a battery)
Highly repetitive motions	Repeating the same motion with the neck, shoulders, elbows, wrists, or hands (excluding keying activities) with little or no variation every few seconds, more than 2 hours total per day
	Performing intensive keying more than 4 hours total per day
Repeated impacts	Using the hand (heel/base of palm) or knee as a hammer more than 10 times per hour, more than 2 hours total per day
Frequent, awkward, or heavy lifting	Lifting object weighing more than 75 pounds once per day or more than 55 pounds more than 10 times per day
	Lifting objects weighing more than 10 pounds if done more than twice per minute, more than 2 hours total per day
	Lifting objects weighing more than 25 pounds above the shoulders, below the knees, or at arms length more than 25 times per day
Moderate to high hand-arm vibration	Using impact wrenches, carpet strippers, chain saws, percussive tools (jack hammers, scalers, riveting or chipping hammers) or other tools that typically have high vibration levels, more than 30 minutes total per day
	Using grinders, sanders, jigsaws, or other hand tools that typically have moderate vibration levels more than 2 hours total per day

often occurs with lateral head movement in non-radicular radiating pain.[28] Limitation in range of motion of the neck (especially extension) with radiating symptoms and/or a positive Sperlings test (cervical extension with some sidebend and contralateral rotation) can help determine if cervical radiculopathy is present.[32]

Nontraumatic neck disorders, which occur frequently, involve primarily neck-shoulder muscles. According to Washington State Fund workers' compensation data, between 1998 and 2006, the annual incidence of neck disorders was 31.5 per 10,000 full-time equivalent employees (FTEs). The annual incidence of neck pain lasting more than 1 week in office environments is about 34%.

Table 20-5 summarizes risk factors for neck and neck/shoulder disorders. Among office workers, women report neck pain about six times as frequently as men. The combination of high mental stress and limited physical exercise increases risk about six-fold. Several work factors have been associated with time away from work due to neck pain, including jobs that involve prolonged flexion and rotation of the neck and jobs that involve a limited role in decision-making.[33]

Among nurses, increased risk of neck/shoulder pain occurs with patient-handling tasks involving pushing/pulling and reaching. When a worker's history of neck/shoulder complaints are combined with a physical exam revealing pressure tenderness, prevalence is about 7% and annual incidence about 2%. Workers who perform highly repetitive shoulder work (16 to 40 movements per minute) and/or forceful work have two to four times the risk.[14,19,34] Prolonged neck flexion and lack of recovery time from highly repetitive work also increase risk. Perceived job demands almost double the risk. Those experiencing a recent increase in exposure (prolonged work using monitors, keyboards, and mice, or work above the shoulder) are more likely to seek healthcare than those

Table 20-5. Risk Factors for Nontraumatic Neck and Neck/Shoulder Disorders

Individual factors	Age
	Female gender (may be a function of gender segregation)
	Little physical exercise
Physical work factors	Prolonged seated work
	Neck flexion, rotation
	Prolonged shoulder shrugging
	Repetitive shoulder or hand work
	Inappropriate keyboard location
Psychosocial factors	Low decision latitude
	High demands
	High mental stress
Jobs with high-risk activities	Dental workers
	Microscopists
	Video display terminal workers
	Surgeons
	Nurses/nursing assistants
	Electronics assemblers

Table 20-6. Risk Factors for Nontraumatic Shoulder Disorders

Individual factors	Age
	Obesity
	Male gender
	Lack of physical exercise
Physical work factors	Repetitive shoulder work
	Repetitive hand work with tools
	High hand force
	Working above shoulder height
	Working in a bent posture
	Physically strenuous work
	Shoulder angle greater than 45° static or repetitively
Psychosocial factors	Low decision latitude
	Monotonous work
	Mental stress
	High job demands
	Depression
Jobs with high-risk activities	Truck drivers
	Carpenters
	Welders
	Drywall installers
	Meatpacking
	Assembly workers
	Masons
	Nursing assistants
	Freight handlers
	Garbage collectors

who have been exposed long term, suggesting a short induction time.

Shoulder Disorders

Rotator cuff tendonitis is one of the most frequent and costly upper-extremity disorders associated with work. In Washington State from 1998 through 2007, the average cost of a compensable workers' compensation claim for rotator cuff tendonitis was $35,000, largely due to extensive lost worktime and frequent surgery.

Rotator cuff disease generally occurs after intensive activity of the shoulder, followed by remission with rest or treatment. Symptoms can become constant, especially with activities that are overhead and require arm strength. Slow onset of localized pain that increases with activity suggests rotator cuff tendonitis, especially when pain is above or lateral to the shoulder. In contrast, sudden onset of pain suggests a traumatic fracture, dislocation, or rotator cuff tear.

Table 20-6 summarizes risk factors for shoulder disorders. Rotator cuff disease is more common in men and after age 40 (with onset generally around age 55). Repetitive overhead activities and sports predispose to rotator cuff tendonitis. In working populations, repetitive, prolonged, and forceful shoulder work increases the risk of shoulder tendonitis three-fold.[19,33,35] Exposure thresholds may be different for men and women.

Risk increases among men who spend 2 or more hours daily with repeated or sustained shoulder abduction greater than 90°; risk increases among women with shoulder abduction greater than 60°. Both men and women are at increased risk when a task is highly repetitive (occurring four or more times daily).[36]

Half of individuals with shoulder tendonitis due to repetitive work recover within 10 months, but recovery slows with increasing age. Newly employed workers are at increased risk of shoulder pain if they are lifting heavy weights, lifting with one hand, lifting above shoulder height, or pushing or pulling heavy loads. Monotonous work and depression may be independent risk factors but not as important as repetitive use of tools or low decision latitude.[37]

Bicipital tendonitis, which is less common than rotator cuff tendonitis, presents with pain in the anterior shoulder, occasionally radiating down to the elbow. It is aggravated by shoulder flexion, forearm supination, or elbow flexion with forceful exertions. In the early stages, pain is worst at onset and completion of an activity, gradually becoming constant. On physical exam, pain in the bicipital groove is exacerbated with resisted arm flexion with a supinated forearm and full elbow extension or on resisted supination.

Elbow and Forearm Disorders

Epicondylitis is characterized by pain at muscle–tendon junctions or insertion points of forearm flexor (medial) or extensor (lateral) tendons. Pain is usually localized around the epicondyle, but it may radiate distally to the forearm. Lateral epicondylitis ("tennis elbow") is more frequently reported than medial epicondylitis ("golfer's elbow"). Lateral epicondylitis results from inflammation at the muscular origin of forearm extensors, leading to microscopic tears and subsequent fibrosis. Medial epicondylitis involves primarily the flexor/pronator muscles at their origin on the anterior medial epicondyle. Concurrent compression of the ulnar nerve in or around the medial epicondyle groove has been estimated to occur in half of the cases. Epicondylitis can occur in data-entry operators; longer duration of keyboarding and unsupported awkward postures increases their risk. Industrial workers, primarily those using forceful twisting (supination/pronation) motions, such as in using screwdrivers, are also at increased risk for epicondylitis. Reducing force requirements of a job, implementing frequent "microbreaks," and varying tasks that use different muscle groups ("active breaks") can usually reduce the incidence and severity of epicondylitis.

Repetitive forceful stress at the musculotendinous junction and its origin at the epicondyle can cause acute tendonitis—which may progress to chronic tendonitis (tendinosis) due to failure of tendon healing. Peak incidence occurs in workers 20 to 49 years old; males account for two-thirds of the cases. Onset can accompany an acute injury, but more commonly it is associated with repetitive use of the extensor/supinator or flexor/pronator muscles. Work activities, such as using a screwdriver or hammer, increase risk. Frequency of forceful exertions as well as the combination of supination and lifting increase risk.[38]

With repetitive work, the incidence of lateral epicondylitis is approximately 11 per 10,000

Table 20-7. Risk Factors for Nontraumatic Elbow/Forearm Disorders

Individual factors	Age
	Other work-related musculoskeletal disorders
Physical work factors	Driving screws
	Tightening with force
Psychosocial factors	Low discretion
	High demands
	High mental stress
Jobs with high-risk activities	Carpenters
	Machinists
	Laborers
	Plumbers
	Assembly work with hand tools
	Hairdressers
	Drywall installers
	Hand packers
	Electricians
	Bus drivers
	Welders
	Grinders/polishers
	Butchers/meatcutters
	Kitchen/food preparation

FTEs, with an average of 271 days away from work per claim and an annual cost in the United States exceeding $12 million.[34] It increases with age, number of other upper-limb diagnoses, and "turn-and-screw" motions.[38,39] The amount of time spent in forceful exertion (lifting or using a power grip) while in pronation (45° or more) are important predictors of lateral epicondylitis.[40] Forceful work increases risk. Medial epicondylitis is often found with other upper-limb disorders in working populations. Approximately 80% of patients recover within 3 years. Table 20-7 summarizes risk factors for elbow and forearm disorders.

Diagnostic criteria include intermittent to continuous pain in the epicondylar area, pain on resisted lateral wrist extension of the wrist, or resisted medial pronation of the wrist. Symptoms often last up to 1 year, irrespective of treatment. They are exacerbated by forceful gripping activities. Poor prognoses are associated with intensive manual work and high baseline pain.

Hand and Wrist Disorders

The most frequent chronic WMSD hand and wrist diagnoses are tendonitis and CTS (Figure 20-2). The incidence of workers' compensation claims

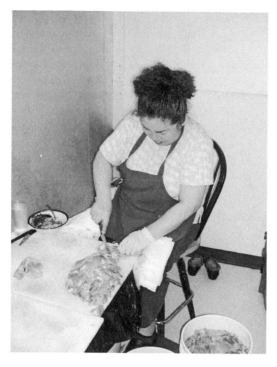

Figure 20-2. Woman in Nicaragua cutting meat. A high degree of hand force and frequent repetition combine to make this a high-risk job for development of carpal tunnel syndrome and tendonitis. In addition, this woman faces the potential hazards of cuts and neck strain. (Photograph by Barbara Silverstein.)

Table 20-8. Risk Factors for Nontraumatic Carpal Tunnel Syndrome and Tendonitis

Individual factors	Age
	Obesity
	Female gender
	Pregnancy
	Rheumatoid arthritis, diabetes, hypothyroidism, hypertension
Physical work factors	High-force, highly repetitive work, hand-arm vibration
	Repetitive pinching tightening/ holding with force
	Repetitive hitting
Psychosocial factors	Low discretion
	Low job satisfaction
	High demands
	Poor social support
	High mental stress
Jobs with high-risk activities	Meatcutting
	Lumber turners
	Food processors
	Carpenters
	Assembly work with hand tools
	Foundry workers
	Hairdressers
	Kitchen workers
	Laborers
	Machine operators
	Sewing operators
	Hand packing
	Typist
	Stock handler/bagger
	Roofers

for all nontraumatic upper-extremity disorders in the United States is 32.4 per 10,000 FTEs, with a median of 10 days away from work.[1] Table 20-8 summarizes risk factors for CTS and tendonitis.

Carpal Tunnel Syndrome

Carpal tunnel syndrome, which is characterized by pain, paresthesias, and/or weakness in the median nerve distribution of the hand, is due to entrapment of the median nerve in the carpal tunnel at the wrist. Diagnostic criteria include symptoms in the median nerve distribution of the hand and abnormal conduction of the median nerve across the wrist.

The most important workplace physical factor associated with the occurrence of CTS is forceful hand exertion; hand exertion force, repetitive forceful exertions, and more time spent in forceful exertion are all important risk factors,[41] as are sustained awkward wrist postures (likely ones that also require forceful hand exertions) and hand-arm vibration. The more these factors

occur simultaneously, the greater the risk.[20] Epidemiological studies have not determined that CTS is associated with computer work,[42,43] but many studies have relied on self-reports of keyboard and mouse use and on overall daily computer use. Meatpackers, assembly-line workers, construction workers, and other workers with repeated or sustained high-force and high-repetition tasks are at much higher risk for CTS than office workers. Carpal tunnel syndrome has been associated with hand-arm vibration,[44] but it is difficult to separate vibration from high hand force. (See Chapter 12B.) When workers are exposed to high force and high repetition simultaneously, CTS risk increases dramatically.[41,44]

Personal risk factors include diabetes, obesity, rheumatoid arthritis, older age, pregnancy, and female gender. In work-related CTS, the gender difference may be due to a greater willingness of women to report symptoms[14] or women working at a greater level of their physical capacity—that is, the same work task requires a higher percentage of maximum voluntary muscle contraction in women than in their male counterparts.

Ulnar nerve entrapment in the Guyon canal at the wrist, which usually presents as motor impairment, is much less frequently reported than median nerve entrapment in the carpal tunnel. Cubital tunnel syndrome (frequently called "student's elbow" or "Saturday night palsy") results from compression of the ulnar nerve due to prolonged weight bearing on the elbow; there is some evidence that prolonged elbow flexion is also a risk factor. Radial nerve entrapment, which is less common than ulnar nerve entrapment, may be related to repetitive upper-arm activities requiring gripping and squeezing, especially with repetitive or forceful supination.

Hand and Wrist Tendonitis/Tenosynovitis

Tendonitis causes pain over the tendon close to where it is inserted in the muscle and can cause mild swelling over the tendon. Tendonitis worsens with repetitive forceful motion. Similar to CTS, the highest risk of hand and wrist tendonitis is associated with a combination of high hand force, repetitive forceful exertions, or a high percentage of work time spent in forceful hand exertions.[45] There are various types of tendonitis associated with the various tendons in the hand and wrist. *DeQuervain's tendonitis*, the most common type, presents with a history of repetitive pinching and pain along the radial aspect of the wrist below the base of the thumb (elicited with the Finkelstein test— passive ulnar deviation with the thumb inside a closed fist). Tendonitis worsens with activity and improves with rest. "Trigger finger" (volar flexor tenosynovitis) presents with tenderness at the proximal end of the tendon sheath, in the distal palm, and with a catching of the tendon when the finger is flexed. There is frequently palpable tendon thickening and nodularity.

The case in Box 20-3 illustrates the intermittent and progressive nature of most work-related disorders of the upper extremity, especially CTS.

The goals of treatment for neck and upper extremity MSDs are elimination or reduction in symptoms and impairment as well as return to work under conditions that will protect health. These goals can be most easily achieved by early and conservative treatment. Early treatment of WMSDs is less difficult and less costly, often reduces the need for surgical procedures, decreases absence from work, shortens stressful exposures, and increases effectiveness of treatment. Early interaction among the clinician, the worker, and the employer facilitates safe and successful return to work. This ergonomics approach has been successful for workers compensation' claimants for upper-limb problems.[5-7]

In addition to engineering changes, restricted duty, job rotation, or temporary transfer may be effective. For job rotation or temporary transfer to be effective, the new job duties must result in a net reduction in level of exposure for the targeted body region/diagnosis. It is often necessary to conduct an evaluation of the new duties to determine whether a reduction in exposure will occur. The magnitude of reduction required to facilitate recovery often is not known. In general, the more severe the disorder, the greater the reduction in magnitude and duration of exposure that will be required. Workers should be removed from the workplace only in severe cases or after less drastic measures have failed to be effective.

Splints and other immobilization devices may provide rest to the symptomatic region of the body. However, they may increase the level of exposure if workers must resist devices to perform regular job tasks. Workers may also adapt to wearing a splint by altering their work activities in a way that leads to substantial stress on another part of the arm, such as the elbow or shoulder. Immobilization or prolonged rest may have direct adverse effects if either leads to muscle atrophy. As a result, careful monitoring is indicated for workers on restricted duty, temporarily transferred to another job, or wearing immobilization devices. In addition, because it is difficult to predict the clinical course of these conditions and because the empiric basis of many treatments is poorly understood, frequent follow-up is desirable.

With early treatment and reduced or eliminated exposure, many of these conditions resolve within a few weeks. People with moderately severe CTS improve better with surgery than with splinting.[46]

With conservative treatment and appropriate workplace adjustments, most workers with

Box 20-3. Carpal Tunnel Syndrome Case

A 31-year-old, right-handed man had been employed in a variety of automobile manufacturing jobs for 13 years. Two years ago, he switched to a new plant and was assigned to a job that required him to manipulate a spot-welding machine beneath cars moving overhead. He completed four welds/minute on each car. The metal handles of the spot welder required substantial force for appropriate positioning, and they were manually repositioned four times/car. The worker's wrists were in extreme extension for a substantial portion of the job cycle.

When the worker started on this job, the work shift was 9 hours for 6 days per week. After 3 weeks on the job, he noted that he had pain in both wrists, numbness and tingling in the first four fingers of his left hand, at first only at night, a few nights each week, after he had fallen asleep. When he awoke at night with the numbness, it was alleviated by shaking his hands. Gradually, over the next several months, the numbness and pain worsened in both frequency and intensity. His left hand would feel numb by the end of the work shift, and any time he was driving his hands would become numb. Because he liked his job and did not want to be placed on restriction, which would mean he could not work overtime, he decided to visit his private physician rather than the company physician. He also was not sure that the company physician would be very sympathetic to his complaints.

The physician found on physical examination that the worker had decreased sensitivity to light touch in the left index and middle fingers and a positive wrist flexion-nerve compression test of the left hand. She suspected CTS and believed that the disorder might be work-related because the patient was young, male, and had no other risk factors, such as diabetes, past history of wrist fracture, or recent trauma to the wrist. The physician discussed job changes with the patient. She also prescribed wrist splints to be used at night.

The splints relieved some of the nighttime numbness for a period. However, over the next 6 months, the symptoms became present most of the time, and he thought that his left hand was becoming weaker. Similar symptoms also developed in his right hand.

The patient felt he could no longer do his job and returned to his physician who ordered nerve conduction tests that showed slowing of median sensory nerve impulse conduction in the carpal tunnel, more so on the right than the left. She referred him to a hand surgeon.

One year after the problem was first noted, the worker had surgery, first on the left hand and then on the right. After surgery, the company placed him in a transitional work center for a 3-month period, where he worked at his own pace and had no symptoms. He then returned to the assembly line with the restriction that he not use welding guns or air-powered hand tools. When he worked on the line, he occasionally had symptoms, but they were substantially less intense and less frequent than before.

He later transferred to a warehouse, because he felt that he would have a better chance of avoiding long layoffs there. His job required use of a stapling gun to seal packages. Three weeks after beginning this job, his symptoms began to return with their former intensity. Through ordinary channels, he immediately sought and was given a transfer to a position driving a forklift truck. This change reduced, but did not eliminate, his symptoms. Currently, he has numbness, tingling, and pain in the fingers of both hands about twice a month. Playing volleyball usually triggers a severe attack. With the use of nighttime splints, he can sleep through most nights without awakening. Although he believes that his hands are weaker than before the symptoms developed, he is still able to perform his job. He has decided that he will continue working as long as the symptoms remain at no more than the present level.

---

upper-extremity WMSDs can return to work. However, a small percentage develop chronic symptoms that are difficult to treat; in these cases, physical capabilities of the worker, work demands, and psychosocial factors strongly influence whether the person can return to work.[6] The ways in which these factors interact are complex. The recognition of psychosocial factors—such as supervisory and peer support and negative self-fulfilling beliefs of the worker, the employer, or the clinician—is important and should not lead to ignoring the role of occupational physical exposures or to "blaming the victim." When the latter occurs, delayed recovery is often attributed to personal weakness, low job satisfaction, or desire for secondary gain. Critical to prevention of these persistent cases is

early intervention—an important reason to promote early reporting of symptoms.

Comprehensive programs to address physical reconditioning of workers, psychosocial factors, and workplace factors, such as ongoing exposure, have been developed.[47] A contract between the worker and the clinician should be established early, explicitly aiming to return the worker safely to work.

LOW BACK PAIN

Low back pain is common among workers who typically present with nonspecific discomfort or sciatica. It is second only to respiratory illnesses as a symptom for physician visits. In the

United States and other high-income countries, about 75% of adults will experience a significant episode of low back pain at some time. More than 22 million cases of back pain that last at least 1 week or more occur annually in the United States, resulting in almost 150 million days away from work.[48]

Low back pain is a major cause of disability, limitation of activity, and economic loss. Disability due to low back pain is influenced by the physical condition of the affected person, medical care, the work environment, the workers' compensation system, and other factors. In the United States in 2015, the incidence of non-fatal occupational low back disorders was 17.3 per 10,000 FTEs, with a median of 7 days of lost time at work. (See Table 20-2.)

Back pain can be categorized by symptoms, medical treatment, and/or disability. Relatively few people with low back pain see a healthcare provider, and most of these encounters do not lead to a change in the person' work status. Very few people with low back pain develop long-term disability. In a given individual, onset, severity, reporting, and prognosis of low back pain may be influenced by many work and nonwork factors. Personal risk factors for low back pain in a patient do not rule out work-related risk factors and vice-versa.

Etiology

Low back pain is associated with work-related lifting, forceful movements, whole body vibration,[49] heavy physical work, and work in awkward postures (bending and twisting).[34,47,50] Psychosocial factors, such as job satisfaction, personality traits, perception of intensified workload, and job control, are associated with low back pain.[51]

Jobs requiring frequent lifting of objects weighing 25 pounds or more seem to be associated with an increase in risk, as are sudden and unexpected maximal lifting.[52] The effect of lifting may be modified by individual fitness and strength; by the rate, position, and height of the lifting task; and the distance of the lifted object to the spine—and the weight of the object lifted, the greatest factor affecting the mechanical strain of lifting. The exposure to vibration that accompanies motor vehicle operation (4 to 6 Hz) is also a risk factor for low back pain.[49] Truck

Table 20-9. Jobs with High-Risk Activities for Sciatica, Washington State Fund Workers' Compensation Claims, 1993–2001

Nursing aides/orderlies	Nurses
Truck drivers	Construction laborers
Carpenters and apprentices	Garbage collectors
Maids and housekeeping cleaners	Glaziers
Drywall installers	Freight/stock handlers
Carpet installers	Brick masons

drivers, manual-material handlers, and nursing personnel have high rates of compensable back pain. Hospital workers, especially nurses, nursing aides, and others who lift and move patients, have high rates of disabling low back disorders.[53] (See Table 20-9.)

The frequency and severity of low back pain are also associated with many personal factors, including age, gender, physical fitness, lumbar mobility and strength, tobacco use, physical activity outside of work, past history of low back disorders, and congenital anomalies, such as spondylolisthesis.[54,55]

Diagnosis and Evaluation

Low back pain may arise from (a) any of the structures comprising the lumbosacral spine and associated soft tissues or (b) abdominal, retroperitoneal, or pelvic structures. It may result from local or systemic processes. Even with clinical tests and imaging procedures, the causes of most episodes of low back pain are not clear and the vast majority of patients cannot be given a precise anatomical diagnosis—with pain typically assumed to be related to soft tissue injury or degenerative changes. Nonspecific terms, such as *sprain* or *strain*, are commonly used to describe the etiology of low back pain.

If low back pain is related to work, it is important to identify any work exposures that may need to be modified to facilitate the patient's recovery and prevent recurrence or occurrence in other workers. Evaluation should address these questions:

- How is the pain related to work?
- Is the pain caused by a serious local condition, such as a fracture, or by a systemic disease?

- Is there compromise of neurological structure or function that may require evaluation by a surgeon?
- Are there social or psychological factors that may amplify or prolong the pain?
- What is the patient's fitness or capacity for future work?[56]

The history should elicit information on:

- The patient's work activities, including awkward or static postures, lifting requirements, other forceful movements, whole body vibration, and need for back bending and twisting
- Monotonous work, job control, job satisfaction, and social support
- Temporal relationship of pain to work or other activities
- Other precipitating factors
- Previous low back disorders
- Onset and time course of symptoms
- Any functional limitations
- Location of symptoms, including radiation of pain to or paresthesias in the distal lower extremity
- Alcohol or drug abuse
- Symptoms of depression.

The history should attempt to identify factors that increase the likelihood of a serious disorder:

- History of trauma
- Age over 50 or under 20
- History of malignancy or immune system compromise
- Pain that worsens with lying in the supine position
- Recent onset of bowel or bladder dysfunction, or "saddle anesthesia"
- Severe or progressive neurologic impairment of the legs.[54]

The history may identify factors that amplify or prolong pain and are amenable to specific intervention, and may provide information that can facilitate the person's eventual return to work.

The physical examination should seek signs suggestive of a serious medical condition. A baseline physical examination allows clinical progression to be assessed. Beginning with the patient disrobed and standing, the alignment, curvature, and symmetry of the spine, pelvis, and lower extremities are evaluated. Range of motion of the lumbosacral spine is assessed in flexion and extension. Visual estimation of range of motion is adequate for general clinical purposes, although goniometers, which precisely measure angles, can be used for more accurate measurement. Measurement of minimal distance from fingertips to floor is useful to assess lumbar and hip mobility. Lateral bending can assess symmetry and any effect of bending on symptoms. Toe raises, heel walking, and standing on one leg (Trendelenburg test) help evaluate muscle weakness in the legs. A thorough neurologic examination must be performed on patients with sciatica or leg complaints. Unfortunately, most of the items commonly assessed on physical examination have limited prognostic significance and limited reproducibility among different examiners.[57]

Diagnostic tests play a limited role in initial evaluation. While X-rays of the lumbosacral spine can be helpful in evaluating chronic or recurrent low back pain, they should be performed for acute back pain only to help determine if a fracture or a systemic disorder is present when either is suggested by the history. For patients age 20 to 50 with nonradicular back pain and no suggestive history of potentially serious underlying condition, it is generally appropriate to wait 4 weeks before considering X-rays. If symptoms have not improved in 4 weeks, plain X-rays of the lubosacral spine should be performed—along with a complete blood count and other tests to determine if an occult neoplasm or osteomyelitis is present.[57,58] If a neoplasm or osteomyelitis is suspected but not detected on the plain X-rays, a bone scan or magnetic resonance imaging (MRI) of the spine should be performed.

Patients with radicular back pain will generally derive little benefit from early diagnostic imaging, since many of them will have spontaneous resolution of symptoms and early surgical intervention is usually indicated only with severe or progressive neurologic deficits. Patients with persistent or progressive neurologic deficits and a physical examination consistent with nerve-root impingement should be referred for an MRI to evaluate the anatomic basis of nerve-root symptoms. Patients with more ambiguous nerve-root involvement may benefit from electromyography (EMG) to determine whether nerve root impingement is present. Interpretation of an MRI can be challenging because a substantial proportion of people *without* back pain have disc abnormalities that are seen with MRI; among asymptomatic adults, about 22% to 40% have MRI evidence of disc herniation and about 24% to 79% have evidence of a bulging disc.[59] Therefore, anatomic abnormalities seen on MRI must be evaluated in the clinical context.

Older adults with symptoms suggestive of spinal stenosis (pain or paresthesias in the legs relieved by spinal flexion, or pseudoclaudication) should be evaluated by computed tomography (CT) or MRI; EMG may be useful to determine the extent of neurologic impairment.

LOWER-EXTREMITY DISORDERS

Work-related musculoskeletal disorders of the lower extremities have received relatively little attention. Studies of work-related lower-extremity disorders have mostly focused on traumatic injuries and osteoarthritis. Although disorders such as achilles tendonitis, plantar fasciitis, and tarsal tunnel syndrome have been recognized as the result of chronic overuse in athletes, they have not been well characterized among workers. Knee bursitis seems to be associated with kneeling work; for example, laying of floors has been recognized as a work task associated with a high rate of knee bursitis and other disorders of the lower extremities. There is no clear evidence demonstrating that occupational exposures cause other foot and ankle disorders.

In the United States, the rate of nonfatal occupational injuries of the lower extremities is 24.9 per 10,000 FTEs, with a median of 12 days away from work. The rate for nonfatal occupational knee injuries is 9.6 per 10,000 FTEs, with a median of 17 days away from work (Table 20-2). Occupations with high rates of workers' compensation claims for nontraumatic knee disorders are carpentry and floor work, plumbing, residential construction, and roofing, and, for knee tendonitis/bursitis, high rates are experienced in those working in carpentry and floor work, plumbing, electrical work, masonry/stonework/tile setting, and roofing.

The best-studied WMSD of the lower extremities is osteoarthritis of the hip and knee. Osteoarthritis is the most prevalent joint disease, the most common disabling medical condition among older adults and a leading cause of disability among people during their working years.[60] It can affect one or several joints, commonly the hips, knees, shoulders, and fingers. Among persons age 55 or older, 5% to 15% have evidence of hip osteoarthritis; knee osteoarthritis is even more common. Osteoarthritis varies in severity, from evidence only on X-rays to severe limitations of working abilities and daily activities. Osteoarthritis is the leading indication for hip and knee replacement. Most cases of osteoarthritis are idiopathic and the processes of disease development are not well understood. Heavy physical work is a risk factor for developing osteoarthritis of the hip.[60-62] Repeated heavy lifting and frequent climbing of stairs are associated with an increased risk of osteoarthritis requiring hip replacement. Osteoarthritis of the knee is associated with occupations requiring frequent knee bending, squatting, heavy lifting, and frequent climbing of stairs.[63,64]

PREVENTION

Preventive measures based on ergonomic interventions are largely experience-based and have not been comprehensively evaluated in the peer-reviewed publications. However, several systematic reviews of ergonomics programs have been performed and summarized,[65,66] leading to best practices that are based on integrated approaches to hazard control rather than specific ergonomic tools. To be successful, ergonomic programs should be:

- Supported by organizational policy
- Implemented with broad-based ergonomics training, rather than focused on a few tools or tasks
- Committed to providing workers appropriate equipment and tools for performing their jobs safely.

Reduction in exposures is the most important approach to prevention. This approach often requires changes in the work station, work process, or use of tools. Appropriate interventions must be specific to the physical exposures and biomechanical risk factors encountered in a particular workplace (Figure 20-3).

It is useful to consider the relationships among the various factors in the work environment that may contribute to either increased or reduced risk. A model has been developed that analyzes the relationship among the

environment, organization, technology, tasks, and workers (Figure 20-4).[67]

For example, hot environments may increase metabolic load, which, in turn, may make it more difficult for a worker to successfully complete a physically demanding task (Chapters 12B and 29). The organization of work may involve severe structural constraints, leaving workers with no opportunity to change postures or movements. A task may involve heavy lifting from the floor; a tool may have too large a handle, requiring a more forceful grip. Attention

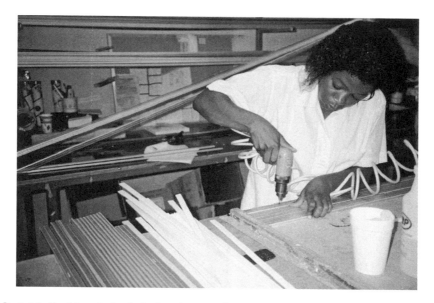

Figure 20-3. In jobs like this, reducing the load on the wrist, elbow, and shoulder can be accomplished by one or more of the following three methods: changing the tool, reorienting it (from vertical to horizontal or vice versa), and changing the height of the work station—either elevating the worker or lowering the piece being worked on. (Courtesy of Washington Industrial Safety and Health Act Services Demonstration Project.)

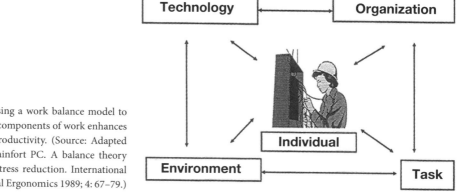

Figure 20-4. Using a work balance model to integrate all of the components of work enhances both health and productivity. (Source: Adapted from Smith MJ, Sainfort PC. A balance theory of job design for stress reduction. International Journal of Industrial Ergonomics 1989; 4: 67–79.)

to how these components of work interact can identify risk factors for MSDs or approaches for reducing risks.

Ergonomic principles must be adapted to fit the specific characteristics of each work environment. They should be viewed as a guide, rather than a blueprint. Chapter 9 describes the range of ergonomics measures that can be taken to reduce WMSDs and acute traumatic injuries, while improving both productivity and the quality of processes and products.

In addition to these engineering controls, there is evidence to support the effectiveness of administrative controls (changing workplace culture), modification of individual risk factors through exercise programs, and the use of programs utilizing a combined approach. Multidisciplinary, participatory approaches that involve employers and employees appear to be successful and foster compliance and acceptance of changes.[68] Sometimes administrative changes, such as work restrictions or job rotation, are useful alternatives, either as preventive or therapeutic interventions. However, most job rotation practices have not been able to produce sufficient effects to control WMSDs in the United States.[69,70] Administrative controls need to be carefully designed by ergonomists. Use of some types of personal protective equipment, such as palm pads and knee pads, are effective. However, lumbar corsets and back belts do not seem to be effective in reducing the occurrence of low back pain due to facilitating the deconditioning of muscles that stabilize the spine.[71]

To reduce exposure, the first step required for instituting changes in workstations or work processes is to analyze the specific characteristics of suspected high-risk jobs. Although an industrial engineer or occupational health or safety professional with ergonomics training can conduct the job review, involvement of those persons who are most knowledgeable about the job is critically important. Operators and supervisors with limited technical training can successfully identify many of the hazardous aspects of a specific job; specific solutions may not be effective or may not be accepted without the involvement of such persons in the job review and development of solutions.

The ACGIH Threshold Limit Value for Hand Activity Level[72] is useful for assessing risk in jobs looking at force and repetition. The Strain Index[73] for the distal upper extremity and Rapid Upper Limb Assessment[74] tools are useful in performing quick risk assessments. The NIOSH Lifting Equation[75] and the ACGIH TLV for Lifting[76] provide guidance on acceptable lifting, depending on weight, location of the load, and frequency of handling.

After a job analysis has identified the potentially hazardous exposures associated with a particular job, specific solutions should be solicited from those who are knowledgeable about the job. With limited training in the control principles (discussed in the next section), engineers, production employees, and front-line supervisors often propose the most useful methods for eliminating hazardous risk factors. If several factors are present, it can be difficult to determine which is the most detrimental. Where possible, integrated solutions should be developed that reduce multiple risk factors at the same time.

Control of repetitiveness, forcefulness, awkward posture, mechanical stress, vibration, and cold are often possible, as illustrated next.

Control of Repetitiveness

1. Use mechanical assists and other types of automation (For example, in packing operations, use a device, rather than the hands, to transfer parts.)
2. Rotate workers among jobs that require different types of motions (Rotation must be viewed as a temporary administrative control, one used only until a more permanent solution can be found.)
3. Implement horizontal work enlargement by adding different elements or steps to a job, especially steps that do not require the same motions as the current work cycle
4. Increase rest allowances or decrease production standards (Managers rarely look favorably on this control strategy.)
5. Design a tool for use in either hand and one for which fingers are not used for triggering motions.

Control of Forcefulness

1. Decrease the weight held in the hand by providing adjustable fixtures to hold parts

being worked on. Many conventional balancers are available to neutralize tool weight. Articulating arms are used in many plants to hold and manipulate heavy tools into awkward positions.

2. Control torque reaction force in powered hand tools by using torque reaction bars, torque-absorbing overhead balancers, and mounted nut-holding devices. Control the time that a worker is exposed to torque reaction by using shut-off rather than stall powered tools. Avoid jerky motions by hand-held tools.

3. Design jobs so that a power grip rather than a pinch can be used whenever possible. (The maximum voluntary contraction in a power grip is approximately three times greater than in a pinch.)

4. Increase the coefficient of friction on hand tools to reduce slipperiness, such as by use of plastic sleeves that can be slipped over metal handles of tools.

5. Design jobs so that slides or hoists are used to move parts or people, to reduce the amount of lifting, handling, or carrying of parts by the worker (Figure 20-5).

Control of Awkward Posture

The primary method for reducing awkward postures is to design adjustability of position into the job (Figure 20-6). Wrist, elbow, and shoulder and back postures required on a job often are determined by the height of the work surface with respect to the location of the worker. A tall worker may use less wrist flexion or ulnar deviation than a shorter worker. In addition, awkward postures can be reduced by the following procedures:

1. Alter the location or method of the work. For example, in automotive assembly operations, changing the line location at which a specific part is installed may result in easier access.

2. Redesign tools or change the type of tool used. For example, when wrist flexion occurs with a piston-shaped tool that is used on a horizontal surface, correction may involve use of an in-line type tool or lowering of the workstation.

3. Alter the orientation of the work. Often tilting work to an angle will reduce awkward

posture of the neck, shoulder, wrists, and/or back.

4. Avoid job tasks that require shoulder abduction or forward flexion greater than 45°, elbow flexion greater than 110°, wrist flexion more than 20°, or extension greater than 30°, or frequent neck rotation, flexion, or extension.

5. Provide support for the forearm when precise finger motions are required, to reduce static muscle loading in the arm and shoulder girdle.

Control of Vibration

1. Do not use impact wrenches or piercing hammers

2. Use balancers, isolators, and damping materials

3. Use handle coatings that attenuate vibrations and increase the coefficient of friction to reduce strength requirements

4. Reduce exposure below ISO standard[77] or Washington State ergonomics standard, Appendix B,[78] using alternative tools. (See Chapter 12B.)

Control of Mechanical Contact Stress

1. Round or flare the edges of sharp objects, such as guards and container edges

2. Use different types of palm-button guards, which allow room for the operator to use the button without contact with the guard

3. Use palm pads, which may provide some protection until tools can be developed to eliminate hand hammering

4. Use compliant cushioning material on handles or increase the length of the handles to cause the force to dissipate over a greater surface of the hand

5. Use different-sized tools for different-sized hands

6. Avoid narrow tool handles that concentrate large forces onto small areas of the hand.

Control of Cold and Use of Gloves

1. Properly maintain power tool air hoses to eliminate cold exhaust air leaks onto the workers' hands or arms.

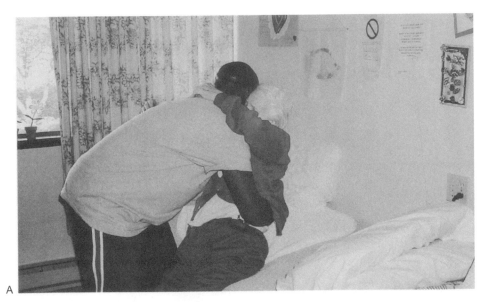

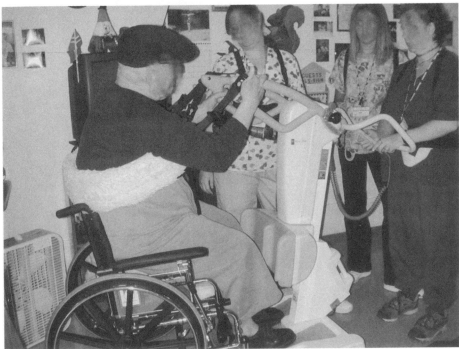

Figure 20-5. Risk of low-back injury can be reduced by using an electrical lifting device to reduce load and awkward postures. The photographs demonstrate lifting a patient without such a device (A) and with one (B). (Photographs by Barbara Silverstein.)

2. Provide a variety of styles and sizes of gloves to ensure proper fit of gloves. Although gloves may protect hands from cold exposures and cuts, they often decrease grip strength (requiring more forceful exertion), decrease tactile sensitivity, decrease manipulative ability, increase space requirements, and increase the risk of becoming caught in moving parts.

3. Cover only that part of the hand that is necessary for protection. Examples include use of safety tape for the fingertips with

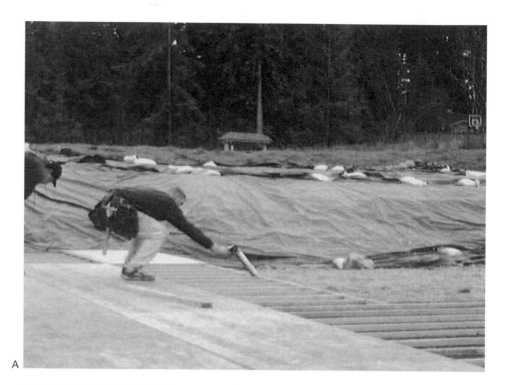

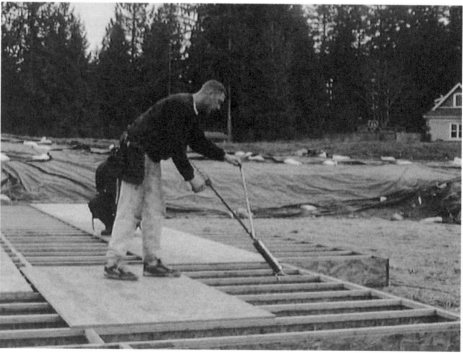

Figure 20-6. (A) Traditional methods of applying glue to floor posts. (B) New method using commercially available extended gun ($50 retail). A handle was added to the gun to reduce hand/wrist fatigue (parts less than $10). Job times were the same for each of the two methods. (Photographs by Barbara Silverstein.)

fingerless gloves and use of palm pads for the palm.

Other Preventive Measures

A conditioning process, which provides a period of time during which workers can gradually adapt their muscles and tendons to new demands, can be a useful approach for workers in forceful or repetitive jobs. Exercise programs that combine aerobic conditioning with specific strengthening of the back and legs may reduce the frequency of recurrence of low back pain.

Training of new workers in the most efficient and least stressful ways of performing their jobs may also be useful. For example, a cake decorator who chooses to decorate five cakes at a time will rotate through the different tasks (and physical requirements) associated with baking and decorating the cakes, incorporating more active breaks than the cake decorator who chooses to decorate 20 cakes at one time, thereby repeating the same step of the process 20 times before moving on to another task.

Similarly, workers with symptoms may, with training, be able to adapt an equally efficient but less stressful work method. However, lifting education programs have generally been ineffective at reducing the frequency of low back pain, likely because the training programs are done without first reducing the lifting task to a safe level of work. This finding highlights the importance of first reducing physical exposures, then training workers on how to optimize their choices in how they perform the work.

Many other training activities have not been evaluated specifically. Several employers, perceiving long-term benefits from a "phasing-in period," have established transitional or training areas where employees may work at a reduced pace for a limited time. In a survey of 5,000 employers in Washington State, among those who used preventive strategies, a larger percentage reported decreased number and severity of MSDs with engineering and administrative measures, such as task variety and reduced overtime, than with strictly personal controls, such as exercise programs and personal protective equipment.

Development of a preplacement screening processes to identify those persons who are at unusually high risk for development of an MSD is the least desirable prevention strategy. Such post-offer preplacement (POPP) screening shifts the cost of reducing the incidence of WMSDs onto workers (who are denied employment or placement) and increases the costs of the hiring and replacement processes. Studies of POPP screening for CTS, for example, have all shown that POPP screening has poor predictive value, is not cost-effective for employers, and may result in denial of employment to many workers who would not have developed CTS.[79] If POPP screening is implemented, it should be used only to document a workers baseline function (in case of a future injury) and to prioritize worker-specific training needs or phase-in periods.

Similarly, preplacement screening with low back X-rays should not be done, as plain X-rays are not a useful predictor of future low back disorders. Preplacement screenings are most effective in jobs where there is a high risk of serious injury or death.

REFERENCES

1. Bureau of Labor Statistics. Nonfatal occupational injuries and illnesses requiring days away from work, 2015. Available at: http://www.bls.gov/news.release/osh2.nr0.htm. Accessed November 30, 2016.
2. The 2016 Liberty Mutual Safety Index. Available at: https://www.libertymutualgroup.com/about-liberty-mutual-site/research-institute-site/Documents/2016%20WSI.pdf. Accessed October 24, 2016
3. Wuellner SE, Adams DA, Bonauto DK. Unreported workers compensation claims to BLS survey of occupational injuries and illnesses: Establishment factors. American Journal of Industrial Medicine. 2016; 59: 274–289.
4. Evanoff B, Abedin S, Grayson D, et al. Is disability underreported following work injury? Journal of Occupational Rehabilitation 2002; 12: 139–150.
5. Loisel P, Gosselin L, Durand P, et al. Implementation of a participatory ergonomics program in the rehabilitation of workers suffering from subacute back pain. Applied Ergonomics 2001; 32: 53–60.
6. Arnetz BB, Sjogren B, Ryden B, et al. Early workplace intervention for employees with musculoskeletal-related absenteeism: A prospective controlled intervention study.

Journal of Occupational and Environmental Medicine 2003; 45: 499–506.

7. Rystrom CM, Eversmann WW Jr. Cumulative trauma intervention in industry: A model program for the upper extremity. In ML Kasdan (ed.). Occupational hand and upper extremity injuries and disease. Philadelphia: Hanley and Belfus, 1991, pp. 489–505.

8. Glass LS. Occupational medicine practice guidelines: Evaluation and management of common health problems and functional recovery in workers (2nd ed.). Beverly Farms, MA: OEM Press, 2004.

9. Pérez-Merino L, Casajuana MC, Bernal G, et al. Evaluation of the effectiveness of three physiotherapeutic treatments for subacromial impingement syndrome: A randomised clinical trial. Physiotherapy. 2016; 102: 57–63.

10. Waddell G, Burton AK. Occupational health guidelines for the management of low back pain at work: evidence review. Occupational Medicine (London) 2001; 51: 124–135.

11. Williams RM, Westmorland M. Perspectives on workplace disability management: A review of the literature. Work 2002; 19: 87–93.

12. Loisel P, Lemaire J, Pointras S, et al. Cost benefit and cost effectiveness analysis of a disability prevention model for back pain management: A six year follow-up study. Occupational and Environmental Medicine 2002; 59: 807–815.

13. Melhorn JM, Wilkinson L, Gardner P, et al. An outcomes study of an occupational medicine intervention program for the reduction of musculoskeletal disorders and cumulative trauma disorders in the workplace. Journal of Occupational and Environmental Medicine 1999; 41: 833–846.

14. Silverstein B, Fan ZJ, Smith CK, et al. Gender adjustment or stratification in discerning upper extremity musculoskeletal disorder risk? Scandinavian Journal of Work, Environment & Health 2009; 35: 113–126.

15. Descatha A, Roquelaure Y, Evanoff B, et al. Predictive factors for incident musculoskeletal disorders in an in-plant surveillance program. Annals of Occupational Hygiene 2007; 51: 337–344.

16. Hakkanen M, Viikari-Juntura E, Martikainen B. Incidence of musculoskeletal disorders among newly employed manufacturing workers. Scandinavian Journal of Work, Environment & Health 2001; 27: 381–387.

17. Stauber WT. Factors involved in strain-induced injury in skeletal muscles and outcomes of prolonged exposures. Journal of Electromyography and Kinesiology 2004; 14: 61–70.

18. Barr, AE, Barbe N, Clark BD. Work related musculoskeletal disorders of the hand and wrist: epidemiology, pathophysiology, and sensorimotor changes. Journal of Orthopedics and Sports Physical Therapy 2004; 34: 610–627.

19. Silverstein B, Bao SS, Fan ZJ, et al. Rotator cuff syndrome: Personal, work-related psychosocial and physical load factors. Journal of Occupational and Environmental Medicine 2008; 50: 1062–1076.

20. Armstrong T, Dale AM, Franzblau A, et al. Risk factors for carpal tunnel syndrome and median neuropathy in a working population. Journal of Occupational and Environmental Medicine 2008; 50: 1355–1364.

21. Gardner BT, Dale AM, Descatha A, et al. Natural history of upper extremity musculoskeletal symptoms and resulting work limitations over 3 years in a newly hired working population. Journal of Occupational and Environmental Medicine 2014; 56: 588–594.

22. Schleifer LM, Ley R, Spalding TW. A hyperventilation theory of job stress and musculoskeletal disorders. American Journal of Industrial Medicine 2002; 41: 420–432.

23. Smith CK, Silverstein BA, Fan ZJ, et al. Psychosocial factors and shoulder symptom development among workers. American Journal of Industrial Medicine 2009; 52: 57–68.

24. Harris-Adamson C, Eisen EA, Dale AM, et al. Personal and workplace psychosocial risk factors for carpal tunnel syndrome: A pooled study cohort. Occupational and Environmental Medicine 2013; 70; 529–537.

25. Harris-Adamson C, Eisen EA, Neophytou A, et al. Biomechanical and psychosocial exposures are independent risk factors for carpal tunnel syndrome: Assessment of confounding using causal diagrams. Occupational and Environmental Medicine 2016; 73: 727–734.

26. Bernard B. Musculoskeletal disorders and workplace factors: A critical review of epidemiologic evidence for work-related musculoskeletal disorders of the neck, upper extremity, and low back (NIOSH Pub. No. 97-141). Cincinnati, OH: NIOSH, 1997.

27. Rempel D, Evanoff B, Amadio PC, et al. Consensus criteria for the classification of carpal tunnel syndrome in epidemiologic studies. American Journal of Public Health 1998; 88: 1447–1451.

28. Sluiter JK, Rest KM, Fringes-Dresden MHW. Criteria document for evaluating the work-relatedness of upper extremity musculoskeletal disorders. Scandinavian Journal of Work, Environment & Health 2001; 27: 1–102.

29. Helliwell PS, Bennett RM, Littlejohn G, et al. Towards epidemiological criteria for soft tissue disorders of the arm. Occupational Medicine 2003; 53: 313–319.

30. Harrington JM, Birrell CL, Gompertz D. Surveillance case definitions for work-related upper limb pain syndromes. Occupational and Environmental Medicine 1998; 55: 264–271.

31. Washington State Department of Labor and Industries Caution Zone Checklist. Available at: http://www.lni.wa.gov/safety/SprainsStrains/evaltools/CautionZones2.pdf. Accessed October 24, 2016.

32. Caridi JM, Pumberger M, Hughes AP. Cervical radiculopathy: A review. Hospital for Special Surgery 2011; 7: 265–272.

33. Ariens GA, Bongers PM, Hoogendorn WE, et al. High physical and psychosocial load at work and sickness absence due to neck pain. Scandinavian Journal of Work, Environment & Health 2002; 28: 221–231.

34. Silverstein B, Adams D. Work-related musculoskeletal disorders of the neck, back and upper extremity in Washington State 1997–2005. Technical Report 40-1-2007. Olympia: Washington State Department of Labor and Industries, 2007.

35. Frost P, Bonde J, Mikkelsen S, et al. Risk of shoulder tendinitis in relation to shoulder loads in monotonous repetitive work. American Journal of Industrial Medicine 2002; 41: 11–18.

36. Roquelaure Y, Bodin J, Ha C, et al. Personal, biomechanical, and psychosocial risk factors for rotator cuff syndrome in a working population. Scandinavian Journal of Work, Environment & Health 2011; 37: 502–511.

37. Leclerc A, Chastang JF, Niedhammer I, et al. Incidence of shoulder pain in repetitive work. Occupational and Environmental Medicine 2004; 61: 33–44.

38. Fan ZJ, Silverstein B, Bao S, et al. Quantitative exposure-response relations between physical workload and prevalence of lateral epicondylitis in a working population. American Journal of Industrial Medicine 2009; 52: 479–490.

39. Leclerc A, Landre MF, Chastang JF. Upper limb disorders in repetitive work. Scandinavian Journal of Work, Environment & Health 2001; 27: 268–278.

40. Fan J, Silverstein BA, Bao S, et al. The association between combination of hand force and forearm posture and incic. Human Factors 2014; 56: 151–1r.

41. Harris-Adamson C, Eisen EA, Kapellusch J, et al. Biomechanical risk factors for carpal tunnel syndrome: A pooled study of 2474 workers. Occupational and Environmental Medicine 2015; 72: 33–41.

42. Mattioli S, Violante FS, Bonfiglioli R. Upper-extremity and neck disorders associated with keyboard and mouse use. Handbook of Clinical Neurology 2015; 131: 427–433.

43. Andersen JH, Fallentin N, Thomsen JF et al. Risk factors for neck and upper extremity disorders among computers users and the effect of interventions: An overview of systematic reviews. PLoS One 2011; 6: e19691.

44. van Rijn RM, Huisstede BMA, Koes BW, et al. Associations between work-related factors and the carpal tunnel syndrome: A systematic review. Scandinavian Journal of Work, Environment & Health. 2009; 35: 19–36.

45. Harris C, Eisen EA, Goldberg R, et al. 1st place, PREMUS best paper competition: Workplace and individual factors of wrist tendinosis among blue-collar workers—the San Francisco study. Scandinavian Journal of Work, Environment & Health 2011; 37: 85–98.

46. Gerristen AA, de Vet HC, Scholten RJ. Splinting vs. surgery in the treatment of carpal tunnel syndrome: A randomized controlled trial. Journal of the American Medical Association 2002; 288: 1245–1251.

47. Eakin JM, Clark J, MacEachen E. Return to work in small workplaces: Sociological perspective on employers' and workers' experience with Ontario's strategy of self-reliance and early return (Working Paper 206). Toronto: Institute for Work and Health, 2003.

48. Guo HR, Tanaka S, Halperin W, et al. Back pain prevalence in US industry and estimates of lost workdays. American Journal of Public Health 1999; 89: 1029–1035.

49. Waters TR, Genaidy A, Barriera Viruet H, et al. The impact of operating heavy equipment vehicles on lower back disorders. Ergonomics 2008; 51: 602–636.

50. National Research Council and Institute of Medicine. Musculoskeletal disorders and the workplace: low back and upper extremities. Washington, DC: National Academy Press, 2001.

51. Sterud T, Tynes T. Work-related psychosocial and mechanical risk factors for low back pain: A 3-year follow-up study of the general

working population in Norway. Occupational and Environmental Medicine 2013; 70: 296–302.

52. Waters TR, Lu ML, Piacitelli LA et al. Efficacy of the revised NIOSH lifting equation to predict risk of low back pain due to manual lifting: Expanded cross-sectional analysis. Journal of Occupational and Environmental Medicine 2011; 53: 1061–1067.

53. Marras WS, Davis KG, Kirking BC, et al. A comprehensive analysis of low-back disorder risk and spinal loading during the transferring and repositioning of patients using different techniques. Ergonomics 1999; 42: 904–926.

54. Deyo RA, Rainville J, Kent DL. What can the history and physical examination tell us about low back pain? Journal of the American Medical Association 1992; 268: 760–765.

55. Dempsey PG, Burdorf A, Webster BS. The influence of personal variables on work-related low back disorders and implications for future research. Journal of Occupational and Environmental Medicine 1997; 38: 748–759.

56. Deyo RA, Weinstein JN. Low back pain. New England Journal of Medicine 2001; 344: 363–370.

57. Johanning E. Evaluation and management of occupational low back disorders. American Journal of Industrial Medicine 2000; 37: 94–111.

58. Straiger TO, Paauw DS, Deyo RA, et al. Imaging studies for acute low back pain. Postgraduate Medical Journal 1999; 105: 161–172.

59. Deyo RA. Magnetic resonance imaging of the lumbar spine. Terrific test or tar baby? New England Journal of Medicine 1994; 331: 115–116.

60. Parniapour M, Nordin M, Skovron ML. Environmentally induced disorders of the musculoskeletal system. Medical Clinics of North America 1990; 74: 347–359.

61. Vingard E, Alfredsson L, Malchau H. Osteoarthritis of the hip in women and its relation to physical workload at work and in the home. Annals of the Rheumatic Disease 1997; 56: 293–298.

62. Yoshimura N, Sasaki S, Iwasaki K, et al. Occupational lifting is associated with hip osteoarthritis: A Japanese case-control study. Journal of Rheumatology 2000; 27: 434–440.

63. Sandmark H, Hogstedt C, Vingard E. Primary osteoarthritis of the knee in men and women as a result of lifelong physical load from work. Scandinavian Journal of Work, Environment & Health 2000; 26: 20–25.

64. Ezzat AM, Li LC. Occupational physical loading tasks and knee osteoarthritis: A review of the evidence. Physiotherapy Canada 2014; 66: 91–107.

65. Amick BC III, Brewer S, Tullar JM, et al. Musculoskeletal disorders. March 1, 2009. Available at: http://www.allbusiness.com/labor-employment/workplace-health-safety-occupational/12275746-1.html. Accessed June 30, 2009.

66. Rivilis I, Van Eerd D, Cullen K, et al. Effectiveness of participatory ergonomic interventions on health outcomes: A systematic review. Applied Ergonomics 2008; 39: 342–358.

67. Smith MJ, Sainfort PC. A balance theory of job design for stress reduction. International Journal of Industrial Ergonomics 1989; 4: 67–79.

68. Evanoff B, Bohr P, Wolf L. Effects of a participatory ergonomics team among hospital orderlies. American Journal of Industrial Medicine 1999; 33: 358–365.

69. Bao SS, Kapellusch JM, Merryweather AS, et al. Relationships between job organizational factors, biomechanical and psychosocial factors. Ergonomics 2016; 59: 179–194.

70. Bao SS, Kapellusch JM, Merryweather AS, et al. Impact of work organizational factors on carpal tunnel syndrome and epicondylitis. Journal of Occupational and Environmental Medicine 2016; 58: 760–764.

71. van Duijvenbode I, Jelle ma P, van Poppel M, et al. Lumbar supports for prevention and treatment of low back pain. Cochrane Database of Systematic Reviews 2008: CD001823. doi: 10.1002/14651858.

72. Kapellusch JM, Gerr FE, Malloy EJ, et al. Exposure-response relationships for the ACGIH TLV for hand activity level: Results from a pooled data study of carpal tunnel syndrome. Scandinavian Journal of Work, Environment & Health 2014; 40: 610–620.

73. Moore JS, Garg A. The strain index: A proposed method to analyze jobs for risk of distal upper extremity disorders. American Industrial Hygiene Association Journal 1995; 56: 443–458.

74. McAtamney L, Corlett EN. RULA: A survey method for the investigation of work-related upper limb disorders. Applied Ergonomics 1993; 24: 91–99.

75. Waters TR, Putz-Anderson V, Garg A, et al. Revised NIOSH equation for the design and evaluation of manual lifting tasks. Ergonomics 1993; 36: 749–776.

76. American Conference of Governmental Hygienists. Lifting TLV-NIE. Cincinnati, OH: ACGIH, 2003, pp. 115–119.

77. American Conference of Governmental Hygienists. Hand arm (segmental) vibration.

In: ACGIH TLVs and BEIs. Cincinnati,
OH: ACGIH Worldwide, 2005, pp. 122–125.

78. Washington State Department of Labor and
Industries. WAC 296-62-051, Ergonomics.
Olympia: Author, 2000.

79. Dale AM, Gardner BT, Zeringue A, et al.
The effectiveness of post-offer pre-placement
nerve conduction screening for carpal tunnel
syndrome. Journal of Occupational and
Environmental Medicine 2014; 56: 840–847.

FURTHER READING

Cohen AL, Gjessing CC, Fine LJ, et al. Elements
of ergonomics programs: A primer based on
workplace evaluations of musculoskeletal
disorders. National Institute of Occupational
Safety and Health Pub. No. 97-117. Cincinnati,
OH: NIOSH, 1997.
*This publication describes the basic elements
of a workplace ergonomics program aimed
at preventing WMSDs. Essential program
elements are addressed, including management
commitment, worker participation, training,
and procedures for identifying, evaluating, and
controlling risk factors This primer includes
a collection of techniques, methods, reference
materials, and sources for other information that
can help in program development.*

Kuorinka I, Forcier L (eds.). Work-
related musculoskeletal disorders
(WMSDs): A reference book for prevention.
London: Taylor & Francis, 1995.
*This 1995 IRSST publication provides a useful
review of earlier literature on WMSDs and
physical exposures. The authors summarize much
information in a concise and readable format.*

Marras WS. The working back: A systems view.
New York: Wiley, 2008.
*This book uses a multidisciplinary perspective
to address the mechanisms influencing low back
pain in the workplace and means to preventing
this common condition. The book indicates
how various influences and risk factors can
be considered collectively in defining risk and
planning preventive efforts.*

National Research Council. Musculoskeletal
disorders in the workplace: Low back and upper
extremities. Washington, DC: National Academy
Press, 2001.
*A comprehensive review of the scientific literature
on the relationship between work and MSDs
of the low back and upper extremities. Major
sections include discussions of epidemiology,
tissue pathology, biomechanics, and interventions.
Summary tables provide descriptive synopses of
key studies. The list of references is extensive.*

Violante F, Armstrong T, Kilbom A. Occupational
ergonomics: Work related musculoskeletal
disorders of the upper limb and back.
London: Taylor & Francis, 2000.
*This book provides a concise overview of
ergonomics and occupational MSDs. Topics
covered include the epidemiology of MSDs,
psychosocial issues, job analysis and design,
case definitions for musculoskeletal problems,
biomechanical models, and regulatory issues.*

21

Cancer

Elizabeth Ward

Cancer encompasses a broad spectrum of diseases that arise in various organs and tissues throughout the body and have in common the uncontrolled growth of abnormal and potentially lethal cells that lose their differentiation and survive for abnormally long periods. Cancer originates with changes in DNA, or gene expression, that may be triggered by endogenous products of metabolism or exogenous chemicals; physical agents, such as ionizing radiation; or biologic agents, such as viruses, other microorganisms, or their products, such as aflatoxin. Inherited genetic factors play a role in susceptibility to cancer, often by influencing how the body responds to an environmental carcinogen (gene–environment interaction). The human health effects of many recognized environmental carcinogens were first documented through studies of occupational groups with heavy, prolonged exposure.

Cancer is a major public health problem in the United States and throughout the world. Each year, approximately 1.6 million U.S. residents are diagnosed with invasive cancer, and approximately 596,000 die of various cancers. Cancer accounts for almost one-third of deaths in the United States, second only to heart disease. Among men, prostate cancer has the highest incidence, followed by lung cancer and colorectal cancer; among women, breast cancer has the highest incidence, followed by lung cancer and colorectal cancer. In both sexes, the three most common cancer sites account for over half of new cases.[1] Since survival is worse for lung cancer than for other common cancers, lung cancer is the most common cause of cancer death among both men and women.

In the United States and other high-income countries (HICs), cancer incidence and mortality patterns shifted dramatically during the 20th century (Figure 21-1). Most notably, lung cancer in men increased sharply after World War II, peaked in the early 1990s, and declined steadily thereafter; lung cancer in women rose later and only recently began to plateau. These trends largely reflect (a) the introduction of manufactured tobacco products early in the 20th century and (b) differences in men and women in the increase and decline of tobacco smoking. Stomach cancer, one of the major cancers early in the 20th century, declined steadily during the century, probably due to advances in food preservation, increased availability of fresh fruits and vegetables, and decreases in the prevalence of

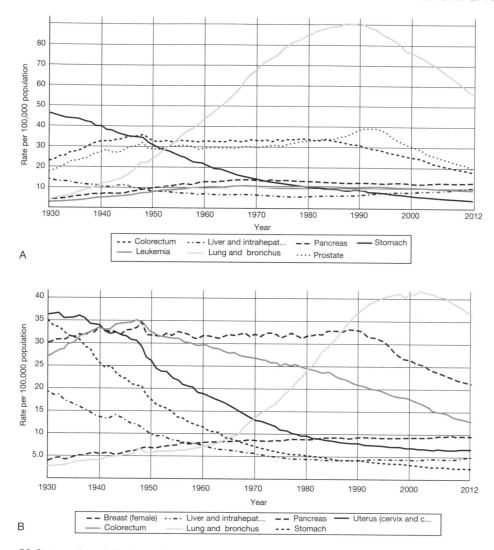

Figure 21-1. Age-adjusted death rates (per 100,000 population) for selected cancers, United States, 1930–2012: (A) males and (B) females. (Source: American Cancer Society)

Helicobacter pylori infection. Cervical and colorectal cancer incidence and mortality rates have declined in the United States because of screening and removal of premalignant lesions, early detection, and treatment.

The global burden of cancer is significant. In 2012, an estimated 14.1 million people were newly diagnosed with cancer and 8.2 million people died from cancer.[2] In HICs, the most common types of cancer are lung and bronchus, colon and rectum, breast, and prostate; in low- and middle-income countries (LMICs), the most common types of cancer are lung and

bronchus, stomach, liver, and breast (Table 21-1). The most common preventable causes of cancer in the United States and other HICs are cigarette smoking and obesity resulting from dietary patterns and physical inactivity. Other important causes of cancer are occupational exposures, viruses and other biologic agents, reproductive factors, consumption of alcohol, environmental pollution, and ionizing and ultraviolet radiation. In LMICs, infectious agents play a greater role in causation of cancer overall. Among the frequent cancers in men and women in LMICs are stomach cancer associated with *H. pylori* infection,

Table 21-1. Ten Leading Sites of New Cancer Cases and Deaths, Developed and Developing Countries, 2012 (in Thousands)

Developed Countries

Estimated New Cases		Estimated Deaths	
Males	Females	Males	Females
Prostate: 759	Breast: 794	Lung, bronchus, and trachea: 417	Lung, bronchus, and trachea: 210
Lung, bronchus, and trachea: 490	Colon and rectum: 338	Colon and rectum: 176	Breast: 198
Colon and rectum: 399	Lung and bronchus: 268	Prostate: 142	Colon and rectum: 158
Urinary bladder: 196	Corpus uteri: 168	Stomach: 107	Pancreas: 91
Stomach: 175	Ovary: 100	Pancreas: 93	Stomach: 68
Kidney: 125	Stomach: 100	Liver: 80	Ovary: 66
Non-Hodgkin lymphoma: 102	Thyroid: 93	Urinary bladder: 59	Liver: 43
Melanoma of the skin: 99	Pancreas: 93	Esophagus: 56	Leukemia: 40
Pancreas: 77	Melanoma of the skin: 92	Leukemia: 51	Cervix uteri: 36
Liver: 81	Non-Hodgkin lymphoma: 89	Kidney: 48	Corpus uteri: 35
All sites:* 3,244	All sites:* 2,832	All sites:* 1,592	All sites:* 1,287

Developing Countries

Estimated New Cases		Estimated Deaths	
Males	Females	Males	Females
Lung, bronchus, and trachea: 751	Breast: 883	Lung, bronchus, and trachea: 682	Breast: 324
Liver: 462	Cervix uteri: 445	Liver: 441	Lung, bronchus, and trachea: 281
Stomach: 456	Lung, bronchus, and trachea: 225	Stomach: 362	Cervix uteri: 230
Prostate: 353	Colon and rectum: 276	Esophagus: 225	Stomach: 186
Colon and rectum: 347	Stomach: 221	Colon and rectum: 198	Liver: 182
Esophagus: 255	Liver: 186	Prostate: 166	Colon and rectum: 163
Urinary bladder: 134	Corpus uteri: 152	Leukemia: 100	Esophagus: 104
Oral cavity: 131	Ovary: 139	Pancreas: 81	Ovary: 86
Leukemia: 120	Thyroid: 137	Non-Hodgkin lymphoma: 75	Leukemia: 74
Non-Hodgkin lymphoma: 116	Esophagus: 153	Oral cavity: 675	Pancreas: 65
All sites:* 4,184	All sites:* 3,831	All sites:* 3,062	All sites:* 2,261

* Excludes nonmelanoma skin cancer.

Source: American Cancer Society. Global cancer facts & figures (3rd ed.). Atlanta: American Cancer Society; 2015.

liver cancer associated with hepatitis B virus and hepatitis C virus infection, and cervical cancer caused by human papilloma virus infection. However, incidence rates of lung, colorectal, breast and prostate cancer are increasing in many LMICs, while rates of infection-related cancers are declining.[2] It is predicted that the burden of cancer and other chronic diseases will continue to increase in LMICs due to increases in cigarette smoking and changes in dietary and physical activity patterns.

People have been exposed to carcinogenic agents in their environment, and cancer has been observed throughout human history. However, industrialization and growth of the chemical industry in early 20th century created opportunities for concentrated, high-level exposures among working populations. Exposures included (a) naturally occurring substances that for the first time were mined and milled for industrial uses, such as asbestos and uranium; (b) substances extracted from natural sources, such as benzene from petroleum; and (c) newly synthesized substances, such as vinyl chloride. Due to large increases in cancer risk associated with high-level industrial exposures from the middle to the end of the 20th century, case reports and epidemiologic studies documented high risks of

(a) bladder cancer among dye workers exposed to the aromatic amines β-naphthylamine and benzidine, (b) lung cancer among uranium miners exposed to radon, (c) lung and skin cancer in workers exposed to arsenic, and (d) lung cancer and pleural and peritoneal mesothelioma among workers exposed to asbestos.

Development of experimental models for carcinogenesis led to formal bioassay programs at the National Cancer Institute and the National Toxicology Program (NTP). These testing programs confirmed both the high correlation between carcinogenicity in experimental models and human carcinogenicity and the scientific basis for prevention of widespread human exposure to carcinogens through toxicologic testing and regulation. Occupational epidemiology studies, many of which were initiated in the 1970s and 1980s, documented the carcinogenicity of asbestos, benzene, beryllium, bis-chloromethyl ether (BCME), coke oven emissions, vinyl chloride, and some other widely used substances.

The proportion of new cancers and deaths in the United States and worldwide that are related to occupational and environmental carcinogens is not precisely known. In 1981, it was estimated that 4% of all cancer deaths in the United States were due to occupational exposures; a more recent estimate is 2.4% to 4.8%. Table 21-2 provides estimates of the number of occupationally related cancer deaths in the United States for selected cancers and illustrative exposures for 1997, the most recent year for which these estimates have been made.[3,4] In Great Britain, it was estimated that, in 2004, 8% of cancer deaths among men and 1.5% among women were attributable to occupational carcinogens.[5] Globally, an estimated 10% of lung cancer deaths, 2% of leukemia deaths, and nearly 100% of mesothelioma deaths are attributable to occupation—with occupational exposures resulting, in the year 2000, in 102,000 deaths from lung cancer, 7,000 from leukemia, and 43,000 from mesothelioma.[6]

OCCUPATIONAL AND ENVIRONMENTAL CARCINOGENS

Although there has been much progress in the recognition and control of carcinogenic hazards

in the United States and many other HICs, some of the earliest recognized occupational carcinogens continue to be widely used and inadequately controlled in much of the world today. Lung cancer accounts for more than half of occupational cancer cases worldwide, and asbestos is, by far, the most important exposure accounting for lung cancer.[7] The World Health Organization (WHO) estimates that 125 million people worldwide are exposed to asbestos at work,[8] despite the recognition of asbestos-related cancers and lung disease for more than 60 years. In addition, excess risks of lung cancer and mesothelioma, an extremely rare cancer of the pleura and peritoneum strongly associated with asbestos, have continued for decades after asbestos exposure was reduced or eliminated. In the United States, where use of asbestos peaked in the 1970s (Figure 21-2), an estimated 27.5 million workers were exposed to asbestos from 1940 to 1979, including 18.8 million exposed to more asbestos than the equivalent exposure from 2 months work in primary manufacturing or insulation.[9] It was projected that annual mortality from asbestos-related diseases in the United States would peak in the year 2000 at about 9,700 deaths (including approximately 3,000 from mesothelioma and 4,700 from lung cancer), then decline, but remain substantial, for another three decades. The projections were fairly accurate for mesothelioma death rates, which decreased from 11.3 per million in 2001 (representing 2,509 deaths) to 10.7 per million in 2010 (representing 2,745 deaths).[10] There has been increasing evidence for associations between asbestos exposure and cancer of other sites, including laryngeal, ovarian, esophageal, stomach, and colorectal cancers.[11]

Production of asbestos globally was estimated at about 2 million metric tons in 2016, down from a peak of over 4.5 million tons in 1975. In 2016, Russia accounted for nearly half of global production, followed by China, Brazil, and Kazakhstan.[12] Countries with the greatest consumption of asbestos in 2013 were China, India, Indonesia, Russia, and Brazil.[13] Occupational and environmental exposures in LMICs have not been well documented, but they may equal or exceed exposures in HICs when they began to industrialize. In South Africa, which mined asbestos minerals throughout most of the 20th century, high prevalence of asbestos-related

Table 21-2. Estimated Number of Occupationally Related Cancer Deaths for Selected Cancers and Illustrative Exposures, United States, 1997

Cause of Death and Exposure	Number of Deaths*	Estimated Number of Exposed Workers	Estimated Percentage Exposed	Relative Risk	Estimated Proportion (Percent) Due to Occupational Exposures (Attributable Fraction)	Estimated Number of Occupationally Related Cancer Deaths
Lung cancer	91,289 (M); 61,877 (F)	NA		NA	6.3–13.0 (combined)	9,677–19,901
Chemical exposures†					6.1–17.3 (M); 2 (F)	6,807–17,031
Environmental tobacco smoke ("never-smokers" only, 10% of all lung cancer deaths)					0.6 (M+F)	870
Indoor radon at work					1.3 (M+F)	2,000
Bladder cancer	7,638 (M); 3,897 (F)	NA		NA	7–19 (M); 3–19 (F)	651–2,191
Mesothelioma	2,081 (M); 548 (F)	NA		NA	85–90 (M); 23–90 (F)	1,895–2,366
Leukemia	19,038 (M+F)				0.8–2.8 (combined)	152–533
Benzene		1,000,000	0.72	2–4	0.8–2.0	
Ethylene oxide		1,000,000	0.72	1.1–3.5	0–1.6	
Ionizing radiation (100+mSv)		61,700	0.04	1.3–2.1	<0.05	
Ionizing radiation (50–100 mSv)		70,900	0.05	1.1–1.4	<0.05	
Laryngeal cancer	3,016 (M)				1.0–20.0 (combined)	30–603
Sulfuric acid		3,000,000	4.4	1.1–5.0	0.4–15.0	
Mineral oils		4,400,000	6.4	1.1–2.0	0.6–6.0	
Skin cancer	1,407 (M)				1.5–6.0 (combined)	21–84
Polycyclic aromatic hydrocarbons		8,222,800	12.0	1.1–1.5	1.2–5.7	
Arsenic		240,000	0.36	2	0.1	
Sinonasal (SN) and nasopharynx (NP) cancer	303 (SN) (M) 436 (NP) (M)				33.0–46.0 (SN) and 30.0–42.0 (NP)	231–322 (SN and NP)
Wood dust		4,515,200	6.8	3.1 (SN); 2.4 (NP)	12.5 (SN); 8.7 (NP)	
Nickel compounds		4,000,000	6.0	2.2	6.7 (SN and NP)	
Hexavalent chromium		3,400,000	5.2	5.2–10.8	18.0–33.8 (SN and NP)	
Kidney cancer	7.131					
Coke production		520,000	0.76	2	0.0–2.3	0–164
Liver cancer	7,283					
Vinyl chloride		320,000	0.48	2.5	0.4–1.1	29–80
Total occupationally related cancer deaths						12,086–26,244

Note. F = female; M = male, NA = not applicable.

* Attributable fractions taken from the literature; see text.

† Including chemicals, metals, fibers, fumes, and particulates.

diseases and significant environmental contamination resulted from early use of open-pit mining, widespread use of a manual process (cobbing) to separate asbestos from rock, frequent employment of women and children in asbestos industries, inadequate dust control in mines and mills, and widespread dumping of tailings near population settlements.[14,15] Hazardous working conditions in the asbestos industry persisted because of the poverty and isolation of

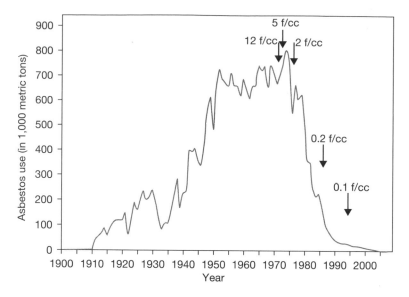

Figure 21-2. Asbestos use and permissible exposure limits (PELs), United States, 1900–2007. Arrows indicate year when Occupational Safety and Health Administration PELs were implemented (such as 12 fibers per cubic centimeter [f/cc] in 1971 and 0.1 f/cc in 1994). (Source: Centers for Disease Control and Prevention. Malignant mesothelioma mortality-United States, 1999–2005. Morbidity and Mortality Weekly Report 2009; 58: 393–396.)

the mining regions; the apartheid system, which allowed few employment opportunities for black workers and forced many into migrant labor; and the weakness of government regulation. Since transition to majority rule in 1994, there have been serious efforts by the South African government to assess exposure, involve affected communities in decision-making, and raise public awareness about asbestos-induced diseases. Production and export of asbestos ended in South Africa in 2003, and in 2008 a complete ban on the use, manufacture, or processing of asbestos was officially announced by the South African government.[14]

India remains a major importer but only a minor producer of asbestos. Expansion of the asbestos industry in India in the 1990s was associated with drastic reductions in import tariffs on raw asbestos and asbestos-containing products. Exposures there occur in mining, milling, manufacturing of asbestos cement and asbestos textiles, and shipbreaking.[16] India is currently a major producer of asbestos cement and pipes.[17] Half of the nearly 700 ships that are scrapped worldwide each year are broken down in India. Each ship contains about 5.5 tons of asbestos, which is then resold to manufacture insulation and roofing materials. Dusty conditions,

inadequate control technology, and lack of personal protective equipment are common.[16-18] In 2006, WHO stated that the most efficient way to eliminate asbestos-related diseases is to ban the use of all forms of asbestos; more than 50 countries, including South Africa, have done so, while the United States and India have not.[16]

Although use of asbestos was phased out in the United States more than three decades ago, clinicians can expect to see patients who have a history of work with high levels of asbestos exposure. Guidelines for medical surveillance of asbestos-exposed workers as well as diagnosis and attribution of asbestos-related diseases have recently been updated by an international expert panel.[19] A map of county-level death rates for mesothelioma can help alert clinicians to geographical areas with increased rates of asbestos-related diseases from shipbuilding, mining, and/or other asbestos-using industries (Figure 21-3). Ongoing asbestos exposure is still possible and likely for individuals involved in renovation and demolition of buildings constructed before the mid-1970s. Rescue and recovery workers at the World Trade Center site in the aftermath of the 9/11 attacks and residents of Lower Manhattan were potentially exposed to asbestos, since asbestos was used

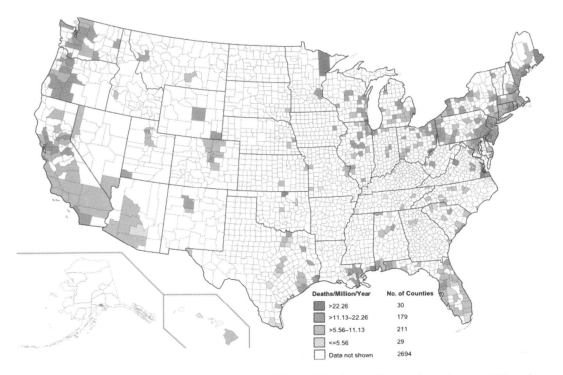

Deaths/Million/Year	No. of Counties
>22.26	30
>11.13–22.26	179
>5.56–11.13	211
<=5.56	29
Data not shown	2694

Figure 21-3. Age-adjusted death rates for malignant mesothelioma (all sites) per million population, by county, U.S. residents age 15 and older, 2000–2009. Age-adjusted rates have not been calculated for counties with less than 10 reportable deaths, and for split/merged counties incorporated for less than the entire time interval (see http://wwwn.cdc.gov/eworld/Appendix/CountyEquivalents). See http://wwwn.cdc.gov/eworld/Home/About for information about data sources, methods, ICD codes, and limitations. (Source: National Institute for Occupational Safety and Health. Work-related lung disease surveillance system (eWoRLD). 2014-805. U.S. Department of Health and Human Services, Centers for Disease Control and Prevention, National Institute for Occupational Safety and Health, Respiratory Health Division, Morgantown, WV, 2014. Available at: https://wwwn.cdc.gov/eworld/Data/805. Accessed on November 8, 2016.)

in the construction of the first 40 floors of the North Tower.[20]

Cancers related to asbestos are not confined to workers with high exposure. Mesotheliomas have been observed among household members of asbestos workers and in residents of asbestos-contaminated communities. For example, vermiculite ore from a mine that operated near Libby, Montana, from the early 1920s until 1990 was contaminated with asbestos, during which time it was given free of charge to the community and used extensively in gardens, driveways, public areas, and homes. Fifteen deaths from mesothelioma were identified among workers who mined, milled, and processed vermiculite in Libby and 11 individuals with mesothelioma were identified who did not have occupational exposure. (Two had household exposure to workers and nine had environmental exposure.)[21,22] A subsequent study found a 50-fold increase in asbestosis mortality among Libby,

Montana, residents who had not been occupationally exposed to asbestos.[23] An investigation of 70 communities across the United States that received asbestos-contaminated vermiculite ore from this mine found 11 communities with excess rates of mesothelioma.[24]

Many mesothelioma cases have also been observed among family members of workers at, and community residents near, an asbestos mine in western Australia. Among the 3,000 women and girls who lived in the mining and milling town of Wittenoom between 1943 and 1992, 40 deaths from mesothelioma had occurred by 2004, representing 8% of total deaths.[25] Mesotheliomas have also been observed in areas of Turkey, Greece, Corsica, New Caledonia, and Cyprus where asbestos and asbestos-like materials present in soil are used to whitewash interior walls of houses. Residents of these areas also have a high prevalence of pleural plaques, a nonspecific effect often due to asbestos exposure.[26,27]

A study of patterns of mesothelioma mortality in two counties in Nevada found a much higher than expected ratio of female-to-male deaths and an elevated proportion of deaths age under age 55, suggesting nonoccupational asbestos exposure that might be related to deposits of carcinogenic fibrous minerals.[28]

Although some aspects of the history of occupational and environmental cancer related to asbestos are unique, this history has much in common with other occupational and environmental carcinogens and allows some important generalizations to be made:

- As is the case with asbestos-associated lung cancers, most cancers caused by occupational or environmental exposures are pathologically and clinically indistinguishable from cancers not caused by these exposures. Therefore, unless elevated risks are exceptionally high, a large and carefully designed epidemiologic study is necessary to determine whether cancer rates are elevated and associated with specific exposures.

- For most carcinogens and most cancer types, the latency period between onset of exposure and diagnosis of cancer is often long, with excess disease rates peaking 30 to 40 years after onset of population exposure. Therefore, epidemiologic studies require accurate and complete records of people who were exposed decades ago. In addition, exposure is often widespread before definitive epidemiologic studies can be done.

- Many occupational carcinogens have other toxic effects often associated with high-level exposure, including pleural plaques and fibrotic lung disease in asbestos workers, myelosuppression in workers exposed to benzene, and liver fibrosis and acroosteolysis (clubbing of the fingers) in workers exposed to vinyl chloride.

- Although exposure to recognized occupational carcinogens has been curtailed in the United States and Western Europe, production and use has shifted to LMICs, where there is limited documentation of both asbestos exposure and occurrence of cancer and other occupationally related diseases.

- Although it is often difficult to detect cancer caused by very low exposures to environmental carcinogens in epidemiologic studies, exposures of the general population to known carcinogens occur and may contribute to cancer incidence and mortality. Such exposures may be localized, such as occurred in communities near asbestos mines and mills, or widespread, such as exposure to low levels of benzene, which is a constituent of cigarette smoke, gasoline vapor, and gasoline engine exhaust.

THE MOLECULAR BASIS OF CANCER

Even among people exposed to high levels of carcinogens for long periods, not all of them develop cancer. Despite their greatly increased relative risk of lung cancer, not all lifetime heavy smokers develop lung cancer, and some non-smokers with no known risk factors develop lung cancer. Both inherited genes and environmental factors play roles in cancer development. Multiple events occurring in a probabilistic fashion may influence whether a person develops cancer. A study of twins concluded that environmental factors are the principal cause of most cancers, with a significant role of heritable factors for prostate cancer (42% of the risk possibly explained by inherited genes), colorectal cancer (35%), and breast cancer (27%).[29]

Carcinogenesis is characterized by four stages: initiation, promotion, malignant transformation, and tumor progression. Initiation occurs when a carcinogen interacts with DNA, most often by forming an adduct between the chemical carcinogen or one of its functional groups and a nucleotide in DNA, or by producing a strand break. If the cell divides before the damage is repaired, an alteration can become permanently fixed as a heritable error that will be passed on to daughter cells. Such heritable changes in DNA structure are called *mutations*. Many mutations have no apparent effect on gene function. However, when mutations occur in critical areas of genes that regulate cell growth, cell death, or DNA repair, they may predispose clonal expansion and accumulation of further genetic damage. *Promoters* are substances or processes that contribute to clonal expansion by stimulating initiated cells to replicate, forming benign tumors or hyperplastic lesions. Promotion is thought to be completely reversible. The process of promotion does not cause heritable alterations or mutations. It stimulates cell turnover, so that mutated cells can exploit their selective growth advantage and proliferate, increasing the probability that a cell will acquire additional mutations and become malignant. Unlike promotion, the end result of malignant transformation is irreversible. Tumor progression involves the further steps of local invasion and/or metastasis.

Many carcinogens are able to form DNA adducts, either because they are intrinsically reactive or are activated, through metabolism, to a DNA-reactive form. Classes of organic compounds associated with cancer include alkylating agents, arylalkylating agents, and arylhydroxylamines. Alkylating agents are chemicals that attach alkyl groups, such as methyl or ethyl groups, to nucleotides to form DNA adducts. Examples of carcinogens in this group include nitrosamines and aflatoxin B_1, a potent liver carcinogen that can contaminate food products. Arylalkylating agents can transfer aromatic or multiringed compounds to a nucleotide to form an addict. Examples of such compounds include polycyclic aromatic hydrocarbons (PAHs), such as benzo(a)pyrene. Arylhydroxylamines are chemicals that transfer aromatic amines to nucleotides to form adducts. Examples of such compounds include the aromatic amines β-naphthylamine and benzidine, which have been responsible for very high rates of bladder cancer among exposed workers. Certain inorganic metals and minerals show carcinogenic activity in people and/or animals, including arsenic, nickel, hexavalent chromium, and asbestos.

The mechanisms of carcinogenesis of particles and fibers include both primary genotoxicity through generation of reactive oxygen species and secondary genotoxicity through particle-induced inflammation. Particles may also carry mutagens to the surface and/or inside of cells. Ionizing radiation is a classic cancer initiator.

The mechanism of carcinogenesis from ionizing radiation is believed to involve formation of mutagenic oxygen free radicals in the shell of hydration surrounding DNA. Once formed, the reactive oxygen species, such as hydroxyl radicals and hydrogen peroxide, can induce strand breaks and more than 30 different DNA adducts as well as DNA-protein cross-links. Unrepaired or misrepaired DNA double-strand breaks are thought to be the principal lesions responsible for induction of genetic damage by ionizing radiation in mammalian cells. while base damage is generally the predominant mechanism for the production of such damage by chemical carcinogens.[30] (See Chapter 12D.)

Metabolic activation is necessary to convert some chemicals to forms that can bond with DNA. For some well-studied chemical carcinogens, the metabolic pathways leading to activation or deactivation influence both target organ specificity and individual susceptibility. Genetic polymorphisms in metabolic enzymes are likely to affect susceptibility to occupational and environmental carcinogens. Studies have examined variation in (a) genes, such as CYP1A1, that code for cytochrome P-450s; (b) intracellular proteins involved in the metabolism of carcinogenic PAHs to epoxides; (c) GSTM1 that codes for a cytosolic enzyme glutathione-S-transferase M1, which can conjugate epoxides of PAHs and aflatoxin; and (d) N-acetyltransferase 2 (NAT2), which codes for the N-acetylation phenotype associated with metabolism of some carcinogenic aromatic amines. After a carcinogen has reached and interacted with cellular DNA, the carcinogenic process may be arrested by DNA repair or promoted by factors that increase cell replication or interfere with the programmed death of damaged cells (apoptosis). Thus, the outcome of a carcinogen–DNA interaction may be influenced by factors such as cell division, clonal expression, loss of tumor suppressor function, and other genetic and epigenetic factors.

Although many mutations probably have no effect on cells, mutations occurring in genes that regulate cell growth are the first step in the evolution of a cancer cell. More than 100 genes can convert normal rodent cells in tissue culture to a transformed phenotype with abnormal growth characteristics in cell culture and the ability to form tumors when explanted into immunocompromised rodents. These dominant transforming genes, called *oncogenes*, encode proteins involved in signal transduction or cell-cycle regulation. Mutations in these genes may trigger production of oncogenic proteins that increase the proliferation of cells that express them. A set of recessive tumor suppressor genes has been identified. Deletion, point mutation, or inactivation of both gene copies allows cells to proliferate unregulated or with reduced restraints.

An oncogene is an altered form of a normal cellular gene called a *proto-oncogene*. Proto-oncogenes encode proteins that participate in the regulation of growth and/or differentiation of normal cells and are involved at various levels in signaling from the extracellular compartment to the nucleus. One of the best-studied examples is the ras oncogene, which was first identified in rat sarcomas. The ras oncogene can be activated by PAHs, N-nitroso compounds, and ionizing radiation and has been found in a wide variety of human cancers, including bladder cancer, lung cancer, and other cancers that are caused by occupational and environmental exposure.

Tumor suppressor genes, or anti-oncogenes, are also important. Ordinarily these function to regulate cell growth and stimulate terminal differentiation or trigger apoptosis of damaged cells. When inactivated, they fail to perform these functions, allowing neoplastic transformation to proceed. A prominent example is the p53 gene, located on chromosome 17. Mutations in the p53 gene have been identified in many cancers, including those of the colon, lung, liver, esophagus, and breast; lymphohematopoietic malignancies; and the Li-Fraumeni syndrome of familial multiple cancer susceptibility. Carcinogenic exposures such as aflatoxin and HBV have been associated with specific mutations on the p53 gene, suggesting that some carcinogens may leave a unique genomic "signature."

Epigenetic mechanisms for deactivation of tumor suppressor genes include methylation of DNA in the gene promoter region, a characteristic that has been observed in many cancers. Abnormal promoter hypermethylation can have the same effect as a coding region mutation in inactivating a tumor suppressor gene.[31]

Once a cell is initiated, clonal expansion may occur through a variety of mechanisms. Initiated cells may be more responsive to growth stimulation, may be unable to terminally differentiate, or may become resistant to apoptosis. Clonal expansion increases the probability that cells with critical mutations will acquire additional genetic damage needed for malignant transformation.

The events involved in progression are less well understood than those involved in initiation or promotion. During progression, populations of tumor cells undergo further selection, and the genome becomes unstable, causing chromosomal alterations with increasing frequency. As the progression phase ends, tumor cells have converted to the neoplastic phenotype, characterized by autonomous growth and ability to erode normal tissue barriers.

Endogenous factors, such as hormones, inflammation, and the by-products of metabolism, are major sources of initiating and promoting events.[32] Reactive oxygen species, including superoxide, hydrogen peroxide, and hydroxyl radicals, and singlet oxygen, generated by normal cellular processes, including respiration, inflammation, and phagocytosis, have the ability to induce mutations. Endogenous DNA lesions are genotoxic and induce mutations that are commonly observed in mutated oncogenes and tumor suppressor genes.[33] The levels of oxidative DNA damage reported in many tissues or in animal models of carcinogenesis exceed the levels of lesions induced by exposure to exogenous carcinogenic compounds. Oxidative DNA damage is probably important in the etiology of many human cancers, but we do not know the precise role that it plays in carcinogenesis and how it synergizes with other forms of genetic and epigenetic events to accelerate cell transformation and malignant transformation. The association of cancer with chronic inflammatory diseases, such as gastritis, chronic hepatitis, ulcerative colitis, and pancreatitis, may result from generation of reactive oxygen species.[32]

Endogenous and exogenous hormones also play a role in the development of cancer, and there is increasing use of hormonal medications for chemoprevention and treatment of cancer. Although metabolites of estradiol and estrone are genotoxic, a major action of these hormones is to accelerate the accumulation of somatic genetic errors. Endogenous and exogenous hormones play an especially important role in development of cancers of the breast, endometrium, ovary, and prostate. Higher cumulative exposure to endogenous estrogen and many ovulating cycles (associated with earlier menarche, later menopause, and lower parity) increase breast cancer risk among women, as does use of combined estrogen and progesterone hormonal therapy for menopausal symptoms. Hormonal medications may have opposing effects in different organs. Oral contraceptives cause a small increase in breast cancer but a large decrease in ovarian cancer. Tamoxifen, a weak estrogen agonist, is effective in treatment of breast cancer and in the prevention of breast cancer for high-risk women, but it increases the risk of endometrial cancer.

IDENTIFICATION OF POTENTIAL CARCINOGENS

Substances that have been formally classified as carcinogens are those in which adequate toxicologic and epidemiologic studies have documented a carcinogenic hazard. Although high-quality epidemiologic data provide a strong basis for hazard identification and risk assessment, it is often not possible to conduct definitive studies in humans. There are many animal carcinogens for which definitive epidemiologic studies cannot be performed due to multiple and/or poorly characterized exposures, use in small workplaces, and/or other limitations. Thus, the prevention of occupational and environmental cancer must often rely on extrapolation of findings in toxicological studies to predict effects in humans and establish limits for human exposure. Although the 2-year rodent bioassay has been the "gold standard" for toxicological testing of carcinogenicity for hazard identification and risk assessment, the time and expense of rodent bioassays severely limits the number of agents that are tested. There are more than 100,000 chemicals used in commerce, and only a small fraction has been adequately tested for cancer and other toxic effects. Therefore, the development of testing methods that are highly predictive of cancer in humans should be given high priority.

Predictions Based on Chemical Structure

Knowledge about the relationship of chemical structure and carcinogenic activity can be used to identify potential chemical carcinogens. Computerized databases of carcinogenic and noncarcinogenic chemicals have been developed to relate structure to carcinogenic activity. Using results of rodent bioassays of more than 300 chemicals, a list of chemical structures that correlate with tumorigenicity in rodent tests has been developed. These characteristics, or "structural alerts," indicate chemicals that should be tested extensively and monitored for evidence of carcinogenicity. However, studies comparing the results of widely used computer databases with the results of in-vivo studies have found limited concordance.[34]

Toxicological Testing

Short-Term Tests for Mutagenicity

Because many known carcinogens are mutagens, short-term tests for genotoxicity have played an important role in the screening of chemicals for potential carcinogenicity. Among these, the Ames assay has been the best studied and most extensively used. This test uses special strains of *Salmonella typhimurium* bacteria that are deficient in DNA repair and cannot grow in the absence of histidine. Cultures of *S. typhimurium* are treated with several dose levels of the chemical being tested. Growth of a cell culture in the absence of histidine indicates a mutation causing reversion to the histidine-positive phenotype. Homogenates of mammalian liver, which promote metabolic activation, may be added to the incubation mixture to allow detection of carcinogens that require metabolic activation. In-vitro mammalian cell mutation assays also exist, including the mouse lymphoma L5178Y assay and the Chinese hamster ovary assay. Other short-term tests involve both in-vitro and in-vivo (in animals) induction of chromosome aberrations, sister chromatid exchanges, and micronuclei.

The concordance between short-term tests of mutagenicity and the results of chronic bioassays (animal tests) depends on the databases selected for comparison. In general, the concordance has declined over time as an increasing proportion of nongenotoxic carcinogens have been tested in rodent bioassays. An analysis of 59 chemicals classified by the International Agency for Research on Cancer (IARC) as human carcinogens (Group 1) or probable human carcinogens (Group 2A) that had been tested for mutagenicity by multiple methods found positive results for 67% in the Salmonella assay and 93% in in-vivo or in-vitro mammalian tests.[35] It is been recommended that screening protocols for genetic effects in vitro include tests for both (a) gene mutation in Salmonella and/or mammalian cells and (b) chromosome aberrations and numerical chromosome changes (aneuploidy) in mammalian cells.[36,37] Some carcinogens are not detected by mutagenicity assays, including hormonal carcinogens, some metals, agents that have a mode of action involving multiple target organs, and agents with a nongenotoxic mode of action.

Chronic Two-Year Bioassay

The "gold standard" for determining the potential carcinogenic activity of a chemical is the 2-year bioassay in rodents. This assay involves test groups of 50 rats and 50 mice of both sexes and at two or three doses of the test agent. In the United States, the B6C3F1 mouse and the F344 rat are commonly used. At about 8 weeks of age, test animals are placed on the test agent (or placebo) for the remaining 96 weeks of their lifespans. The test agent may be administered in feed, by gavage (forced feeding), or by inhalation. The maximum dose level used in a 2-year bioassay is determined by the *estimated maximally tolerated dose* (MTD), usually derived from a 90-day study. The MTD is defined by the Environmental Protection Agency (EPA) as "the highest dose that causes no more than a 10% weight decrement, as compared to appropriate control groups; and does not produce mortality, clinical signs of toxicity, or pathological lesions (other than those that may be related to a neoplastic response) that would be predicted to shorten the animal's natural lifespan." Controversy exists around the use of the MTD, with some scientists claiming that it is not high enough to elicit the anticipated effects, while others voicing concern that the MTD is too high, it may overwhelm host defenses against low exposure levels, and may induce cancer because of toxicity and abnormal cell proliferation. In any case, high exposure levels are necessary to provide meaningful results without requiring studies that are prohibitively large and costly.

Even with the use of high exposure levels, the high cost of 2-year bioassays, estimated to be over $1 million per chemical, limits the number of tests that can be conducted. Over the past two decades, there has been considerable interest in the development and application of short-term or accelerated cancer bioassays using genetically modified (GM) animals that exhibit high sensitivity to chemically induced cancers.[38] GM animals have an alteration in a gene critical for tumorigenesis that by itself would not induce cancer within a 6- to 12-month assay period but would cause a rapid induction of tumors or a decrease in latency upon exposure to a carcinogen. Such GM animals are playing an increasingly important role in the safety evaluation and risk evaluation of chemical carcinogens. However, current models seem to be more reliable in identifying noncarcinogenic agents than in detecting carcinogenic agents, and no single GM model can be relied upon to detect all trans-species and human carcinogens. Using more than one GM model can improve ability to detect carcinogens, but it is likely that there are trans-species and human carcinogens that operate through mechanisms that will not be detected using the current GM approaches.[38] Therefore, the 2-year bioassay remains the only widely accepted indicator of carcinogenic potential to humans by international and national health and regulatory agencies.

Many substances that are carcinogenic in rodent bioassays have not been adequately studied in humans, usually because an adequate study population has not been identified. Among the substances that have proven carcinogenic in animals, all have shown positive results in well-conducted 2-year bioassays. Moreover, between 25% and 30% of established human carcinogens were first identified through animal bioassays. Since animal tests necessarily use high-dose exposures, in most cases human risk assessment requires extrapolating the exposure–response relationship observed in rodent bioassays at higher doses to predict effects in humans at lower doses. Typically, regulatory agencies in the United States have adopted the default assumption that no threshold level of exposure exists for carcinogenesis. For some chemicals, mechanistic hypotheses have been advanced to suggest that there may be a threshold, but for most carcinogens, it is considered to be not feasible to generate empirical data on the exposure–response curves at low levels to confirm or refute these hypotheses. Although the presence or absence of carcinogenicity is similar across many species, the target organ affected by cancer may vary, largely because of differing metabolic pathways, in different species. Benzidine, for example, causes bladder cancer in humans, hepatomas in mice, and intestinal tumors in rats. IARC is presently creating a database of tumor sites in humans and animal studies that will be useful in evaluating tumor site concordance.[39]

Toxicogenomics and High-Throughput Screening

The potential to use toxicogenomic technologies to identify potential human carcinogens and to prioritize substances for 2-year cancer bioassays has been of great interest. Incorporation of toxicogenomics into screening tests involves measuring gene, protein, or metabolite changes in response to specific doses of an administered test compound at a specific time point, with or without the parallel development of more traditional markers of toxicity. Toxicogenomic technologies include technologies that analyze DNA sequences (genomics), messenger RNA expression (transcriptomics), proteins in living systems (proteomics), and small-molecule components of living systems (metabolomics). They are used to yield data that can integrate toxicant-specific alterations in gene, protein, and metabolite expression with phenotypic responses of cells, tissues, and organisms.[40] These approaches may be especially useful to identify nongenotoxic carcinogens, define groups of substances that may have similar toxicity because they elicit similar cellular responses, and reflect the contemporary understanding that carcinogens can act through multiple modes of action and mechanisms.

Toxicity Testing in the 21st Century (Tox21), a multiagency collaboration in the United States, was established to use high-throughput screening to identify patterns of compound-induced biological response, characterize toxicity and disease pathways, facilitate cross-species extrapolation, model low-dose extrapolation, prioritize compounds for more extensive toxicological evaluation (either in vitro or in vivo) and develop predictive models for biological response in humans.[41] The first phases of Tox21 were built on in-vitro high-throughput assays, using gene or protein-reporter constructs after short-term chemical exposure in order to robotically screen hundreds—and now thousands—of chemicals. These automated in-vitro assays have focused on activation of nuclear receptors and assays measuring activation of specific cellular stress-response pathways. Continuing development of Tox21 will incorporate toxicogenomic methods to address some limitations of the existing systems and enhance the ability of extrapolating high-throughput results to human toxicity and disease.[42]

Classification of Carcinogens

In 1969, IARC initiated its monograph program to evaluate the carcinogenic risk of chemicals to humans and to produce monographs on individual chemicals. (Information on the program can be obtained at http://monographs.iarc.fr/.) The program assembles international groups of experts to critically review and evaluate evidence on the carcinogenicity of a wide range of human exposures. Published data regarding an agent, mixture, or exposure circumstance are reviewed to determine the level of evidence for carcinogenicity in humans and experimental animals.

The criteria for sufficient evidence of carcinogenicity are quite stringent. For humans, sufficient evidence for carcinogenicity requires that "a positive relationship has been observed between the exposure and cancer in studies in which chance, bias and confounding could be ruled out with reasonable confidence." For animals, sufficient evidence for carcinogenicity requires "an increased incidence of malignant neoplasms in (a) two or more species of animals or (b) in two or more independent studies in one species carried out at different times or in different laboratories or under different protocols. An increased incidence of tumors in both sexes of a single species in a well-conducted study, or a single study in one species or sex, when malignant neoplasms occur to an unusual degree can also provide sufficient evidence for carcinogenicity in animals."[41] Based on separate evaluations of carcinogenicity in humans and experimental animals, the agent, mixture, or exposure circumstance is classified into one of five groups:

> *Group 1—Carcinogenic to humans*: This category is used when there is sufficient evidence of carcinogenicity in humans. In exceptional circumstances, an agent may be placed in this category when evidence of

carcinogenicity in humans is less than sufficient but there is sufficient evidence of carcinogenicity in animals and strong evidence in
exposed humans that the agent acts through
a relevant mechanism of carcinogenicity.

Group 2A—Probably carcinogenic to humans:
This category is used when there is limited
evidence of carcinogenicity in humans
and sufficient evidence for carcinogenicity in animals. In some cases, an agent may
be placed in this category when there is
inadequate evidence of carcinogenicity in
humans and strong evidence of carcinogenicity in animals and strong evidence that
carcinogenesis is mediated by a mechanism that also operates in humans.

Group 2B—Possibly carcinogenic to humans:
This category is used for agents for which
there is limited evidence of carcinogenicity in humans and less than sufficient evidence of carcinogenicity in animals, or
inadequate evidence for carcinogenicity in
humans, but sufficient evidence of carcinogenicity in animals.

*Group 3—Not classifiable as to its carcinoge-
nicity in humans.*

Group 4—Probably not carcinogenic to humans.

Using this classification, IARC has evaluated
over 1,003 chemicals, industrial processes, and
personal habits. It has classified 120 agents, mixtures, and exposure circumstances in Group 1, 81
in Group 2A, 299 in Group 2B, 502 in Group 3,
and 1 in Group 4. Tables 21-3 and 21-4 list agents,
mixtures, and exposure circumstances (such as
industrial processes) in Group 1 and Group 2A
for which exposures are predominantly occupational or environmental. In 2012, IARC convened
two workshops in which 10 key characteristics of
human carcinogens were identified. These characteristics can be used to identify and categorize
scientific findings related to cancer mechanisms
when assessing whether an agent is a potential
human carcinogen (Table 21-5).[43]

Starting with Monograph 112, IARC working groups have applied these characteristics
in their review of potential carcinogens.[44] They
have also used results of Tox21 and ToxCast (a
high-throughput screening and computational
toxicology program of the EPA), in addition to
more traditional in-vitro and in-vivo test results,
to evaluate the presence or absence of these

characteristics. In order to do this, the IARC
Monograph 112 Working Group mapped the
821 available assay endpoints in the ToxCast/
Tox21 database to the key characteristics of
known human carcinogens, based on the biological target being probed by each assay. The
consensus assignments comprised 263 assay
end-points that mapped to 7 of the 10 "key
characteristics." The Working Group then determined whether a chemical was "active" or "inac-
tive" for each of the selected assay endpoints. The
relative effects of the agents for which ToxCast/
Tox21 data were available were compared with
those of 178 chemicals selected from the more
than 800 chemicals previously evaluated in the
IARC Monographs that had been screened by
the ToxCast/Tox21. The results were presented
as a rank order of all compounds arranged in
the order of their relative effect and were used to
systematically assess the strength of the evidence
that the agent exhibits each of key characteristics. For example, for diazinon, one of the agents
evaluated in Monograph 112, the evidence for
the carcinogenic mechanisms of genotoxicity
and oxidative stress were found to be strong and
likely to operate in humans; however, in contrast,
evidence for receptor-mediated mechanisms,
effects on proliferation, and immunosuppression was considered weak. These findings contributed to the overall evaluation of diazinon as
probably carcinogenic to humans (Group 2A).

The NTP also has a systematic process for
evaluating human carcinogens, which classifies
agents, mixtures of substances, and exposure circumstances as "known to be human carcinogens"
or "reasonably anticipated to be human carcinogens." The *14th Report on Carcinogens*, issued by
NTP in 2016, listed 62 substances as "known to
be human carcinogens" and 186 as "reasonably
anticipated to be human carcinogens."[45]

GENE–ENVIRONMENT INTERACTION

In recent decades, there has been increasing
interest in understanding genetic factors
that influence cancer development. A *gene–
environment* interaction can be defined as "a
different effect of an environmental exposure on
disease risk in persons with different genotypes"
or equivalently "a different effect of a genotype on disease risks in persons with different

Table 21-3. Definite Human Carcinogens with Potential for Occupational or Environmental Exposure (IARC Group 1)*

Exposures	Examples of Occurrence	Tumor Sites or Types for Which There Is Sufficient Evidence in Humans	Other Sites or Types with Limited Evidence in Humans
Aflatoxins (naturally occurring mixtures of)	Gravins, peanuts (farmworkers)	Liver	
4-Aminobiphenyl	Dye and rubber industry	Bladder	
Arsenic and arsenic compounds	Insecticides, nonferrous metal smelting, mining and milling of ores containing arsenic	Lung, skin, urinary bladder	Kidney, liver, prostate
Asbestos (chrysotile, crocidolite, amosite, tremolite, actinolite, and anthrophyllite)	Mining and milling, insulation, shipyard workers, sheet metal workers, asbestos cement industry	Lung, mesothelioma, larynx, ovary	Colorectum, pharynx, stomach
Benzene	Chemical industry	ANLL	ALL, CLL, MM, NHL
Benzidine	Rubber and dye industries	Bladder	
Benzidine-based dyes	Coloring paper, textiles, and leather		
Beryllium and beryllium compounds	Beryllium extraction and processing, aircraft and aerospace industries, electronics and nuclear industries	Lung	
1,3-butadiene	Chemical and rubber industries	Hematolymphatic organs	
Bis(chloromethyl) ether (BCME) and chloromethyl methyl ether (CMME)	Chemical industry	Lung	
Cadmium and cadmium compounds	Metalworking industry, batteries, soldering, coatings	Lung	Prostate, kidney
Chromium (VI) compounds	Chromate production plants, dyes and pigments, plating and engraving, chromium ferro-alloy production, stainless steel welding	Lung	Nasal cavity and paranasal sinuses
Coal, indoor emissions from household combustion of	Residential use of coal for heating and cooking	Lung	
Coal tar pitches	Coal distillation	Skin, scrotum, lung, bladder	
Coal tars	Coal distillation	Skin, lung	
1,2-Dichloropropane	Solvent and chemical intermediate	Biliary tract (Cholangiocarcinoma)	
Dioxin (2,3,7,8-tetrachlorodibenzo-dioxin)	Herbicide production and application	All sites combined, lung	
Dyes metabolized to benzidine	Dye production; textile dyeing		
Engine exhaust, diesel	Transportation, trucking, mining	Lung	
Erionite	Environmental (Turkey)	Mesothelioma	
Ethylene oxide	Sterilant in healthcare settings; chemical component		Lymphoid tumors (NHL, MM, CLL), breast
Fluoro-edenite (fibrous amphibole)	Naturally occurring mineral in regions of Italy	Mesothelioma	
Formaldehyde	Production, pathologists, medical laboratory technicians, plastics, textile industry	Nasopharyngeal, leukemia	Sinonasal
Gallium arsenide	Used in high-speed semiconductors, high-power microwaves, fiberoptics		

(continued)

Table 21-3. (Continued)

Exposures	Examples of Occurrence	Tumor Sites or Types for Which There Is Sufficient Evidence in Humans	Other Sites or Types with Limited Evidence in Humans
Hepatitis B and C virus	Healthcare settings	Liver	
HIV	Healthcare settings	Sarcoma	
Ionizing radiation (all types)	Fallout from nuclear explosions and reactor accidents	Lung, bone, leukemia, thyroid	
Leather dust	Footwear production, leather tanning and processing	Nasal cavity and paranasal sinuses	
Lindane	Agricultural workers, pesticide applicators	Non-Hodgkin lymphoma	
4,4-methylenebis (chloroaniline)	Curing agent in polyurethane industry		
Mineral oils	Machining, jute processing	Skin	
Mustard gas	Production, war gas	Lung	Larynx
2-Naphthylamine	Rubber and dye industries	Bladder	
Neutrons	Radiation workers	Unknown	
Nickel compounds	Nickel refining and smelting	Lung, nasal cavity, and paranasal sinuses	
Outdoor air pollution	General population, roadway and transportation workers	Lung	
Outdoor air pollution, particulate matter in	General population, roadway and transportation workers	Lung	
Pentachlorophenol	Used historically as a wood preservative and insecticide; environmental contaminant	Non-Hodgkin lymphoma	
Phosphorus-32, as phosphate	Phosphate mining and processing	Lung	
Plutonium	Plutonium production workers	Lung, liver, bone	
Polychlorinated biphenyls (PCBs)	Used historically in dielectric fluids in capacitors and transformers; environmental and food contaminant	Malignant melanoma	Non-Hodgkin lymphoma, breast
Radium-224, -226, and -228 and their decay products	Uranium mining and milling	Bone, mastoid process, paranasal sinus	
Radon-226 and its decay products	Indoor environments, mining	Lung	Leukemia
Schistosoma hematobium infection	Farming and other outdoor work in endemic areas	Bladder	
Shale oils	Energy production	Skin	
Silica dust, crystalline, in the form of quartz or crystobalite	Hard rock mining, sandblasting, glass and porcelain manufacturing	Lung	
Solar radiation	Outdoor work	Skin	Eye, lip
Soots	Chimneys, furnaces	Skin, lung	
Mists from strong inorganic acids	Metal, fertilizer, battery, and petrochemical industries	Larynx, lung, possibly nasal sinus	
Talc (with asbestiform fibers)	Talc mining, pottery manufacturing	See asbestos	
Ortho-toluidine	Production of dyes, pigments, and rubber chemicals	Bladder	
Trichloroethylene	Metal degreasing	Kidney	
Ultraviolet radiation from welding	Construction, manufacturing, repair trades	Ocular melanoma	
Vinyl chloride	Plastic industry	Angiosarcoma of the liver, hepatocellular carcinoma	
Welding fumes	Construction, manufacturing, repair trades	Lung	Kidney
X- and gamma radiation	Medical, nuclear fuel cycle	Many sites, including leukemia, thyroid, breast	

(continued)

Table 21-3. (Continued)

Exposures	Examples of Occurrence	Tumor Sites or Types for Which There Is Sufficient Evidence in Humans	Other Sites or Types with Limited Evidence in Humans
Wood dust	Wood and furniture industries	Nasal cavity and paranasal sinuses, nasopharynx	

Industrial Processes and Exposure Circumstances
Acheson process, occupational exposure
Aluminum production
Auramine production
Boot and shoe manufacturing and repair
Chimney sweeping
Coal gasification
Coal tar distillation
Coke production
Furniture and cabinet making
Glass, making of
Hematite mining (with radon exposure)
Involuntary smoking (exposure to secondhand or environmental tobacco smoke)
Iron and steel founding
Isopropyl alcohol production (strong acid process)
Magenta manufacturing
Painter (occupational exposure as)
Paving and roofing with coal tar pitch
Rubber manufacturing industry
Sandblasting
UV tanning devices
Welding

Note. IARC = International Agency for Research on Cancer; ALL = acute lymphocytic leukemia; ANLL = acute non-lymphocytic leukemia; CLL = chronic lymphocytic leukemia; MM = multiple myeloma; NHL = non-Hodgkin lymphoma; STS = soft tissue sarcoma.
Source: Current as of July 7, 2017. Up-to-date IARC evaluation data can be found at the IARC website, http://www.iarc.fr, or more specifically at the Monographs Database Web page, http://193.51.164.11/.

Table 21-4. Probable Human Occupational Carcinogens with Potential for Occupational or Environmental Exposure (IARC Group 2A)*

Exposures	Illustrative Examples of Occurrence
Acrylamide	Polyacrylamide manufacturing
Benz[a]anthracene	Coal distillation
Biomass fuel (primarily wood), indoor emissions from household combustion of	Indoor environments using biomass fuel
Bitumens, oxidized, and their emissions	Roofing
Captofol	Fungicide
alpha-Chlorinated toluenes	Plastics industry
4-Chloro-ortho-toluidine	Dye and chlordimeform manufacture
Cobalt metal with tungsten carbide	Alloy production
Creosotes	Wood preservatives
Cyclopenta[cd]pyrene	Engine exhaust
DDT (4,4-Dichlorodiphenyltrichloroethane)	Insecticide
Diazinon	Insecticide
Dibenz[a,h]anthracene	Coal distillation
Dibenzo[a,l]pyrene	Wood and coal combustion, engine exhaust
Dichloromethane	Solvent, paint stripper, degreaser
Dieldrin, and aldrin metabolized to dieldrin	Insecticide

(continued)

Table 21-4. (Continued)

Exposures	Illustrative Examples of Occurrence
Diethyl sulfate	Petrochemical industry
Dimethylcarbamoyl chloride	Chemical manufacturing
Dimethylhydrazine, 1,2-	Rocket propellants and fuels, boiler water treatments, chemical reactants, medicines, cancer research
Dimethyl sulfate	Former war gas, now used in chemical industry
Epichlorhydrin	Resin manufacturing, solvent.
Ethylene dibromide	Fumigant, gasoline additive
Glycidol	Chemical intermediate, sterilant
Glyphosate	Herbicide
Hydrazine	Foaming agent, rocket fuels, chemical industry
Indium phosphide	Electronics and semiconductor production
High-temperature frying, emissions from	Commercial cooking settings
Lead compounds, inorganic	Batteries, lead alloys
N-nitrosodiethylamine	Solvent
Malathion	Insecticide
2-Mercaptobenzothiazole	Rubber manufacturing
6-Nitrochrysene	Present in diesel exhaust
1-Nitropyrene	Present in diesel exhaust
2-Nitrotoluene	Chemical intermediate used in dye production
N-nitrosodimethylamine	Solvent
Non-arsenical insecticides (occupational exposures in spraying and application of)	Agriculture
Polybrominated biphenyls	Flame retardants, electrical equipment
1,3-Propane sultone	Chemical intermediate
Silicon carbide whiskers	Used in aluminium and other composite materials
Styrene-7,8-oxide	Chemical industry
Tetrachlorethylene	Dry cleaning
Tetrabromobisphenol A	Flame retardant
3,3′,4,4′-Tetrachloroazobenzene	Byproduct of manufacturing and contaminant of some herbicides
Tetrafluoroethylene	Synethesis of polymers
1,2,3-Trichloropropane	Pesticide; rubber manufacturing; solvent
Tris(2,3-dibromopropyl)phosphate	Flame retardant, polystyrene foam manufacturing
Ultraviolet radiation A, B, and C	Outdoor work
Vinyl bromide	Plastic industry
Vinyl fluoride	Chemical industry
Exposure Circumstances	
Art glass, glass containers, and pressed ware (manufacture of)	
Carbon electrode manufacture	
Dry cleaning (occupational exposures in)	
Hairdresser or barber (occupational exposure as a)	
Petroleum refining (occupational exposures in)	
Shift work that involves circadian disruption	

Note. IARC = International Agency for Research on Cancer.
Source: Current as of July 7, 2017. Up-to-date IARC evaluation data can be found at the IARC website, http://www.iarc.fr, or more specifically at the Monographs Database Web page, http://193.51.164.11/.
* Other probable carcinogens, including medications (especially cancer chemotherapeutic agents, a risk for healthcare workers), infectious agents, and foods, are classified in Group 2A but are not listed here.

environmental exposures."[46] Assessing gene–environment interactions may be important in conducting studies to identify human carcinogens and in identifying population subgroups with greatest cancer susceptibility and potential to benefit from interventions.[46] There have been relatively few examples of well-established gene–environment interactions in cancer, although the

number of publications on this subject is growing rapidly.[47] Among the most well-established gene–environment interactions are genetic polymorphisms in xenobiotic-metabolizing enzymes and cancer of the urinary bladder.

The potential for exposure to certain aromatic amines to cause large excesses in bladder cancer was recognized in the first half of the 20th

Table 21-5. Key Characteristics of Carcinogens

Characteristic	Examples of relevant evidence
1. Is electrophic or can be metabolically activated	Parent compound or metabolite with an electrophilic structure (such as epoxide or quinone), formation of DNA and protein adducts
2. Is genotoxic	DNA damage (DNA strand breaks, DNA-protein cross-links, or unscheduled DNA synthesis), intercalation, gener mutations, cytogenetic changes (such as chromosome aberrations or micronuclei)
3. Alters DNA repair or causes genomic instability	Alterations of DNA replication or repair (such as topoisomerase II, base-excision, or double-strand break repair)
4. Induces epigenetic alterations	DNA methylation, histone modification, microRNA expression
5. Induces oxidative stress	Oxygen radicals, oxidative stress, oxidative damage to macromolecules (such as DNA or lipids)
6. Induces chronic inflammation	Elevated white blood cells, myeloperoxidase altered cytocine and/or chemokine production
7. Is immunosuppressive	Decreased immunosurveillance, immune system dysfunction
8. Modulates receptor-mediated effects	Receptor activation or inactivation (such as ER, PPAR, or AhR) or modulation of endogenous ligands (including hormones)
9. Causes immortalization	Inhibition of senescence, cell transformation
10. Alters cell proliferation, cell death or nutrient supply	Increased proliferation, decreased apoptosis, changes in growth factors, energetics and signaling pathways related to cellular replication or cell cycle control, angiogenesis

Note. AhR = arylhydocarbon receptor; ER = estrogen receptor; PPAR = peroxisome proliferator-activated receptor.
Source: Smith MT, Guyton KZ, Gibbons CF, et al. Key characteristics of carcinogens as a basis for organizing data on mechanisms of carcinogenesis. Environmental Health Perspectives 2016; 124: 713–721.

century when reports began to accumulate about excess numbers of bladder cancers occurring in dye-manufacturing industries. Occupational exposures that are considered to have sufficient evidence for carcinogenicity to the uninary bladder in humans include 4-aminobiphenyl, benzidine, 2-naphthalamine, and *ortho*-toluidine.[48,49]

Multiple metabolic pathways are involved in the activation of aromatic amines to DNA-reactive intermediates in the human bladder. Metabolism begins in the liver with either (a) N-oxidation by cytochrome P-450-associated enzymes, which activates the parent compound to a highly electrophilic form, or (b) N-acetylation by NAT2, which reduces the availability of parent compound that can undergo N-oxidation. Individuals with the NAT2 slow-acetylator genotype exposed to 2-naphthylamine or 4-aminobiphenyl have an increased risk for bladder cancer.

Tobacco smoke is a major nonoccupational source of exposure to carcinogenic aromatic amines. Smokers with NAT2 slow-acetylation genotypes demonstrate higher relative and absolute risks for bladder cancer compared with those with rapid/intermediate-acetylation genotypes.[50] Smokers with a homozygous deletion of glutathione-*S*-gene (GSTM1), which is responsible for detoxification of another class of carcinogens found in tobacco smoke (PAHs), also have an increased risk of bladder cancer compared to those with genotypes containing at least one functional allele.[51]

Genetic variations in xenobiotic pathway genes (cytochrome P-450s (CYPs), glutathione transferases (GSTs), and (NATs) modify the relationship between hair dye use and risk of non-Hodgkin lymphoma (NHL) for women who started using dyes before 1980 when these products contained carcinogenic aromatic amines.[52] This relationship was also found to be modified by polymorphisms in DNA repair genes. For example, one study examined seven genes related to double-strand break repair, including BRCA1 and BRCA2, six genes involved in the nucleotide excision pathway, four genes involved in the base-excision repair pathway, and one gene that can repair alkylated bases in DNA. The study found significant associations between polymorphisms in several genes and follicular lymphoma, the NHL subtype that is most strongly associated with use of hair dye.[53]

In contrast to studies of the relationship between polymorphisms in xenobiotic metabolizing enzymes and DNA repair genes, which were hypothesis-driven, advances in technology have enabled genome-wide association studies (GWAS) using case-control designs. Such studies may identify new genetic loci that influence disease risk, which can be subject to further investigation to determine their functional significance. GWAS studies require large sample sizes and often involve consortia, which include data from multiple studies.[54]

CARCINOGENS AND PUBLIC HEALTH

Cancer Risk Assessment

In contrast to the IARC and NTP processes that focus on *hazard identification, risk assessment* is a procedure for characterizing and quantifying the amount of harm expected to result from an exposure. This process was developed in the 1970s as regulatory agencies attempted to (a) set permissible levels of exposure, based on acceptable levels of risk, and (b) quantify the amount of benefit that would be expected from regulation at a specific level. While risk assessment is a generic process that can be applied to any risk, including nonmalignant diseases, it is discussed in this chapter because it arose in the context of cancer risk.

The four basic components of risk assessment, which were described by the National Research Council in 1983, can be applied specifically to cancer:

- *Hazard identification* involves a review of the relevant biologic and chemical information bearing on whether an agent may cause cancer.
- *Dose–response assessment* involves quantifying a dosage and evaluating its relationship to the incidence of a specific cancer.
- *Exposure assessment* involves making qualitative or quantitative estimates of the magnitude, duration, and route of exposure.
- *Risk characterization* integrates and summarizes the three preceding elements. Presented with assumptions and uncertainties, it provides an estimate of the risk to public health and a framework to define the significance of the risk.

In risk characterization, the exposure level that will lead to a particular magnitude of risk is estimated using mathematical models. Different models, based on different biological

assumptions, yield different results. Since risk assessment always involves some estimates, uncertainty factors are often used to introduce margins of safety. Physiologically based pharmacokinetic (PBPK) models have been used to (a) refine predictions made when extrapolating animal data to humans and (b) assess the human relevance of certain animal tumors.

Risk assessment offers a quantitative approach to assessing the risk of exposures. If the aim of public policy is to control rather than eliminate carcinogenic exposures, then risk assessment provides a framework for deciding how much exposure to permit. Risk assessment is transparent; the assumptions used are generally made explicit. However, critics point out that many of these assumptions, such as cross-species extrapolation and linear extrapolation to low doses, do not eliminate important scientific uncertainties. In addition, risk assessment is typically performed on one substance at a time, while actual exposures do not occur in isolation. Finally, risk assessment raises ethical concerns, because those who bear the risk are generally not those who benefit from production of a substance being evaluated and they are usually not well represented in quantifying and allocating risk.

Cancer Clusters

A *cluster* is an unusual aggregation of cases of disease, injury, or death that have occurred together in time and space. Although clusters may be identified by surveillance performed by health professionals, more often suspected clusters are reported to public health agencies by concerned citizens. (See Chapter 6.) Responses to inquiries about perceived environmental clusters may consume substantial resources of public health agencies, yet they rarely lead to the identification of etiologic agents. Those clusters that have identified previously unrecognized carcinogens have been clusters of extremely rare diseases and/or clusters of disease in well-defined populations. Historically, the investigation of occupational cancer clusters has led to the identification of several human carcinogens. For example, the associations between vinyl chloride monomer and angiosarcoma of the liver and between BCME and oat cell carcinoma of the lung were each first suspected by recognizing a cluster of cases at a single company.

Occupational Cancer Clusters

Although investigations of occupational cancer clusters have sometimes led to identification of new hazards, more often concerns about clusters arise from misperceptions of normal patterns of cancer incidence or mortality in working populations. Overall, 44% of U.S. men and 37% of U.S. women will be diagnosed with cancer at some time in their lifetimes;[1] thus, occurrence of multiple cancers in a specific group of workers is not uncommon. To respond quickly to concerns about cancer clusters and to monitor and detect any unusual mortality patterns, some large corporations have developed databases for surveillance of deaths among workers. Optimally, a file can be developed of all workers employed by a company in a given period of time, who can then be followed to determine vital status (if they are alive or dead) and causes of death. Surveillance systems based on death certificates alone (proportionate mortality ratio analyses) have also been used. Ideally, work history and exposure information should be included in surveillance databases, so that the rate and causes of death of workers with and without exposures of concern can be analyzed. However, if this is not feasible, nested case-control studies can be performed to evaluate job and exposure histories for cancers or other diseases that appear to be in excess.

When concern about a cancer cluster arises in a company with an ongoing surveillance program, it may be possible to determine fairly quickly whether the number of cases or deaths exceeds the number that would be expected. (See Chapter 5.) In the absence of a surveillance system, investigation of a cancer cluster in the workplace involves a number of steps:

1. Obtain a list of cancer cases on which the suspicion is based, with as much work history and clinical information as possible, including the date of onset of each cancer and date of hire at the plant for each cancer patient. Cancers diagnosed before or shortly after hire should be excluded from consideration.
2. Determine whether cancers are primary or secondary, especially for sites such as liver and brain, where metastatic lesions are common. A suspected cluster based on a variety of common cancer types arising at expected ages is less likely to be occupationally related than a cluster of one type of cancer, especially if the latter is (a) at an uncommon anatomical site, (b) of an uncommon histological type, or (c) occurring at younger ages than expected. Similarly, a suspected cluster arising from individuals with diverse jobs and exposures is less likely to be occupationally associated than one arising among workers employed in the same department or with similar exposures. Often, occupational cancer clusters represent cases from current, former, and retired workers.
3. Estimate the number of expected cases in the population at risk, which might include all workers employed at the facility from the time it opened. The number of expected deaths from any specific cancer in a population depends on the total number of workers, when they were hired, their age at hire, and gender and race distribution. It is difficult to estimate this number accurately without conducting a full cohort mortality study.
4. Develop information about the workplace exposures at present and in the past. In those workplaces with exposures to confirmed or suspected carcinogens, there should be heightened concern.
5. Obtain advice from experts early in the process to ensure that planned investigations are designed well and will be likely to yield useful information. This process should be open, with involvement of management and nonmanagement personnel and experts who are considered to be objective and credible. (See Chapter 5.)

Community Cancer Clusters

Each year, state and local health departments in the United States respond to more than 1,000 inquiries about suspected cancer clusters. Most states have developed a stepwise approach to triage requests from the public, using established criteria to determine their response. Most of the inquiries about cancer clusters to state health departments are situations that are clearly not clusters and can be resolved by telephone. For the remainder, follow-up is needed, first to confirm the number of persons affected, their ages, type of cancer, dates of diagnosis, and other factors and then to compare cancer incidence in the affected population with "background" rates in state tumor registries.

Not all suspected cancer clusters can or should be investigated extensively. Increasingly, epidemiologic studies of the community are only conducted when the following conditions are met:

1. The observed number of cases of a specific type of cancer statistically significantly exceeds the number expected.
2. Either the type of cancer or age at onset is highly unusual.
3. The population at risk can be defined.
4. Prolonged exposures to known or suspected carcinogens at levels that exceed environmental limits can be documented.

Rigorous documentation and investigation of a cancer cluster is generally an expensive, multiyear process, complicated by anxiety and pressure to generate information quickly. For example, in 1999, what appeared to be an excessive number of children diagnosed with leukemia while living in Churchill County, Nevada, was brought to the attention of the Nevada State Health Department. After an extensive case-finding effort, it was confirmed that, between 1997 and 2002, 16 children who lived in the county at the time of, or prior to, diagnosis developed leukemia. Among the 16 children, 11 lived in the county at the time of diagnosis, whereas only 1 case in a child residing in the county would have been expected. Statistical testing indicated that the likelihood that this cluster was a random event was very small. Although the number of childhood leukemia cases was unusual, the distribution of leukemia cell types was not. The Nevada State Health Department, in collaboration with the Centers for Disease Control and Prevention (CDC) and other agencies, collected air, water, soil and dust samples from almost 80 homes and tested samples for heavy metals, pesticides, polychlorinated biphenyls, and volatile organic compounds. Environmental samples were also tested for radon and other radioactive elements. Levels of most contaminants measured were not elevated, compared with national referent data or existing environmental standards. None of the measured contaminants were associated with the occurrence of childhood leukemia. There also were investigations of records of historical exposures in the community and possible exposures from a nearby naval air station. Although elevated levels of arsenic and tungsten were found in the municipal water supply, an expert panel concluded that this was not a likely explanation for the childhood leukemia cluster, because arsenic does not seem to be related to childhood leukemia and elevated levels of tungsten are found in many parts of Nevada. Continued investigation has not identified any exposures likely to be associated with increased risk of childhood leukemia.[55]

The CDC and the Council of State and Territorial Epidemiologists provides detailed guidelines for local and state health departments on the management and investigation of clusters of cancer and other diseases reported by the public.[56] Perhaps the most important challenge for public health agencies is to communicate effectively with the public. Informed clinicians can plan an important role by helping to educate patients and their families about cancer and by contributing to public debate and decision-making.

PREVENTING OCCUPATIONAL CANCER

Eliminating or reducing exposure to known or potential carcinogens is central to the prevention of occupational cancer. As described in Chapters 4 and 8, the best approaches to controlling exposure to hazardous substances in the workplace are (a) to eliminate exposure altogether by substitution or (b) to minimize exposure by engineering controls, such as process enclosure and ventilation. For example, benzene, which causes leukemia and other diseases, has been substituted by toluene and other organic solvents for many of its former uses. Exposure to vinyl chloride monomer, which causes angiosarcoma of the liver and other diseases, was greatly reduced by enclosing the processes where it had been present. Less desirable, but necessary in some settings such as hazardous work clean-up activities, is the use of personal protective equipment (PPE). However, establishment of an adequate program using PPE requires considerable expertise, training, and management commitment. Technical issues include the proper type of dermal and respiratory protection, requirements for fit-testing of respirators, training, maintenance, and monitoring of compliance. Personal protective equipment is uncomfortable to wear, may allow an exposure to hazardous substances if it malfunctions, and may even present its own hazards, such as hyperthermia from working in whole-body protective clothing. Therefore, process changes and environmental controls are almost always preferable to controlling exposure with PPE.

Other aspects of primary prevention include worker training and product labeling to increase awareness of workplace hazards and training to minimize exposures. Well-designed environmental monitoring programs should be established in workplaces where potential carcinogens are present to ensure effective exposure control. In settings where exposure to a potential carcinogen or other hazardous substance may occur through multiple routes, such as the respiratory system and the skin, biological monitoring of exposure should be considered to ensure adequate control.

Secondary prevention by cancer screening may be warranted for populations of workers with known or suspected increased cancer risks. Screening tests for early detection of bladder cancer have been employed for workers exposed to carcinogenic aromatic amines, such as β-naphthylamine, benzidine, and 4-aminobiphenyl. The two methods most commonly used are urinalysis for microscopic hematuria and urine cytology. Hematuria is relatively sensitive in detecting both superficial and invasive bladder cancer, but its low specificity results in a high false-positive rate, requiring many invasive studies on healthy individuals. Urine cytology has good sensitivity and specificity for high-grade bladder cancer but poor sensitivity for low-grade, papillary lesions. Early detection may not produce a survival advantage for patients whose disease is detected through such screening. However, highly effective treatment exists for both low-grade and high-grade

lesions detected at an early stage. More advanced screening techniques using molecular biomarkers have been successful in predicting risk of bladder cancer in a cohort of benzidine-exposed workers.[57]

A large randomized control trial in the United States demonstrated that screening with the use of low-dose computed tomography (CT) reduces mortality from lung cancer,[58] and in 2014 the U.S. Preventive Services Task Force recommended annual screening for adults age 50 to 89 years who have a 30-pack-year smoking history and currently smoke or have quit within the past 15 years.[59] Lung CT screening should also be considered for individuals with an increased risk of lung cancer due to occupational exposure, such as asbestos-exposed workers.[60]

OCCUPATIONAL AND ENVIRONMENTAL CANCER: SELECTED TOPICS

Environmental causes of cancer are highly diverse, including biological, physical (radiological), and chemical hazards. The topics covered in detail in the next sections were selected based on the magnitude of impact on human cancer to illustrate a diversity of exposures and exposure circumstances and to highlight emerging or newly recognized hazards.

Hepatocellular Carcinoma: Hepatitis B and C Viruses and Aflatoxin

An estimated 782,500 new liver cancer cases and 745,500 deaths occurred globally during 2012, with China accounting for about 50% of the cases and also about 50% of the deaths. The vast majority (70% to 90%) of liver cancers are hepatocellular carcinomas (HCCs). Liver cancer rates are the highest in East and Southeast Asia and Northern and Western Africa and lowest in South Central Asia and Northern, Central, and Eastern Europe (Figure 21-4).[2,61] In the United States, the liver cancer incidence rate from 2008 to 2012 was 11.4 per 100,000 for males and 3.9 per 100,000 for females. HCC incidence and mortality have been increasing in the United States since 1973.[62] Major risk factors for HCC globally are chronic infection with hepatitis B

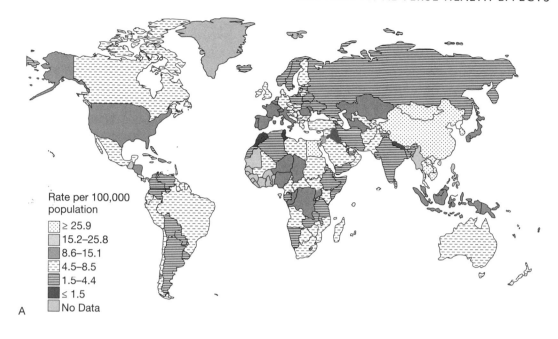

Rate per 100,000
population

≥ 25.9
15.2–25.8
8.6–15.1
4.5–8.5
1.5–4.4
≤ 1.5
No Data

A

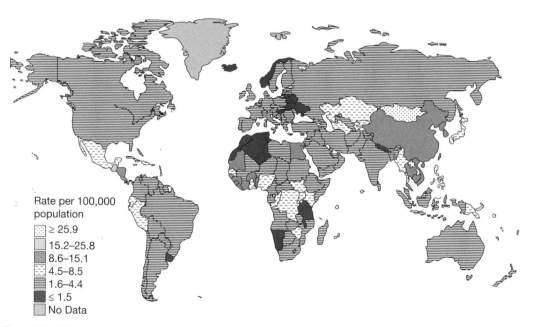

Rate per 100,000
population

≥ 25.9
15.2–25.8
8.6–15.1
4.5–8.5
1.6–4.4
≤ 1.5
No Data

B   *Per 100,000, age standardized to the World Standard Population.

Figure 21-4. International variation in liver cancer incidence rates, 2012: (A) males, and (B) females. (Source: American Cancer Society. Global cancer facts and figures [3rd edition]. Atlanta: American Cancer Society, 2015.)

virus (HBV) or hepatitis C virus (HCV) and exposure to aflatoxins as food contaminants. Hepatitis B virus accounts for the majority of HCC cases in LMICs, while HCV infection plays a more prominent role in HICs.[61] In the

United States, an estimated 850,000 to 2.2 million persons are living with chronic HBV infection,[24,25] and from 2.7 to 3.5 million persons are living with chronic HCV infection.[62] (See Chapters 13 and 27.)

Carriage of HBV is defined as the presence of the hepatitis B surface antigen (HBsAg) in the blood for 6 months or longer. HBsAg is produced by replication of HBV virus in hepatocytes. Carriage of HBV has been associated with a 50-fold increased risk of HCC.[63] The highest HBV carrier rates occur in Africa, China, and Oceania (excluding Australia and New Zealand). The main determinant of HBV carriage is age at infection, with infection in utero or during the first 5 years of life associated with much greater rates of carriage than infection later in life. Approximately 90% of infants infected in utero or around the time of birth and 25% of those infected during the first 5 years of life become carriers, while fewer than 5% of those infected past the age of 10 years become carriers.

In contrast, about 80% of all HCV infections result in carriage. Direct transmission by blood contamination, usually though a needle, is the most important mode of transmission, resulting in a high prevalence among intravenous drug users and onset of infection mainly among teenagers and young adults in most of the world. Many people are unaware of their infection, and the CDC and U.S. Preventive Services Task Force now recommend screening all persons born between 1945 and 1965 to identify those with HCV infection. Although this birth cohort compromises approximately 25% of the U.S. population, it accounts for approximately 75% of all HCV infections in the United States.[64]

The risk of HBV carriage is greatly decreased by HBV vaccination within 48 hours after birth. Risk is further diminished by administration of hepatitis B immune globulin (HBIG) to infants with carrier mothers. However, since HBIG is expensive to manufacture, public health programs in Asia and Africa only use hepatitis B vaccine. By the end of 2016, a total of 190 countries had introduced the HBV vaccine into their national infant immunization schedules, with many countries achieving more than 80% coverage for the full recommended dose.[61,65] It is unlikely that a vaccine against HCV will be developed in the near future since HCV is an RNA virus that shows marked genetic heterogeneity, although new antiviral therapies may prevent chronic infection among those with acute infection. Preventive measures include screening for HCV in donated blood and emphasis on clean, safe needle use.

Occupational exposures to percutaneous injuries are a potential source of infections with bloodborne pathogens among healthcare workers (see Chapters 13 and 32C). Although strategies are available to prevent infections due to sharps injuries, they have not been widely implemented in LMICs. It is estimated that in the year 2000 worldwide, 16,000 new HCV infections and 66,000 new HBV infections may have occurred due to percutaneous injuries.[66]

One way to decrease of HCC is by reducing contamination of food supplies with aflatoxins, which are mycotoxins (toxic fungal metabolites) produced by *Aspergillis flavus* and *A. parasiticus*. Aflatoxin contamination of foods occurs mainly in LMICs with hot, humid climates. It is found on a variety of oilseeds and cereal crops. Often the regions with high exposure are the same as those with high HBV infection rates. Aflatoxins are potent hepatocarcinogens. Hepatitis B virus and aflatoxin have a synergistic effect on HCC risk.[63] A variety of measures can reduce aflatoxin contamination, including pre- and postharvest crop management and dietary change. These measures are especially important in parts of the world where there is a high prevalence of HBV and HCV carriers.

Treatments are now available that can reduce the risk of HCC development for HBV and HBC carriers but may not be widely available outside of HICs; even within HICs, cost may be a barrier for some treatments.

Indoor Air Pollution from Burning Solid Fuels

Household use of solid fuels for cooking and heating is thought to be an important cause of lung cancer among nonsmoking women in LMICs. Globally, almost 3 billion people rely for their primary source of domestic energy on solid fuels, including coal and biomass (fuel from wood, charcoal, crop residues, and dung) often in open fireplaces or in poorly functioning earth or metal stoves. Combustion is incomplete and results in substantial emissions that contain particles, carbon monoxide, nitrous oxides, sulfur oxides (primarily from coal), formaldehyde, and polycyclic organic matter, including carcinogens such as benzo(a)pyrene. Indoor emissions from household combustion of coal increase lung cancer risk—an exposure classified as a Group 1 carcinogen by IARC, and IARC has classified household combustion of biomass fuel (mainly wood) as probably carcinogenic to humans (Group 2A). Indoor air pollution is responsible annually for an estimated 3.8 million premature deaths globally, most of which are from acute and chronic respiratory disease. [67] The proportion of households relying mainly on solid fuels for cooking decreased from 62% in 1980 to 41% in 2010, but, due to population growth, the number of exposed persons has remained stable at about 2.8 million. Solid fuel use is most prevalent in Africa and Southeast Asia, where over 60% of households cook with solid fuels.[68]A recent meta-analysis that included 18 case-control studies found evidence that exposure to indoor air pollution increased risk not only for lung cancer, but also for several other cancers, including cervical, oral, nasopharyngeal, pharyngeal, and laryngeal cancer.[69]

Radon

Environmental (indoor) radon exposure is second only to cigarette smoking as a leading cause of lung cancer. Radon (radon-222) is a naturally occurring decay product of radium-226, the fifth daughter of uranium-238. Two of the decay products of radon-222 emit alpha particles, which are highly effective at damaging tissues. Both uranium-238 and radium-226 are present in most soils and rocks, although concentrations vary widely (Figure 21-5). Radon exposure in homes and workplaces is largely a result of radon-contaminated gas arising from soil. Although radon is ubiquitous in indoor and outdoor air and also in the air of underground passages and mines, its concentration is increased by the presence of a rich source and by low ventilation of air in contact with the source.

Radon, unlike exposure to cigarette smoke, is naturally occurring and cannot be completely eliminated from homes and workplaces. Within buildings, radon levels are usually highest in the basement due to its proximity to the ground, from which radon-containing soil gas diffuses. Thus, people who spend much of their time in basements, at home or at work, face a greater

potential for exposure. The EPA sets action levels for concentration of radon in homes and provides information about how it is measured and how levels can be reduced, such as by installing ventilation.

Exposure to radon among miners is associated with an increase in lung cancer risk.[70] Studies have consistently demonstrated a linear increase in lung cancer risk with increasing cumulative exposure to radon. Although the increase in relative risk per unit exposure is higher for people who have never smoked than for smokers, the increase in absolute risk is much higher for smokers.

Since average radon exposures among miners have been about 10-fold greater than average indoor exposures, extrapolation of risk assessments from studies in miners to the lung cancer risk for people exposed to radon in their homes may be unreliable. To study the relationship between residential radon exposure and lung cancer risk, several case-control studies in the general population were initiated in the 1980s. Meta-analyses and collaborative analyses of these case-control studies found statistically significant exposure–response trends that are similar to (a) exposure–response trends extrapolated from higher dose exposures among miners and (b) relative risks computed directly from studies of miners with low cumulative exposures.[71-73] An estimated 10% to 15% of lung cancer deaths in the United States have been attributed to radon (among "ever-smokers" and "never-smokers" combined).[74] Most radon-related lung cancers occur among ever-smokers. However, an estimated 2,100 to 2,900 of the 11,000 deaths from lung cancer among nonsmokers in the United States each year are thought to be radon-related. The geologic potential for radon exposure differs throughout the United States (Figure 21-5). Approximately one-third of radon-induced lung cancer could be prevented if homes with radon concentrations exceeding the EPA action level of 4 picocuries/L in air could reduce radon concentrations below that level.

Environmental Tobacco Smoke (Passive or Involuntary Smoking)

Involuntary smoking consists of exposure to a complex mixture of chemicals generated during

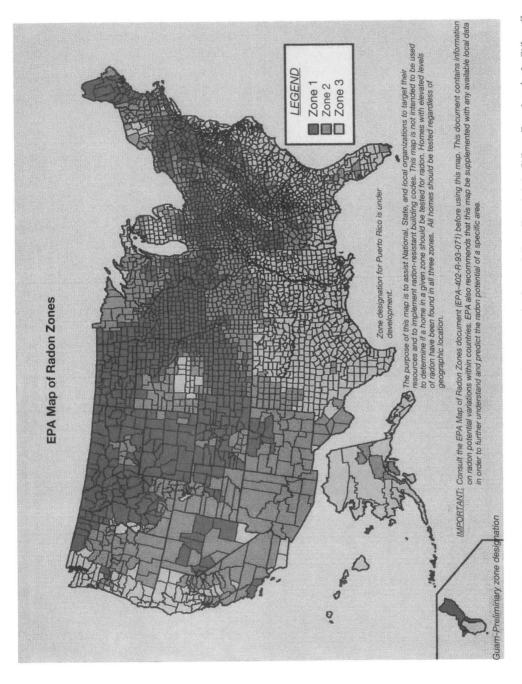

Figure 21-5. Radon zones, United States. Counties with predicted average indoor radon screening levels > 4 pCi/L are Zone 1, 2–4 pCi/L are Zone 2, and < 2 pCi/L are Zone 3. (Source: U.S. Environmental Protection Agency. Available at https://www.epa.gov/sites/production/files/2015-07/documents/zonemapcolor.pdf. Accessed on February 27, 2017.)

* Other carcinogens, including medications (especially cancer chemotherapeutic agents, a risk for healthcare workers), foods, tobacco, and viruses, are classified as IARC Group 1 carcinogens but are not listed here.

* Other probable carcinogens, including medications (especially cancer chemotherapeutic agents, a risk for healthcare workers), infectious agents, and foods, are classified in Group 2A but are not listed here.

the burning of tobacco products. It contains sidestream smoke—the material emitted from smoldering tobacco products between puffs—as well as exhaled mainstream smoke. Compounds identified in tobacco smoke include recognized carcinogens, such as 4-aminobiphenyl, arsenic, and benzo(a)pyrene. Numerous studies and meta-analyses have documented increased risk from lung cancer among nonsmokers exposed to environmental tobacco smoke (ETS), also known as secondhand smoke, in the workplace and home. A large prospective study found that 16% of lung cancer in never-smokers and 24% in ex-smokers are attributable to ETS mainly due to work-related exposure.[75] The same study also found an association between exposure to ETS in childhood and increased risk of lung cancer in adulthood.

In response to the health effects associated with cigarette smoking and exposure to ETS, many countries and U.S. states have enacted smoke-free policies, including legislative and other measures to protect against harmful exposure to secondhand smoke. An IARC working group concluded that (a) these policies substantially decrease secondhand smoke exposure; (b) smoke-free workplaces decrease the prevalence of adult smoking and decrease cigarette consumption in continuing smokers; and (c) voluntary smoke-free home policies decrease children's secondhand smoke exposure, decrease adult smoking, and decrease youth smoking. Substantial progress has been made in reducing exposures to ETS. Self-reported ETS at home declined between 2000 and 2010, from 24% to 8.2% for children and from 12.1% to 4.4% for adults. From 1992–1993 to 2010–2011, the percentage of households where no adult was allowed to smoke inside the home at any time (households that adopted a smoke-free home rule) increased from 43% to 83%.[76,77]

Shift Work and Circadian Rhythm Disruption

Long-term occupational exposure to light at night and circadian rhythm disruption appears to increase breast cancer risk. Disruption of other hormonal pathways may also lead to increased risk of cancer. An IARC working group concluded that "shift work that involves circadian disruption is probably carcinogenic to humans"[78]—a finding based on limited evidence from epidemiologic studies and sufficient evidence from animal studies.[79,80] A recent meta-analysis of 28 studies found a significant association between circadian disruption and breast cancer risk; each 10-year increment of shift work was associated with 16% higher risk of breast cancer.[80] There is increasing evidence that prostate cancer is associated with proxies of circadian disruption and sleep loss.[81] Several studies have found associations between working night shifts and ovarian cancer.[82,83]

Animal studies have investigated the effect of constant light, dim light at night, simulated chronic jet lag, or circadian timing of carcinogens; most have shown a major increase in tumor incidence.[78] Other studies found a tumorigenic effect of reduced nocturnal melatonin secretions or removal of the pineal gland (where melatonin is produced). Disruption of the circadian system by exposure to light at night results in alteration of sleep-activity patterns, suppression of melatonin production, and deregulation of circadian genes involved in cancer-related pathways. Inactivation of the circadian period gene, Per2, promotes tumor development in mice; in human breast and endometrial tumors, expression of PERIOD genes is inhibited.[78] Suppressed melatonin may also result in increased levels of estrogen, thereby inducing tumors in hormone-sensitive organs, such as the breast.

Although investigation of the role of environmental lighting and circadian rhythm disruption is a relatively new area of research, it is of direct importance in the workplace since 15% to 20% of workers in the United States and Europe are engaged in shift work that involves night work. In addition, one of the defining features of the human environment for the past 120 years has been artificial electric lighting. Changes in the light-dark cycle related to artificial lighting in HICs in the 20th century may have contributed to increasing incidence of breast, colon, prostate, and other cancers.[84] (See Chapter 14.)

Nanoparticles

In the past decades, increasing numbers of workers have been involved with the production, use, and disposal of nanoparticles, which are defined as being under 100 nm at their largest dimension. (See Chapter 8.) There are a wide variety of such particles, for which varying physiochemical features (size, shape, composition, charge, crystallinity, solubility, added functional groups, and impurities) can lead to different toxicologic potential. Because development of nanomaterials is new, most exposures occur in pilot or start-up facilities in a wide range of manufacturing and materials sectors.[85,86] Although toxicologic data involving nanoparticles are limited, studies suggest that some materials that are relatively nontoxic in larger particles are highly toxic or carcinogenic in nanoparticles.

Uses of carbon nanotubes have been rapidly increasing in electronics, optics, drug-delivery devices, protective clothing, strengthening of sports equipment, and research. Concerns about the carcinogenicity of carbon nanotubes have been raised because the shape and dimensions of the carbon fibers are similar to those of asbestos. One study has shown that carbon nanotubes cause in the abdominal mesothelium of mice pathological changes similar to those caused by asbestos. More research is needed to determine what types of carbon fibers cause the greatest risk, the extent of exposure needed to produce a carcinogenic effect, and whether exposed humans develop nonmalignant lung disease, lung cancer, or mesothelioma. A precautionary approach has been advocated to decrease the possibility of health risks to exposed workers until more definitive research is completed.[87]

CASE STUDIES IN OCCUPATIONAL AND ENVIRONMENTAL CANCER

CASE 1

A computer company has a site with 4,200 employees engaged in research and development, manufacturing, sales and service, and repairs. The human resources director is interested in cancer prevention. What are the most important measures an employer can implement to prevent cancer?

Comment: The first priority of the employer is to ensure that any exposure to potential carcinogens in the workplace is minimized or eliminated. In addition to compliance with regulatory requirements, companies should ensure that appropriate experts review toxicological data on all chemicals used, select the least toxic products, and implement proper exposure controls and monitoring for all potentially toxic substances. Several substances used in the microelectronics industry have recently been evaluated by IARC. It classified gallium arsenide as a Group 1 carcinogen and indium phosphide as a Group 2A carcinogen. Substances with evidence of carcinogenicity in animals should be treated as potentially carcinogenic to humans, and appropriate exposure monitoring and control should be implemented, even if not required by regulations. Engineering controls are generally preferred over PPE for exposure control. Depending on the nature and extent of chemical exposures, consideration should be given to change rooms, on-site laundering of work clothing, and other precautions to minimize potential transport of hazardous substances outside the workplace. Health and safety committees, with representation of management and nonmanagement personnel, should review workplace health and safety procedures, prioritize issues, and coordinate measures to inform and educate workers.

Employers can reduce the risk of cancer among all employees by offering health insurance benefits that include coverage for smoking cessation and all recommended types of cancer screening. If employees are or may be at increased risk of cancer due to work exposure, the possibility of offering additional cancer screening should be considered. Regardless of occupational factors, opportunities exist for cancer control and health promotion through workplace programs.

Cigarette smoking and obesity are the two most important causes of cancer in the general population in the United States. Smoke-free workplaces reduce exposure of nonsmokers to ETS, encourage smokers to decrease smoking or quit, and reduce the potential for exposure to workplace chemicals through hand-to-mouth contact while smoking. Transition to a smoke-free workplace should be accompanied by support to help smokers quit, including counseling services and pharmacotherapy. The workplace may also be used to promote healthy diets and physical activity. Provision of healthy food choices in workplace cafeterias may encourage healthy eating habits. On-site exercise facilities or subsidies for health-club memberships can encourage physical activity. (See Chapter 10.)

CASE 2

A 44-year-old flight attendant is concerned about breast cancer due to her occupation. Is her concern justified?

Comment: Almost all epidemiologic studies performed on flight attendants have shown a significant excess risk of breast cancer. [88] Occupational exposures that might explain this increased risk include cosmic radiation and circadian rhythm disruption. Although radiation exposures among flight crew members are not routinely monitored, those who regularly fly long distance at high altitudes or on flight routes near the North Pole or South Pole may have higher exposure to ionizing radiation than the average U.S. radiation worker. (See Chapter 12D.) Flight attendants who work during pregnancy may exceed the International Commission on Radiation Protection recommended limit of 1 mSv to the conceptus during pregnancy. Many flight attendants also experience circadian rhythm disruption on flights that cross multiple time zones or occur overnight. The possibility that the increased risk of breast cancer among flight attendants is related to circadian rhythm disruption is supported by a consistent finding of increased breast cancer risk among other groups of female night workers and studies in experimental animals documenting increased tumor incidence associated with circadian rhythm disruption. Despite increasing evidence for increased risk of breast cancer among flight attendants and the possible role of circadian rhythm disruption, it is still not certain if this association is causal, in

part because of the complexity of separating the influence of occupational and nonoccupational risk factors for breast cancer.

Important breast cancer risk factors in the general population include a family history of breast cancer in a parent or sibling, nulliparity, older age at first birth, earlier age at menarche, later age at menopause, use of hormone replacement therapy, and obesity. Although many of these risk factors are not readily modifiable, women interested in reducing their breast cancer risk should be encouraged to maintain a healthy body weight, engage in regular physical activity, and minimize alcohol consumption. The American Cancer Society recommends that women of average risk begin annual clinical breast exam and mammography at age 45 and inform their physician promptly about any changes in their breasts between exams. A woman's personal risk profile for breast cancer should be determined based on family history and other factors. Additional options, including enhanced screening and chemoprophylaxis, should be offered to high-risk women who meet established criteria.

CASE 3

A 67-year-old machinist is diagnosed with rectal cancer. He asks his surgeon if his work exposure to metalworking fluids could have caused it. He wonders whether his son, who now works as a machinist, is at increased risk.

Comment: Millions of gallons of metalworking fluids are used each day in the United States for cutting, milling, drilling, stamping, and grinding. More than 1 million workers are engaged in these activities and potentially exposed to metalworking fluids by inhalation and dermal contact. Metalworking fluids are complex mixtures of chemicals that are classified into three major types: straight oils, soluble oils, and semisynthetic metalworking fluids. The identity and proportion of chemical species in these mixtures are dependent on several factors, including the manufacturer and the cooling and lubrication requirements of the machining process. In addition, several additives are used in metalworking fluids to extend their operational lifespan, and other substances contaminate the complex mixture during manufacturing. The three major types of metalworking fluids are as follows:

1. *Straight oils* are composed primarily of solvent-refined petroleum oils. Before the 1940s, metalworking fluids were predominantly straight oils. In 1984, untreated and mildly treated mineral oils containing PAHs were classified by IARC as human carcinogens. Highly refined petroleum oils (lubricant base oils) continue to be used in lower production operations and those requiring lubrication. Straight oils may contain elemental sulfur, sulfur compounds, and chlorinated compounds, such as chlorinated paraffins, some of which are carcinogenic.
2. *Soluble oils* are combinations of highly refined mineral oils (30% to 85%) and emulsifiers, and they are typically diluted with water at ratios of 1 part concentrate to 5 to 40 parts water. Semi-synthetic metalworking fluids contain a lower proportion of lubricant base oils (5% to 30%), a higher proportion of emulsifiers, and 30% to 50% water.
3. *Synthetic oils* contain no petroleum oils and may be water soluble or water dispersible. They are composed of water with additives, including buffers, such as ethanolamines.

Exposures to metalworking fluids have been associated with increased risks of cancers of several sites, including stomach, esophagus, lung, prostate, brain, colon, rectum, and the hematopoietic system. The specific metalworking fluid constituents or contaminants responsible for increased risks for specific cancers remain under investigation.[89]

Several studies have reported an association between exposure to metalworking fluids and rectal cancer. A comprehensive study of the health effects of exposure to metalworking fluids found a significant association between exposure to straight oils and rectal cancer, with a two-fold increased risk among workers with a cumulative exposure of over 3 mg/m³-years. Risk was greatest for those hired before 1970, perhaps reflecting either less carcinogenicity of more modern metalworking fluids or the relatively short follow-up of workers hired

after 1970. More recent studies have found increased rectal cancer risk associated with exposure to soluble and synthetic oils as well. [89] While it is plausible that exposure to metalworking fluids may have contributed to the development of rectal cancer in this machinist, it is unclear whether his son will be at risk as a result of present-day metalworking fluid exposures. Over the past several decades, substantial changes have been made in metalworking, including changing the types of metalworking fluids used; reducing potentially carcinogenic contaminants, such as nitrosamine precursors; and reducing exposure concentrations through process changes and engineering controls—all of which may decrease the risk of rectal cancer among more recent workers. Given that the specific constituent of metalworking fluids responsible for the increased risk of rectal cancer is unknown, increased risk of rectal cancer for workers who began exposure recently cannot be ruled out. Metalworking fluids have been nominated for toxicologic testing by the National Toxicology Program, with the goal of better understanding the carcinogenicity of formulations currently used. The son's individual risk of developing colorectal cancer also depends on whether there have been other family members diagnosed with colorectal cancer at a young age and whether he has certain specific diseases that increase colorectal cancer risk. Colorectal cancer screening can both detect cancer at an early stage and prevent it by removing adenomatous polyps. Screening for colorectal cancer is recommended for the general population starting at age 50, with earlier and enhanced screening recommended for those at high risk.

CASE 4

A study found that 10 current and former workers at a chemical manufacturing plant with 5,000 workers have developed brain cancer over the past 10 years. The workers' union requests an investigation and asks whether an exposure at our plant is causing brain cancer and what should be done.

Additional investigation identifies two additional cases, for a total of 12. No medical records are available for three of the 12. Five appear to have died of brain cancer, and four appear to have been diagnosed with benign brain tumors. While case confirmation continues, another worker is diagnosed with brain cancer. The local newspaper interviews this worker's wife and writes a story suggesting a company conspiracy to cover up a brain cancer epidemic. Concern begins to center around a plant department with historical exposure to nitrosamines and many other chemicals.

Union and management agree to bring in outside consultants to review the case and exposure information. The consultants state that it is unclear whether the observed cases represent an excess. The number of brain cancer deaths does not greatly exceed the number that might be expected from studies of other cohorts of workers. However, since ascertainment of cases was not done systematically, it is not known if all brain cancer cases have been identified. The consultants agree that, while brain cancer clusters have been reported in the chemical industry, limited evidence exists for an association between specific chemical exposures and brain cancer. They further agree that, given the wide variety of chemical processes present at the plant, retrospective exposure assessment would be very time consuming and expensive.

Comment: The best way to approach a possible brain cancer excess at the workplace is to conduct a cohort mortality study. In this situation, such a study could be done quickly if it was confined to employees working there on or after January 1, 1978. Since that date, employees' work histories and demographic information have been computerized and can be linked with the National Death Index, which can provide accurate information on deaths throughout the United States since 1978. The consultants request a comprehensive industrial hygiene survey, which will be performed by an independent contractor to ensure that current exposure protection is adequate.

The consultants agree to reconvene after the study is completed to review its results. If the study confirms excess mortality from brain cancer, further studies may be indicated to identify high-risk departments and processes. If not, the consultants would recommend that the company continue to conduct mortality surveillance for this cohort of workers.

RESEARCH AND POLICY PRIORITIES

A major challenge is to develop better data to evaluate the hazards of chemicals, mixtures, and exposure circumstances in IARC Groups 2A and 2B and others with some evidence of carcinogenicity in animal or human studies. Historically, many of the recognized human carcinogens were identified in occupational cohorts where very high exposures resulted in very high relative risks. The changing nature of the workplace and increasing complexity of exposures have made such occupational epidemiology studies more difficult (Chapter 5). As a result of regulatory and voluntary controls, exposure levels and attendant risks are much lower than in the past. Many exposures are mixtures, and many occupations involve exposure to an ever-changing and diverse array of substances. These changes create the need for more sensitive measures to detect cancer risks in occupational populations. For example, studies may need to incorporate quantitative estimates of risk for multiple exposure agents, examine possible interaction between occupational and nonoccupational exposures, and consider the use of biomarkers to better define intermediate markers related to exposure and biologic effects.

The potential for biomarkers to play a role in improving understanding of human cancer risks has been recognized but not fully exploited. Biomarkers can play an important role in understanding a number of stages in the process through which exogenous exposures result in cancer, including internal dose, biologically effective dose, early biologic effect, altered structure and function, premalignant changes, and clinical disease. Biomarker data have been used by IARC to support classification of ethylene oxide and 2,3,7,8-tetrachlorodibenzodioxin (dioxin) as Group 1 carcinogens, in the absence of definitive evidence of increases in cancer incidence or mortality from epidemiologic studies. Incorporation of biomarkers of genetic susceptibility may play a role in studies of potential occupational and environmental carcinogens. However, current scientific knowledge about genetic susceptibility to environmental and occupational cancer is too limited for clinical application.

There is much scientific controversy and debate about the extrapolation of effects in animals to humans, especially concerning (a) low levels of human exposure and (b) the strength of evidence that certain mechanisms of action in rodents are not applicable in humans. This controversy and debate, while highly technical, have practical consequences for the classification of, and exposure control for, chemicals of public health importance. Research conducted to clarify these issues must be objective and supported, at least in part, by public and private institutions with no financial interest in the outcome. In addition, scientific and government agencies considering these issues should ensure representation from all perspectives, including labor, management, and affected communities.

The Precautionary Principle is aimed at avoiding possible harm associated with suspected, but not definite, environmental risks. In the face of scientific uncertainty about potential carcinogens, it has been advanced to provide a framework within which to consider public health actions. It provides justification for acting in the face of uncertain knowledge to address potential risks from specific environmental exposures. The Precautionary Principle states that appropriate public health action should be taken in response to limited evidence of likely and substantial harm, when that evidence is plausible and credible. The burden of proof is shifted from demonstrating the presence of risk to demonstrating its absence.

Clinicians' roles in confronting occupational cancer vary. They should maintain a high index of suspicion of occupational causes of cancer when treating patients. Clinicians should work to identify past exposures, using the patient's knowledge, toxicological resources, consultants, and other sources of information. In cases of ongoing exposures, clinicians should help to reduce or eliminate hazardous exposure. Finally, clinicians should educate patients, employee and employer groups, and communities about the hazards of carcinogenic exposures and ways to prevent them.

REFERENCES

1. Siegel RL, Miller KD, Jemal A. Cancer statistics, 2016. CA: A Cancer Journal for Clinicians 2016; 66: 7–30.

2. Torre LA, Siegel RL, Ward EM, Jemal A. Global cancer incidence and mortality rates and trends—An update. Cancer Epidemiology, Biomarkers & Prevention 2016; 25: 16–27.

3. Doll R, Peto R. The causes of cancer: Quantitative estimates of avoidable risks of cancer in the United States today. Journal of the National Cancer Institute 1981; 66: 1191–1308.

4. Steenland K, Burnett C, Lalich N, et al. Dying for work: The magnitude of US mortality from selected causes of death associated with occupation. American Journal of Industrial Medicine 2003; 43: 461–482.

5. Rushton L, Hutchings S, Brown T. The burden of cancer at work: Estimation as the first step to prevention. Occupational and Environmental Medicine 2008; 65: 789–800.

6. Driscoll T, Takala J, Steenland K, et al. Review of estimates of the global burden of injury and illness due to occupational exposures. American Journal of Industrial Medicine 2005; 48: 491–502.

7. Straif K. The burden of occupational cancer. Occupational and Environmental Medicine 2008; 65: 787–788.

8. World Health Organization. Elimination of asbestos-related diseases. Updated March 2014. Available at: http://www.who.int/ipcs/assessment/public_health/Elimination_asbestos-related_diseases_EN.pdf?ua=1. Accessed November 18, 2016.

9. Nicholson WJ, Perkel G, Selikoff IJ. Occupational exposure to asbestos: Population at risk and projected mortality—1980–2030. American Journal of Industrial Medicine 1982; 3: 259–311.

10. Centers for Disease Control and Prevention, National Institute for Occupational Safety and Health. Malignant mesothelioma: Mortality data. Available at: https://wwwn.cdc.gov/eworld/Grouping/Malignant_mesothelioma/100. Accessed October 16, 2016.

11. Straif K, Benbrahim-Tallaa L, Baan R, et al. A review of human carcinogens—Part C: Metals, arsenic, dusts, and fibres. Lancet Oncology 2009; 10: 453–454.

12. U.S. Geological Survey. Mineral commodities summaries, January 2016. Available at: http://minerals.usgs.gov/minerals/pubs/commodity/asbestos/mcs-2016-asbes.pdf. Accessed October 31, 2016.

13. Virta RL, Flanagan DM. Asbestos (advance release). In: USGS 2014 minerals yearbook, December 2015. Available at: http://minerals.usgs.gov/minerals/pubs/commodity/asbestos/myb1-2014-asbes.pdf. Accessed October 31, 2016.

14. Harington JS, McGlashan ND, Chelkowska EZ. South Africa's export trade in asbestos: Demise of an industry. American Journal of Industrial Medicine 2010; 53: 524–534.

15. Braun L, Greene A, Manseau M, et al. Scientific controversy and asbestos: Making disease invisible. International Journal of Occupational and Environmental Health 2003; 9: 194–205.

16. Frank AL, Joshi TK. The global spread of asbestos. Annals of Global Health 2014; 80: 257–262.

17. Dave SK, Beckett WS. Occupational asbestos exposure and predictable asbestos-related diseases in India. American Journal of Industrial Medicine 2005; 48: 137–143.

18. Ansari FA, Ahmad I, Ashquin M, et al. Monitoring and identification of airborne asbestos in unorganized sectors, India. Chemosphere 2007; 68: 716–723.

19. Vainio H, Oksa P, Tuomi T, et al. Helsinki Criteria update 2014: Asbestos continues to be a challenge for disease prevention and attribution. Epidemiologia e prevenzione. 2016; 40: 15–19.

20. Landrigan PJ, Lioy PJ, Thurston G, et al. Health and environmental consequences of the world trade center disaster. Environmental Health Perspectives 2004; 112: 731–739.

21. Sullivan PA. Vermiculite, respiratory disease, and asbestos exposure in Libby, Montana: Update of a cohort mortality study. Environmental Health Perspectives 2007; 115: 579–585.

22. Whitehouse AC, Black CB, Heppe MS, et al. Environmental exposure to Libby Asbestos and mesotheliomas. American Journal of Industrial Medicine 2008; 51: 877–880.

23. Naik SL, Lewin M, Young R, et al. Mortality from asbestos-associated disease in Libby, Montana 1979–2011. Journal of Exposure Science and Environmental Epidemiology 2017; 27: 207–213.

24. Horton DK, Bove F, Kapil V. Select mortality and cancer incidence among residents in various U.S. communities that received asbestos-contaminated vermiculite ore from Libby, Montana. Inhalation Toxicology 2008; 20: 767–775.

25. Reid A, Berry G, Heyworth J, et al. Predicted mortality from malignant mesothelioma among women exposed to blue asbestos at Wittenoom, Western Australia. Occupational and Environmental Medicine 2009; 66: 169–174.

26. Osman E, Hasan B, Meral U, et al. Recent discovery of an old disease: Malignant pleural mesothelioma in a village in south-east Turkey. Respirology 2007; 12: 448–451.

27. Constantopoulos SH. Environmental mesothelioma associated with tremolite asbestos: Lessons from the experiences of Turkey, Greece, Corsica, New Caledonia and Cyprus. Regulatory Toxicology and Pharmacology 2008; 52: S110–S115.

28. Baumann F, Buck BJ, Metcalf RV, et al. The presence of asbestos in the natural environment is likely related to mesothelioma in young individuals and women from southern Nevada. Journal of Thoracic Oncology 2015; 10: 731–737.

29. Lichtenstein P, Holm NV, Verkasalo PK, et al. Environmental and heritable factors in the causation of cancer—Analyses of cohorts of twins from Sweden, Denmark, and Finland. New England Journal of Medicine 2000; 343: 78–85.

30. Drdina DJ. Ionizing radiation. In: WK Hong, RC BastJr, WN Hait, et al (eds.). Holland-Frei Cancer Medicine (8th ed.). Shelton, CT: People's Medical Publishing House, 2010, pp. 248–261.

31. Herman JG, Baylin SB. Gene silencing in cancer in association with promoter hypermethylation. New England Journal of Medicine 2003; 349: 2042–2054.

32. Jackson AL, Loeb LA. The contribution of endogenous sources of DNA damage to the multiple mutations in cancer. Mutation Research 2001; 477: 7–21.

33. Marnett LJ. Oxyradicals and DNA damage. Carcinogenesis 2000; 21: 361–370.

34. Mayer J, Cheeseman MA, Twaroski ML. Structure-activity relationship analysis tools: Validation and applicability in predicting carcinogens. Regulatory Toxicology and Pharmacology 2008; 50: 50–58.

35. Waters MD, Stack HF, Jackson MA. Genetic toxicology data in the evaluation of potential human environmental carcinogens. Mutation Research 1999; 437: 21–49.

36. Ashby J, Waters MD, Preston J, et al. IPCS harmonization of methods for the prediction and quantification of human carcinogenic/mutagenic hazard, and for indicating the probable mechanism of action of carcinogens. Mutation Research 1996; 352: 153–157.

37. Eastmond DA, Hartwig A, Anderson D, et al. Mutagenicity testing for chemical risk assessment: Update of the WHO/IPCS Harmonized Scheme. Mutagenesis 2009; 24: 341–349.

38. Eastmond DA, Vulimiri SV, French JE, Sonawane B. The use of genetically modified mice in cancer risk assessment: Challenges and limitations. Critical Reviews in Toxicology 2013; 43: 611–631.

39. Baan R, Grosse Y, Lajoie P, et al. The IARC Monographs workshops: Tumour concordance between humans and experimental animals and mechanisms involved in human carcinogenesis. Available at: https://monographs.iarc.fr/ENG/Publications/TumourConcordancePoster2012.pdf. Accessed November 8, 2016.

40. Guyton KZ, Kyle AD, Aubrecht J, et al. Improving prediction of chemical carcinogenicity by considering multiple mechanisms and applying toxicogenomic approaches. Mutation Research 2009; 681: 230–240.

41. Tice RR, Austin CP, Kavlock RJ, Bucher JR. Improving the human hazard characterization of chemicals: A Tox21 update. Environmental Health Perspectives 2013; 121: 756–765.

42. Merrick BA, Paules RS, Tice RR. Intersection of toxicogenomics and high throughput screening in the Tox21 program: An NIEHS perspective. International Journal of Biotechnology 2015; 14: 7–27.

43. Smith MT, Guyton KZ, Gibbons CF, et al. Key characteristics of carcinogens as a basis for organizing data on mechanisms of carcinogenesis. Environmental Health Perspectives 2016; 124: 713–721.

44. International Agency for Research on Cancer. IARC monographs on the evaluation of carcinogenic risks to human: Some organophosphate insecticides and herbicides: Diazinon, glyphosate, malathion, parathion, and tetrachlorvinphos (Volume 112). 2015. Available at: http://monographs.iarc.fr/ENG/Monographs/vol112/mono112-08.pdf. Accessed November 9, 2016.

45. National Toxicology Program. 14th report on carcinogens. Research Triangle Park, NC: U.S. Department of Health and Human Services, 2016. Available at: https://ntp.niehs.nih.gov/pubhealth/roc/index-1.html. Accessed November 18, 2016.

46. Boffetta P, Winn DM, Ioannidis JP, et al. Recommendations and proposed guidelines for assessing the cumulative evidence on joint effects of genes and environments on cancer occurrence in humans. International Journal of Epidemiology 2012; 41: 686–704.

47. Garcia-Closas M, Rothman N, Figueroa JD, et al. Common genetic polymorphisms modify the effect of smoking on absolute risk of bladder cancer. Cancer Research 2013; 73: 2211–2220.

48. Cogliano VJ, Baan R, Straif K, et al. Preventable exposures associated with human cancers. Journal of the National Cancer Institute 2011; 103: 1827–1839.

49. List of classifications by cancer sites with sufficient or limited evidence in humans, Volumes 1 to 117. Adapted from Table 4 in Cogliano VJ, Baan R, Straif K, et al. Preventable exposures associated with human cancers. Journal of the National Cancer Institute 2011; 103: 1827–1839. Available at: https://monographs.iarc.fr/ENG/Classification/Table4.pdf Accessed November 6, 2016.

50. Figueroa JD, Han SS, Garcia-Closas M, et al. Genome-wide interaction study of smoking and bladder cancer risk. Carcinogenesis 2014; 35: 1737–1744.

51. Engel LS, Taioli E, Pfeiffer R, et al. Pooled analysis and meta-analysis of glutathione S-transferase M1 and bladder cancer: A HuGE review. American Journal of Epidemiology 2002; 156: 95–109.

52. Zhang Y, Hughes KJ, Zahm SH, et al. Genetic variations in xenobiotic metabolic pathway genes, personal hair dye use, and risk of non-Hodgkin lymphoma. American Journal of Epidemiology 2009; 170: 1222–1230.

53. Guo H, Bassig BA, Lan Q, et al. Polymorphisms in DNA repair genes, hair dye use, and the risk of non-Hodgkin lymphoma. Cancer Causes Control. 2014; 25: 1261–1270.

54. Burgio MR, Ioannidis JP, Kaminski BM, et al. Collaborative cancer epidemiology in the 21st century: The model of cancer consortia. Cancer Epidemiology, Biomarkers & Prevention 2013; 22: 2148–2160.

55. Rubin CS, Holmes AK, Belson MG, et al. Investigating childhood leukemia in Churchill County, Nevada. Environmental Health Perspectives 2007; 15: 151–157.

56. Abrams B, Anderson H, Blackmore C, et al. Investigating suspected cancer clusters and responding to community concerns: Guidelines from CDC and the Council of State and Territorial Epidemiologists. Morbidity and Mortality Weekly Report 2013; 62: 1–14.

57. Hemstreet GP 3rd, Yin S, Ma Z, et al. Biomarker risk assessment and bladder cancer detection in a cohort exposed to benzidine. Journal of the National Cancer Institute 2001; 93: 427–436.

58. Patel AR, Wedzicha JA, Hurst JR. Reduced lung-cancer mortality with CT screening. New England Journal of Medicine 2011; 365: 2035; author reply 2037–2038.

59. Moyer VA. Screening for lung cancer: U.S. Preventive Services Task Force recommendation statement. Annals of Internal Medicine 2014; 160: 330–338.

60. Markowitz S. Asbestos-related lung cancer and malignant mesothelioma of the pleura: Selected current issues. Seminars in Respiratory and Critical Care Medicine 2015; 36: 334–346.

61. Torre LA, Bray F, Siegel RL, et al. Global cancer statistics, 2012. CA: A cancer Journal for Clinicians 2015; 65: 87–108.

62. Ryerson AB, Eheman CR, Altekruse SF, et al. Annual report to the nation on the status of cancer, 1975-2012, featuring the increasing incidence of liver cancer. Cancer 2016; 122: 1312–1337.

63. Wild CP, Hall AJ. Primary prevention of hepatocellular carcinoma in developing countries. Mutation Research 2000; 462: 381–393.

64. Carter W, Connelly S, Struble K. Reinventing HCV treatment: Past and future perspectives. Journal of Clinical Pharmacology 2017; 57: 287–296.

65. Loharikar A, Dumolard L, Chu S, et al. Status of new vaccine introduction — worldwide, September 2016. Morbidity and Mortality Weekly Report 2016; 65: 1136–1140.

66. Prüss-Ustün A, Rapiti E, Hutin Y. Estimation of the global burden of disease attributable to contaminated sharps injuries among health-care workers. American Journal of Industrial Medicine 2005; 48: 482–490.

67. World Health Organization. Household air pollution and health (Fact sheet No. 292), Updated February 2016. Available at: http://www.who.int/mediacentre/factsheets/fs292/en/. Accessed July 7, 2017.

68. Bonjour S, Adair-Rohani H, Wolf J, et al. Solid fuel use for household cooking: Country and regional estimates for 1980–2010. Environmental Health Perspectives 2013; 121: 784–790.

69. Josyula S, Lin J, Xue X, et al. Household air pollution and cancers other than lung: A meta-analysis. Environmental Health 2015; 14: 24.

70. Schubauer-Berigan MK, Daniels RD, Pinkerton LE. Radon exposure and mortality among white and American Indian uranium miners: An update of the Colorado Plateau cohort. American Journal of Epidemiology 2009; 169: 718–730.

71. Darby S, Hill D, Deo H, et al. Residential radon and lung cancer—Detailed results of a collaborative analysis of individual data on 7148 persons with lung cancer and 14,208 persons without lung cancer from 13 epidemiologic studies in Europe. Scandinavian Journal of Work, Environment & Health 2006; 32: 1–83.

72. Lubin JH. Studies of radon and lung cancer in North America and China. Radiation Protection Dosimetry 2003; 104: 315–319.

73. Krewski D, Lubin JH, Zielinski JM, et al. A combined analysis of North American case-control studies of residential radon and lung cancer. Journal of Toxicology and Environmental Health, Part A 2006; 69: 533–597.

74. Committee on Health Risks of Exposure to Radon. Health effects of exposure to radon. BEIR VI. Washington, DC: National Academy Press, 1999.

75. Vineis P, Hoek G, Krzyzanowski M, et al. Lung cancers attributable to environmental tobacco smoke and air pollution in non-smokers in different European countries: A prospective study. Environmental Health 2007; 6: 7.

76. Yao T, Sung HY, Wang Y, et al. Sociodemographic differences among U.S. children and adults exposed to secondhand smoke at home: National Health Interview Surveys 2000 and 2010. Public Health Reports 2016; 131: 357–366.

77. King BA, Patel R, Babb SD, et al. National and state prevalence of smoke-free rules in homes with and without children and smokers: Two decades of progress. Preventive Medicine 2016; 82: 51–58.

78. Straif K, Baan R, Grosse Y, et al. Carcinogenicity of shift-work, painting, and fire-fighting. Lancet Oncology 2007; 8: 1065–1066.

79. Megdal SP, Kroenke CH, Laden F, et al. Night work and breast cancer risk: A systematic review and meta-analysis. European Journal of Cancer 2005; 41: 2023–2032.

80. He C, Anand ST, Ebell MH, et al. Circadian disrupting exposures and breast cancer risk: A meta-analysis. International Archives of Occupational and Environmental Health 2015; 88: 533–547.

81. Sigurdardottir LG, Valdimarsdottir UA, Fall K, et al. Circadian disruption, sleep loss, and prostate cancer risk: A systematic review of epidemiologic studies. Cancer Epidemiology, Biomarkers & Prevention 2012; 21: 1002–1011.

82. Carter BD, Diver WR, Hildebrand JS, et al. Circadian disruption and fatal ovarian cancer. American Journal of Preventive Medicine 2014; 46: S34–S41.

83. Bhatti P, Cushing-Haugen KL, Wicklund KG, et al. Nightshift work and risk of ovarian cancer. Occupational and Environmental Medicine 2013; 70: 231–237.

84. Stevens RG, Blask DE, Brainard GC, et al. Meeting report: The role of environmental lighting and circadian disruption in cancer and other diseases. Environmental Health Perspectives 2007; 115: 1357–1362.

85. Schulte P, Geraci C, Zumwalde R, et al. Sharpening the focus on occupational safety and health in nanotechnology. Scandinavian Journal of Work, Environment & Health 2008; 34: 471–478.

86. Schulte PA, Schubauer-Berigan MK, Mayweather C, et al. Issues in the development of epidemiologic studies of workers exposed to engineered nanoparticles. Journal of Occupational and Environmental Medicine 2009; 51: 323–335.

87. The Lancet Oncology. Space elevators, tennis racquets, and mesothelioma. Lancet Oncology 2008; 9: 601.

88. Schubauer-Berigan MK, Anderson JL, Hein MJ, et al. Breast cancer incidence in a cohort of U.S. flight attendants. American Journal of Industrial Medicine 2015; 58: 252–266.

89. Friesen MC, Costello S, Thurston SW, Eisen EA. Distinguishing the common components of oil- and water-based metalworking fluids for assessment of cancer incidence risk in autoworkers. American Journal of Industrial Medicine 2011; 54: 450–460.

FURTHER READING

National Toxicology Program. Report on carcinogens (14th edn.). Research Triangle Park, NC: Department of Health and Human Services, 2016.
Includes 248 listings of agents, substances, mixtures, and exposure circumstances that are known or reasonably anticipated to cause cancer in humans.

International Agency for Research on Cancer. IARC monographs on the evaluation of carcinogenic risks to humans. Lyon, France: IARC.
The IARC Monographs identify environmental factors that can increase the risk of human cancer. These include chemicals, complex mixtures, occupational exposures, physical agents, biological agents, and lifestyle factors. Evaluations are based on interdisciplinary working groups of expert scientists who review the published studies and evaluate the weight of evidence that an agent can increase the risk of cancer.

Rushton L. The global burden of occupational disease. Current Environmental Health Reports 2017; doi: 10.1007/s40572-017-0151-2.
An updated estimate of the global burden of occupational disease.

Stewart BW, Bray F, Forman D, et al. Cancer prevention as part of precision medicine: 'Plenty to be done'. Carcinogenesis 2016; 37: 2–9.
Recent review on multidisciplinary approaches for research on cancer prevention, and multisectoral involvement in developing and applying interventions to address the cancer burden.

22

Respiratory Disorders

Crystal M. North and David C. Christiani

CASE 1

A 60-year-old man, who had been a sand-blaster, was hospitalized for the third time in 4 months for shortness of breath. Three years before, he began having shortness of breath and a fast heart rate with moderate exertion. These symptoms increased over the next several months. He was evaluated by the company physician, who told him that he had "bad lungs" but gave him no treatment.

Two years before, his shortness of breath on exertion worsened, and he was hospitalized. Arterial blood gases were PaO_2 87 mm Hg and $PaCO_2$ 31 mm Hg on room air. A chest X-ray showed multiple interstitial nodules. Forced vital capacity (FVC) was 73% of predicted. Diffusing capacity was normal. Tuberculosis smear, culture, and cytology of bronchial washings were all negative. He was sent home without therapy and was told not to return to work. He has not worked since.

Seven months ago, he developed a cough, occasionally productive of thin, clear to grayish sputum, and then was admitted to the hospital three more times for increasing shortness of breath. Since the last hospitalization 1 month ago, he has been continuously dependent on oxygen and has remained in bed most of the time.

The patient had smoked one pack of cigarettes per day for 5 years, until quitting 20 years ago. He had no history of asthma, pneumonia, surgery, or allergies.

For 23 years, he operated a sandblasting machine in a basement room (20 by 40 feet). Dust escaped continuously through crevices of the sandblasting unit, and much dust escaped every time he opened the door of the unit to remove and install a piece to be blasted. The windows were closed. An exhaust fan in a wall did not seem to remove any dust. A room fan, installed to circulate the air in the room, often did not work. The patient wore a helmet with a cloth apron that covered his shoulders. When the air in the room was very dusty, he breathed from a tank of compressed air that he wore.

Physical examination revealed a thin man in moderate respiratory distress, sitting hunched over, gasping for breath, with grunting expirations. Pulse was 110, respiratory rate 40, blood pressure 110/80, and temperature 98°F. Lung and heart examinations were normal, except for a systolic ejection murmur and an increased second heart sound over the pulmonic valve area. He had clubbed fingernails and cyanosis. Arterial blood gases on room air revealed significant hypoxemia (PaO_2 39 mm Hg, $PaCO_2$ 38 mm Hg). A chest X-ray showed diffuse, interstitial, small, rounded densities throughout both lung fields and hilar fullness. These densities were judged to be "q"-sized with a 2/2 profusion in all lung fields, using the International Labour Organization (ILO) nomenclature for chest radiographs.[1] The diagnosis of silicosis was made. He remained completely disabled and died 3 months later.

This case is a severe case of pneumoconiosis, an occupational respiratory disease. Workplace exposure responsible for such chronic disabling lung disease occurs gradually over long periods. At first, exposures do not result in acute symptoms, but, once symptoms do appear, often little can be done beyond palliative treatment. Unless discovered very early in their course, most work-related respiratory diseases are not curable. Disease prevention is therefore critically important.

Occupational lung disease was observed in ancient times—in the writings of Hippocrates and in pictographs from Egypt. Some of these chronic diseases are still present. At this time, estimates of the prevalence and incidence of occupational respiratory disease suggest that only a small fraction of chronic occupational respiratory disease is correctly identified as associated with work.

Pneumoconioses and occupational asthma are work-related respiratory diseases that often are not correctly diagnosed. For example, approximately 8% of U.S. residents have physician-diagnosed asthma, but a much larger proportion of people *report* either asthma or wheezing, cough, or other symptoms of bronchial hyper-responsiveness. Physicians who see workers reporting wheezing should diagnose the problem and determine whether it is related to work.

EVALUATION OF INDIVIDUALS

Evaluations of pulmonary response to occupational and environmental exposures should include the following: (a) a complete history, including occupational and environmental exposures, tobacco use, and respiratory symptoms (Chapter 4); (b) a physical examination, with special attention to breath sounds; (c) a chest X-ray, with attention to parenchymal and

pleural opacities; and (d) pulmonary function tests.

History

Review of symptoms should include questions on chronic cough, chronic sputum production, shortness of breath (dyspnea), wheezing unrelated to respiratory infections, chest tightness, and chest pain. In occupational asthma and pulmonary edema, symptoms may peak 8 to 16 hours after exposure. Understanding symptom periodicity and timing is important. Respiratory symptoms during the workweek that improve on weekends or holidays strongly suggest an occupational disease. Recognizing the temporal relationships of symptoms with non-occupational exposures may be more difficult, since these exposures may be occurring daily in the home environment. Use of the American Thoracic Society (ATS) Respiratory Symptom Questionnaire[2] has been helpful in systematically obtaining information on respiratory symptoms, both for clinicians and epidemiologists.

Physical Examination

The most remarkable finding in most people with occupational and environmental respiratory disease is the relative absence of physical signs. However, auscultation can reveal important diagnostic clues. Fine rales may be heard at the lung bases, often at end-inspiration; they are more common in asbestosis than in other interstitial lung diseases. Hearing wheezes and understanding their temporal relationship to exposure may help in evaluating suspected cases of occupational and environmental asthma. A pleural rub may be heard as a result of a pleural reaction caused by exposure to asbestos. Clubbing of the digits, a nonspecific sign, may be seen rarely in advanced lung diseases, including asbestosis, bronchial carcinoma, and idiopathic pulmonary fibrosis. Signs of right ventricular heart failure, such as pedal edema, may indicate severe lung disease.

Chest X-ray

A chest X-ray should be taken when malignancy, pneumoconiosis, hypersensitivity pneumonitis, or most other lung disorders are suspected. For cases of occupational airways disease, such as work-related asthma (WRA), chest X-rays are rarely helpful. For suspected cases of pneumoconiosis, a trained "B reader" should interpret the X-ray, using the ILO system for pneumoconiosis (Table 22-1).[1] The ILO system permits semiquantitative interpretation of chest X-rays to identify early evidence and progression of parenchymal and pleural disease. It focuses on size, shape, concentration (profusion), and distribution of small parenchymal opacities as well as distribution and extent of pleural thickening or calcification. Rounded opacities in the upper lung fields are usually associated with silicosis, whereas linear (irregular) opacities in the lower lung fields are usually associated with asbestosis. Deviations from these patterns are common; for example, silicosis and coal workers' pneumoconiosis (CWP) can be associated with irregular

Table 22-1. Schematic of International Labour Organization Classification System for Chest X-Rays*

I. Size and Shape of Small Opacities

Rounded Opacities†		Irregular Opacities	
p	≤ 1.5 mm diameter	s	Fine linear opacities > 1.5 mm width
q	1.6–3.0 mm diameter	t	Medium opacities 1.6–3.0 mm width
r	3.1–10.0 mm diameter	u	Coarse, blotchy opacities 3.1–10.0 mm width

II. Concentration (Profusion) and Distribution

Small Opacities

Major Categories		Minor Divisions			Distribution‡	
0	Small opacities absent or less than category 1 Normal lung markings visible	0/–	0/0	0/1	RU RM	LU LM
1	Small opacities present but few Normal lung markings usually visible	1/0	1/1	1/2	RL	LL
2	Small opacities numerous Normal lung markings partially obscured	2/1	2/2	2/3		
3	Small opacities very numerous Normal lung markings totally obscured	3/2	3/3	3/+		

Large Opacities

A	One or more opacities with greatest summed diameter 1–5 cm
B	One or more opacities larger or more than Category A. Total area < equivalent of right upper zone
C	One or more opacities. Total area exceeds equivalent of right upper zone

III. Pleural Thickening§

Width		Extent		Calcification	
A	Maximum up to 5 mm	1	Up to 1/4 lateral wall	1	One or several regions summed diameter ≤ 2 cm
B	Maximum 5–10 mm	2	1/4–1/2 lateral wall	2	One or several regions summed diameter 2–10 cm
C	Maximum > 10 mm	3	Exceeds 1/2 lateral wall	3	One or several regions summed diameter > 10 cm

* In addition to these scores, the reader is guided in scoring technical quality of the X-ray (good, acceptable, poor, unacceptable) and in identifying other relevant features (such as bullae, cancer, abnormal cardiac size, emphysema, fractured rib, pneumothorax, tuberculosis).

† Size recorded by two letters to distinguish single type from mixed type. For example, q/q if only q opacities are present, but q/t if q opacities predominate but t are also present.

‡ Recorded by dividing lungs into three regions per side and checking all regions containing the designated small opacities.

§ Width estimated only if seen in profile. Extent estimated as maximum length of thickening (profile or face on). Calcification site (diaphragm, wall, other) and extent are noted separately for two sides.

opacities. In addition, workers exposed to mixed dusts, such as silica and asbestos, can present with mixed rounded and irregular opacities in any or all lung fields. The ILO system has the advantage of using a standardized set of comparison radiographic films, which can be used to classify X-rays at one point in time or to follow an individual or a population for change over time.

Although chest X-rays present evidence of abnormality, they do not provide information on disability or impairment and do not necessarily correlate well with pulmonary function test findings. A person with severe obstructive disease may show little evidence of it on a chest X-ray. In contrast, a person exposed chronically to iron oxide or tin oxide may show a dramatically abnormal chest X-ray but little if any pulmonary inflammatory reaction or lung function abnormality. Additionally, conventional chest X-rays may prove to be insensitive to subtle lung abnormalities. Although the ILO system was developed for epidemiologic studies and not for clinical evaluation of individuals, it may be an important facet to the posteroanterior chest X-ray interpretation by describing types of opacities and their distribution, both of which may be characteristic of a specific pneumoconiosis.

High-resolution computed tomography (HRCT) scanning has dramatically improved physicians' ability to detect and classify subtle lung diseases that are not seen, or only minimally visible, on conventional chest X-rays (Figure 22-1). While there is currently no standardized method for using computed tomography in classification of the pneumoconioses, the National

Institute for Occupational Safety and Health (NIOSH) has published federal regulations for the use of digital chest images in the evaluation of pneumconioses.[1]

Pulmonary Function Tests

Pulmonary function tests, required for medical surveillance by some Occupational Safety and Health Administration (OSHA) standards, are used commonly and are reliable, reproducible, and easy to perform. In a well-equipped pulmonary function laboratory, spirometry, lung volume determinations, gas exchange analyses, and exercise testing can be performed with relative ease. In a physician's office, only spirometry is readily and inexpensively performed; it does, however, provide much useful information. Most cases of respiratory disease yield abnormal test results or accelerated decline in pulmonary function within the "normal" ranges before onset of clinical symptoms, especially if individuals are followed at regular 1- to 3-year intervals. Although pulmonary function tests may demonstrate several patterns of abnormalities, one cannot rely on them alone to determine etiology. Hospital-based tests, such as lung volume determinations, gas exchange analyses, exercise tests, and bronchial challenge tests, can help in refining a diagnosis.

Basic tests of pulmonary function can be obtained with a simple portable spirometer. Test results are derived from the volume-time and flow-volume curves (Figure 22-2). Although several different measurements can be derived from the forced expiratory curve, the simplest and the most generally useful ones for evaluating occupational or environmental respiratory disease are (a) FVC, (b) forced expiratory volume in the first second of forced expiration (FEV_1), and (c) the ratio of FEV_1 to FVC. The peak expiratory flow rate (PEFor PEFR) is a measurement that is most useful when tested serially over time, such as throughout the workday or workweek. While PEF can be determined by spirometry, workers can also measure and record their own PEFs using a simple hand-held peak flow meter (see section on "Work-Related Asthma" later in this chapter). A simple scheme for the interpretation of spirometric measurements is shown in Table 22-2. Results are compared with predicted values

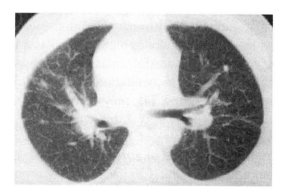

Figure 22-1. High-resolution computed tomograph of lungs of a man with silicosis.

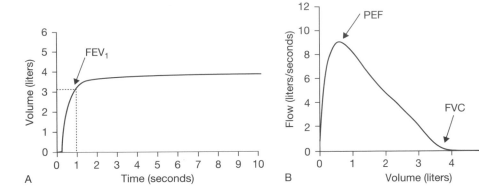

Figure 22-2. Normal spirogram. (A) Volume-time curve and (B) Flow-volume curve. FEV1, forced expiratory volume in the first second; FVC, forced vital capacity; PEF, peak expiratory flow. (Source: Adapted from Townsend MC. ACOEM position statement. Spirometry in the occupational setting. American College of Occupational and Environmental Medicine. Journal of Occupational and Environmental Medicine 2000; 42: 228–245.)

Table 22-2. Spirometry Interpretation

Type of Response	Percentage Predicted*			Response to Inhaled Bronchodilators
	FEV_1	FVC	FEV_1/FVC %	
Normal	≥80%	≥80%	≥70%	—
Obstructive	<80%	≥80%[†]	<70%	±
Restrictive	≥80%	<80%	≥70%	—
Mixed	<80%	<80%	<70%	±

Note. FEV_1 = forced expiratory volume in 1 second; FVC = forced vital capacity.
* Predicted FEV_1 and FVC based on Knudson RJ, Lebowitz MD, Holberg CJ, et al. Changes in the normal maximal expiratory flow volume curve with growth and aging. American Review of Respiratory Disease 1983; 127: 725.
[†] Severe obstruction can result in reduction of FVC also.

based on gender, ethnicity, age, and height, all of which have been derived from a population of asymptomatic, nonsmoking adults. Results are then expressed as a percent predicted of the expected value.

Criteria for the proper performance and evaluation of spirometry are based on ATS recommendations.[3–5] Many types of equipment are marketed to provide these tests, yet several have been inadequately standardized. The ATS guidelines on the standardization of spirometry include recommendations on instrument reliability and test performance.[3,4]

The pneumoconioses silicosis and asbestosis are considered *restrictive* diseases because they result in reduction in total lung capacity. In the absence of significant airways disease, flow rates are maintained and may even be above normal because of decreased lung compliance with increased elastic recoil. In contrast, CWP and occupational asthma are more often *obstructive* lung diseases, with decreased airflow and normal or increased lung volumes. In many lung diseases, when multiple environmental exposures (including tobacco smoke) have occurred, a *mixed restrictive-obstructive* pattern is frequently present. Some mineral dusts, such as asbestos and coal dust, alone can cause a mixed restrictive-obstructive pattern, because of damage to both the lung parenchyma and the airways.

EVALUATION OF GROUPS

It may not be until a group of individuals is evaluated that a respiratory disease can be associated with work or the ambient environment. For example, an occupational physician in Missouri recognized a group of eight workers in the community who had developed fixed obstructive lung disease after working at a microwave popcorn plant.[6] He reported this finding to the local health department, which led to an intensive investigation and recognition that bronchiolitis obliterans—now also colloquially known as *popcorn worker's lung disease*—can be caused by workplace exposures; this disorder is now a major focus in occupational medicine and the subject of a NIOSH initiative. (See the section on "Occupational Airways Disease.")

Comparisons with baselines should be performed whenever possible to permit evaluation of change over time in individuals or a group compared to a measured, rather than a predicted value. Decrements in lung function, development of respiratory symptoms, and recognition of chest X-ray abnormalities are often far more significant when internally compared to previous examinations rather than externally compared

to other individuals or groups. Any worker who may be exposed in the future to respiratory hazards at work should have a baseline pulmonary function test before potential exposure.

The major types of respiratory response to external agents are summarized in Tables 22-3 and 22-4. Occupational lung cancer is discussed in Chapter 21, and work-related infectious diseases of the respiratory tract are discussed in Chapter 13. Air pollution is discussed in Chapter 15.

ACUTE IRRITANT RESPONSES

Irritation in the upper respiratory tract is frequently associated with symptoms due to regional inflammation. Nasal and paranasal sinus irritation can cause congestion that may result in severe frontal headaches, nasal obstruction, runny nose, sneezing, and nosebleeds. Throat inflammation is commonly reported as a dry cough. Laryngeal inflammation can cause

Table 22-3. Major Types of Occupational Pulmonary Disease

Pathologic Function Process	Example of Disease or Exposure	Clinical History	Physical Examination	Chest X-ray	Pulmonary Function Pattern
Fibrosis	Silicosis	Dyspnea on exertion, cyanosis, shortness of breath	Clubbing	Nodules	Restrictive or mixed obstructive and restrictive
	Asbestosis	Dyspnea on exertion, cyanosis, shortness of breath	Clubbing, rales	Linear pleural plaques, calcifications	DLCO normal or decreased
Reversible airway obstruction (mucous plugging, asthma)	Byssinosis, isocyanate asthma, irritant asthma (RADS)	Cough, chest tightness, shortness of breath, asthma attacks	↑Respiratory rate, wheeze	Usually normal	Normal or obstructive with bronchodilator improvement Normal or high DLCO
Emphysema	Cadmium poisoning (chronic)	Cough, sputum, dyspnea	↑Respiratory rate, ↑ expiratory phase	Hyperaeration, bullae	Obstructive low DLCO
Granulomatous lung disease	Beryllium disease	Cough, weight loss, shortness of breath	↑Respiratory rate	Small nodules	Usually restrictive with low DLCO
Bronchiolitis obliterans	Flavoring or flavoring ingredients	Cough, chest tightness, shortness of breath, fixed airway obstruction	↑Respiratory rate, ↑ expiratory phase	Usually normal	Obstructive without bronchodilator improvement DLCO normal
Pulmonary edema	Smoke inhalation (firefighter or house fire victim)	Frothy, bloody sputum production	Coarse, bubbly rales	Diffuse air space opacity	Usually restrictive with decreased DLCO Hypoxemia at rest

Note. DLCO = diffusing capacity of the lung for carbon monoxide; RADS = reactive airways dysfunction syndrome.

Table 22-4. Common Environmental Pollutants with Respiratory Effects

Pollutant	Common Sources	Health Effects
Sulfur oxides	Coal and oil power plants Oil refineries, smelters Stoves burning wood, coal, kerosene Industrial chemical manufacture	Throat irritation Exacerbation of asthma, chronic bronchitis, and other respiratory illnesses with significant airflow obstruction
Particulates	Motor vehicle exhaust Fossil-fuel power plants Heavy construction Natural sources, such as volcanoes, bushfires, windblown dust, and oceans	Increased susceptibility to lung infections Exacerbation of asthma, chronic bronchitis, and other respiratory illnesses with significant airflow obstruction
Oxides of nitrogen	Motor vehicle exhaust Fossil-fuel power plants Oil refineries	Throat irritation Lung injury Exacerbation of asthma and COPD Increased susceptibility to lung infections
Ozone	Motor vehicle exhaust Ozone generators Aircraft cabins Power plants	Throat irritation Lung injury Exacerbation of asthma and COPD Increased susceptibility to lung infections
Carbon monoxide	Motor vehicle exhaust Fossil-fuel burning Kerosene space heaters Incinerators Industrial equipment	Hypoxia leading to heart and nervous system damage, death
Polycyclic aromatic hydrocarbons	Surface runoff from roads and land surfaces Sewage effluents Diesel exhaust Cigarette smoke Stove smoke	Lung cancer
Radon	Soil, rock, and groundwater	Lung cancer
Asbestos	Asbestos mines and mills Insulation Building materials	Mesothelioma Lung cancer Asbestosis
Arsenic	Copper smelters Cigarette smoke Pressure-treated wood Pesticides	Lung cancer

hoarseness and, if severe, may result in laryngeal spasms associated with glottal edema, severe anxiety, shortness of breath, and cyanosis.

In the lower airways, in contrast, acute symptoms are often due to bronchospasm. In asthma, there is also thickening of the basement membrane, mucosal edema and infiltration with inflammatory cells, mucus hypersecretion and plugging from proliferation of goblet cells, and increased presence of smooth muscle at preterminal bronchioles.

Occupational asthma is being recognized more frequently. Precipitating agents number over 300 and include industrial cleaning products, such as glutaraldehyde and bleach, soldering fluxes, and epoxy resins (Table 22-5). In addition, many irritant substances not usually associated with asthma can produce bronchial hyperreactivity when high levels of exposure have occurred. Single high-dose exposure to irritants such as ammonia or chlorine can result in nonspecific bronchial hyperreactivity, referred to as *reactive airways dysfunction syndrome (RADS)* or *irritant-induced asthma*, which may persist for months to years or may never fully resolve. It is not clear if chronic low-dose irritant exposures can also *cause* RADS or work-related asthma WRA, although irritants can *exacerbate* pre-existing RADS or asthma.

Pulmonary edema and pneumonitis can occur following acute irritation of the deep respiratory tract. Pulmonary edema occurs

Table 22-5. Selected Causes of Occupational Asthma*

Agents	Occupations
High–Molecular-Weight Compounds	
Animal products: dander, excreta, serum, secretions, fish glue	Animal handlers, laboratory workers, veterinarians, bookbinders, postal workers
Plants: grain, dust, flour, tobacco, tea, hops, latex, cotton, coffee beans	Grain handlers, tea workers, textile workers, bakers and workers in natural oil manufacturing and in tobacco, food processing, and healthcare workers
Enzymes: B. subtilis, pancreatic extracts, papain	Bakers and workers in the detergent, pharmaceutical, trypsin, fungal amylase, and plastic industries
Dyes: anthraquinone, carmine, paraphenyl diamine, henna extract	Fabric and fur dyers, beauticians
Other: crab, prawn	Crab and prawn processors
Low–Molecular-Weight Compounds	
Diisocyanates: toluene diisocyanate, methylene diphenyl diisocyanate	Polyurethane industry workers, roofers, insulators, painters, plastics workers, workers using varnish, and foundry workers
Anhydrides: phthallic and trimellitic anhydrates	Epoxy resin and plastics workers
Wood dust: oak, mahogany, California redwood, western red cedar	Carpenters, sawmill workers, and furniture makers
Metals: platinum, nickel, chromium, cobalt, vanadium, tungsten carbide	Platinum- and nickel-refining workers and hard-metal workers, platers, and welders
Soldering fluxes	Solderers
Drugs: penicillin, methyldopa, tetracyclines, cephalosporins, psyllium, organophosphates	Pharmaceutical and healthcare industry workers and farmworkers
Other organic chemicals: urea formaldehyde, dyes, formalin, azodicarbonamide, hexachlorophene, ethylene diamine, dimethyl ethanolamine, polyvinyl, chloride pyrolysates	Workers in chemical, plastic, and rubber industries; hospitals; laboratories; foam insulation, manufacture; food wrapping; and spray painting

* Mechanism believed to be immunoglobulin E–mediated for high-molecular-weight compounds and for some low-molecular-weight compounds. The immunologic mechanism for asthma from many low-molecular-weight substances remains undefined.

following extravasation of fluid and cells from the pulmonary capillary bed into the alveoli. Primary pulmonary edema is due to direct toxic action on the capillary walls. For example, exposure to ozone or oxides of nitrogen, common in industrial settings, can cause pulmonary edema. This response can be immediate, such as when a trapped worker cannot escape from a place of high exposure, or delayed, when exposure is lower. In contrast to pulmonary edema, pneumonitis is an inflammation of the lung parenchyma in which cellular infiltration rather than fluid extravasation predominates. It can be caused by exposure, such as to beryllium or cadmium.

Factors Involved in Toxicity

The most widespread causes of acute responses are irritant gases. Water is a major constituent of the respiratory tract lining, and solubility of these gases in water is the most significant factor influencing their site of action. Gases with high solubility act on the upper respiratory tract within *seconds*. For example, fatal epiglottic edema has been associated with irritants of high solubility, such as ammonia, hydrochloric acid, and hydrofluoric acid. In contrast, moderately soluble gases act on both the upper and lower respiratory tract within *minutes*. Chlorine gas, fluorine gas, and sulfur dioxide are irritants of this type, producing both upper respiratory irritation and bronchoconstriction. The low-solubility irritants, such as ozone, oxides of nitrogen, and phosgene, are most insidious. With few warning signs, they penetrate to the deep portions of the respiratory tract and act predominantly on the alveoli *6 to 24 hours* after exposure. Because of this considerable delay in onset of symptoms, individuals can be exposed to large amounts of these irritants without any warning symptoms.

Other factors influencing the site of action of an irritant gas are intensity and duration of exposure. The amount of exposure depends not only on air concentrations but also on work effort. A worker with a sedentary job exposed to a given concentration of a respiratory irritant receives a much lower dose than a worker with an active job requiring rapid breathing and a high minute ventilation (the product of tidal volume and respiratory rate).

A final element that influences the site of action is interaction, such as synergism or antagonism. Sulfur dioxide and water droplets are synergistic, combining to deliver a sulfuric acid–like vapor to the respiratory tract. Ammonia and sulfur dioxide, however, are antagonistic and together produce less response than either can individually. The presence of a carrier, such as an aerosol, may increase the effect of an irritant gas. For example, sulfur dioxide may cause a moderate effect and a sodium chloride aerosol no effect on the respiratory tract; however, concurrent respiratory exposure to both of these substances may result in a marked effect because the aerosol delivers the sulfur dioxide more deeply into the lung.

Highly Soluble Irritants

Primary examples of highly soluble irritants are (a) ammonia, used as a soil fertilizer and in the manufacture of dyes, chemicals, plastics, and explosives; in tanning leather; and as a household cleaner; (b) hydrochloric acid (hydrogen chloride), used in chemical manufacturing, electroplating, and metal pickling; and (c) hydrofluoric acid (hydrogen fluoride), used predominantly for etching and polishing of glass, as a chemical catalyst in the manufacture of plastics, as an insecticide, and for removal of sand from metal castings in foundry operations.

The primary physical effects of highly water-soluble irritants are first perception of their odors and then irritation of the eyes, the nose, and sometimes the throat. In high doses, the respiratory rate can increase and bronchospasm can occur. Lower respiratory tract effects, however, do not occur unless the person is severely overexposed or trapped in an environment. The irritant effects are powerful and usually provide adequate warning to prevent overexposure of people free to escape from exposure. The history and physical examination are the most important parts of evaluating people exposed to irritants. Pulmonary function tests may show

significant airflow limitation, reflecting bronchospasm shortly after exposure. Chest X-rays are not helpful unless there is pulmonary edema.

Management of reactions to these irritants is immediate removal of the worker and, if breathing is labored or hypoxemia is present, administration of oxygen. If severe exposure or loss of consciousness occurs, observation in a hospital for development of pulmonary edema is advisable.

Prevention of exposures relies on proper industrial hygiene practices with local exhaust ventilation as an essential component. Respirators should be used only as a temporary control measure in an emergency. If respirators are required to prevent overexposure, workers must be trained in their proper use and maintenance.

CASE 2

A 25-year-old man came to the emergency room with acid burns. Before taking a job as an electroplater 5 weeks before, he was in perfect health. On the first day at this job, he developed itching. He then developed sores, which healed with scars, at sites of splashes of workplace chemicals. After 4 days on this job, he developed a runny nose, throat irritation, and a productive cough. He also noted some shortness of breath at work.

His work involved dipping metal parts into tanks containing chrome solutions and acid. He wore a paper mask (disposable respirator), rubber gloves, and an apron but no eye protection. Although heavy fumes were present in the $60 \times 20 \times 14$-foot room, there was no ventilation. None of the other eight workers in the room seemed to have similar medical problems.

Past history revealed three prior hospitalizations for pneumonia but not asthma or allergies. He smoked about four cigarettes a day.

From age 16 to 18, he worked as a sheet metal punch-press operator for a tool and dye company. At age 18, he worked as a drip-pan cleaner for a soup company. From age 19 to 21, he was a student in an auto mechanic school. From age 21 to 24, he occasionally worked as a gas station attendant.

Physical examination was normal, except for multiple areas of round, irregularly shaped, depigmented, 1 mm atrophic scars on both forearms and exposed areas of the anterior thorax and face; a 4 mm, rounded, punched-out ulcer, with a thickened, indurated, undermined border and an erythematous base on his left cheek; an erythematous pharynx; and bilateral conjunctivitis. His nasal septum was not perforated. Patch tests with dichromate, nickel, and cobalt were all negative. A chest X-ray was normal.

He was diagnosed with irritation and inflammation of the upper respiratory tract and an irritant contact dermatitis, both due to chromic acid mist. His symptoms resolved with removal from exposure. Periodic medical monitoring was advised to provide early diagnosis of a possible cancer of the nasal sinuses, for which he may be at increased risk because of his chromium exposure. Finally, a follow-up industrial hygiene survey of the workplace was initiated to control exposures for the other exposed workers.

Many small electroplating firms have no local ventilation over open vats of chromic and other acids. Frequently, a high level of chrome or other metals in the fumes is liberated when metal parts are immersed for plating. Chrome and chromic acid mist are local irritants. Primarily in hexavalent forms, chromium is considered to be a carcinogen; epidemiologic studies have shown an elevated lung cancer risk among exposed workers.[7] (See Chapter 21.)

Moderately Soluble Irritants

The moderately soluble irritants include chlorine, fluorine, and sulfur dioxide. Chlorine is widely used in the chemical industry to synthesize various chlorinated hydrocarbons, whereas outside the chemical industry its major use is in water purification and as a bleach in the paper industry. Fluorine is used in the conversion of uranium tetrafluoride to uranium hexafluoride, in the development of fluorocarbons, and as an oxidizing agent. Fluoride is used in the electrolytic manufacture of aluminum, as a flux in smelting operations, in coatings of welding rods, and as an additive to drinking water. Sulfur dioxide is commonly used as a disinfectant, a fumigant, and a bleach for wood pulp, and it is formed as a by-product of coal burning, smelter processes, and the paper industry. Sulfur dioxide is a colorless, highly water-soluble gas, and hence it affects mostly the upper respiratory tract and has limited deposition in the lower airways. However,

during exercise, the resultant increased minute ventilation may result in greater lower airway deposition than what would be usually expected. When sulfur dioxide is released into the atmosphere, it combines with water, metals, and other pollutants to form aerosols, most importantly sulfuric acid, metallic acids, and ammonium sulfates. These aerosols induce asthmatic responses.

Particulate air pollution, consisting of particles suspended in the air after various forms of combustion or other industrial activity, increases morbidity and mortality.[8] In contrast to particles greater than 10 μm in diameter, particles less than 2.5 μm in aerodynamic diameter ($PM_{2.5}$) are carried deep into the lungs and are more likely to be deposited in the lower airways.

These irritants, like the highly soluble ones, initially cause irritation of mucous membranes, often manifested by persistent cough. Acute symptoms are usually of short duration. Low levels of continuous exposures, which are better tolerated than exposures to highly soluble irritants, can nevertheless cause decreased pulmonary function.[9]

In addition, these irritants can lead to other health problems. Chlorine gas can corrode teeth, and fluorine can cause chemical skin burns. Chronic exposure to fluoride is associated with increased bone density, cartilage calcification, discoloration of teeth in children, and possibly rheumatologic syndromes, such as seronegative arthritis. (However, fluoride applied topically or added to water supplies has been demonstrated to reduce dental caries in children.) Sulfur dioxide exposure can cause bronchospasm, especially in people with asthma, and may eventually contribute to chronic obstructive pulmonary disease. Management and prevention are similar to that for disorders due to highly soluble irritants. Pulmonary function tests, especially spirometry, are recommended in surveillance programs for individuals with chronic exposure.

Low-Solubility Irritants

Usually, the effects of irritants with low solubility are mild throat irritation and occasional headache. Much more significant is pulmonary edema, which manifests 6 to 24 hours after exposure, preceded by symptoms of bronchospasm, such as chest tightness and wheezing

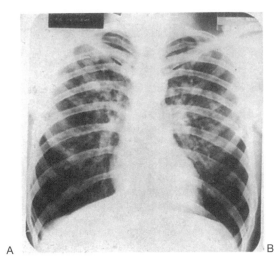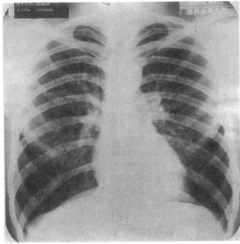

A   B

Figure 22-3. Chest X-rays in a copper minerL (A) 24 hours after overexposure to oxides of nitrogen, pulmonary edema is evident. (B) One week after exposure, there is resolution of pulmonary edema. (Courtesy of the late Benjamin G. Ferris, M.D., Harvard School of Public Health, Boston, Massachusetts.)

(Figure 22-3). Although management and prevention are similar to those for highly soluble irritants, overnight observation of patients is frequently necessary, when excess exposure has occurred, because of the insidious onset of pulmonary edema.

Two of the most commonly produced industrial and urban pollutants are ozone and oxides of nitrogen, which are usually produced by the action of sunlight on the waste products of the internal combustion engine. Both are present in welding fumes and therefore are found in many work environments. Ozone is used as a disinfectant; as a bleach in the food, textile, and pulp and paper industries; and as an oxidizing agent. Oxides of nitrogen are used in chemical and fertilizer manufacture and in metal processing and cleaning operations.

Of great concern are unburned hydrocarbons and nitrogen dioxide, which are the main constituents of smog, commonly seen in Los Angeles, Mexico City, Bangkok, and other large cities. Levels are usually lowest in the morning, are highest at midday, and taper off after sunset. Higher levels are found in the summer, when sunlight is more intense and temperatures are higher. (See Chapter 15.)

Ozone and oxides of nitrogen are relatively insoluble in water and therefore reach deeper into the respiratory tract as compared with sulfur dioxide and other gases. Chronic exposure to oxides of nitrogen may result in bronchiolitis obliterans, an obstructive deficit on spirometry, and a chest X-ray with evidence of pulmonary edema and bilateral patchy airspace opacities.

Silo filler's disease results from exposures to oxides of nitrogen in the upper chambers of grain silos due to anaerobic fermentation of green silage. Its brownish color is an important warning sign for farmers. Acute overexposure and death have resulted from inadequately ventilated silos.

Exposure to ozone levels, even below the U.S. National Ambient Air Quality Standard of 70 ppb for 8 hours, has resulted in symptoms and decreases in peak expiratory flow. These exposure levels are lower than in Los Angeles and the northeastern part of the United States.

The Environmental Protection Agency (EPA) has developed the Air Quality Index (AQI), which gives a numeric score (0 to 500) for air quality on a given day. The AQI considers five major pollutants: ozone, sulfur dioxide, nitrogen dioxide, carbon monoxide, and particulate pollution. An AQI is calculated for each; the reported AQI is the highest of these five scores. Values between 101 and 150 have been designated "unhealthy for sensitive groups." The EPA defines "sensitive groups" as persons with heart or lung disease, older adults, and children. People who are active outdoors may also be sensitive to ozone. On days with high AQIs, those who are in sensitive groups are advised to stay indoors, close car windows, and use air conditioning to protect against exposure and adverse effects of ozone and other pollutants. AQIs above 150 are considered "unhealthy" for the general public, and those above 300 are considered "hazardous." More information on ambient ozone and on air quality standards can be found at http://www.airnow.gov.

NONIRRITANT EXPOSURES

Carbon Monoxide

Carbon monoxide is emitted mainly from internal combustion engines used in motor vehicles. Other causes of exposure include incomplete combustion of coal, paper, wood, oil, gas, or any other carbonaceous material. Carbon monoxide adversely affects blood oxygenation. The affinity of carbon monoxide for hemoglobin is about 200 times more than the affinity of oxygen for hemoglobin, thus severely reducing the ability of the blood to transport oxygen. Carbon monoxide can cause severe hypoxia, resulting in fatal neurological and cardiac consequences, and chronic exposure has been shown to be associated with increased hospitalizations in people with pre-existing lung disease.[10] (See Chapters 11, 23, and 26.)

AIR POLLUTION

Indoor Air Pollution

The World Health Organization estimates that 4.3 million die annually due to indoor air pollution, with women and children dying at higher rates than men. Indoor air pollution is widespread in low- and middle-income countries (LMICs) because of burning biomass fuels indoors for cooking and heating. Biomass fuels, which include crop residues, charcoal, firewood, and animal dung, are inexpensive but highly polluting materials that are frequently used by poor people living in rural areas. Concentrations

of particulate matter, carbon monoxide, and air pollutants from burning biomass are often orders of magnitude higher than levels in international health standards. For example, the EPA 8-hour time-weighted average standard for carbon monoxide exposure is 9 ppm, compared to a mean 24-hour carbon monoxide concentration of 500 ppm in homes where biomass is used for cooking.[11] Indoor air pollution is associated with increased risks for malignancies, lung disease, cardiovascular disease, cerebrovascular disease, cataracts, adverse pregnancy outcomes, and respiratory illness in young children.[12]

Residents of high-income countries are also exposed to high levels of indoor pollution, usually due to tight building construction and use of building materials and furnishings that emit high levels of volatile organic compounds. Indoor air pollution in homes and non-factory public buildings, such as office buildings, schools, and hospitals, can cause mucous-membrane irritation, pulmonary and cardiovascular disorders, and death.

Outdoor Air Pollution

Outdoor air pollution, which has contributed to pulmonary disease since the first use of coal in the 14th century, substantially increased during the Industrial Revolution in the 1800s in high-income countries. In contrast, LMICs are now experiencing substantially increasing levels of outdoor air pollution, due largely to automobiles and inadequate regulations.

Outdoor air pollution is associated with increased mortality, as determined by many prospective studies since the early 1990s.[13,14] A recent study, for example, found associations between mortality and chronic exposure to both ozone and $PM_{2.5}$, with ozone contributing specifically to mortality from respiratory disease.[15] (See Chapter 15.) Acute and chronic morbidity and mortality have occurred during and after the serious pollution episodes in Donora, Pennsylvania, in 1948; in London in 1952; and during and after the World Trade Center attack in New York in 2001.

The public health impact of air pollution on children has been substantial.[16] Both outdoor and indoor air pollution increases (a) the incidence of acute respiratory hospital admissions in children, (b) school absences, and (c) medication use in children with asthma, and it decreases peak flow rates in otherwise normal children.

CHILDHOOD ASTHMA

Asthma, a leading cause of chronic childhood illness, is a major cause of childhood disability and lost days from school.[17-19] In the United States, an estimated 6.5 million children have active asthma at any given time, and 9 million children have been diagnosed with asthma at some point in their childhood. About 3% of ambulatory visits and emergency-department visits by children are for asthma.

Childhood asthma prevalence in the United States more than doubled between 1980 and the mid-1990s. Although overall prevalence appears to have plateaued since 1999, overall healthcare utilization for asthma has continued to increase, and asthma-related mortality remains elevated in certain ethnic groups.

There are well-documented racial disparities in childhood asthma prevalence and severity in the United States. African-American, Native-American, and Puerto Rican and other Hispanic children have a higher prevalence of asthma than Caucasian children. Emergency-department visits, hospitalizations, and deaths due to asthma are much more frequent among African-American children than among any other group of children; African-American children die from asthma at six times the rate of Caucasian children. Rates of ambulatory-care visits by African-American children are lower than those for children of other racial groups.

Some of these disparities arise from differences in environmental risk factors. Early exposure to some allergens may increase risk of asthma. However, early exposure to animal dander, such as among children living on farms, may decrease risk of asthma. Exposure of inner-city children to dust mites and cockroach antigen appears to increase the risk of developing asthma.[20] History of severe viral respiratory illness, especially with respiratory syncytial virus (RSV), is another risk factor. However, asthmatic children seem to be predisposed to severe viral respiratory illnesses, so RSV may be unmasking pre-existing disease.

Environmental tobacco smoke and both outdoor and indoor air pollution exacerbate, and may also possibly cause, childhood asthma. High prenatal exposure to nitrous oxide, carbon monoxide, and PM_{10} is associated with decreased pulmonary function in newborns. Higher childhood exposure to nitrous oxide, carbon monoxide, ozone, and particulate matter is associated with similar adverse effects.[21,22] Concentrations of sulfur dioxide are associated with infant mortality.[23]

Genetic or other mechanisms may also contribute to asthma risk. Atopy is a risk factor for asthma; some children have eczema or allergic rhinitis before they develop asthma. Atopy tends to be inherited; family history of atopy and/or asthma has also been used in predicting a child's risk of asthma.

The clinical course of childhood asthma varies. Some children have resolution of lung function abnormalities without recurrence in adulthood; others have persistent asthma without remission. Atopy and a low FEV_1/FVC ratio at age 18 may be independent predictors of relapse.[24] Severe or inadequately treated asthma in childhood can result in lifelong impairment in lung function, primarily due to airway damage. Inadequately treated asthma leads to persistent airways inflammation. Over time, persistent airways inflammation results in structural changes, including increased mass of smooth muscle and enlargement of mucous glands, which together lead to luminal narrowing and fixed obstruction, which is not responsive to inhaled medications. Therefore, asthma exacerbated by work exposures may sometimes be partially attributed to asthma during childhood. (See Chapter 30.)

In caring for adults and children with asthma, one should take a complete occupational and environmental history in order to identify and then reduce exposures that trigger or exacerbate symptoms (Chapter 4). Questions should focus on type of housing, presence of smokers in the household, infestations with insects or rodents, mold or musty odors, visible water damage, pets, and other family members affected with asthma. Educating parents on how to reduce their children's exposures to allergens can help improve prognosis. Nongovernmental organizations and government agencies offer free educational materials for caregivers and others.[25]

OCCUPATIONAL AIRWAYS DISEASE

CASE 3

An 18-year-old woman, with an 8-week history of wheezing, a productive cough, and shortness of breath and a 1-day history of cyanosis of her fingertips, presents to an emergency department. She had begun working at a tool supply and manufacturing company 9 weeks before—1 week before her symptoms began. Her usual job was grinding carbide-steel drill bits. Part of her work involved sharpening drill bits on a machine that generated copious metal dust, often covering the machine and her face, hands, and clothes. There was no exhaust ventilation, and no respiratory protection was provided.

After her respiratory symptoms began 8 weeks before, she was temporarily assigned to cleaning drill bits in a solvent bath. On this job, she felt lightheaded but had no difficulty breathing. After a long holiday weekend, she was again assigned to drill-bit grinding and, after several hours, developed a cough. The next day, the cough worsened and she experienced shortness of breath, prompting a second visit to her physician. When she improved from that episode, she returned to work again and experienced exacerbation of coughing and shortness of breath, prompting her emergency-department visit.

Past medical history revealed childhood seasonal rhinitis but no asthma, eczema, or other allergies. There was no family history of allergies or asthma.

Physical examination revealed a pulse rate of 128 and a respiratory rate of 40. She had cyanosis of the lips and fingertips. Chest examination revealed diffuse bilateral wheezes and use of accessory muscles for breathing.

Arterial blood gases on room air at rest revealed a markedly low PaO_2 (39 mm Hg). Spirometry revealed a normal FVC but a markedly abnormal FEV_1 (53% of predicted). A chest X-ray was normal. White blood cell count was elevated at 11,200 cells/mm^3, with increased eosinophils (10%). She was treated with oxygen, bronchodilators, and steroids. She improved clinically and by the second day her FEV_1 had improved to 82% of predicted.

Her physician learned from the state occupational safety and health agency that carbide-steel bit alloys contain nickel, cobalt, chromium, vanadium, molybdenum, and tungsten and that grinding these bits can produce cobalt and tungsten carbide dusts, which can cause pulmonary sensitization.

The diagnosis in this case was occupational asthma. No specific agent was confirmed to be responsible, but the presence of tungsten carbide and cobalt dusts indicated that they probably caused her asthma. Since changing jobs, she has felt well and has not had further bronchospasm.

Work-Related Asthma

More than 25 million Americans have physician-diagnosed asthma.[19] Globally, an estimated 330 million people have asthma. Between 9% and 15% of new-onset adult asthma in industrialized countries is attributable to occupational factors.[26,27] *Work-related* asthma (WRA), which is induced by inhalation exposure in the workplace, is the most frequently diagnosed occupational lung disease in industrialized countries, including the United States.[28] Work-related asthma includes asthma developing de novo in the workplace (*occupational asthma*) as well as pre-existing asthma that is triggered or exacerbated by workplace exposures (*work-exacerbated asthma*).[29] Work-exacerbated asthma affects about 20% of persons with pre-existing asthma.[30]

A wide variety of materials and circumstances can cause occupational asthma (Table 22-5). In addition to occupational exposures, asthma can be triggered in the workplace by exertion, cold air, tobacco smoke, and other factors. All people with asthma are at risk for work-exacerbated asthma, which can be induced by chemical, physical, or biologic factors.

Immunologic WRA, the most frequent form of WRA, accounts for more than 90% of cases. Primary causative agents are high-molecular-weight (HMW) compounds, usually proteins of animal or vegetable origin. Most HMW compounds result in an immunoglobulin E (IgE)-mediated reaction, the typical allergic or atopic immune response. Common examples of HMW triggers include latex and animal dander. Immunologic WRA can also be triggered by low-molecular-weight (LMW) compounds. Some LMW compounds (such as diisocyanates and platinum) act through an IgE-mediated mechanism, but most LMW compounds (such as glutaraldehyde) act through non-IgE-mediated mechanisms. There is always a latency period between exposure and development of immunologic WRA as the immune system becomes primed. Latency periods among compounds vary widely, from hours to months or longer. Once a worker is sensitized, the exposure needed to produce symptoms typically becomes increasingly smaller. Atopy is a risk factor for immunologic WRA caused by HMW compounds. However, atopy is not a good predictor of sensitization.[31]

Nonimmunologic WRA accounts for less than 10% of WRA cases. It differs from immunologic WRA in that no immune sensitization occurs, and therefore no latency period is necessary. Nonimmunologic WRA may occur after a single high-level exposure to a workplace irritant, such as hydrochloric acid or other acids and chlorine bleach or other bases. Some compounds that can cause sensitization are also irritants at certain concentrations. For example, glutaraldehyde may cause immunologic WRA in some workers and a nonimmunologic irritant response in others. Many irritants also cause skin reactions, which, in turn, can increase the risk for immunologic WRA. Many workers are exposed to both irritants and sensitizers; if an irritant causes skin breakdown, a worker may have increased exposure to a sensitizer through areas of open skin. (See Chapter 25.)

A diagnosis of WRA should be considered in all workers with new-onset asthma and those with previously quiescent or well-controlled asthma who experience increased symptoms of asthma. Diagnosis of occupational asthma depends greatly on the occupational history and the symptom history, which is more sensitive than specific. Workers report wheezing, chest tightness, shortness of breath, or cough as typical symptoms, although nasal and sinus symptoms may also occur. Symptoms may develop during the workday and improve in the evening away from work. Symptoms may also worsen throughout the workweek and improve over weekends or vacations. Some responses are delayed, however, and workers may report symptoms primarily at night or on weekends, with fewer symptoms at work. If exposure has

been prolonged, symptoms may be persistent, losing any temporal pattern with work. In addition, removal from exposure does not always lead to complete recovery. One meta-analysis estimated that only 32% of workers have complete symptomatic recovery after cessation of exposure to the causative agent.[32] This meta-analysis also found that older age and a longer period of symptomatic exposure were negative prognostic indicators for recovery.

A high suspicion for WRA should prompt a thorough exposure history, including exposures at previous jobs. Making a diagnosis of WRA can be challenging. The American College of Chest Physicians (ACCP) has published recent guidelines on diagnosis and management of WRA, including a useful flowsheet for clinical evaluation.[27] Diagnostic workup begins with confirming asthma using pre- and post-bronchodilator spirometry testing or by methacholine challenge testing if spirometry is normal. Once asthma is confirmed, a relationship to work, and ideally to a specific workplace exposure, should be sought. Establishing a relationship of asthma to work can include serial measurements of PEFR throughout the day using a hand-held flow meter. For example, a worker can measure PEFR four times daily (on both workdays and other days) for 2 weeks, which may help establish a clear pattern. Alternatively, workers can have office-based spirometry performed on them before and after work shifts in a company-based or other occupational medicine clinic. A decrease of at least 300 mL, or 10%, of the FEV_1 (measured as the mean of the two best of three acceptable results each time) between the beginning and end of the first shift of the workweek suggests a work-related effect.

To establish a relationship with a specific exposure, blood tests (such as IgE specific to the suspected exposure) or skin-prick testing using the suspected substance can be helpful. Unfortunately, such testing is not available for most exposures, and positive serum or skin testing does not diagnose WRA due to that exposure—it only establishes sensitization to an exposure. Many more workers are sensitized than have symptoms or disease. However, the ACCP recommends that such additional testing be done whenever available because the more positive findings that can be established, including work-related symptoms or positive methacholine challenge, the more certain the relationship to work becomes.[27]

Although it is done elsewhere in the world, specific inhalation challenge testing is not typically available in the United States because of risk of anaphylaxis or other serious reactions. In a specific challenge test, the suspected exposure (instead of methacholine) is inhaled to provoke bronchospasm.

Acute care for those with attacks of WRA is the same as for any other cases of asthma. Long-term management, however, almost always requires removal from exposure, which is especially critical in immunologic WRA since even very low levels of exposure can trigger symptoms in a sensitized worker. Pharmacologic management of chronic disease is also similar to that of asthma not related to work. Close monitoring of symptoms and lung function should be maintained for a person who must continue exposure to a suspected offending agent.

Finally, when a diagnosis of WRA cannot be established, other related conditions need to be considered, including vocal cord dysfunction, eosinophilic bronchitis, upper respiratory tract irritation, hypersensitivity pneumonitis, and psychogenic factors. However, asthma (including WRA) can coexist with these other conditions.

Occupational Chronic Obstructive Pulmonary Disease

Occupational exposures may be a much more important contributor to the development of chronic obstructive pulmonary disease (COPD) than previously recognized. Up to 15% of cases of COPD can be attributed to occupational exposures to various vapors, gases, dusts, and fumes. Some workplace factors may even double the risk of COPD.[33]

Chronic bronchitis is probably the most frequent chronic respiratory response to external agents. A clinical diagnosis must satisfy the following ATS criteria: a recurrent productive cough occurring 4 to 6 times a day at least 4 days of the week, for at least 3 months during the year and at least 2 consecutive years. In contrast, *simple bronchitis* is defined as the production of phlegm on most days for as much

as 3 months of the year. The excess mucus production associated with bronchitis often causes airflow obstruction. Chronic bronchitis is frequently superimposed on other respiratory diseases due to cigarette smoke and/or occupational hazards, including mineral dusts and fumes (such as from coal, fibrous glass, asbestos, metals, and oils); organic dusts (such as from cotton and grains); irritants (such as ozone and oxides of nitrogen); plastic compounds (such as phenolics and isocyanates); acids; and smoke (such as from fires).

Flavorings-Related Lung Disease

In 2000, an occupational physician reported eight cases of bronchiolitis obliterans in former workers of a Missouri microwave popcorn plant.[6] Four of these individuals were awaiting lung transplantation. NIOSH conducted medical and environmental examinations that identified diacetyl (2,3-butanedione), a chemical used in butter flavoring, as the responsible agent.[34] Additional affected workers were identified at the plant and in California,[6] the United Kingdom, and elsewhere. Since some affected workers had been employed by plants that made artificial flavoring, NIOSH named this clinical entity *flavorings-related lung disease*—also known as *flavorings-related bronchiolitis obliterans* and *popcorn worker's lung disease.*[35] Diacetyl is also found in other flavorings, including coffee flavoring[36] and many e-cigarette flavorings.[37] E-cigarette use is increasing, especially among young people. Based on the research previously in this chapter, people who smoke e-cigarettes with diacetyl-based flavorings are at increased risk for flavorings-related lung disease.

Symptoms include nonproductive cough, wheezing, dyspnea on exertion, and occasionally fever, night sweats, and weight loss. Symptoms generally develop and worsen gradually. Periods away from work generally do not improve symptoms.

Diagnostic evaluation includes an occupational history, with a focus on diacetyl exposure if flavorings-related lung disease is suspected. Spirometry usually reveals fixed obstruction (a reduction in both FEV_1 and FEV_1/FVC that do not reverse with bronchodilator administration). Lung volume testing may show hyperinflation, since air-trapping is a key feature of bronchiolitis obliterans. Unlike emphysema or various causes of interstitial lung disease, the diffusing capacity is usually normal. Imaging tends to be normal, or it shows only hyperinflation or air-trapping. High-resolution computer tomography sometimes reveals thickened airway walls. Most cases recognized thus far have not responded to medical treatment. More information on this disease can be found on the NIOSH website.[38]

HYPERSENSITIVITY PNEUMONITIS

Hypersensitivity pneumonitis (HP), previously known as extrinsic allergic alveolitis, refers to reactions associated with the most illustrative of all occupational disease names (Table 22-6). Hypersensitivity pneumonitis results from an immunologic response to inhaled antigens from organic or LMW compounds, commonly fungi or thermophilic bacteria that are present in a surprisingly wide variety of settings. Generally, these antigens are less than 3 μm in diameter, enabling them to deposit deep in the terminal bronchioles and alveoli, where the reaction occurs. These antigens are then cleared via lymphatic channels that drain into the hilar lymph nodes, inducing the immunologic response,

which is mediated by immunoglobulin G. The immune response is also characterized by complement activation and stimulation of alveolar macrophages. Repeated exposure to the antigen can lead to fibrosis. Once hypersensitivity is established, small doses of antigen may trigger episodes of alveolitis.[39]

A worker with HP typically has shortness of breath and a nonproductive cough but little or no wheezing. In acute episodes, sudden onset of respiratory symptoms, fever, and chills is dramatic. Physical examination may reveal rapid breathing, fine basilar rales, and hypoxemia. Pulmonary function tests may show marked reduction in lung volumes consistent with restrictive disease. Arterial blood gas measurements generally show an increased alveolar–arterial oxygen difference and a reduced diffusing capacity. Other diagnostic testing for HP may include measuring specific antibodies (precipitins) in serum, which are highly sensitive but not specific, and demonstrating a serum antibody response, which alone is not itself diagnostic. A conventional chest X-ray and HRCT can be helpful in acute episodes by revealing patchy infiltrates or a diffuse, fine micronodular shadowing. Radiographic findings are often evanescent, however, and are therefore easily missed in acute episodes. Bronchoalveolar lavage fluid

Table 22-6. Examples of Hypersensitivity Pneumonitis

Disease	Antigenic Material	Antigen
Farmer's lung	Moldy hay or grain	
Bagassosis	Moldy sugar cane	Thermophilic actinomycetes
Mushroom worker's lung	Mushroom compost	
Humidifier fever	Dust from contaminated air conditioners or furnaces	
Maple bark disease	Moldy maple bark	*Cryptostroma* species
Sequoiosis	Redwood dust	*Graphium* species, Pallurlaria
Bird fancier's lung	Avian droppings or feathers	Avian proteins
Pituitary snuff taker's lung	Pituitary powder	Bovine or porcine proteins
Suberosis	Moldy cork dust	*Penicillium* species
Paprika splitter's lung	Paprika dust	*Mucor stolonifer*
Malt worker's lung	Malt dust	*Aspergillus clavatus* or *Aspergillus fumigatus*
Fishmeal worker's lung	Fishmeal	Fishmeal dust
Miller's lung	Infested wheat flour	*Sitophilus granarius* (wheat weevil)
Stipatosis	Esparto fibers	*Aspergillus fumigatus*
Metalworking fluid–associated hypersensitivity pneumonitis	Metalworking fluid (coolants)	*Mycobacterium chelonae* *Pseudomonas nitroreducens*
Furrier's lung	Animal pelts	Animal fur dust
Coffee worker's lung	Coffee beans	Coffee bean dust
Chemical worker's lung	Urethane foam and finish	Isocyanates (such as toluene diisocyanate), anhydrides

may show lymphocytosis with a predominance of CD8 T cells. Biopsies generally reveal poorly formed granulomata and nonspecific findings, such as bronchiolitis, lymphocyte infiltration, foamy macrophages, and areas of fibrosis.

If the worker is removed from exposure, symptoms and signs usually disappear in 1 to 2 weeks. In severe cases, corticosteroid treatment is required. If repeated exposures occur, especially at relatively low levels that cause only mild symptoms, a more chronic disease may develop. The worker may be unaware of the association of symptoms with work exposure because symptoms can be similar to a persistent or intermittent case of the flu. Over a period of months, however, there is usually gradual onset of dyspnea, which can be accompanied by weight loss and lethargy. Physical examination findings are similar to those in the acute reaction, although the individual may appear less acutely ill and may demonstrate finger clubbing. The chest X-ray, however, is more suggestive of chronic interstitial fibrosis and pulmonary function tests show a restrictive defect. The disease may progress to severe dyspnea, and the end result can resemble idiopathic pulmonary fibrosis (IPF), both clinically and histologically. The risk of fibrosis may partly depend on host factors, including genetic markers. Familial forms of HP tend to present at younger ages than nonfamilial forms and may phenotypically appear similar to IPF.[40]

Prevention rests on removal from exposure. This can be more readily accomplished than with asthma because environmental controls can focus on the elimination of conditions that foster bacterial or fungal growth. Process changes may also be necessary to prevent antigen production, and local exhaust ventilation, rather than, or in conjunction with, personal protective equipment (masks) should be used.

Hypersensitivity Pneumonitis Associated with Metalworking Fluids

Cases of HP have been described in numerous workers as shown in Table 22-6. One of the most common causes is in workers' exposure to metalworking fluids (coolants) contaminated with microbial flora.[41] Exposed workers have also developed other occupational lung diseases,

such as WRA. The metalworking fluids implicated in such outbreaks are water-based, and microbial flora contaminants have appeared to be the causative agents. Sputum cultures of those affected in these outbreaks have revealed gram-positive bacteria and strains of *Pseudomonas* and, most consistently, "rapid-growing" nontuberculous mycobacterial (NTMB) species, especially *Mycobacterium chelonae* or *Mycobacterium immunogenum*. Outbreaks of skin disease have also been reported, consistent with the spectrum of NTMB-caused disease.

BYSSINOSIS AND OTHER DISEASES CAUSED BY ORGANIC DUSTS

Some types of airway constriction are believed to be due to direct toxic effects on the airways. Byssinosis (meaning "white thread" in Greek) is associated with exposure to cotton, hemp, and flax processing. It has been called "brown lung" (a misnomer because the lungs are not brown), analogous to the term "black lung" used to describe CWP.

Byssinosis has been shown to develop in response to dust exposure in cotton processing, but prevalence can range from 2% to 50%. It is especially prevalent among cotton workers in the initial, very dusty operations where bales are broken open, blown (to separate impurities from fibers), and carded (to arrange the fibers into parallel threads). A lower prevalence of disease occurs in workers in the spinning, winding, and twisting areas, where dust levels are lower. The lowest prevalence of byssinosis has been found among weavers, who experience the lowest dust exposure. Processing of cloth is practically free of cotton dust, as in the manufacture of denim, which is washed during dyeing before thread is spun. Byssinosis has also been described in nontextile sectors where cotton is processed, such as cottonseed oil, cotton-waste utilization, and garneting (bedding and batting) industries. The same syndrome has been shown to occur in workers exposed in processing soft hemp, flax, and sisal.

Byssinosis is characterized by shortness of breath and chest tightness. These symptoms are most prominent on the first day of the workweek or after being away from the workplace over an extended period of time (which explains why it is sometimes called "Monday morning tightness"). No previous exposure is necessary for symptoms to develop. Symptoms are often associated with changes in pulmonary function. Characteristically, there is a decrease in FEV_1 during the Monday work shift or during the first day back at work after at least 2 consecutive days off. Because workers do not normally lose lung function during a workday, an acute loss of at least 10% or 300 mL (whichever is greater) in an individual, or 3% or 75 mL (whichever is greater) in a group of 20 or more workers, can be considered significant enough to require further investigation. Over time, cotton dust workers have an accelerated decrement in FEV_1, consistent with fixed airflow obstruction and chronic obstructive lung disease. Diagnosis is based mainly on symptoms; no characteristic examination or chest X-ray findings are associated with byssinosis. Therefore, the patient should be questioned systematically about symptoms.

It is assumed that byssinosis progresses if duration of exposure to sufficiently high dust levels is prolonged. Mild or early byssinosis is probably reversible if exposure ceases, but long-standing disease is irreversible. People with severe byssinosis are rarely seen in an industrial survey because they are too disabled to work. The end stage of the disease is fixed airway obstruction with hyperinflation and air-trapping. Cigarette smokers are at increased risk of irreversible byssinosis.

Much research has been done on possible etiologic mechanisms and effects. Extracts of cotton bract, a leaf-like part of the cotton flower, have been shown to release pharmacologic mediators, such as histamine, and prostaglandins. It seems likely that the mechanism of byssinosis involves stimulation of the same inflammatory receptors by endotoxin and by cotton dust. Gram-negative bacterial endotoxin contaminates cotton fiber, and aqueous extracts of endotoxin have produced acute symptoms and lung function declines.

Two other respiratory conditions are associated with work in the cotton industry:

1. *Mill fever*: This self-limited condition usually begins on first exposure to a cotton-dust environment. It lasts for 2 or 3 days and has no known sequelae. It is a flu-like illness characterized by headache, malaise, and fever—symptoms similar to metal fume fever and polymer fume fever. Mill fever is probably related to gram-negative bacterial material in mill dust; it usually affects workers only once, but after prolonged absence from a mill, re-exposure may trigger another attack. This syndrome is also referred to as organic dust toxic syndrome, a form of inhalation fever.

2. *Weaver's cough*: Weavers have experienced outbreaks of acute respiratory illness characterized by a dry cough, although their dust exposure is comparatively low. It may result from sizing material or from mildewed yarn that is sometimes found in high-humidity weaving rooms.

Other organic/vegetable materials are associated with obstructive respiratory diseases, including flax (baker's asthma), swine confinement buildings (acute airflow obstruction), and wood dust (asthma and chronic airflow obstruction). It appears that chronic exposure to organic dusts can result in both acute and chronic lung disease.[42]

PNEUMOCONIOSES

Pulmonary fibrosis is a well-documented environmental and work-related chronic pulmonary reaction. This condition, which varies according to inciting agent, intensity, and duration of exposure, is generally referred to as a pneumoconiosis. It is usually due to an inorganic dust or coal that must be of respirable size (less than 5 μm) to reach terminal bronchioles and alveoli. Dust of this size is not visible, and so its presence may not be recognized by workers. There are two typical patterns of fibrosis: (a) localized and nodular, usually peribronchial, fibrosis and (b) diffuse interstitial fibrosis. Both lead to a restrictive lung disease pattern on spirometry. The clinical features of all pneumoconioses are similar: initial nonproductive cough, shortness of breath of increasing severity, and, in the later stages, productive cough, distant breath sounds, and signs of right heart failure. The pneumoconioses are often associated with obstructive airways disease caused by the same agents or concomitant cigarette smoking during a working lifetime.

Silicosis

Crystalline silica (SiO_2) is a major component of the earth's crust. Therefore, exposure occurs in a wide variety of settings, such as mining, quarrying, stone cutting and grinding (Figure 22-4); foundry operations; ceramics and vitreous enameling; use of fillers for paints and rubber; and hydraulic fracking for natural gas extraction.

OSHA estimates that almost 2 million U.S. workers are exposed to silica. An estimated 12 million Chinese workers are exposed to silica. China recorded more than 500,000 cases of silicosis between 1991 and 1995. In recent years, the number of silicosis cases in China has been increasing rapidly, while the latency period between exposure and diagnosis of disease has been decreasing.[43] Reported silicosis cases are decreasing in the United Kingdom, where 100 new cases were reported in 2013 and 2014 combined, compared with 1,164 in 2002.[44] In the United States, silica-related deaths are decreasing, although more than 100 deaths occurred in 2010.[45] Evolving knowledge of the risk of silica exposure led OSHA to decrease the permissible exposure limit to 50 μg of respirable crystalline silica per cubic meter of air.[46]

Silicosis occurs more frequently in the upper lobes of the lungs, with nodules varying in size from microscopic to 6 mm in diameter. In severe cases, nodules coalesce and become fibrotic masses several centimeters in diameter. Nodules are firm and intact with a whorled pattern and rarely cavitate. Microscopically, the nodules are hyalinized, with a well-organized circular pattern of fibers in a cellular capsule. The amount of fibrosis appears proportional to the free silica content and to the duration of exposure. Fibrosis progresses even after removal from exposure. Except in acute silicosis, symptoms usually do not occur until 10 to 20 years after initiation of exposure. Evidence of pathologic response to silica exposure exists well before symptoms occur.

Evaluation of workers exposed to silica includes lung function tests (that may show reduced FVC or total lung capacity or mixed obstructive and restrictive patterns and reduced diffusing capacity), a chest X-ray (that may appear more abnormal than the lung function tests), and determination of (a reduced) hemoglobin oxygen saturation on exercise. As the disease progresses, there can be decreased oxygen saturation at rest and reduced total lung capacity. The chest X-ray usually shows rounded opacities, localized initially to the upper lung fields. The size and distribution of these opacities increase over time, and "eggshell" calcification of hilar lymph nodes occurs in some cases.

Chronic silicosis is classified either as simple or complicated, although there is a continuum between these two forms of the disease. The simple form is noted on the chest film by the presence of multiple, small, round opacities, usually in the upper zones. The concentrations of these opacities are used in classifying simple silicosis (ILO profusion categories 1 to 3).[1] Although simple silicosis alone is not a common cause of

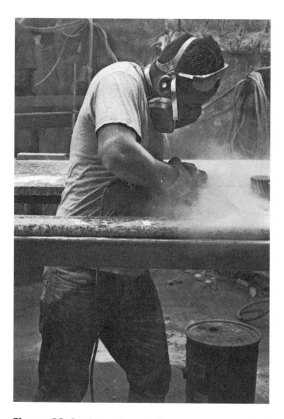

Figure 22-4. This worker grinding a countertop made of quartz is heavily exposed to crystalline silica. (Photograph by Earl Dotter.)

disability, it can contribute to disability as well as progress to complicated silicosis. In progressive massive fibrosis (PMF), several of the simple nodules appear to aggregate and produce larger conglomerate lesions, which enlarge and encroach upon the vascular bed and airways (ILO parenchymal categories A, B, and C). The extent of lung function impairment appears directly related to the radiographic size of the lesions and is most severe in categories B and C.

An important complication of silicosis is tuberculosis (TB). There is an increased incidence of TB among workers in the mining, quarrying, and tunneling industries and in steel and iron foundries. Workers exposed to silica may be at increased risk of TB, even in the absence of radiographic evidence for silicosis. Infections with atypical mycobacteria, such as *Mycobacterium kansasii* and *Mycobacterium avium-intracellulare*, can also occur and are related to the geographic distribution of these organisms. (See Chapter 13.) Treatment for such cases may require more vigorous drug treatment than for TB cases without silicosis. No relationship has yet been shown between silicosis and cigarette smoking. Another potential complication of silica exposure is lung cancer. Epidemiologic studies have demonstrated a link between silica exposure and lung cancer, and the International Agency for Research on Cancer (IARC) has classified silica as a Group 1 carcinogen.

Prevention of silicosis focuses on reduction of exposure through wet processes, isolation of dusty work, and local exhaust ventilation. Annual TB screening by purified protein derivative (PPD) skin testing or, if the PPD is positive, chest radiography is essential in silica-exposed workers. There is an ongoing national effort in the United States to eliminate silica in all sandblasting operations. Manual sandblasting has been banned in the United States and most European countries, but it is still practiced widely in LMICs. New uses of manual sandblasting, such as denim processing in the apparel industry, has increased the number of workers exposed to silica; for example, in Bangladesh, an estimated 2.2 million denim-processing workers are exposed. Elimination of silica from individual work practices could substantially reduce the at-risk population.

Acute silicosis, a distinct entity, is a devastating disease. It is due to extraordinarily high exposures to small silica particles (1 to 2 μm). These exposures occur in abrasive sandblasting and in the production and use of ground silica. In one of the most tragic industrial disasters in U.S. history, approximately 3,000 miners employed to build the Hawk's Nest Tunnel through Gauley Mountain in West Virginia, starting in 1927, were exposed to massive amounts of silica due, in part, to the mineral content of the rock they were cutting. No personal protective equipment was provided or used. According to a monument erected by the West Virginia Department of Culture and History, there were 109 workers, mainly black migrant workers, who died. Congressional hearings later revealed that 476 workers had died, and the number may have actually been higher. (See Chapter 2.)

Symptoms of acute silicosis include dyspnea progressing rapidly over a few weeks, weight loss, productive cough, and sometimes pleuritic pain. Diminished resonance on percussion of the chest and rales on auscultation can be found. Lung function tests show a marked restrictive defect, with a substantial decrement in total lung capacity. The chest X-ray has a diffuse ground-glass, or miliary TB–like appearance, rather than the appearance in classic nodular silicosis. The pathologic process in this disease is characterized by a widespread fibrosis, with a diffuse interstitial, macroscopic appearance, and a microscopic appearance and chemical constituency resembling pulmonary alveolar proteinosis but with doubly refractile particles of silica lying free within the alveolar exudate. Disease onset usually occurs 6 months to 2 years after initial exposure. Acute silicosis is often fatal, usually within 1 year of diagnosis.

Diatomaceous earth is an amorphous silica material mined predominantly in the western United States. It is used as a filler in paints and plastics, as a heat and acoustic insulator, as a filter for water and wine, and as an abrasive. In contrast to the various forms of crystalline silica, amorphous silica has relatively low pathogenicity. However, some processes using diatomaceous earth include heating (calcinating) it to remove organic material. This heating process can produce up to 60% crystalline silica as cristobalite, which is highly fibrogenic. Exposure to this form of diatomaceous earth, therefore, must be treated the same as exposure to crystalline silica.

Silica appears in a wide variety of minerals in different combined forms known as silicates. Many of these silicates, such as asbestos, kaolin, and talc, also cause pneumoconiosis, but the types of pneumoconiosis that they produce have features distinct from those of silicosis.

Asbestos is the most widespread and best known of the silicates. It causes asbestosis and several types of cancers. (See Chapter 21.)

Asbestosis

Asbestos is a fibro-silicate that appears in nature in four major types (chrysotile, crocidolite, amosite, and anthophyllite) that produce similar chronic respiratory reactions. All four types are comprised of fibers that are indestructible at temperatures as high as 800°C. Use and production of these materials greatly increased in the 20th century. According to the EPA, U.S. consumption peaked in 1973 at 885,000 tons. While asbestos is no longer produced in the United States, an estimated 360 metric tons were imported in 2015 for use in the chloralkali industry, and in manufacturing roofing, coatings, friction products, and other materials.

OSHA estimated that, in 2016, there were 1.3 million U.S. workers in construction and general industry who were still potentially exposed to asbestos. OSHA also estimated that a total of 27 million U.S. workers had been occupationally exposed to asbestos between 1940 and 1979. Asbestos has been used in a variety of applications: asbestos cement products (tiles, roofing, and drain pipes), floor tile, insulation and fireproofing (in construction and shipbuilding), textiles (for heat resistance), asbestos paper (in insulating and gaskets), and friction materials (brake linings and clutch pads) (Figure 22-5). Probably the most hazardous current exposures occur in repair and demolition of buildings and ships and in a variety of maintenance jobs where exposures may be unsuspected by the workers. In the United States and many other countries, the construction industry is the major source of asbestos exposure to workers, mainly from disrupting previously installed asbestos products. (See Chapter 32B.)

The effect of asbestos exposure in the community can be significant, as seen in Libby, Montana.

Strip mining, transportation, and processing of vermiculite ore containing asbestiform minerals was conducted in and around Libby from 1923 until 1990. As a result, asbestos-related lung diseases have been observed in Libby residents and workers at the mine. Numerous potential exposure sources existed, including direct exposure at work or in the community, use of vermiculite ore waste at home, and inadvertent exposure of family members via dust brought home on workers' clothes, skin, and hair. Among former workers at the Libby mine, 29% had pleural changes consistent with asbestos exposure in 2004–2005, compared to 2% in 1980. These pleural changes are directly related to cumulative fiber exposure.[47] (See Chapter 21.)

The main symptoms of asbestosis are cough and shortness of breath, which may be more severe than the appearance of the chest X-ray might indicate. In 20% of those affected, basilar rales are present, heard best at end inspiration or early expiration. Pleural rubs and pleural effusions can occur. Benign asbestos effusions can occur less than 10 years after initial exposure, and they are generally small and unilateral and may resolve spontaneously. They can, however, be associated with pain and fever. Although not common, pleuritic pain or chest tightness is more frequent in asbestos-related disease than in other pneumoconioses. Pleural effusion or pleuritic pain in a person with a history of asbestos exposure should always prompt an evaluation for mesothelioma.

Pathologically, the lung appears macroscopically as a small, pale, firm, and rubbery organ with fibrotic adherent pleura. The cut surface shows patchy to widespread fibrosis, and the lower lobes are more frequently affected than the upper. The microscopic appearance is characterized by interstitial fibrosis. Chest X-rays show widespread irregular (linear) opacities, more common in the lower lung fields.

Asbestos (ferruginous) bodies can be seen microscopically in sputum and lung tissue. These are dumbbell-shaped bodies, 20 to 150 μm in width, that appear to be fibers covered by a mucopolysaccharide layer. Iron pigment (from hemoglobin breakdown) makes them appear golden brown. They are not diagnostic of asbestos-related disease, but, when present even in small numbers in sputum or

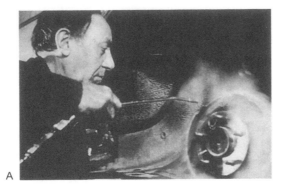

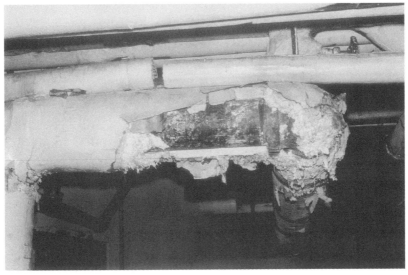

Figure 22-5. Examples of occupational exposure to asbestos: (A) Brake mechanic exposed to asbestos fibers while using compressed air to clean brake drum. (Photograph by Nick Kaufman.) (B) Exposed asbestos pipe insulation. (Photograph by Earl Dotter.)

tissue sections, they indicate substantial occupational exposure to airborne asbestos fibers. Most urban dwellers in industrialized countries have a measurable asbestos burden, but the concentrations of asbestos bodies in nonoccupationally (or paraoccupationally) exposed populations are orders of magnitude lower than in those with occupational exposures. In the "background" population of urban dwellers, 50 to 100 microscopic sections of lung would have to be searched to find a single asbestos body, whereas people with very early asbestosis have asbestos bodies in nearly every section. Those with more severe asbestosis usually have many asbestos bodies per section. Asbestos bodies may also be found in other parts of the body besides the lungs; they form round fibers that are transported by lung lymphatics into the circulation.

A particular feature of asbestos exposure, unlike other pneumoconioses, is the frequent presence of asbestos-induced circumscribed pleural fibrosis, known as pleural plaques, which are sometimes the only evidence of exposure. These plaques can calcify, may be bilateral, and are located more commonly in the parietal pleura. Sometimes, these plaques may provide evidence for prior asbestos exposure or help explain why pulmonary function tests are abnormal (Figure 22-6).

Pleural plaques are one manifestation of the rather marked pleural reaction to asbestos fibers. Other such evidence seen on chest X-rays is a "shaggy"-appearing cardiac or diaphragmatic

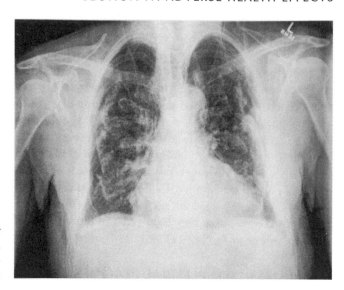

Figure 22-6. Calcified plaques in a worker who had been heavily exposed to asbestos. (Source: Parkes WR. Occupational lung disorders (4th ed.). Boca Raton, FL: CRC Press, 2017.)

border. An early, nonspecific sign is a blunted costophrenic angle. Diffuse pleural thickening also occurs, probably less commonly than the more specific pleural plaques. Asbestos-induced diffuse visceral pleural fibrosis may also occur and may impair lung function. Advanced pleural fibrosis may act like a cuirass, severely constricting breathing and leading to respiratory failure.

The evaluation of an individual suspected of having asbestosis includes determining whether there has been a history of exposure; a physical examination to ascertain whether rales are present; a chest X-ray, which may show irregular linear opacities and a variety of pleural reactions; and pulmonary function tests, which may show evidence of restrictive disease and a decreased diffusing capacity. In addition, the peribronchiolar fibrosis may have an obstructive component. Hence, in both nonsmokers and smokers with asbestosis (as with all pneumoconioses), a mixed restrictive–obstructive pattern may be seen.

Asbestosis, like silicosis, may progress after removal from exposure. Asbestos exposure, even without asbestosis, carries with it the added risk of mesothelioma of the pleura or peritoneum, lung cancer, and cancers of the gastrointestinal tract and other organs. (See Chapter 21.) Prevention focuses on substitution with materials such as fibrous glass, use of wet processes to reduce dust generation, local exhaust ventilation to capture the dust that is generated, and respiratory protection. Exposed persons who smoke should be advised to stop smoking, in part

because the risk factors of cigarette smoking and asbestos for lung cancer (but not for mesothelioma) are synergistic—that is, the risk of both exposures is greater than the sum of the risks of each exposure alone.

In 2004, the ATS published an official statement on the diagnosis and initial management of nonmalignant disease related to asbestos.[48] Nonmalignant asbestos-related disease includes asbestosis,; pleural plaques, thickening, or fibrosis; benign asbestos pleural effusion; and airflow obstruction. This statement outlines diagnostic criteria, recommended clinical evaluation, expected disease outcomes, and implications of diagnosis for patient management. The statement is available online at the ATS website (http://www.thoracic.org).

Pneumoconioses Due to Talc and Kaolin

Talc is a hydrated magnesium silicate that occurs in a variety of natural forms. The two major types are nonfibrous and fibrous. The nonfibrous forms, such as those found in Vermont, are free of both crystalline silica and fibrous asbestos tremolite; the fibrous forms, such as those found in New York State, can contain up to 70% fibrous material, including amphibole forms of asbestos. Talc exposures occur mainly during its use as an additive to paints and as a lubricant in the rubber industry, especially in inner tubes. Evidence suggests that high doses of nonfibrous talc or moderate doses of fibrous talc accumulated over a long time can result in chronic respiratory disease known as talcosis, with the same symptoms as other pneumoconioses.

Pathologically, the macroscopic appearance of the lung is characterized by poorly structured nodules, unlike the firm nodules of silicosis or the diffuse fibrosis of asbestosis. The microscopic appearance consists of ill-defined nodules with some diffuse interstitial fibrosis. Evaluation of people exposed to talc includes pulmonary function tests and chest X-rays. Chest X-rays may show both nodular and linear opacities and also pleural plaques. Studies addressing the possibility of a cancer risk associated with fibrous talc exposure found a four-fold increase in risk of lung cancer in New York State talc miners.

Kaolin (China clay) is a hydrated aluminum silicate found in the United States (in a band from Georgia to Missouri), India, and China. It is used in ceramics; as a filler in paper, rubber, paint, and plastic products; and as a mild soap abrasive. Kaolin is not particularly hazardous in the mining processes because it is usually a wet ore and mined by jet-water mining techniques.

The pneumoconiosis resulting from chronic exposures to kaolin dust (kaolinosis) produces no unique clinical features. Pathologically, the macroscopic appearance is one of immature silicotic nodules, although conglomerate nodules may appear. Pleural involvement occurs only if the lung is massively involved. The microscopic appearance consists of nodules with randomly distributed collagen.

Coal Workers' Pneumoconiosis

In the United States until the 1960s, coal workers' respiratory disease was considered a variant of silicosis and was often known as an anthracosilicosis. It is now clear that CWP is an etiologically distinct entity that can be induced by both coal dust and pure carbon. Coal workers' pneumoconiosis exists both in uncomplicated and complicated forms; the latter, known as progressive massive fibrosis (PMF), is the most severe and disabling form of the disease. Although exposure to coal dust occurs most commonly in underground mines, there is also some exposure in handling and transport of coal. Significant exposure also occurs in the trimming or leveling

of coal in ships when preparing material for transport.

Uncomplicated CWP increases the likelihood for future development of the complicated form. Diagnoses of CWP have relied primarily on chest X-rays, which show nodular opacities of less than 1 cm (mostly less than 3 mm) in diameter. Progressive massive fibrosis, in contrast, is seen on chest X-rays as the development of conglomerations of these small opacities to sizes greater than 1 cm in diameter.

In the early stages, CWP is asymptomatic. Initial symptoms are dyspnea on exertion with progressive reduction in exercise tolerance. As nodular conglomeration begins and PMF is diagnosed, symptoms become more severe, with marked exertional dyspnea, severe disability, or total incapacity. With PMF, copious black sputum is often produced. There is general agreement that PMF leads to premature disability and death. No such agreement, however, exists for the impact of simple CWP.

Coal dust also contributes independently to the disability observed in coal workers through the production of chronic bronchitis, airway obstruction, and emphysema. The occurrence of bronchitis and loss of pulmonary function are both dose-dependent on coal dust exposure, in smokers and nonsmokers. With CWP, chest x-rays show widely distributed, small, round opacities.

The greater the intensity and duration of exposure (cumulative exposure), the more likely it is that a miner will get one of these diseases. Concomitant silicosis can occur as well if the quartz content of the coal is high. These two diseases may present in any combination.

Pathologically, CWP appears macroscopically as soft, black, indurated nodules. Microscopic observation shows dust in and around macrophages near respiratory bronchioles. Nodules show random collagen distribution, and the lung shows centrilobular emphysema.

In PMF, the large conglomerate masses have variable shapes and do not respect the architecture of the lung. The surfaces are hard, rubbery, and black, and cavitation often occurs (Figure 22-7). Microscopically, the appearance is not distinct from the simple nodules. Chest X-rays show large conglomerate opacities (Figure 22-8).

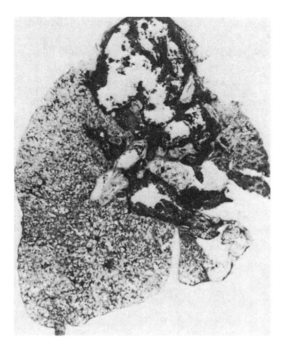

Figure 22-7. Gough section of lung of coal worker with 18 years of mining experience completed 20 years before death. It shows cavitation as well as centrilobular emphysema, which was present in both lungs. (Courtesy of J.C. Wagner, MRC Pneumoconiosis Unit, Llandough Hospital, Penarth, Wales, United Kingdom.)

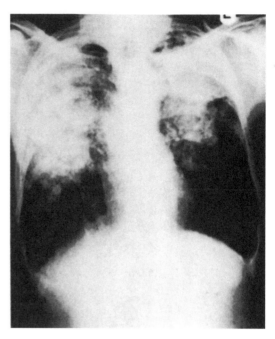

Figure 22-8. Chest X-ray of coal worker whose lung section appears in Figure 22-7, taken 2 weeks before death. The appearance is classic for progressive massive fibrosis with larger conglomerate masses in both lung fields. (Courtesy of J.C. Wagner, MRC Pneumoconiosis Unit, Llandough Hospital, Penarth, Wales, United Kingdom.)

Although evaluation for CWP is the same as for the other pneumoconioses, a particular feature affecting evaluation is the Federal Mine Safety and Health Act of 1977, which prescribes what types of abnormalities make a person eligible for disability benefits. Because these are subject to continuous revision, consultation with the Mine Safety and Health Administration in the U.S. Department of Labor is advisable. Miners have special rights to a low-dust environment with increased medical monitoring if they are found to have CWP, and they have the right to permanent removal from the high-dust environment with wage retention. These rights are unique among workers in the United States, although arguably such an approach should be applied in the prevention of all pneumoconioses. (See Chapter 3.)

Rheumatoid pneumonconiosis (Caplan syndrome), occurs when pneumoconiosis (silicosis, asbestosis, or CWP) is accompanied by rheumatoid arthritis. First described in 1953 by Dr. Anthony Caplan in a group of 51 Welsh coal miners, Caplan syndrome is defined by an increased number of nodules relative to others with pneumoconiosis but less respiratory impairment in many cases. Radiographically, there are multiple well-defined bilateral nodules or masses, primarily peripheral in distribution. The pathologic appearance is that of alternate black and gray-white bands of material in conglomerate masses that frequently cavitate or calcify. Patients also have rheumatoid arthritis clinically, and they usually have positive serologies for rheumatoid disease as well.

Flock Worker's Lung

An emerging pneumoconiosis is chronic interstitial lung disease in workers employed in the nylon flocking industry. Index cases were first described in plants in Rhode Island and Canada in the early 1990s.[49,50] Since then, more cases have been reported. Processes in the flocking industry include cutting nylon tow (cables of synthetic monofilaments), flocking the cut fibers (applying them to an adhesive-coated substrate), dying the nylon flock, and other finishing processes. Environmental studies of flocking plants have identified multiple airborne exposures, including bioaerosols, nylon fibers, and tannic acid. Prior to cutting and flocking, the nylon polyamide fibers were believed by manufacturers to be of nonrespirable size, but air sampling conducted by NIOSH has revealed long, thin, respirable-size nylon particles. While there are still additional candidate exposures, the respirable fibers are currently believed to be the causative agent in flock worker's lung.[51]

In the initial case series, median latency was 6 years from date of hire to onset of symptoms.[50] Most common clinical symptoms include dry cough and dyspnea. Chest X-ray and HRCT findings have included patchy infiltrates with a "ground-glass" appearance and occasional areas of fibrosis. Bronchoalveolar lavage fluid often has a high proportion of eosinophils. The most consistent histopathologic findings of lung biopsy specimens have been a pattern of nonspecific interstitial pneumonia, lymphoid nodules, and lymphocytic bronchiolitis without evidence of granulomata. However, other patterns, including bronchiolitis obliterans organizing pneumonia, can occur. The long-term clinical course of this disease can be complete resolution, persistent interstitial lung disease with pulmonary function abnormalities, or progressive lung function decline and ultimate death.[52]

CHRONIC BERYLLIUM DISEASE

Chronic beryllium disease (CBD), the most well-known and best-characterized occupational granulomatous lung disease, is a systemic disease that affects the lungs more than other organs. It develops in workers who make metal alloys containing beryllium, a strong, lightweight, nonmagnetic metal used in industries such as aerospace and defense, high-end audio and electronics equipment, and design of nuclear weapons. Workers are exposed by inhaling beryllium-containing dust, which can result in immune sensitization in susceptible workers. Sensitization can then progress to CBD, but not all sensitized workers develop symptomatic disease.

A *granuloma* is a cellular immune response to an inciting agent in which immune cells organize into microscopic clusters or nodules. Macrophages or multinucleated giant cells (fused macrophages) are at the core of the granuloma, and other immune cells, such as lymphocytes and neutrophils, as well as fibroblasts and collagen may also be present. Granulomata can be the result of infectious agents, usually *Mycobacterium tuberculosis* or NMTB, or non-infectious agents.

Chronic beryllium disease may be clinically indistinguishable from sarcoidosis, an idiopathic systemic granulomatous disease that also affects the lung disproportionately. Serum angiotensin converting enzyme levels may be elevated, as in sarcoidosis, although this is not a highly sensitive test in either disease. A more specific test to determine cell-mediated immunity to beryllium is the beryllium lymphocyte proliferation test (BeLPT) on peripheral lymphocytes or lymphocytes from bronchoalveolar lavage samples. The BeLPT is a highly specific and sensitive test for sensitization to beryllium, but it alone is not diagnostic of CBD. Transbronchial or surgical lung biopsies or samples of affected lymph nodes will show noncaseating (nonnecrotic) granulomata, which, together with evidence of sensitization to beryllium (such as a positive BeLPT), are generally diagnostic of CBD.[53]

As in sarcoidosis, the pattern of pulmonary function testing can be extremely variable. Most patients with CBD develop restrictive disease, often with impaired gas exchange marked by a decrease in diffusing capacity. However, obstructive disease, isolated gas exchange abnormalities, and normal pulmonary function tests can all be seen. Chest X-rays or computed tomography scans frequently show hilar and/or mediastinal lymphadenopathy, as in sarcoidosis, and a variety of parenchymal findings, such as nodules and opacities with a "ground-glass" appearance.

Genetic polymorphisms in the major histocompatibility (MHC) complex have been identified as a major susceptibility factor for sensitization to beryllium. In a small series of CBD cases and controls, polymorphisms in the human leukocyte antigen gene HLA-DPB1 have been identified as conferring susceptibility, but up to 25% of people with CBD do not carry this genetic variation.[54,55] MHC (HLA) Class II antigens are involved in the T cell response to external antigens. T cells are also part of the immune response that results in granuloma formation. Although the BeLPT is recommended for monitoring workers at increased risk for disease or potentially exposed to higher beryllium levels,[53] genetic testing of prospective workers remains a controversial ethical question and, thus far, has not been used routinely to identify workers at risk for beryllium sensitization and thus CBD.

MISCELLANEOUS INORGANIC DUST DISORDERS

Fibrous glass and related products, referred to as synthetic vitreous fibers (SVFs), manmade vitreous fibers, manmade mineral fibers, or very fine vitreous fibers, have been used for insulation purposes for over 80 years. More recently, they have played an important role as an asbestos substitute. Synthetic vitreous fibers are amorphous silicates with a length-to-diameter ratio of greater than 3:1. They are made mainly from rock, slag, glass, or kaolin clay, and they can be divided into three main groups: mineral wool, fibrous glass, and ceramic fiber.

Synthetic vitreous fibers can induce skin, eye, and upper respiratory tract irritant responses. There have been few case reports of pulmonary disease due to SVF exposure. In general, respiratory symptoms are absent or mild, and chest X-rays and pulmonary function tests are normal. Limited studies of workers exposed to fine-diameter fibers have revealed evidence of irregular opacities consistent with pneumoconiosis. An excess of pleural changes (especially pleural plaques) and mild respiratory symptoms without abnormalities in lung function have been demonstrated in workers involved in the production of refractory ceramic fibers.[56] There is growing concern about the possible carcinogenicity of these very fine fibers. IARC has classified special-purpose glass fibers, such as E-glass and "475" glass fibers, and also ceramic fibers as possibly carcinogenic to humans, and it has determined that insulation glass wool, continuous glass filament, rock (stone) wool, and slag wool are not classifiable as to their carcinogenicity to humans. Studies of workers exposed to glass wool, continuous glass filament, rock (stone), and slag wool have not provided consistent evidence of an association between exposure to fibers and risk for lung cancer or mesothelioma. There is limited epidemiological data to permit an adequate evaluation of the cancer risk associated with exposure to refractory ceramic fibers. In chronic inhalation studies, ceramic fibers produce an increase in the incidence of mesothelioma in hamsters and an increased incidence of lung tumors in rats. Because of persistent uncertainties, occupational exposures to SVFs should be lowered as much as possible with engineering controls, proper worker training, and safe work practices.

Individual exposures to iron dusts, particularly those resulting from steel-grinding operations, welding, or foundry work, are common. The only clinical effect of pure iron oxide exposure is a reddish-brown coloring of the sputum. Lung function tests show no clinical abnormality, whereas chest X-rays show many small (0.5 to 2.0 mm) opacities without confluence. Lung sections show macrophages laden with iron dust but without fibrosis or cellular reaction. With removal from further iron oxide dust exposure, the radiographic abnormalities slowly resolve. Similar results can be seen in exposures to tin, barium, and antimony.

ACKNOWLEDGMENTS

Cases 1 and 2 are courtesy of Stephen Hessl, MD, Daniel Hryhorczuk, MD, and Peter Orris, MD, Section on Occupational Medicine, Cook County Hospital, Chicago, Illinois. Case 3 is courtesy of the late James Keogh, MD, University of Maryland School of Medicine, Baltimore (unpublished curriculum materials).

REFERENCES

1. International Labor Organization. Guidelines for the use of the ILO International Classification of Radiographs of Pneumoconioses, revised edition 2011. Available at: http://www.ilo.org/safework/info/publications/WCMS_168260/lang--en/index.htm. Accessed November 14, 2016.
2. Ferris BG. Epidemiology Standardization Project (American Thoracic Society). American Review of Respiratory Disease. 1978; 118: 1–120.

3. Miller MR, Crapo R, Hankinson J, et al. General considerations for lung function testing. European Respiratory Journal 2005; 26: 153–161.

4. Miller MR, Hankinson J, Brusasco V, et al. Standardisation of spirometry. European Respiratory Journal 2005; 26: 319–338.

5. Hankinson JL, Odencrantz JR, Fedan KB. Spirometric reference values from a sample of the general U.S. population. American Journal of Respiratory and Critical Care Medicine 1999; 159: 179–187.

6. Centers for Disease Control and Prevention. Fixed obstructive lung disease in workers at a microwave popcorn factory—Missouri, 2000–2002. Morbidity and Mortality Weekly Report 2002; 51: 345.

7. International Agency for Research on Cancer. IARC Monographs on the Evaluation of Carcinogenic Risks to Human: Chromium, nickel and welding (Vol. 49). Lyon, France: IARC, 1990. Available at: https://monographs.iarc.fr/ENG/Monographs/vol49/mono49.pdf. Accessed November 14, 2016.

8. Villeneuve PJ, Goldberg MS, Krewski D, et al. Fine particulate air pollution and all-cause mortality within the Harvard Six-Cities Study: Variations in risk by period of exposure. Annals of Epidemiology 2002; 12: 568–576.

9. Rice MB, Ljungman PL, Wilker EH, et al. Long-term exposure to traffic emissions and fine particulate matter and lung function decline in the Framingham heart study. American Journal of Respiratory and Critical Care Medicine 2015; 191: 656–664.

10. Moore E, Chatzidiakou L, Kuku MO, et al. Global associations between air pollutants and chronic obstructive pulmonary disease hospitalizations: A systematic review. Annals of the American Thoracic Society 2016; 13: 1814–1827.

11. Bruce N, Perez-Padilla R, Albalak R. Indoor air pollution in developing countries: A major environmental and public health challenge. Bulletin of the World Health Organization 2000; 78: 1078–1092.

12. Dherani M, Pope D, Mascarenhas M, et al. Indoor air pollution from unprocessed solid fuel use and pneumonia risk in children aged under five years: A systematic review and meta-analysis. Bulletin of the World Health Organization 2008; 86: 390–398C.

13. Pope CA 3rd, Thun MJ, Namboodiri MM, et al. Particulate air pollution as a predictor of mortality in a prospective study of U.S. adults. American Journal of Respiratory and Critical Care Medicine 1995; 151: 669–674.

14. Chen H, Goldberg MS, Villeneuve PJ. A systematic review of the relation between long-term exposure to ambient air pollution and chronic diseases. Reviews on Environmental Health 2008; 23: 243–297.

15. Jerrett M, Burnett RT, Pope CA 3rd, et al. Long-term ozone exposure and mortality. New England Journal of Medicine 2009; 360: 1085–1095.

16. World Health Organization. Effects of air pollution on children's health and development: A review of the evidence. 2005. Available at: http://www.euro.who.int/__data/assets/pdf_file/0010/74728/E86575.pdf. Accessed November 14, 2016.

17. Akinbami LJ. The state of childhood asthma, United States. 1980–2005. 2006. Available at: http://www.cdc.gov/nchs/data/ad/ad381.pdf. Accessed November 14, 2016.

18. Akinbami LJ, Moorman JE, Garbe PL, Sondik EJ. Status of childhood asthma in the United States, 1980–2007. Pediatrics 2009; 123: S131–S145.

19. Akinbami LJ, Moorman JE, Bailey C, et al. Trends in asthma prevalence, health care use, and mortality in the United States, 2001–2010. NCHS Data Brief 2012; 94: 1–8.

20. Stewart LJ. Pediatric asthma. Primary Care 2008; 35: 25–40, vi.

21. Mortimer K, Neugebauer R, Lurmann F, et al. Air pollution and pulmonary function in asthmatic children: effects of prenatal and lifetime exposures. Epidemiology 2008; 19: 550–557; discussion 561–552.

22. Rice MB, Rifas-Shiman SL, Litonjua AA, et al. Lifetime exposure to ambient pollution and lung function in children. American Journal of Respiratory and Critical Care Medicine 2016; 193: 881–888.

23. Schwartz J. Air pollution and children's health. Pediatrics 2004; 113: 1037–1043.

24. Gelfand EW. Pediatric asthma: A different disease. Proceedings of the American Thoracic Society 2009; 6: 278–282.

25. The National Environmental Education Foundation. Available at: http://www.neefusa.org/resources/publications.htm. Accessed October 24, 2016.

26. Mapp CE, Boschetto P, Maestrelli P, Fabbri LM. Occupational asthma. American Journal of Respiratory and Critical Care Medicine 2005; 172: 280–305.

27. Tarlo SM, Balmes J, Balkissoon R, et al. Diagnosis and management of work-related asthma: American College Of Chest Physicians Consensus Statement. Chest 2008; 134: 1S–41S.

28. Dodd KE, Mazurek JM. Asthma among employed adults, by industry and occupation – 21 states, 2013. Morbidity and Mortality Weekly Report 2016; 65: 1325–1331.

29. Friedman-Jimenez G, Harrison D, Luo H. Occupational asthma and work-exacerbated asthma. Seminars in Respiratory and Critical Care Medicine 2015; 36: 388–407.

30. Henneberger PK, Redlich CA, Callahan DB, et al. An official American Thoracic Society statement: Work-exacerbated asthma. American Journal of Respiratory and Critical Care Medicine 2011; 184: 368–378.

31. Malo JL, Tarlo SM, Sastre J, et al. An official American Thoracic Society Workshop report: Presentations and discussion of the fifth Jack Pepys Workshop on Asthma in the Workplace. Comparisons between asthma in the workplace and non-work-related asthma. Annals of the American Thoracic Society 2015; 12: S99–S110.

32. Rachiotis G, Savani R, Brant A, et al. Outcome of occupational asthma after cessation of exposure: a systematic review. Thorax 2007; 62: 147–152.

33. Omland O, Wurtz ET, Aasen TB, et al. Occupational chronic obstructive pulmonary disease: A systematic literature review. Scandinavian Journal of Work, Environment & Health 2014; 40: 19–35.

34. Kreiss K, Gomaa A, Kullman G, et al. Clinical bronchiolitis obliterans in workers at a microwave-popcorn plant. New England Journal of Medicine 2002; 347: 330–338.

35. Holden VK, Hines SE. Update on flavoring-induced lung disease. Current Opinion in Pulmonary Medicine 2016; 22: 158–164.

36. Bailey RL, Cox-Ganser JM, Duling MG, et al. Respiratory morbidity in a coffee processing workplace with sentinel obliterative bronchiolitis cases. American Journal of Industrial Medicine 2015; 58: 1234–1245.

37. Allen JG, Flanigan SS, LeBlanc M, et al. Flavoring chemicals in e-cigarettes: Diacetyl, 2,3-pentandeione, and acetoin in a sample of 51 products, including fruit-, candy- and cocktail-flavored e-cigarettes. Environmental Health Perspectives 2016; 124: 733–739.

38. National Institute for Occupational Safety and Health. Flavorings-related lung disease. January 2016. Available at: https://www.cdc.gov/niosh/topics/flavorings/. Accessed October 24, 2016.

39. Selman M, Pardo A, King TE Jr. Hypersensitivity pneumonitis: Insights in diagnosis and pathobiology. American Journal of Respiratory and Critical Care Medicine 2012; 186: 314–324.

40. Okamoto T, Miyazaki Y, Tomita M, et al. A familial history of pulmonary fibrosis in patients with chronic hypersensitivity pneumonitis. Respiration: International Review of Thoracic Diseases 2013; 85: 384–390.

41. Burge PS. Hypersensitivity pneumonitis due to metalworking fluid aerosols. Current Allergy and Asthma Reports 2016; 16: 59. doi:10.1007/s11882-016-0639-0.

42. Christiani DC. Organic dust exposure and chronic airway disease. American Journal of Respiratory and Critical Care Medicine 1996; 154: 833–834.

43. Ding Q, Schenk L, Hansson SO. Occupational diseases in the people's Republic of China between 2000 and 2010. American Journal of Industrial Medicine 2013; 56: 1423–1432.

44. Health and Safety Executive. Pneumoconiosis (excluding asbestosis) in Great Britain 2014. Available at: www.hse.gov.uk/statistics/causdis/pneumoconiosis/. Accessed October 23, 2016.

45. Bang KM, Mazurek JM, Wood JM, et al. Silicosis mortality trends and new exposures to respirable crystalline silica—United States, 2001–2010. Morbidity and Mortality Weekly Report 2015; 64: 117–120.

46. Occupational Safety and Health Administration. Occupational exposure to respirable crystalline silica. Final rule. Federal Register 2016; 81: 16285–16890.

47. Rohs AM, Lockey JE, Dunning KK, et al. Low-level fiber-induced radiographic changes caused by Libby vermiculite: A 25-year follow-up study. American Journal of Respiratory and Critical Care Medicine 2008; 177: 630–637.

48. American Thoracic Society. Diagnosis and initial management of nonmalignant diseases related to asbestos. American Journal of Respiratory and Critical Care Medicine 2004; 170: 691–715.

49. Centers for Disease Control and Prevention. Chronic interstitial lung disease in nylon flocking industry workers—Rhode Island, 1992–1996. Morbidity and Mortality Weekly Report 1997; 46: 897.

50. Kern DG, Crausman RS, Durand KT, et al. Flock worker's lung: Chronic interstitial lung disease in the nylon flocking industry. Annals of Internal Medicine 1998; 129: 261–272.

51. Kern DG, Kuhn C 3rd, Ely EW, et al. Flock worker's lung: Broadening the spectrum of clinicopathology, narrowing the spectrum of suspected etiologies. Chest 2000; 117: 251–259.

52. Turcotte SE, Chee A, Walsh R, et al. Flock worker's lung disease: Natural history of cases

and exposed workers in Kingston, Ontario. Chest 2013; 143: 1642–1648.

53. Balmes JR, Abraham JL, Dweik RA, et al. An official American Thoracic Society statement: Diagnosis and management of beryllium sensitivity and chronic beryllium disease. American Journal of Respiratory and Critical Care Medicine 2014; 190: e34–e59.

54. Richeldi L, Sorrentino R, Saltini C. HLA-DPB1 glutamate 69: A genetic marker of beryllium disease. Science 1993; 262: 242–244.

55. Snyder JA, Demchuk E, McCanlies EC, et al. Impact of negatively charged patches on the surface of MHC class II antigen-presenting proteins on risk of chronic beryllium disease. Journal of the Royal Society Interface 2008; 5: 749–758.

56. Utell MJ, Maxim LD. Refractory ceramic fiber (RCF) toxicity and epidemiology: A review. Inhalation Toxicology 2010; 22: 500.

FURTHER READING

Cherniack M. Hawk's Nest incident: America's worst industrial disaster. New Haven, CT: Yale University Press, 1989.
Description of a large outbreak of acute silicosis related to industrial exposure, which led

ultimately to the inclusion of pneumoconiosis in workers' compensation systems.

Muzaffar SA, Christiani DC. Frontiers in occupational and environmental lung disease research. Chest 2012; 141: 772–781.
A review of current research and developments on the horizon.

Newman Taylor A, Cullinan P, Blanc, P, Pickering A (eds.). Parkes' Occupational Lung Disorders (4th ed.). Boca Raton, FL: CRC Press, 2016.
Excellent and current textbook on occupational lung disease.

Seaman DM, Meyer CA, Kanne JP. Occupational and environmental lung disease. Clinics in Chest Medicine 2015; 36: 249–268.
An excellent summary of the topic.

Cullinan P, Muñoz X, Suojalehto H, et al. Occupational lung diseases: From old and novel exposures to effective preventive strategies. Lancet Respiratory Medicine 2017; 5: 445–455.
An excellent global summary, which includes recommendations for research, surveillance, and other action of reduce the burden of occupational lung diseases.

Swidey N. Trapped under the sea: One engineering marvel, five men, and a disaster ten miles into the darkness. New York: Crown Publishing, 2014.
Vivid account of deaths among tunnel workers exposed to carbon monoxide.

23

Neurological Disorders

Margit L. Bleecker

Acute or subacute occupational exposure to high levels of neurotoxic compounds, which occurred in the past and resulted in unique presentations of neurological disorders, occur infrequently today. Some examples included the "mad hatter" syndrome associated with inorganic mercury, overt parkinsonism with manganese, wrist drop with inorganic lead, dementia with repeated exposure to high levels of mixed solvents, and spastic paraparesis (stiff legs due to involvement of corticospinal tract) with tri-o-cresyl phosphate exposure. Although neurotoxic workplace exposures have become more controlled, overexposure may still occur when there are deficiencies in ventilation, faulty heating systems leading to carbon monoxide exposure, and use of inappropriate personal protective equipment or other control measures. Nevertheless, lower levels of exposure to neurotoxic compounds may cause nonspecific symptoms, such as headache, fatigue, dizziness, mental confusion, poor memory, decreased concentration, tremor, alteration in mood, imbalance, and paresthesias. In some cases, disappearance or decrease of symptoms when exposure ceases, such as on weekends and holidays, leads to initial suspicion that workplace exposure is responsible for the nonspecific symptoms. Some potential neurological manifestations of occupational exposure to neurotoxic compounds are summarized in Table 23-1.

CASE STUDY

Since 1999, there have been reports of occupational overexposure to 1-bromopropane, an organobromine solvent that has been used increasingly over the past 20 years as a substitute for chlorofluorocarbons, such as methylene chloride, perchloroethylene, and trichloroethylene, all of which deplete the strastopheric ozone layer. 1-bromopropane is also preferred because methylene chloride and trichloroethylene are potent carcinogens and nonhalogenated hydrocarbon alternatives are highly flammable. 1-bromopropane is used as a degreaser for metals, plastics, electronic, and optical components; as a solvent in spray adhesive; in drycleaning; in the production of asphalt, aircraft maintenance, and synthetic fibers; and as an intermediate in pharmaccutical synthesis. Only ACGIH has recommended 0.1 ppm (0.5 mg/m^3) as a time-weighted average guideline for air exposure.[1]

Six workers in a furniture factory who had been exposed to 1-bromopropane vapors from spray adhesives developed severe neurotoxicity.[2] The index case was a 29-year-old woman who worked full-time for 4 years gluing foam cushions, when she developed distal leg numbness and pinprick paresthesias, then leg weakness requiring assistance to walk. Her serum bromide level was 170 mg/dL (reference range: 0–40 mg/dL). Examination revealed spastic and weak legs, clonus at the knees and ankles, a Babinski's sign, and a stocking distribution of decreased vibration, proprioception, and light touch. Her gait showed a spastic paraparesis with scissoring (crossing one's legs when walking due to increased adductor tone in thighs). The rest of the examination was normal. Nerve conduction studies (electromyography) were normal, but the motor distal latencies of the peroneal and ulnar nerves were at the upper limits of normal. Other causes of spastic paraparesis were not found despite extensive serum, cerebrospinal fluid, and imaging tests. Magnetic resonance imaging (MRI) of the brain and cervical and thoracic spine were normal.

Ventilation at the factory had been from a tabletop fan at each station, which workers had turned off a month before to conserve heat. Even though respirators approved by the National Institute for Occupational Safety and Health and latex gloves were available, workers chose not to use them. Four of the other five affected workers had worked full-time for at least 3 years before developing similar symptoms, and the sixth affected worker had worked there for the previous 3 months and also 3 months during the previous year. Five of the six affected workers had some improvement but were left with persistent motor and sensory abnormalities, headaches, and cognitive changes; the sixth worker became asymptomatic.

These cases demonstrate the involvement of both (a) the central nervous system (CNS), with headache, depressed mood, cognitive impairment, spasticity, hyperreflexia, clonus, Babinski's sign and gait ataxia, and (b) the peripheral nervous system (PNS), with sensory loss in a stocking-glove distribution and weakness. The CNS involvement accounted for poor recovery; peripheral nerves regenerate as reflected by these workers' improvement in sensory and motor exams. Nerve biopsy from another case of 1-bromopropane intoxication found an axonopathy.[3]

Table 23-1. Illustrative Potential Neurologic Manifestations of Occupational Exposure to Neurotoxins

Manifestation	Agents
Ataxic gait	Acrylamide
	1-Bromopropane
	Chlordecone (Kepone)
	n-Hexane
	Manganese
	Mercury
	Methyl n-butyl ketone
	Organophosphates
	Tri-o-cresyl phosphate
Flaccid bladder and/or sexual dysfunction	Dimethylaminopropionitrile (DMAPN)
	Lead
Constricted visual fields	Mercury
Cranial neuropathy	Carbon disulfide
	Dichloroacetylene
Headache	1-Bromopropane
	Carbon monoxide
	Chlordecone (Kepone)
	Lead
	Toluene
Impaired visual acuity	Carbon disulfide
	n-Hexane
	Lead
	Mercury
	Methanol
	Styrene
	Toluene
Myoclonus	Methyl bromide
Opsoclonus	Chlordecone (Kepone)
Ototoxicity	Carbon disulfide
	Carbon monoxide
	Lead
	Mercury
	Hydrocarbons
	Thallium
Parkinsonism	Carbon disulfide
	Carbon monoxide
	Hydrocarbons
	Manganese
	Pesticides
Seizures	Benzene hexachloride (Lindane)
	Methyl bromide
Spastic paraparesis	1-Bromopropane
	Tri-o-cresyl phosphate
Tremor	Carbon disulfide
	Carbamates
	Chlordecone (Kepone)
	Hydrocarbons
	Lead
	Manganese
	Mercury
	Organophosphates

TOXIC NEUROPATHIES

No etiology can be found for about 30% of patients with peripheral neuropathies.[4,5] A variety of chemicals can cause toxic neuropathies. However, in approaching a patient with a possible toxic neuropathy, a clinician must consider the evidence that the exposure in question can cause a peripheral neuropathy, as described previously, as well as the following:

- Pre-existing neuropathies caused by diabetes mellitus or other disorders increase the susceptibility to a neurotoxic exposure.[6]
- Peripheral nerves may be compromised by pre-existing or new nerve entrapment syndromes that can accentuate the effect of the neurotoxic agent.[7,8]
- Aging makes the nervous system more vulnerable to neurotoxic exposures; metabolic changes that account for adverse effects from neurotoxic exposure occur more readily, and regeneration from peripheral nerve damage occurs more slowly.[9]

Toxic peripheral neuropathies affect the longest axons. Symptoms are usually sensory, begin in the feet, and eventually involve the hands—in the classic *stocking-glove distribution*. Symptoms vary and include tingling, pins-and-needles sensation (parasthesia), numbness, a burning sensation, pain, and misperception of sensory stimuli (dysesthesia). (There are exceptions, such as lead neuropathy, which involves the most active motor units and presents with weakness resulting in wrist drop.[10]) Involvement of the autonomic nervous system is uncommon, although it is a major component of the toxic neuropathy associated with β-dimethylaminopropionitrile (DMAPN), which presented primarily with neurogenic bladder dysfunction.[11]

Surveillance for peripheral neuropathies in the workplace is best accomplished using a validated symptom questionnaire and a quantitative measure of nerve function, such as vibration, which reflects damage to the larger myelinated nerve fibers—those most commonly affected in toxic neuropathies.[12] In order to avoid multiple comparisons—and thereby improve the ability to detect impairment—a case definition of peripheral neuropathy should be used.[13] Nerve conduction studies are still considered the "gold standard" to document pathology in peripheral nerves: they require no participation by the patient; they only examine the largest, most rapidly conducting axons (the A-beta fibers); and they require a trained individual to perform them. Patients with axonopathies, the most common form of toxic neuropathies, have normal conduction velocities as long as some large axons are preserved, but the amplitude of the response (which reflects the number of axons recruited into the response) will be decreased due to the loss of axons. Nerve conduction studies may demonstrate abnormalities in sensory nerve fibers at a time when no clinical sensory loss is present.[14] Quantitative sensory testing studies require minimal training to administer, but participation by the patient is needed. Depending upon what modality is measured (vibration, temperature, or pain threshold), one can examine the integrity of nerve fibers of different sizes.

NEUROPATHOLOGY

In axonopathies, protein synthesized in the perikaryon is not transported down the axon, resulting in *dying-back* degeneration of the most distal part of the axon. This damage occurs at the distal end of axons in both the CNS and PNS (*central-peripheral distal axonopathy*), which usually occurs in the longest and largest nerve fibers.[15] Because of interference with axonal transport, swellings filled with neurofilaments develop on the proximal side of the node of Ranvier. When these become large, such as in hexacarbon neuropathy, retraction of myelin creates secondary demyelination, which slows nerve conduction velocity.[16]

NEUROBEHAVIORAL TESTING

As was demonstrated by the index case in the 1-bromopropane case study, workers exposed to neurotoxicants experience a variety of symptoms. With 1-bromopropane exposure, the patient experienced new memory loss, depressed mood, and daily headache 2 years after the acute exposure had ceased.

Neuropsychological testing often plays an important role in evaluating patients with neurobehavioral impairments possibly associated with exposure to neurotoxicants. Neuropsychological tests are administered by paper and pencil or on a computer. When neuropsychological batteries are administered to exposed *populations*, they usually require approximately 1 hour as they are usually detecting subclinical abnormalities that may be associated with exposure but are not capable of providing a clinical diagnosis. By contrast, neuropsychological testing of an individual in a clinical setting requires many hours to more accurately define the areas of impairment and other factors that may contribute to the performance. Table 23-2 summarizes cognitive domains commonly affected by neurotoxicant exposure and neuropsychological tests that are used to evaluate these domains. The cognitive domains most sensitive to demonstrate exposure-related impairment are attention/concentration, verbal and visual memory, working memory/executive function, visuospatial skills (visuoperception/visuoconstruction), motor functioning, and mood/affect. Two examples of tasks for attention include learning an increasing length of numbers and performing a timed test of connecting circles in a specified order. Another test for attention/concentration abilities measures response time to seeing a visual stimulus shown at different time intervals. An example of a visuoperception/visuocontruction task involves placing red and white blocks in increasingly difficult geometric designs, a task that requires speed and accuracy. Some motor tasks assess speed and manual dexterity, such as measuring time to place ridged pegs into slotted holes with different orientations. Some tasks measure sustained attention and visuomotor speed, such as entering as quickly as possible the appropriate symbol below rows of numbers, using a key that matches number and symbol. Working memory/executive function refers to the ability to remember something and then to manipulate it, such as remembering a list of numbers and then presenting them in reverse order—a task that involves executive functions, such as planning and organization.

In order to attribute poor performance in a variety of cognitive domains to an exposure, there must be measures on *hold tests*, the results of which are resistant to the effects of a neurotoxicant exposure and therefore reflect premorbid abilities. In Table 23-2 these are listed under "General intelligence" and reflect measures of overlearned abilities, such as reading skills and vocabulary. Therefore, if vocabulary is borderline or low-average for age and education, it should not be surprising that some measures in other areas may also be borderline or low-average and not necessarily an outcome of exposure.

It is unusual to have new memory loss begin 2 years after cessation of solvent exposure when mental status was normal at the time of initial hospitalization, as demonstrated in the case study. However, the presence of depressed mood 2 years later is a common persistent complaint with exposure to neurointoxicants, which may cause slowed mental processing and mild attentional deficits and may mimic dementing conditions.[17] Depressed mood may be a direct consequence of solvent exposure but also, as in this case, related to the ongoing disability of spastic paraparesis requiring a cane for walking. When somatic symptoms, such as headache, fatigue, and dizziness, and cognitive complaints persist, the clinician should consider the presence of depression. In some cases, depending upon the type and circumstances of exposure, symptoms of posttraumatic stress disorder or generalized anxiety may be present and interfere with performance on neuropsychological testing. When health outcome information is available on the Internet without any relationship to dose, fear of what will happen following an exposure to a neurointoxicant is greatly exacerbated. This can lead individuals who have smelled a solvent to believe they have brain damage, when, in fact, they do not because the odor threshold for the solvent is much lower than the threshold limit value (TLV) for air concentration—considered to be a safe level of exposure.

When neurobehavioral test batteries are administered to populations with occupational exposure to neurotoxicants, the significant dose-effect relationships usually reflect performance within the normal range and therefore would be considered a "subclinical manifestation of CNS dysfunction."[18] In contrast, *impaired*

Table 23-2. Cognitive Domains Commonly Affected by Neurointoxicant Exposure

Domain	Tests	Metals	Solvents	Other
General intelligence	Wechsler Adult Intelligence Scale IV Picture Completion Information Vocabulary Wide Range Achievement Test 4 Reading North American Adult Reading Test			
Attention/Concentration	Digit Span Forward Digit Symbol Trail Making Test A Simple Visual Reaction Time	Lead Mercury	1-Bromopropane Carbon disulfide Methyl chloride Styrene Toluene White spirits Xylene	Carbon monoxide Ethylene oxide
Verbal memory	Logical Memory Rey Auditory Verbal Learning Test	Lead	White spirits	Carbon monoxide Ethylene oxide
Visual memory	Benton Visual Retention Visual Reproduction	Mercury	1-Bromopropane White spirits	Carbon monoxide Ethylene oxide
Working memory/ Executive functioning	Digit Span Backwards Stroop Trail Making Test B	Lead Manganese	1-Bromopropane White spirits	Carbon monoxide
Visuoperception/ Visuoconstruction	Block Design Hooper Visual Organization Test Rey–Osterrieth Complex Figure Test Digit Symbol	Lead Mercury	Carbon disulfide Styrene Toluene White spirits	Carbon monoxide Organophosphates
Motoric functioning	Finger-Tapping Test Grooved Pegboard	Lead Mercury	1-Bromopropane Carbon disulfide Methyl chloride Styrene Toluene White spirits	Carbon monoxide
Mood/Affect	Beck Anxiety Inventory Beck Depression Inventory II Minnesota Multiphasic Personality Inventory-3 Profile of Mood Scale Posttraumatic Stress Disorder Scale	Lead Manganese Mercury	1-Bromopropane Carbon disulfide Methyl alcohol Methyl chloride Styrene Toluene White spirits	Carbamates Carbon monoxide Organochlorines Organophosphates
General cognitive screening	Cognistat Mini-Mental State Exam Montreal Cognitive Assessment	Lead		

Note. Details of tests, including administration, interpretations, neuropathology, and diagnostic issues, are provided in Lezak MD, Howieson DB, Loring DW (eds.). Neuropsychology assessments (4th ed.). New York: Oxford University Press, 2004, pp. 329–333.

performance is defined on the basis of a clinical neuropsychological evaluation of an individual that is one to two standard deviations below what is expected for that individual.

Too often there are no data on the degree of exposure; therefore, assumptions have to be made indirectly based on such information as symptoms at the time of exposure, duration of symptoms, and content of safety data sheets. For some neurotoxicants, such as carbon monoxide, much is known about the association of air levels and biomarkers (such as carboxyhemoglobin) and their association with symptoms or clinical findings. Because significant solvent exposure is usually associated with headaches, the onset of headaches that is temporarily associated with solvent exposure may serve as an indirect indicator of exposure when biomarkers or air levels are not available. Headaches caused by occupational solvent exposure improve when exposure ceases, leading to improvement during time away from work. Therefore, when headaches persist for years after cessation of exposure, it is important to search for comorbid conditions, such as depression.

CLINICAL EVALUATION

The following steps should be considered when clinically evaluating patients with exposure to neurotoxicants:

- Review all active medical problems and their severity, as well as medications taken on a regular basis
- Ask about time of onset and duration of symptoms in relation to exposure (With chronic solvent exposure, the latency for toxic neuropathies may be as long as 10 years. For acute exposure to high solvent concentrations, symptoms such as headaches, dizziness, and fatigue may begin immediately and resolve when exposure ceases.)
- If an occupational cause is suspected, ask about potential exposures and use of personal protective equipment
- Determine if other workers from the same area have similar complaints
- Note that neurological findings on physical examination must be biologically plausible in order to be associated with exposure (For example, since toluene affects the CNS but not the PNS, the presence of a peripheral neuropathy after toluene exposure must be due to another etiology.)
- Become familiar with the epidemiological literature concerning the alleged exposure as it helps to determine where the neurological examination should be focused and expanded (Some mental status screening tools can provide a more comprehensive assessment of cognitive performance than the simple Mini-Mental State Examination. For toxic neuropathies, measures of quantitative sensory examination, such as vibration threshold, can be followed over time.)
- When examining a group of workers with different levels of exposure (as determined by biomarkers, air levels, job title, and/or years employed), determine if a dose–response (exposure–effect) relationship is present
- When an individual patient is clinically examined in the absence of exposure data, consider relying on improvement of signs and symptoms when exposure ceases in order to determine an association between exposure and the disorder (This may take a long time since nerve conduction studies in patients with toxic neuropathies may take up to a year before improvement is seen. One must remember that the PNS has the ability to regenerate, while the CNS does not; therefore, for example, signs attributed to damage in spinal cord pathways may become more prominent as a patient with toxic neuropathy recovers.)
- Consider and rule out other plausible etiologies before concluding that a specific exposure caused the disorder.

ILLUSTRATIVE NEUROTOXINS

Carbon Monoxide

Carbon monoxide (CO) is a colorless, odorless, nonirritant gas that binds to hemoglobin with an affinity 200 times greater than oxygen to form carboxyhemoglobin (COHb). Decreased oxygen-carrying capacity results in tissue hypoxia. At COHb levels of 1% to 5%, tissue hypoxia is prevented by increased blood flow and increased oxygen extraction.[19] With higher COHb levels, adverse effects are more serious (Table 23-3). If loss of consciousness and hypotension occur, there may be delayed neurologic sequelae, presenting 2 to 40 days later due to diffuse demyelination in the brain; however, signs and symptoms are reversible in most cases.[20,21] (See Chapters 11 and 26.)

When there is incomplete combustion of hydrocarbons, often due to poorly functioning heating systems and inadequate ventilation of flame-based heating sources, CO may be released and cause adverse health effects. This situation can occur when gasoline-powered machines are used indoors;[22] propane-powered forklifts are operated in warehouses[23] or propane-powered

Table 23-3. Human Response with Varying Levels of Carboxyhemoglobin

COHb	Findings in Humans
<1%	Endogenous carbon monoxide from catabolism of hemoglobin; at these concentrations carbon monoxide has many neuroprotective effects.
1%–9%	Normal levels in tobacco smokers; chest pain and decreased exercise duration with ischemic heart disease
15%–20%	Headache; changes in visual evoked potentials
20%–30%	Severe headache, dizziness, nausea, fatigue; impaired manual dexterity
30%–40%	Severe headache, nausea, vomiting, increased heart and respiratory rate, loss of consciousness with hypotension
40%–50%	Coma and seizures, hypotension
60%–70%	Lethal if untreated

ice-resurfacing machines are operated in skating rinks,[24] and when gasoline-powered generators are used after loss of power, especially when they are improperly located or have inadequate ventilation.[25]

Carbon monoxide in the atmosphere is higher with heavy traffic. It is even higher in tunnels and parking garages. Explosives used in surface blasting may produce CO through detonation. While smoking, smokers are exposed to 400 to 500 ppm CO, resulting in 3% to 8% COHb, which may increase to 15% in heavy smokers, compared to 1% to 3% in nonsmokers. In the workplace, the TLV for carbon monoxide is 25 ppm (30 mg/m³), which yields a 3.5% level of COHb.

Onset of symptoms (headache, dizziness, nausea, fatigue, confusion, and memory problems) generally occurs above a COHb of 20%.[26,27] However, when people with cardiovascular disease are exposed to CO, their exercise duration is decreased due to chest pain at COHb concentrations of 2.7% to 5%.[28] At 20% to 30% COHb, a psychometric test 1 month after exposure found no significant difference for memory attention, executive function, or reaction time.[29]

Chronic intermittent exposure to CO around 106 ppm has been found to be associated with significant impairment by neuropsychological testing in several functional domains, including executive function, visuospatial judgment, organization, psychomotor speed, and attention.[30]

The biological half-life of COHb when breathing room air is 4 to 6 hours. This decreases to 40 to 60 minutes with breathing 100% oxygen and further to 15 to 30 minutes with hyperbaric oxygen treatment.

Lead

Many different types of workers are occupationally exposed to lead (Figures 23-1A and B). Blood lead levels (BLLs), which reflect recent lead exposure, have a half-life of 25 to 35 days. They are used to determine if lead-exposed workers are being excessively exposed at work. (The biological exposure index for lead, a guideline value used to assess biological monitoring results, is 200 µg/L [20 µg/dL].) Cumulative lead exposure can be measured determining bone lead concentration using X-ray fluorescence. Bone lead concentration is much more closely associated with neurobehavioral impairment than BLL testing is.[31-33] Lead in bone, which accounts for 90% to 95% of total body burden of lead, has a half-life of 25 to 35 years. The adverse neurobehavioral effects of lead are associated with cumulative lead exposure but not with BLLs.

Classically, lead neuropathy was associated with a motor neuropathy, manifest by wrist drop in battery workers. It was usually accompanied by other effects of lead, such as anemia and abdominal pain. Frequent involvement of the upper extremities was unusual since toxic peripheral neuropathies typically begin in the longest and largest nerve fibers with initial symptoms in the toes. The underlying pathology was loss of large fibers without demyelination.[34] The weakness in the upper extremities was related to frequently used muscles.[10] Occupational lead neuropathy so severe that it causes wrist drop is virtually nonexistent now.

Since the mid-1980s, the neuropathic changes associated with chronic lead exposure appear to primarily involve sensory nerve fibers. A threshold effect for changes in nerve

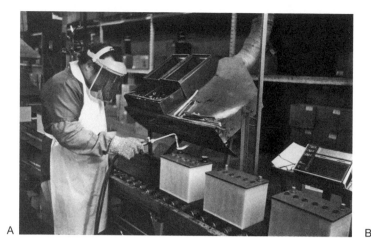
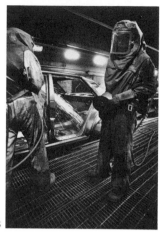

Figure 23-1. Current work practice rules require significant personal and environmental protection in situations of lead exposure: (A) Lead battery worker is protected mainly by local exhaust ventilation. (B) Automobile lead grinder is protected by air-supplied hood and floor exhaust ventilation. (Photographs by Earl Dotter.)

conduction studies has been found at a BLL of 40 µg/dL.[35]

The subclinical effects in the PNS are often accompanied by subclinical effects in performance on neuropsychological batteries in many cognitive domains (Table 23-2). The most consistent abnormal findings with lead exposure are with fine motor performance and visuomotor tasks. Higher performance on a measure of cognitive reserve (reading achievement test) has been shown to protect against the effects of chronic lead exposure on measures of cognitive performance but not on motor performance.[36]

In addition to these adverse health effects, lead exposure causes ototoxicity, as measured by auditory-evoked potentials in the brainstem.

Organic Solvents

Organic solvents, which are volatile liquids at room temperature, are strongly lipophilic, enabling their easy access to the CNS and PNS. N-hexane and methyl n-butyl ketone, both of which are hexacarbon solvents, are metabolized to 2,5-hexanedione, causing a toxic neuropathy by interfering with fast axonal transport. Glue sniffers who use n-hexane develop a toxic neuropathy characterized by distal weakness, muscle atrophy, loss of ankle reflexes, and sensory loss. As they recover from the peripheral

neuropathy, pyramidal tract signs are unmasked, reflecting the "dying-back" process in the CNS.[16] Nerve conduction velocity is slowed because of the myelin retraction around the large multifocal swelling in the distal axons.

In the leather shoe industry, exposure to n-hexane in glues resulted in motor and sensory signs. After removal from exposure, there was deterioration (*coasting*) for several months believed to be caused by storage of n-hexane in lipid-rich organs.[37] Methyl ethyl ketone added to n-hexane and methyl n-butyl ketone potentiated metabolism to the active metabolite 2,5-hexanedione, resulting in outbreaks of peripheral neuropathies.[38,39]

A study in paint manufacturing plants estimated lifetime exposure to a mixture of aliphatic and aromatic hydrocarbons; it demonstrated that among workers a dose–effect relationship between exposure and vibration threshold in the feet, even though workers had no symptoms of peripheral neuropathy.[40,41]

In the 1980s, there was concern that long-term exposure to solvents could result in a syndrome of neuropsychiatric symptoms, including memory impairment, difficulty concentrating, fatigue, personality changes, headache, and irritability.[42-45] This syndrome is now known as *chronic solvent-induced encephalopathy* (CSE).[46,47] The diagnosis relies on verifying substantial long-term exposure to neurotoxic solvents, nonspecific signs and symptoms (with onset before cessation of exposure), and exclusion of other organic brain syndromes and primary psychiatric diseases. Neuropsychological impairment is the hallmark of CSE, which usually consists of an irreversible cognitive disorder accompanied by a mood disorder, mainly depression or anxiety. A study found that solvent-exposed workers are more likely to have excessive alcohol consumption and alcoholism.[47] Neuropsychological tests reveal impairments in attention, speed of information processing, short-term memory, and motor performance.[46] The diagnosis of CSE is not confirmed until a 1- to 2-year period of follow-up has been completed.

In order to determine if CSE existed in the United States, 187 solvent-exposed workers in the paint manufacturing industry were examined. Solvent exposure was based on 13 to 15 years of personal breathing zone samples.[40] After adjusting for confounders, analysis of neuropsychological test results found that there were significant exposure-effect relationships between solvent exposure and abnormalities on several neuropsychological tests.[41] Higher levels of exposure were not associated with increased headaches, fatigue, difficulty concentrating, short-term memory loss, or irritability.[48] The performance scores on both the neuropsychological and neuropsychiatric effects were within normal limits. In sum, the observed effects were subclinical and have not been shown to progress with ongoing low-level exposure to solvents.

One important difference between workers with CSE and workers in this paint manufacturing industry study is that workers with CSE are exposed to higher levels of solvents, resulting in symptoms at the time of exposure.

Manganese

Manganese, which is used to harden steel and is present in welding fumes, can cause a syndrome similar to Parkinson disease. High occupational manganese exposure in mines in Chile in the early 1950s caused parkinsonism—with dystonia, emotional lability, gait disturbance, and psychosis ("manganese madness").[49] Symptoms in manganese-induced parkinsonism are usually symmetric in onset, with bradykinesia,

propensity to fall backward, gait disturbance ("cock walk"), and dystonia; there is no resting tremor. In contrast, symptoms of idiopathic Parkinson disease begin asymmetrically, with tremor, rigidity, and bradykinesia on one side. Manganese-induced parkinsonism does not improve with cessation of exposure and, in contrast to Parkinson disease, does not respond to levodopa.[50]

A study of manganese-exposed welders found a 10-fold significantly elevated prevalence of parkinsonism compared to the general population.[51] In a group of shipyard welders, the prevalence of parkinsonism was 15.6%, compared to 0% in comparison workers.[52] The uptake pattern on positron emission tomography scan, which showed significantly lower uptake in the caudate nucleus, may be an early (asymptomatic) marker of manganese neurotoxicity. The classic finding with manganese neurotoxicity on MRI has been T1-weighted hyperintensities within the globus pallidus, which could be quantitated with the *pallidal index* (ratio of signal intensity over globus pallidus compared to reference white matter).[53] An increased pallidal index was found in asymptomatic manganese-exposed workers that correlated with cumulative manganese exposure. These results were strengthened by increasing the intensity measures to include combined basal ganglia, caudate nucleus, and posterior putamen.[54] Expanding MRI imaging to include functional MRI facilitates detection of preclinical abnormalities in manganese-exposed workers and potentially identification of at-risk workers.[55,56]

Age of onset of parkinsonism in manganese-exposed workers is, on average, younger (46 years) than the onset age of Parkinson disease (63 years).[57] Parkinsonism in populations exposed to the fuel additive methylcyclopentadienyl manganese tricarbonyl (MMT) have earlier onset, a more severe clinical course, and earlier mortality than patients with Parkinson disease.[58]

More research is needed in this area of subclinical neurobehavioral abnormalities associated with neurotoxic exposure to determine if reversibility occurs when exposure ceases and if these preclinical/subclinical changes alter the slope of age-related changes in the nervous system.

REFERENCES

1. Occupational Safety and Health Administration. Hazard Alert: 1-Bromopropane (Publication Number 2013-150). 2014. Available at: https://www.osha.gov/dts/hazardalerts/1bromopropane_hazard_alert.html. Accessed January 27, 2017.

2. Majersik J, Caravati EM, Stephens JD. Severe neurotoxicity associated with exposure to the solvent 1-bromopropane (n-propyl bromide). Clinical Toxicology 2007; 45: 270–276.

3. Samukawa M, Ichihara G, Oka N, et al. A case of severe neurotoxicity associated with exposure to 1-bromopropane, and alternative to ozone-depleting or global warning solvents. Archives of Internal Medicine 2012; 172: 1257–1260.

4. Prineas J. Polyneuropathies of undetermined cause. Acta Neurologica Scandinavica 1970; 44: 3–72.

5. Dyck PJ, Oviatt KF, Lambert RH. Intensive evaluation of referred unclassified neuropathies yield improved diagnosis. Annals of Neurology 1981; 10: 222–226.

6. Chaudhry V, Chaudhry M, Crawford TO, et al. Toxic neuropathy in patients with pre-existing neuropathy. Neurology 2003; 60: 337–340.

7. Hopkins A. Experimental lead poisoning in the baboon. British Journal of Industrial Medicine 1970; 27: 130–140.

8. Bleecker ML, Ford DP, Vaughan CG, et al. Effects of lead exposure and ergonomic stressors on peripheral nerve function. Environmental Health Perspectives 2005; 113: 1730–1734.

9. Fullerton PM. Toxic chemicals and peripheral neuropathy. Proceedings of the Royal Society of Medicine 1969; 62: 201–210.

10. Cantarow A, Trumper M. Lead poisoning. Baltimore, MD: Williams & Wilkins, 1944.

11. Keogh JP, Pestronk A, Wertheimer D, et al. An epidemic of urinary retention caused by dimethylaminopropionitrile. Journal of the American Medical Association 1980; 243: 746–749.

12. Buchanan D, Jamal GA, Pilkington A, et al. Clinical validation of methods of diagnosis of neuropathy in a field study of United Kingdom sheep dippers. Occupational and Environmental Medicine 2002; 59: 442–446.

13. Gerr F, Letz R. Epidemiological case definitions of peripheral neuropathy: Experience from two neurotoxicity studies. Neurotoxicity 2000; 21: 761–768.

14. LeQuesne PM. Electrophysiological investigation of toxic neuropathies in man. 6th International Congress of EMG. Acta Neurologica Scandinavica 1979; 60: 54–55.

15. Spencer PS, Schaumburg HH. Central-peripheral distal anoxopathy—The pathology of dying-back polyneuropathies. In: Zimmerman HM (ed.). Progress in neuropathology. New York: Grune & Stratton, 1976, pp. 253–295.

16. Korobkin R, Asbury AK, Sumner AJ, et al. Glue-sniffing neuropathy. Archives of Neurology 1975; 219: 158–162.

17. Lezak MD, Howieson DB, Loring DW (eds.). Neuropsychology assessment (4th ed.). New York: Oxford University Press, 2004, pp. 329–333.

18. White RF, Kengel M, Grashow R. Neurotoxicology. In: Parsons MW, Hammeke TA (eds.). Clinical neuropsychology: A pocket handbook for assessment (3rd ed.). York, PA: American Psychological Association, 2014, pp. 338–363.

19. Benignus VA, Muller KE, Malott CM. Dose-effects functions for carboxyhemoglobin and behavior. Neurotoxicology and Teratology 1990; 12: 111–118.

20. Choi IS. Delayed neurological sequelae in carbon monoxide intoxication. Archives of Neurology 1983; 40: 433–435.

21. Lin WC, Lu CH, Lee WC, et al. White matter damage in carbon monoxide intoxication assessed in vivo using diffusion tensor MR imaging. American Journal of Neuroradiology 2009; 30: 1017–1021.

22. Centers for Disease Control and Prevention. Unintentional carbon monoxide poisoning from indoor use of pressure washers—Iowa, January 1992–January 1993. Morbidity and Mortality Weekly Report 1993; 42: 777–779, 785.

23. Fawcett TA, Moon RF, Fracica PJ, et al. Warehouse workers' headache, carbon monoxide poisoning from propane-fueled forklifts. Journal of Occupational Medicine 1992; 34: 12–15.

24. Centers for Disease Control and Prevention. Carbon monoxide poisoning at an indoor ice arena and bingo hall—Seattle 1996. Morbidity and Mortality Weekly Report 1996; 45: 265–267.

25. Centers for Disease Control and Prevention. Carbon monoxide poisoning after two major hurricanes—Alabama and Texas, August–October 2005. Morbidity and Mortality Weekly Report 2006; 55: 236–239.

26. Schulte JH. Effects of mild carbon monoxide intoxication. Archives of Environmental Health 1963; 7: 524–530.

27. Benignus VA, Kafer ER, Muller KE, et al. Absence of symptoms with carboxyhemoglobin levels of 16-23%. Neurotoxicology and Teratology 1987; 9: 345–348.

28. Department of the Environment. Expert panel on air quality standards: Carbon monoxide. London: HMSO, 1994.

29. Deschamps D, Geraud C, Julien H, et al. Memory one month after acute carbon monoxide intoxication: A prospective study. Occupational and Environmental Medicine 2003; 60: 212–216.

30. Prockop LD. Carbon monoxide brain toxicity: Clinical, magnetic resonance imaging, magnetic resonance spectroscopy, and neuropsychological effects in 9 people. Journal of Neuroimaging 2005; 15: 144–149.

31. Lindgren KN, Masten VL, Ford DP, et al. Relation of cumulative exposure to inorganic lead and neuropsychological test performance. Occupational and Environmental Medicine 1996; 53: 472–477.

32. Bleecker ML, Lindgren KN, Ford DP. Differential contribution of current and cumulative indices of lead dose to neuropsychological performance by age. Neurology 1997; 48: 639–645.

33. Schwartz B, Lee BK, Lee GS, et al. Associations of blood lead, dimercaptosuccinic acid-chelatable lead, and tibia lead with neurobehavioral test scores in South Korean lead workers. American Journal of Epidemiology 2001; 153: 453–464.

34. Buchthal F, Behse F. Electrophysiology and nerve biopsy in men exposed to lead. British Journal of Industrial Medicine 1979; 26: 135–147.

35. Ehle A. Lead neuropathy and electrophysiological studies in low level lead exposure: A critical review. Neurotoxicology 1986; 7: 203–216.

36. Bleecker ML, Ford DP, Celio MA, et al. Impact of cognitive reserve on the relationship of lead exposure and neurobehavioral performance. Neurology 2007; 69: 470–476.

37. Passero S, Battistini N, Cioni R, et al. Toxic polyneuropathy of shoe workers in Italy: A clinical, neuropsychological and follow up study. Italian Journal of Neurological Sciences 1983; 4: 463.

38. Altenkirch H, Mager J, Stoltenburg G, et al. Toxic polyneuropathies after sniffing a glue thinner. Journal of Neurology 1977; 214: 137–152.

39. Saida K, Mendell JR, Billmaier DJ, et al. Peripheral changes induced by methyl n-butyl ketone and potentiation by methyl ethyl ketone. Journal of Neuropathology and Experimental Neurology 1976; 35: 207–224.

40. Ford, DP, Schwartz BS, Powell S, et al. A quantitative approach to the characterization of cumulative and average solvent exposure in paint manufacturing plants. American Industrial Hygiene Association Journal 1991; 52: 226–234.

41. Bleecker ML, Bolla KI, Agnew J, et al. Dose-related subclinical neurobehavioral effects of chronic exposure to low levels of organic solvents. American Journal of Industrial Medicine 1991; 19: 715–728.

42. Seppalainen AM, Lindstrom K, Martelin T. Neuropsychological and psychological picture of solvent poisoning. American Journal of Industrial Medicine 1980; 1: 31–42.

43. Elofsson S, Gamberale F, Hinmarsh T, et al. Exposure to organic solvents: A cross-sectional epidemiologic investigation on occupationally exposed car and industrial spray painters with special reference to the nervous system. Scandinavian Journal of Work, Environment & Health 1980; 6: 239–273.

44. Errebo-Knudsen EO, Olsen F. Organic solvents and presenile demmntia (the painter's syndrome): A critical review of the Danish literature. Science of the Total Environment 1986; 48: 45–67.

45. Gade A, Mortensen EL, Bruhn P. "Chronic painter's syndrome": A reanalysis of psychological test data in a group of diagnosed cases, based on comparisons with matched controls. Acta Neurologica Scandinavica 1988; 77: 293–306.

46. van Valen E, van Thriel C, Akila R, et al. Chronic solvent-induced encephalopathy: European concensus of neuropsychological characteristics, assessment, and guidelines for diagnostics. NeuroToxicology 2012; 33: 710–726.

47. Saino MA. Neurotoxicity of solvents. In: Lotti M, Bleecker ML (eds.). Handbook of clinical neurology, Volume 131, 3rd Series. London: Elsevier, 2015, pp. 93–110.

48. Bolla KI, Schwartz BS, Agnew J, et al. Subclinical neuropsychiatric effects of chronic low-level solvent exposure in US paint manufacturers. Journal of Occupational Medicine 1990; 32: 671–677.

49. Rodier J. Manganese poisoning in Moroccan miners. British Journal of Industrial Medicine 1955; 12: 21–35.

50. Lu CS, Huang CC, Chu NS, et al. Levodopa failure in chronic manganism. Neurology 1994; 44: 1600–1602.

51. Racette NA, Tabbal SD, Jennings D, et al. Prevalence of parkinsonism and relationship to exposure in a large sample of Alabama welders. Neurology 2005; 64: 230–235.

52. Racette BA, Criswell SR, Lundin JI, et al. Increased risk of parkinsonism associated with welding exposure. NeuroToxicology 2012; 33: 1356–1361.

53. Kim Y, Kim KS, Yang JS, et al. Increase in signal intensities on T1-weighted magnetic resonance images in symptomatic manganese-exposed workers. NeuroToxicology 1999; 20: 901–907.

54. Criswell SR, Perlmutter JS, Haung JL, et al. Basal ganglia intensity indices and diffusion weighted imaging in manganese-exposed welders. Occupational and Environmental Medicine 2012; 69: 437–443.

55. Chang Y, Lee JJ, Seo JH, et al. Altered working memory process in the manganese-exposed brain. NeuroImage 2010; 53: 1279–1285.

56. Chang Y, Song HJ, Lee JJ, et al. Neuroplastic changes within the brains of manganese-exposed welders: Recruiting additional neural resources for successful motor performance. Occupational and Environmental Medicine 2010; 67: 809–915.

57. Racette BA, McGee-Minnich L, Moerlein SM, et al. Welding-related parkinsonism: Clinical features, treatment, and pathophysiology. Neurology 2001; 56: 8–13.

58. Finkelstein MM, Jerrett M. A study of the relationships between Parkinson's disease and markers of traffic-diverted and environmental manganese air pollution in two Canadian cities. Environmental Research 2007; 104: 420–432.

FURTHER READING

Feldman RG. Occupational & environmental neurotoxicology. Philadelphia: Lippincott–Raven, 1999.
This book is valuable for a historical perspective. It provides descriptions of neurologic disorders due to higher exposures than occur today.

Lotti M, Bleecker ML (eds.). Handbook of clinical neurology. Vol. 131: Occupational neurology, 3rd Series.London: Elsevier, 2015.
This book provides a broad coverage of occupational disorders due to neurotoxicants, including movement disorders, cognitive change, sensory system impairment, the effect on the nervous system of ergonomic stressors, and traumatic brain injury/concussion. Underlying pathophysiology is discussed.

Spencer PS, Schaumburg HH. Ludolph AC (eds.). Experimental and clinical neurotoxicology. New York: Oxford University Press, 2000.
This reference text is an extensive compilation of neurotoxic chemicals and mixtures. The strength of association of each substance with its proposed biological action and its clinical neurological effect is assessed.

White RF, Kengel M, Grashow R. Neurotoxicology. In: Parsons MW, Hammeke TA (eds.). Clinical neuropsychology: A pocket handbook for assessment (3rd ed.). York, PA: American Psychological Association, 2014, pp. 338–363.
This chapter provides a succinct approach to neurotoxicology for the neuropsychologist. Differences in the approaches of epidemiology and clinical neuropsychology are highlighted. The role of co-morbidities is also addressed.

24

Reproductive and Developmental Disorders

Linda M. Frazier and Deborah Barkin Fromer

The overall proportion of adverse reproductive outcomes that is attributable to known reproductive toxicants is thought to be relatively low. However, as detection methods in reproductive toxicology and epidemiology have become more sensitive, adverse effects have been noted at lower exposure levels than previously and for additional agents. In some jobs and geographic areas, many individuals are exposed to agents that are known or suspected reproductive toxicants. Significant exposures to hazardous chemicals may occur in the workplace due to lack of protective equipment, inadequate training, and failure to provide uncontaminated washing facilities. Hazardous chemicals and polluting technologies are often used in the workplace because they are cheaper than safer alternatives. Reproductive and developmental toxicant exposure may also occur at home, through hobbies, household repairs, consumer products, food, or drinking water. For example, polybrominated diphenyl ethers (PBDEs), which are flame retardants that are extensively used in consumer products in the United States, may cause development neurotoxicity.[1]

Historically, birth defects caused by pharmaceuticals ingested during early pregnancy served to disprove the then-prevailing belief that the placenta acted as a protective barrier for the fetus. These pharmaceuticals included thalidomide, which caused limb malformations and other anomalies, and diethylstilbestrol (DES), which caused uterine malformations and vaginal cancer in prenatally exposed women. Mercury and polyhalogenated biphenyl exposures from contaminated food caused severe birth defects in infants, even when their mothers were relatively asymptomatic. In 1977, occupational exposure to dibromochloropropane (DBCP) caused male infertility and alterations in the sex ratio of offspring (see Box 24-1 and Figure 24-1), demonstrating that reproductive toxicity could affect both women and men.[2]

PRECONCEPTION

Most reproductive studies, whether in laboratory animals or in epidemiologic studies of men and women, examine the effects of toxicant exposure that begins before conception and continues throughout gestation. Organohalide compounds, such as polychlorinated biphenyls (PCBs), 2,3,7,8-tetrachlorodibenzo-p-dioxin (TCDD), DDT, and

Box 24-1. DBCP: A Potent Male Reproductive Toxicant

Barry S. Levy

In 1977, a small group of men in a northern California pesticide formulation plant noticed that few of them had recently fathered children. A strong association was found between decreased sperm count and exposure to dibromochloropropane (DBCP), a brominated organochlorine that had been used as a nematocide since the mid-1950s. Testicular biopsies showed the seminiferous tubules to be the site of action and spermatogonia to be the target cell. The relation between reduced sperm count and exposure to DBCP, both in its manufacture and in its use, was confirmed in other studies in the United States and abroad. Follow-up of workers after cessation of exposure showed that spermatogenic function eventually recovered in those less severely affected. However, many of the azoospermic men remained so for many years after cessation of exposure.

Much DBCP was exported by U.S.-based multinational corporations to developing (low- and middle-income) countries. A substantial amount of this pesticide was exported even after DBCP was banned in the United States. Workers exposed to DBCP in developing countries were not informed of its hazards, trained in its use, or provided personal protective equipment to safeguard themselves adequately (Figure 24-1). In one study of approximately 26,400 DBCP-exposed workers in developing countries who sued U.S. companies, 24% were azoospermic and 40% were oligospermic. A symposium with five articles on DBCP, including a report on this study of DBCP-exposed workers, has been published.[1]

Reference

1. Levy BS, Levin JL, Teitelbaum DT (Guest Editors). DBCP-induced sterility and reduced fertility among men in developing countries: A case study of the export of a known hazard (Symposium). International Journal of Occupational and Environmental Health 1999; 5: 115–153.

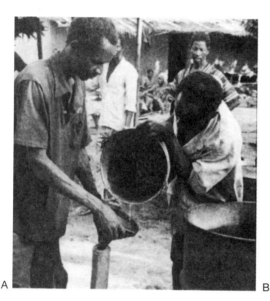 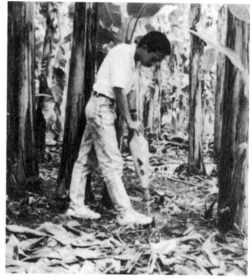

A   B

Figure 24-1. Many workers in low-income countries became sterile from exposure to DBCP, even after it was banned in the United States. (A) Simulation of worker pouring DBCP solution, which he had mixed with a stick in a 55-gallon drum, into an applicator. (B) Simulation of worker injecting DBCP solution around the roots of a banana tree. (Photographs by Barry S. Levy.)

PBDEs, cause ongoing exposure because they persist in fatty tissues.[1,3] If a woman has been heavily exposed to lead in the past, a significant amount is stored in bone and can be released into her blood during pregnancy at levels that adversely affect neurologic development of the fetus (Figure 24-2).[4]

Genetic toxicity is a mechanism by which reproductive and developmental processes are harmed. Using bacterial assays, increased mutagenic activity has been detected in the urine of

workers exposed to anesthetic gases, chemotherapeutic agents, and epichlorohydrin. Increased frequencies of chromosomal aberrations have been reported in radiation workers and in workers exposed to chemicals, such as benzene, styrene, ethylene oxide, epichlorohydrin, arsenic, chromium, and cadmium.

Structural chromosomal abnormalities in the fetus may have no adverse effects or may be associated with birth defects, mental retardation, and other health problems. Numerical chromosomal

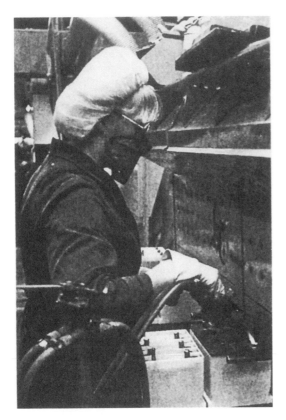

Figure 24-2. Adequate control of lead exposure for all workers requires a high level of engineering control and may also require personal protective equipment. Because U.S. law prohibits exclusion of pregnant women from lead work, controls must be sufficient to protect the fetus as well. (Source: Zenz C. Occupational medicine: Principles and practical applications. Chicago: Year Book, 1975. Reproduced with permission.)

abnormalities (aneuploidy) are a major cause of spontaneous abortion. For aneuploidies that are compatible with life, infants often suffer physical, behavioral, and intellectual impairments. Structural and numerical chromosomal abnormalities may originate in either the male or female gamete.[5,6]

Workplace Exposures among Men

Increased rates of pregnancy loss have been reported in the wives of men who are occupationally exposed to lead, inorganic mercury, organic solvents, pesticides, and other agents (Table 24-1). Male exposure to DBCP and possibly other toxicants can cause altered sex ratio in offspring, usually a deficit of male children.[7]

Certain paternal occupations may increase the risk for congenital malformations, low birthweight, neurodevelopmental disorders, and childhood cancers.

Workplace exposures can be taken into the home on a worker's skin, hair, or contaminated clothing or shoes, causing secondary (para-occupational) exposure to spouses and children. Sperm production may be harmed directly (by injuring testicular cells) or indirectly (by interfering with the hormonal regulation of spermatogenesis). As long as the stem cell precursors are spared, the reduction in sperm production may be reversible over time.

In addition to DBCP, ethylene dibromide, another pesticide, has been associated with decreased sperm velocity, motility, and viability. Occupational exposure (verified by urine tests) to ethyl parathion and methamidophos, both organophosphate pesticides, has resulted in aneuploidy in sperm cells, suggesting a genetic mechanism by which paternal exposure to these compounds could cause birth defects.[8]

Other pesticides have also been linked to paternally mediated reproductive problems.[9] Spontaneous abortion risk was increased two-fold if husbands applied herbicides but was increased five-fold if they applied herbicides and did not wear protective equipment during application.[10] In another study, concentration of DDT metabolites in body fat was demonstrated to have a dose–response relationship with birth defects in offspring of men who applied this insecticide in a malaria control program.[11]

Among the toxic metals, lead has been most intensively studied. Lead may have a direct toxic effect on the gonads and may also impair reproductive endocrine function. Paternal lead exposure has been associated with low birthweight among offspring, mainly when the father's exposure level is high, of long duration, or combined with other exposures, such as organic solvents. In lead-exposed men, blood lead levels above 40 µg/dL reduce sperm counts and impair sperm motility and morphology.[12]

Chemicals have differing potencies for producing adverse reproductive effects. The glycol ether 2-methoxyethanol (ethylene glycol monomethyl ether) is an organic solvent that causes testicular atrophy and disruption of the

Table 24-1. Selected Workplace Exposures with Suspected Effects on Male Reproductive Function

Adverse Effects	Examples*
Decreased libido, hormonal alterations	Lead, mercury, manganese, carbon disulfide, estrogen agonists (such as polychlorinated biphenyls, organohalide pesticides); workers manufacturing oral contraceptives
Spermatotoxicity	DBCP, lead, carbaryl, toluenediamine and dinitrotoluene, ethylene dibromide, plastic production (styrene and acetone), ethylene glycol monoethyl ether, perchloroethylene, mercury, heat, military radar, kepone, bromine, radiation (Chernobyl), carbon disulfide, 2,4-dichlorophenoxy acetic acid (2,4-D), welding
Spontaneous abortion in partner	Solvents, lead, mercury; workers in rubber and petroleum industries
Altered sex ratio in offspring	DBCP, TCDD
Congenital malformations in offspring	Pesticides, chlorphenates, solvents; firefighters, painters, welders, auto mechanics, motor vehicle drivers, sawmill workers and workers in aircraft, electronics and forestry and logging industries
Low birthweight or preterm birth in offspring	Lead
Neurobehavioral disorders in offspring	Alcohols, cyclophosphamide, ethylene dibromide, lead
Childhood cancer in offspring	Solvents, paints, pesticides, petroleum products; welders, auto mechanics, motor vehicle drivers, machinists and workers in aircraft and electronics industries.

Note. DBCP = dibromochloropropane; TCDD = 2,3,7,8-Tetrachlorodibenzo-*p*-dioxin.
* Some human evidence, albeit limited, has linked each health outcome with the occupations listed and with workplace exposure to at least one of the agents listed; for other agents, animal evidence is available.

Table 24-2. Selected Workplace Exposures with Suspected Effects on Female Reproductive Function

Adverse Effects	Examples*
Subfecundity	Certain herbicides, fungicides and organic solvents, mercury, nitrous oxide; agricultural workers, hairdressers, semiconductor manufacture, woodworkers, dental assistants
Menstrual dysfunction	Lead, mercury, shift work, antineoplastic drugs; hairdressers using chemicals, agricultural workers, athletes, dancers
Spontaneous abortion	Organic solvents such as perchloroethylene, glycol ethers, toluene, xylene, formalin, chloroform, lead, mercury, nitrous oxide, ethylene oxide, antineoplastic drugs, certain pesticides; semiconductor or shoe manufacture workers, laboratory workers, dental assistants, nurses, pharmacists, agricultural workers
Congenital malformations in offspring	Mixed organic solvents, trichloroethylene, halogenated aliphatic solvents, glycol ethers, aliphatic aldehydes or acids, lead, antineoplastic drugs, propellants, dyes, pigments; agricultural workers, hairdressers, housekeepers
Hypertensive disorders of pregnancy	Organic solvents
Low birthweight	Lead, prolonged standing, frequent shift changes. Possibly ethylene oxide, aromatic amines, chlorophenols
Infectious sequelae	Fetal carrier state (hepatitis B, human immunodeficiency virus), fetal morbidity/mortality (rubella, varicella-zoster, human parvovirus B19), serious maternal pneumonia (varicella-zoster)
Contamination of breast milk	Most agents entering the mother's bloodstream can be found in breast milk
Neurobehavioral disorders in offspring	Lead, mercury, possibly organic solvents

* Some human evidence, albeit limited, has linked each health outcome with the occupations listed and with workplace exposure to at least one of the agents listed; for other agents, animal evidence is available.

seminiferous tubules; it has been associated with decreased sperm counts in exposed men. A similar solvent, 2-ethoxyethanol (ethylene glycol monoethyl ether) requires a dose 10-fold higher than 2-methoxyethanol to cause these effects.

Workplace Exposures among Women

Women's fertility can be impaired by toxic occupational exposures in the periconceptual period (Table 24-2). Women who work in agricultural occupations, especially if they mix and apply herbicides or fungicides, have increased rates of fertility problems. Subfecundity has also been identified among women who work intensively with organic solvents in semiconductor manufacture, in woodworking, and in dental offices that handle mercury or nitrous oxide without optimal industrial hygiene measures.[13,14]

Disturbances in ovulation can manifest as menstrual dysfunction. Menstrual disorders have been reported among female agricultural workers, women employed in lead battery plants, female workers exposed to metallic mercury, cosmetologists (who may be exposed to formaldehyde, ethyl acetate, or other chemicals), and shift workers. Antineoplastic drugs disrupt ovarian function not only in cancer patients but also in nurses who handle these drugs without adequate safety precautions.[15]

Exposure to Environmental Pollutants

Doses from exposures to contaminants in food, water, soil, or air are often much lower than doses from highly contaminated workplaces. Nevertheless, adverse reproductive and developmental effects have been linked to certain environmental pollutants, especially those that bioaccumulate (Table 24-3).

Table 24-3. Selected Environmental Pollutants Associated with Adverse Reproductive and Developmental Effects

Agents	Sources*	Adverse Effects
2,3,7,8-tetrachlorodibenzo-p-dioxin	Industrial releases, food chain	Worsened semen parameters, altered sex ratio, immune system disorders, altered timing of puberty, endometriosis, various cancers in laboratory animals
Pesticides such as DDT, dieldrin, mirex, lindane, methoxyclor, and chlordecone	Food chain, household contamination	Early pregnancy loss, male urogenital defects, low birthweight, neurobehavioral disorders, immune system disorders, possibly childhood cancer, earlier menopause
Polychlorinated biphenyls	Fish with high oil content, such as salmon, trout or mackerel; fatty foods, household contamination	Endometriosis, subfecundity, reduced birthweight, immune system disorders
Polybrominated diphenyl ethers	Household dust contaminated with flame retardants from textiles, polyurethane foam and plastics; food chain	Neurobehavioral impairment
Perfluorooctane sulfonate, perflurooctanoic acid	Drinking water, household dust contaminated with stain-resisting agents applied to textiles, industrial releases	Neurobehavioral impairment
Human estrogens, bisphenol A	Drinking water contaminated with pharmaceuticals from human and animal waste, food stored in polycarbonate or epoxy resin containers	Reduced male fertility, altered prostate and mammary development, earlier puberty in girls
Phthalates, parabens	Body care products, cosmetics, sunscreen	Worsened semen parameters
Trihalomethanes	Drinking water purified by processes, such as chlorination	Spontaneous abortion, low birthweight
Lead	Paint containing lead (used for home interiors in the United States until the 1970s), homes and yards contaminated by leaded gasoline exhaust, industrial releases	Pregnancy-induced hypertension, preterm birth, fetal growth restriction, immune system disorders, neurobehavioral impairment
Arsenic	Drinking water	Spontaneous abortion, preterm birth
Methylmercury	Large predatory fish, such as shark, swordfish, king mackerel, and tilefish; industrial releases	Birth defects, neurobehavioral impairment
Polyaromatic hydrocarbons, particulates, other air pollutants	Motor vehicles, solid fuel used to heat homes or cook, industrial emissions	Early pregnancy loss, low birthweight, immune system disorders

* Exposure to many of these pollutants may also occur during breastfeeding.

Endocrine-disrupting chemicals may affect function of reproductive other hormones. Human estrogens can be pollutants; after routine wastewater treatment, the effluent contains residual amounts of estradiol, estrone, and other pharmaceuticals that frequently enter the water supply from human and livestock waste.

Women's fertility can be impaired by endometriosis, which has been induced in monkeys by TCDD. A significant exposure–response relationship has been found between PCBs and phthalate esters and severity of endometriosis.[16]

Bisphenol A is present in more than 90% of school-age children and adults in the United States. Low doses of this substance have been associated with adverse reproductive outcomes, such as reduced sperm counts and miscarriages.[17] People are exposed to bisphenol A when it leaches into food and beverages from containers manufactured with polycarbonate plastics and epoxy resins.

Male fertility can be affected by pollutants through processes that span generations. Exposure of pregnant rats during fetal testicular development to vinclozolin, an antiandrogen, or methoxyclor, an estrogenic pesticide, reduces sperm production in offspring. These offspring transmit the impairment to subsequent generations through an epigenetic mechanism mediated by DNA methylation.[18] Chemicals can also alter ovarian gene expression.

During the past 40 years, average sperm counts have decreased in several geographic regions, and rates of hypospadias, cryptorchidism, and testicular cancer have risen.[19] Pollutants with estrogenic or antiandrogenic properties are suspected of causing these changes because they can cause these problems in laboratory animals. For example, in one study, serum TCDD levels were associated with reduced semen parameters in men who had been environmentally exposed to TCDD during infancy or early childhood.[20] TCDD suppresses activity of androgens, which are necessary for stimulating Sertoli cell proliferation in the testicles during infancy and early childhood. One systematic review and meta-analysis[19] focused on longitudinal studies that evaluated data from prenatal or perinatal pollutant measurements in

biological materials (maternal blood or urine, placenta, fat tissue, amniotic fluid, cord blood, or breast milk). Although the researchers did not demonstrate a clear increase in any single male reproductive disorder associated with suspected endocrine disruptors, prenatal DDE exposure increased the risk for the composite outcome of having one of three disorders (cryptorchidism, hypospadias, or testicular cancer). On the other hand, the increase in testicular cancer incidence from 1960 to 2014 was confined to males 15 to 29 years of age in Nordic countries, suggesting that exposures during childhood and adolescence may be as important as prenatal exposures.[21] Case-control studies showing higher blood levels of pollutants, such as chlordane and PCBs, near the time of testicular cancer diagnosis support this hypothesis.

Pollutants may adversely affect reproductive outcomes by mechanisms other than endocrine disruption. For example, polycyclic aromatic hydrocarbons (PAHs)—products of fossil-fuel combustion and tobacco smoke—can cause oocyte destruction and ovarian failure in mice. Maternal PAH exposure has been associated with birth defects, such as neural tube defects, in a region that was polluted from burning coal; women with high placental PAH levels had a 10-fold increase in risk for having a child with a neural tube defect.[22]

PREGNANCY

Working women have better pregnancy outcomes than unemployed women, especially in high-income countries—likely the result of healthy behaviors, such as avoidance of smoking and alcohol during pregnancy and the economic benefits derived from working, such as better nutrition and improved access to healthcare. However, some employment-related exposures increase the risk for adverse pregnancy outcomes (Table 24-2).

Fetal development is rapid during the first weeks of gestation, before a woman knows she is pregnant. The critical period for development of the heart, central nervous system, limbs, and kidneys begins at 3 to 4 weeks gestation. A hazardous exposure can disrupt the complex process of DNA transcription, protein synthesis, and signal transduction, as well as cell division, differentiation, and migration. The second and third trimesters are characterized by significant growth of the fetus and by differentiation and maturation of organ systems. Therefore, exposure to toxic agents after the first trimester can still cause problems in the developing fetus.

Miscarriage (Spontaneous Abortion)

Hazardous exposures cause early fetal loss in laboratory animal studies. Epidemiologic studies have demonstrated associations between miscarriage in humans and embryotoxic exposures. These exposures include organic solvents, such as chloroform, methyl alcohol, methylene chloride, and perchloroethylene, in occupations that include dry-cleaning, semiconductor or shoe manufacture, and laboratory work. Metals, such as lead and mercury, and anesthetic gases, such as enflurane, halothane, and nitrous oxide, are embryotoxic. Certain pharmaceuticals handled by healthcare workers, such as antineoplastic agents, pentamidine, ganciclovir, and ribavirin are embryotoxic in animals. Environmental pollutants, including polybrominated biphenyls, PAHs, and some pesticides (such as chlordecone, chlorpyrifos, and lindane) can cause fetal loss.

Healthcare workers may be exposed to antineoplastic drugs or sterilizing agents, such as ethylene oxide; poorly controlled exposure to these agents has been associated with increased miscarriage rates.[23] Exposure to lead, even at moderate levels, has been associated with spontaneous abortion. Heavy contamination with mercury from gold and mercury mines in low- and middle-income countries has caused miscarriage and fetal neurotoxicity.[24]

Women in agricultural families may have an increased risk for miscarriage. Although many of the highly toxic, chlorinated hydrocarbon pesticides have been banned from use in the United States and European countries, these chemicals are still applied widely in low- and middle-income countries and persist in the environment. Higher serum levels of DDT metabolites correlate with higher rates of spontaneous abortion.[25] Studies examining the effects of drinking-water contaminants on fetal loss have yielded

mixed results; however, high exposures to chlorination byproducts ((trihalomethanes) and arsenic have been associated with high risk of spontaneous abortion.[26,27]

Birth Defects

Many of the same exposures that increase risk for miscarriage increase risk for congenital anomalies. Infants born to women exposed during pregnancy to halogenated aliphatic solvents, glycol ethers, and benzene and other organic solvents may be at increased risk for development of major congenital malformations, including orofacial clefts.[28,29]

Maternal lead exposure may increase the risk for neural tube defects, perhaps by interfering with folate metabolism. Agricultural work by pregnant women has been linked to risk of limb defects. Other maternal exposures that may increase risks for birth defects include aliphatic aldehydes or acids, antineoplastic drugs, propellants, dyes and pigments, work as a hairdresser or housekeeper, and professional application of pesticides in the home.

Ionizing radiation exposure may occur among healthcare workers or flight crews. Substantially higher radiation doses are required to induce birth defects than those received in usual occupational settings. Selected healthcare workers may be at risk for acquiring infections in the workplace during pregnancy that can cause congenital anomalies (Table 24-2).

Endocrine-disrupting pollutants have been associated with increased rates of urogenital genital malformations in boys. Although results are not completely consistent, some studies based on biologic monitoring of exposures have confirmed associations between tissue levels of endocrine-disrupting chemicals and hypospadias and cryptorchidism.[19]

Low Birthweight

Low birthweight may occur due to preterm birth or fetal growth restriction. For many infants born with very low birthweight, early delivery was required because of pregnancy complications, such as placental abruption or eclampsia. Maternal exposure to organic solvents at work has been associated with preeclampsia and other causes of preterm birth (Table 24-2). Pregnancy-induced hypertension has been linked to lead exposure from air pollution; blood lead levels above 10 µg/dL increase this risk. A study in a community with a secondary lead smelter found that placental lead levels were higher in infants who were preterm.[30]

The risk for having a small-for-gestational-age infant increases in jobs requiring prolonged standing (more than 6 hours), frequent heavy lifting, irregular shifts, or job stress combined with low social support—especially when three or all four of these characteristics are present.[31] Modest off-duty exercise among healthy pregnant women does not increase this risk. Fetal growth restriction is also associated with intensive exposure to many of the chemicals that increase the risk for spontaneous abortion. Simultaneous exposure may occur to multiple workplace chemicals; for example, exposures in the rubber industry include nitrosamines, phthalates, and PAHs. If both parents work in the rubber industry, reduction in birthweight is equivalent to the effect of maternal smoking.[32]

Air pollution has been associated with low birthweight, although the magnitude of risk is small for low-level exposures and some studies have not found this association. In the Czech Republic, among 108,173 births, preterm birth rates increased 18% for every 50 µg/m³ increase in total suspended particulates and 27% for every 50 µg/m³ increase in sulfur dioxide.[33] Fetal growth restriction is also increased by prolonged exposure to environmental tobacco smoke, especially if this is combined with exposure to highly polluted outdoor air. Many studies show that certain gene polymorphisms reduce the ability to detoxify tobacco smoke and other hazardous chemicals, and this may explain differences in susceptibility to adverse reproductive outcomes from these exposures.

Contamination of drinking water with benzene or chlorinated solvents has been associated with low birthweight in several populations. Some studies show no relationship between birthweight and halogenated by-products from water purification, but trihalomethane levels above regulatory limits (> 80 µg/L) increase the risk of fetal growth restriction.[34] Maternal plasma PCB levels are associated with reduced birthweight. Dietary sources of PCBs include fish with high oil content (Table 24-3). Consuming four meals of fish with high oil content per month correlates with a 50% increase in maternal PCB levels.[35]

Developmental Immunotoxicity

The fetal immune system, which develops in a coordinated process involving the thymus, liver, and bone marrow, produces specialized clones of cells primed to respond to foreign antibodies and other threats. The immune system develops in stages throughout pregnancy and postnatal life. The impact of toxicant exposure varies according to the timing of exposure. Consequences include increased susceptibility to infections, greater risk for allergies, and increased occurrence of asthma, childhood leukemia, and auto-immune diseases, such as type 1 diabetes and autoimmune thyroid disorders.[36] The developing immune system is less able to withstand toxic exposures than the adult immune system. TCDD administered to pregnant rats and mice causes atrophy of the fetal thymus at lower doses than are required for the same effect to occur in adult animals; prenatal TCDD exposure in laboratory animals also alters the development and function T-lymphocyte lineages and increases the risk for later autoimmunity. Children exposed to maternal smoking prenatally have an increased risk of developing asthma. PCBs reduce infant responses to the measles-mumps-rubella vaccine. Agents that damage the fetal immune system in laboratory animals include mercury, lead, cadmium, DDT, diazinon, chlordane, methoxychlor, and bisphenol A.

Breastfeeding

In 1951, DDT was found in breast milk. Since then, many other chemical contaminants have been found in breast milk, including heavy metals (mercury, lead, cadmium, and arsenic) organic solvents, organochlorine insecticides (DDT, chlordane, dieldrin, aldrin, heptachlor, hexa-chlorobenzene, and hexachlorocyclohexane), and other environmental chemicals with high lipid solubility and long half-lives (PCBs, furans, TCDD, and PBDEs). Although breast milk can deliver significant amounts of these chemicals to an infant, some studies have demonstrated that the benefits of breastfeeding outweigh the risks of chemical contaminants.[37] Since the 1970s, levels of DDT metabolites have declined in breast milk in countries where they have been banned or regulated, such as the United States, Canada, and the nations of Western Europe.[38] Unlike DDT, PBDEs remain in widespread use in the United States. Breast milk from U.S. mothers has PDBE levels that are 10 times higher than those in Europe, where PBDEs are more highly regulated.[1]

LATENT EFFECTS

There are several well-documented examples of prenatal exposures that produce effects that are more prominent during childhood or adulthood than during infancy.

Childhood

Neurobehavioral effects from prenatal toxicant exposures can be detected in newborns, but important effects may not manifest themselves until later in childhood. Lead exposure is the best documented toxic risk factor for childhood neurobehavioral problems. (See Chapters 23 and 30.) Low-level lead exposure during brain development is associated with childhood problems in memory, learning, and behavior, all of which may persist through adolescence. Studies in laboratory animals demonstrate that gestational exposure to lead without postnatal exposure is sufficient to cause persistent learning and memory deficits.[39]

Because mercury is a developmental neurotoxicant that bioaccumulates in fish, health agencies have recommended that pregnant and lactating women limit their consumption of fish, especially large predatory species (Table 24-3). Blood mercury levels in about 8% of U.S. women of childbearing age exceed the dose recommended by the Environmental Protection Agency.

Occupational exposure to organic solvents in the prenatal period has been associated with decreased neurobehavioral performance during childhood. A study demonstrated that 3- to 7-year-old children whose mothers worked with organic solvents during pregnancy scored lower than controls on tests of language and

graphomotor skillse and more often exhibited problem behaviors.[40] Deficits in color vision, which in adults have been linked with occupational exposure to organic solvents, occur more frequently among children whose mothers were exposed to organic solvents during pregnancy.

Environmental exposure to PCBs impairs neurodevelopment in children. PBDEs produce hyperactivity and impair learning and memory in rodents.[1] Interference with thyroid hormone function by these compounds may contribute to their neurotoxicity. Higher perfluorooctane sulfonate levels in maternal blood during pregnancy increase risk for hyperactivity and child behavior problems.[41] Reducing air pollution can improve children's neurologic development. When a coal-burning power plant in China was closed, DNA adducts from PAHs decreased from 0.32 to 0.20 adducts/10^8 nucleotides and the proportion of 2-year-olds who had delayed motor development decreased from 15% to 5%.[42]

Exposure to endocrine-disrupting chemicals alters the timing of puberty in humans and laboratory animals.[43] Lead and TCDD delay the onset of puberty in girls and boys, whereas higher DDT, PCB, PBDE, and bisphenol A levels are associated with earlier onset of puberty only in girls. Adolescents with substantially delayed or accelerated puberty may experience psychosocial problems. Early puberty reduces adult height by prematurely ending long bone growth, and younger age at menarche increases the risk of breast cancer.

Diethylstilbestrol (DES) was the first major agent found to cause transplacental carcinogenesis in humans—a phenomenon that is well documented in laboratory animals for a variety of carcinogens. The National Toxicology Program (NTP) and the International Agency for Research on Cancer (IARC) have determined that several pesticides banned from use in LMICs, such as mirex, heptachlor, hexachlorobenzene, and DDT, are carcinogenic. NTP and IARC are concerned that several pesticides that remain in common use, such as ethylene dibromide and lindane, may be carcinogenic to humans. A prospective study of 17,357 children found that the rate of childhood cancer was almost doubled among children whose fathers did not use chemically resistant gloves when handling pesticides.[44]

Adulthood

Some toxicant exposures during prenatal development cause malignant and nonmalignant disorders that may not become evident until adulthood. Drinking water contaminated with arsenic has been associated with bronchiectasis and lung cancer among adults who had been exposed prenatally and during early childhood.[45] Similar findings have been noted in controlled experiments with mice. In-utero exposure to estrogenic compounds alters mammary development and may increase the risk for breast cancer.[46] Prenatal exposure to endocrine disruptors has been associated with testicular cancer and possibly with increased risk for prostate cancer.[17,19]

Obesity during adulthood may be increased by early life exposure to endocrine-disrupting chemicals. Studies in rodents have shown that gestational exposures to endocrine-disrupting compounds, such as bisphenol A, DES, and PCBs are associated with obesity in adulthood.[17,47] Epidemiologic studies have linked endocrine disruptors to obesity and other adverse effects when exposure occurs throughout the life cycle. However, early lifetime exposure is especially likely to cause obesity because it induces epigenetic changes associated with later development of obesity and an increase in the fat cell pool by preferential differentiation of stem cells into fat-storage cells.[47]

Smokers enter menopause sooner than nonsmokers; when tobacco exposure occurs only during the prenatal period, the risk for early menopause is also increased.[48] Premature ovarian senescence has been demonstrated in animals exposed to TCDD and PCBs during gestation.

Nervous system effects are produced in children by fetal exposure to many chemicals found in the environment and workplace. These findings have led to concerns that early life exposure to endocrine disruptors and neurotoxicants may increase the risk for neurodegenerative disorders that occur with aging.[49] (See Chapter 30.)

EVALUATION AND CONTROL OF RISK

Reproductive processes are vulnerable to environmental and occupational hazards in men and women. However, it is often difficult to determine the precise cause of a couple's subfecundity, a child's congenital anomaly, or other health problems because (a) precise assessment of exposures is difficult, (b) other health problems may contribute to these reproductive outcomes, and (c) data from research is imperfect and incomplete.

To assess reproductive risk from a potential exposure, four questions are relevant:

1. **What is the agent?** The names of chemicals can be found on product labels and safety data sheets. Although researching this information is often laborious, it is necessary.

2. **Is exposure actually occurring, and, if so, what are the dose and the timing of exposure?** Exposure to an agent does not necessarily lead to entry into the body. Exposure level is affected by how the agent is handled, what engineering controls have been implemented, and what protective equipment has been used. Toxicant levels can sometimes be measured in blood or body fluids. Inhalational exposures can be estimated with air samples. Skin contact can result in high doses of chemicals being absorbed through the skin, even if air levels are low. A birth defect known to develop at gestational week 7 could not have been caused by an acute exposure that occurred only in the third trimester. Spermatogenesis takes about 70 days to complete, so the critical period for genotoxic male exposures is thought to be about 2 to 3 months before conception.

3. **Is there evidence to suggest that a particular agent causes adverse reproductive or developmental effects?** A comprehensive literature review or consultation with an expert in reproductive hazard assessment is needed to answer this question.

4. **Given the available evidence, does the agent pose a significant reproductive or developmental risk?** Available data can help estimate the degree of risk. A mildly elevated blood lead level during pregnancy, for example, will not lead to severe mental retardation. It is important to place the potential exposure in context, taking into account other concurrent exposures as well

as biologic risks, including parental age, medical problems (such as poorly controlled diabetes mellitus), medications (such as certain antiepileptic, psychotropic, and anticoagulant drugs), substance use or abuse, and family history of heritable syndromes.

Data from animal research and epidemiologic studies have demonstrated that certain occupational and environmental exposures are associated with adverse reproductive or developmental outcomes (Tables 24-1, 24-2, and 24-3). A precautionary approach is warranted, emphasizing avoidance of hazardous exposures beginning in the preconception period for men and women. The following case illustrates this approach.

CASE STUDY

A 27-year-old-man presented for medical evaluation because of inability to conceive with his 25-year-old wife for 13 months. In his job at an automobile repair shop, he disassembled radiators with an oxygen-acetylene torch and resoldered them with lead-tin solder. There was no ventilation of his dusty work station. His wife washed his workclothes, which were laden with lead dust, at home. The medical workup of his wife's infertility revealed no abnormalities. A semen analysis indicated that his sperm count was in the extreme lower end of the normal range (18 million sperm/ml), as well as mildly abnormal motility and morphology. His blood lead level (BLL) was 63 μg/dL and his wife's BLL was 22 μg/dL.

This man had lead poisoning from exposure to lead fumes and dust. Washing of his workclothes most likely accounted for his wife's elevated BLL.

Sometimes it is difficult to determine if a fertility problem is related to a toxicant exposure, although causality is suggested by improvement in sperm indices after reduction or removal of the exposure. Because of the OSHA lead standard, this man was eligible for medical removal from occupational exposure, without loss of wages or benefits, because his BLL was over 60 μg/dL. An OSHA workplace inspection could have identified control measures to protect all workers. The man should have been evaluated by a physician with expertise in treating lead poisoning. The couple should have

been counseled about the hazards of lead and ways to minimize exposures through safer work practices and prevention of home contamination with workplace lead dust. The couple should use contraception until their BLLs fall to 10 μg/dL or lower, a level that should not be exceeded during pregnancy.

REFERENCES

1. Costa LG, Giordano G. Developmental neurotoxicity of polybrominated diphenyl ether (PBDE) flame retardants. Neurotoxicology 2007; 28: 1047–1067.
2. Levy BS, Levin JL, Teitelbaum DT (eds.). DBCP-induced sterility and reduced fertility among men in developing countries: A case study of the export of a known hazard. International Journal of Occupational and Environmental Health 1999; 5: 115–150.
3. Mitro SD, Johnson T, Zota AR. Cumulative chemical exposures during pregnancy and early development. Current Environmental Health Reports 2015; 2: 367–378.
4. Miranda ML, Edwards SE, Swamy GK, et al. Blood lead levels among pregnant women: Historical versus contemporaneous exposures. International Journal of Environmental Research and Public Health 2010; 7: 1508–1519.
5. Mattison DR. Environmental exposures and development. Current Opinion in Pediatrics 2010; 22: 208–218.
6. Demarini DM. Declaring the existence of human germ-cell mutagens. Environmental and Molecular Mutagenesis 2012; 53: 166–172.
7. Terrell ML, Hartnett KP, Marcus M. Can environmental or occupational hazards alter the sex ratio at birth? A systematic review. Emerging Health Threats Journal 2011; 4: 10.3402/ehtj.v4i0.7109.
8. Perry MJ. Effects of environmental and occupational pesticide exposure on human sperm: A systematic review. Human Reproduction Update 2008; 14: 233–242.
9. Hanke W, Jurewicz J. The risk of adverse reproductive and developmental disorders due to occupational pesticide exposure: An overview of current epidemiological evidence. International Journal of Occupational Medicine and Environmental Health 2004; 17: 223–243.
10. Arbuckle TE, Savitz DA, Mery LS, Curtis KM. Exposure to phenoxy herbicides and the risk of spontaneous abortion. Epidemiology 1999; 10: 752–760.

11. Salazar-Garcia F, Gallardo-Diaz E, Ceron-Mireles P, et al. Reproductive effects of occupational DDT exposure among male malaria control workers. Environmental Health Perspectives 2004; 112: 542–547.

12. Jensen TK, Bonde JP, Joffe M. The influence of occupational exposure on male reproductive function. Occupational Medicine (London) 2006; 56: 544–553.

13. Chen PC, Hsieh GY, Wang JD et al. Prolonged time to pregnancy in female workers exposed to ethylene glycol ethers in semiconductor manufacturing. Epidemiology 2002; 13: 191–196.

14. Olfert SM. Reproductive outcomes among dental personnel: A review of selected exposures. Journal of the Canadian Dental Association 2006; 72: 821–825.

15. Chasle S, How CC. The effect of cytotoxic chemotherapy on female fertility. European Journal of Oncology Nursing 2003; 7: 91–98.

16. Reddy BS, Rozati R, Reddy S, et al. High plasma concentrations of polychlorinated biphenyls and phthalate esters in women with endometriosis: A prospective case control study. Fertility and Sterility 2006; 85: 775–779.

17. Hutz RJ, Carvan MJ, Larson JK, et al. Familiar and novel reproductive endocrine disruptors: Xenoestrogens, dioxins and nanoparticles. Current Trends in Endocrinology 2014; 7: 111–122.

18. Guerrero-Bosagna C, Skinner MK. Environmentally induced epigenetic transgenerational inheritance of male infertility. Current Opinion in Genetics and Development 2014; 26: 79–88.

19. Bonde JP, Flachs EM, Rimborg S, et al. The epidemiologic evidence linking prenatal and postnatal exposure to endocrine disrupting chemicals with male reproductive disorders: A systematic review and meta-analysis. Human Reproduction Update 2017; 23: 104–125.

20. Mocarelli P, Gerthoux PM, Patterson DG Jr, et al. Dioxin exposure, from infancy through puberty, produces endocrine disruption and affects human semen quality. Environmental Health Perspectives 2008; 116: 70–77.

21. Giannandrea F, Fargnoli S. Environmental factors affecting growth and occurrence of testicular cancer in childhood: An overview of the current epidemiological evidence. Children 2017; 4:1. doi:10.3390/children4010001.

22. Yuan Y, Jin L, Wang L, et al. Levels of PAH-DNA Adducts in placental tissue and the risk of fetal neural tube defects in a Chinese population. Reproductive Toxicology 2013; 37: 70–75.

23. Lawson CC, Rocheleau CM, Whelan EA, et al. Occupational exposures among nurses and risk of spontaneous abortion. American Journal of Obstetrics and Gynecology 2012; 206:327.e1–327.e8.

24. Maramba NP, Reyes JP, Francisco-Rivera AT, et al. Environmental and human exposure assessment monitoring of communities near an abandoned mercury mine in the Philippines: A toxic legacy. Journal of Environmental Management 2006; 81: 135–145.

25. Korrick SA, Chen C, Damokosh AI, et al. Association of DDT with spontaneous abortion: A case-control study. Annals of Epidemiology 2001; 11: 491–496.

26. Stillerman KP, Mattison DR, Giudice LC, et al. Environmental exposures and adverse pregnancy outcomes: A review of the science. Reproductive Sciences 2008; 15: 631–650.

27. Milton AH, Smith W, Rahman B, et al. Chronic arsenic exposure and adverse pregnancy outcomes in Bangladesh. Epidemiology 2005; 16: 82–86.

28. Cordier S, Garlantézec R, Labat L, et al. Exposure during pregnancy to glycol ethers and chlorinated solvents and the risk of congenital malformations. Epidemiology 2012; 23: 806–812.

29. Desrosiers TA, Lawson CC, Meyer RE, et al. Maternal occupational exposure to organic solvents during early pregnancy and risks of neural tube defects and orofacial clefts. Occupational and Environmental Medicine 2012; 69: 493–499.

30. Baghurst PA, Robertson EF, Oldfield RK, et al. Lead in the placenta, membranes, and umbilical cord in relation to pregnancy outcome in a lead-smelter community. Environmental Health Perspectives 1991; 90: 315–320.

31. Croteau A, Marcoux S, Brisson C. Work activity in pregnancy, preventive measures, and the risk of delivering a small-for-gestational-age infant. American Journal of Public Health 2006; 96: 846–855.

32. Jakobsson K, Mikoczy Z. Reproductive outcome in a cohort of male and female rubber workers: A registry study. International Archives of Occupational and Environmental Health 2009; 82: 165–174.

33. Bobak M. Outdoor air pollution, low birth weight, and prematurity. Environmental Health Perspectives 2000; 108: 173–176.

34. Hoffman CS, Mendola P, Savitz DA, et al. Drinking water disinfection by-product exposure and fetal growth. Epidemiology 2008; 19: 729–737.

35. Halldorsson TI, Thorsdottir I, Meltzer HM, et al. Linking exposure to polychlorinated biphenyls with fatty fish consumption and reduced fetal growth among Danish pregnant women: A cause for concern? American Journal of Epidemiology 2008; 168: 958–965.

36. Hertz-Picciotto I, Park HY, Dostal M, et al. Prenatal exposures to persistent and non-persistent organic compounds and effects on immune system development. Basic and Clinical Pharmacology and Toxicology 2008; 102: 146–154.

37. Ribas-Fito N, Cardo E, Sala M, et al. Breastfeeding, exposure to organochlorine compounds, and neurodevelopment in infants. Pediatrics 2003; 111: e580–e585.

38. Smith D. Worldwide trends in DDT levels in human breast milk. International Journal of Epidemiology 1999; 28: 179–188.

39. Yang Y, Ma Y, Ni L, et al. Lead exposure through gestation-only caused long-term learning/memory deficits in young adult offspring. Experimental Neurology 2003; 184: 489–495.

40. Pelé F, Muckle G, Costet N, et al. Occupational solvent exposure during pregnancy and child behaviour at age 2. Occupational and Environmental Medicine 2013; 70: 114–119.

41. Høyer BB, Ramlau-Hansen CH, Obel C, et al. Pregnancy serum concentrations of perfluorinated alkyl substances and offspring behaviour and motor development at age 5–9 years—A prospective study. Environmental Health 2015; 14: 2. doi:10.1186/1476-069X-14-2.

42. Perera F, Lu TY, Zhou ZJ, et al. Benefits of reducing prenatal exposure to coal-burning pollutants to children's neurodevelopment in China. Environmental Health Perspectives 2008; 116: 1396–1400.

43. Jacobson-Dickman E, Lee MM. The influence of endocrine disruptors on pubertal timing. Current Opinion in Endocrinology, Diabetes and Obesity 2009; 16: 25–30.

44. Flower KB, Hoppin JA, Lynch CF, et al. Cancer risk and parental pesticide application in children of agricultural health study participants. Environmental Health Perspectives 2004; 112: 631–635.

45. Vahter M. Health effects of early life exposure to arsenic. Basic Clinical Pharmacology and Toxicology 2008; 102: 204–211.

46. Fenton SE, Birnbaum LS. Timing of environmental exposures as a critical element in breast cancer risk. Journal of Clinical Endocrinology and Metabolism 2015; 100: 3245–3250.

47. Nappi F, Barrea L, Di Somma C, et al. Endocrine aspects of environmental "obesogen" pollutants. International Journal of Environmental Research and Public Health 2016; 13: 765. doi:10.3390/ijerph13080765.

48. Strohsnitter WC, Hatch EE, Hyper M, et al. The association between in utero cigarette smoke exposure and age at menopause. American Journal of Epidemiology 2008; 167: 727–733.

49. Weiss B. Endocrine disruptors as a threat to neurological function. Journal of the Neurological Sciences 2011; 305: 11–21.

FURTHER READING

Chevrier C, Dananche B, Bahuau M, et al. Occupational exposure to organic solvent mixtures during pregnancy and the risk of non-syndromic oral clefts. Occupational and Environmental Medicine 2006; 63: 617–623.
A case-control study of exposure to chlorinated solvents, possible association between oral clefts and glycol ethers, petroleum solvents, and aliphatic alcohols.

Frazier LM, Hage ML (eds.). Reproductive hazards of the workplace. New York: John Wiley & Sons, 1998.
This text provides practical strategies for assessing and managing occupational reproductive and developmental risks. It reviews chemicals and other common hazards in the workplace.

Hauser R, Meeker JD, Duty S, et al. Altered semen quality in relation to urinary concentrations of phthalate monoester and oxidative metabolites. Epidemiology 2006; 17: 682–691.
Abnormally low sperm concentration was 3.3 times more common among men whose urinary monobutyl phthalate level was high.

Qin X, Wu Y, Wang W, et al. Low organic solvent exposure and combined maternal infant gene polymorphisms affect gestational age. Occupational and Environmental Medicine 2008; 65: 482–487.
A genetic epidemiology study of birth outcomes among a cohort of 1,113 women who worked for a large petrochemical company. Gestation was significantly shorter when the mother had organic solvent exposure and both she and her infant lacked certain cytochrome P450 genes that help detoxify chemicals.

Shepard TH, Lemire RJ. Catalog of teratogenic agents (12th ed.). Baltimore: Johns Hopkins University Press, 2007.
This book describes more than 3,000 agents, including pharmaceuticals, chemicals, environmental pollutants, food additives, household products, viruses, and genes, that cause heritable syndromes or congenital anomalies. It also includes overviews of clinical and experimental teratology.

25

Skin Disorders

Loren C. Tapp and Boris D. Lushniak

The skin plays an important role in providing a protective, living barrier between the external environment of the world around us and the internal environment of the human body. As a first-line protective barrier, the cutaneous surface is also subject to the hostile forces of the external environment and, as such, can be directly injured or damaged by these environmental forces.

In general, the causes of environmental skin disorders can be grouped into the following categories:

1. *Physical insults*: Friction, pressure, trauma, vibration, heat, cold, variations in humidity, radiation (ultraviolet, visible, infrared, and ionizing), and electric current
2. *Biological causes*: Plants, bacteria, rickettsiae, viruses, fungi, protozoa, parasites, and arthropods
3. *Chemical insults*: Water, inorganic acids, alkalis, salts of heavy metals, aliphatic acids, aldehydes, alcohols, esters, hydrocarbons, solvents, metallo-organic compounds, lipids, aromatic and polycyclic compounds, resin monomers, and proteins.

These insults are present in every aspect of our environment and can affect the skin in the home setting, during outdoor and leisure activities, while involved in hobbies, and in the work environment. Occupational dermatology is the facet of dermatology that deals with skin diseases whose etiology or aggravation is related to some exposure in the workplace. The role of a healthcare practitioner involved in occupational dermatology is not only to diagnose and treat patients but also to determine the etiology of occupational skin diseases and make recommendations for their prevention. Making the diagnosis and offering treatment, determining etiology, and recommending preventive measures all can be difficult undertakings.

Environmental and occupational skin diseases can manifest themselves in a variety of ways. This chapter emphasizes skin conditions caused by environmental agents that have a direct effect on the skin. These include irritant contact dermatitis, allergic contact dermatitis, contact urticaria, skin infections, skin cancers, and a large group of miscellaneous skin diseases. Certain common skin diseases, such as atopic dermatitis and psoriasis, are exacerbated by environmental factors, but their etiology remains unclear and they are not covered here.

CONTACT DERMATITIS

Contact dermatitis is the most common occupational and environmental skin disease. Epidemiologic data show that contact dermatitis comprises 90% to 95% of all occupational skin diseases.[1,2] *Contact dermatitis*—both irritant and allergic—is an inflammatory skin condition caused by skin contact with an exogenous agent or agents, with or without a concurrent exposure to a contributory physical agent, such as ultraviolet light. It can result from a nonimmunologic reaction to chemical irritants (irritant contact dermatitis) or from an immunologic reaction to allergens (allergic contact dermatitis). Irritant contact dermatitis is a cutaneous inflammation resulting from a direct cytotoxic effect of a chemical or physical agent, while allergic contact dermatitis is a type IV, delayed or cell-mediated, immune reaction. There are over 57,000 chemicals reported to cause skin irritation, but only 4,350 chemicals are known skin allergens.[3] These are mostly confined to small-molecular-weight chemicals that act as haptens, and usually only a small percentage of people are susceptible to them.

In acute contact dermatitis, the skin initially turns red and can develop small, oozing vesicles and papules. After several days, crusts and scales form. Stinging, burning, and itching may accompany the skin lesions. With no further contact with the etiologic agent, the dermatitis usually disappears in 1 to 3 weeks. With chronic exposure, deep fissures, scaling, and hyperpigmentation can occur. Exposed areas of the skin, such as hands and forearms, which have the greatest contact with irritants or allergens, are most commonly affected. Over 80% of occupational contact dermatitis involves the hands.[4,5] If the agent gets on clothing, it can induce dermatitis at areas of greatest contact, such as thighs, upper back, armpits, and feet. Dusts can produce dermatitis at areas where the dust accumulates and is held in contact with the skin, such as under the collar and belt line, at the tops of socks or shoes, and in flexural areas, such as the antecubital and popliteal fossae. Mists can produce a dermatitis on the

face and anterior neck. Irritants and allergens can be transferred to remote areas of the body, such as the trunk or genitalia, by unwashed hands or from areas of accumulation, such as under rings or interdigital areas. It is often impossible to clinically distinguish irritant contact dermatitis from allergic contact dermatitis, as both can have a similar appearance and both can be clinically

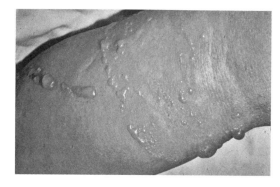

Figure 25-1. Acute contact dermatitis from exposure to ethylene oxide, a strong irritant.

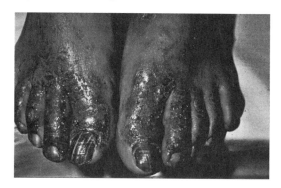

Figure 25-2. Subacute dermatitis from the rubber accelerator mercaptobenzothiazole, which is found in the rubber in a work boot.

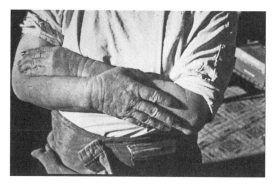

Figure 25-3. Chronic dermatitis from exposure to kerosene, a solvent that was used for cleaning the skin.

evident as an acute, subacute, or chronic condition (Figures 25-1, 25-2, and 25-3).

Public Health Importance

Measures of the public health importance of a disease include the absolute number of cases, the incidence rate, the prevalence (rate), the economic impact of the disease, and the prognosis and preventability of the disease.[6]

Specific national data sources on contact dermatitis are limited. In the United States, data from the National Ambulatory Medical Care Survey, a national probability sample survey of nonfederal office–based physicians, showed that in 2012 skin rash was the principal reason for 12.5 million patient visits—1.3% of all visits for that year.[7] Based upon previous surveys, it is estimated that approximately one-half of these visits would have had a diagnosis of contact dermatitis or other eczemas.

In 2010, the National Health Interview Survey (NHIS) included an Occupational Health Supplement, which included questions on dermatitis. The survey consisted of personal interviews of people in randomly selected households. For 17,524 workers participating in the NHIS, the overall prevalence was 9.8% for all dermatitis; 5.6% of these cases were attributed to work by health professionals. Projecting these results to the U.S. working population resulted in an estimate of 15.2 million workers with dermatitis and 850,000 workers with work-related dermatitis.[8]

Specific national occupational disease and illness data are available from the U.S. Bureau of Labor Statistics (BLS), which conducts annual surveys of approximately 200,000 employers selected to represent all private industries in the United States.[9] All occupational skin diseases or disorders, including contact dermatitis, are tabulated in this survey. Bureau of Labor Statistics data show that occupational skin diseases consistently accounted for 30% to 45% of all cases of occupational illnesses from the 1970s through the mid-1980s, and in recent years accounted for 15 to 18% of all occupational illness.[9] A decline in this proportion may be partially related to an increase seen in disorders associated with repeated trauma.

Table 25-1. Reported Incidence of Occupational Skin Diseases, United States, 2002–2014

Year	Number (in thousands)	Rate (per 100,000)
2002	44.9	51
2003	43.4	49
2004	38.9	44
2005	40.1	44
2006	41.4	45
2007	35.3	37
2008	35.8	38
2009	25.9	29
2010	24.9	29
2011*	–	–
2012*	–	–
2013	26.0	28
2014	21.8	23

* Bureau of Labor Statistics data from 2011 and 2012 contain incorrect national-level estimates and are not shown. http://www.bls.gov/bls/errata/iif_errata_1014.htm

Bureau of Labor Statistics data for occupational skin diseases for 2002 to 2014 are shown in Table 25-1. In 2014, the BLS estimated 21,800 cases of occupational skin diseases or disorders in the U.S. workforce.[9] However, because of BLS survey limitations, it has been estimated that the number of actual occupational skin diseases may be 10 to 50 times higher than that reported by the BLS.[10] This increase would potentially raise the number of occupational skin disease cases to between 218,000 and 1.1 million per year. In 2014, BLS data showed an annual incidence rate of 23 cases per 100,000 workers.[9]

In 2010, the Occupational Health Supplement of the NHIS indicated that the period prevalence for occupational contact dermatitis occurring in the preceding year was 0.55%. Projecting these results to the U.S. working population resulted in an estimate of almost 850,000 people with occupational contact dermatitis and a 1-year period prevalence of 550 per 100,000 workers for the year.[8] The numbers and rates in the BLS and NHIS surveys are not directly comparable because they rely on different information sources with different ascertainment methods and different case definitions.

The economic impact of a disease can be measured by the direct costs of medical care and workers' compensation or disability payments, and the indirect costs associated with lost workdays and lost productivity. The Safety and Health Assessment and Research for

Prevention (SHARP) program analyzed data from Washington State workers' compensation dermatologic claims and work-related skin diseases reported through SHARP's "sentinel provider network" from 1993 through 1997. During these 5 years, close to 5,000 claims were accepted for work-related skin disorders and 42,471 lost workdays (days away from work) were reported, costing more than $1.6 million in time loss payments and $1.5 million in medical bills. Comparison with provider network data estimated that compensation data underrepresents the number of work-related skin disorders by more than four-fold.[11]

An analysis of Oregon workers' compensation claims data for 1990 through 1997 estimated the average claim rate of occupational dermatitis to be 5.7 per 100,000 workers. In this 8-year period, 727 workers' compensation claims were filed for occupational dermatitis, of which 611 were determined to be compensable. The total cost of all dermatitis claims was $2.2 million, averaging about $270,000 annually. Oregon claim rates are lower than other states since reporting is not mandatory unless the incident requires 3 or more days of disability leave, illnesses and injuries from self-employed workers, such as hairdressers, are not reported. The average cost per claim was $3,552, and the average disability time was 24 days.[12]

A review of 2007 BLS data showed that, of the 35,300 reported cases of occupational skin diseases, 5,640 (16%) resulted in days away from work.[9] The median time away from work was 4 days, but 22% of lost-workday cases had 11 or more days away from work. Of those with days away from work, 64% had a diagnosis of dermatitis. In 2014, of the 21,800 skin disease cases, 3,210 (15%) resulted in days away from work. Of these cases, 2,320 (72%) had a diagnosis of acute dermatitis, with a median of 2 days lost, and the remaining 890 cases were reported as skin and subcutaneous tissue disorders.[9] An additional 30 cases had a diagnosis of chronic dermatitis.[9]

Studies on the prognosis of occupational contact dermatitis stress the importance of primary prevention. A questionnaire survey of 124 patients 5 years after they were initially diagnosed with irritant hand dermatitis found 18% with low, 50% with medium, and 32% with severe hand dermatitis. Severity was measured by self-reported frequency of relapses,

frequency of dermatologist visits, and use of topical corticosteroids.[13] A questionnaire survey of 540 patients 1 year after initial diagnosis of occupational hand dermatitis found 41% were improved and 25% had persistently severe or aggravated symptoms. Poor prognosis was associated with the presence of atopic dermatitis and being 25 years of age or older. Prognosis was not affected by whether the dermatitis was irritant or allergic. Those with severe occupational hand dermatitis at baseline had a higher risk of taking sick leave and job loss in the following year than those with mild cases. The study found no significant improvement in the disease after the change of job. Severe impairment of quality of life at baseline was a strong predictor of prolonged sick leave, but the presence of depression did not affect prolonged sick leave.[14] A study that followed patients with occupational allergic contact dermatitis 2 years after diagnosis found that 89% had persistent dermatitis and that workers who had changed jobs improved significantly more frequently than those who did not.[15]

Persistent postoccupational dermatitis (PPOD) can occur following allergic or irritant contact dermatitis. Persistent postoccupational dermatitis begins as a clear-cut occupational contact dermatitis, initially gets better when removed from exposure, but with time the capacity for resolution is lost and persistent dermatitis develops. Predictive factors for PPOD include duration of disease, inability to avoid causative agents, and age.[16] Widespread hand dermatitis on initial examination was found to be the greatest factor for a poor long-term prognosis; other important factors identified include young age at onset of hand dermatitis, history of childhood eczema, and contact allergy.[17] Outcomes may or may not be influenced by leaving the dermatitis-provoking job. In addition, many skin disorders, including contact dermatitis, have been shown to have a significant impact on quality of life.[18-21]

Over the years, there have been changes in the epidemiology of occupational skin diseases. A decrease in the absolute number of cases and in the incidence rate in the BLS survey from the 1970s to the early 21st century may be attributable to several factors, including changes in industry and industrial practices, increased awareness and preventive measures, and possible underreporting, underrecognition, and misclassification. Still, occupational contact dermatitis remains a relatively common disease with a noteworthy public health impact. These factors, along with the potential chronicity of the disorder, its effect on an individual's vocational and avocational activities, and its preventability make occupational contact dermatitis a disease of public health importance.

Population at Risk and Etiologic Agents

There are many occupations that have unique exposures resulting in occupational contact dermatitis. Total numbers and incidence rates of occupational dermatologic conditions, by major industry division, based on the BLS survey for 2014 are shown in Table 25-2.[9] The greatest number of cases of occupational skin diseases is seen in education and health services, but the highest incidence rate is seen in the category natural resources and mining.

In 2010, the NHIS found that the occupational groups with the highest prevalence of dermatitis included healthcare, personal care, and service workers; workers in life, physical, and social sciences; and workers in the arts, entertainment, and recreation industries.[8] Of all accepted workers' compensation claims for occupational contact dermatitis in Oregon, the occupations with highest claim rates were farming, fishing, and forestry workers (18.2%); machine operators and assemblers (16.5%); service-related workers

(15.3%); laborers (13.7%); precision production crafts workers (8.0%); and protective services workers (5.7%), followed by technicians and related support workers, transportation and material movers, and professional specialty, administrative support, executive, administrative, and sales employees.[12] Self-employed individuals, such as hairdressers and cosmetologists, are not represented in these claims.

The etiology of irritant contact dermatitis is often multifactorial, but the most common skin irritant is wet work, defined as exposure of skin to liquid for more than 2 hours per day, use of occlusive gloves for more than 2 hours per day, or frequent hand cleaning.[22,23] Other common causes of irritant contact dermatitis include soaps and detergents, solvents, food products, cleaning agents, plastics and resins, petroleum products and lubricants, metals, and machine oils and coolants.[22,23] Frictional irritant contact dermatitis can be caused from low humidity, heat, paper, tools, metals, fabrics, plastics, fibrous glass and other particulate dusts, cardboard, and other exposures.[24,25] Causes of allergic contact dermatitis include plants (poison ivy, poison oak, and poison sumac), metallic salts, germicides, plastic resins, rubber additives, and fragrances.[26] The skin patch test allergens found to be most relevant in North American dermatologic patients along with potential sources of exposure are shown in Table 25-3.[27] Recent studies of North American food service workers who were dermatologic patients found 55% with allergic contact dermatitis; most frequent allergens included thiuram mix and carba mix found in gloves.[28] Among North American hairdressers and cosmetologists who were dermatologic patients, 73% were diagnosed with allergic contact dermatitis; relevant occupational allergens included glyceryl thioglycolate, p-phenyldiamine, nickel sulfate, and 2-hydroxyethyl methacrylate found in hair and nail products.[29] Among North American mechanics and repairers who were dermatologic patients, rubber accelerators (from gloves and auto parts) and methylchlorisothiazolinone/methylisothiazolinone (a preservative in oils, lubricants, solvents, and fuels) were the most comment occupationally related allergens.[30] A study of workers' compensation records in Portland, Oregon, from 2005 to 2014 found that the most relevant skin allergens in

Table 25-2. Incidence of Occupational Skin Diseases, by Industry Sector, 2014

Industry	Number	Rate (per 100,000)
Natural resources and mining	1,000	55
Education and health services	6,100	40
Manufacturing	4,400	36
Leisure and hospitality	3,000	32
Construction	1,100	20
Professional and business services	2,100	15
Trade/transport/utilities	3,100	14
Other services	300	11
Financial activities	400	6
Information	100	5
Total	**21,600**	**23**

Table 25-3. North American Contact Dermatitis Group Patch-Test Results, Ranked by Relevance, 2013–2014[27]

Test Substance	Common Sources	Rank
Methylisothiazolinone 0.2% aq	Biocides, cosmetics, toiletries	1
Nickel sulfate 2.5% pet	Metals, jewelry	2
Fragrance mix I 8% pet	Toiletries, scented products	3
Methylchlorisothiazolinone/ methylisothiazolinone 0.01% aq	Biocides, cosmetics, toiletries	4
Myroxylon pereirae (Balsam of Peru) 25% pet	Skin and haircare products	5
p-Phenylenediamine 1% pet	Hair dyes, leather	6
Fragrance mix II 14% pet	Toiletries, scented products	7
Formaldehyde 2% aq	Textiles, skincare products	8
Lanolin alcohol 50% pet	Skincare products	9
Iodopropynyl butylcarbamate 0.5% pet	Paints, skincare and haircare products	10
Formaldehyde 1% aq	Textiles, skincare products	11
Bacitracin 20% pet.	Topical medicaments	12
Quaternium-15 2% pet	Cosmetics, sunscreens	13
Cinnamic aldehyde 1% pet	Scented toiletries	14
Carba mix 3% pet	Rubber, pesticides	15
Propylene glycol 100% aq	Cosmetics, topical medications	16
Methyldibromoglutaronitrile/ phenoxyethanol 2.0% pet	Biocides, skincare products	17
Cobalt chloride 1% pet	Metals, jewelry	18
Neomycin 20% pet.	Topical medicaments	19
OPDMA 0.1% aq		20

Note. Relevance was based on the Significance-Prevalence Index Number (SPIN), a weighted calculation depending on degree of certainty ascribed to relevance.

SPIN calculation = (proportion of population allergic) × (1 × $R_{definitive}$ + 0.66 × $R_{probable}$ + 0.33 × $R_{possible}$) × 100.

aq = in aqueous solution; pet = in petrolatum.

patients with occupational hand dermatitis who had been skin-patch tested were thiuram mix, carba mix, potassium dichromate, epoxy resin, chloroxylenol PCMX, formaldehyde, and Quaternium-15.[31] In healthcare workers with occupational contact dermatitis who were skin-patch tested, thiuram mix was the most common relevant allergen.[31]

Diagnosis

The environmental cause or work-relatedness of contact dermatitis may be difficult to determine. The accuracy of the diagnosis is related to the skill level, experience, and knowledge of the health professional who makes the diagnosis and confirms the relationship with environmental or workplace exposures. Guidelines are available for assessing the work relatedness of dermatitis, but even with guidelines the diagnosis may be difficult.[2,32] The diagnosis is based on the medical and occupational histories and physical findings. The importance of

the patient's history of exposures and disease onset is clear. Standardized questionnaires for surveying work-related skin diseases are available and can be helpful in the workplace.[33] In irritant contact dermatitis, there are no additional confirmatory tests. Patch tests may be used to distinguish allergic contact dermatitis from irritant contact dermatitis.[23] In many instances, allergic contact dermatitis can be confirmed by skin patch tests using specific standardized allergens or, in some circumstances, by provocation tests with nonirritating dilutions of industrial contactants. Irritant contact dermatitis may be overestimated (and allergic contact dermatitis underestimated) due to time, expense, and availability of skin patch testing; physician experience; and the limited availability of allergens in the United States.[34] Skin patch tests should only be conducted by healthcare professionals trained in conducting and interpreting the tests. Skin patch tests should never be conducted with unknown substances.

Answers to the following questions can help determine work-relatedness:

1. Is the clinical appearance consistent with contact dermatitis?
2. Are there workplace exposures to potential cutaneous irritants or allergens?
3. Is the anatomic distribution of dermatitis consistent with cutaneous exposure in relation to the job task?
4. Is the temporal relationship between exposure and onset consistent with contact dermatitis?
5. Are nonoccupational exposures excluded as probable causes?
6. Does dermatitis improve away from the exposure to the suspected irritant or allergen?
7. Do patch tests or provocation tests identify a probable causal agent?[32]

Prevention

Strategies in the prevention of occupational contact dermatitis include the following:

- Identifying irritants and allergens
- Substituting chemicals that are less irritating or allergenic
- Establishing engineering controls to reduce exposure
- Utilizing personal protective equipment (PPE), such as gloves and special clothing
- Emphasizing personal and occupational hygiene
- Providing educational programs to increase awareness in the workplace[35]

Chemical changes in industrial materials have been beneficial. For example, the addition of ferrous sulfate to cement to reduce the hexavalent chromium content has been effective in reducing occupational allergic contact dermatitis in Europe. Protective gloves can reduce or eliminate skin exposure to hazardous substances if used correctly, but they may actually cause or worsen hand dermatitis (by permeation and penetration) if selected poorly and used improperly (by contamination).[36] The use of PPE may occlude irritants or allergens next to the skin, and PPE components may directly irritate the skin, so the correct use of PPE is at least as important as its selection.[37] Similarly, the excessive pursuit of personal hygiene in the workplace may actually lead to misuse of soaps and detergents, resulting in irritant contact dermatitis. Proper handwashing methods and adequate moisturizing is valuable in preventing contact dermatitis.[5] The effectiveness of barrier creams is controversial since there are limited data on the protective nature of these topical products during actual working conditions involving high-risk exposures. Educating the workforce about skin care, exposures, and PPE use is an especially important measure in the prevention of occupational contact dermatitis.[38-40]

CONTACT URTICARIA

Urticaria is defined as the transient appearance of elevated, erythematous pruritic wheals or serpiginous exanthem, usually surrounded by an area of erythema. In addition, areas of macular erythema or erythematous papules may also be present. These skin lesions appear and peak in minutes to hours after the etiologic exposure, and individual lesions usually disappear within 24 hours. Urticarial lesions usually involve the trunk and extremities, although they can involve any epidermal or mucosal surface. Large wheal formation, where the edema extends from the dermis into the subcutaneous tissue, is referred to as angioedema. This condition is more commonly seen in the more distensible tissues, such as the eyelids, lips, earlobes, external genitalia, and mucous membranes.

Urticarial lesions can be classified in one or more of the following categories based upon characteristic features:

1. *Duration or chronicity*: Acute or chronic
2. *Clinical distribution of the lesions or the extradermal manifestation*: Localized, generalized, or systemic associated with rhinitis, conjunctivitis, asthma, or anaphylaxis
3. *Etiology*: Idiopathic or cause-specific
4. *Routes of exposure*: Direct contact, inhalation, or ingestion
5. *Mechanisms*: Nonimmunologic, immunologic, or idiopathic

Acute urticaria ranges from a single episode to recurrences over a period of less than 6 weeks. Common causes of acute urticaria include insect bites or stings and food or drug allergies. Chronic urticaria occurs daily, or almost daily, over a period longer than 6 weeks. Food, drugs, and infections can also be causes of chronic urticaria. However, in the chronic form, the exact causative agents may never be identified. In most cases of urticaria, the cause is unknown.

Occupational urticaria is presumed or proven to be caused by exposure to one or more substances or physical agents in the workplace. Occupational urticaria may be acute or chronic, localized or generalized, or associated with systemic manifestations, such as asthma. In occupational settings, direct contact with substances, and possibly inhalation, may be the most common routes of exposure inducing urticaria. The pathologic mechanisms may be nonimmunologic, immunologic, or not known.[41] *Contact urticaria* is defined as urticaria that occurs after direct skin contact with a substance. Another type of immediate skin reaction, "*protein contact dermatitis*," has clinical features of both immediate and delayed hypersensitivity and is associated with atopy. Pruritis, erythema, and urticarial or vesicular lesions occur within 30 minutes of contact with proteins (fruits, vegetables, spices, plants, grains, enzymes, or animal proteins) followed by eczematous dermatitis. Protein contact dermatitis typically affects the hands.[41-45] Urticarias that result from nonchemical exposures are commonly classified as *physical urticarias*. These include mechanical urticarias, caused by trauma, pressure, friction, and vibration, and urticaria resulting from local exposure to water or to physical agents, such as cold, heat, and solar radiation.

Public Health Importance

Data specific for environmental and occupational urticaria are limited. In 2014, the BLS estimated 21,800 cases of occupational skin diseases or disorders in the U.S. workforce.[9] Further information is available on the 2,320 cases that involved days away from work. Of this subgroup, 60 (2.6%) had urticaria/hives. Their median time away from work was 1 day. Among 19 patients with contact urticaria to occupational natural rubber latex, all had persistent skin symptoms 2 years after diagnosis and only 42% reported improvement; these patients had a poorer prognosis than occupational allergic contact dermatitis patients.[15]

Population at Risk and Etiologic Agents

In general, risk factors for contact urticaria include a history of atopy; a compromise to the barrier function of intact skin due to conditions such as eczema, abrasions, and ulcers; and, in some cases, occupation. Based upon reviews of epidemiologic studies, exposures, and patterns seen in case reports, several occupations may be at higher risk for the development of contact urticaria. These include food handlers, cooks, caterers, and bakers; healthcare workers, dental professionals, and pharmaceutical industry workers; animal handlers, such as laboratory workers and veterinarians; gardeners, florists, woodworkers, and agricultural workers; and hairdressers.

For food handlers, cooks, caterers, and bakers, the following foods have been reported to induce contact urticaria: apples, bananas, beans, beer, caraway seeds, carrots, eggs, endives, fish, garlic, grains, kiwi fruit, lettuce, meat (beef, chicken, lamb, liver, pork, and turkey), milk, onions, olives, peaches, potatoes, rice, shellfish, spices, strawberries, and tomatoes.[41,42,44,46-49] Bakers can develop contact urticaria and other systemic symptoms after exposure to rye, wheat, barley, oat, and buckwheat flours, cinnamon, vanillin, and additive flour enzymes, such as alpha-amylase.[41,42,44,47]

In healthcare, dental, and pharmaceutical environments, dermal exposure to a variety of medications or chemical disinfectants can put workers at risk. Exposures that can cause contact urticaria include aminothiazole, bacitracin, benzocaine, cephalosporins, chloramine, chloramphenicol, chlorhexidine, chlorocresol, ethylene oxide, gentamicin, neomycin, nitrogen mustard, penicillin, pentamidine isethionate, phenothiazines, piperacillin, rifamycin, and streptomycin.[41,42,48,49] Recent studies have found that the increased use of nonpowdered latex gloves and nonlatex gloves in healthcare settings have resulted in fewer cases of natural rubber latex allergy, at one time an important cause of contact urticaria in healthcare professionals.[50–52]

Contact urticaria has been found to be caused by animal hair, dander, placenta, saliva, seminal fluid, amniotic fluid, milk, blood, insects, and bacterial and fungal enzymes.[41,42,53] Slaughterhouse workers, laboratory workers, veterinarians and related workers, and dairy farmers are at risk for developing contact urticaria when exposed to these allergens.

Certain woods and plants can cause contact urticaria. These include elm, larch, mahogany, mulberry, obeche (African maple), and teak woods; and plants, such as algae, cacti, *Cannabis sativa*, chrysanthemum, *Ficus benjamina* (weeping fig), lilies, *Limonium tataricum, Phoenix canariensis* (canary palm), tobacco, tulips, and fungi (shiitake mushrooms). High-risk occupations include agricultural workers, carpenters, florists, gardeners, and woodworkers. Caterpillar hair, insect stings, and moths can also cause contact urticaria in outdoor workers. Agricultural workers may also be exposed to fertilizers and pesticides, some of which can cause contact urticaria.[41,42] Hair-bleaching products, such as ammonia persulfate, are common nonprotein substances that can cause contact urticaria in hairdressers.[41,54]

A variety of industrial chemicals can cause contact urticaria, including acrylic monomers (plastics), polyfunctional aziridine hardener (aziridine reacted with a multifunctional acrylic), aliphatic polyamines (epoxy resins), alkyl-phenol novolac resin, ammonia, castor bean (fertilizers), diethyltoluamide (DEET), formaldehyde (used in clothing, leather, fumigation, and resins), isocyanates, lindane (a parasiticide), paraphenylenediamine, phenylmercuric priopionate (an antibacterial fabric softener), plastic additives (such as butylhydroxytoluene and oleylamide), reactive dyes, sodium sulfide (used in photographs, dyes, and tanning), sulfur dioxide, vinyl pyrrolidone, xylene, and other solvents.[41,42,48,49] Contact urticaria can occur with exposure to a variety of metal salts, including chromium, cobalt, iridium, nickel, platinum, and rhodium.[42]

Diagnosis

The diagnosis of environmental or occupational urticaria is based on the medical and exposure history, physical findings, and in vitro or in vivo testing. Proving etiology or work-relatedness may be difficult. Suggested criteria include the following:

1. Documentation of urticaria by physical examination
2. Exposure to an agent known or presumed to cause urticaria
3. A temporally consistent relationship between exposure and onset of urticaria (usually 30 to 60 minutes)
4. Associated medical symptoms and localization of urticaria consistent with the route and body location of exposure
5. Resolution of the urticaria away from the exposure
6. Exclusion of nonenvironmental or nonoccupational causes
7. Medical testing results indicating allergy to a substance in the environment or workplace. Useful medical tests include the open or closed patch test, prick or scratch test, and tests demonstrating specific immunoglobulin E to suspect occupational antigens, such as by radioallergosorbent (RAST) assays. Evaluating with both prick and patch testing has been recommended.[41,47,55]

Prevention

Strategies in the prevention of environmental and occupational urticaria overlap with those strategies used in the prevention of contact dermatitis and include:

- Identifying allergens
- Substituting with chemicals that are nonallergenic
- Implementing engineering controls to reduce exposure
- Utilizing PPE, such as gloves and special clothing
- Emphasizing personal and occupational hygiene
- Establishing educational programs to increase awareness in the workplace.

DERMATOLOGIC INFECTIOUS DISEASES

Environmental or occupational dermatologic infectious diseases are diseases that result from exposure to an infectious agent found in the environment or workplace and have a major manifestation on the skin surface. (Secondarily infected wounds are not discussed here.) Many environmental and occupational dermatologic infectious diseases cause not only cutaneous signs and symptoms but also systemic effects. Exposure can occur through direct skin contact (epicutaneous), by inoculation (percutaneous), or via the respiratory system (inhalational).

Public Health Importance

Epidemiologic data specifically related to environmental or occupational dermatologic infectious diseases are very limited. Other than limited descriptions in case presentations, case studies, and epidemic investigation reports, little is known about the epidemiology of most of these diseases in the United States. In many cases, it is difficult to definitively prove that the disease process is occupationally related. There is limited information on occupational dermatologic infectious diseases in the BLS data. In 2014, there were an estimated 21,800 cases of occupational skin diseases or disorders, or 2.3 per 10,000 workers.[9] Infections of the skin and subcutaneous tissue accounted for 3.4%, or 740 cases (0.1 per 10,000 workers). Most of these cases were listed as cellulitis or abscess (480).[9] Median time away from work was 7 days. In 2014, under a separate category of infectious and parasitic diseases, the BLS recorded 1,020 cases that resulted in at least 1 day away from work.[9] Few diagnoses were listed in this category, but diagnoses with potential skin manifestations included scabies/chiggers/mites (470) and viral diseases accompanied by exanthem (120), which included chickenpox (90) and herpes zoster (20).

Population at Risk and Etiologic Agents

Environmental and occupational dermatologic infectious diseases can be grouped by etiologic agent into categories: bacterial, rickettsial, viral, superficial fungal, subcutaneous fungal, systemic fungal, and parasitic.[56] In general, risk of infection can be associated with individual susceptibility, including factors such as immune status and trauma to the skin breaching its protective barrier; the distribution of the pathogen in the environment; and exposure to the pathogen, considering its reservoir, mode of transmission, and conditions in which the pathogen thrives. Reservoirs of the pathogens include people, such as coworkers, clients, patients, or children; animals and animal products; soil and plant materials; ticks and insects; and water and marine life. Conditions in which pathogens can thrive and increase susceptibility include wet conditions, such as wet work, and hot and humid environments. The environmental and occupational dermatologic infectious diseases associated with these sources and conditions are listed in Table 25-4. In addition, laboratory personnel working directly with pathogens are at risk of infection. There has also been concern over possible work-duty exposures for first responders and healthcare professionals during a bioterrorist attack.

Diagnosis

In many cases, it is often difficult to prove definitively the environmental or occupational relatedness of the disease process. Questions to be answered by the clinician include the following:

1. Is the patient's condition a dermatologic infectious disease?
2. Is the organism found in the patient's environment?
3. Was there an opportunity for the person to become infected in the workplace or general environment?
4. What other exposures, such as recreational activities, must be considered?

Diagnosis is disease-specific and therefore beyond the scope of this chapter.

Prevention

Clinicians should view each case of a potential environmental or occupational dermatologic

Table 25-4. Exposures Associated with Dermatologic Infectious Diseases

People, Patients, and Children	Animal and Animal Products	Soil and Plants
Tuberculosis (cutaneous)	Anthrax	Anthrax
Methicillin-resistant *Staphylococcus aureus*	Brucellosis	Dermatophytes (geophilic)
	Cat scratch disease	Chromomycosis
Herpetic whitlow	Erysipeloid	Mycetoma
Warts	*Mycobacterium bovis*	Sporotrichosis
Measles	Tularemia	Blastomycosis
Rubella	Methicillin-resistant *Staphylococcus aureus*	Paracoccidioidomycosis
Chickenpox	Orf	Cutaneous larva migrans
Herpes zoster (shingles)	Milker's nodules	
Hand-foot-mouth disease	Monkeypox	**Wet Work and Hot and Moist Environments**
Erythema infectiosum (fifth disease)	Warts	Candidiasis
Dermatophytes (anthropophilic)	Dermatophytes (zoophilic)	Dermatophytoses
Scabies	Mites	Tinea versicolor
Ticks and Insects	**Water, Marine, Fish, and Shellfish Exposures**	
Lyme disease	Erysipeloid	
Tularemia	*Mycobacterium marinum* granuloma	
Rocky Mountain spotted fever	Tularemia	
Typhus	*Vibrio vulnificus* infection	
Ehrlichiosis	*Aeromonas hydrophila* infection	
Leishmaniases	*Photobacterium (Vibrio) damsela* infection	
	Vibrio parahaemolyticus infection	
	Pseudomonas aeriginosa infection	
	Warts	
	Cercarial dermatitides	

Source: Wawrose, DJ, Lushniak, BD. Occupational infectious diseases with dermatologic features. In Wright WE (ed.). Occupational and environmental infectious diseases (2nd ed.). Beverly Farms, MA: OEM Press, 2009, pp. 404–421.

infectious disease from a broader public health perspective as a potential sentinel health event. This recognition and resultant action by clinicians, in appropriate consultation with public health officials, could lead to potential disease prevention in other people. This can only occur with proper diagnosis, a high level of suspicion by the clinician in suspecting environmental or workplace exposures, ultimate confirmation of the association to the exposures that caused the disease, and implementation of measures to reduce these exposures. If successful, this approach would lead to the prevention of relapses and of new cases of dermatologic infectious diseases.

SKIN CANCER

In 1775, Sir Percival Pott in England first made the link between occupational exposures (soot clinging to skin in chimney sweeps) and skin cancer (squamous cell carcinoma of the scrotum). In 1894, Dr. Paul Unna in Germany drew attention to the association between chronic sun exposure and skin cancers in outdoor workers, such as farmers and sailors.

Skin cancers include melanoma, basal cell carcinoma, and squamous cell carcinoma. Excessive sun exposure is associated with premature skin aging, actinic keratosis, and skin cancer.[57] Nonionizing ultraviolet radiation (UVR) from the sun is the primary cause of skin cancer, in general, and is also the primary cause of occupational skin cancer. The International Agency for Research on Cancer has concluded that there is sufficient evidence to establish UVR as a human carcinogen. In addition, a variety of chemical exposures may play a role in the etiology of skin cancers.

Public Health Importance

Melanoma is the least prevalent of the three skin cancers, but it carries the greatest risk of fatality, accounting for 73% of skin cancer deaths in the United States. The American Cancer Society estimated that, in 2016, over 76,000 people in the United States would be diagnosed with melanoma and over 10,000 would die of this disease.[58] Melanoma is likely to be related to excessive sun exposure, although the relationship is complex; it seems to be associated with severe sunburns during childhood. Basal cell carcinoma and squamous cell carcinoma are more clearly related to sun exposure, probably as a result of cumulative, chronic exposure. Basal cell and squamous cell skin cancers are, by far, the most common cancers in the United States, with over 5 million new cases and about 2,000 deaths each year.[58]

Population at Risk and Etiologic Agents

Implicated etiologies for skin cancers include non-ionizing radiation from sunlight exposure and other sources of UVR, ionizing radiation, and thermal and chemical stimuli. Outdoor workers may receive up to six to eight times the dose of UVR compared to indoor workers,[59,60] and rates for some skin cancers among outdoor workers have been associated with cumulative UVR exposure.[61] Studies have found an increased risk of skin cancer among agricultural workers, welders, watermen, police officers, physical education teachers, pilots, and cabin attendants.[62] According to the BLS, in 2015, over 3% of the workforce (more than 4 million workers) were included in occupations frequently associated with outdoor work: construction, farm, and forestry workers; fishing workers; gardeners; groundskeepers; mail carriers; amusement/recreation attendants; and surveying and mapping workers.[9] There are likely many more workers occupationally exposed to UVR from sunlight as well as artificial sources, such as welding arcs. In addition, workers exposed to ionizing radiation and chemical agents, such as polycyclic aromatic hydrocarbons, arsenic, alkylating agents, and nitrosamines, may be at increased risk of skin cancer. Arsenic intoxication, which can result from ingestion of contaminated well water, has resulted in hyperpigmentation, palmar and plantar arsenical keratoses, and superficial squamous cell and basal cell carcinomas. Other risk factors for skin cancers include fair skin types, fair hair, having many moles or nevi,

family history of skin cancer, sunburn in childhood or adolescence, a weakened immune system, and older age.[58,63]

Diagnosis and Treatment

Diagnosis is based upon history, physical findings, and pathology results. Treatment of specific skin cancers, which is beyond the scope of this chapter, depends on the specific type of skin cancer, size, depth, and location of the lesion, and evidence of metastases.

Prevention

The strategies of prevention are primarily based on preventing excessive UVR exposure.[64] This can be accomplished by limiting exposure to sunlight, introducing changes in practices to limit sun exposure during peak UVR hours (10 A.M. to 4 P.M.), wearing UVR-protective clothing and wide-brimmed hats; generously applying broad-spectrum, water-resistant sunscreens that block both UVA and UVB; and wearing UV-blocking sunglasses. Limiting skin exposure to chemicals known to play a role in skin cancer is also important.

The *2014 Surgeon General's Call to Action to Prevent Skin Cancer* emphasized the importance of workplace exposures and advocated for increasing the availability of sun protection for outdoor workers, integrating sun safety into workplace health education and promotion programs, and incorporating sun safety into workplace policies and safety training.[65]

In many areas, the National Weather Service, in cooperation with the Environmental Protection Agency, issues daily predictions for UVR exposure. The daily UV Index, reported on a scale from <2 (very low) to 11+ (very high), is part of selected local weather broadcasts and can be used to warn outdoor workers and others of potential high-exposure days, when prevention strategies should be emphasized.

OTHER ENVIRONMENTAL AND OCCUPATIONAL SKIN DISEASES

Many other skin diseases may be related to environmental and occupational exposures (Table 25-5).

Table 25-5. Other Environmental and Occupational Skin Diseases and Examples of Associated Exposures

Condition	Associated Exposures
Hyperkeratoses/calluses/fissuring/ blistering	Mechanical trauma
Burns	Heat, electricity, radiation, acids, alkalis
Frostbite/immersion foot, chilblain	Cold, moist environments
Folliculitis/furuncles and acneform dermatoses	Oils, greases
Chloracne	Chlorinated hydrocarbons
Photodermatitis (phototoxic and photoallergic)	Plants, coal tar, creosote, fragrances
Depigmentation/leukoderma	Phenols, hydroquinones
Hyperpigmentation/occupational melanosis	Coal tar pitch
Skin discolorations	Silver, gold
Occupational Raynaud disease/vibration white finger	Tools causing hand-arm vibration
Miliaria rubra/prickly heat	Hot, humid work environments
Asteatotic eczema/winter eczema	Cool, dry work environments
Granulomatous dermatoses	Beryllium, zirconium
Ulcerative lesions	Chromium, chemical burns
Connective tissue disorders such as scleroderma	Silica, vinyl chloride
Nail disorders	Mechanical trauma, contact dermatitis, infections
Alopecia	Chlorbutadine, dimethylamine

Other skin diseases may not be caused by occupational exposures, but they may be exacerbated by such exposures. Examples include lesions of psoriasis produced at sites of skin friction or injury, rosacea exacerbated by heat, and wet work initiating dyshidrotic eczema.

CONCLUSION

Environmental and occupational skin diseases include allergic contact dermatitis, irritant contact dermatitis, contact urticaria, a variety of infectious diseases, skin cancers, and other diseases. Thorough investigations of workers with occupational skin diseases can be difficult. Workers should be encouraged to report all potential work-related skin problems to their employers and to their physicians. Because the work-relatedness of skin diseases may be difficult to prove, each person with possible work-related skin problems needs to be fully evaluated by a physician, preferably one familiar with occupational and dermatological conditions. A complete evaluation includes a full medical and occupational history and a review of exposures. The National Institute for Occupational Safety and Health is revamping its skin notations for use in distinguishing between systemic, localized, and sensitizing health effects of dermal chemical exposures.[66] A complete evaluation also includes a physical examination;

diagnostic tests, such as skin patch tests to detect causes of allergic contact dermatitis; and follow-up to assess the clinical course of the affected person. Individuals with occupational skin diseases should be protected from exposures to presumed causes or exacerbators of the disease. In some cases of allergic contact dermatitis and contact urticaria, workers may have to be reassigned to areas where exposure is minimal or nonexistent.

Environmental and occupational skin diseases have a major public health impact. They are common, often have a poor prognosis, and result in a substantial economic impact for both affected individuals and society as a whole. Importantly, these diseases are amenable to public health interventions.

AUTHORS' NOTE

The findings and conclusions in this chapter are those of the authors and do not necessarily represent the views of the National Institute for Occupational Safety and Health or the University of Maryland.

REFERENCES

1. Lushniak BD. Occupational contact dermatitis. Dermatologic Therapy 2004; 17: 272–277.

2. Ingber A, Merims S. The validity of the Mathias criteria for establishing occupational causation and aggravation of contact dermatitis. Contact Dermatitis 2004; 51: 9–12.

3. De Groot AC. Patch testing (3rd ed.). Wapserveen, The Netherlands: Acdegroot Publishing, 2008.

4. Flyvholm MA, Bach B, Rose M, Jepsen KF. Self-reported hand eczema in a hospital population. Contact Dermatitis 2007; 57: 110–115.

5. Warshaw E, Lee G, Storrs FJ. Hand dermatitis: A review of clinical features, therapeutic options, and long-term outcomes. American Journal of Contact Dermatitis 2003; 14: 119–137.

6. Lushniak BD. The importance of occupational skin diseases in the United States. International Archives of Occupational and Environmental Health 2000; 76: 325–330.

7. Centers for Disease Control and Prevention, National Center for Health Statistics. National Ambulatory Medical Care Survey: 2012 State and National Summary Tables. Available at: http://www.cdc.gov/nchs/data/ahcd/namcs_summary/2012_namcs_web_tables.pdf. Accessed November 21, 2016.

8. Luckhaupt SE, Dahlhamer JM, Ward BW, et al. Prevalence of dermatitis in the working population, United States, 2010 National Health Interview Survey. American Journal of Industrial Medicine 2013; 56: 625–634.

9. Bureau of Labor Statistics. Occupational injuries and illnesses in the United States. U.S. Department of Labor, Bureau of Labor Statistics. Available at: http://www.bls.gov/iif/oshsum.htm. Accessed October 18, 2016.

10. Mathias CGT. The cost of occupational skin disease. Archives of Dermatology 1985; 121: 332–334.

11. Sama SR, Bushley A, Cohen M, et al. Work-related skin disorders in Washington State, 1993–1997. Safety and Health Assessment and Research for Prevention, Washington State Department of Labor and Industries, Report 36-4-1998, 1998.

12. McCall BP, Horwitz IB, Feldman SR, Balkrishnan R. Incidence rates, costs, severity, and work-related factors of occupational dermatitis: A workers' compensation analysis of Oregon, 1990–1997. Archives of Dermatology 2005; 141: 713–718.

13. Jungbauer FH, van der Harst JJ, Groothoff JW, Coenraads PJ. Skin protection in nursing work: Promoting the use of gloves and hand alcohol. Contact Dermatitis 2004; 51: 135–140.

14. Cvetkovski RS, Zachariae R, Jensen H, et al. Prognosis of occupational hand eczema: A follow-up study. Archives of Dermatology 2006; 142: 305–311.

15. Clemmensen KKB, Caroe TK, Thomsen SF, et al. Two-year follow-up survey of patients with allergic contact dermatitis from an occupational cohort: Is the prognosis dependent on the omnipresence of the allergen? British Journal of Dermatology 2014; 170: 1100–1105.

16. Sajjachareonpong P, Cahill J, Keegel T, et al. Persistent post-occupational dermatitis. Contact Dermatitis 2004; 51: 278–283.

17. Meding B, Wrangsjo K, Jarvholm B. Fifteen-year follow-up of hand eczema: Predictive factors. Journal of Investigative Dermatology 2005; 124: 893–897.

18. Lan CC, Feng WW, Lu YW, et al. Hand eczema among University Hospital nursing staff: Identification of high-risk sector and impact on quality of life. Contact Dermatitis 2008; 59: 301–306.

19. Fowler JF, Ghosh A, Sung J, et al. Impact of chronic hand dermatitis on quality of life, work productivity, activity impairment, and medical costs. Journal of the American Academy of Dermatology 2006; 54: 448–457.

20. Cvetkovski RS, Rothman KJ, Olsen J, et al. Relation between diagnoses on severity, sick leave and loss of job among patients with occupational hand eczema. British Journal of Dermatology 2005; 152: 93–98.

21. Kadyk DL, McCarter K, Achen F, Belsito DV. Quality of life in patients with allergic contact dermatitis. Journal of the American Academy of Dermatology 2003; 49: 1037–1048.

22. Slodownik D, Lee A, Nixon R. Irritant contact dermatitis: A review. Australasian Journal of Dermatology 2008; 49: 1–9.

23. Chew AI, Maibach HI. Occupational issues of irritant contact dermatitis. International Archives of Occupational and Environmental Health 2003; 76: 339–346.

24. McMullen E, Gawkrodger DJ. Physical friction is under-recognized as an irritant that can cause or contribute to contact dermatitis. British Journal of Dermatology 2006; 154: 154–156.

25. Morris-Jones R, Robertson SJ, Ross JS, et al. Contact dermatitis and allergy: dermatitis caused by physical irritants. British Journal of Dermatology 2003; 147: 270–275.

26. Mathias CGT. Prevention of occupational contact dermatitis. Journal of the American Academy of Dermatology 1990; 23: 742–748.

27. DeKoven JG, Warshaw EM, Belsito DV, et al. North American Contact Dermatitis Group

patch-test results, 2013–2014. Dermatitis 2016; 28: 33–46.

28. Warshaw EM, Kwon GP, Mathias CGT, et al. Occupationally related contact dermatitis in North American food service workers referred for patch testing, 1994–2010. Dermatitis 2013; 24: 22–26.

29. Warshaw EM, Wang MZ, Mathias CGT, et al. Occupational contact dermatitis in hairdressers/ cosmetologists: Retrospective analysis of North American Contact Dermatitis Group data, 1994–2010. Dermatitis 2012; 23: 258–268.

30. Warshaw EM, Hagen SL, Sasseville D, et al. Occupational contact dermatitis in North American mechanics and repairers referred for patch testing: Retrospective analysis of cross-sectional data from the North American Contact Dermatitis Group 1998 to 2014. Dermatitis 2016; 28: 47–57.

31. Coman G, Zinsmeister C, Norris P. Occupational contact dermatitis: workers' compensation patch test results of Portland, Oregon, 2005–2014. Dermatitis 2015; 26: 276–283.

32. Mathias CGT. Contact dermatitis and workers' compensation—Criteria for establishing occupational causation and aggravation. Journal of the American Academy of Dermatology 1989; 20: 842–848.

33. Susitaival P, Flyvholm MA, Meding B, et al. Nordic occupational skin questionnaire (NOSQ-2002): A new tool for surveying occupational skin diseases and exposure. Contact Dermatitis 2003; 49: 70–76.

34. Kucenic MJ, Belsito DV. Occupational allergic contact dermatitis is more prevalent than irritant contact dermatitis: A 5-year study. Journal of the American Academy of Dermatology 2002; 46: 695–699.

35. National Institute of Occupational Safety and Health. Proposed national strategy for the prevention of leading work-related diseases and injuries—dermatological conditions. DHHS (NIOSH) Publication 89-136. Cincinnati, OH: Author, 1988.

36. Foo CC, Goon AT, Leow YH, Goh CL. Adverse skin reactions to personal protective equipment against severe acute respiratory syndrome: A descriptive study in Singapore. Contact Dermatitis 2006; 55: 291–294.

37. Kwon S, Campbell LS, Zirwas MJ. Role of protective gloves in the causation and treatment of occupational irritant contact dermatitis. Journal of the American Academy of Dermatology 2006; 55: 891–896.

38. Weisshaar E, Radulescu M, Bock M, et al. Educational and dermatological aspects of secondary individual prevention in healthcare workers. Contact Dermatitis 2006; 54: 254–260.

39. Loffler H, Bruckner T, Diepgen T, Effendy I. Primary prevention in health care employees: A prospective intervention study with a 3-year training period. Contact Dermatitis 2006; 54: 202–209.

40. Schwanitz HJ, Riehl U, Schlesinger T, et al. Skin care management: Educational aspects. International Archives of Occupational and Environmental Health 2003; 76: 374–381.

41. Holness DL, Arrandale VH, Mathias CGT. Occupational urticarial and allergic contact dermatitis. In: Malo JL, Chan-Yeung M, Bernstein DI (eds.). Asthma in the workplace (4th ed.). Boca Raton, FL: CRC Press, Taylor & Francis, 2013, pp. 418–433.

42. Gimenez-Arnau A, Maurer M, De La Cuadra J, Maibach H. Immediate contact skin reactions, an update of contact urticaria, contact urticarial syndrome and protein contact dermatitis—"A Never Ending Story." European Journal of Dermatology 2010; 20: 552–562.

43. Killig C, Werfel T. Contact reactions to food. Current Allergy and Asthma Reports 2008; 8: 209–214.

44. Amaro C, Goossens A. Immunological occupational contact urticaria and contact dermatitis from proteins: A review. Contact Dermatitis 2008; 58: 67–75.

45. Doutre MS. Occupational contact urticaria and protein contact dermatitis. European Journal of Dermatology 2005; 15: 419–424.

46. Williams JDL, Lee AYL, Matheson MC, et al. Occupational contact urticaria: Australian data. British Journal of Dermatology 2008, 159: 125–131.

47. Usmani N, Wilkinson SM. Allergic skin disease: Investigation of both immediate- and delayed-type hypersensitivity is essential. Clinical and Experimental Allergy 2007; 37: 1541–1546.

48. Reitschel RL, Fowler JF. Contact urticaria. In: Reitschel RL, Fowler JF (eds.). Fisher's contact dermatitis (6th ed.). Hamilton, Ontario: BC Decker, 2008, pp. 615–633.

49. Taylor JS, Leow YH, Fisher AA. Contact urticaria. In Adams RM (ed.). Occupational skin disease (3rd ed.). Philadelphia: W.B. Saunders, 1999, pp. 111–134.

50. Suneja T, Belsito DV. Occupational dermatoses in health care workers evaluated for suspected allergic contact dermatitis. Contact Dermatitis 2008; 58: 285–290.

51. Filon FL, Radman G. Latex allergy: A follow up study of 1040 healthcare workers. Occupational and Environmental Medicine 2006; 63: 121–125.

52. Taylor JS, Erkek E. Latex allergy: Diagnosis and management. Dermatologic Therapy 2004; 17: 289–301.

53. Foti C, Antelmi A, Mistrello G, et al. Occupational contact urticaria and rhinoconjunctivitis from dog's milk in a veterinarian. Contact Dermatitis 2007; 56: 169–171.

54. Bensefa-Colas L, Telle-Lamberton M, Faye S, et al. Occupational contact urticarial: Lessons from the French National Network for Occupational Disease Vigilance and Prevention (RNV3P). British Journal of Dermatology 2015; 173: 1453–1461.

55. Holness L, Mace SR. Results of evaluating health care workers with prick and patch testing. American Journal of Contact Dermatitis 2001; 12: 88–92.

56. Wawrose DJ, Lushniak, BD. Occupational infectious diseases with dermatologic features. In Wright WE (ed.). Occupational and environmental infectious diseases (2nd ed.). Beverly Farms, MA: OEM Press, 2009, pp. 404–421.

57. Gallagher RP, Lee TK. Adverse effects of ultraviolet radiation: A brief review. Progress in Biophysics and Molecular Biology 2006; 92: 119–131.

58. American Cancer Society website. Available at: http://www.cancer.org/cancer/index. Accessed November 21, 2016.

59. Holman CDJ, Gibson IM, Stephenson M, et al. Ultraviolet radiation of human body sites in relation to occupation and outdoor activity: field studies using personal UVR dosimeters. Clinical and Experimental Dermatology 1983; 8: 869–871.

60. Hammond V, Reeder AI, Gray A. Patterns of real-time occupational ultraviolet radiation exposure among a sample of outdoor workers in New Zealand. Public Health 2009; 123: 182–187.

61. Vitasa BC, Taylor HR, Strickland PT, et al. Association of nonmelanoma skin cancer and actinic keratosis with cumulative solar exposure in Maryland watermen. Cancer 1990; 65: 2811–2817.

62. Ramirez CC, Federman DG, Kirsner RS. Skin cancer as an occupational disease: The effect of ultraviolet and other forms of radiation. International Journal of Dermatology 2005; 44: 95–100.

63. Leiter U, Eigentler T, Garbe C. Epidemiology of skin cancer. Advances in Experimental Medicine and Biology 2014; 810: 120–140.

64. Glanz K, Buller DB, Saraiya M. Reducing ultraviolet radiation exposure among outdoor workers: State of the evidence and recommendations. Environmental Health 2007; 6: 22.

65. U.S. Department of Health and Human Services. The Surgeon General's Call to Action to Prevent Skin Cancer. Washington, DC: U.S. Department of Health and Human Services, Office of the Surgeon General, 2014.

66. National Institute for Occupational Safety and Health. Current intelligence bulletin 61: A strategy for assigning new NIOSH skin notations. DHHS (NIOSH) Publication No. 2009–147. Cincinnati, Ohio: NIOSH, 2009.

FURTHER READING

National Institute for Occupational Safety and Health. Occupational dermatoses. Available at: http://www.cdc.gov/niosh/topics/skin/occderm-slides/ocderm.html.
NIOSH offers this occupational dermatoses photolibrary and program for physicians on its website.

Adams RM. Occupational skin disease (3rd ed.). Philadelphia: WB Saunders, 1999.

Honari G, Taylor SJ; Sood A. Occupational skin diseases due to irritants and allergens. In: Goldsmith LA, Katz SI, Gilchrest BA, et al. (eds.). Fitzpatrick's dermatology in general medicine (8th ed). New York: McGraw-Hill, 2012, Chapter 211.

Holness DL, Arrandale VH, Mathias CGT. Occupational urticarial and allergic contact dermatitis. In: Malo JL, Chan-Yeung M, Bernstein DI (eds.). Asthma in the workplace (4th ed.). Boca Raton, FL: CRC Press, Taylor & Francis. 2013, pp. 418–433.

Johansen JD, Frosch PJ, Lepoittevin JP (eds.). Contact dermatitis (5th ed.). Berlin: Springer-Verlag, 2011.

Marks JG, Elsner P, DeLeo VA. Contact and occupational dermatology. St. Louis MO: Mosby, 2002.

Reitchel RL, Fowler JF. Fisher's contact dermatitis (6th ed.). Hamilton, Ontario: BC Decker, 2008.

Rustemeyer T, Elsner P, John SM, Maibach HI (eds.). Kanerva's occupational dermatology. Berlin: Springer-Verlag, 2012.

Wawrose DJ, Lushniak, BD. Occupational infectious diseases with dermatologic features. In Wright WE (ed.). Occupational and environmental infectious diseases (2nd ed.). Beverly Farms, MA: OEM Press, 2009, pp. 404–421.
These eight books and book chapters are excellent references on occupational and environmental skin disorders

26

Cardiovascular Disorders

Kenneth D. Rosenman

The mortality rate for cardiovascular disease (CVD) has continued to decrease in the United States, falling 29% between 2003 and 2013.[1] However, CVD is still the most frequent cause of death (accounting for 31% of deaths), with, on average, more than 2,200 dying daily.[1] The National Heart Lung and Blood Institute estimates that 82.6 million U.S. residents have CVD, including 76.4 million with hypertension and 16.3 million with coronary heart disease.[2] Each year, about 1.2 million Americans are diagnosed with a myocardial infarction, 795,000 with a stroke, and 670,000 with congestive heart failure.[2]

There are many risk factors for coronary heart disease, including dyslipidemia, cigarette smoking, hypertension, diabetes, and obesity. The etiology of most cases of hypertension is unknown; less than 10% have known causes.

Occupational and environmental exposure to specific chemicals and physical and psychological stressors are risk factors for CVD. An estimated 5% to 19% of CVD cases are attributed to occupational and environmental factors,[3] including psychological strain (in jobs with high job demand and low job control or poor effort-reward balance), shift work, noise, environmental (secondhand) tobacco smoke, particulates, carbon monoxide (CO), lead (Figure 26-1), and organic solvents. Cardiovascular disease is so prevalent that, even if the percentage of CVD attributable to occupational and environmental factors were less than 5% to 19%, many people would still develop CVD due to these factors.

Clinicians need to consider occupational and environmental exposures when evaluating CVD in workers, such as auto mechanics with angina pectoris who may be exposed to CO from car exhaust. Inadequate consideration of occupational and environmental factors may delay diagnosis or result in death.[4, 5]

CORONARY ARTERY DISEASE

Occupational factors may trigger an acute coronary event, such as a myocardial infarction or an arrhythmia. Prolonged exposure may cause CVD by promoting development of atherosclerosis. (See Table 26-1.) The following sections describe some of these factors.

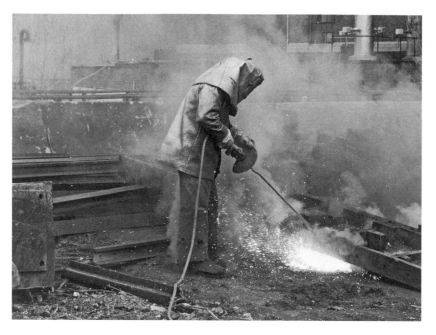

Figure 26-1. This worker is exposed to lead by cutting metal that has a lead-based coating.

Table 26-1. Illustrative Occupational and Environmental Risk Factors for Cardiovascular Disease

Disease	Risk Factor
Coronary artery disease	
Angina/Myocardial infarction	Carbon disulfide
	Carbon monoxide
	Decreased lung function
	Nitrates
	Particulates
	Psychological strain (high work demand and low job control)
	Secondhand tobacco smoke
Sudden death	All causes above for angina/ myocardial infarction plus:
	Cold or hot workplaces
	Fluorocarbons
	Solvents
Cardiomyopathy	Arsenic
	Cobalt
Hypertension	Carbon disulfide
	Lead
	Noise
Arrhythmias	Carbon monoxide
	Fluorocarbons
	Solvents
Peripheral vascular disease/ Claudication	Arsenic
	Carbon monoxide
	Vibration
Cor pulmonale	Fibrogenic dusts

Carbon Disulfide

Exposure to carbon disulfide, a solvent that is used in manufacturing other chemicals, is usually limited to chemical manufacturing facilities (Figure 26-2). It causes atherosclerosis by affecting lipoproteins, blood pressure, arterial elastic properties, and oxidative stress.[6] (Other solvents have not been found to increase atherosclerosis, although some cause arrhythmias and have been associated with sudden death.) Workers manufacturing viscose rayon, who use carbon disulfide, are at increased risk for coronary artery disease. In animal studies, high-fat diets increase the atherosclerotic effect of carbon disulfide, which appears to be reversible with cessation of exposure.[7] The permissible exposure limit (PEL) of the Occupational Safety and Health Administration (OSHA) (20 ppm) does not adequately protect against the development of atherosclerosis.[8]

Carbon Monoxide

Carbon monoxide exposure is produced by combustion, such as with the burning of gasoline, diesel fuel, propane, coal, natural gas,

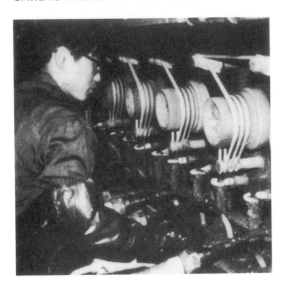

Figure 26-2. A worker tends machines that spool rayon thread from carbon disulfide. Worker exposure to carbon disulfide was high until this process was enclosed, which reduced worker exposure and, by recycling the carbon disulfide, saved the company a substantial amount of money. (Photograph by Barry S. Levy.)

wood, oil, or tobacco. Acute manifestations of coronary artery disease may occur after CO exposure. Carbon monoxide can be fatal when combustion occurs in an enclosed area, such as a gasoline-powered washer used in a basement, a diesel-powered electricity generator used without adequate ventilation during a blackout, or a propane forklift used in a warehouse. Because the incidence of CO toxicity increases during cold weather when furnaces are used and doors and windows are closed, CO toxicity is more frequent in colder latitudes.

Compared to oxygen, CO has 200 times higher affinity for hemoglobin, forming carboxyhemoglobin (COHb), and 50 times higher affinity for myoglobin. In addition, CO shifts the oxyhemoglobin curve to the left, which reduces oxygen delivery to tissues, inhibits mitochondrial enzymes, impairs oxygen diffusion into mitochondria, and increases platelet adhesiveness. Animal studies suggest that CO directly affects (a) cells, with increased oxidant production and lipid preoxygenation, and (b) the heart, with decreased cardiac output, increased myocardial lactate production, and a decreased threshold for ventricular fibrillation.

Carboxyhemoglobin can be measured in either arterial or venous blood or by a specialized pulse CO-oximeter.[*] Carboxyhemoglobin has a cherry red color, which can be seen in mucous membranes—a specific, but not sensitive, sign. Carboxyhemoglobin is produced endogenously from the normal breakdown of hemoglobin. It is increased by hemolysis from any cause. Induction of hepatic cytochrome oxidase activity from medications also may increase endogenous COHb production. Normal levels of COHb are less than 1%. Ambient air pollution can increase COHb to 1.7%. Therefore, less than 2% is typically used as a laboratory reference range for COHb. Interpretation of a patient's COHb needs to take into account both the duration of time since exposure to CO and whether the patient received treatment, such as oxygen in the ambulance on the way to the emergency department. The normal half-life of COHb is 4 to 6 hours on room air; 40 to 80 minutes on 100% oxygen; and 15 to 30 minutes with hyperbaric oxygen.

At the OSHA workplace PEL for CO (50 ppm), COHb levels increase to as high as 7.4%. Average COHb levels are 4.7% in cigarette smokers, 2.9% in cigar smokers, and 2.2% in pipe smokers. It is unusual for cigarette smokers to have COHb levels greater than 10%. Exposure to environmental (secondhand) tobacco smoke increases COHb levels by 0.5% to 1.0%. Carbon-monoxide detectors for home use are designed to prevent acute CO poisoning. The alarm only sounds when a specific level of CO is reached in the air for a minimum amount of time: 400 ppm for 4 to 15 minutes, 150 ppm for 10 to 50 minutes, or 70 ppm for 6 to 240 minutes. Therefore, a person could have a COHb level as high as 10% with the alarm not sounding. The relationship between airborne CO and blood COHb levels is shown in Table 26-2.

Carboxyhemoglobin levels increase with length of exposure. If the concentration of CO in the air is constant, an equilibrium in a person's COHb level will be reached. At rest, this

---

* Oxygen saturation is overestimated by (a) all pulse oximeters in the presence of COHb and (b) in measurements of arterial blood gases, where the value for oxygen saturation is calculated from the arterial oxygen content and the reduction in hemoglobin-binding sites available to oxygen (because of the presence of COHb is not included in the equation to calculate oxygen saturation).

Table 26-2. Air Levels of Carbon Monoxide Corresponding to Blood Levels of Carboxyhemoglobin

Concentration of Carboxyhemoglobin (%)	Carbon Monoxide (ppm)	Comments
<1	0	Endogenous production from breakdown of hemoglobin
<2	9	EPA's ambient air 8-hour standard
2.2*	400***	Pipe smoker
2.9*	400***	Cigar smoker
4.7**	400***	Cigarette smoker
5.4	35	EPA's ambient air 1-hour ceiling standard
7.4	50	OSHA's workplace 8-hour TWA standard

Note. EPA = Environmental Protection Agency; OSHA = Occupational Safety and Health Administration; TWA = time-weighted average.
* Average values.
** Average value, range 1% to 10%.
*** With intermittent smoking, inhaled concentration of carbon monoxide is less.

equilibrium is achieved in 8 hours. With exercise and increased pulmonary ventilation, equilibrium is achieved sooner. After exposure to the solvent methylene chloride (used in paint and bathtub glaze–stripping products), which is uniquely metabolized to CO, levels of COHb may reach 12%.

Levels of COHb below 30% are associated with headache, nausea, and weakness. Levels of COHb that are 30% or higher are associated with decreased mental alertness and weakness, with increasing likelihood of collapse and coma as levels increase. Myocardial injury, reflected by electrocardiogram (EKG) changes or increases in myocardial enzymes, occurs in over one-third of patients with CO poisoning severe enough to be treated with hyperbaric oxygen.[9]

Workplace standards that allow COHb levels up to 7.4% are not protective for individuals with coronary artery disease. Levels of 2% to 4% can reduce the time to anginal chest pain, can cause ST segment changes on EKG in those with coronary artery disease and can cause claudication in those with peripheral vascular disease. Levels of 5% and higher can increase cardiac enzymes and arrhythmias,[10] whereas levels of 6% and higher can increase the frequency of ventricular premature contractions[11] and levels of 10% and higher can cause myocardial infarctions.

The evidence that CO chronically promotes the development of atherosclerosis is not as strong as the evidence that it causes acute CVD events. Animal studies have shown that CO causes increased vascular permeability, arterial wall hypoxia, and platelet adhesiveness—all of which can accelerate atherosclerosis. Epidemiologic studies of firefighters and foundry workers who had been exposed to CO demonstrated increased risk of coronary events while they were employed, which decreased with cessation of exposure. Similarly, studies have shown a decrease in both hospitalizations and deaths from myocardial infarction after enactment of smoke-free workplace laws.[12] Studies have shown an increased risk of coronary events when a person is a smoker and that the risk decreases when he or she quits—but not to the level of risk of those who never smoked.

Decreased Lung Function

Decreased forced expiratory volume in 1 second (FEV_1) is a risk for coronary artery disease[13]—a risk that is distinct from the risk of right-sided heart failure (cor pulmonale) due to lung disease. This risk might be due to a hypoxic effect on the heart from lung disease or to substances causing inflammation of the lungs and vascular endothelium.

Hot and Cold Temperatures

Working in either a hot or cold environment has triggered acute coronary events in people with underlying coronary artery disease. This is consistent with population studies that show that CVD deaths and hospitalizations increase during the winter and during heat waves.[14-16] Cardiovascular disease mortality above normal during a heat wave is followed by CVD mortality below normal after the heat wave, indicating a shift in the time of death in people with significant underlying CVD—without an actual change in the overall mortality rate.[15,16]

Physiologic changes, such as vasospasm in cold weather or peripheral dehydration and increased blood viscosity in hot weather, coupled with increased physical activity at work, can trigger a coronary event in someone with pre-existing coronary atherosclerosis. In addition, endothelial dysfunction appears to increase as ambient temperature increases. Evidence suggests that long-term work in a cold environment increases the risk of coronary artery disease. (See Chapters 12B and 29.)

Lead

Increased CVD mortality has been reported in individuals with elevated blood lead levels (BLL).[17] This association may be due to increases in blood pressure, homocysteine concentration, and/or heart rate variability.[18] (See Chapters 11, 23, 28, and 30 for further discussion of lead.)

Nitrates

Monday morning death (sudden cardiac death after a weekend away from work exposure) was first described among workers in the explosives manufacturing industry during the 1930s.[19] Death was caused by rebound vasospasm in the coronary arteries from withdrawal from exposure to nitrates, which can occur with exposure to ammonium and sodium nitrate, ethylene glycol dinitrate, nitroglycerin, dinitroluene, and trinitroluene. (These chemicals can also cause methemoglobinemia.) Increased CVD mortality from myocardial infarction and stroke has been reported in long-term workers in the explosives industry who are exposed to nitrates, perhaps because they develop rebound vasospasm when away from work.[20]

Powder head is a related phenomenon in which workers develop headaches on weekends away from work due to withdrawal from occupational nitrate exposure. To prevent headaches, workers have placed a few grains of explosive powder in their hatbands throughout the weekend in order to maintain exposure to nitrates.

Particulates

Particulate air pollution, due to combustion, can be toxic to the cardiovascular system. Exposure to fine particulates, mainly from power plants and motor vehicles, is widespread in the general population. Exposure to fine particulates (less than 2.5 μm in aerodynamic diameter, or $PM_{2.5}$) is associated with acute and chronic coronary artery disease.[21,22] Fine particulates cause changes in heart rate variability, arterial dysfunction, and inflammation in old and young people as well as animals. Specific metals, such as nickel or vanadium, in fine particulates are thought to play an important role in causing these toxic effects.

Reducing the levels of fine particulates can have huge benefits. For example, a decrease of 10 μg/m³ can increase life expectancy by 0.6 year.[21] Ambient air standards in the United States allow fine particulates up to a 15 μg/m³ annual average and a 35 μg/m³ average in a 24-hour period. Of all U.S. residents, 17% live in nonattainment areas for the annual standard and 30% live in nonattainment areas for the 24-hour standard. The 15 μg/m³ annual average is not adequately protective. Since particulate levels are lower indoors, patients with coronary artery disease should reduce their activity and time spent outdoors if the air quality index is high.[23]

Workers who are exposed to fine particulates, such as vehicle mechanics or welders, have decreased heart rate variability.[24] (Decreased heart rate variability is associated with increased CVD mortality.) Workers exposed to diesel exhaust, such as coal miners, truck drivers, and construction workers, have increased coronary artery disease.[25,26] Ground-level ozone air pollution may increase CVD mortality.

Psychosocial Factors

Two models have been used to investigate the role of work stress in causing heart disease. The job strain model hypothesizes that work in high-demand jobs with low job-decision latitude increases the risk of heart disease, while high levels of job control negate the adverse effects of a demanding job. The effort-reward imbalance model assumes that work in jobs with high effort but inadequate reward increases the risk of heart disease. In the effort-reward imbalance model, an additional risk factor is overcommitment, characterized by a set of attitudes, behaviors, and emotions reflecting excessive striving in combination with a desire to be approved of and esteemed. One study concluded that 7% to 16% of CVD is secondary to the stress of jobs with high demand and low decision latitude.[27] Many, but not all, studies support job strain as an important CVD risk factor. Studies showing that interventions to decrease job strain and/ or increase decision latitude decrease CVD are needed to both establish a causal association and indicate how to reduce the adverse effect.[28] The mechanism of such an association may be mediated through known cardiac risk factors. For example, bus drivers who are at increased risk of CVD mortality also have an increased prevalence of hypertension. Their job has a high demand to remain on schedule but an inability to control traffic or road conditions. Further studies to examine the interaction between genetic polymorphism and job strain in predicting CVD risk are needed. (See Chapter 14.)

There are marked differences in cardiac risk factors by industry and occupation.[29] The use of occupation as a marker of socioeconomic status and, therefore, as a surrogate for lifestyle habits known to be cardiac risks—rather than as a marker for some psychological or environmental risk factor associated with the occupation—has complicated (a) interpretation of why workers in certain occupations have higher rates of CVD and (b) the development of effective interventions.[30] Worksite wellness programs can be targeted to occupations or industries with a high prevalence of risky lifestyles by educating individual workers on CVD risks, implementing preventive measures (such as eliminating unhealthy snacks from workplace vending machines), and/or addressing systemic issues (such as occupational stress and hazardous exposures). (See Chapter 10.)

Shift Work

The metabolic syndrome (abdominal obesity, dyslipidemia, elevated blood pressure, insulin resistance, and a prothrombotic and proinflammatory state) has been associated with shift work, including in healthcare workers (see Chapter 14).[31,32] It is unclear if shift work causes increased prevalence of CVD risk factors or if individuals of a certain socioeconomic status who have a higher prevalence of CVD risk factors are more likely to perform shift work. Either way, clinicians need to consider CVD risk factors in shift workers. In addition, control of insulin-dependent diabetics is more difficult in shift workers. Forward rotating shifts have been shown to alleviate daytime sleepiness and reduce systolic blood pressure.[33] Further research is needed to evaluate the health effects of different rotating shift schedules.[34]

Another factor to be considered in the effect of work schedules is the number of hours worked per week. A meta-analysis controlling for known CVD risk factors found an association between both stroke and coronary heart disease and working 55 or more hours per week.[35]

Sedentary Work

Studies showing decreased CVD in individuals who exercise regularly have been based on nonwork aerobic activity. This protective effect has not been consistently found in association with physical activity at work.[36,37] This difference between work and nonwork physical activity has been attributed to (a) the nature of activity at work, which is less likely to be aerobic, and (b) an inverse relationship between high physical work activity and decreased time or interest to perform aerobic physical activity outside of work.

Firefighters

Potential CVD risk factors for firefighters include strenuous work in a hot environment, exposure to fine particulates, occupational stress, and exposures to acrolein (an aldehyde in smoke) and CO. The risk of death from coronary heart disease is increased 12 to 136 times during firefighting as compared with nonemergency periods.[38] Even in healthy firefighters, ST-segment changes occur during fire suppression.[39] Previous coronary artery disease, hypertension, and cigarette smoking are independent predictors of fatal heart attacks during active firefighting.[40] However, career firefighters have not been shown to have more coronary heart disease than other groups of workers.

ARRHYTHMIAS

All types of arrhythmias, including supraventricular and ventricular rhythms, those due to sick sinus syndrome and heart block, and atrioventricular junctional and escape rhythms, have been associated with exposure to CO and organic solvents. About half of cardiac deaths occur suddenly, and arrhythmias (with or without underlying coronary artery disease) are a major cause. For 2 million Americans hospitalized annually, an arrhythmia is a discharge diagnosis.

Solvents are used as carriers for other substances that are insoluble in water, as chemical intermediates in manufacturing, and as fuels. Commonly used organic solvents that can cause arrhythmias include benzene, xylene, tetrachloroethylene, trichloroethylene, trichloromethane, and fluorocarbons. (See Chapter 11.)

Arrhythmias from exposure to solvents have occurred in manufacturing, dry-cleaning (with tetrachloroethylene exposure), laboratory-based pathology, and pesticide spraying (with exposure to the solvent carrier in pesticide spray). Exposure can also occur among people outside of work, who are using cleaning products or other household products. Even higher levels of exposure occur among individuals who abuse commercial or household products to create euphoria, delusions, sedation, and hallucinations.

Animal models, used to assess the ability of specific organic solvents to directly affect myocardial tissue and to increase sensitivity to catecholamines, have shown (a) initiation of an arrhythmia is based on the threshold concentration, not the duration of exposure; (b) sensitization to catecholamines continues as long as the solvent is present in the blood, even after the solvent is no longer being inhaled; (c) halogenated derivatives of aliphatic hydrocarbons, such as trichloroethane, are more toxic than unsubstituted hydrocarbons, such as ethane; (d) combined exposure to noise and fluorocarbons has a greater effect than fluorocarbon exposure alone; and (e) solvents have a negative inotropic effect on the heart.

Epidemiologic studies of workers exposed to fluorocarbons have not shown increased arrhythmias under "normal working conditions," a finding consistent with the animal studies that a threshold concentration, which may vary among individuals, needs to be reached. Since the solvent concentration in the blood is the immediate precipitating factor, arrhythmias may occur after exposure has ceased but before blood concentrations have fallen, such as on the way home from work.

Dizziness, headaches, lightheadedness, and nausea may occur as direct effects of exposure to any solvent, even in the absence of an arrhythmia. In addition, eye or nose irritation or sore throat, possibly with a reddened mucosa or a runny nose, may be found on physical examination. Abnormalities in kidney and/or liver function may occur as a result of exposure to particular solvents, although the use of many of the solvents with organ-specific toxicity, such as benzene, carbon tetrachloride, or chloroform, has been markedly reduced. Measurement of solvents in blood, exhaled air, or as a metabolite in urine is possible but often not readily available in clinical practice. A history of recurrent sensation of skipped heart beats or palpitations, chest discomfort, dyspnea, or syncope that occurs at work or shortly after work can be assessed by continuous EKG monitoring, coupled with assessment of location and activity of any arrhythmias that are detected.

Some medications are known to inhibit the human Ether-a-go-go Related Gene (hERG), which codes for the potassium-ion channel, and thereby cause prolongation of the QT interval on EKG. Although new medications are screened to determine if they target this gene, no such testing has been done on new or existing workplace chemicals.

CARDIOMYOPATHY

The most common cause of cardiomyopathy is atherosclerosis. However, as described next, cardiomyopathy has occurred in two outbreaks among people who drank beer to which arsenic or cobalt had been added. Cardiomyopathy has also been associated with work in hot or cold environments.

Arsenic was inadvertently added to beer in England in the early 1900s, causing many cases of cardiomyopathy.[41] However, no cases of work-related cardiomyopathy have ever been reported due to arsenic exposure.

Four work-related cardiomyopathy cases have been reported from cobalt exposure.[42] Long-term work-related exposure to cobalt alters left-ventricle relaxation and filling.[43] In the 1960s in the United States, Canada, and Belgium, hundreds of cardiomyopathy cases were reported due to ingestion of beer after 8 mg of cobalt was added as a foam stabilizer; case-fatality rates were as high as 22%.[44] Cobalt was prescribed for anemia in the 1950s at much higher daily doses (150 mg) but did not cause cardiomyopathy. The interaction among cobalt, alcohol, and the protein-poor diet of heavy beer drinkers was presumed to be the mechanism for the toxicity, which may explain why very few work-related cases have been reported due to work exposure. Workers involved in the manufacture or machining of tungsten carbide products are likely to be exposed to cobalt. A newly identified source of exposure has been the use of metal-on-metal hip implants, which use a cobalt-chromium alloy.[45]

A study in Japan showed that workers in hot or cold environments were at increased risk for idiopathic dilated cardiomyopathy.[46] A reversible interstitial myocarditis has been reported among children with lead poisoning from ingesting paint chips but not among adults with work exposure to lead.[47]

HYPERTENSION

Lead

Low levels of lead exposure have been associated with an increase in blood pressure. Below a BLL of 25 µg/dL, for each doubling of the BLL, the systolic blood pressure, on average, increases 1 to 2 mm, and the diastolic blood pressure increases—but to a lesser degree.[48] In the United States, with the elimination of lead from gasoline and indoor residential paint in the 1970s, the average BLL of the population fell to below 2 µg/dL. (See Figure 11-7 in Chapter 11.) OSHA allows BLLs as high as 60 µg/dL.

The effect of lead on increasing blood pressure in workers is not as dramatic as might be expected, since above 25 µg/dL the effect of lead

on blood pressure levels off. Blood pressure correlates better with chronic measurements of lead exposure, such as with X-ray fluorescence of lead in tibial bone, than with BLLs. One study estimated there would be 24,000 fewer myocardial infarctions a year in the United States if BLLs were reduced by half.[49] Adult exposure to lead is most common in the manufacture of car batteries, removal of lead paint from metal structures (such as bridges or water towers), removal of lead paint from homes built before 1978, manufacture of brass or bronze (which contain 8% to 10% lead), and the use of lead bullets in indoor firing ranges (See Chapter 11).

Noise

Exposure to excessive noise is common. Sudden acute exposure to noise increases epinephrine levels, vascular restriction, heart rate, and blood pressure—although with repeated exposure these acute effects are attenuated. Nevertheless, there is much evidence that occupational and community noise exposure increases blood pressure. One study found that, for each 5-decibel increase in occupational noise exposure, there is a 0.51 mm Hg increase in systolic blood pressure and a 1.14 increased relative risk for hypertension.[50] The noise level of heavy city traffic is 85 dB, which is the 8-hour time-weighted average in the workplace at which OSHA requires implementation of a hearing conservation program with education, audiometry (measurement of hearing acuity), and hearing protection. For comparison, the noise level for power tools and chain saws range from 95 to 110 dB, and a gunshot creates noise in the range of 140 dB. (See Chapter 12A.)

In studies investigating the association between noise level and blood pressure, individuals have their blood pressure and noise exposure measured simultaneously throughout a 24-hour period,[51] or individuals with a history of noise exposure are assessed over a period of years for the occurrence of hypertension or a change in their blood pressure.[52] The effect of noise on causing hypertension in a community setting (not limited to a work shift) appears to be even greater, with a relative risk in one study of 1.26.[50] No controlled studies have been performed assessing the effect on reducing noise exposure in those with elevated blood pressure.

PERIPHERAL VASCULAR DISEASE AND RAYNAUD DISEASE

Arsenic

Peripheral vascular disease prevalence and CVD mortality are higher in people who live in areas of Chile and Taiwan where levels of arsenic in drinking water from natural rock sediment range from 0.80 to 1.82 ppm. The Environmental Protection Agency (EPA) standard for levels of arsenic in drinking water is less than 0.01 ppm (10 ppb). In the United States, areas of the Midwest, New England, and the Southwest have had levels above the EPA standard but generally at levels below 0.1 ppm—well below the levels found in Chile and Taiwan. However, even at these lower levels, increased fatal and nonfatal CVD has been reported.[53] The increased prevalence of peripheral vascular disease in Taiwan was reversed after the water source was changed and the arsenic level reduced.[54] Arsenic in drinking water also causes hyperpigmentation, keratosis of the skin, and skin cancer. The pathological changes seen in people living in these communities in Chile and Taiwan were either arteriosclerosis or thromboangiitis obliterans.

In animal studies, arsenic induces inflammation, increases coagulation, and inhibits nitric oxide synthetase. Long-term exposure to arsenic may increase risk factors for atherosclerosis, including diabetes and hypertension. In the past, Raynaud disease (peripheral vasospasm) was seen in vineyard workers exposed to inorganic arsenic pesticides, which are no longer used.

Cadmium and Lead

Cadmium and lead exposure have been reported to increase the risk for peripheral vascular disease.[55]

Carbon Monoxide

People with peripheral vascular disease who were exposed to CO had reduced time to the development of claudication in a controlled exercise study.

Cold

Fish filleters who process large quantities of wet and cold fish have increased risk for Raynaud disease (Figure 26-3).

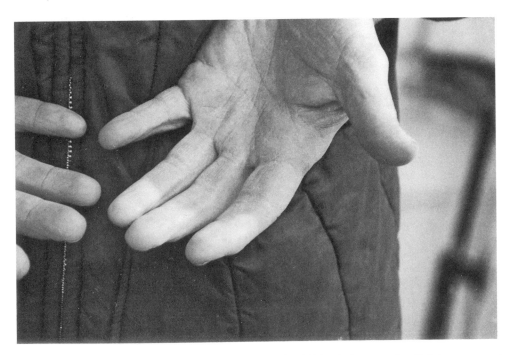

Figure 26-3. Supermarket worker with blanching fingertips of his left hand, demonstrating digital vasospasm due to Raynaud disease. His job included entering a large walk-in freezer to obtain food to stock shelves.

Vibration

The use of handheld equipment, such as chain saws, jack hammers, chippers, and grinders—especially when used under cold, wet conditions—increases the incidence of Raynaud disease. Prevalence has been as high as 50% to 80% in some groups of workers. Since this type of equipment is often noisy, there is also an association between Raynaud disease and hearing loss.

Once Raynaud disease develops, just the sound of the vibrating equipment may induce vasospasm. Even the use of equipment with one hand may induce vasospasm in the other hand. The pathophysiology of Raynaud disease amplifies the effect of norepinephrine constrictor receptors on vascular smooth muscle cells. With chronic exposure to vibration, fibrosis develops and blood viscosity increases. (See Chapter 12B.)

Preventive measures include (a) engineering changes to reduce the need for handheld tools; (b) designing of handheld tools so that they vibrate less; and (c) changing work practices, including ensuring proper maintenance of handheld equipment, taking rest breaks, learning to grasp vibrating tools as lightly as possible, and providing warm clothing and gloves in cold weather.

Vinyl Chloride

In the past, vinyl-chloride manufacturing workers who cleaned vinyl-chloride reaction kettles developed severe peripheral vascular disease in their fingers with acro-osteolysis (destruction of bone in the distal phalanges).

COR PULMONALE

Cor pulmonale is defined as enlargement of the right ventricle secondary to lung disease. Destruction and/or vasoconstriction of pulmonary arterioles due to hypoxia may occur as a result of exposure to silica or other fibrogenic dusts or exposure to chlorine gas or other occupational causes of obstructive lung disease. (See Chapter 22.)

IMPAIRMENT AND DISABILITY

Heart disease is a common cause for disability in the Social Security Disability Insurance program, in which degree of impairment—and not cause—is used to determine eligibility. In contrast, in state-based workers' compensation systems, compensation for heart disease is uncommon for workers other than police and firefighters. Most states have *heart laws* for police officers and firefighters. These laws, which generally predated medical studies on job strain or specific workplace exposures, such as particulates, are based on the perceived occupational stress and strain experienced by police officers and firefighters. The heart laws for public safety officers in individual states vary but differ from workers' compensation laws for other workers, which require physicians to state that conditions are caused by work within a reasonable degree of medical probability (more likely than not) for a condition to be considered work-related. Heart laws, in contrast, presume that heart disease in police officers and firefighters *is* work-related; they either (a) require employers who wish to contest such a workers' compensation claim to prove that the case of heart disease is not related to work or (b) do not allow employers to use evidence of previous heart disease. For other workers, chronic work stress and/or strain is usually not considered sufficient for a person to be eligible for workers' compensation from heart disease; instead unusual work stress or strain, in comparison to the worker's stress or strain outside of work, is required to qualify for compensation from an acute cardiac illness at work.

There is a comprehensive guide to determine fitness to return to work after a myocardial infarction or a cardiac procedure.[56] There are specific medical requirements for airplane pilots and truck drivers that must be met at time of entry into these occupations and periodically thereafter. These medical requirements include evaluation for CVD. None of the guidelines or requirements for fitness to work includes consideration of specific workplace exposures, such as CO, organic solvents, or hot or cold environments. Since workers with underlying heart disease are at greater risk from these exposures, clinicians should consider these workplace exposure factors when assessing a patient's fitness to return to work. Evaluation of a patient's risk factors for CVD may also be useful in predicting which truck drivers will be involved in motor vehicle crashes[57] and in evaluating general fitness for work.[58]

Clinicians should also consider the use of various medications in patients with heart disease that would increase their risk of an adverse event. These medications include (a) diuretics and beta blockers in workers exposed to heat, such as furnace operators as well as construction and landscape workers on hot summer days, and (b) vasodilators taken by workers in the explosives manufacturing industry.

REFERENCES

1. Mozaffarian D, Benjamin EJ, Go AS, et al. Executive summary: Heart disease and stroke statistics—2016 update: A report from the American Heart Association. Circulation 2016; 133: 447–454.
2. National Heart Lung and Blood Institute. NHLBI morbidity and mortality chart book. 2012 Available at: http://www.nhlbi.nih.gov/files/docs/research/2012_ChartBook_508.pdf Accessed August 19, 2016.
3. Steenland K, Burnett C, Lalich N, et al. Dying for work: The magnitude of US mortality from selected causes of deaths associated with occupation. American Journal of Industrial Medicine 2003; 43: 461–482.
4. Stewart RD, Hake CL. Paint remover hazard. Journal of the American Medical Association 1976; 235: 398–401.
5. Mevorach D, Heyman SN. Clinical problem solving pain in the marriage. New England Journal of Medicine 1995; 332: 48–50.
6. Luo JC, Chang HY, Chang SJ, et al. Elevated triglyceride and decreased high density lipoprotein level in carbon disulfide workers in Taiwan. Journal of Environmental Medicine 2003; 45: 73–78.
7. Nurminen M, Hernberg S. Effects of intervention on the cardiovascular mortality of workers exposed to carbon disulfide: A 15-year follow up. British Journal of Industrial Medicine 1985; 42: 32–35.
8. Gelbke HP, Göen T, Mäurer M, et al. A review of health effects of carbon disulfide in viscose industry and a proposal for an occupational exposure limit. Critical Review of Toxicology 2009; 39: 1–126.
9. Satran D, Henry CR, Adkinson C, et al. Cardiovascular manifestations of moderate to severe carbon monoxide poisoning. Journal of the American College of Cardiology 2005; 45: 1513–1516.
10. Elsasser S, Mall T, Grossenbacher M, et al. Influence of carbon monoxide on the early course of acute myocardial infarction. Intensive Care Medicine 1995; 21: 716–722.
11. Dahms TE, Younis LT, Wiens RD, et al. Effects of carbon monoxide exposure in patients with documented cardiac arrhythmias. Journal of the American College of Cardiology 1993; 21: 442–450.
12. Dove MS, Dockery DW, Mittleman MA, et al. The impact of Massachusetts' smoke-free workplace laws on acute myocardial infarction deaths. American Journal of Public Health 2010; 100: 2206–2212.
13. Sin DD, Wu LL, Paul Man SF. The relationship between reduced lung function and cardiovascular mortality. Chest 2005; 127: 1952–1959.
14. Nayha S. Cold and the risk of cardiovascular disease. A review. International Journal of Circumpolar Health 2002; 61: 373–380.
15. Braga AL, Zanobetti A, Schwartz J. The effect of weather on respiratory and cardiovascular deaths in 12 U.S. cities. Environmental Health Perspectives 2002; 110: 859–863.
16. Phung D, Thai PK, Guo Y, et al. Ambient temperature and risk of cardiovascular hospitalization: An updated systematic review and meta-analysis. Science of the Total Environment 2016; 550: 1084–1102.
17. Navas-Acien A, Guallar E, Silbergeld EK, Rothenberg SJ. Lead exposure and cardiovascular disease-a systematic review. Environmental Health Perspectives 2007; 115: 472–482.
18. Chen CC, Yen HW, Lo YH, et al. The association of prolonged QT interval on electrocardiography and chronic lead exposure. Journal of Occupational and Environmental Medicine 2013; 55: 614–619.
19. RuDusky BM. Acute myocardial infarction secondary to coronary vasospasm during withdrawal from industrial nitroglycerine exposure—A case report. Angiology 2001; 52: 143–144.
20. Reeve G, Bloom T, Rinsky R, Smith A. Cardiovascular disease among nitroglycerin-exposed workers. American Journal of Epidemiology 1983; 188: 418.
21. Pope CA III, Ezzati M, Dockery DW. Fine particulate air pollution and life expectancy

in the United States. New England Journal of Medicine 2009; 360: 376–386.

22. Samet JM, Rappold A, Graff D, et al. Concentrated ambient ultra-fine particle exposure induces cardiac changes in young health volunteers. American Journal of Respiratory and Critical Care Medicine 2009; 179: 1034–1042.

23. AirNow. Available at: www.airnow.gov. Accessed September 28, 2016.

24. Umukoro PE, Fan T, Zhang J, et al. Long-term metal PM 2.5 exposures decrease cardiac acceleration and deceleration capacities in welders. Journal of Occupational and Environmental Medicine 2016; 58: 227–231.

25. Laden F, Hart JE, Smith TJ, et al. Cause-specific mortality in the unionized U.S. trucking industry. Environmental Health Perspectives 2007; 115: 1192–1196.

26. Toren K, Bergdahl IA, Nilsson T, et al. Occupational exposure to particulate air pollution and mortality due to ischemic heart disease and cerebrovascular disease. Occupational and Environmental Medicine 2007; 64: 515–519.

27. Johnson JV, Stewart W, Hall EM, et al. Long-term psychosocial work environmental and cardiovascular mortality among Swedish men. American Journal of Public Health 1996; 86: 324–331.

28. Bonde JP, Munch-Hansen T, Agerbo E, et al. Job strain and ischemic heart disease: A prospective study using a new approach for exposure assessment. Journal of Occupational and Environmental Medicine 2009; 51: 732–738.

29. Shockey TM, Sussell AL, Odom EC. Cardiovascular health status by occupational group—21 states, 2013. Morbidity and Mortality Weekly Report 2016; 65: 793–798.

30. MacDonald LA, Cohen A, Baron S, et al. Occupation as socioeconomic status or environmental exposure? A survey of practice among population-based cardiovascular studies in the United States. American Journal of Epidemiology 2009; 169: 1411–1421.

31. Pietroiusti A, Neri A, Somma G, et al. Incidence of metabolic syndrome among night shift health care workers. Occupational and Environmental Medicine 2010; 67: 54–57.

32. DeBacquer D, VanRisseghem M, Clays E, et al. Rotating shift work and the metabolic syndrome: A prospective study. International Journal of Epidemiology 2009; 38: 848–854.

33. Viitasalo K, Kuosma E, Laitinen J, et al. Effects of shift rotation and the flexibility of a shift system on daytime alertness and cardiovascular risk factors. Scandinavian Journal of Work, Environment & Health 2008; 34: 198–205.

34. Wang A, Arah OA, Kauhanen J, et al. Shift work and 20-year incidence of acute myocardial infarction: Results from the Kuopio Ischemic Heart Disease Risk Factor Study. Occupational and Environmental Medicine 2016; 73: 588–594.

35. Kivimäki M, Jokela M, Nyberg ST, et al. Long working hours and risk of coronary heart disease and stroke: A systematic review and meta-analysis of published and unpublished data for 603,838 individuals. Lancet 2015; 386: 1739–1746.

36. Rothenbacher D, Hoffmeister A, Brenner H, et al. Physical activity, coronary heart disease, and inflammatory response. Archives of Internal Medicine 2003; 163: 1200–1205.

37. van Uffelen JG, Wong J, Chau JY, et al. Occupational sitting and health risks: A systematic review. American Journal Preventive Medicine 2010; 39: 379–888.

38. Kales SN, Soteriades ES, Christophi CA, et al. Emergency duties and deaths from heart disease among firefighters in the United States. New England Journal of Medicine 2007; 356: 1207–1215.

39. Al-Zaiti S, Rittenberger JC, Reis SE, et al. Electrocardiographic responses during fire suppression and recovery among experienced firefighters. Journal of Occupational and Environmental Medicine 2015; 57: 938–942.

40. GeibeJr, Holder J, Peeples L, et al. Predictors of on-duty coronary events in male firefighters in the United States. American Journal of Cardiology 2008; 101: 585–589.

41. Reynolds ES. An account of the epidemic outbreak of arsenical poisoning occurring in beer drinkers in the north of England and midland countries in 1900. Lancet 1901; 1: 166–170.

42. Jarvis JQ, Hammond E. Meier R, et al. Cobalt cardiomyopathy. Journal of Occupational Medicine 1992; 34: 620–626.

43. Linna A, Oksa P, Groundstroem K, et al. Exposure to cobalt in the production of cobalt and cobalt compounds and its effect on the heart. Occupational and Environmental Medicine 2004; 61: 877–885.

44. Morin YL, Foley AR, Martineau G, et al. Quebec beer-drinkers' cardiomyopathy.

Canadian Medical Association Journal 1967; 97: 881–883.

45. Allen LA, Ambardekar AV, Devaraj KM, et al. Clinical problem-solving: Missing elements of the history. New England Journal of Medicine 2014; 370: 559–566.

46. Miura K, Nakagawa H, Toyoshuma H, et al. Environmental factors and risk of idiopathic dilated cardiomyopathy: A multi-hospital case-control study in Japan. Circulation Journal 2004; 68: 1011–1017.

47. Silver W, Rodriguez-Torres R. Electrocardio-graphic studies in children with lead poisoning. Pediatrics 1968; 41: 1124–1127.

48. Glenn BS, Stewart WF, Links JM, et al. The longitudinal association of lead with blood pressure. Epidemiology 2003; 14: 30–36.

49. Schwartz J. Lead, blood pressure, and cardiovascular disease in men and women. Environmental Health Perspectives 1991; 91: 71–75.

50. VanKemper EE, Kruize H, Boshuizen HC, et al. The association between noise exposure and blood pressure and ischemic heart disease: A meta-analysis. Environmental Health Perspectives 2002; 110: 307–317.

51. Chang TY, Su TC, Lin SY, et al. Effects of occupational noise exposure on 24-hour ambulatory vascular properties in male workers. Environmental Health Perspectives 2007; 115: 1660–1664.

52. Sbihi H, Davics HW, Demers PA. Hypertension in noise-exposed sawmill workers: A cohort study. Occupational and Environmental Medicine 2008; 65: 643–646.

53. Moon KA, Guallar E, Umans JG, et al. Association between exposure to low to moderate arsenic levels and incident cardiovascular disease: A prospective cohort study. Annals of Internal Medicine 2013; 159: 649–659.

54. Pi J, Yamauchi H, Sun G, et al. Vascular dysfunction in patients with chronic arsenosis can be reversed by reduction of arsenic exposure. Environmental Health Perspectives 2005; 113: 339–341.

55. Navas-Acien A, Selvin E, Sharrett AR, et al. Lead, cadmium, smoking, and increased risk of arterial disease. Circulation 2004; 109: 3196–3201.

56. Rondinelli RD, Genovese E, Katz RT et al. The cardiovascular system. In: RD Rondinelli (ed.). Guides to the evaluation of permanent impairment (6th ed.). Chicago: American Medical Association, 2008, pp. 47–76.

57. Ronna BB, Thiese MS, Ott U, et al. The association between cardiovascular disease risk factors and motor vehicle crashes among professional truck drivers. Journal of Occupational and Environmental Medicine 2016; 58: 828–832.

58. Palladino R, Caporale O, Nardone A, et al. Use of Framingham risk score as a clinical tool for the assessment of fitness for work: Results from a cohort study. Journal of Occupational and Environmental Medicine 2016; 58: 805–809.

FURTHER READING

Ernst A, Zibrak JD. Carbon monoxide poisoning. New England Journal of Medicine 1998; 339: 1603–1608.
Good review of carbon monoxide poisoning.

Hansson GK. Inflammation, atherosclerosis, and coronary artery disease. New England Journal of Medicine 2005; 352: 1685–1695.
Good review of inflammation and atherosclerosis, which is relevant to a number of occupational exposures.

Kivimäki M, Virtanen M, Elovainio M, et al. Work stress in the etiology of coronary heart disease—a meta-analysis. Scandinavian Journal of Work, Environment & Health 2006; 32: 431–442.
Meta-analysis on work stress and cardiovascular disease.

Li J, Loerbroks A, Angerer P. Physical activity and risk of cardiovascular disease: what does the new epidemiological evidence show? Current Opinions in Cardiology 2013; 28: 575–583.
Summary of recent prospective studies on the risk of CVD in relationship to both leisure and occupational physical activity.

NTP monograph on health effects of low-level lead. June 13, 2012. Available at: http://ntp.niehs.nih.gov/ntp/ohat/lead/final/monographhealtheffectslowlevellead_newissn_508.pdf. Accessed August 24, 2016.
Comprehensive review of literature on adverse health effects of lead to both children and adults.

Skogstad M, Johannessen HA, Tynes T, et al. Systematic review of the cardiovascular effects of occupational noise. Occupational Medicine (London) 2016; 66: 10–16.
Good review of noise exposure related to cardiovascular disease and hypertension.

Speyer FE, Wegman DH, Raminey A. Palpitation rates associated with fluorocarbon exposure in hospital setting. New England Journal of Medicine 1975; 292: 624–626.

Example of report of arrhythmia associated with solvent exposure in hospital workers.

Thurston GD, Burnett RT, Turner MC, et al. Ischemic heart disease mortality and long-term exposure to source-related components of U.S. fine particle air pollution. Environmental Health Perspectives 2016; 124: 785–794.

Study showing that a reduction in particulates from coal burning would have the greatest benefit in reducing mortality from heart disease.

Vetter C, Devore EE, Wegrzyn LR, et al. Association between rotating night shift work and risk of coronary heart disease among women. JAMA 2016; 315: 1726–1734.

A recent prospective study showing a small, but significantly increased, risk of CVD with longer duration of shift work.

27

Liver Disorders

Barry S. Levy

Many chemical, biological, and physical factors can adversely affect the liver. There are many potential occupational and environmental exposures to these factors. It is often challenging to recognize occupationally and environmentally related liver disorders because liver disorders are frequently attributed to other commonly occurring factors, such as ingestion of ethyl alcohol.

FUNCTIONS OF THE LIVER

The liver is the main organ for metabolizing foreign substances (xenobiotics). (See Chapter 7.) The liver maintains homeostasis by processing nutrients, such as glycogen and other carbohydrates, lipids, and dietary amino acids. It also filters particles; bioactivates or detoxifies various substances, such as steroid hormones and xenobiotics; synthesizes proteins, such as albumin and clotting factors; and forms and secretes bile.[1] The liver plays a major role in defending the body against invasive microorganisms. It has an unusual capacity for growth and regeneration.

The liver receives about 75% of its blood supply from the portal vein, which carries xenobiotics absorbed by the small intestine, and 25% of its blood supply from the hepatic artery. Xenobiotics that are metabolized in the liver and excreted in the bile may be further metabolized in the intestine and reabsorbed, increasing the exposure of the liver to potential toxicants.

TYPES OF LIVER DAMAGE

Types of hepatobiliary injury (damage) include death of hepatocytes, fatty infiltration (steatohepatitis), canalicular cholestasis, bile duct damage, immune-mediated responses, sinusoidal disorders, fibrosis and cirrhosis, and tumors.[1] Acute disease is generally reversible, often without evidence of residual damage. Chronic liver disease may arise from repeated bouts of acute disease or from an insult that causes persistent damage. Although inflammatory mediators that respond to toxic intermediary compounds are formed to scavenge cellular debris, they may also lead to hepatic fibrosis and ultimately cirrhosis with impaired hepatic function and portal hypertension.

ASSESSMENT OF LIVER DAMAGE

The most commonly used indicators of hepatocellular injury are enzymes that leak from injured or necrotic hepatocytes, raising levels of these enzymes in the blood. Alanine aminotransaminase (ALT) and aspartate transaminase (AST) are the enzymes that are most commonly measured. In general, toxins and obesity are associated with a serum AST:ALT ratio less than 1, and alcoholic liver disease is associated with a serum AST:ALT ratio greater than 2. While these enzymes have high sensitivity, they have low specificity for liver damage. Nonhepatic sources can contribute to serum elevations of these enzymes; both of these enzymes are found in skeletal and cardiac muscle, ALT is found in the kidneys, and AST is found in red blood cells. The serum level of gamma-glutamyl transpeptidase (GGTP) is more specific for liver disease than ALT or AST, but it is so sensitive that it is often increased when no liver disease is apparent. Serum alkaline phosphatase levels are useful diagnostic tools; in cholestatic liver disease, they are higher than AST and ALT levels, and in infiltrative liver disease, they are elevated while AST and ALT levels are generally near normal. Serum bilirubin levels may also be helpful; an elevated serum level of conjugated bilirubin suggests liver disease, whereas an elevated serum level of unconjugated bilirubin suggests hemolysis or Gilbert syndrome.

The synthetic function of the liver is measured by clotting tests and blood protein levels, as well as by more sophisticated tests that measure the ability of the liver to metabolize or clear specific agents after administration of a challenge dose. Ultrasound measurement of fat deposition and ultrasound or magnetic resonance imaging to measure degree of fibrosis are noninvasive procedures to determine the presence and degree of liver disease.

Liver biopsy remains the gold standard for diagnosis and prognosis of liver disease, although it is invasive and can result in adverse effects. Some scoring systems based on pathology examination of liver tissue can be used for determining diagnosis and prognosis of liver disease. These are based on descriptions of necro-inflammatory activity and the degree of fibrosis to distinguish ongoing activity found in chronic active hepatitis (chronic aggressive hepatitis) from chronic persistent hepatitis. Persistently elevated markers of liver injury, such as ALT and AST, suggest aggressive disease.

CAUSES OF OCCUPATIONAL AND ENVIRONMENTAL LIVER DISORDERS

Infectious Agents

Viral hepatitis, especially with hepatitis B virus (HBV) and hepatitis C virus (HCV), has been a major risk for workers in healthcare,[2] solid-waste management,[3] and other occupations. The introduction and widespread use of HBV vaccine has markedly decreased the risk of HBV infection in many of these workers. (See Chapter 13.) A recent systematic review and meta-analysis of 44 studies on HCV in healthcare workers reported that high- and moderate-quality studies found a significantly increased risk among healthcare workers (odds ratio [OR] = 1.6), especially medical and laboratory staff, compared to control populations; the risk was even higher among health professionals who had high probability of blood contact (OR = 2.7).[2]

Some cases of hepatitis E virus (HEV) may also be occupationally related. A recent meta-analysis of 12 cross-sectional studies found a significant association between occupational exposure to swine and HEV infection, with crude odds ratios ranging from 1.47 to 8.09. The authors concluded that much evidence supports that swine and possibly other animals are a reservoir of HEV infection.[4]

Workers who have contact with specific species of animals are at increased risk of infectious diseases that may affect the liver. Those who have contact with small mammals, such as mice and rabbits, may be at risk for leptospirosis. Workers exposed to sheep, goats, or cattle may be at risk for brucellosis. Both leptospirosis and brucellosis can cause granulomatous hepatitis, as can tuberculosis, schistosomiasis, histoplasmosis, and other infectious diseases possibly related to occupational or environmental exposures.

Hepatotoxins

The liver receives ingested substances via the portal vein as well as inhaled and dermally absorbed substances via the hepatic artery. More than 100 industrial chemicals can be acutely hepatotoxic in experimental animals or humans. Potentially hepatotoxic exposures also include ethyl alcohol, some prescription or over-the-counter medications, some herbal medicines, and some recreational drugs. (See Table 27-1.) Acetaminophen overdose, which may occur at relatively low doses if accompanied by regular alcohol use, is the most frequent cause of fulminant liver failure in the United States. Recognition of this condition and early appropriate treatment may be life-saving.[5] Clinicians treating patients who are experiencing pain, including those who have work-related injuries, should advise them to reduce alcohol intake.

Metabolic reactions may make chemicals more or less hepatotoxic. (See Chapter 7.) The most important family of enzymes catalyzing metabolism of xenobiotics are the cytochrome P450 enzymes. Liver enzymes can be induced by a variety of agents, increasing the ability to process similar agents; they can be inhibited directly or inhibited competitively by agents that compete for enzyme sites. Various exposures may interact to increase the likelihood of adverse hepatic effects, such as certain chemicals interacting with ethyl alcohol. Nonalcoholic fatty liver disease is the most common liver disorder in the United States and other high-income countries, where obesity, type 2 diabetes mellitus, dyslipidemia, and the metabolic syndrome are prevalent.[6] The presence of nonalcoholic fatty liver disease may also increase the adverse effects of hepatotoxic chemicals.[7]

The intensity and duration of hepatotoxin exposure predict the severity of outcome. For example, low-level exposure to hepatotoxins of short duration may cause a transient elevation of AST and ALT, reflecting reversible cellular

Table 27-1. Illustrative Chemical Agents That Have Caused Occupational Hepatic Disorders

Types of Agents	Examples	Illustrative Hepatic Disorders
Naturally occurring chemicals		
Mycotoxins	Aflatoxins	Hepatocellular carcinoma, acute and chronic hepatitis
Plant toxins	Cycasin, safrole	Acute hepatic injury
Bacterial toxins	Exotoxins and endotoxins	Acute cholestatic injury
Mushroom toxins	Phalloidins	Acute cholestatic injury
Algae toxins	Microcystin	Acute and chronic hepatic injury
Synthetic compounds		
Alcohol	Ethyl alcohol	Fatty liver, cirrhosis
Pesticides	Dichlorodiphenyltrichloroethane (DDT), Kepone, chlorobenzene	Fatty liver, chronic hepatic injury
Aromatic amines	Methylene dianiline	Acute cholestatic injury
	2-Acetylaminofluorene	Hepatic injury
Halogenated hydrocarbons	Carbon tetrachloride, trichloroethane	Fatty liver, cirrhosis
	Vinyl chloride	Hepatic angiosarcoma, toxicant-associated fatty liver disease, sinusoidal endothelial damage
	Chloroform	Acute hepatic injury
Chlorinated aromatics	Polychlorinated biphenyls, tetrachlorodibenzo-p-dioxin	Acute and chronic hepatic injury
Nitroalkanes and nitroaromatics	Trinitroluene, dimethylnitrosamine, trinitrophenol	Fatty liver, acute and subacute hepatic injury
Metals and metalloids	Arsenic	Acute hepatic injury, cirrhosis, hepatic angiosarcoma
	Beryllium, copper	Hepatic granulomata
	Chromium	Cholestatic injury
	Phosphorus	Acute hepatic injury, cholestatic injury

Source: Adapted from Wang J-S, Groopman JD. Hepatic disorders, in BS Levy, DH Wegman (eds.). Occupational health: Recognizing and preventing work-related disease and injury (4th ed.). Philadelphia: Lippincott Williams & Wilkins, 2000, p. 632.

damage. Higher-level and longer-duration exposures are more likely to cause widespread necrosis.

Carbon tetrachloride is a hepatotoxin thought to produce toxicity through intermediary metabolites, with free radical formation leading to lipid peroxidation, leading to permeability of plasma membranes, leading to disturbances of cell homeostasis, and eventually leading to cell death. In parallel, substantial mitochondrial damage occurs, releasing more inflammatory mediators, including agents that lead to apoptosis rather than necrotic cell death. Low-level, long-term exposure to carbon tetrachloride (and other agents) may lead to acute and chronic cell injury with fatty deposition, which may increase susceptibility to other hepatotoxins.

Toxic hepatitis can be caused by a variety of chemicals. Occupational exposure, via inhalation and skin absorption, to some organic solvents can cause toxic hepatitis.[8] Organic solvents are widely used in many industrial processes, including degreasing, metal processing, manufacturing and spraying of paint, and manufacturing and maintenance of automobiles and aircraft. The main pathogenic processes by which solvent-induced liver damage occurs are thought to be inflammation, cytochrome P450 dysfunction, dysfunction of mitochrondria, and oxidative stress.[8] Hepatotoxic organic solvents include trichloroethylene,[9,10] carbon tetrachloride,[11-13] and chloroform[12]; there is also evidence that tetrachloroethylene, xylene, toluene, and 1,1,1-trichloroethane are toxic to the liver.[14] Many other chemicals have been demonstrated to cause hepatotoxicity in experimental animals but not, or not consistently, in humans.

Occupational exposure to specific hepatotoxins, including vinyl chloride monomer (VCM), has been causally associated with toxicant-associated fatty liver disease and a more severe form known as toxicant-associated steatohepatitis.[15] Vinyl chloride monomer has also been causally associated with a form of non-cirrhotic portal hypertension related to sinusoidal endothelial damage.[16]

Two studies have indicated that serum perfluorooctanoic acid concentration is associated with modest increases in liver enzymes. The magnitude of effect was not consistent between these studies.[17]

Halothane, a halogenated hydrocarbon widely used in the past as an anesthetic, can cause acute hepatitis in a small percentage of people due to a hypersensitive immune response.

Physical Agents

Occupational or environmental exposure to two physical agents, extreme heat and ionizing radiation can cause liver disorders. Acute liver failure is relatively frequent during heat stroke, which can cause centrilobular necrosis and cholestasis.

Ionizing radiation can induce radiation hepatitis, also known as radiation-induced liver disease. A mean dose of 30 Gy is generally considered safe, but lower radiation doses may cause it in people with abnormal liver function. Survivors often develop cirrhosis.

Carcinogens

A number of agents can cause liver cancer or bile duct cancer (Table 27-2). Occupational or environmental exposures can occur with most of these agents.

Vinyl chloride monomer, which has been designated as a Group 1 carcinogen by the International Agency for Research on Cancer, is a well-established cause of angiosarcoma of the liver, a rare tumor. The association between VCM and angiosarcoma of the liver was first reported in 1974, when initially three, then seven, cases were recognized in workers at a factory with 270 employees that manufactured polyvinyl chloride (PVC) and other copolymers of VCM.[18,19] Review of pathologic material from these workers and four others with hepatic disease revealed portal fibrosis and atypical sinusoidal lining cells.[19] Polyvinyl chloride, a polymerized form of VCM, is used extensively in the plastics industry.

Exposure to inorganic arsenic has also been associated with liver cancer. A recent meta-analysis of 12 studies concerning inorganic arsenic exposure via drinking water found a significant association between inorganic arsenic exposure and liver cancer mortality (meta-standardized mortality ratio = 1.80).[20]

More than 4 billion people are dietarily exposed to aflatoxins, a well-established cause of hepatocellular carcinoma (HCC), the most

Table 27-2. Agents Classified by the International Agency for Research on Cancer as Carcinogenic for Liver or Bile Duct Cancer*

Carcinogenic Agents with Sufficient Evidence in Humans	Agents with Limited Evidence in Humans
Aflatoxins	Androgenic (anabolic) steroids
Alcoholic beverages	Arsenic and inorganic arsenic compounds
Clonorchis sinensis (Human liver fluke)	Betel quid without tobacco
1,2-Dichloropropane	DDT
Estrogen-progestogen contraceptives	Dichloromethane (Methylene chloride)
Hepatitis B virus	HIV, type 1
Hepatitis C virus	*Schistosoma japonicum*
Opisthorchis viverrini (Southeast Asian liver fluke)	Trichloroethylene
Plutonium	X-radiation, gamma-radiation
Thorium-232 and its decay products	
Tobacco smoking (in smokers and in smokers' children)	
Vinyl chloride	

* Either with "sufficient" or with "limited" evidence. This table does not include factors not covered in the IARC Monographs, notably genetic traits, reproductive status, and some nutritional factors.
Source: International Agency for Research on Cancer. List of classification by cancer sites with sufficient or limited evidence in humans, Volumes 1–117. Available at: https://monographs.iarc.fr/ENG/Classification/Table4.pdf. Accessed July 6, 2017.

common type of liver cancer. A recent systematic review and meta-analysis found that, in 17 studies from locations in China, Taiwan, and sub-Saharan Africa (where there is high exposure to dietary aflatoxins), the population attributable risk of aflatoxin-related HCC was 17% overall and 21% in HBV-positive populations.[21]

ACKNOWLEDGMENT

The author thanks Michael Hodgson, MD, and Rosemary Sokas, MD, MOH for their contributions in the development of this chapter.

REFERENCES

1. Jaeschke H. Toxic responses of the liver. In CD Klaassen (ed.). Casarett and Doull's toxicology: The basic science of poisons (8th ed.). New York: McGraw Hill Education, 2013, pp. 642–644.
2. Westermann C, Peters C, Lisiak B, et al. The prevalence of hepatitis C among healthcare workers: A systematic review and meta-analysis. Occupational and Environmental Medicine 2015; 72: 880–888.
3. Corrao CRN, Del Cimmuto A, Marzuillo C, et al. Association between waste management and HBV among solid municipal waste workers: A systematic review and meta-analysis of observational studies. Scientific World Journal Oct 9; 2013: 692083. doi: 10.1155/2013/692083.
4. De Schryver A, De Schrijver K, Francois G, et al. Hepatitis E virus infection: An emerging occupational risk? Occupational Medicine 2015; 65: 667–672.
5. Yoon E, Babar A, Choudhary M, et al. Acetaminophen-induced hepatotoxicity: A comprehensive update. Journal of Clinical and Translational Hepatology 2016; 4: 131–142.
6. Lazo M, Hernaez R, Eberhardt MS, et al. Prevalence of nonalcoholic fatty liver disease in the United States: The Third National Health and Nutrition Examination Survey, 1988–1994. American Journal of Epidemiology 2013; 178: 38–45.
7. Hodgson M, van Thiel DH, Goodman-Klein B. Obesity and hepatotoxins as risk factors for fatty liver disease. British Journal of Industrial Medicine 1991; 48: 690–695.
8. Malaguarnera G, Cataudella E, Giordano M, et al. Toxic hepatitis in occupational exposure to solvents. World Journal of Gastroenterology 2012; 18: 2756–2766.
9. Agency for Toxic Substances and Disease Registry. Toxicological profile for trichloroethylene (Update). Atlanta: ATSDR, 1997.
10. U.S. Environmental Protection Agency. Trichloroethylene health risk assessment: Synthesis and characterization. External Review Draft/600/P-01/002A. Washington, DC: EPA, 2001.

11. Clawson GA. Mechanisms of carbon tetrachloride hepatotoxicity. Pathology and Immunopathology Research 1989; 8: 104–112.

12. Plaa GL. Chlorinated methanes and liver injury: Highlights of the past 50 years. Annual Review of Pharmacology & Toxicology 2000; 40: 42–65.

13. Brattin WJ, Glende EA Jr, Recknagel RO. Pathological mechanisms in carbon tetrachloride hepatotoxicity. Journal of Free Radicals in Biology & Medicine 1985; 1: 27–38.

14. Brautbar N, Williams John II. Industrial solvents and liver toxicity: Risk assessment, risk factors and mechanisms. International Journal of Hygiene and Environmental Health 2002; 205: 479–491.

15. Wahlang B, Beier JI, Clair HB, et al. Toxicant-associated steatohepatitis. Toxicologic Pathology 2013; 41: 343–360.

16. Sherman M. Vinyl chloride and the liver. Journal of Hepatology 2009; 51: 1074–1081.

17. Steenland K, Fletcher T, Savitz DA. Epidemiologic evidence on the health effects of perfluorooctanoic acid (PFOA). Environmental Health Perspectives 2010; 118: 1100–1108.

18. Creech JL Jr, Johnson MN. Angiosarcoma of liver in the manufacture of polyvinyl chloride. Journal of Occupational Medicine 1974; 16: 150–151.

19. Falk GH, Creech JL, Heath CW Jr, et al. Hepatic disease among workers at a vinyl chloride polymerization plant. JAMA 1974; 230: 59–63.

20. Wang W. Cheng S, Zhang D. Association of inorganic arsenic exposure with liver cancer mortality: A meta-analysis. Environmental Research 2014; 135: 120–125.

21. Liu Y, Chang C-C, Marsh GM, Wu F. Population attributable risk of aflatoxin-related liver cancer: Systematic review and meta-analysis. European Journal of Cancer 2012; 48: 2125–2136.

FURTHER READING

Zimmerman HJ. Hepatotoxicity: The adverse effects of drugs and other chemicals on the liver (2nd ed.). Philadelphia: Lippincott Williams & Wilkins, 1999.
A comprehensive textbook on hepatotoxicity, with excellent chapters on occupational and environmental hepatotoxicity.

Zimmerman HJ, Lewis JH. Chemical- and toxin-induced hepatotoxicity. Gastroenterology Clinics of North America 1995; 24: 1027–1045.

Malaguarnera G, Cataudella E, Giordano M, et al. Toxic hepatitis in occupational exposure to solvents. World Journal of Gastroenterology 2012; 18: 2756–2766.

Brautbar N, Williams J 2nd. Industrial solvents and liver toxicity: Risk assessment, risk factors and mechanisms. International Journal of Hygiene and Environmental Health 2002; 205: 479–491.

Wahlang B, Beier JI, Clair HB, et al. Toxicant-associated steatohepatitis. Toxicological Pathology 2013; 41: 343–360.
Useful review articles.

28

Kidney Disorders

Virginia M. Weaver, Bernard G. Jaar, and Jeffrey J. Fadrowski

Acute and chronic exposures to nephrotoxic agents in the workplace or the general environment can cause kidney disorders. High-level, short-term nephrotoxicant exposures may result in acute conditions. Chronic, lower-level exposures, especially when present with diabetes or other risk factors, may cause or contribute to chronic kidney disease (CKD), which increases morbidity as well as all-cause and cardiovascular mortality.[1]

Globally, from 1990 to 2010, CKD accounted for the third largest increase in years of life lost due to premature mortality (after HIV/AIDS and diabetes).[2] In the United States, CKD is estimated to affect more than 15% of noninstitutionalized adults.[3] In 2014, there were almost 700,000 U.S. residents with end-stage renal disease (ESRD) requiring dialysis or transplantation, an increase of 74% since 2000,[4] largely due to increased obesity and resultant diabetes and hypertension. Care for ESRD patients resulted in Medicare expenditures of $32.8 billion in 2014.[4]

ASSESSMENT OF KIDNEY FUNCTION

Endogenous markers, such as serum creatinine and cystatin C, are useful estimates of glomerular filtration rate (GFR), but their value is limited by non-renal factors that also influence their serum levels. For example, serum creatinine levels are partly related to muscle mass since creatinine is a metabolite of creatine in myocytes. Measurement of creatinine clearance eliminates the need to account for the impact of muscle mass on serum creatinine but presents the practical challenge of a 24-hour urine collection. Therefore, GFR-estimating equations (eGFR), which combine serum creatinine (or cystatin C) with age, gender, and other variables, are the most commonly used measures of kidney function. Above-normal serum creatinine (or cystatin C) or below-normal eGFR indicate decreased kidney function. Albuminuria is an early marker for kidney disease that also predicts CKD progression as well as cardiovascular and all-cause mortality.[1]

Significant kidney injury may occur before eGFR declines. In addition, estimates of GFR are less accurate at levels greater than 60 ml/min/1.73 m². Urinary early biological effect (EBE) markers have been studied as more sensitive indicators of kidney damage; however, other than albuminuria, few such markers have been validated prospectively, especially in populations exposed to nephrotoxicants. Beta-2-microglobulin, a low-molecular-weight protein whose presence in urine indicates proximal tubular damage, is a validated marker for high-level cadmium exposure,[5,6] although instability at urine pH levels less than 6 makes its use challenging.

In addition, at the lower toxicant exposure levels in many high-income countries, associations between urinary EBE markers and nephrotoxicants may be due to co-excretion because many of these markers are proteins and nephrotoxicants are often bound to proteins in the body.[7,8] Unexpected research results based on eGFRs have also been reported recently. Examples include positive associations between urine metals and eGFR,[9] with results that differ based on the method used to adjust the metal for urine concentration or by the eGFR equation used;[10-12] blood and urinary cadmium levels that are associated in opposite directions with eGFR;[13] and associations with measured, but not predicted, toxicant levels.[14] These data suggest that kidney function and/or processing may influence biomarker levels.[15]

Due to these concerns, this chapter emphasizes longitudinal research and clinical outcomes with less weight on studies that rely on exposure and EBE outcomes when both are measured in urine and on studies with cross-sectional designs. Animal data are also discussed since, despite interspecies differences and higher levels of exposure, experimental design is a key strength rarely possible in human research.

ACUTE KIDNEY INJURY

High-level exposure to some chemicals can cause acute kidney injury. For example, acute tubular necrosis can be caused by ethylene glycol ingestion due to calcium oxalate crystals in the renal tubules and by arsine, which causes hemolytic anemia that leads to tubular damage. Acute high-level exposure to lead in children can cause Fanconi syndrome, in which proximal tubular injury results in excretion of low-molecular-weight proteins, glucose, and other small molecules, which are normally absorbed by the proximal tubules.

In 2008, an epidemic of acute kidney injury in Chinese infants and young children was linked to the ingestion of milk powder adulterated with melamine, a synthetic chemical with a high nitrogen content that falsely elevates protein levels. Urinary tract injury arises from stones containing melamine and uric acid.[16] The Chinese Ministry of Health reported that, as of December 2008, almost 300,000 children were affected, resulting in 51,900 hospitalizations and six deaths.[17] Among the affected children, 8% had persistent kidney abnormalities 1 year after diagnosis.[18] In response to this epidemic, the World Health Organization's tolerable daily intake for melamine was lowered with similar responses by governments of the United States, the European Union, and China.[19]

CHRONIC KIDNEY DISEASE

Globally, diabetes and hypertension are the main risk factors for CKD. In chronic, high-level exposures, nephrotoxicants can cause CKD; at lower levels of exposure, these agents may contribute to CKD when combined with other risk factors.

Glomerular Disease

Workers exposed to crystalline silica, such as in mining and sandblasting, have an increased risk for glomerulonephritis and Goodpasture's syndrome.[20,21] An association between occupational silica exposure and CKD has also been reported in one study.[22] Solvents have been implicated as a cause of glomerulonephritis.[23] Patients with glomerulonephritis who are occupationally exposed to solvents progress to ESRD faster than those without such exposure.[24]

Chronic mercury exposure infrequently causes nephrotic syndrome, characterized by immune-complex-mediated glomerular damage and excretion of 3.5 or more grams of protein daily. Personal use of skin-lightening creams and occupational exposure to mercury vapor can cause this disorder.[25] Chronic mercury exposure can also cause proximal tubular damage.

Chronic Tubulointerstitial Disease: Metals

Arsenic

Increased mortality rates for kidney disease have been reported in ecologic studies,[26] with decreased mortality after arsenic levels in drinking water were reduced.[27] A prospective cohort study of more than 10,000 participants in Bangladesh found a positive association between change in urinary arsenic concentration and incidence of proteinuria.[28] A prospective study of more than 3,000 Native Americans found an increased incidence of CKD associated with baseline urinary arsenic concentration.[29] Experimental studies in animals have also reported adverse effects of arsenic on the kidney.[26] However, in recent cross-sectional analyses, higher urinary arsenic levels were associated with higher eGFR.[29,30] Epidemiologic research on the kidney impact of arsenic has been summarized in a recent review, which concluded that additional prospective studies are needed to determine a threshold for adverse kidney effects.[26]

Cadmium

Cadmium bioaccumulates in the kidney, where it targets the proximal tubules, causing tubulointerstitial fibrosis. High-level exposure to cadmium via ingestion of rice irrigated with industrially polluted water resulted in an outbreak of itai-itai ("ouch-ouch") disease in Japan starting in the early 1900s. Cadmium exposure was extremely high; urinary cadmium levels were often greater than 20 μg/g creatinine.[31,32] (In contrast, the geometric mean urinary cadmium in the 2011–2012 U.S. National Health and Nutrition Examination Survey was only 0.22 μg/g creatinine.[33]) Osteomalacia and osteoporosis with secondary fractures and severe pain were prominent features of those affected in this outbreak. Proximal tubular injury, assessed with urinary EBE markers, was common. Although based on small numbers, increased mortality from kidney disease was observed.[6,34] A few reports of CKD[35] and ESRD[36] have also been published.

Persistent elevations in urinary EBE markers have been observed in workers with chronic, high-level exposure to cadmium.[5] Some workers have had kidney stones or evidence of CKD.[5,37,38] The Occupational Safety and Health Administration (OSHA) requires biological monitoring with urinary beta-2-microglobulin and blood and urinary cadmium for workers exposed at or above the action level. The OSHA

Cadmium Biological Monitoring Advisor eTool is a useful online calculator to determine mandatory actions, including additional medical evaluations that are required by OSHA.[39] Given the impact of multiple risk factors on kidney disease, exposure to cadmium should be minimized in people with CKD, regardless of its cause, or with CKD risk factors, such as diabetes.

For many years, regulatory agencies, when setting standards, have considered kidney dysfunction as the most sensitive indicator of the adverse effects of cadmium. Setting exposure limits has become increasingly important because of widespread, low-level cadmium in the food chain from phosphate fertilizer that is naturally contaminated with cadmium.[40] However, determining risk at low levels of exposure is difficult due to limited prospective data and recent concerns that associations between urine cadmium, a commonly used measure of cumulative exposure, and urinary EBE markers that are proteins may reflect co-excretion rather than nephrotoxicity.[7,8]

Lead

Lead targets the proximal tubules. The presence of intranuclear inclusion bodies, containing lead-protein complexes, in the proximal tubular cells is an early finding in acute, high-level lead poisoning (blood lead level [BLL] over 100 μg/dL),[41] which now occurs rarely in high-income countries. Fanconi syndrome may occur, with excretion of low-molecular-weight molecules. Chronic lead poisoning with BLL greater than 60 μg/dL may result in lead nephropathy with chronic interstitial nephritis, characterized by contracted, fibrotic kidneys; decreased GFR; and, frequently, hypertension and gout.[42]

An epidemic of ESRD occurred in Queensland, Australia, from 1915 to 1935, when survivors of childhood lead poisoning died from kidney failure as young adults.[43] An epidemic of lead poisoning related to artisanal mining of lead-rich gold ore occurred in Nigeria in 2010, with an estimated 400 or more deaths in children.[44] In this epidemic, prechelation geometric mean BLL was 149 μg/dL for the children initially tested.[44]

With moderate to high levels of lead exposure, decreased creatinine clearance,[42] mortality from kidney disease[45] and, in animal studies, decreased GFR and pathology consistent with lead nephropathy have been reported.[46] Relevant data on lead effects across the range of exposures include the following:

- A study of over 58,000 U.S. men found a significantly increased risk for incident ESRD at a BLL greater than 51 µg/dL (in those with 5 or more years of follow-up).[47]
- A prospective study found that higher baseline tibia lead levels, reflecting an increased body burden of lead, were significantly associated with a greater increase in serum creatinine in individuals with diabetes or hypertension.[48]
- Increased risk in children associated with maternal erythrocyte lead has been observed.[49]
- Case-control studies have reported an increased risk for ESRD associated with prior environmental lead exposure[50] but not CKD from occupational lead exposure, defined using an expert rating method based on job history.[51]
- An association with CKD progression has been observed in prospective data in environmentally exposed patients[52] but not in those occupationally exposed.[51,53]
- Randomized experimental trials from one medical center have reported that chelation with EDTA slows CKD progression in environmentally exposed adults.[54]
- Increased serum creatinine was observed in an animal model of lead exposure from birth to postpuberty;[55] to our knowledge, this effect was observed at the lowest BLL in an animal model (7.5 µg/dL).
- An ecological study found that declining kidney disease mortality rates between 1981 and 2007 in Taiwan were significantly associated with decreasing lead emissions following phase-out of leaded gasoline.[56]

Overall, prospective data support lead as a risk factor for CKD, especially in the presence of other CKD risk factors. Globally, lead exposure is generally decreasing while other CKD risk factors, such as diabetes, are increasing. The risk of lead-related nephrotoxicity, therefore, is a function of these two trends.

Under the OSHA Lead Standard, BLL monitoring is mandated for workers exposed above the action level (30 µg/m^3 averaged over an 8-hour period). Kidney function monitoring (with blood urea nitrogen, serum creatinine, and urinalysis) is required in medical examinations triggered by BLLs, symptoms, and other criteria. Early detection of lead nephrotoxicity is difficult since tubular injury has few initial signs or symptoms. Exposure should be minimized, especially in workers with underlying CKD, regardless of cause, or with common CKD risk factors, such as diabetes mellitus. (See Chapters 11, 23, and 30 for further discussion of lead.)

Other Causes of CKD

Aristolochic acid, a naturally occurring toxin found in plants of the Aristolochia genus, has been identified as the cause of interstitial nephritis, following ingestion of Chinese herbal medications in diet clinics, and of Balkan endemic nephropathy. [57,58] Both disorders, which present as chronic tubulointerstitial disease, increase risk for urothelial carcinoma.

Recent research that has evaluated the potential for nephrotoxicity from other agents includes the following:

- A prospective study of 669 participants found that exposure to fine particulate matter in ambient air was associated with lower eGFR.[59]
- A cross-sectional study of associations between measured and model-predicted serum perfluorooctanoic acid (PFOA) concentrations and eGFR in 9,600 children observed an association between higher measured PFOA and lower eGFR, which was not present with predicted PFOA levels.[14] The authors noted the potential for reverse causality to explain these findings.

Perfluoroalkyl acids and some additional toxicants, including phthalates, bisphenol A, dioxins, furans, polycyclic aromatic hydrocarbons, and polychlorinated biphenyls, were recently reviewed for their potential to cause adverse kidney effects.[60] Depending on the agent, increased albuminuria, increased blood pressure, increased serum uric acid, and both increased and decreased eGFR were reported in the studies discussed in the review.

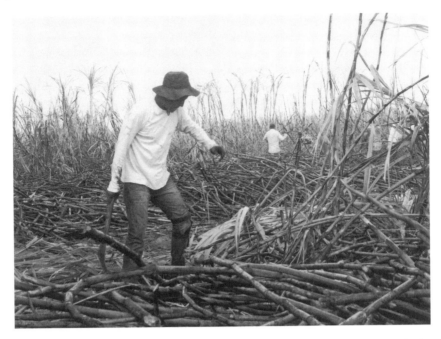

Figure 28-1. Sugarcane workers in El Salvador are at increased risk for chronic kidney disease of unknown etiology. (Photograph by Aaron Sussell.)

Chronic Kidney Disease of Unknown Etiology

In the past two decades, an epidemic of CKD of unknown etiology (CKDu) in young and middle-age adults has been reported in some countries in Central America, Sri Lanka, the state of Andhra Pradesh in India, and the El-Minia Governorate in Egypt.[61] Men employed in agricultural jobs are at highest risk, and commonly implicated causes of CKD, such as diabetes and hypertension, are generally absent. Kidney biopsies have shown interstitial fibrosis and tubular atrophy, along with glomerular damage that may be secondary or part of the primary process.[61] It is uncertain whether outbreaks in different locations reflect the same disease process.

Due to lack of dialysis and kidney transplantation in the affected areas, the case-fatality rate is high. Mortality rates from renal failure in men in Nicaragua and El Salvador are seven to nine times higher than they are in the United States.[62] In Central America, CKDu has caused an estimated 20,000 deaths.[63] Therefore, CKDu has probably caused far more deaths and years of life lost than any of the other kidney disorders described in this chapter.

The Second International Research Workshop on Mesoamerican Nephropathy, in 2015, concluded that the CKDu observed in Central America, called *Mesoamerican nephropathy*, is an occupational disease.[64] Several potential causes of CKDu have been considered.[65] Physically demanding work in hot environments resulting in recurrent dehydration is a leading etiologic possibility, especially in Central America.[66] Supporting this possibility, a study of dehydration in rodents reported increased serum creatinine, proximal tubular injury, and interstitial fibrosis.[67] Decline in eGFR over the course of a harvesting season occurred in sugarcane workers (Figure 28-1).[68] A cross-shift study of agricultural workers in the United States found evidence of acute kidney injury in 12% of 295 workers; risk was significantly associated with payment of workers on a piece-rate basis.[69] Multiple mechanisms may be involved as recurrent kidney injury from dehydration progresses to CKD.[70] Agrochemicals, such as pesticides and herbicides, and water contaminants have been a major focus of etiologic research in Sri Lanka.[71,72] Infections are also possible causes, given the geographic locations where CKDu has been reported. The Consortium for the Epidemic of Nephropathy in Central America and Mexico, is an international organization that connects researchers and healthcare professionals who are studying potential causes of CKDu and providing assistance to affected patients.

Various interventions are being implemented. The Worker Health and Efficiency Program in El Salvador is aimed at reducing heat stress and dehydration in sugarcane workers, utilizing the OSHA Water.Rest.Shade. program,[73] along with a machete modification.[74,75] Clean water programs are being implemented in Sri Lanka.

REFERENCES

1. Levey AS, de Jong PE, Coresh J, et al. The definition, classification, and prognosis of chronic kidney disease: A KDIGO Controversies Conference report. Kidney International 2011; 80: 17–28.
2. Lozano R, Naghavi M, Foreman K, et al. Global and regional mortality from 235 causes of death for 20 age groups in 1990 and 2010: A systematic analysis for the Global Burden of Disease Study 2010. Lancet 2012; 380: 2095–2128.
3. Centers for Disease Control and Prevention. Chronic Kidney Disease (CKD) Surveillance Project. Available at: https://nccd.cdc.gov/ckd/detail.aspx?Qnum=Q8. Accessed September 9, 2016.
4. United States Renal Data System, USRDS 2016 annual data report. Bethesda, MD. Available at: https://www.usrds.org/2016/view/Default.aspx. Accessed November 29, 2016.
5. Roels HA, Van Assche FJ, Oversteyns M, et al. Reversibility of microproteinuria in cadmium workers with incipient tubular dysfunction after reduction of exposure. American Journal of Industrial Medicine 1997; 31: 645–652.
6. Nishijo M, Morikawa Y, Nakagawa H, et al. Causes of death and renal tubular dysfunction in residents exposed to cadmium in the environment. Occupational and Environmental Medicine 2006; 63: 545–550.
7. Chaumont A, Nickmilder M, Dumont X, et al. Associations between proteins and heavy metals in urine at low environmental exposures: Evidence of reverse causality. Toxicology Letters 2012; 210: 345–352.
8. Akerstrom M, Sallsten G, Lundh T, Barregard L. Associations between urinary excretion of cadmium and proteins in a nonsmoking population: Renal toxicity or normal physiology? Environmental Health Perspectives 2013; 121: 187–191.
9. Shelley R, Kim NS, Parsons P, et al. Associations of multiple metals with kidney outcomes in lead workers. Occupational and Environmental Medicine 2012; 69: 727–735.
10. Weaver VM, Garcia Vargas G, Silbergeld EK, et al. Impact of urine concentration adjustment method on associations between urine metals and estimated glomerular filtration rates (eGFR) in adolescents. Environmental Research 2014; 132: 226–232.
11. Weaver VM, Kim N-S, Lee B-K, et al. Differences in urine cadmium associations with kidney outcomes based on serum creatinine and cystatin C. Environmental Research 2011; 111: 1236–1242.
12. You L, Zhu X, Shrubsole MJ, et al. Renal function, bisphenol A, and alkylphenols: Results from the National Health and Nutrition Examination Survey (NHANES 2003-2006). Environmental Health Perspectives 2011; 119: 527–533.
13. Buser MC, Ingber SZ, Raines N et al. Urinary and blood cadmium and lead and kidney function: NHANES 2007-2012. International Journal of Hygiene and Environmental Health 2016; 219: 261–267.
14. Watkins DJ, Josson J, Elston B, et al. Exposure to perfluoroalkyl acids and markers of kidney function among children and adolescents living near a chemical plant. Environmental Health Perspectives 2013; 121: 625–630.
15. Weaver VM, Kotchmar DJ, Fadrowski JJ, Silbergeld EK. Challenges for environmental epidemiology research: Are biomarker concentrations altered by kidney function or urine concentration adjustment? Journal of Exposure Science and Environmental Epidemiology 2016; 26: 1–8.
16. Hau AK, Kwan TH, Li PK. Melamine toxicity and the kidney. Journal of the American Society of Nephrology 2009; 20: 245–250.
17. Gossner CM, Schlundt J, Ben Embarek P, et al. The melamine incident: Implications for international food and feed safety. Environmental Health Perspectives 2009; 117: 1803–1808.
18. Wang PX, Li HT, Zhang L, Liu J-M. The clinical profile and prognosis of Chinese children with melamine-induced kidney disease: A systematic review and meta-analysis. Biomed Research International 2013; 2013: http://dx.doi.org/10.1155/2013/868202.
19. Dalal RP, Goldfarb DS. Melamine-related kidney stones and renal toxicity. Nature Reviews Nephrology 2011; 7: 267–274.

20. Dahlgren J, Wardenburg M, Peckham T. Goodpasture's syndrome and silica: A case report and literature review. Case Reports in Medicine 2010; doi:10.1155/2010/426970.

21. Calvert GM, Steenland K, Palu S. End-stage renal disease among silica-exposed gold miners: A new method for assessing incidence among epidemiologic cohorts. JAMA 1997; 277: 1219–1223.

22. Vupputuri S, Parks CG, Nylander-French LA, et al. Occupational silica exposure and chronic kidney disease. Renal Failure 2012; 34: 40–46.

23. Min B, Kim G, Kang T, et al. IgA nephropathy in a laboratory worker that progressed to end-stage renal disease: A case report. Annals of Occupational and Environmental Medicine 2016; 28: 35. doi 10.1186/s40557-016-0118-z.

24. Jacob S, Hery M, Protois JC, et al. Effect of organic solvent exposure on chronic kidney disease progression: The GN-PROGRESS cohort study. Journal of the American Society of Nephrology 2007; 18: 274–281.

25. Li SJ, Zhang SH, Chen HP, et al. Mercury-induced membranous nephropathy: Clinical and pathological features. Clinical Journal of the American Society of Nephrology 2010; 5: 439–444.

26. Zheng L, Kuo CC, Fadrowski J, et al. Arsenic and chronic kidney disease: A systematic review. Current Environmental Health Reports 2014; 1: 192–207.

27. Chiu HF, Yang CY. Decreasing trend in renal disease mortality after cessation from arsenic exposure in a previous arseniasis-endemic area in southwestern Taiwan. Journal of Toxicology and Environmental Health A 2005; 68: 319–327.

28. Chen Y, Parvez F, Liu M, et al. Association between arsenic exposure from drinking water and proteinuria: Results from the Health Effects of Arsenic Longitudinal Study. International Journal of Epidemiology 2011; 40: 828–835.

29. Zheng LY, Umans JG, Yeh f, et al. The association of urine arsenic with prevalent and incident chronic kidney disease: Evidence from the strong heart study. Epidemiology 2015; 26: 601–612.

30. Weidemann D, Kuo CC, Navas-Acien A, et al. Association of arsenic with kidney function in adolescents and young adults: Results from the National Health and Nutrition Examination Survey 2009-2012. Environmental Research 2015; 140: 317–324.

31. Nogawa K, Kobayashi F, Honda R. A study of the relationship between cadmium concentrations in urine and renal effects of cadmium. Environmental Health Perspectives 1979; 28: 161–168.

32. Nogawa K, Kido T. Biological monitoring of cadmium exposure in itai-itai disease epidemiology. International Archives of Occupational and Environmental Health 1993; 65: S43–S46.

33. Centers for Disease Control and Prevention. Fourth National Report on Human Exposure to Environmental Chemicals, updated tables. Atlanta: Department of Health and Human Services, 2015. Available at: http://www.cdc.gov/biomonitoring/pdf/FourthReport_UpdatedTables_Feb2015.pdf. Accessed November 30, 2016.

34. Li Q, Nishijo M, Nakagawa H, et al. Relationship between urinary cadmium and mortality in habitants of a cadmium-polluted area: A 22-year follow-up study in Japan. Chinese Medical Journal 2011; 124: 3504–3509.

35. Nogawa K. Biologic indicators of cadmium nephrotoxicity in persons with low-level cadmium exposure. Environmental Health Perspectives 1984; 54: 163–169.

36. Kido T, Nogawa K, Ishizaki M, et al. Long-term observation of serum creatinine and arterial blood pH in persons with cadmium-induced renal dysfunction. Archives of Environmental Health 1990; 45: 35–41.

37. Piscator M. Long-term observations on tubular and glomerular function in cadmium-exposed persons. Environmental Health Perspectives 1984; 54: 175–179.

38. Jarup L, Persson B, Edling C, Elinder CG. Renal function impairment in workers previously exposed to cadmium. Nephron 1993; 64: 75–81.

39. United States Department of Labor. elaws: Employment laws assistance for workers & small businesses—OSHA Cadmium Biological Monitoring Advisor. Available at: http://www.dol.gov/elaws/cadmium.htm. Accessed November 30, 2016.

40. European Food Safety Authority. Cadmium dietary exposure in the European population. EFSA Journal 2012; 10: 1–37.

41. Weaver V, Jaar B. Lead nephropathy and lead-related nephrotoxicity. In D. Basow (ed.). UpToDate. Waltham, MA: UpToDate:.

42. Wedeen RP, Malik DK, Batuman V. Detection and treatment of occupational lead nephropathy. Archives of Internal Medicine 1979; 139: 53–57.

43. Inglis JA, Henderson DA, Emmerson BT. The pathology and pathogenesis of chronic lead nephropathy occurring in Queensland. Journal of Pathology 1978; 124: 65–76.

44. Tirima S, Bartrem C, von Lindern I, et al. Environmental remediation to address childhood lead poisoning epidemic due to artisanal gold

mining in Zamfara, Nigeria. Environmental Health Perspectives 2016; 124: 1471–1478.

45. Steenland K, Selevan S, Landrigan P. The mortality of lead smelter workers: An update. American Journal of Public Health 1992; 82: 1641–1644.

46. Khalil-Manesh F, Gonick HC, Cohen AH, et al. Experimental model of lead nephropathy. I. Continuous high-dose lead administration. Kidney International 1992; 41: 1192–1203.

47. Chowdhury R, Darrow L, McClellan W, et al. Incident ESRD among participants in a lead surveillance program. American Journal of Kidney Disease 2014; 64: 25–31.

48. Tsaih SW, Korrick S, Schwartz J, et al. Lead, diabetes, hypertension, and renal function: The Normative Aging Study. Environmental Health Perspectives 2004; 112: 1178–1182.

49. Skröder H, Hawkesworth S, Moore SE, et al. Prenatal lead exposure and childhood blood pressure and kidney function. Environmental Research 2016; 151: 628–634.

50. Sommar JN, Svensson MK, Björ BM, et al. End-stage renal disease and low level exposure to lead, cadmium and mercury: A population-based, prospective nested case-referent study in Sweden. Environmental Health 2013; 12:9.

51. Evans M, Fored CM, Nise G, et al. Occupational lead exposure and severe CKD: A population-based case-control and prospective observational cohort study in Sweden. American Journal of Kidney Diseases 2010; 55: 497–506.

52. Yu CC, Lin JL, Lin-Tan DT. Environmental exposure to lead and progression of chronic renal diseases: A four-year prospective longitudinal study. Journal of the American Society of Nephrology 2004; 15: 1016–1022.

53. Chowdhury R, Mukhopadhyay A, McClellan W, et al. Survival patterns of lead-exposed workers with end-stage renal disease from Adult Blood Lead Epidemiology and Surveillance program. American Journal of the Medical Sciences 2015; 349: 222–227.

54. Lin-Tan DT, Lin JL, Yen TH, et al. Long-term outcome of repeated lead chelation therapy in progressive non-diabetic chronic kidney diseases. Nephrology Dialysis Transplantation 2007; 22: 2924–2931.

55. Berrahal AA, Lasram M, El Elj N, et al. Effect of age-dependent exposure to lead on hepatotoxicity and nephrotoxicity in male rats. Environmental Toxicology 2011; 26: 68–78.

56. Wu W-T, Tsai P-J, Yang Y-H, Wu T-N. Health impacts associated with the implementation of a national petrol-lead phase-out program (PLPOP): Evidence from Taiwan between 1981 and 2007. Science of the Total Environment 2011; 409: 863–867.

57. De Broe ME. Chinese herbs nephropathy and Balkan endemic nephropathy: Toward a single entity, aristolochic acid nephropathy. Kidney International 2012; 81: 513–515.

58. Gokmen MR, Cosyns JP, Arlt VM, et al. The epidemiology, diagnosis, and management of aristolochic acid nephropathy: A narrative review. Annals of Internal Medicine 2013; 158: 469–477.

59. Mehta AJ, Zanobetti A, Bind MA, et al. Long-term exposure to ambient fine particulate matter and renal function in older men: The Veterans Administration Normative Aging Study. Environmental Health Perspectives 2016; 124: 1353–1360.

60. Kataria A, Trasande L, Trachtman H. The effects of environmental chemicals on renal function. Nature Reviews Nephrology 2015; 11: 610–625.

61. Weaver VM, Fadrowski JJ, Jaar BG. Global dimensions of chronic kidney disease of unknown etiology (CKDu): A modern era environmental and/or occupational nephropathy? BMC Nephrology 2015; 16: 145.

62. Pan American Health Organization. Visualizing renal failure and chronic kidney diseases age-standardized mortality rate in countries of the Americas, 2000–2009. Non-communicable diseases and mental health. Available at: http://ais.paho.org/phip/viz/nmh_renalfailure_ckd_visualization.asp. Accessed November 30, 2016.

63. Ramirez-Rubio O, McClean MD, Amador JJ, Brooks DR. An epidemic of chronic kidney disease in Central America: An overview. Journal of Epidemiology and Community Health 2013; 67: 1–3.

64. Second International Research Workshop on Mesoamerican Nephropathy. Mesoamerican nephropathy. 2016. Available at: http://www.regionalnephropathy.org/wp-content/uploads/2016/08/MeN-2015-Scientific-Report-high-resolution_final.pdf. Accessed January 9, 2017.

65. Weiner DE, McClean MD, Kaufman JS, Brooks DR. The Central American epidemic of CKD. Clinical Journal of the American Society of Nephrology 2013; 8: 504–511.

66. Glaser J, Lemery J, Rajagopalan B, et al. Climate change and the emergent epidemic of CKD from heat stress in rural communities: The case for heat stress nephropathy. Clinical Journal of the American Society of Nephrology 2016; 11: 1472–1483.

67. Roncal Jimenez CA, Ishimoto T, Lanaspa MA, et al. Fructokinase activity mediates dehydration-induced renal injury. Kidney International 2014; 86: 294–302.

68. Laws RL, Brooks DR, Amador JJ, et al. Changes in kidney function among Nicaraguan sugarcane workers. International Journal of Occupational and Environmental Health 2015; 21: 241–250.

69. Moyce S, Joseph J, Tancredi D, et al. Cumulative incidence of acute kidney injury in California's agricultural workers. Journal of Occupational and Environmental Medicine 2016; 58: 391–397.

70. Roncal-Jimenez C, Lanaspa MA, Jensen T, et al. Mechanisms by which dehydration may lead to chronic kidney disease. Annals of Nutrition and Metabolism 2015; 66: 10–13.

71. Jayatilake N, Mendis S, Maheepala P, Mehta FR. Chronic kidney disease of uncertain aetiology: Prevalence and causative factors in a developing country. BMC Nephrology 2013; 14: 180. doi: 10.1186/1471-2369-14-180.

72. Levine KE, Redmon JD, Elledge MF, et al. Quest to identify geochemical risk factors associated with chronic kidney disease of unknown etiology (CKDu) in an endemic region of Sri Lanka: A multimedia laboratory analysis of biological, food, and environmental samples. Environmental Monitoring and Assessment 2015; 188: 548. doi:10.1007/s10661-016-5524-8.

73. Occupational Safety and Health Administration. Work.Rest.Shade. Available at: https://www.osha.gov/SLTC/heatillness/index.html?utm_source=Twitter. Accessed November 30, 2016.

74. La Isla Foundation. The WE Program—"WE Can End CKDnT" Video. Available at: https://laislafoundation.org/the-we-program-we-can-end-ckdnt-video/. Accessed November 30, 2016.

75. Bodin T, García-Trabanino R, Weiss I, et al. Intervention to reduce heat stress and improve efficiency among sugarcane workers in El Salvador: Phase 1. Occupational and Environmental Medicine 2016; 73: 409–416. doi:10.1136/oemed-2016-103555.

FURTHER READING

Weaver VM, Fadrowski JJ. Kidney disease in children and the environment. In: PJ Landrigan, RA Etzel (eds.) Textbook of children's environmental health. New York: Oxford University Press, 2014, pp. 447–457.
This chapter provides an overview of environmental exposures that cause kidney disease in children.

Weaver VM, Fadrowski JJ, Jaar BG. Global dimensions of chronic kidney disease of unknown etiology (CKDu): A modern era environmental and/or occupational nephropathy? BMC Nephrology 2015; 16: 145.
This review discusses the potential for outbreaks of chronic kidney disease of unknown etiology to be related to a common occupational or environmental factor. The review also notes that none of the toxicants implicated in past epidemics of kidney disease appears to be the primary cause of the current outbreaks.

Weiner DE, McClean MD, Kaufman JS, Brooks DR. The Central American epidemic of CKD. Clinical Journal of the American Society of Nephrology 2013; 8: 504–511.
This review provides a detailed discussion of the various possible causes of chronic kidney disease of unknown etiology studied to date.

SECTION V

AN INTEGRATED APPROACH TO PREVENTION

29

Climate Change

Barry S. Levy and Jonathan A. Patz

Climate change—or, more accurately, climate disruption—is having profound environmental and health consequences.[1-3] In this chapter, we review the environmental and occupational health consequences of climate change and describe approaches to mitigation of emissions of greenhouse gases (GHGs, the primary cause of climate change) and to adaptation, which aims to minimize the consequences of climate change.

Climate change has been defined as "a change of climate which is attributed directly or indirectly to human activity that alters the composition of the global atmosphere and which is in addition to the natural climate variability observed over comparable time periods."[4] *Climate* is distinct from *weather*. *Climate* is defined as "the average course or condition of the weather at a place usually over a period of years as exhibited by temperature, wind velocity, and precipitation."[5] In contrast, *weather* is defined as "the state of the air and atmosphere at a particular time and place: the temperature and other outside conditions (such as rain, cloudiness, etc.) at a particular time and place."[5] Climate scientists frequently use a period of 30 years to distinguish between *climate* and *weather*.

Climate change, which can be caused by natural variability or human activity, is a function of the balance between incoming (solar) short-wave radiation and outgoing (infrared) long-wave radiation. This balance is affected by the earth's atmosphere in a manner similar to that of the glass greenhouse (or a car's windshield), which allows sunlight to enter and then traps the heated air from rising and mixing with cooler air aloft.

Over the past several decades, emissions and airborne concentrations of carbon dioxide, methane, nitrous oxide, and other GHGs have continued to increase substantially. Carbon dioxide concentrations in the atmosphere began increasing soon after the beginning of the Industrial Era (Figure 29-1).[6] Concentrations of carbon dioxide, methane, and nitrous oxide in the atmosphere are now higher than their highest concentrations recorded over the past 800,000 years. Countries emitting the most GHGs generally suffer less consequences than those emitting the least GHGs. (Figure 29-2).

Environmental consequences of climate change include increases in (a) temperature as well as frequency, severity, and/or duration of heat waves; (b) heavy precipitation events;

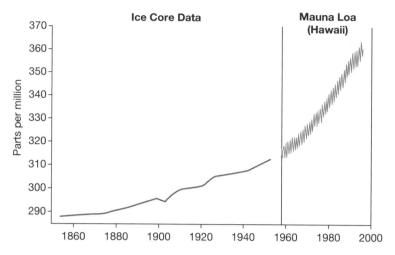

Figure 29-1. Carbon dioxide concentrations in the atmosphere (in parts per million), 1860–2000. Concentrations from 1860 to approximately 1960 are based on ice core data. Concentrations since approximately 1960 are based on continual measurements by scientists at an observatory on Mauna Loa, Hawaii, reflecting vegetation absorbing carbon dioxide each spring and releasing carbon dioxide into the atmosphere each autumn. (Source: White House Initiative on Global Climate Change. The greenhouse effect and historical emissions. http://clinton4.nara.gov/Initiatives/Climate/greenhouse.html. Accessed February 28, 2017.)

(c) intensity and/or duration of drought; (d) intense tropical cyclone activity; and (e) sea level. Other environmental consequences include shrinking of glaciers and polar ice caps, increases in chemical pollutants and aeroallergens in the ambient air, increased acidity of oceans, and ecosystem changes that reduce biodiversity.

The Intergovernmental Panel on Climate Change (IPCC), a scientific body under the auspices of the United Nations, provides objective data on climate change and its impacts. The IPCC has performed comprehensive assessment of (a) changes that have already occurred and the human contribution to these changes (Table 29-1) and (b) the likelihood of further changes (Table 29-2).[7] Virtually all climate scientists are convinced that climate change is caused by human activity, primarily from use of fossil fuels but also by industrial processes, agricultural activities, and deforestation.

The IPCC has determined that warming of the earth since the 1950s has been "unequivocal" and "unprecedented," and it has attributed this warming, with 95% certainty, to human activity. Average surface temperature increased 0.85°C (1.53°F) between 1880 and 2012.[8] IPCC has predicted that during the 2081–2100 period, the temperature on the earth's surface will increase between an average of 1.0° and 3.7°C (1.8° and 6.7°F). In the United States, the frequency of daily temperatures over 38°C (100°F) is anticipated to increase substantially; temperature levels that now occur once in 20 years could occur every 2 years.[9] Extreme heat events (heat waves) are becoming more frequent, more severe, and longer in duration.[9] In tropical areas, increased temperature is making outdoor work extremely difficult. Some locations may become uninhabitable because of extreme heat.

Throughout the world, El Niño-related variability of precipitation will likely intensify; in many dry regions, mean precipitation will decrease. In the United States, it is expected that precipitation will become less frequent but more intense.[9] Heavy rainfall episodes are likely to occur more frequently because warmer air holds more water vapor. Episodes of heavy rainfall are most likely to cause adverse health impacts through flooding, causing injuries as well as cases of gastrointestinal illness due to sewage contamination of drinking water. Globally, between 1980 and 2009, at least 2.8 billion people were adversely affected and more than 500,000 died as a result of floods. In coming years, floods are anticipated to increase throughout the world.

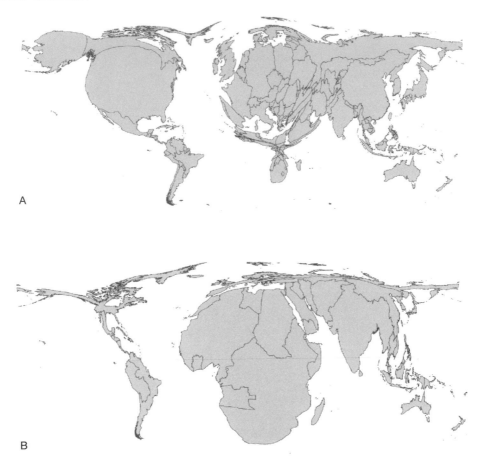

Figure 29-2. Global maps demonstrating (A) relative proportions of GHG emissions by country and (B) magnitude and severity of the consequences of climate change by country. (Source: Patz JA, Gibbs HK, Foley JA, et al. Climate change and global health: Quantifying a growing ethical crisis. EcoHealth 2007; 4: 397–405. doi.10.1007/s10393-007-0141-1.)

While there is some uncertainty regarding whether the frequency of all hurricanes and cyclones will increase, there is evidence that the frequency of more extreme hurricanes has already increased, with resultant adverse health consequences. Because of warmer ocean-surface temperatures, hurricanes are likely to become more intense.

Inadequate rainfall together with extreme heat events will likely result in droughts of increasing frequency, severity, and duration. These droughts threaten food security and cause adverse consequences for health, nutrition, and economic well-being in many regions of the world.

Climate change is anticipated to increase the occurrence of wildfires due to increased temperatures together with decreased rainfall. Wildfires create air contamination with fine particulate matter, which causes irritation of the respiratory tract and exacerbation of chronic lung disorders.

Additive effects can occur due to the combination of climate change and poor land-use policies. For example, as human populations extend into flood plains and vulnerable coastal areas, the consequences of floods and coastal storm surges tend to increase. In areas where there has been deforestation, heavy rainfall is much more likely to increase landslides. The impact of Hurricane Katrina on New Orleans in 2005 was probably heightened by previous recession of coastal wetlands, which therefore provided less buffering from storm surges.

Global mean sea level has increased approximately 20 cm (8 inches) during the past century— far more than in the previous 2,000 years. By 2100, sea level is projected to rise, mainly due to

Table 29-1. Assessment That Various Changes Have Occurred and of a Human Contribution to Observed Changes

Phenomenon and Direction of Trend	Assessment that Changes Occurred (Typically Since 1950 Unless Otherwise Indicated)	Assessment of a Human Contribution to Observed Changes
Warmer and/or fewer cold days and nights over most land areas	Very likely	Very likely
Warmer and/or more frequent hot days and nights over most land areas	Very likely	Very likely
Warm spells/heat waves: Frequency and/or duration increases over most land areas	Medium confidence on a global scale Likely in large parts of Europe, Asia, and Australia	Likely
Heavy precipitation events: Increase in frequency, intensity, and/or amount of heavy precipitation	Likely more land areas with increases than decreases	Medium confidence
Increases in intensity and/or duration of drought	Low confidence on a global scale Likely changes in some regions	Low confidence
Increases in intense tropical cyclone activity	Low confidence in long term (centennial) changes Virtually certain in North Atlantic since 1970	Low confidence
Increased incidence and/or magnitude of extreme high sea level	Likely (since 1970)	Likely

Source: Intergovernmental Panel on Climate Change. Climate change 2014: Impacts, adaptation, and vulnerability. Cambridge, UK: Cambridge University Press, 2014.

Table 29-2. Assessment of the Likelihood of Further Changes in the Early and Late 21st Century

Phenomenon and Direction of Trend	Early 21st Century	Late 21st Century
Warmer and/or fewer cold days and nights over most land areas	Likely	Virtually certain
Warmer and/or more frequent hot days and nights over most land areas	Likely	Virtually certain
Warm spells/heat waves: Frequency and/or duration increases over most land areas	Not formally assessed	Very likely
Heavy precipitation events: Increase in the frequency, intensity, and/or amount of heavy precipitation	Likely over many land areas	Very likely over most of the midlatitude land masses and over wet tropical regions
Increases in intensity and/or duration of drought	Low confidence	Likely (medium confidence) on a regional to global scale
Increases in intense tropical cyclone activity	Low confidence	More likely than not in the Western North Pacific and North Atlantic
Increased incidence and/or magnitude of extreme high sea level	Likely	Very likely

Source: Intergovernmental Panel on Climate Change. Climate change 2014: Impacts, adaptation, and vulnerability. Cambridge, UK: Cambridge University Press, 2014.

thermal expansion and melting of glaciers, by 26 to 63 cm (about 10.1 to 24.6 inches).[7] Sea level rise will worsen storm surges and coastal erosion. It threatens to inundate small island nations in the Pacific Ocean and to damage farmland in Bangladesh and other low-lying countries. In addition, sea level rise causes salinization of groundwater in coastal areas, thereby increasing risk of hypertension among local residents who drink this water.[10]

ADVERSE HEALTH CONSEQUENCES

Climate change is having profound health consequences, which are likely to become more severe and more widespread in coming decades. Direct public health consequences of climate change include heat-related disorders; respiratory and allergic disorders; vector-borne, waterborne, and foodborne infectious diseases; and health impacts of extreme weather events. Climate change can also cause indirect health consequences, including reduced food security, distress migration, and collective violence. In addition, all of the environmental and health consequences of climate change can adversely affect the mental health of individuals, communities, and entire nations.

Heat-Related Disorders

Heat-related disorders related to climate change receive the most attention during heat waves (often defined as periods of 5 or more days when ambient temperatures exceed the average maximum for the 1961–1990 period by 5°C [9°F]). Serious heat waves throughout the world have caused much morbidity and mortality. In a 1995 heat wave in Chicago, more than 700 people died, and in a 1999 heat wave there, 80 people died. In 2003, an extended heat wave in Europe claimed the lives of more than 70,000 people, 15,000 of them in France alone. In 2014 in India, more than 2,500 people died during a heat wave. Risk factors for morbidity and mortality during heat waves include older age, living alone, residence in public housing, absence of air conditioning, homelessness, and working outdoors.[9]

Also of great significance are the impacts of heat on health as well as work, human performance, and daily life in warm periods other than heat waves.[11] These impacts will increase over time. Weather conditions will be less suitable for outdoor work, with labor production likely falling 20% by the 2050s.[12] The Middle East, Southeast Asia, and Central America are likely to be especially impacted.[13] In addition, outdoor athletic events will be adversely affected; by 2085, it is projected that only 8 of 543 cities outside of Western Europe would meet the low-risk category for holding the Summer Olympics.[14]

Acute health effects of heat exposure include heat exhaustion, heat rash, heat syncope, dehydration, and potentially fatal heat stroke, as well as complications of common chronic diseases, such as diabetes mellitus and heart, lung, and kidney disease. Chronic health effects of heat exposure include chronic kidney disease due to repeated dehydration, birth defects in offspring of women who work in physically demanding jobs, and exacerbation of diabetes and heart, lung, and kidney disease.

People living in urban areas may face greater health consequences resulting from heat waves due partially to the *urban heat island effect*. This phenomenon develops because cities generate and retain heat due to dark surfaces on roads, parking lots, and roofs, which absorb and retain heat more readily. By radiating heat at night, urban heat islands increase nighttime temperatures. Measures to prevent or minimize heat-related disorders during heat waves include the identification of high-risk groups and development of preparedness plans, including heat-warning systems, emergency response protocols, and plans to move high-risk individuals to cooler indoor places during heat waves.

Respiratory and Allergic Disorders

Respiratory and allergic disorders are increasing as a result of climate change:

- With warming of the atmosphere, concentrations of ground-level ozone increase, causing respiratory tract irritation and exacerbation of asthma.[15]
- Particulate matter in smoke from wildfires causes or exacerbates respiratory symptoms, especially in people with asthma,

chronic obstructive pulmonary disease, and other chronic respiratory disorders.[16]

- Increased pollen production and longer pollen seasons are causing symptoms that are more severe and lasting longer in people with allergic rhinitis.[17]

Infectious Diseases

Vector-borne, waterborne, and foodborne infectious diseases are increasing as a result of climate change.

Vector-borne Diseases

Climate change, in combination with international trade and travel, is widening the geographic distribution of mosquitoes, ticks, and other vectors that carry disease agents. Warmer temperatures are also facilitating transmission of vector-borne diseases at high altitudes in tropical areas. Disease agents transmitted by vectors include the West Nile, Zika, dengue, Rift Valley fever, and Japanese encephalitis viruses as well as *Plasmodium falciparum* (the parasite that causes malaria). Diseases transmitted by mosquitoes may occur more frequently because warmer temperature increases (a) the number of days when mosquitoes are active, (b) the rate at which they reproduce, and (c) their metabolism, causing them to feed on blood more frequently.[18]

Waterborne Diseases

The occurrence of waterborne diseases is influenced by climate change. Floods and increased surface-water runoff from extremes of the hydrologic cycle increase the possibility of sewage contamination of drinking water. Some studies have demonstrated a temporal association between heavy downpours and acute gastrointestinal illness. In addition, during droughts people often find it difficult to access safe drinking water and they often drink water that has been contaminated with pathogens or toxic substances, such as pesticides.[19,20]

Foodborne Diseases

As a result of climate change, foodborne diseases due to bacteria will likely increase because high temperatures increase growth and persistence of pathogenic bacteria in food. In addition, if contaminated water is used to prepare food, the risk of foodborne disease is increased.

Extreme Weather Events

Climate change is increasingly associated with extreme weather events, which can cause adverse health effects, including:

- Fatal and nonfatal injuries during the events and their aftermath
- Waterborne disease (as already described)
- Damage to farmland and related infrastructure, causing food shortages and malnutrition, decreased access to safe drinking water, and distress migration and its health consequences
- Socioeconomic and political instability, which may lead to collective violence and other public health problems.

In the United States between 1980 and 2016, there were 203 weather and climate disasters, such as tropical cyclones (hurricanes) and other severe storms, floods, and droughts that each resulted in $1 billion or more in damage. These disasters caused an average of 260 deaths annually (mainly from severe storms and heat waves related to drought) and cost an annual average of about $320 billion.[21]

Indirect Health Consequences

Indirect health consequences due to climate change occur as a result of food insecurity, distress migration, and collective violence. These consequences are far more likely to occur in low- and middle-income countries than in high-income countries.

Food Insecurity

Availability of food is likely to decrease as a result of drought and flooding, seawater incursion into coastal farmlands and aquifers, and possibly increased diseases affecting crops. The IPCC has projected that during the next few decades global food demand will increase (perhaps as much as 14% per decade) and global food production will decrease (perhaps as much as 2% per decade).[22] Some recent studies suggest that the concentration of essential micronutrients in food, such as iron and zinc, may decrease. There are likely to be marked increases in food prices, leading to higher rates of childhood malnutrition and, in some places, food riots. In addition, many people, especially subsistence farmers, rural pastoralists, and others living close to the land in low-income countries, will be forced to change their traditional dietary patterns. By some estimates, climate change will create, by 2050, as many as 25 million more malnourished children under the age of 5—mainly in low-income countries.[23,24]

Distress Migration

Climate change is likely to cause displacement of millions of people. Decreased food security, rising sea level, reduced access to safe water, and the threat of collective violence will force many people to leave their homes and communities, becoming internally displaced persons within their own countries or refugees in other countries. Some projections indicate that there could be as many as 25 million to 50 million "climate refugees" by 2050.[25]

Collective Violence

Collective violence represents another set of indirect health consequences due to climate change.[26] The World Health Organization defines *collective violence* as "the instrumental use of violence by people who identify themselves as members of a group . . . against another group or set of individuals in order to achieve political, economic, or social objectives." Collective violence includes war and other forms of armed conflict; genocide, torture, and other forms of state-sponsored violence; and gang warfare and other forms of organized violent crime.

The weight of evidence from many studies in different time periods and many geographic locations demonstrates that collective violence can be associated with climate change, primarily due to socioeconomic and political instability that climate change can cause.[27] Several different factors can lead to this instability, including increased temperature, extremes of precipitation (with associated floods and droughts), damage to farmland and resultant crop failures, and, as a consequence, food shortages, loss of farm-related income, and distress migration.[28]

Climate change can multiply risks of conflict from many causes, including disputes over land ownership and political power, social and economic issues, and ethnic hatred. Much research, including two large meta-analyses,[29,30] have demonstrated that when the temperature is hot and/or precipitation is extreme, social stability is likely to decrease and conflict is likely to increase. Scarcity of food, safe water, and other essentials for life can increase the risk of violence.

Climate change contributed to the development of the civil war in Syria. From 2006 to 2009, a severe drought in Syria turned approximately 60% of the land to desert and caused the death of up to 80% of cattle. Hundreds of thousands of farmers and their family members, most of them from ethnic minorities, migrated to cities, where they experienced discrimination as well as mistreatment by the government of President Bashar al-Assad. Resultant political and social instability contributed to the start of the civil war, which has since caused more than 500,000 deaths and uprooted more than 11 million people—more than 6 million have been internally displaced and 5 million have fled to other countries.[31-33]

Human Rights and Social Justice

Climate change contributes to human rights violations and social injustice at the global, national, and local levels.

At the global level, there is social injustice on a large scale. Those countries with the most GHG emissions generally suffer the least consequences of climate change and those countries with the least GHG emissions suffer the most consequences.[34] For example, in a recent year, per-capita GHG emissions in the United States and several other high-income countries were about 10-fold greater than those in low-income countries. As climate change continues, economies of high-income countries will likely prosper while those of low-income countries will likely suffer, with decreasing annual economic growth rates—mainly due to very high temperature; heavy reliance of sectors exposed to extreme weather variability, such as agriculture and natural resource extraction; and limited air-conditioning, insurance systems, and other forms of risk management.[35] (See Figure 29-2.)

At the national and local levels, climate change has a disproportionate effect on those living in poverty, minorities, women, children, older people, those with chronic diseases or disabilities, people living in areas with climate-sensitive diseases (such as diarrhea and malaria), those with poor access to safe food and drinking water, and people with inadequate access to health services.[36]

ADDRESSING CLIMATE CHANGE

The main ways of addressing climate change are mitigation and adaptation. *Mitigation*, which is a form of primary prevention, includes policies and actions to stabilize or reduce the emission of GHGs. *Adaptation*, which is a form of secondary prevention, includes policies and actions to reduce the impact of climate change.

Mitigation

Mitigation includes policies concerning energy, transportation, food and agriculture, and land use designed to reduce atmospheric concentrations of GHGs. Energy policies can promote development and use of renewable energy, encourage decreased production and use of fossil fuels, and reduce overall energy demand.[37] In the United States, use of wind and solar power is rapidly increasing.[38] (Despite the benefits of wind power, workers who install and maintain wind turbines may face occupational safety risks, as shown in Figure 29-3.) Transportation policies can promote fuel efficiency of vehicles, use of public transportation, and active transport (walking and bicycling) (Figure 29-4).[39] Food and agriculture policies can promote sustainable practices, enhance food security, decrease consumption of meat (which causes a relatively large carbon footprint), promote growth and consumption of fruits and vegetables, and decrease emissions of methane, a highly potent GHG.[40] Growth of corn and other crops to produce biofuels can provide benefits, but may reduce land available for growing food crops, thereby driving up food prices. Land-use policies, by protecting existing forests and promoting growth of new forests, can maintain or increase carbon sinks, which absorb carbon dioxide from the atmosphere.

Mitigation can produce many health co-benefits. For example, reducing the use of fossil fuels decreases air pollution and improves health. Promoting active transport reduces GHG emissions, increases physical activity, and helps prevent cardiovascular disease.[41]

Adaptation

Health professionals can promote and engage in adaptation measures, such as:

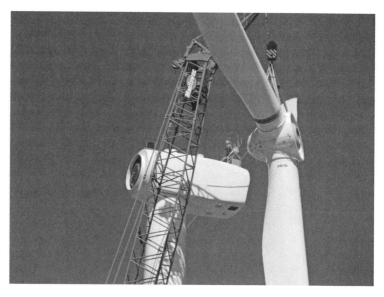

Figure 29-3. Worker atop a large wind turbine. (Photograph by Frank Wenzel.)

- Educating and raising awareness of peers, policymakers, and the general public about climate change and its adverse consequences
- Performing surveillance for emerging vector-borne diseases and other health consequences of climate change

- Assessing vulnerability of various populations at risk of the consequences of climate change
- Building resilience of individuals, organizations, and communities
- Promoting collaboration among community groups and other nongovernmental

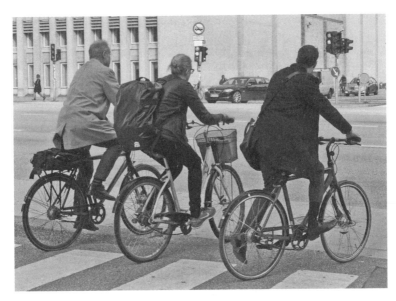

Figure 29-4. Bicyclists in Copenhagen. (Photograph by Barry S. Levy.)

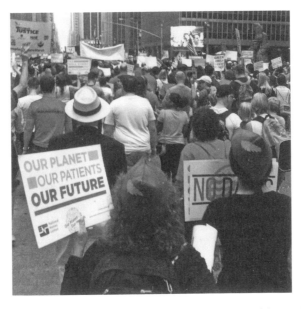

Figure 29-5. People's Climate March in New York in 2014. (Photograph by Jonathan A. Patz.)

organizations, government agencies, and others to prepare for the adverse health consequences of heat waves, increased transmission of vector-borne diseases, and extreme weather events

• Promoting and participating in research on the health effects of climate change and on evaluating policies and other measures to address climate change.[42]

Individuals can address climate change by (a) insulating their homes and limiting heating and air-conditioning; (b) using active transport or public transportation or carpooling; (c) eating less red meat and more fruits and vegetables; and (d) becoming more engaged in climate change issues, such as by supporting the work of nongovernmental organizations and becoming involved in political activity.[43] (See Figure 29-5.)

In addition, individuals, especially health professionals, can play important roles in informing policymakers and the general public about the health consequences of climate change, necessary for developing the popular and political will to address climate change. (See Figure 29-6.) This is especially important in the United States, where many people do not believe that climate change (or global warming) is real or that human activity is an important cause of it.

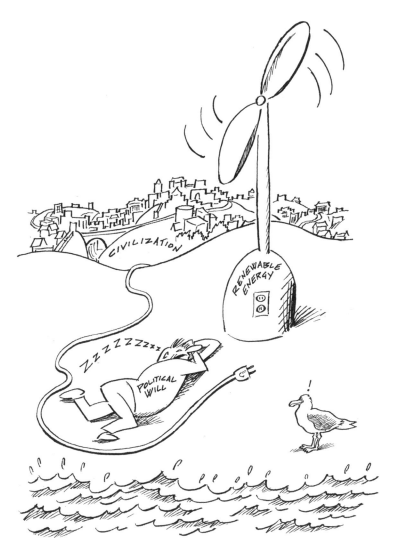

Figure 29-6. How long dare we wait? (Drawing by Nick Thorkelson.)

Studies have shown that:

- 13% of the U.S. population ("the alarmed") are highly engaged in global warming, are changing their behaviors, and strongly support vigorous national policies to address it.
- 31% ("the concerned") are less certain of their conclusions about global warming, less personally engaged, less likely to be changing their behaviors, and slightly less supportive of policies to address it.
- 23% ("the cautious") are less certain that human activity is the cause of global warming but show moderate support for policies to address it.
- 7% ("the disengaged") have not thought much about global warming, but they show moderate support for climate change policies.
- 13% ("the doubtful") do not recognize global warming as a threat.
- 13% ("the dismissive") have concluded that global warming is not happening and believe that policies to address it are misguided at best.[44]

Health professionals and others can inform people about the relevance of climate change to health by communicating the following five key messages:

- Climate change is real.
- Climate change is the result of human activity.
- There is consensus among climate scientists that human-caused climate change is happening.
- Climate change is harmful to people.
- People can take actions that will limit climate change.[45,46]

International agreements can facilitate and support national policies and programs to address climate change. At the United Nations Climate Change Conference (COP21) in Paris in December 2015, representatives of 196 countries, in the Paris Climate Agreement, committed to reducing GHG emissions. In addition, at COP21 high-income countries committed to making major financial contributions to assist low-income countries in addressing climate change.[47]

As of mid-2017, the new U.S. administration announced plans to withdraw its support for the Paris Climate Agreement and began reducing funding for research on climate change and for implementation of policies to address it. However, at the same time, government agencies, nongovernmental organizations, academic institutions, business organizations, and other entities at the state and local level were increasing their work in addressing climate change.

REFERENCES

1. Levy BS, Patz JA. (eds.) Climate change and public health. New York: Oxford University Press, 2015.
2. Levy BS, Patz JA. Climate change, human rights, and social justice. Annals of Global Health 2015; 81: 310–322.
3. Patz JA, Frumkin H, Holloway T, et al. Climate change: Challenges and opportunities for global health. JAMA 2014; 312: 1565–1580.
4. United Nations Framework Convention on Climate Change. Full text of the convention. 1992. Available at: https://unfccc.int/resource/docs/convkp/conveng.pdf. Accessed February 27, 2017.
5. Merriam-Webster Dictionary. Climate. Available at: http://www.merriam-webster.com/dictionary/climate. Accessed February 27, 2017.
6. White House Initiative on Global Climate Change. The greenhouse effect and historical emissions. Available at: http://clinton4.nara.gov/Initiatives/Climate/greenhouse.html. Accessed February 28, 2017.
7. Intergovernmental Panel on Climate Change. Climate change 2014: Impacts, adaptation, and vulnerability. Cambridge, UK: Cambridge University Press, 2014.
8. Stocker TF, Qin D, Plattner GK, et al. (eds.). Summary for policymakers. In: IPCC. Climate change 2013: The physical science basis. Contribution of Working Group I to the Fifth Assessment Report of the Intergovernmental Panel on Climate Change. Cambridge, UK: Cambridge University Press, 2013.
9. Basu R. Disorders related to heat waves. In BS Levy, JA Patz (eds.). Climate change and public health. New York: Oxford University Press, 2015, pp. 87–103.
10. Khan AE, Scheelbeek PFD, Shilpi AB, et al. Salinity in drinking water and the risk of (pre) eclampsia and gestational hypertension in coastal Bangladesh: A case-control study. PLoS One 2014; 9: e108715. doi:10.1371/journal.pone.0108715.

11. Kjellstrom T, Lemke B, Otto PM, et al. Heat impacts on work, human performance, and daily life. In BS Levy, JA Patz (eds.). Climate change and public health. New York: Oxford University Press, 2015, pp. 73–86.

12. Dunne JP, Stouffer RJ, John JG. Reductions in labour capacity from heat stress under climate warming. Nature Climate Change 2013; 3: 563–566.

13. Kjellstrom T, Kovats SR, Lloyd SJ, et al. The direct impact of climate change on regional labor. Archives of Environmental and Occupational Health 2009; 64: 217–227.

14. Smith KR, Woodward A, Lemke B, et al. The last summer Olympics? Climate change, health and work outdoors. Lancet 2016; 388: 642–644.

15. U.S. Environmental Protection Agency. 2013 final report: Integrated science assessment for ozone and related photochemical oxidants (Report No.: EPA 600/R-10/076F). Research Triangle Park, NC: Office of Research and Development, EPA, 2013. Available at: http://cfpub.epa.gov/ncea/isa/recordisplay.cfm?deid=247492. Accessed March 1, 2017.

16. U.S. Environmental Protection Agency. 2009 final report: Integrated science assessment for particulate matter (Report No.: EPA/600/R-08/139F). Washington, DC: EPA, 2009. Available at: https://cfpub.epa.gov/ncea/risk/recordisplay.cfm?deid=216546. Accessed March 1, 2017.

17. Ziska LH. Aeroallergens and climate change (textbox). In BS Levy, JA Patz (eds.). Climate change and public health. New York: Oxford University Press, 2015, pp. 113–114.

18. Reisen WK. Landscape epidemiology of vector-borne diseases. Annual Review of Entomology 2010; 55: 461–483.

19. Shrestha S, Babel MS, Pandey VP (eds.). Climate change and water resources. Boca Raton, FL: CRC Press, 2014.

20. Grover VI (ed.). Impact of climate change on water and health. Boca Raton, FL: CRC Press, 2012.

21. NOAA National Centers for Environmental Information. U.S. billion-dollar weather and climate disasters. Available at: https://www.ncdc.noaa.gov/billions/. Accessed February 27, 2017.

22. Intergovernmental Panel on Climate Change. Climate change and food security. In: IPCC. Climate change 2014: Impacts, adaptation, and vulnerability. Contribution of Working Group II to the Fifth Assessment Report of the Intergovernmental Panel on Climate Change, 2014. Available at:

http://www.climatechangefoodsecurity.org/ipcc_ar5.html. Accessed February 1, 2017.

23. Black RE, Victora GC, Walker SP, et al. Maternal and child undernutrition and overweight in low-income and middle-income countries. Lancet 2013; 382: 427–451.

24. Horton S, Steckel RH. Global economic losses attributable to malnutrition in 1990–2000 and projections to 2050. In B Lomborg (ed.). How much have global problems cost the world? Cambridge, UK: Cambridge University Press, 2013.

25. McMichael C, Barnett J, McMichael AJ. An ill wind? Climate change, migration, and health. Environmental Health Perspectives 2012; 120: 646–654.

26. Levy BS, Sidel VW (eds.). War and public health (2nd ed.). New York: Oxford University Press, 2008.

27. Levy BS, Sidel VW, Patz JA. Climate change and collective violence. Annual Review of Public Health 2017; 38: 241–257.

28. Homer-Dixon TF. Environment, scarcity, and violence. Princeton, NJ: Princeton University Press, 1999.

29. Hsiang SM, Burke M, Miguel E. Quantifying the influence of climate on human conflict. Science 2013; 341: 1235367. doi.10.1126/science.1235367.

30. Hsiang SM, Burke M. Climate, conflict, and social stability: What does the evidence say? Climatic Change 2014; 123: 39–55.

31. Barnard A. Death toll from war in Syria now 470,000, group finds. The New York Times, February 11, 2016. Available at: https://www.nytimes.com/2016/02/12/world/middleeast/death-toll-from-war-in-syria-now-470000-group-finds.html?_r=0. Accessed February 27, 2017.

32. Syria Regional Refugee Response. Regional overview. Available at: http://data.unhcr.org/syrianrefugees/regional.php. Accessed February 27, 2017.

33. United Nations Office for the Coordination of Humanitarian Affairs. Syrian Arab Republic. Available at: http://www.unocha.org/syria. Access February 27, 2017.

34. Patz JA, Gibbs HK, Foley JA, et al. Climate change and global health: Quantifying a growing ethical crisis. EcoHealth 2007; 4: 397–405. doi.10.1007/s10393-007-0141-1.

35. Moore FC, Diaz DB. Temperature impacts on economic growth warrants stringent mitigation policy. Nature Climate Change 2015; 5: 127–131.

36. McMichael AJ, Campbell-Lendrum K, Kovats S, et al. Global climate change. In M Ezzati, AD Lopez, A Rodgers, CJL Murray (eds.). Comparative quantification of health risks: Global and regional burden of disease attributable to selected major risk factors (Vol. 2). Geneva: World Health Organization, 2004, pp. 1543–1650.

37. Haines A, Smith KR, Anderson D, et al. Policies for accelerating access to clean energy, improving health, advancing development, and mitigating climate change. Lancet 2007; 370: 1264–1281.

38. U.S. Energy Information Administration. Frequently asked questions: What is U.S. electricity generation by energy source? (Last updated: April 1, 2016). Available at: https://www.eia.gov/tools/faqs/faq. cfm?id=427&t=3. Accessed February 27, 2017.

39. Transportation Research Board. Policy options for reducing energy use and greenhouse gas emissions from U.S. transportation. 2001. Available at: http://onlinepubs.trb.org/ onlinepubs/sr/sr307.pdf. Accessed March 1, 2017.

40. Stull VJ, Patz JA. Agriculture policy. In BS Levy, JA Patz (eds.). Climate change and public health. New York: Oxford University Press, 2015, pp. 319–342.

41. Haines A, McMichael AJ, Smith KR, et al. Public health benefits of strategies to reduce greenhouse-gas emission: Overview and implications for policy makers. Lancet 2009; 374: 2104–2114.

42. Frumkin H, Hess J, Luber G, et al. The public health response to climate change. American Journal of Public Health 2008; 98: 435–445.

43. Union of Concerned Scientists. Cooler, smarter: Practical steps for low-carbon living. Washington, DC: Island Press, 2012.

44. Roser-Renouf C, Leiserowitz A, Maibach E, et al. Global warming's six Americas, 2014. Yale University and George Mason University. New Haven, CT: Yale Project on Climate Change Communication, 2015.

45. Leiserowitz A, Maibach E, Roser-Renouf C, et al. Climate change in the American mind: Americans' global warming beliefs and attitudes in April, 2014. New Haven, CT: Yale University and George Mason University, Yale Project on Climate Change Communication, 2013. Available at: http://environment.yale.edu/ climate-communication/article/Behavior-April-2013. Accessed March 1, 2017.

46. Maibach EW, Nisbet M, Baldwin P, et al. Reframing climate change as a public health issue: An exploratory study of public reactions. BMC Public Health 2010; 10: 299.

47. Davenport C, Gillis J, Chan S, Eddy M. Paris Climate Change Conference 2015: Inside the Paris climate deal. New York Times, December 12, 2015. Available at: https://www.nytimes. com/news-event/un-climate-change-conference. Accessed March 1, 2017

FURTHER READING

Intergovernmental Panel on Climate Change. Climate change 2013: The physical science basis. Cambridge, UK: Cambridge University Press, 2013.

Intergovernmental Panel on Climate Change. Climate change 2014: Impacts, adaptation, and vulnerability. Cambridge, UK: Cambridge University Press, 2014.
Two comprehensive reports by the Intergovernmental Panel on Climate Change.

Gore A. An inconvenient sequel: Truth to power. New York: Rodale, 2017.
A well-illustrated recent book on climate change and its consequences, which is designed for the general public and policymakers.

Butler CD (ed.). Climate change and global health. Oxfordshire, UK: CABI, 2014.

Levy BS, Patz JA. (eds.) Climate change and public health. New York: Oxford University Press, 2015.

Luber G, Lemery J. Global climate change and human health: From science to practice. San Francisco: Jossey-Bass, 2015.
Three informative books on climate change and its wide range of health consequences.

Watts N, Adger WN, Agnolucci P, et al. Health and climate change: Policy responses to protect public health. Lancet 2015; 386: 1861–1914.

Watts N, Adger WN, Ayeb-Karlsson S, et al. The Lancet Countdown: Tracking progress on health and climate change. Lancet 2017; 389: 1151–1164.
Important reports on the work of international multidisciplinary collaborations among academic institutions and practitioners from many countries.

30

Children's Environmental Health

Philip J. Landrigan

Children's environmental health is the branch of pediatric medicine and public health that studies the influence of the environment on children's health, development, and risk of disease.[1] It considers environmental exposures during pregnancy as well as exposures in infancy, childhood, and adolescence. It studies parental environmental and occupational exposures that may influence the health of children. And it traces the influence of early-life environmental exposures on health and development throughout the lifespan—from conception, to infancy, to childhood and adolescence, and throughout adult life.[2]

The core concept of children's environmental health is that children are unique. Because they are passing through the early, formative stages of human development, children are qualitatively and quantitatively different from adults in their patterns of exposure and in their vulnerabilities to environmental hazards.[3] The health consequences of environmental exposures in infancy and childhood are often very different from the consequences of exposures later in life.

Children's environmental health, which is highly interdisciplinary, considers the environment broadly. It recognizes that childhood environments are complex, comprised of many layers and changes over the course of a child's development. It therefore studies the influences of chemical exposures in early life on children's health,[4] the nutritional environment in the womb,[2] the built environment,[5] stress,[6] and the social environment.[7] It studies interactions among these multiple environments at different life stages, considering a broad view of all childhood exposures, termed the *exposome*. It examines interactions among environmental exposures, poverty, and social injustice. And it examines environmental influences on the human genome and *epigenome*, defined as the network of chemical compounds surrounding DNA that modify the genome without altering DNA sequences and have a role in determining which genes are active in a particular cell.

Children's environmental health translates research findings into evidence-based plans for disease prevention and protection of children's health. Its ultimate goals are to safeguard children's health and to improve the environments where children live, learn, and play.

Four great challenges confronting children's environmental health are:

- Increasing rates of noncommunicable diseases among children globally, for which environmental exposures are partly responsible
- Children's exposure to thousands of inadequately tested chemicals of unknown hazard
- The global movement of toxic chemicals and hazardous waste from high-income countries to low- and middle-income countries (LMICs)
- Inadequate training of physicians and other health professionals in environmental medicine, which results in missed diagnoses of environmental disease in children and lost opportunities for treatment and prevention.

HISTORICAL ORIGINS OF CHILDREN'S ENVIRONMENTAL HEALTH

Children's environmental health arose in the second half of the 20th century through a convergence of scientific insights from research in three disciplines: pediatric toxicology, nutritional epidemiology, and the social sciences.

The Contributions of Pediatric Toxicology

Pediatric toxicology, the study of the effects of toxic chemicals on children's health, is the oldest of these three disciplines. It derives many of its approaches and methodologies from toxicology and occupational medicine. Pediatric toxicology arose from clinical and epidemiologic studies of epidemics due to dissemination of toxic chemicals, inadequately tested pharmacologic agents, and other hazards into the environment where children were exposed. These epidemics, which typically involved acute, high-dose exposures, included:

- Lead poisoning among children in Queensland, Australia, in 1904, due to lead-based paint ingested by children playing on painted verandas.
- Leukemia in Hiroshima and Nagasaki, Japan, among children who had been

exposed to ionizing radiation from atomic bombs. Incidence began to increase 2 to 3 years afterward, peaked about 7 years afterward, and then declined. Risk was highest in those children who were most heavily exposed.
- Microcephaly among infants in Hiroshima and Nagasaki who had been exposed to ionizing radiation in utero in the first trimester of pregnancy, which was due to radiation injury to the developing brain. There was no comparable damage observed in adults.
- Mercury poisoning, manifested by cerebral palsy, mental retardation, and seizures among children in Minamata, Japan, a remote fishing village where pregnant women ingested fish that were heavily contaminated with methylmercury.[8] The source was a chemical factory that had discharged mercury-containing waste into Minamata Bay. The mothers were not physically affected.
- Phocomelia, a previously rare birth defect of the limbs, in Europe in the 1950s and 1960s.[9] Clinical and epidemiologic studies found that the affected babies had been exposed in utero to thalidomide, a sedative prescribed to women during the first trimester of pregnancy to alleviate morning sickness. More than 10,000 cases were reported globally—8,000 in Germany alone—before thalidomide was removed from the market and the epidemic ended. Thalidomide was most harmful when taken between days 34 and 50 of gestation, precisely the time when the limbs form. Depending upon the timing of exposure, thalidomide was found also to be associated with defects of the eyes, ears, heart, and gastrointestinal and urinary tracts, as well as with autism.
- Adenocarcinoma of the vagina among young women who were exposed in utero to diethylstilbestrol, a synthetic estrogen that had been prescribed to their mothers to prevent miscarriage.[10] Incidence peaked in the years immediately after puberty. Mothers were physically unaffected.

Investigation of these epidemics and related research established three fundamental principles of children's environmental health:

1. Toxic chemicals can cross the placenta and cause fetal injury, dispelling the myth that the placenta provides an impervious barrier of protection.
2. In-utero and early-life exposures to toxic chemicals and other environmental hazards can have devastating effects on children that are potentially lifelong.
3. Infants and young children (but not adults) have windows of vulnerability to toxic chemicals that are developmentally determined—in which even extremely small exposures can cause profound damage.

These epidemics occurred during the period when concern about the environment was first emerging in the United States. Especially important was the publication in 1962 of Rachel Carson's *Silent Spring*, which described widespread contamination of the environment with DDT and other pesticides and the consequent near extinction of the bald eagle and the osprey. Publication of *Silent Spring* marked the birth of the Environmental Movement and was among the major factors that led to creation of the Environmental Protection Agency (EPA).

The Contributions of Nutritional Epidemiology

Nutritional epidemiology is the second area of scientific research that led to the development of children's environmental health. In the 1980s, Professor David Barker and his colleagues at the University of Southampton in England began conducting research that revealed the influence of the nutritional environment in utero on children's health.[2] After they observed that places in England and Wales where infant mortality was highest in the early 1900s had very high mortality rates from heart disease 60 to 70 years later, they hypothesized that undernutrition in utero might explain this finding. To test this hypothesis, they conducted a long-term cohort study of 5,000 men and found that those who had a low birthweight or had suffered undernutrition during infancy had increased rates of cardiovascular disease, hypertension, diabetes, and renal disease in adulthood.[11] These findings were corroborated by studies of infants born to mothers who had survived a famine in the Netherlands during World War II, when Nazi occupiers reduced daily caloric intake to starvation levels; these infants developed markedly increased rates of obesity, diabetes, and heart disease in adulthood.

Professor Barker's studies gave rise to the *developmental origins of health and disease hypothesis* (DOHAD).[12] The biological basis for DOHAD is that risk of disease across the lifespan is shaped by an adaptive response to the early-life environment. Known as *fetal programming*, this response is established during windows of vulnerability in early development, mainly in utero, when biologic systems are immature and highly malleable. Once established, fetal programming can persist and can become manifest at any point in life—even after many years or decades of latency—thereby influencing health and risk of disease throughout the lifespan. Epigenetic modification of fetal gene expression, based on metabolic cues received from the mother during pregnancy, may be a mechanism of fetal programming that at least partly accounts for Professor Barker's observations and for the developmental origins of adult disease.

The Contributions of Social Science Research

Epidemiologic research in the social sciences is the third area of scientific inquiry that contributed to the development of children's environmental health.[7] This research found that (a) exposure in utero to maternal stress and (b) exposure in early childhood to traumatic events, such as extreme violence, child abuse, rape, and incest, can increase risk of disease throughout the lifespan.[13] This research demonstrated that psychosocial stress in early life is associated with a wide range of physical and mental illnesses, including asthma and obesity in childhood and depression, cardiovascular disease, and autoimmune disease in adulthood.

A theoretical framework known as *stress-health paradigm* helps to explain the connections between psychosocial stress in early life and the later appearance of disease.[14] In this framework, psychosocial stress in early life is viewed as a toxic exposure that can permanently disrupt biologic systems during early periods of developmental plasticity. Pathologic hyperactivation of the hypothalamic–pituitary–adrenocortical axis appears to mediate this disruption.[15] It leads to altered functioning of the autonomic nervous system and then to excessive cortisol secretion, which appear to become permanently programmed, possibly through epigenetic modification of gene expression.[16] These changes, in turn, increase risk for (a) permanent alteration of immune and inflammatory processes and (b) persistently disrupted emotional regulation and hyperreactivity to stress. All of these factors increase risk of disease throughout life and predispose to self-destructive behaviors that further impair health, such as smoking and excessive risk-taking.[13]

Synthesis of Areas of Research

Concerning children's health and development, there are striking similarities among the findings derived from pediatric toxicology, nutritional epidemiology, and social science research. Studies in each of these three disciplines have shown that exposures to adverse environmental influences during windows of vulnerability in early life have the potential to produce disease and dysfunction not only in childhood but also throughout the lifespan—a recognition that is bridging these previously separate areas of research and practice.[17] This recognition has led to transdisciplinary research, suggesting that interactions and synergies may operate among different types of environmental insults in early development, such as between the adverse health effects of lead exposure and social stressors.

REPORT ON DIETARY PESTICIDES

In 1993, the publication of *Pesticides in the Diets of Infants and Children*, a report by the U.S. National Academy of Sciences (NAS), accelerated the development of children's environmental health.[3] This report demonstrated that children are much more heavily exposed and more sensitive to pesticides and other toxic chemicals than adults. Its authors summarized their findings by stating, "Children are not little adults." This report identified four attributes of children that account for their heightened susceptibility:

1. Children breathe more air, drink more water, and eat more food than adults on a

per-kilogram body-weight basis and therefore have proportionately greater exposures to pesticides and other toxic chemicals.

2. Their metabolic pathways are immature, and therefore they are less able to rapidly detoxify and excrete many toxic chemicals.

3. Their delicate developmental processes are easily disrupted. During windows of vulnerability in early child development, which have no counterpart in adults, exposure to even very low doses of toxic chemicals or other environmental hazards can increase disease risk across the lifespan.

4. Children have more future years than adults when they can develop long-lasting diseases that may be caused by harmful exposures in early life.

The NAS report also found that U.S. federal pesticide laws were not adequately protecting children's health, and it recommended improved legislation.

The NAS report greatly increased awareness of U.S. policymakers about the vulnerability of infants and children to pesticides and other toxic chemicals in the environment. It led to passage, in 1996, of the Food Quality Protection Act, the only federal environmental law with explicit provisions for the protection of children. The law led to the establishment within EPA of the Office of Children's Health Protection and to a Presidential Executive Order that required all U.S. federal agencies to consider children's special susceptibilities in all new regulations. In addition, it led, in 1997, to the Miami Declaration on Children's Environmental Health, a multinational pledge to make the protection of children's health against environmental threats a global priority.

GROWTH OF RESEARCH

The NAS report also stimulated an increase in U.S. federal investment in research on children's environmental health. As a result, there has been enormous growth in children's environmental health over the past two decades:

- A national network of Children's Environmental Health and Disease Prevention Research Centers was established, which has led to the discovery of many risk factors for environmental diseases in children, including developmental neurotoxicants, endocrine disruptors, and respiratory toxicants.[18]

- A network of clinically-oriented Pediatric Environmental Health Specialty Units (PEHSUs) was established, initially in the United States and then in Canada, Mexico, Argentina, Uruguay, and Spain.
- National and international conferences that have established and refined a research agenda for children's environmental health, including sessions at the annual meeting of the International Society for Environmental Epidemiology.
- *Environmental Health Perspectives*, the journal of the National Institute of Environmental Health Sciences, has established a special section in each monthly issue devoted to children's environmental health.
- The American Academy of Pediatrics has published three editions of the *Handbook of Pediatric Environmental Health* ("The Green Book").[19]
- The *Textbook on Children's Environmental Health* was published.[1]
- Training programs have been launched to educate pediatricians and research scientists in children's environmental health.
- Major prospective birth-cohort studies have been initiated in many countries to discover associations between environmental exposures in early life and children's health. To further increase statistical power for discovering environmental causes of rare diseases, data from several of these studies are being pooled by the International Agency for Research on Cancer (IARC) through its International Childhood Cancer Consortium.

THE CURRENT STATUS OF CHILDREN'S ENVIRONMENTAL HEALTH

The ambient environment in high-income countries has dramatically improved over the past century, and children's health in these countries has dramatically improved during this period. The childhood mortality rates have decreased by over 50%; infant mortality rates have decreased by over 90%. Life expectancy at birth has doubled. Despite AIDS and other emerging infections during recent decades, infectious diseases are no longer dominant causes of childhood morbidity and mortality. The principal serious illnesses in U.S. children now are noncommunicable diseases—the *new pediatric morbidity*.[20] Even in LMICs, the proportion of morbidity and mortality in children due to noncommunicable diseases is steadily increasing.

This shift in morbidity and mortality from mainly infectious to noncommunicable diseases—the *epidemiological transition*—was largely due to major improvements in the environment: the delivery of safe drinking water, the provision of safe and nutritious food, treatment of sewage, control of insect vectors, and construction of safer homes. These environmental improvements, collectively termed the *exposure transition*,[21] have been major drivers of this transition, especially before the availability of vaccines, antibiotics, and other modern methods of treatment and prevention. The decline in mortality in infectious diseases in the United States began in the 1860s, soon after construction of major urban water systems and almost 80 years before the discovery of penicillin. Among the major, noncommunicable diseases of children in the United States are:

- Asthma, whose frequency has doubled since 1980. It is the leading cause of pediatric hospitalization and school absenteeism. Prevalence has risen especially rapidly among poor children of color residing in inner cities.
- Birth defects, which are now the leading cause of infant mortality. Certain birth defects, such as hypospadias, have markedly increased.
- Neurodevelopmental disorders, such as dyslexia, mental retardation, attention deficit hyperactivity disorder, and autism, which affects 5% to 10% of the 4 million infants born each year in the United States.
- Leukemia and brain cancer in children and testicular cancer in adolescents, all of which have increased in reported incidence since the 1970s, despite declining mortality.

Table 30-1. Selected Associations Between Prenatal Exposures and Disorders or Impairment in Childhood and Adulthood

Period of Exposure	Exposure	Disorder or Impairment	Reference
Childhood	Secondhand smoke (environmental tobacco smoke)	Asthma in children	22
Childhood	Particulate air pollution	Asthma in children	23–25
Infancy	Particulate air pollution	Sudden infant death syndrome	26
Early childhood	Early-life exposure to lead	Neurodevelopmental impairment (with reduction of IQ, shortening of attention span, and disruption of behavior) in children	27
Childhood	Polychlorinated biphenyls	Neurodevelopmental impairment (with reduction of IQ) in children	28
Childhood	Methylmercury	Neurodevelopmental impairment (with reduction of IQ and shortening of attention span) in children	29
Prenatal	Ethyl alcohol	Neurodevelopmental impairment (with reduction of IQ and disruption of behavior) in children	30
Prenatal	Nicotine	Preterm birth and diminished IQ	31
Prenatal	Arsenic or manganese	Neurodevelopment impairment (with reduction of IQ) in infants	32, 33
Prenatal	Organophosphates	Neurodevelopmental impairment (with reduction of IQ and behavioral disruption) in children and abnormalities in brain structure and function in children	34–37
Prenatal	Phthalates or bisphenol A	Neurodevelopmental impairment (with reduction of IQ and behavioral disruption) in children	38, 39
Prenatal	Brominated flame retardants	Neurodevelopmental impairment (with persistent reduction of IQ and disruption of behavior) in children	40

- Cancer, which is now the second leading cause of death in U.S. children, surpassed only by traumatic injuries.
- Preterm birth, the incidence of which has increased by 27% since 1981.
- Obesity, which since the 1970s has in prevalence, and its consequence, type 2 diabetes, which has approximately doubled since then.

Due to markedly increased research, evidence is mounting that harmful environmental exposures are important contributors to the causation of noncommunicable diseases in children. Prospective epidemiological studies of birth cohorts have found associations between prenatal exposures and disease in both childhood and adulthood. Examples are shown in Table 30-1.[22-40]

The built environment is a source of both health and disease risk for children. A higher proportion of children in the United States than ever before live in cities and suburbs. Characteristics of the built environment, such as inadequate safe-play spaces, sidewalks and bicycle paths, and availability of wholesome food in "urban food deserts," may influence diet, activity patterns, and ultimately risk for obesity and type 2 diabetes in children.[5] (See Chapter 34.)

PREVENTION OF ENVIRONMENTAL DISEASE IN CHILDREN

The discovery of environmental causes of disease in children has led to successful prevention of disease. Examples include:

- Removal of lead from gasoline brought about a 90% reduction in blood lead levels of U.S. children.[41] (See Figure 11-7 in Chapter 11.)
- A ban on polychlorinated biphenyl (PCB) production, which was part of the Toxic Substances Control Act, led to reductions of PCB blood levels in children and the number of children suffering from PCB-induced loss of intelligence.
- Elimination of residential uses of organophosphate pesticides led to fewer infants born with low birthweight and small head circumference.
- Reduction in children's exposure to arsenic in water led to lower risk of skin and liver cancer.
- Reduction in children's exposure to urban air pollution led to lower rates of childhood asthma and improvement of lung function.[42]

These successful preventive measures benefitted not only children's health but also the economy. Improvements in air quality in the United States led to estimated benefits (mainly savings in healthcare expenses) of almost $30 for every $1 invested. Removal of lead from gasoline not only reduced lead poisoning by over 90% but also returned an estimated $200 billion of increased productivity to the U.S. economy in each year since 1980, reflecting the increased intelligence, creativity, and economic productivity of children not cognitively impaired by lead.[41]

CHILDREN'S EXPOSURES TO SYNTHETIC CHEMICALS

Despite advances in children's environmental health, children are still exposed to thousands of synthetic chemicals whose hazards are unknown. More than 85,000 chemicals have been registered with EPA.[4] These chemicals are used in millions of consumer products, including food packaging, building materials, fuels, cleaning products, cosmetics, medicinal products, toys, and baby bottles. Most of these chemicals have been created during the past 50 years.

Children are extensively exposed to these chemicals, as documented by national biomonitoring surveys conducted by the Centers for Disease Control and Prevention (CDC), which have detected measurable quantities of over 200 synthetic chemicals in the blood or urine of almost all U.S. residents and in the breast milk of nursing mothers.[43,44] Most of these chemicals have not undergone even minimal assessment for potential toxicity. Only about 20% have been screened for their potential to disrupt early human development or to cause disease in infants and children.[3] Almost nothing is known about the potential effects of children's simultaneous exposure to multiple chemicals.

Without studies to investigate adverse effects associated with specific chemical exposures, silent disease and subclinical dysfunction can go unrecognized for many years. A dramatic example is the "silent epidemic" of childhood lead poisoning that occurred among millions of U.S. children exposed, from the 1940s to the 1970s, to lead that was added to gasoline (Figure 30-1).[41] Many of those children suffered brain injury with reduction of IQ before the hazard was recognized and lead was removed from gasoline. Examples of other substances that were widely used before they were adequately tested with tragic consequences include asbestos, DDT, thalidomide, PCBs, diethylstilbestrol, and chlorofluorocarbons. If thalidomide had caused a 10-point loss of IQ instead of obvious birth defects of the limbs, it might still be on the market.

A recurrent theme in these tragedies was that, with little or no premarket assessment, newly synthesized chemicals, or new uses for chemicals frequently used before, were enthusiastically marketed by corporations and widely used by consumers, resulting in wide dissemination in the environment. Then, years afterward, they were found to have adverse health effects. Chemicals were presumed to be safe, without systematic assessment of their potential toxicity.

In addition, early warnings were ignored, delaying control measures, sometimes for

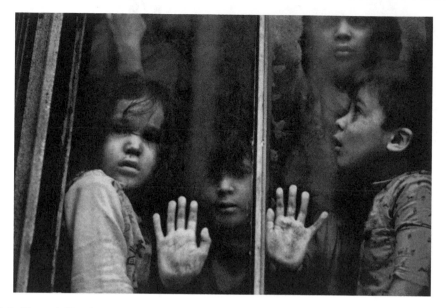

Figure 30-1. Young children living in inner-city tenement buildings, as shown here, are at high risk for childhood lead poisoning. Surveillance programs can help identify children at high risk and help to design and implement intervention and other preventive measures. (Photograph by Earl Dotter.)

decades. In some instances, corporations with vested interests in protecting markets for hazardous materials, such as lead and asbestos, actively opposed measures to investigate and control children's exposures to these materials. These corporations used highly sophisticated disinformation campaigns to confuse the public and to discredit science, attacking pediatricians and environmental scientists who called attention to the health risks of these materials.

A major unanswered question in children's environmental health is: Are there additional chemicals in wide use that pose unrecognized hazards to children's health? About 12 chemicals, based on clinical and epidemiologic studies, are known to be developmental neurotoxicants in children. However, another 200 chemicals cause neurotoxicity in adults, and another 1,000 cause neurotoxic effects in experimental animals.[45] It is not known how many of these additional 1,200 chemicals, some of which are widely used, may pose neurotoxic hazards to infants and children.

To address the problem of exposure of infants, young children, and pregnant women to inadequately tested chemicals, legislators in many countries have developed health-protective laws that overturn the presumption that chemicals

are safe until proven to cause harm. These laws require that (a) chemicals already in use be tested to determine if they are safe, beginning with those deemed to pose the greatest hazard, and (b) new chemicals be demonstrated to be safe before they are allowed to be sold.

In 2007, the European Union enacted the Registration, Evaluation, Authorisation and Restriction of Chemical Substances (REACH) legislation, which requires industry to generate substantial data on potential risks of commercial chemicals and to register this information in a central database. The European Union has been using this information to develop regulations intended to protect children's health, including bans and restrictions of certain potentially toxic products, such as phthalates in children's toys.

The U.S. Congress passed bipartisan chemical safety legislation in 2016—the Frank R. Lautenberg Chemical Safety for the 21st Century Act. It requires the EPA to:

- Evaluate existing chemicals for safety, within clear and enforceable time frames
- Establish a process to prioritize existing chemicals for evaluation
- Use new risk-based standards to evaluate the safety of chemicals, rather than

risk-benefit analyses or the costs of protective measures
- Take action to address unreasonable risks within 2 years (or 4 years, if an extension is needed)
- Make an affirmative finding on the safety of a new chemical or significant new use of an existing chemical before selling it is permitted.

The act provides increased public access to information on chemical safety and consistent funding for the EPA to assume its new responsibilities.[46]

Compliance with these new legislative mandates in Europe and the United States will require the development and deployment of new approaches to toxicity testing of chemicals that are more efficient and less costly than traditional whole-animal testing. The National Institute of Environmental Health Sciences and the EPA, through its Tox 21 program, is developing such approaches, which (a) incorporate new technologies, such as exposure modeling, use of sensors, biomonitoring, "omics" technologies, novel computational methods, "big data" mining, and bioinformatics, and (b) integrate toxicologic findings with genomic and health outcome data, as is currently done by IARC in its assessment of the potential carcinogenicity of chemicals.

In addition, to protect children against toxic chemicals in the environment, formation of a clearinghouse for developmental toxicity has been proposed. Operating in parallel with IARC,[47] it would assess industrial chemicals for developmental toxicity using a precautionary approach that emphasizes prevention. It would assess chemicals for developmental toxicity in the same way that IARC assesses chemicals for carcinogenicity. It would facilitate and coordinate epidemiological and toxicological studies and promote preventive measures.

THE GLOBAL EXPORT OF TOXIC CHEMICALS

Globalization of commerce has encouraged the relocation of polluting industries, such as chemical manufacturing, pesticide production, and waste recycling, to LMICs.[48] These industries are now booming in LMICs, where labor costs are low and environmental regulation, worker protection, and public health infrastructure are often minimal. Workers and community residents in these countries are increasingly exposed to multiple pollutants, including hazardous wastes, often under unpredictable circumstances. The patterns of environmental contamination in high-income countries and LMICs, which had been very different, are becoming more similar. As an example, cardiovascular disease is now a leading cause of morbidity and mortality in India and China, and two-thirds of all cancers globally occur in LMICs.

Examples of health and environmental catastrophes caused by toxic chemical pollution in LMICs have included:

- The Bhopal disaster in India in 1984, in which thousands of people were killed and injured (many of them developed chronic respiratory or other disorder) by a massive methyl isocyanate release into the environment by a chemical explosion in a pesticide manufacturing plant (This is an example of both the global export of toxic chemicals as well as expansion of production at a plant with poor safety measures.)
- The continuing annual export of 2 million tons of newly produced asbestos, mainly from Russia, Kazakhstan, Brazil, and China, to LMICs (There, it is largely used in construction, leading to exposure of workers and community residents, including young children.)
- Informal recycling of car batteries in megacities in LMICs, resulting in occupational, "take-home" (paraoccupational), and community exposure to lead (This has occurred when workers have not been provided with changing and showering facilities at their workplaces and, therefore, carry lead or other contaminants home on their clothing, shoes, skin, or hair, causing toxic effects in their children and other family members.)
- Releases of mercury to the environment from artisanal gold mining, often near rural villages and urban communities where pregnant women and young children have been exposed

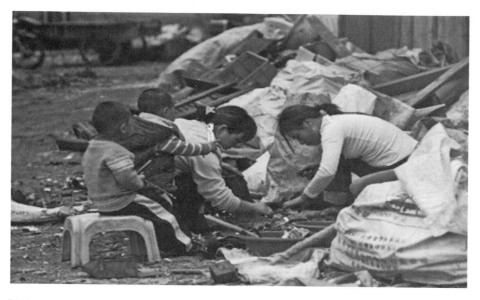

Figure 30-2. Children at an e-waste recovery site, South China. (Photograph by Pure Earth, a New York-based nongovernmental organization dedicated to remediating hazardous waste site in low- and middle-income countries.)

- The annual export to LMICs of 45 million tons of e-waste, with children often employed as pickers and sorters at e-waste recovery sites (Figure 30-2). (Children are exposed at these sites to lead, rare earth elements, beryllium, polychlorinated biphenyls, and dioxins.)

TRAINING NEEDS

Physicians and other healthcare providers play critical roles in recognizing, treating, and preventing environmental disorders in children. Alert clinicians can identify new associations between environmental exposures and disorders in children and can thereby help prevent additional cases.

Informed suspicion is central to diagnosing environmentally-related illness. Clinicians need to recognize that any child may have an illness that is caused or exacerbated by an environmental exposure. Because diseases of environmental origin in children seldom have unique characteristics, the environmental history, supplemented by laboratory testing, is the principal diagnostic tool. (See Chapter 4.)

Unfortunately, environmental diseases in children are underdiagnosed and many are incorrectly ascribed to other causes. Most physicians and other healthcare providers have not been adequately trained to take an environmental history or to recognize environmental exposures as a cause of illness in children. Inadequate professional education is at the root of this problem. Of 127 medical schools responding to a 1988 survey by the Association of American Medical Colleges, only two reported having a required course in environmental and occupational health.[49] As a result, many physicians do not obtain environmental histories from their patients and lack a logical framework for assessing the significance of environmental exposures even when patients report them. This problem was documented by a 2006 survey of pediatricians in New York State, which found that most pediatricians stated that the role of environment in children's health is significant but that they had low confidence in their own ability to deal with environmental threats to children's health such as pesticides, mercury, and mold.[50]

To assist clinicians in making diagnoses of environmental disease in children, the following approach to obtaining a history of environmental exposure has been developed,[51] recognizing that it is impossible to obtain a detailed exposure history for every patient. Clinicians should routinely ask the following screening questions to every new patient and every patient with a new disease:

1. In the history of the present illness:
   - Do you think that the child's illness was caused by an environmental exposure?
   - Did symptoms begin shortly after the child moved to a new home, school, or day-care center?
   - Did symptoms abate during a school vacation period and then recur after the child returned to school?
   - Were symptoms temporally related to an event, such as application of pesticides, a spill of chemicals, or an episode of heavy air pollution?
   - Were there similar cases of illness among other children in the same school or same community?

2. In the social and family history:
   - Where does the child attend school or day care?
   - What industrial facilities are near the child's home and school?
   - What are the parents' occupations?
   - Might a parent be inadvertently bringing toxic materials home from work on their workclothes, shoes, hair, or skin?

3. In the review of systems:
   - Has the child ever been exposed to lead, chemicals, pesticides, or other environmental hazards?

If any suspicious information is elicited in the screening interview, the clinician should either obtain a more detailed exposure history and/or refer the child for evaluation to one of the federally supported PEHSUs across the United States. (Information on the nearest PEHSU is available at: http://www.pehsu.net/.) In addition, in California and New York, state-supported Centers of Excellence in Children's Environmental Health provide clinical and nonclinical consultations as well as "second opinions." Some of the PEHSUs and Centers of Excellence can arrange home visits to assess suspected environmental hazards. Some state and local health departments and the CDC can assess environmental exposures and assist in the diagnosis and treatment of environmental disease in children.

REFERENCES

1. Landrigan PJ, Etzel RA (eds.). Textbook of children's environmental health. New York: Oxford University Press, 2013.
2. Barker DJ. The developmental origins of adult disease. Journal of the American College of Nutrition 2004; 23: 588S–595S.
3. National Academy of Sciences. Pesticides in the diets of infants and children. Washington, DC: National Academies Press, 1993.
4. Landrigan PJ, Goldman L. Children's vulnerability to toxic chemicals: A challenge and opportunity to strengthen health and environmental policy. Health Affairs 2011; 30: 842–850.
5. Jackson RJ, Sinclair S. Designing healthy communities. San Francisco: Jossey-Bass, 2011.
6. Wright RJ. Psychological stress: A social pollutant that may enhance environmental risk. American Journal of Respiratory and Critical Care Medicine 2011; 184: 752–754.
7. National Academy of Sciences. From neurons to neighborhoods: The science of early childhood development. Washington, DC: National Academies Press, 2000.
8. Harada H. Congenital Minamata disease: Intrauterine methylmercury poisoning. Teratology 1978; 18: 285–288.
9. Lenz W. Chemicals and malformations in man. In: Second International Conference on Congenital Malformation. New York: International Medical Congress, 1963, pp. 263–276.
10. Herbst AL, Hubby MM, Azizi F, et al. Reproductive and gynecologic surgical experience in diethylstilbestrol-exposed daughters. American Journal of Obstetrics & Gynecology 1981; 141: 1019–1028.
11. Barker DJ, Winter PD, Osmond C, et al. Weight in infancy and death from ischaemic heart disease. Lancet 1989; 2: 577–580.
12. Barker DJP, Eriksson JG, Forsen T, et al. Fetal origins of adult disease: Strength of effects and biological basis. International Journal of Epidemiology 2002; 31: 1235–1239.
13. Felitti VJ, Anda RF, Nordenberg D, et al. Relationship of childhood abuse and household dysfunction to many of the leading causes of death in adults: The Adverse Childhood Experiences (ACE) study. American Journal of Preventive Medicine 1998; 14: 245–258.
14. Garbarino J. Raising children in a socially toxic environment. San Francisco: Jossey-Bass, 1995.
15. Johnson SB, Riley AW, Grange DA, et al. The science of early life toxic stress for pediatric practice and advocacy. Pediatrics 2012; 131: 319.

16. Skinner MK. Role of epigenetics in developmental biology and transgenerational inheritance. Birth Defects Research, Part C: Embryo Today 2011; 93: 51–55.

17. Heindel JJ, Balbus J, Birnbaum L, et al. Developmental origins of health and disease: Integrating environmental influences. Endocrinology 2015; 156: 3416–3421.

18. Gray K, Lawler CP. Strength in numbers: Three separate studies link in utero organophosphate pesticide exposure and cognitive development. Environmental Health Perspectives 2011; 119: 326–329.

19. Etzel RA, Balk SJ, American Academy of Pediatrics, Council on Environmental Health. Pediatric environmental health (3rd ed.). Elk Grove Village, IL: American Academy of Pediatrics, 2012.

20. Haggerty R, Rothman J. Child health and the community. New York: John Wiley & Sons, 1975.

21. Smith KR, Ezzati M. How environmental health risks change with development: The epidemiologic and environmental risk transitions revisited. Annual Review of Environment and Resources 2005; 30: 291–333.

22. Salam MT, Li YF, Langholz B, et al. Early-life environmental risk factors for asthma: Findings from the Children's Health Study. Lancet 2004; 363: 119–125.

23. Gauderman WJ, Avol E, Gilliland F, et al. The effect of air pollution on lung development from 10 to 18 years of age. New England Journal of Medical 2004; 351: 1057–1067.

24. Friedman MS, Powell KE, Hutwagner L, et al. Impact of changes in transportation and commuting behaviors during the 1996 Summer Olympic Games in Atlanta on air quality and childhood asthma. JAMA 2001: 285; 897–905.

25. Suh HH, Bahadori T, Vallarino J, Spengler JD. Criteria air pollutants and toxic air pollutants. Environmental Health Perspectives 2000; 108: 625–633.

26. Woodruff, T. Grillo J, Schoendorf C. The relationship between selected causes of postneonatal infant mortality and particulate air pollution in the United States. Environmental Health Perspectives 1997; 105: 608–612.

27. Budtz-Jørgensen E, Bellinger D, Lanphear B, et al. An international pooled analysis for obtaining a benchmark dose for environmental lead exposure in children. Risk Analysis 2013; 33: 450–461.

28. Jacobson JL, Jacobson SW. Intellectual impairment in children exposed to polychlorinated biphenyls in utero. New England Journal of Medicine 1996; 335: 783–789.

29. Grandjean P, Weihe P, White RF, et al. Cognitive deficit in 7-year old children with prenatal exposure to methylmercury. Neurotoxicology and Teratology 1997; 19: 417–428.

30. Barr HM, Streissguth AP. Identifying maternal self-reported alcohol use associated with fetal alcohol spectrum disorders. Alcoholism: Clinical and Experimental Research 2001; 25: 283–287.

31. England LJ, Aagaard K, Bloch M, et al. Developmental toxicity of nicotine: A transdisciplinary synthesis and implications for emerging tobacco products. Neuroscience & Biobehavorial Reviews 2016; 72: 187–189.

32. Wasserman GA, Liu X, Parvez F, et al. Water arsenic exposure and intellectual function in 6-year-old children in Araihazar, Bangladesh. Environmental Health Perspectives 2007; 115: 285–289.

33. Khan K, Factor-Litvak P, Wasserman GA, et al. Manganese exposure from drinking water and children's classroom behavior in Bangladesh. Environmental Health Perspectives 2011; 119: 1501–1506.

34. Rauh V, Arunajadai S, Horton M, et al. 7-year neurodevelopmental scores and prenatal exposure to chlorpyrifos, a common agricultural pesticide. Environmental Health Perspectives 2011; 119: 1196–1201.

35. Bouchard MF, Chevrier J, Harley KG, et al. Prenatal exposure to organophosphate pesticides and IQ in 7-year old children. Environmental Health Perspectives 2011; 119: 1189–1195.

36. Engel SM, Wetmur J, Chen J, et al. Prenatal exposure to organophosphates, paraoxonase 1, and cognitive development in childhood. Environmental Health Perspectives 2011; 119: 1182–1188.

37. Rauh VA, Perera FP, Horton MK, et al. Brain anomalies in children exposed prenatally to a common organophosphate pesticide. Proceedings of the National Academy of Sciences 2012; 109: 7871–7876.

38. Engel SM, Miodovnik A, Canfield RL, et al. Prenatal phthalate exposure is associated with childhood behavior and executive functioning. Environmental Health Perspectives 2010; 118: 565–571.

39. Braun JM, Kalkbrenner AE, Calafat AM, et al. Impact of early-life bisphenol A exposure on behavior and executive function in children. Pediatrics 2011; 128: 873–882.

40. Herbstman JB, Sjodin A, Kurzon M, et al. Prenatal exposure to PBDEs and neurodevelopment. Environmental Health Perspectives 2010; 118: 712–719.

41. Grosse SD, Matte T, Schwartz J, et al. Economic gains resulting from the reduction in children's blood lead in the United States. Environmental Health Perspectives 2002; 110: 721–728.

42. Gauderman WJ, Urman R, Avol E, et al. Association of improved air quality with lung development in children. New England Journal of Medicine 2015; 372: 905–913.

43. Centers for Disease Control and Prevention. National Report on Human Exposure to Environmental Chemicals. Atlanta: CDC, 2016. Available at: http://www.cdc.gov/exposurereport/. Accessed November 30, 2016.

44. Woodruff TJ, Zota AR, Schwartz JM. Environmental chemicals in pregnant women in the US: NHANES 2003–2004. Environmental Health Perspectives 2011; 119: 878–885.

45. Grandjean P, Landrigan PJ. Developmental neurotoxicity of industrial chemicals: A silent pandemic. Lancet 2006; 368: 2167–2178.

46. U.S. Environmental Protection Agency. The Frank R. Lautenberg Chemical Safety for the 21st Century Act. Available at: https://www.epa.gov/assessing-and-managing-chemicals-under-tsca/frank-r-lautenberg-chemical-safety-21st-century-act. Accessed November 30, 2016.

47. Grandjean P, Landrigan PJ. Neurobehavioural effects of developmental toxicity. Lancet Neurology 2014; 13: 330–338.

48. Laborde A, Tomasina F, Bianchi F, et al. Children's health in Latin America: The influence of environmental exposures. Environmental Health Perspectives 2015; 123: 201–209.

49. Association of American Medical Colleges. 1989–1990 AAMC curriculum directory. Washington, DC, 1989.

50. Trasande L, Boscarino J, Graber N, et al. The environment in pediatric practice: A study of New York pediatricians' attitudes, beliefs, and practices towards children's environmental health. Journal of Urban Health 2006; 83: 760–772.

51. Goldman RH, Peters JM. The occupational and environmental health history. JAMA 1981; 246: 831–2836.

FURTHER READING

Etzel RA, Balk SJ (editors). Handbook of pediatric environmental health (3rd ed.). Elk Grove Village, IL: American Academy of Pediatrics, 2012.
A ready reference for office or clinic use. Known as the "Green Book," it is the counterpart to the

American Academy of Pediatrics Handbook of Pediatric Infectious Diseases, known as the "Red Book."

Landrigan PJ, Etzel RA (eds.). Textbook on children's environmental health. New York: Oxford University Press, 2013.
An authoritative reference work suitable for college or postgraduate courses or for deeper reading by health professionals.

OTHER RESOURCES

Academic Pediatric Association, Special Interest Group on Environmental Health. Available at: http://www.ambpeds.org/specialInterestGroups/sig_env_health.cfm
A discussion group that convenes at pediatric meetings and posts relevant information on the Internet.

American Academy of Pediatrics, Council on Environmental Health. Available at: https://www.aap.org/en-us/about-the-aap/Committees-Councils-Sections/Council-on-Environmental-Health/Pages/default.aspx.
The American Academy of Pediatrics' highest-level advisory group on children's environmental health, it issues official position statements on topics in children's environmental health on behalf of the Academy.

Children's Environmental Health Network. Available at: http://cehn.org/wordpress/.

Environmental Health Perspectives. Available at: http://ehp.niehs.nih.gov/.
This peer-reviewed, open-access journal of the National Institute of Environmental Health Sciences regularly publishes articles on topics in children's environmental health.

International Society for Children's Health and the Environment. Available at: http://www.ische.ca/.

International Society for Environmental Epidemiology. Available at: http://www.iseepi.org/.
The ISEE presents multiple reports on topics on children's environmental health at its annual scientific meeting.

International Network on Children's Health, Environment and Safety. Available at: http://inchesnetwork.net/.
A global network of physicians and health scientists dedicated to advancing children's environmental health.

World Health Organization. Network of Collaborating Centres for Children's

Environmental Health. Available at: http://www.niehs.nih.gov/research/programs/geh/partnerships/network/index.cfm.
A global network of designated academic centers that work in close collaboration with the World Health Organization to advance scientific knowledge and build professional capacity in children's environmental health.

31

Protecting Disaster Rescue and Recovery Workers

Dori B. Reissman, Maryann M. D'Alessandro, Lisa Delaney, and John Piacentino

This chapter describes worker protection strategies and health surveillance activities in terms of temporal phases of disaster and emergency management. Disaster safety management capacities and coordination plans must be developed before a disaster occurs to deal with the complexities of hazard assessment and control, worker education and training, worker illness and injury surveillance, and access to healthcare services. These activities are performed by diverse groups of occupational and environmental health professionals.

INTRODUCTION

Defining Disaster

A *disaster* is defined as a serious disruption in the functioning of society that poses a significant level of threat to life, health, property, or the environment and requires outside assistance to manage or cope with it.[1] There are several ways of classifing disasters and crisis events. Disasters may be caused by human action or by forces of nature, including extreme weather events (such as hurricanes, tornados, and cyclones), geological disturbances (such as earthquakes and volcanic eruptions), and epidemics of disease (such

as of Ebola virus disease). A *complex humanitarian disaster* is a situation in which populations are displaced due to armed conflict, dramatic political change, or other causes.[2] Technological or industrial disasters may occur from human neglect, error, or by deliberate and harmful actions.

Hazard assessment is of prime importance for all types of disasters. Common hazards to anticipate in planning include:

- Bulky or sharp debris
- Fallen trees
- Downed but energized power lines
- Weakening and possible collapse of structures
- Displaced wild animals, such as rodents, reptiles, and insects
- Chemical or gas releases, such as from broken pipelines or storage containers
- Bloodborne pathogens from injured and bleeding victims, including those infected with HIV and hepatitis C virus
- Flooding and destructive forces of water
- Water damage and mold
- Fires with heavy smoke and dust
- Diesel exhaust from large equipment used during prolonged recovery activities.

Box 31-1. Framework of the U.S. Federal Government Response to Disasters

The National Preparedness System outlines an organized process for all people in a community to engage in preparedness activities and achieve the National Preparedness Goal.[1,2] The five mission areas of preparedness are Prevention, Protection, Mitigation, Response, and Recovery. Each mission area is comprised of core capabilities organized by a planning framework with a unified approach and common terminology.

The National Response Framework (NRF) aligns key federal coordinating roles and responsibilities for emergency response in a scalable fashion. It operates in partnership with state and local government agencies, nongovernmental organizations, and the private sector.[3] In 2016, the NRF was updated to emphasize that a whole community works together, integrating all sectors, to meet the needs of those affected by disasters.[4]

The NRF has a Worker Safety and Health Support Annex, coordinated by the Occupational Safety and Health Administration.[5] Expert technical assistance comes from industrial hygienists, sanitary engineers, occupational medicine physicians and nurses, and other health and safety professionals.

The scope of activities within this annex addresses capabilities to identify, characterize, and control health and safety hazards, the use of personal protective equipment (PPE), on-scene worker risk communication, training, and medical evaluation. Technical assistance can also be requested concerning long-term medical surveillance, immunizations and prophylaxis, and support of the psychological resiliency of emergency response workers. All response operations use an incident command system (ICS) that is coordinated by the National Incident Management System (NIMS), which emphasizes local control of an incident with support from federal and state government agencies. This system provides a "consistent approach to operational structures and supporting mechanisms, and an integrated approach to resource management."[6]

The National Oil and Hazard Substances Pollution Contingency Plan (NCP) governs the national response capability and overall coordination for oil spills and hazardous substance releases. The U.S. Coast Guard is the lead agency when a discharge occurs in a coastal zone, whereas the Environmental Protection Agency (EPA) is the lead agency when spills occur inland. The NCP is a part of the National Response System, which involves multilayered networks of federal, state, local, and tribal government agencies as well as industry. The system includes the National Response Center, On-Scene Coordinator, the National Response Team, and Regional Response Teams.

References

1. Federal Emergency Management Agency. National Preparedness Goal. Washington, DC: Federal Emergency Management Agency, 2016. Available at: https://www.fema.gov/national-preparedness-goal. Accessed November 15, 2016.
2. Federal Emergency Management Agency. National Preparedness System. Washington, DC: Federal Emergency Management Agency, 2016. Available at: https://www.fema.gov/national-preparedness-system. Accessed November 15, 2016.
3. U.S. Department of Homeland Security. Homeland Security Presidential Directive 5. Washington, DC: U.S. Department of Homeland Security, 2003. Available at: https://www.dhs.gov/publication/homeland-security-presidential-directive-5. Accessed November 29. 2016.
4. U.S. Department of Homeland Security. National response framework. Washington, DC: U.S. Department of Homeland Security, 2016. Available at: https://www.fema.gov/media-library-data/1466014682982-9bcf8245ba4c60c120aa915abe74e15d/National_Response_Framework3rd.pdf. Accessed November 15, 2016.
5. U.S. Department of Homeland Security. Worker Safety and Health Support Annex. Washington, DC: U.S. Department of Homeland Security, 2008. Available at: https://www.fema.gov/pdf/emergency/nrf/nrf-support-wsh.pdf. Accessed November 15, 2016.
6. Federal Emergency Management Agency. National incident management system. Washington, DC: U.S. Department of Homeland Security, Federal Emergency Management Agency, 2016. Available at: https://www.fema.gov/national-incident-management-system. Accessed November 15, 2016.

National planning has also considered terrorism scenarios involving chemical, biological, radioactive, nuclear, or explosive (CBRNE) substances, which could cause massive disruption or destruction.

The framework of the U.S. federal government response to disasters is described in Box 31-1.

Events Influencing Policy and Research for Worker Protection

Large-scale and complex disasters occurring in 2001 highlighted the need to organize disaster safety management and ensure that worker safety and health is integrated into the management of incidents.[3-6] On September 11, 2001 (9/11), terrorists hijacked and crashed four commercial jet airplanes, two into the Twin Towers of the World Trade Center, one into the Pentagon, and one into a field in Pennsylvania.[7] Hundreds of firefighters were killed while attempting to rescue thousands of people below the point of building impacts, causing intense emotions among the response community.[3] Erratic credentialing procedures, personal protective equipment (PPE) supply shortages and design challenges, disrupted telecommunication systems, faulty instrument readings (due to intense smoke), and the lack of unified authority thwarted efforts to characterize the environmental contamination and better inform efforts to protect workers.[3,4] Inconsistent interpretation of environmental sampling data and advice about safe exposure thresholds emerged, creating confusion, distress, and mistrust of the public institutions managing risk and uncertainties. Shortcomings in on-scene safety information, training, and enforcement made it difficult to control internal perimeters or hazard zones established to differentiate needs for training, fit-testing and proper use of PPE, and practices for worker protection (see Figure 31-1).[4]

In 2011, President Barack Obama signed into law the James Zadroga 9/11 Health and Compensation Act of 2010, which established the World Trade Center Health Program.[8] This federally funded healthcare entitlement, exposure registry, and research program has since been extended to 2090. Healthcare services are delivered through a "center-of-excellence" model, with standardized annual medical monitoring examinations and expert treatment services for qualifying conditions. Program beneficiaries include eligible responders, clean-up workers, and others adversely impacted by the 9/11 disaster. The program also conducts health surveillance and research addressing emerging conditions that may be linked with 9/11 exposure, atypical disease mechanisms leading to treatment resistance, and health burdens impacting the quality of life over time.[9]

Soon after 9/11, journalists in Florida and New York and U.S. senators received postal letters containing anthrax spores mixed in a powder-like substance, leading to a massive public health and law enforcement effort to tracke these bioterrorism events. Investigations found that anthrax spores were contaminating postal-service hubs that process mail throughout the Washington, DC–New York City corridor. The risk of fulminant disease from anthrax infection led to mass distribution of antibiotics, including for workers wearing PPE, lest there be undetected breaches.[10] There was confusion about divergent methodologies and authorities for measuring and interpreting environmental and occupational exposure to the anthrax-laden powder. These events led to planning for CBRNE scenarios and worker protection to be ready to

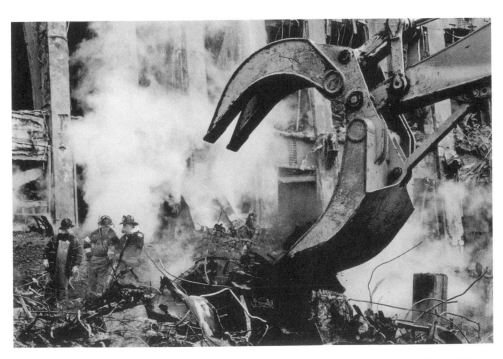

Figure 31-1. Recovery workers at the World Trade Center site in September 2001. (Photograph by Earl Dotter.)

deal with terrorism from such agents. Federal resources supported these efforts, and the Department of Homeland Security was established, headed by a cabinet-level secretary.[11]

These events stimulated research at the National Institute for Occupational Safety and Health (NIOSH), including on personal protective technology. Contributing to national preparedness for emergency responders, NIOSH published seven special test procedures for respiratory protective devices (RPDs) for chemical, biological, radiological, and nuclear hazards.[12] Advances in research are enabling sensors to indicate when the air-filtering cartridge of an RPD has reached the end of its service life and needs to be changed.[13] In addition, since 2005, NIOSH has funded a standing committee on PPE for workplace safety and health to enable input of stakeholders on PPE research, standards development, and user guidance.[14]

In 2003, the emergence of severe acute respiratory syndrome (SARS) threatened healthcare workers in Southeast Asia and Canada, challenging healthcare institutions and government agencies to improve infection control and respiratory protection for emerging pathogens.[15] Subsequent outbreaks of influenza spurred greater attention to pandemic influenza preparedness, due to the susceptibility of human populations and variations in viral transmission and pathogenicity.[16] The possibility of an impending pandemic stimulated the public health community to address the readiness of the healthcare sector to respond to a pandemic. Readiness concerns included appropriate selection and use of PPE, optimization of vaccination campaigns, and pre- and postexposure prophylaxis. Innovations in PPE are needed to reduce fit-testing requirements for RPDs and improve their comfort and tolerability in healthcare settings.[17,18] More work needs to done to assess how well PPE conforms to design specifications after market. Risk-based, evidence-driven guidance needs to be applied to link workplace hazards during an emergency response to appropriate standards and to identify the appropriate PPE to meet standards to keep workers safe.

In 2005, Hurricane Katrina led to the inundation of New Orleans, unmasking many health and response disparities. Lessons from this disaster led to the Post-Katrina Emergency Management Reform Act of 2006, which reorganized the Federal Emergency Management Agency and expanded its authority to address gaps in emergency response.[19,20]

In 2010, millions of gallons of oil spilled into the Gulf of Mexico after the Deepwater Horizon oil drilling rig exploded and sank. Lessons learned from previous responses led to the early development of guidance to protect workers. Near real-time adjustments were made in these recommendations because of timely field assessments of potential hazards on shore and off, including the physical hazards onboard marine vessels, heat stress, chemical dispersants involved in oil containment and cleanup, and the psychosocial hazards attendant to variations in work crews and safety culture.[21-24] Communication of risks to workers was made a top priority, and environmental and health data was made available on the Environmental Protection Agency (EPA) and NIOSH websites throughout the spill response.

A deadly fire and explosion at the West Fertilizer Plant in Texas in 2013, which killed 15 people, injured 260, and caused massive community damage, was determined to have been caused by a failure of proper planning and training.[25] The report of the U.S. Chemical Safety Board on this disaster helped to raise community, labor, industry, and government awareness about the dangers of fertilizer grade ammonium nitrate and the needs for community awareness, storage regulation, and hazardous-materials training for voluntary firefighters.

The epidemic of Ebola virus disease, mainly in 2014, which devastated three countries in West Africa, infected and killed more people—including more healthcare providers—than any previous Ebola outbreak.[26,27] This experience showed that access to PPE is not enough and that policies and procedures need to be in place for training response workers and emergency medical providers in the donning and doffing of PPE.[27,28] Heat stress was an important healthcare worker safety factor in the warm and humid West African climate and could result in problems with coordination and cognitive function leading to errors in judgment and unsafe use of PPE. Given the serious nature of this infection, just-in-time research was performed to provide updated guidance on selection of PPE and use of cooling devices. Research included testing garments for fluid resistance and blood penetration under mechanical pressure and testing the length of time PPE ensembles could be used before core body temperature rose to unsafe levels.[29]

Responses to the 9/11 attacks, Deepwater Horizon oil spill, Ebola virus disease epidemic, and the Zika virus disease outbreak have highlighted the important need for disaster-science research on the health consequences of novel exposures that arise during disaster response and to evaluate the effectiveness of preventive measures.[30-32] Research before, during, and after disasters can lead to improved effectiveness of emergency responses, lower injury and illness occurrence among responders, and inform future response strategies. However, the unpredictability of what emergencies will occur and when makes it difficult to conduct research during disasters. Challenges include lack of baseline health data for responders, access to study populations and the disaster site, and rapid funding mechanisms. Often the most important data, including initial exposure sampling and a roster of responders, is not collected due to the heightened but narrow focus on immediate response and inadequate planning and response culture. Additional operational challenges include obtaining timely approvals from human research subject protection boards and other entities that constrain federal collection of data, such as the Office of Management and Budget, based on the Paperwork Reduction Act of 1980.

NIOSH has recently established the Disaster Science Responder Research Program to enable starting occupational safety and health research quickly after a disaster occurs and to support pre-event disaster research.[32,33]

Description of Emergency Response Workers

Typically, the definition of emergency response workers has included firefighters, emergency medical services workers, and law enforcement personnel. However, depending on the nature and scale of the incident, additional workers contribute to the emergency response activities and include many types of professionals and skilled laborers, including electric utility workers restoring power and road crews freeing up transportation routes blocked by fallen trees and other debris (Box 31-2).[34] For example, during the Deepwater Horizon oil spill, commercial and subsistence fishermen were recruited to assist with the cleanup. Nontraditional responders, who are required for a fast response to emergencies, need additional training. Essential services are those that maintain community operations and minimize disruption from loss of power, sanitation, potable water, safe food and medicine, and needed services (such as transportation). Workers providing essential services during a severe infectious epidemic are likely to function as emergency responders and include healthcare providers, healthcare support personnel, behavioral health and social service personnel, public health investigators, and representatives of nongovernmental faith-based or civic organizations who directly assist affected people. Workers are often untrained for the roles they must perform in response to large-scale disasters, including managing distraught persons in quarantine or

---

Box 31-2. Functions of World Trade Center Responders

Traditional Workers
Emergency service workers
Federal disaster responders
Firefighters
Law enforcement personnel
Urban search and rescue

Nontraditional Workers
Building cleaners
Building trades
Civil service workers

Counselors
Engineers
Environmental assessment workers
Media representatives
Mortuary workers
Nonemergency healthcare workers
Pastoral care workers
Public officials
Sanitation workers
Transport workers
Veterinarians
Volunteers

Source: Moline J, Herbert R, Levin S, et al. WTC medical monitoring and treatment program: Comprehensive health care response in aftermath of disaster. Mount Sinai Journal of Medicine 2008;75: 67–75.

isolation, dependents of essential-service workers, and others, such as children, older people, medically fragile and institutionalized persons, and pets, service animals, and livestock.

DISASTER SAFETY MANAGEMENT

Before a disaster occurs, it is essential to build the capacities and flexibility required to protect disaster-response workers. Collectively, these functions and capabilities have been termed *disaster safety management*.[4] As workers from many disciplines and organizational entities are likely to become involved in disaster response and recovery, the following core tasks must be coordinated:[1,4,22,35]

- Identifying and monitoring site-specific hazards (scientifically measuring and interpreting findings)
- Determining and implementing site-specific exposure control strategies
- Monitoring and reporting health and injury surveillance for disaster workers
- Facilitating worker protection education and training on scene (just in time)
- Ensuring appropriate site access controls and credentialing, especially for unaffiliated volunteers
- Ensuring adequate supply and effective use of PPE
- Ensuring access to appropriate medical and behavioral healthcare services.

Effective worker protection requires coordination and cooperation among all entities involved. Appropriately qualified and experienced occupational safety and health personnel must be assigned to the tasks listed previously. Safety and health plans need to be professionally designed, monitored, and tailored to specific worksite conditions. Controlling exposures to occupational hazards is the fundamental method of protecting workers. Disaster safety management needs to provide ongoing real-time guidance to disaster incident leadership at all levels of government, healthcare, and business sectors to ensure robust standards are met to reliably protect responders. Capacity building occurs both within and across organizations (Table 31-1).

The Emergency Responder Health Monitoring and Surveilliance (ERHMS) system contains specific recommendations and tools for protecting the health and safety of responders in all phases of a response, including predeployment, deployment, and postdeployment (see Figure 31-2).[22] Medical monitoring and surveillance in ERHMS can identify exposures and/or signs and symptoms early in an emergency situation in order to prevent and mitigate adverse physical and psychological effects. Data collected during the response can help identify which, if any, responders would benefit from medical referral and possible enrollment in a long-term health surveillance program.

Occupational Health Surveillance

In its broadest sense, *occupational health surveillance* refers to the "systematic collection, analysis, and interpretation" of health and exposure data for the purposes of identifying cases of occupational illness or disease, monitoring trends of occupational illness or injury, and monitoring exposure to workplace hazards.[36] (See Chapter 6.) Surveillance also includes the

Table 31-1. Building Emergency Response Capacity

Individual	Organizational and Community

• Medical evaluation (physical and mental health)
  • Fitness for duty
  • Medical baseline
• Attainment of credentials
• Education
• Training exercises
• Fitting of PPE ensembles
• Pre-mission briefing
	• Establishment of personnel tracking system
	• Identification of health and safety officers
	• Training exercises
	• Selection and fitting of PPE ensembles
	• Communication and coordination with local, state, and federal emergency response entities

Note. PPE = personal protective equipment.

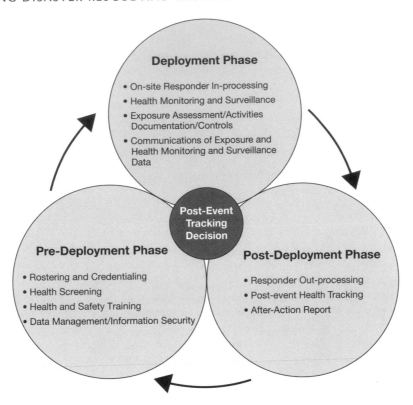

Figure 31-2. Lifecycle of a worker and workforce deploying to a disaster. (Source: U.S. Environmental Protection Agency. Emergency Responder Health Monitoring and Surveillance. National Response Team Technical Assistance Document (TAD). Washington, DC: U.S. Environmental Protection Agency, 2012. Available at https://www.nrt.org/sites/2/files/ERHMS_Final_060512.pdf. Accessed November 29, 2016.)

timely dissemination of information to people who can implement effective prevention and control measures. It is a critical function in protecting emergency response workers and includes activities in both hazard surveillance and medical surveillance. Hazard surveillance, medical surveillance, and screening are also critical functions of the Worker Safety and Health Support Annex and are tied to public health and medical activities (Emergency Support Function No. 8 [ESF8]) of the National Response Framework (Box 31-3).[19]

Hazard Surveillance

Environmental sampling and monitoring are critical functions during disaster response, recovery, and remediation phases of a disaster. The goal of hazard surveillance is to characterize work-related exposures to prevent or control (limit) responder exposures. A good

---

Box 31-3. Public Health and Medical Services (ESF8) from the National Response Framework

- Assessment of public health/medical needs
- Health surveillance
- Medical care personnel
- Health/medical/veterinary equipment and supplies
- Patient evacuation
- Patient care
- Safety and security of drugs, biologics, and medical devices
- Blood and blood products

- Food safety and security
- Agriculture safety and security
- All-hazard public health and medical consultation, technical assistance, and support
- Behavioral healthcare
- Public health and medical information
- Vector control
- Potable water/wastewater and solid waste disposal
- Mass fatality management, victim identification, and decontaminating remains
- Veterinary medical support

archival source of information about prior disasters and associated release of toxic substances is the Hazardous Substances Emergency Events Surveillance System, maintained by the Agency for Toxic Substances and Disease Registry.[37,38] In more defined workplace settings, personal exposure monitoring can be conducted to better assess individual exposures, but this is often not practical in a disaster setting. This hazard information is utilized to develop strategies to limit responder exposures and inform medical surveillance activities.

Medical Surveillance

Medical surveillance is the analysis of health information to identify cases of occupational injury or illness or a change in biological function among workers in order to evaluate workplace controls or identify opportunities for workplace interventions to prevent occupational illness or disease.[36,39] Examples of medical surveillance activities include reviews of (a) Occupational Safety and Health Administration (OSHA)-required injury and illness logs from emergency response operations and (b) health data from predeployment, intradeployment, and postdeployment medical evaluations.

Medical Screening

Medical screening is an initial examination conducted to detect unrecognized disease or organ dysfunction before an individual would normally seek medical care.[36,39] The primary purpose of medical screening is to limit disease progression by providing early diagnosis and treatment as well as by limiting continued hazard exposure. Results can be considered individually or aggregated to create an understanding of novel health effects or novel relationships between exposures and health effects.[40,41]

Varying Roles of Occupational and Environmental Safety and Health Professionals

The occupational or environmental safety and health professional may assume various roles in protecting emergency response workers and/or the general public (Box 31-4). Roles often differ by specific profession (such as physician, nurse, industrial hygienist, or sanitary engineer), credentialing, and experience. The National Incident Management System identifies a safety officer who is responsible for assuring personnel safety, monitoring hazardous and unsafe situations, preparing a site-specific safety and health plan, monitoring the incident, and advising the incident commander. Various roles include scientific exposure assessment and site characterization, design and implementation of hazard control strategies, worker safety education and training, health surveillance, direct patient care, and medical monitoring. In addition, these professionals may provide indirect support to workers through technical consultation, team leadership, or as an official liaison to the disaster safety management infrastructure at varying management levels in the field or at headquarters. Such roles require a working knowledge of data collection and analytical techniques (such as root cause, fault tree analysis, failure mode and effect analysis, and basic statistics) to identify high-risk safety conditions, operations, and practices and develop trend analysis and statistical reports. Knowledge and experience would also be required to manage and lead other safety and health professional staff members, which would include human resource–related activities, work/rest scheduling, task management, conflict negotiation, and other skills pertaining to interpersonal relations, team leadership, and psychological resiliency on scene and postevent.

Under the National Response Framework, the Department of Health and Human Services coordinates federal support for public health and medical activities during a disaster (ESF8; Box 31-3).[1] Environmental and occupational health and safety professionals may also be asked to handle a variety of functions listed in Box 31-5, especially as they pertain to temporary housing (including shelters) and work facilities to ensure safe food, water, waste disposal, shower/wash stations, and vermin control.[35] Understanding the variety and interrelationship of roles will help to ensure coordination during all phases of emergency management (preparedness, response, and recovery).

Box 31-4. Public and Environmental Health
Issues in Disasters

Emergency management and public health share a philosophy of preventing injury and illness whenever possible. In terms of disaster preparedness, a helpful approach is to analyze the systems or pathways of the goods, services, utilities, and linkages that allow a community (or larger population unit) to function. Some experts have termed this a *lifeline vulnerability assessment*.[1] A community is able to function on a daily basis because of its lifelines, albeit the essential infrastructure.

Emergency planners should anticipate the likely disaster hazards that might occur within their jurisdictions, accounting for risks imposed by local industry, commercial transportation routing, population density, economic diversity, land use, and regional weather or geological patterns. The types of hazards include dangerous weather (hurricanes or tornados), earthquakes, flooding (rainfall exceeding river capacity or levee or dam breach), power loss, fire, widespread infectious disease (such as influenza), and industrial or commercial transportation incidents (such as chemical spills and explosions involving toxic materials).

Risk communication is a critical function in disaster response. Information needs to be disseminated to and understood by all persons attempting to gain access to, or remain within, a disaster-stricken area. Carbon monoxide poisoning can occur from power generators (such as for heating) used within enclosed spaces. There are risks of injury from debris strewn about or falling from unprotected heights, or inadequate structural integrity of affected buildings. Downed wires may still be energized, posing threats of electrocution. Wild or stray animals, reptiles, or poisonous insects may be threats. There are risks of serious infection from improper wound care or poor sanitation. In addition, there are risks associated with exposure to extremes in temperature (heat or cold). Guidance should be widely disseminated about proper methods of sanitizing contaminated surfaces, handling flooded ventilation systems, addressing mold problems, recognizing allergies (such as to mold), handling of dangerous power tools (such as chain saws), appropriately using personal protective gear, and disinfecting private well water.

Within the first days to weeks of a disaster, regardless of whether people are living in their primary residences or in shelters, they need access to potable water, safe food, essential medicines, healthcare, housing, electrical power, and proper sanitation. Special populations, such as frail elderly people, children, and rurally isolated people, must be considered. Surveys of the community will be required to ascertain the adequacy of these resources and to identify additional needs for outreach services to assist those less able to mobilize from their homes. Needs assessments are typically conducted within days to weeks of a disaster and involve door-to-door surveys and often a population sampling method.

Other systems also need to be evaluated. Health and safety monitoring within makeshift housing (shelters), evacuation centers, temporary medical facilities, and schools can indicate the magnitude of the disaster impact and can affect how and if people can access necessary resources. Sheltering facilities can be evaluated for potential problems with water or food supply, improper food handling or sanitation practices, and decisions regarding high-occupancy spacing and child safety. Such inspections can identify immediate health and safety threats as well as potential catalysts for problems, including supervision of children and housing and visitation for pets. Understanding the characteristics of the underlying population, in conjunction with the environmental conditions, can drive public health messages. Staff members of facilities will likely also be experiencing stress from the event itself and from the occupancy demands within the facility. Providing risk communication and staff training via a Site Safety Officer or overriding organization (such as the Red Cross or Salvation Army) can help to clarify roles and tasks, cross-training, and control of staff work/rest cycles.

Targeted health screening and disease surveillance measures are needed to monitor population health and to help optimally direct scarce resources. This screening or assessment must be connected to clinical services able to identify and stabilize chronic or newly emerging illnesses, injuries, and mental or behavioral health problems. The event scenario and potential human exposure(s) will inform the content and duration of such health screening and surveillance activities. Shorter term health monitoring in high-occupancy facilities will assist in early detection and mitigation of infectious disease outbreaks. Exposure to certain chemicals or ionizing radiation may require longer term monitoring for latent disease or adverse reproductive impacts.

Reference

1. Johnston D, Becker J, and Cousins J. Lifelines and urban resilience. In D Paton, D Johnston (eds.). Disaster resilience: An integrated approach. Springfield, IL: Charles C. Thomas, 2006. pp. 40–65.

OSHA Standards Applicable to Emergency Response and Preparedness

The Occupational Safety and Health Administration (OSHA) has identified several health and safety standards relevant to emergency preparedness and response activities.[42] Providing a complete list of applicable OSHA standards is impractical. However, many of these standards have special importance to healthcare professionals, given their requirements for medical evaluation and/or medical consultation. Substance-specific standards

Box 31-5. Emergency Response Activities Designed to Protect Worker Safety and Health During the Deployment Period

- Deployment of an appropriately credentialed safety officer
- Establishment of site security and control (perimeter control and designated hazard zones)
- Establishment of evacuation routes and procedures
- Registration of emergency response workers
- Site characterization (potential exposures) and job hazard analysis (personal and environmental sampling and investigation and statistical reporting)
- Design, implementation, and evaluation/continual refinement and communication about the health and safety plan (HASP)

- Official enforcement of the HASP (compliance)
- Establishment and maintenance of OSHA 300 log to report injuries and illnesses
- Monitoring of crew shift length for adequacy of rest, hydration, and nutrition
- Treatment for any emerging physical or mental health problems
- Monitoring for trends with health and injury surveillance
- Reviewing and approving the medical plan, ensuring healthcare services (ICS 206)
- Maintaining a Unit/Activity Log (ICS 214) for OSHA 300 injury/illness reporting
- Supervision of other safety personnel
- Familiarization with process to coordinate with overall disaster response management.

(with medical surveillance components) may also apply depending on whether the incident involves the release of a toxic industrial chemical.

Knowledge of the regulatory requirements for medical evaluation and consultation is essential to effectively protecting worker safety and health. Medical evaluations of emergency response and recovery workers should at least meet applicable regulatory requirements. For example, under the Hazardous Waste Operations and Emergency Response (HAZWOPER) standard, the medical evaluation consists of a medical and work history with special emphasis on symptoms related to (a) the handling of hazardous substances and health hazards and (b) fitness for duty, including the ability to wear any required PPE under conditions that may be expected at the worksite (such as temperature extremes).[43] This standard also describes the frequency of the medical evaluation, such as prior to assignment or as soon as possible upon notification by an employee that he or she has developed signs or symptoms indicating possible overexposure to hazardous substances or health hazards. In addition to developing and conducting medical evaluations, occupational safety and health professionals may also have a role in training workers. For example, under the OSHA Bloodborne Pathogens Standard, training is required for workers with exposure to blood or other potentially infectious materials.[44]

The regulatory requirements for emergency preparedness and response represent the minimum required to protect workers. Many of the applicable OSHA standards were not designed with consideration of the emergency response environment. For example, although emergency response operations have been characterized as noisy, use of hearing protection could adversely impact the ability of emergency responders to communicate with one another.[3,45] Not all responders are equally covered by OSHA standards. For example, state and local government employees performing emergency response, such as firefighters and law enforcement, are not covered by OSHA regulations in jurisdictions without a State Occupational Safety and Health Plan. Finally, additional considerations, such as mental and behavioral health needs, may also be necessary to more fully meet the medical needs of emergency response and recovery workers.

Hazard Control and the Site-Specific Worker Health and Safety Plan

The OSHA HAZWOPER standard (29 CFR 1910.120) requires a written site-specific worker health and safety plan (HASP) for engaging in cleanup operations conducted at uncontrolled hazardous waste sites, corrective actions involving hazardous waste cleanup operations at sites covered by the Resource Conservation and Recovery Act, such as treatment, storage, and disposal and emergency response operations for the release or threatened release of hazardous substances.[43,46-48] (See Chapter 18.) The key elements of the HASP include hazard analysis and site-specific requirements for training, PPE, medical surveillance, air monitoring, site control, decontamination, emergency response plan, confined space entry program, and a spills containment program.

TIME PHASES FOR EMERGENCY AND DISASTER RESPONSE ACTIVITIES

The National Planning Framework organizes emergency and disaster response activities in three functional time phases: *preparedness, response,* and *recovery* (Table 31-2).[1]

1. *Preparedness*: The preparedness phase includes activities related to building capacity in order to effectively respond to an emergency. Planning, training, acquiring equipment, and evaluating the effectiveness of emergency response capabilities through training exercises are all a part of building capacity.
2. *Response*: The response phase begins once an incident has occurred. During this phase, emergency response personnel are deployed to the site of the incident in order to mitigate its effect on life, the environment, property, the economy, and society overall. Responders engaged in immediate

rescue operations tend to take greater risks in the chaotic disaster work setting in the service of saving or sustaining the lives of those directly affected. Little time is available to assess the hazards before rescue efforts begin.

3. *Recovery*: The transition between response and recovery operations may not always be clear. In general, recovery operations begin once immediate lifesaving activities are complete and potentially life-threatening hazards are stabilized. The short-term recovery phase focuses on returning the area involved in the disaster to a functional state of self-sufficiency, with attention given to helping individuals, households, businesses, and critical infrastructure meet basic needs. Depending on the incident, the long-term recovery phase may last for months or even years.

These time phases are useful for characterizing and coordinating the major functional elements of disaster management, such as transportation, communication, and public health and medical services (Boxes 31-3 and 31-5). *Deployment* typically refers to mobilizing assets (resources and capabilities) to help manage the disaster. The assets typically include skilled personnel and specialized equipment. The assets are safely returned as early as possible in the response phase termed *demobilization* to enable resource tracking and accountability for both resources and provisions guiding mutual aid and assistance.

Workers are involved in all of these phases. The charge to the occupational safety and health professional is to protect the health and safety of the workers participating in the emergency response, recovery, remediation, and cleanup activities. Depending on the activity, the occupational safety and health professional may have worker protection responsibilities to an individual worker (such as direct patient care) or to an organization (such as population-based medical monitoring or health surveillance). Many aspects of disaster safety management require diverse skill sets. Qualifications will differ with respect to the tasks required, and expertise from several disciplines will need to be coordinated to ensure that workers are protected.

Table 31-2. Disaster Safety Management Life Cycle

Preparation	• Educate, train, and equip workers (anticipated hazards and command/control operations)
	• Establish medical baseline and readiness to deploy
	• Exercise and evaluate systems
Response	• Assess the situation (identify hazards and control strategies)
	• Deploy resources and capabilities
	• Coordinate activities and functions
	• Demobilize assets (people and equipment)
Recovery	• Short term (identify needs and provide resources)
	• Long term (epidemiological study and medical surveillance)

Individual (Worker) and Organizational (Employer) Preparedness

The workplace can be significantly harmed by a disaster, an act of terrorism, or another traumatic incident. The scope and scale of anticipated events may require a thorough systems-level vulnerability analysis, from raw material supply chains to market delivery of final product or services, including disruption in transportation routes required for workers to be on the job.[48] Preparedness encompasses the period of time before a worker or an organization is engaged in emergency response activities. At the individual level, a worker must acquire and maintain appropriate education, training, and certification (credentials) specific to his or her potential deployment roles. Before disasters lead to lawsuits, emergency responders may feel at risk as targets of future litigation for "on-the-fly" decisions and actions that they must take while in the midst of the emergency response. Medical, emotional, and cognitive readiness are important dimensions of workforce health protection planning.

At the level of organizational preparedness, activities focus on ensuring that qualified workers are ready and appropriately outfitted with personal protective ensembles for deployment. Activities are also designed to build an integrated response capacity within an organization and within a community (Table 31-1). Effective disaster safety management requires appropriate infrastructure and interagency planning and coordination before the emergency arises. Predeployment and preparedness activities shape and influence the overall success of the emergency response efforts and, in turn, the disaster recovery process.

While the field of emergency management encourages an all-hazards approach to planning, it is not uncommon to organize the core plan around the more likely emergency events, such as an industrial explosion or fire, a facility collapse, violence by a disgruntled employee, or a natural disaster that destroys or disrupts business operations, such as by flooding, hurricane-strength winds, or an earthquake. The advent of infectious disease epidemics, such as SARS or H1N1 (swine) influenza, place additional life demands on workers who must care for ill or dependent family members, especially if schools are closed by public health officials to slow down the spread of infection. While business continuity is a key component of such planning, worker safety and health must be incorporated into strategic thinking. The cost of not doing this can be quite high, including loss of specialized workers with a corresponding need to recruit and train new staff members, interim loss of productivity; and workers' compensation costs for job-related injury, illness, or disability, as well as other potentially cascading organizational effects, such as loss of morale.

The day-to-day stress in the workplace can impact health from more cumulative factors within worksites, such as how a job is designed, organizational structure, management style, management and coworker commitment to safe work practices (safety climate), and the availability of adequate resources and support to achieve the mission.[49] (See Chapter 14.) Disasters and large-scale emergencies also create competing life demands on a worker to ensure the safety and welfare of loved ones who may also be affected. Disasters erode normally protective supports, increase the risks of diverse problems, and tend to amplify pre-existing problems of social injustice and inequality within affected populations.[50] The disaster may provoke new social problems for residents and local business employers by separating families, disrupting social support networks, and compromising critical infrastructure, such as the ability to provide essential goods and services (water, food, medical care, power, and housing/facilities).

Integrating Psychological and Behavioral Risk Management

Worker safety and health practitioners must integrate psychological and behavioral risk management strategies into crisis and contingency planning; these require knowledge of the psychological and behavioral consequences of the disaster, terrorism, or other traumatic incident (Box 31-6).[51,52] Traumatic incidents and disaster exposure can increase the risk of distress reactions or dysfunction, behaviors increasing risk to health and safety, or psychiatric illnesses. One

Box 31-6. Lessons Learned from Prior Disaster Response to Anticipate Psychological and Behavioral Health Hazards and Service Needs

- It is difficult to prepare responders for everything they might encounter.
- Even seasoned responders can face situations and issues that cause uneasiness and distress.
- It is not unusual for responders to be asked to work outside their areas of expertise.
- Concerns about family members and friends rank high on responders' lists of priorities.
- Timely, accurate, and candid information should be shared to facilitate decision-making.
- Managers, at every level, need to consider the health, safety, and resiliency of workers on the job as part of situation awareness and for staged planning (which implies needs for occupational health and wellness monitoring).

- Resiliency is an integral component of occupational safety and health, which requires preplanning to maximize worker recovery.
- Self-care plans and peer-support activities are essential to mission completion.
- Everything possible should be done to safeguard responders' physical and emotional health.
- Responders do not need to face response challenges alone. They may share their experiences with friends, teammates, family members, and colleagues.
- It is especially difficult for responders to maintain emotional distance when they witness the deaths of children.
- Organizational differences among groups of responders and cultural differences between victims and responders can impede the timely and efficient provision of emergency services.
- Individuals may be thrust into leadership roles for which they have had little to no formal training.

---

should anticipate needs for psychological interventions in the workplace and plan to ensure that possible intervention measures are based on empirically defensible or evidence-based practices and are conducted by qualified individuals.[53] Interventions include leadership initiatives, administrative policies, and enhancing services by partnering with other organizations that can help provide and/or train others to provide psychosocial support services, such as management of stress, anger, and grief as well as crisis intervention counseling.[54]

Predeployment Medical Evaluation

The fitness-for-duty determination should establish a baseline status and take physical, psychological, and behavioral health into account to determine whether the worker will be able to perform anticipated essential job functions at the disaster site without posing a threat to self, others, or the overall emergency response. This includes an assessment of (a) the adequacy of medical control, (b) fitness, and (c) functional implications for responders with chronic health conditions—especially those related to long work hours, hot environments, disrupted sleep, and nutritional opportunities and when power is in short supply, such as that needed for refrigerated medication or CPAP machines. This determination should be made in compliance with

medical and legal standards, as outlined in the Americans with Disabilities Act.[55] Some emergency response workers may already be enrolled in medical surveillance programs as a part of their routine employment.[56,57]

Emergency Deployment

Emergency deployment encompasses the time period when a worker is actively engaged in responding to an incident. Very little time may be available for preparation of personnel prior to deployment (usually a week or less). Individuals preparing to deploy should receive a premission health and safety briefing that includes guidance about anticipated hazards (physical, chemical, biological, and interpersonal/psychological). Predeployment situational awareness should be provided via updated reports and/or materials designed for rapid dissemination. During the deployment period, characterization of hazards in the environment begins. For example, environmental and personal sampling may be employed to understand the composition and concentration of hazardous materials released in a dust cloud after structural collapse and/or structures may be evaluated for instability. Given that the predeployment medical evaluation is based on an understanding of likely or anticipated hazards, the occupational safety and health professional should gather information about any hazards to which the deployed worker may be exposed. This information will be an essential consideration when designing and implementing a medical screening program for use during the postdeployment period.

Similarly, PPE selection is an iterative process because preselected PPE ensembles may not adequately address unanticipated hazards and because hazards may change as the emergency evolves. In addition, most PPE is designed to function during a short-term incident. However, workers responding to the World Trade Center incident reported equipment failure and fatigue and heat exhaustion due to sustained PPE use during the extended response period.[3] Emergency response personnel are often required to work extended hours in high-risk environments, where alertness and attention to detail are absolute requirements for safe work practices. Elevated stress and fatigue can lead to faulty decision-making, unsafe work behaviors, and increased exposures to health hazards.[58] Optimally, the responder has emergency plans and systems in place to handle concerns about the safety and welfare of family members and other loved ones to avoid both fractured attention on the job and increased likelihood of accidents, improper work practices, and poor decision-making.[59,60]

Demobilization

Demobilization is a process that provides closure to the deployment period for both the responder and the organization. At the individual level, it includes the exit interview for the responder and verifies information collected about possible exposures, health or injury events, and follow-up contact information. Information is shared regarding mission successes and challenges for operational continuity (lessons learned), potential health effects, and available health services and resources. Deployment-related illness and injury data should be aggregated and analyzed with respect to geography, process, and time to help inform the need for postevent medical surveillance or epidemiologic investigation. From the organizational perspective, demobilization focuses on the withdrawal of deployed assets, including workers and their equipment.

Postdeployment

The postdeployment period begins once responders return to their routine work and extends forward in time as long as is practicable to understand health and safety impacts from disaster response work. Characterizing the health and safety impacts from disaster response work is generally accomplished through hazard surveillance combined with follow-up assessment and clinical services, such as physical examinations, medical screening, and psychological resiliency services. Responders should be kept abreast of the availability of these resources, as well as any entitlements or legal rights. Prior responders are encouraged to report and answer surveys regarding emerging adverse health events potentially related to deployment. Under the Worker Safety and Health Annex of the National Response Framework, OSHA has the responsibility to coordinate the federal response in "providing technical assistance, advice, and support for medical surveillance and monitoring as required by regulation (such as asbestos and lead) and evaluating the need for longer term epidemiological follow up and medical monitoring of response and recovery workers."[19]

The need for medical screening or more extensive health surveillance may be triggered through hazard surveillance activities conducted during the response as well as the emergence of concerning health effects in significant numbers of responders. Although it is not possible to describe a medical screening program suitable for all types of emergency response operations, design and implementation should adhere to some standard elements:[36]

- Assessment of workplace hazards
- Identification of target-organ toxicities for each hazard
- Selection of a screening test for each health effect
- Development of action criteria
- Standardization of the testing process
- Performance of testing
- Interpretation of test results
- Test confirmation
- Determination of work status
- Notification
- Diagnostic evaluation
- Evaluation and control of exposure
- Recordkeeping.

The nature of the emergency response environment presents several challenges to successfully designing and implementing an effective medical screening program, as described next.

ASSESSMENT OF WORKPLACE HAZARDS

The hazards of an emergency response may not yet be fully characterized or effectively communicated to clinical occupational safety and health professionals. Given that medical screening is often administered to workers without symptoms or at a point when overt disease is not fully recognized, it is essential that the screening program address likely health effects. Assessments of likely health effects are most reliable when based on knowledge of the hazard exposure.

Identification of Target Organ Toxicities, Selection of Screening Tests, and Development of Action Criteria

Even when hazards have been characterized, they may be diverse and complex. For example, hazard surveillance of the region impacted by hurricanes Katrina, Rita, and Wilma in 2005 identified exposures of noise, dust, asbestos, silica, formaldehyde, and carbon monoxide.[45] The variety of hazard exposures of emergency response workers can lead to an overly broad medical screening evaluation with a consequent decrease in the program's performance with respect to specificity and positive predictive value. Thus, care should be taken to identify target organ toxicities, select appropriate screening tests, and develop action criteria for test results.

Standardization of the Testing Process, Performance, Interpretation of Test Results, and Test Confirmation

Emergency response and recovery operations involve the coordination of multiple worker populations, employers, and organizational authorities. Demobilization of workers from the emergency response environment can include the dispersion of response workers over a large geographic area and/or the distribution of workers among various employers. Differences in geographic distribution and employers can give rise to differences in access to postdeployment medical screening as well as differences in medical personnel performing testing. During the 2014 Ebola virus disease epidemic, the Centers for Disease Control and Prevention recommended that local public health officials monitor healthcare workers, other volunteers, and travelers returning from West Africa and issued specific guidance on how to evaluate screening for Ebola virus disease. Despite these logistical difficulties, elements of the testing process should be standardized to maximize its utility to the medical surveillance program and workers.

Determination of Work Status, Notification, and Diagnostic Evaluation

The decentralization of emergency response workers can also lead to variations in clinical evaluations, such as effectively addressing work status, performing diagnostic evaluations, and notifying workers of clinical results and injury and illness trends. It can also impede the effective communication of hazard surveillance data. Despite these logistical difficulties, determinations of work status, notification, and diagnostic evaluation should be standardized.

Evaluation and Control of Exposure and Recordkeeping

The chaotic nature of the emergency response environment, the diversity of responding entities, and the decentralized worker population postdeployment make accurate evaluation and control of exposures and recordkeeping especially difficult. Basic requirements, such as knowing who worked at the site, how long they worked there, what they did, and whether they wore PPE, are essential to correlating workplace exposures with occupational injury and illness and communicating health and safety information to responding organizations and workers.

Workers engaged in emergency response and recovery activities should receive some level of medical assessment upon demobilization, depending on the nature of the incident and the hazards identified/assumed. The medical baseline established during the predeployment medical evaluation is fundamental to allowing comparisons in health status before and after emergency response operations.

It is also important to establish a site registry of workers that includes a review of site records to help identify who was present, for how long, doing what (job duties and possible exposures), and use of PPE.

ACKNOWLEDGMENT

The authors appreciate the assistance of Emily Hurwitz for background research and editing of references.

The findings and conclusions in this chapter are those of the authors and do not necessarily represent the views of the National Institute for Occupational Safety and Health.

REFERENCES

1. U.S. Department of Homeland Security. National response framework. Washington, DC: U.S. Department of Homeland Security, 2016. Available at: https://www.fema.gov/media-library-data/1466014682982-9bcf8245ba4c60c120aa915abe74e15d/National_Response_Framework3rd.pdf. Accessed November 15, 2016.
2. The SPHERE Project. Humanitarian charter and minimum standards in disaster response. Oxford: Oxfam International, 2004. Available at: http://www.ifrc.org/Docs/idrl/I283EN.pdf. Accessed November 15, 2016.
3. Jackson BA, Peterson DJ, Bartis JT, et al. Protecting emergency responders: Lessons learned from terrorist attacks. Santa Monica, CA: RAND Corporation, 2002. Available at: https://www.rand.org/content/dam/rand/pubs/conf_proceedings/2006/CF176.pdf. Accessed November 15, 2016.
4. Jackson BA, Baker JC, Ridgely MS, et al. Protecting emergency responders, Volume 3: Safety management in disaster and terrorism response. DHHS Publication no. 2004-144. Santa Monica, CA: RAND Corporation for the National Institute for Occupational Safety and Health, 2003. Available at: http://www.cdc.gov/niosh/docs/2004-144/pdfs/2004-144.pdf. Accessed November 15, 2016.
5. LaTourrette T, Peterson DJ, Bartis JT, et al. Protecting emergency responders, Volume 2: Community views of safety and health risks and personal protection needs. Santa Monica, CA: RAND Corporation for the National Institute for Occupational Safety and Health, 2003: Available at: http://www.rand.org/pubs/monograph_reports/MR1646.html. Accessed November 15, 2016.
6. Willis HH, Castle NG, Sloss EM, Bartis JT. Protecting emergency responders, Volume 4: Personal protective equipment guidelines for structural collapse events. Santa Monica, CA: Rand Corporation for the National Institute for Occupational Safety and Health, 2006. Available at: http://www.rand.org/pubs/monographs/MG425/. Accessed November 15, 2016.
7. Lioy P, Weisel C, Millette J, et al. Characterization of the dust/smoke aerosol that settled east of the World Trade Center (WTC) in lower Manhattan after the collapse of the WTC 11 September 2001. Environmental Health Perspectives 2002; 110: 703–714.
8. World Trade Center Health Program. Available at: https://www.cdc.gov/wtc/index.html. Accessed December 21, 2016.
9. National Institute for Occupational Safety and Health. World Trade Center Health Program Research Gateway. Washington, DC: National Institute for Occupational Safety and Health, 2016. Available at: https://wwwn.cdc.gov/ResearchGateway/. Accessed November 15, 2016.
10. Heyman D. Lessons from the anthrax attacks: Implications for U.S. bioterrorism preparedness. Washington, DC: Center for Strategic and International Studies, 2002.
11. Homeland Security Act, Pub. L. No. 107-296 (2002) 116 Stat. 2135. Available at https://www.congress.gov/bill/107th-congress/house-bill/5005. Accessed November 29, 2016.
12. National Institute for Occupational Safety and Health. What's special about CBRN self-contained breathing apparatus (SCBA)? Cincinnati, OH: Author, 2011. Available at: https://www.cdc.gov/niosh/docs/2011-183/pdfs/2011-183.pdf. Accessed November 15, 2016.
13. Occupational Safety and Health Administration. Respiratory protection eTool. Available at: https://www.osha.gov/SLTC/etools/respiratory/change_schedule.html. Accessed November 15, 2016.

14. Standing Committee on Personal Protective Equipment for Workplace Safety and Health. Available at: http://nationalacademies.org/hmd/activities/publichealth/ppeinworkplace.aspx>). Accessed December 21, 2016.

15. Campbell A. Executive summary. The SARS Commission interim report. SARS and public health in Ontario. Ontario: SARS Commission, 2004. Available at: http://www.health.gov.on.ca/english/public/pub/ministry_reports/campbell04/campbell04.html. Accessed November 15, 2016.

16. National Institute for Occupational Safety and Health. Framework for Setting the NIOSH PPT Program Action Plan for Healthcare Worker PPE: 2013–2018. Atlanta: National Institute for Occupational Safety and Health, 2013. Available at http://www.cdc.gov/niosh/docket/review/docket129A/pdfs/HCWRoadmapFrameDocV3_6-7-13.pdf. Accessed November 15, 2016.

17. Radonovich LJ, Baig A, Shaffer RE, et. al. Better respiratory equipment using advanced technologies for healthcare employees (Project B.R.E.A.T.H.E), 2009. Available at: http://www.publichealth.va.gov/docs/cohic/project-breathe-report-2009.pdf. Accessed November 29, 2016.

18. Radanovich LJ, Bessesen MT, Cummings DA, et al. The Respiratory Protection Effectiveness Clinical Trial (ResPECT): A cluster-randomized comparison of respirator and medical mask effectiveness against respiratory infections in healthcare personnel. BMC Infectious Diseases 2016; 16: 243. doi:10.1186/s12879-016-1492-2.

19. U.S. Department of Homeland Security. Worker Safety and Health Support Annex. Washington, DC: U.S. Department of Homeland Security, 2008. Available at: https://www.fema.gov/pdf/emergency/nrf/nrf-support-wsh.pdf. Accessed November 15, 2016.

20. Post-Katrina Emergency Management Reform Act (2006), enacted as Title VI of the Department of Homeland Security Appropriations Act, 2007, Pub. L. No. 109-295, 120 Stat. 1355. Available at https://www.congress.gov/bill/109th-congress/house-bill/5441 and https://www.congress.gov/bill/109th-congress/senate-bill/3721. Accessed November 29, 2016.

21. U.S. Environmental Protection Agency. National Contingency Plan Proposed Rule—Revisions to Ailgn with the National Response Framework. Washington, DC: U.S. EPA, 2016. Available at: https://www.epa.gov/emergency-response/national-contingency-plan-proposed-rule-revisions-align-national-response. Accessed November 15, 2016.

22. U.S. Environmental Protection Agency. Emergency Responder Health Monitoring and Surveillance. National Response Team Technical Assistance Document (TAD). Washington, DC: U.S. Environmental Protection Agency, 2012. Available at https://www.nrt.org/sites/2/files/ERHMS_Final_060512.pdf. Accessed Novermber 29, 2016.

23. Ahrenholz SH, Sylvain DC. Case study: Deepwater Horizon response workers exposure assessment at the source: MC252 well no. 1. Journal of Occupational & Environmental Hygiene 2011; 8: D43–50.

24. Michaels D, Howard J. Review of the OSHA-NIOSH response to the Deepwater Horizon Oil Spill: Protecting the health and safety of cleanup workers. PLoS Current Disasters; July 18, 2012. doi:10.1371/4fa83b757656e.

25. U.S. Chemical Safety and Hazard Investigation Board. West Fertilizer Company Fire and Explosion. Publication No. 2013-02-I-TX. U.S. Chemical Safety and Hazard Investigation Board, 2016. Available at: http://www.csb.gov/west-fertilizer-explosion-and-fire-/. Accessed November 15, 2016.

26. Edmunds KL, Abd Elrahman S, Bell DJ, et. al. Recommendations for dealing with waste contaminated with Ebola virus: A hazard analysis of critical control points approach. Bulletin of the World Health Organization 2016; 94: 424–432.

27. Fischer WA, Weber DJ, Wohl DA. Personal protective equipment: Protecting health care providers in an Ebola outbreak. Clinical Therapeutics 2015; 37: 2402–2410.

28. Fischer WA, Hynes NA, Perl TM. Protecting health care workers from Ebola: Personal protective equipment is critical but is not enough. Annals of Internal Medicine 2014; 161: 753–754.

29. Food and Drug Administration. Personal protective equipment for infection control. Silver Spring, MD: Food and Drug Administration, 2016. Available at: http://www.fda.gov/medicaldevices/productsandmedicalprocedures/generalhospitaldevicesandsupplies/personalprotectiveequipment/default.htm. Accessed November 15, 2016.

30. National Biodefense Science Board. Call to action: Include scientific investigations as an integral component of disaster planning and response. A report from the National Biodefense Science Board. National Biodefense Science Board, 2011. Available at: http://www.phe.gov/Preparedness/legal/boards/nprsb/Documents/nbsbrec14.pdf. Accessed November 15, 2016.

31. Lurie N, Manolio T, Patterson A, et al. Research as a part of public health emergency response. New England Journal of Medicine, 2013; 368: 1251–1255.

32. Boustead A, LaTournette T. NIOSH Disaster Science Research Initiative, Summary of the July 2014 DSRI Workshop. DHHS publication no. PR-1740-NIOSH. Santa Monica, CA: RAND Corporation for the National Institute for Occupational Safety and Health, 2015. Available at: https://www.cdc.gov/niosh/topics/disastersciences/pdfs/niosh-dsri-reportpeerreviewed2015-06-12.pdf. Accessed November 15, 2016.

33. National Institute for Occupational Safety and Health. Disaster Science Responder Research Program. Atlanta: National Institute for Occupational Safety and Health, 2016. Available from: http://www.cdc.gov/niosh/topics/disastersciences/default.html. Accessed November 15, 2016.

34. Moline J, Herbert R, Levin S, et al. WTC medical monitoring and treatment program: Comprehensive health care response in aftermath of disaster. Mount Sinai Journal of Medicine 2008; 75: 67–75.

35. U.S. Army Corps of Engineers. Safety and health requirements manual. Manual No. EM385-1-1. Washington, DC: 2008. Available at: http://www.usace.army.mil/Safety-and-Occupational-Health/Safety-and-Health-Requirements-Manual/. Accessed November 15, 2016.

36. Baker EL, Matte TP. Occupational health surveillance. In: Rosenstock L, Cullen MR, Brodkin CA, Redlich CA (eds.). Textbook of clinical occupational and environmental medicine (2nd ed.). London: Elsevier, 2005, pp. 76–82.

37. Kaye W, Orr M, Wattigney W. Surveillance of hazardous substance emergency events: Identifying areas for public health prevention. International Journal of Hygiene and Environmental Health 2008; 208: 37–44.

38. Agency for Toxic Substances and Disease Registry. Hazardous substances emergency events surveillance. Atlanta: U.S. Department of Health & Human Services, Agency for Toxic Substances and Disease Registry, 2009. Available at: https://www.atsdr.cdc.gov/hs/hsees/. Accessed November 15, 2016.

39. Occupational Safety and Health Administration. Medical screening and surveillance, medical screening. Washington, DC: Occupational Safety and Health Administration, 2007. Available at: https://www.osha.gov/SLTC/medicalsurveillance/. Accessed November 15, 2016.

40. Halperin WE, Ratcliffe J, Frazier TM, et al. Medical screening in the workplace: proposed principles. Journal of Occupational Medicine 1986; 28: 547–552.

41. Mitchell C, Gochfeld M, Shubert J, et al. Surveillance of workers responding under the National Response Plan. Journal of Occupational and Environmental Medicine 2007; 49: 922–927.

42. Occupational Safety and Health Administration. Principal emergency response and preparedness requirements and guidance. Publication No. OSHA 3122-06R. Washington, DC: Occupational Safety and Health Administration, 2004. Available at: https://www.osha.gov/Publications/osha3122.pdf. Accessed November 15, 2016.

43. Occupational Safety and Health Administration. Hazardous waste operations and emergency response (29 C.F.R. 1910.120; 29 C.F.R 1926.65). Washington, DC: Occupational Safety and Health Administration, 1994.

44. Occupational Safety and Health Administration. Bloodborne pathogens (29 C.F.R. 1910.1030). Washington, DC: Occupational Safety and Health Administration, 1991.

45. Occupational Safety and Health Administration. Hurricane exposure and risk assessment matrix for hurricane response and recovery work. Washington, DC: Occupational Safety and Health Administration, 2005. Available at: https://www.osha.gov/SLTC/etools/hurricane/. Accessed November 15, 2016.

46. Occupational Safety and Health Administration. OSHA e-HASP Software—Version 2.0 (e-HASP2). Washington, DC: 2006. Available at https://www.osha.gov/dep/etools/ehasp/. Accessed November 15, 2016.

47. Occupational Safety and Health Administration. Model Health & Safety Plan (HASP) for Clean-up of Facilities Contaminated with Anthrax Spore. Washington, DC: 2016. Available from: https://www.osha.gov/dep/anthrax/hasp/index.html. Accessed November 15, 2016.

48. Federal Emergency Management Agency. Emergency management guide for business and industry. Washington, DC: U.S. Department of Homeland Security, Federal Emergency Management Agency, 1993. Available at: https://www.fema.gov/pdf/library/bizindst.pdf. Accessed November 15, 2016.

49. Hurrell JJ, Kelloway EK. Psychological job stress. In: Rom WN, Markowitz SB (eds.). Environmental and occupational medicine

(4th ed.). Philadelphia: Lippincott, Williams and Wilkins, 2007, pp. 855–866.

50. Inter-Agency Standing Committee. IASC guidelines on mental health and psychosocial support in emergency settings. Geneva: Inter-Agency Standing Committee, 2007. Available at: https://interagencystandingcommittee.org/node/2915. Accessed November 15, 2016.

51. Ursano RJ, Vineburgh NT, Gifford RK, et al. Workplace preparedness for terrorism: Report of findings Alfred P. Sloan Foundation. Bethesda, MD: Center for the Study of Traumatic Stress, 2006. Available at: https://www.cstsonline.org/assets/media/documents/CSTS_report_sloan_workplace_prepare_terrorism_preparedness.pdf. Accessed November 15, 2016.

52. Vineburgh NT, Gifford RK, Ursano RJ, et al. Workplace disaster preparedness and response. In Ursano RJ, Fullerton CS, Weisaeth L, Raphael B (eds.). Textbook of disaster psychiatry. Cambridge, UK: Cambridge University Press, 2007, pp. 265–284.

53. Hobfoll SE, Watson PJ, Ruzek JI, et al. Five essential elements of immediate and mid-term mass trauma intervention: Empirical evidence. Psychiatry 2007; 70: 283–315.

54. Reissman DB, Kowalski-Trakofler K, Katz CR. Public health practice and disaster resilience: A framework integrating resilience as a worker protection strategy. In Southwick S, Charney D, Friedman M, Litz B (eds.). Resilience: Responding to challenges across the lifespan. Cambridge, UK: Cambridge University Press, 2011.

55. Americans with Disabilities Act, as amended 42 U.S.C. 12101 (1990). Available at: https://www.eeoc.gov/laws/statutes/ada.cfm. Accessed November 29, 2016.

56. National Fire Protection Association. NFPA 1582 standard on comprehensive occupational medical program for fire departments. Quincy, MA: National Fire Protection Association, 2007.

57. Goldberg RL, Spilberg SW, Weyers SG. Medical screening manual for California law enforcement. California Commission on Peace Officer Standards and Training. Sacramento: California Commission on Peace Officer Standards and Training, 2005.

58. Caruso CC, Bushnell T, Eggerth D, et al. Long working hours, safety, and health: Toward a national research agenda. American Journal of Industrial Medicine 2006; 49: 930–942.

59. Reissman DB, Watson PJ, Klomp RW, et al. Pandemic influenza preparedness: Adaptive responses to an evolving challenge. Journal of Homeland Security and Emergency Management 2006; 3: 13.

60. Johnston D, Becker J, Cousins J. Lifelines and urban resilience. In D Paton, D Johnston (eds.). Disaster resilience: An integrated approach. Springfield, IL: Charles C. Thomas, 2006, pp. 40–65.

32A

Hazards for Agricultural Workers

Amy K. Liebman and John May

CASE 1

A papermill worker, who was a member of a labor union, severed his flexor tendon. His employer sent him directly to the emergency department, where he was treated immediately and referred to a hand surgeon, who repaired the tendon within 24 hours. The worker filed a workers' compensation claim, and his expenses for medical treatment and lost worktime were covered. The patient was referred to an occupational therapist. The employer made accommodations so the employee could return to work during part of his recovery. The patient fully recovered and was back at his regular job within 3 months.

CASE 2

An "undocumented" migrant farmworker was harvesting broccoli on a cold day, making hundreds of cuts with a sharp knife, when his fingers became numb and he sliced off a fingertip. He was dropped off at the emergency department by his supervisor, who told him to say that he had sustained the injury at home. His employer threatened to call the federal Immigration and Customs Enforcement agency if he told the medical staff that the injury occurred at work. His employer was not required to—and did not—carry workers' compensation insurance, and he did not provide health insurance for workers. The farmworker was treated in the emergency department, where his wound was closed and he was given pain medication that would only last 3 days. No follow-up was scheduled because no local orthopedist accepted patients without health insurance. His employer did not make modified work available and terminated his employment.

These contrasting cases demonstrate that the management of occupational injuries differs depending on union membership, immigration status, type of industry, and workers'-compensation and health-insurance coverage.

FARMWORKERS AND HIRED AGRICULTURAL WORKERS

In the following discussion, *farmer* refers to the farm owner or operator. Unlike many other employment situations, many farmers contribute substantial physical labor and they often personally perform the more complex and dangerous tasks. The farmer employs directly, or contracts for, *agricultural workers (farmworkers)*. On many farms, family members of the farmer as well as other unpaid workers may also contribute substantial labor. *Farmworkers* generally refers to hired workers in crop agriculture who are either *migrant workers* (who move in order to work) or *seasonal workers* (whose employment reflects the seasonal nature of crop agriculture). These workers, who are typically immigrants from Mexico and Central America, often do not have legal authorization to work in the United States. H2-A visas and some other visas are specifically designed to enable agricultural workers to work in the United States for part of a year. In 2014, almost 225,000 H2-A visas were issued to agricultural workers from Mexico.[1] Nevertheless, about half of all farmworkers in the United States do not have authorization to work legally in this country. Beyond crop agriculture, the number of immigrant workers is increasing in animal production. Immigrants comprise more than half of workers now employed in dairy farming. These immigrant workers are less mobile than others because dairy farming is not seasonal.

Demographics

In 2012, the United States had 2.1 million farms, most of them small. Three-quarters of these generate less than $50,000 in sales annually and nearly 60% generate only $10,000. There were 3.3 million *farm operators* (who do farm work or make the day-by-day decisions), nearly one-third of them women, most frequently working as second operators. The average principal operator is a 58-year-old white male. Hired workers, including agricultural service workers, comprise one-third of agricultural labor force. The number of people employed in agriculture as hired workers in the United States decreased from 1,142,000 in 1990 to 1,063,000 in 2012, of whom 576,000 were in full-year positions, 199,000 in part-year positions, and 288,000 in agricultural service positions and brought to farms by contractors.[2] Of these workers, 56% worked in crop agriculture and 44% in livestock. An estimated 28% of hired workers are women.[3] Other estimates of hired agricultural workers suggest as many as 2.4 million workers are employed

in agriculture.[3] While hired workers comprise 33% of people employed on farms, they do an estimated 60% of the work.[4] Nearly 40% of hired agricultural workers live in California, Texas, and southwestern states, and one-fourth live in the Midwest. Immigrant and migrant workers, largely from Mexico and increasingly from Central America, comprise about 72% of the hired agricultural labor force. The average immigrant or migrant worker is 38 years old, has completed an average of 9 years of formal education, and speaks limited or no English. Nearly half of immigrant and migrant workers lack legal authorization to work in the United States.

The proportion of immigrant agricultural workers who regularly move for employment has decreased. Immigrant and migrant workers are at increased risk of occupational injury and death. Foreign-born Hispanic workers, compared to Hispanic workers born in the United States, are at risk of an occupational fatality.[5] Because many workers do not have authorization for employment in the United States, fear of deportation is an important barrier to workplace health and safety. Many workers pay substantial fees to enter the United States and take extreme risks in trying to find gainful employment. These economic and human costs have helped to foster a workforce that is less likely to report workplace health and safety violations and wage violations, and less likely to seek medical attention for an occupational injury or illness. Many agricultural workers enter the United States on H-2A visas, which are directly linked to a specific employer, thereby restricting free movement of labor. Although authorized and covered by workers' compensation, workers on H-2A visas remain vulnerable due to this restriction and their desire to keep their current jobs and return the following year.

Occupational health and safety is adversely impacted by barriers to mobility, differences in language and culture, unfamiliarity with local health services, and limited eligibility to access publicly and privately funded healthcare. These workers often receive limited or no training on how to safely perform their jobs.

Substandard housing represents another set of threats to the health and safety of agricultural workers. Health risks at home include exposure to dilapidated housing structures; exposure to overcrowding; pesticides; substandard or unsafe heating, cooking, and electrical systems; and inadequate or unsafe sanitation and drinking water.[6]

FATAL AND NONFATAL INJURIES

In 2014, there were nearly 480 occupationally related deaths in agriculture in the United States—a rate of 25.6 fatalities per 100,000, compared to 3.4 for all workers.[7] Most of these deaths were caused by transportation hazards (such as tractor rollovers), mechanical issues, and large animals.

The major causes of nonfatal injuries for farmers and hired workers include mechanical hazards, animals, and falls (Figure 32A-1 and Table 32A-1). Recent analyses of data from the Iowa Trauma Registry indicate annual rates for serious but nonfatal injuries between 2005 and 2010 ranging from 30.5 to 81.3 per 100,000.

There are many challenges in obtaining accurate occupational injury data in agriculture.

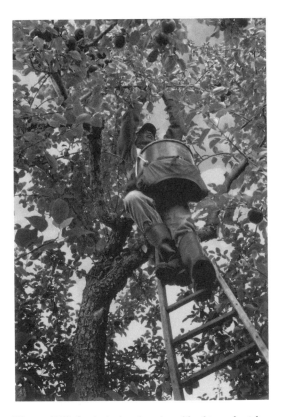

Figure 32A-1. Agricultural workers, like this apple picker, face numerous safety hazards. (Photograph by Earl Dotter.)

Agricultural workers are frequently hired on a part-time basis; they typically have other employment. Therefore, industry and occupation are often recorded inaccurately on death certificates. Accurately counting nonfatal injuries and determining injury rates are far more problematic than counting fatal injuries for several reasons:

- The Bureau of Labor Statistics only counts injuries among employees, not workers who are self-employed workers, as is frequent in farming.
- Small-farm operators and their family members are excluded, despite high injury rates, because the Occupational Safety and Health Administration (OSHA) requires only farms with 11 or more employees to report injuries, thereby excluding over 20% of all farm employees.
- Farm operators both inadvertently and deliberately underreport injuries.
- There is underreporting of injuries to employers by employees, especially immigrant workers.
- The total number of workers (rate denominator) is often not accurate because of undercounting, especially of immigrant workers and, to a lesser degree, the unpaid children and other family members of farm operators.[2]

WORKER PROTECTION REGULATIONS IN AGRICULTURE

Agricultural workers do not have many of the regulatory health and safety protections provided to workers in most other industries in the United States. Hired agricultural workers have been systematically excluded from key labor laws. The National Labor Relations Act (1935) does not enable agricultural workers to bargain collectively, although California and other states have allowed agricultural workers to unionize. The Fair Labor Standards Act (1938) does not require small-farm employers to pay the minimum wage, exempts overtime for all agricultural employees, and permits child labor in agriculture. There have been a few gains for agricultural workers since the 1930s, such

Table 32A-1. Selected Health Effects, Hazards, and Control Strategies in Agriculture

Health Effect	Hazard	Control Strategy
Musculoskeletal disorders	Prolonged stooping; heavy lifting; repetitive movements of the upper extremities during planting, pruning, and harvesting	Ergonomic reengineering of tools and workplace; decrease of weight of loads; job rotation among repetitive and nonrepetitive tasks
Pesticide-related conditions	Mixing, loading, and applying pesticides; working in fields recently sprayed with pesticides; aerial drift of pesticides from adjacent fields; exposure to pesticides in living quarters	Substitution with less toxic substances; adequate protective equipment; training on prevention of pesticide exposures; administrative restrictions on working in fields where exposure may occur
Traumatic injuries	Work-related incidents with tractors and other farm equipment; motor vehicle crashes during transport to and from fields; lacerations from sharp tools for cutting and pruning	Rollover protection on tractors; effective shielding on machinery; effective marking and lighting for roadways; barn design to minimize large animal contacts; safe cutting tools
Respiratory conditions	Airborne exposure to allergic and irritant substances, either naturally occurring in the soil and crops or due to chemical substances	Change process or use moisture to minimize dust generation; optimize ventilation; seek less toxic compounds; remove sensitized workers; respiratory protection
Dermatitis	Skin contact with allergic and irritant substances, either naturally occurring in the soil and crops or in fertilizers and pesticides	Substitution with less toxic materials; use of gloves and sleeves, if indicated; administrative controls to remove sensitized workers from exposure; change out of contaminated clothing
Infectious diseases	Inadequate sanitation facilities; exposure to tuberculosis, sexually transmitted diseases, and other infectious diseases due to living arrangements of migrant workers; exposure to microbial agents in animal work	Improved sanitation facilities; improved housing facilities; improved medical screening and treatment services
Cancer	Exposure to chemical substances in pesticides and other agricultural products; prolonged sun exposure	Substitution with substances that do not cause cancer; protective clothing and sunscreen; administrative controls to limit exposure
Eye conditions	Exposure to dusty conditions; foreign bodies from plant material penetrating the eye	Use of protective eye wear; dust control; pocket containers of saline eyewash
Mental disorders	Long working hours; inadequate pay; social isolation from family and friends	Improved working and housing conditions; availability of mental health services
Heat-related illness	Exposure to hot, humid environments	Ready access to fluids that workers will drink; surveillance of nonacclimated workers; worker and employer education on symptoms; enforced rest in shade with earliest symptoms

Source: Adapted from National Institute for Occupational Safety and Health. New directions in the surveillance of hired farm worker health and occupational safety: A report of the work group convened by NIOSH, May 5, 1995, to identify priorities for hired farm worker occupational health surveillance and research.

as federal regulations limiting employment of children in agriculture. However, U.S. child labor laws provide less protection for children employed in agriculture than for children employed in other industries, such as a minimum permissible work age of 14 in agriculture compared to 16 in other industries. Children as young as 12 may work in agriculture with the consent of their parents. Work tasks designated as hazardous by the federal government can be performed at age 16 in agriculture but not until age 18 in other industries. Other gains include a California law passed in 2016 requiring overtime pay. Despite these gains, systemic agricultural exceptionalism persists, forcing many agricultural workers to remain below the federal poverty level and to endure poor working conditions.

The Occupational Safety and Health Administration has promulgated few regulations to protect hired agricultural workers. In 1987, OSHA promulgated water and sanitation regulations for agricultural workers, but only after farmworker advocates sued the agency. In addition, Congress specifically prohibits OSHA from using federal funds for enforcement activities on farms employing 10 or fewer workers and those not providing worker housing.[8,9]

The Worker Protection Standard (WPS) is the primary regulatory standard protecting hired agricultural workers from pesticide exposure— one of the few worker protection regulations administered by the Environmental Protection Agency (EPA) and its designated state regulatory agencies. The EPA revised the WPS in 2015 to establish parity in protection from chemicals between agricultural workers and those in other industries. The revised WPS requires yearly pesticide safety training, notification of pesticide applications, use of personal protective equipment, restricted-entry intervals following pesticide application, decontamination supplies, and emergency medical assistance. It also prohibits pesticide application and early re-entry by workers younger than 18 years of age.

State laws also generally treat hired agricultural workers less favorably than other workers. For example, workers' compensation laws in most states exclude hired agricultural workers; only 14 states require employers to provide workers' compensation for agricultural workers to the same extent as other workers. However, all farmworkers with H2-A visas must be provided workers' compensation insurance by their employers.[10,11]

A few states, such as California, Oregon, and Washington, provide agricultural workers with strong regulatory protections and occupational health and safety programs. For example, California and Washington require cholinesterase-monitoring programs for workers applying certain pesticides.

THE FARM WORKPLACE

Farm Equipment

Hazardous farm equipment significantly contributes to agricultural injuries. Sturdily constructed implements and tractors are commonly in service for 30 or more years. Because of poor design or poor maintenance, safety features are frequently inadequate. Hazardous tractors represent a major risk; combined Census of Fatal Occupational Injuries data show that, between 1992 and 2005, there were 2,869 deaths in farm tractor–related incidents. The leading cause of these incidents has been tractor overturn due to a high center of gravity, irregular or steep terrain, and absence of rollover protective structures. Absence of effective shielding on other farm devices places workers at risk of rapid entanglement in conveyors, augers, bailers, and power takeoff drives or tractors, resulting in loss of limbs and often death. (See Chapter 19.)

Noise

There are many sources of loud noise in the farm environment, often related to older equipment and absent mufflers. Hearing loss is frequent in middle-aged and older farmers; audiograms tend to indicate high-frequency hearing loss, suggesting noise as the likely cause. (See Chapter 12A.)

Dust

Dust is ubiquitous in the farm environment, including inorganic dust raised from soil by wind or agricultural activities and, more often, predominantly organic dust, containing a blend of plant components, microbes, insects, mites, animal feed, and mammalian hair, dander, and feces. In a small proportion of workers, sensitization to microbial components in barn dust may cause "farmer's lung," a form of hypersensitivity pneumonitis. Farmers who have daily, unprotected dust exposures may develop asthma or agricultural bronchitis, especially if they are engaged in animal husbandry. Symptoms of bronchitis and minor spirometric abnormalities are more common in farmers working with animals than those working solely in crop production.[12] (See Chapter 22.)

WORK IN CROP PRODUCTION

Production of crops and orchard fruit and some horticultural production place workers at increased risk of musculoskeletal disorders due to mechanical and organizational factors. The frequent heavy lifting, prolonged awkward postures (bending, stooping, squatting, or extensive overhead reaching) and rapid, repetitious movements all represent problems for crop workers. Continued cycles in which considerable force is applied and the work phase exceeds the recovery phase increase the risk of musculoskeletal disorders. Hourly 5-minute pauses in work can reduce the risk of musculoskeletal disorders.[13] Piece-rate compensation of workers (based upon harvest production) increases the pace of work, placing workers at increased risk of strains, sprains, and chronic pain from musculoskeletal disorders. (See Chapter 20.)

Crop workers may experience problems related to extensive contact with plant materials. Tobacco pickers often hold freshly picked moist leaves under their arms as they walk along the row. About one-fourth of these workers will, at some time in a picking season, experience nausea, vomiting, abdominal pain, diarrhea, dizziness, palpitations, and/or headache related to transdermal absorption of nicotine (green tobacco sickness). Other types of contact with plant components or with chemicals on plant leaves may induce contact dermatitis, due to irritation or an allergic response. (See Chapter 25.)

Heat and Solar Radiation

Major concerns are heat-induced illness and solar radiation. Between 1992 and 2006, 68 heat-stroke deaths occurred in crop production workers (an annual average rate of 0.39 per 100,000 crop workers). The combination of high ambient temperature, solar radiation, and intense exertion can create a substantial heat load. The body's main defense is evaporative heat loss, the effectiveness of which depends upon the relative humidity and the worker's ability to produce a substantial amount of sweat. Sweat generation, in turn, depends upon adequate hydration and acclimation, which evolves over days to weeks and results in increased fluid intake, reduced fluid loss in the urine, increased blood volume, and enhanced blood flow to the skin. With acclimation, a heat-stressed worker may generate up to 2 L of sweat per hour. Problems arise when humidity reduces the efficiency of sweat

evaporation; intake of fluids is inadequate; medications, caffeine, or alcohol increase fluid loss; and workers are not sufficiently acclimated to the conditions. Workers experiencing cramping, lightheadedness, and decreased sweating are at increased risk of potentially fatal heat stroke; they must be removed from work to a shaded location, given fluids, and possibly cooled with ice.[14] (See Chapter 12C.)

Ultraviolet (UV) light is another hazard for agricultural workers, especially those spending many hours in fieldwork. Farmers have increased rates of solar-related skin problems, ranging from actinic keratoses to frank malignancies, including cancer of the lip. Ultraviolet light contributes to sunburn and eye irritation commonly experienced by field workers. With prolonged exposure to UV light, dust, and wind, workers may develop conjunctivitis, cataracts, and pterygia (benign growths of the conjunctivae). (See Chapters 12D and 25.)

Farmworkers may also experience other types of ocular problems. Their eyes can be injured by direct contact with plants or tree branches or irritated by the spread of plant materials and chemicals from hands to face and eyes. Many agricultural workers have not had their vision tested. For example, despite a high prevalence of visual-acuity complaints, three-fourths of North Carolina crop workers had not undergone previous vision screening; when examined, they had acuity losses in near vision more commonly than in distance vision, at overall rates similar to the general population.[15] Inability to document and address acuity losses in near vision may place some workers at increased risk of injury from sharp knives and hand tools.[15]

Pesticide Exposure

An estimated 2.1 billion pounds of pesticides are used in the United States each year, mostly in agriculture.[16] In 1996 (the year for which the best estimate is available), an estimated 10,000 to 20,000 occupational pesticide poisonings occurred among agricultural workers. More recent estimates are lower but are based on incomplete data. Between 2007 and 2010, there were 644 cases of acute occupational pesticide poisoning among agricultural workers identified in 11 states by the National Institute for Occupational Safety and Health (NIOSH)-sponsored Sentinel Event Notification System for Occupational Risks, for an estimated incidence rate of 18.4 per 100,000.[17] Thirty states require clinicians to report cases of pesticide overexposure.[11] Most overexposures occur not among those applying pesticides but among workers who are inadvertently exposed to pesticides while performing routine farm tasks, such as harvesting and weeding. These overexposures commonly occur when pesticides being sprayed on one field drift into the breathing zone of farmworkers in nearby fields or when workers handle crops with pesticide residues.[18] Although less than one-third of cases of pesticide poisoning lead to lost time from work, it is difficult to determine whether this reflects the affected workers' need to continue working or the mild severity of most cases—or both, given the economic insecurity of most farmworkers.

Accurate clinical diagnosis of pesticide poisoning is based on medical history, physical findings, and laboratory tests. In mild to moderate pesticide overexposures, a nonspecific clinical presentation is common. Few clinical diagnostic tools are readily available. Cholinesterase activity provides a nonspecific marker of overexposure to organophosphate and carbamate pesticides. California and Washington require biomonitoring of cholinesterase activity for pesticide applicators. These biomonitoring programs have helped to reduce overexposure, leading to removal of workers from excessive pesticide exposure. (See Chapter 11.)

Mental Health

Farmers are at high risk for occupational stress and suicide. The greatest job strain, for all workers, including farm owner/operators and hired workers, results from a combination of high psychological demands (such as having to work intensely and quickly) and limited control over key factors at work.[19] The demands of farming are substantial. Often, a massive amount of work—spring planting, successive hay cutting, or crop harvest—must be completed within a relatively short period. While owner/operators have some control over how they address immediate work demands, they may have no control over variables such as weather, crop prices, costs

of inputs, and availability of labor. Hired workers are impacted by the same time demands of planting and harvesting and have less freedom regarding their work conditions (scheduling, subordinate status, and piece-work pay).

Isolation is a major source of stress, especially with the loss of neighboring farms and social structures that previously provided socialization and support in rural environments. Other sources of stress are financial challenges, generational conflict within families regarding management and inheritance of farms, and the impact of occupational injuries on ability to work.[20] Farmers are culturally disinclined to seek medical help, especially assistance for mental health problems, for which resources may be quite limited.

Suicide occurs at high rates among farmers. In 2012, workers in farming, fishing, and forestry had the highest suicide rate (84.5 per 100,000 overall and 90.5 per 100,000 among males) of any occupational group. (For comparison, the rate for the general population was 16.1 suicide deaths per 100,000.)[21] Adverse neurologic effects of some pesticides might contribute to depressive symptoms. A large study demonstrated an association between depression and a history of pesticide poisoning but not between depression and routine use of pesticides.[22]

Immigrant and migrant agricultural workers face many challenges to their mental health, including adverse effects of stress, anxiety, and depression. But research on their mental health is limited, and available data vary widely. Structural and situational stressors that adversely impact their mental health include prolonged separation from family, social isolation, lack of resources, the physical stress of work, discrimination, lack of permanent employment, overcrowded and poor living conditions, and concerns about immigration status. Inadequate services, poverty, and language and cultural differences exacerbate the mental health challenges that they face.[23,24] (See Chapter 14.)

Sexual Harassment and Violence

Sexual harassment and violence in the workplace are other important concerns for agricultural workers. A study of 150 female immigrant and migrant workers in California found that more than 60% had experienced sexual harassment.[25] A study of 20 female agricultural workers in Washington State found that they frequently experienced sexual harassment in the workplace.[26]

Cancer

Agricultural workers have long been concerned about their possible risks for cancer. The most comprehensive study of this subject is the longitudinal Agricultural Health Study, with almost 80,000 participants, mostly Iowa and North Carolina farmers with pesticide certification and their spouses. Begun in the early 1990s, this study has documented exposure to pesticides, gathered genetic material, and tracked incidence of all malignancies and some other disorders in this population. A 2010 report described follow-up of this cohort through 2006—with almost 1 million person-years and 4,000 incident malignancies.[27] Findings included decreased overall incidence of cancer; increased incidence of cancers of the lip, prostate, and ovary; multiple myeloma and several subtypes of non-Hodgkin lymphoma and leukemia in farmers; and a relative increase in the incidence of lung cancer associated with a few specific pesticides, including chlorpyrifos and diazinon.[28] Among the 30,000 spouses tracked in the study, one-fourth of whom reported personal use of organophosphate insecticides, incidence rates of breast, thyroid, and ovarian cancers were elevated.[29] (See Chapter 21.)

Work with Animals

Each year in the United States an estimated 30 to 40 agricultural workers die from incidents related to cattle or horses.[30,31] From 2008 to 2012, an annual average of 39 workers died while working in dairy cattle and milk production.[31] Immigrants comprise 51% of workers on dairy farms, where work processes often put workers in close contact with cattle weighing 1,500 to 2,000 pounds; most nonfatal work injuries on dairy farms are due to interactions with cattle.[32,33] About 6 injuries per 100 full-time workers in dairy-cattle and milk production occurred in 2012, almost twice the average of other

industries in the United States.[34] Dairy workers are also at high risk for developing zoonoses because of their regular contact with animals and animal waste. (See Chapter 13.) Immigrant diary workers often confront greater risks due to language differences, lack of health and safety training, and vulnerabilities due to their undocumented immigration status.[35]

ACKNOWLEDGMENT

Cases 1 and 2 courtesy of Michael Rowland, MD, MPH, Medical Director, Maine Migrant Health Program.

REFERENCES

1. U.S. Department of Homeland Security. Yearbook of immigration statistics: 2014 temporary admissions. Available at: https://www.dhs.gov/yearbook-immigration-statistics. Accessed October 24, 2016.
2. Leigh JP, Du J, McCurdy SA. An estimate of the U.S. government's undercount of nonfatal occupational injuries and illnesses in agriculture. Annals of Epidemiology 2014; 24: 254–259.
3. Carrol D, Gabbard S, Nakamoto J. A changing crop labor force and the implications for health care. Presented at the National Advisory Council on Migrant Health Meeting in San Jose, CA. January 14, 2016.
4. Martin P, Taylor JE. Ripe with change: Evolving farm labor markets in the United States, Mexico, and Central America. Washington, DC: Migration Policy Institute, 2013.
5. U.S. Department of Labor, Bureau of Labor Statistics. Census of fatal occupational injuries charts, 1992–2014 (revised data). Available at: http://www.bls.gov/iif/oshwc/cfoi/cfch0013.pdf. Accessed October 11, 2016.
6. Arcury TA, Weir M, Chen H, et al. Migrant farmworker housing regulation violations in North Carolina. American Journal of Industrial Medicine 2012; 55: 191–204.
7. U.S. Department of Labor, Bureau of Labor Statistics. National census of fatal occupational injuries in 2015. New Release USDL-16-2304, December 16, 2016, pp 4–5. Available at: https://www.bls.gov/news.release/pdf/cfoi.pdf. Accessed January 16, 2017.
8. Liebman AK, Augustave W. Agricultural health and safety: Incorporating the worker perspective. Journal of Agromedicine 2010; 15: 192–199.

9. Schell G. Farmworker exceptionalism under the law: How the legal system contributes to farmworker poverty and powerlessness. In: Thompson CD, Wiggins MF, eds. The human cost of food. Austin: University of Texas Press, 2002, pp. 139–166.

10. Liebman AK, Wiggins MF, Fraser C, et al. Occupational health policy and immigrant workers in the agriculture, forestry, and fishing sector. American Journal of Industrial Medicine 2013; 56: 975–984.

11. Migrant Clinicians Network and Farmworker Justice. Pesticide reporting and workers' compensation in agriculture—Interactive map. Austin, TX: Migrant Clinicians Network. Available at: http://www.migrantclinician.org/issues/occupational-health/pesticides/reporting-illnesses.html. Accessed October 24, 2016.

12. Iversen M, Pedersen B. Relation between respiratory symptoms, type of farming, and lung function disorders in farmers. Thorax 1990; 45: 919–923.

13. Faucett J, Meyers J, Miles J, et al. Rest break interventions in stoop labor tasks. Applied Ergonomic 2007; 38: 219–226.

14. Arbury S, Jacklitsch B, Farquah O, et al. Heat illness and death among workers—United States, 2012–2013. Morbidity and Mortality Weekly Report 2014; 63: 661–665.

15. Quandt SA, Schulz MR, Chen H, Arcury TA. Visual acuity and self-reported visual function among migrant farmworkers. Optometry and Vision Science 2016; 93: 1189–1195.

16. Grube A, Donaldson D, Kiely T, Wu L. Pesticides industry sales and usage: 2006 and 2007 market estimates. Washington, DC: U.S. Environmental Protection Agency, 2011. Available at: http://www.panna.org/sites/default/files/EPA%20market_estimates2007.pdf. Accessed October 24, 2016.

17. Calvert GM, Beckman J, Prado JB, et al. Summary of notifiable noninfectious conditions and disease outbreaks: Acute occupational pesticide-related illness and injury—United States, 2007–2010. Morbidity and Mortality Weekly Report 2015; 62: 5–10.

18. Reeves M, Katten A, Guzman M. Fields of poison 2002: California farmworkers and pesticides. A report by Californians for Pesticide Reform. 2002. Available at: http://www.ufw.org/white_papers/report.pdf. Accessed October 24, 2016.

19. Karasek RA, Theorell T. Healthy work: Stress, productivity and the reconstruction of working life. New York: Basic Books, 1990.

20. May J. Clinically significant occupational stressors in New York farmers and farm families. Journal of Agricultural Safety and Health 1998; 4: 9–14.

21. McIntosh WL, Spies E, Stone DM, et al. Suicide rates by occupational group—17 states, 2012. Morbidity and Mortality Weekly Report 2016; 65: 641–645.

22. Beseler CL, Stallones L, Hoppin JA, et al. Depression and pesticide exposures among private pesticide applicators enrolled in the Agricultural Health Study. Environmental Health Perspectives 2008; 116: 1713–1719.

23. Winkelman SB, Chaney EH, Bethel JW. Stress, depression and coping among Latino migrant and seasonal farmworkers. International Journal of Environmental Research and Public Health 2013; 10: 1815–1830.

24. Grzywacz JG, Quandt SA, Chen H, et al. Depressive symptoms among Latino farmworkers across the agricultural season: Structural and situational influences. Cultural Diversity & Ethnic Minority Psychology 2010; 16: 335–343.

25. Waugh IM. Examining the sexual harassment experiences of Mexican immigrant farmworking women. Violence Against Women 2010; 16: 237–261.

26. Kim NJ, Vásquez VB, Torres E, et al. Breaking the silence: Sexual harassment of Mexican women farmworkers. Journal of Agromedicine 2016; 21: 154–162.

27. Koutros S, Alavanja MC, Lubin JH, et al. An update of cancer incidence in the Agricultural Health Study. Journal of Occupational and Environmental Medicine 2010; 52: 1098–1105.

28. Alavanja MC, Dosemeci M, Samanic C, et al. Pesticides and lung cancer risk in the Agricultural Health Study cohort. American Journal of Epidemiology 2004; 160: 876–885.

29. Lerro CC, Koutros S, Andreotti G, et al. Organophosphate insecticide use and cancer incidence among spouses of pesticide applicators in the Agricultural Health Study. Occupational and Environmental Medicine 2015; 72: 736–744.

30. Langley RL, Morrow WE. Livestock handling—Minimizing worker injuries. Journal of Agromedicine 2010; 15: 226–235.

31. U.S. Department of Labor, Bureau of Labor Statistics. Census of Fatal Occupational Injuries (CFPI)—Current and revised data. September 11, 2014. Retrieved from: http://www.bls.gov/iif/oshwc/cfoi/cftb0277.pdf Accessed October 17, 2016.

32. McCurdy SA, Carroll DJ. Agricultural injury. American Journal of Industrial Medicine 2000; 38: 463–480.

33. Román-Muñiz IN, Van Metre DC, Garry FB, et al. Training methods and association with worker injury on Colorado dairies: A survey. Journal of Agromedicine 2006; 11: 19–26.

34. U.S. Department of Labor, Bureau of Labor Statistics. Occupational injuries/illnesses and fatal injuries profiles [query with NAICS code 11212]. Department of Labor. Available at: http://www.bls.gov/data/#injuries. Accessed October 17, 2016.

35. Liebman AK, Juarez-Carrillo PM, Reyes IA, Keifer MC. Immigrant dairy workers' perceptions of health and safety on the farm in America's Heartland. American Journal of Industrial Medicine 2016; 59: 227–235.

ADDITIONAL RESOURCE

The Centers for Agricultural Disease and Injury Research, Education, and Prevention represent a major effort by NIOSH to protect the health and safety of agricultural workers and their families. These centers were established as part of a Centers for Disease Control and Prevention/ NIOSH Agricultural Health and Safety Initiative in 1990. The centers were established by cooperative agreement to conduct research, education, and prevention projects to address pressing agricultural health and safety problems in the United States. The centers are distributed geographically throughout the United States to be responsive to the agricultural health and safety issues unique to different regions of the country. More information is available at: https://www. cdc.gov/niosh/oep/agctrhom.html.

32B

Hazards for Construction Workers

Gavin H. West and Laura S. Welch

Construction workers build, repair, renovate, modify, and demolish structures—including houses, office buildings, places of worship, factories, hospitals, roads, bridges, tunnels, stadiums, docks, and airports. To understand injury and illness risks in construction work, one must understand the diverse tasks performed by workers in numerous construction trades (Table 32B-1).

Construction often must be done in extreme heat or cold, at night, and in windy, rainy, snowy, or foggy weather. Heat exposure can cause serious adverse health effects, including death. With growing concerns over climate change, the risk of heat-related illness is expected to increase (Chapter 28). Intermittent and seasonal work adds to health and safety risks and to the stress of job insecurity. Episodic employment, frequent change of employer, and continuous change in worksite exposures and ambient conditions make it difficult to document workers' jobs and hazardous exposures. For these reasons, there are only limited data on the nature and magnitude of hazardous exposures in the construction industry.

In developed countries, construction is consistently ranked among the most dangerous occupations. In 2014, 19% of all fatal on-the-job injuries in the United States occurred in construction, although construction accounted for only 5% of total employment.[1-2] Falls are the leading cause of fatal work-related injuries in the industry, accounting for roughly one-third of these deaths and thousands of serious injuries each year. The persistence of these injuries prompted the launch in 2012 of an ongoing national fall prevention campaign, which encourages construction employers (especially residential contractors who have a high risk of falls) to plan ahead to get the job done safely, provide the appropriate equipment, and train everyone to use the equipment correctly.

For nonfatal injuries, the Bureau of Labor Statistics (BLS) reported, in 2015, a rate of 134.8 lost-workday cases per 10,000 full-time-equivalent construction workers, substantially higher than the overall rate of 93.9 for all private-sector industries. Leading causes of injuries with lost workdays (days away from work) among construction workers were overexertion (34%), contact with objects (33%), and falls (24%). Leading specific diagnoses were strains and sprains (34%), fractures (12%), cuts and lacerations (9%), and soreness and pain, excluding back pain (6%).[3]

Table 32B-1. Construction Occupations and Tasks

Boilermakers	Construct, assemble, maintain, and repair stationary steam boilers and boiler house auxiliaries. Work involves use of hand and power tools, plumb bobs, levels, wedges, dogs, or turnbuckles. Assist in testing assembled vessels. Direct cleaning of boilers and boiler furnaces. Inspect and repair boiler fittings, such as safety valves, regulators, automatic-control mechanisms, water columns, and auxiliary machines
Brick masons	Lay and bind building materials, such as brick, structural tile, concrete block, cinder block, glass block, and terracotta block, with mortar and other substances to construct or repair walls, partitions, arches, sewers, and other structures
Carpenters	Construct, erect, install, or repair structures and fixtures made of wood, such as concrete forms; build frameworks, including partitions, joists, studding, and rafters; wood stairways, window and door frames, and hardwood floors. May also install cabinets, siding, drywall and batt or roll insulation
Carpet installers	Lay and install carpet from rolls or blocks on floors. Install padding and trim flooring materials
Cement masons and concrete finishers	Smooth and finish surfaces of poured concrete, such as floors, walks, sidewalks, roads, or curbs using a variety of hand and power tools. Align forms for sidewalks, curbs, or gutters; patch voids; use saws to cut expansion joints
Construction laborers	Perform tasks involving physical labor at building, highway, and heavy construction projects, tunnel and shaft excavations, and demolition sites. May operate hand and power tools of all types: air hammers, earth tampers, cement mixers, small mechanical hoists, surveying and measuring equipment, and a variety of other equipment and instruments. May clean and prepare sites, dig trenches, set braces to support the sides of excavations, erect scaffolding, clean up rubble and debris, and remove asbestos, lead, and other hazardous waste materials
Drywall and ceiling tile installers	Apply plasterboard or other wallboard to ceilings or interior walls of buildings. Apply or mount acoustical tiles or blocks, strips, or sheets of shock-absorbing materials to ceilings and walls of buildings to reduce or reflect sound. Materials may be of decorative quality. Include lathers who fasten wooden, metal, or rockboard lath to walls, ceilings, or partitions of buildings to provide support base for plaster, fire-proofing, or acoustical material
Electricians	Install, maintain, and repair electrical wiring, equipment, and fixtures. Ensure that work is in accordance with relevant codes. May install or service street lights, intercom systems, or electrical control systems
Insulation workers	Apply insulating materials to pipes or ductwork or other mechanical systems to help control and maintain temperature. Also line and cover structures with insulating materials. May work with batt, roll, or blown insulation materials
Operating engineers	Operate one or several types of power construction equipment, such as motor graders, bulldozers, scrapers, compressors, pumps, derricks, shovels, tractors, or front-end loaders to excavate, move, and grade earth, erect structures, or pour concrete or other hard surface pavement. May repair and maintain equipment in addition to other duties
Painters	Paint walls, equipment, buildings, bridges, and other structural surfaces, using brushes, rollers, and spray guns. May remove old paint to prepare surface prior to painting. May mix colors or oils to obtain desired color or consistency
Paperhangers	Cover interior walls and ceilings of rooms with decorative wallpaper or fabric, or attach advertising posters on surfaces, such as walls and billboards. Duties include removing old materials from surface to be papered
Plumbers, pipefitters, and steamfitters	Assemble, install, alter, and repair pipelines or pipe systems that carry water, steam, air, or other liquids or gases. May install heating and cooling equipment and mechanical control systems
Plasterers and stucco masons	Apply interior or exterior plaster, cement, stucco, or similar materials. May also set ornamental plaster
Reinforcing iron and rebar workers	Position and secure steel bars or mesh in concrete forms to reinforce concrete. Use a variety of fasteners, rod-bending machines, blowtorches, and hand tools. Includes rod busters
Roofers	Cover roofs of structures with shingles, slate, asphalt, aluminum, wood, and related materials. May spray roofs, sidings, and walls with material to bind, seal, insulate, or soundproof sections of structures

(continued)

Table 32B-1. (Continued)

Sheetmetal workers	Fabricate, assemble, install, and repair sheetmetal products and equipment, such as ducts, control boxes, drainpipes, and furnace casings. Work may involve any of the following: setting up and operating fabricating machines to cut, bend, and straighten sheetmetal; shaping metal over anvils, blocks, or forms using hammer; operating soldering and welding equipment to join sheetmetal parts; inspecting, assembling, and smoothing seams and joints of burred surfaces. Includes sheetmetal duct installers who install prefabricated sheetmetal ducts used for heating, air conditioning, or other purposes
Stonemasons	Build stone structures, such as piers, walls, and abutments. Lay walks, curbstones, or special types of masonry for vats, tanks, and floors
Structural iron and steel workers	Raise, place, and unite iron or steel girders, columns, and other structural members to form completed structures or structural frameworks. May erect metal storage tanks and assemble prefabricated metal buildings
Terrazzo workers and finishers	Apply a mixture of cement, sand, pigment, or marble chips to floors, stairways, and cabinet fixtures to fashion durable and decorative surfaces
Tile and marble setters	Apply hard tile, marble, and wood tile to walls, floors, ceilings, and roof decks

Source: Bureau of Labor Statistics. Standard occupational classification manual, 1998 revision. Available at: http://stats.bls.gov/soc/socguide.htm.

Construction injuries comprise a disproportionate share of the total costs of occupational injuries in all industries in the United States—almost $13 billion annually. Fatal injuries account for 40% of this cost; nonfatal injuries and illnesses (mainly injuries with lost workdays) account for the rest. On average, the death of a construction worker results in losses of $4 million, and a nonfatal injury with lost workdays costs approximately $42,000. These estimates include (a) direct costs, such as payments for hospitals, physicians, and medicines; (b) indirect costs, such as wage losses, household production losses, and costs of administering workers' compensation; and (c) quality-of-life costs—that is, the value attributed to the pain and suffering that victims and their families experience as a result of injuries or illnesses.[4]

Employers in construction spend more on workers' compensation than employers in any other industry. In 2010 (the most recent year for which data are available), of all employer costs in construction, 4% were spent on workers' compensation—more than double the costs for manufacturing employers and almost three times the average cost for employers in all industries. Other data show that workers' compensation insurance premiums for some occupations are much higher than this average. For example, the median insurance premium rate for roofing in 2011 was $25 for each $100 of payroll.[3] Nevertheless, only 46% of all medical expenses for work-related injuries were paid by workers' compensation—and

only 27% among injured Hispanic construction workers. The remaining amount was paid by workers and their families or by other public or private sources, subsidizing workers' compensation medical coverage in the construction industry by at least $734 million annually.[4-5]

Occupational diseases are also an important cause of morbidity in construction workers. Table 32B-2 summarizes diseases that are sentinel health events that may occur in construction workers and specific hazardous exposures that can lead to these diseases. These sentinel health events help to focus attention on intervention and prevention measures. These hazardous exposures include air contaminants, such as wood dust, abrasive blasting dust, gypsum and alkaline dusts, silica, asbestos, lead, diesel exhaust, and welding fumes.

LEAD AND OTHER HEAVY METALS

Lead exposure and resultant toxicity are especially important problems in the construction industry. (See Chapters 11, 23, 24, and 28.) Excessive lead exposure is associated with several construction tasks, and an estimated 1 million construction workers in the United States are occupationally exposed to lead.[6] More than 80% of these workers are involved in commercial or residential remodeling. Before 1993, the Occupational Safety and Health Administration

Table 32B-2. Sentinel Health Events in Construction

Sentinel Health Event	Industry/Process/Occupation	Agent
Asbestosis	Asbestos industries and utilizers	Asbestos
Bronchitis (acute), pneumonitis, and pulmonary edema due to fumes and vapors	Arc welders, boilermakers	Nitrogen oxides Vanadium pentoxide
Chronic or acute renal failure	Plumbers	Inorganic lead
Contact dermatitis	Cement masons and finishers, carpenters, floor layers	Adhesives and sealants; irritants (such as cutting oils, phenol, solvents, acids, alkalis, detergents); allergens (such as nickel, chromates, formaldehyde, dyes, rubber products)
Extrinsic asthma	Woodworkers, furniture makers	Red cedar (plicatic acid) and other wood dusts
Histoplasmosis	Bridge maintenance workers	*Histoplasma capsulatam*
Inflammatory and toxic neuropathy	Furniture refinishers, degreasing operations	Hexane
Malignant neoplasm of scrotum	Chimney sweeps	Mineral oil, pitch, tar
Malignant neoplasm of nasal cavities	Woodworkers, cabinet and furniture makers, carpenters	Hardwood and softwood dusts Chlorophenols
Malignant neoplasm of trachea, bronchus, and lung	Asbestos industries and utilizers	Asbestos
Malignant neoplasm of nasopharynx	Carpenter, cabinet maker	Chlorophenols
Malignant neoplasm of larynx	Asbestos industries and utilizers	Asbestos
Mesothelioma (malignancy of peritoneum and pleura)	Asbestos industries and utilizers	Asbestos
Noise effects on inner ear	Occupations with exposure to excessive noise	Excessive noise
Raynaud phenomenon (secondary)	Jackhammer operator, riveter	Whole-body or segmental vibration
Sequoiosis	Red cedar mill workers, woodworkers	Redwood sawdust
Silicosis	Sandblasters	Silica
Silicotuberculosis	Sandblasters	Silica + *Mycobacterium tuberculosis*
Toxic encephalitis	Lead paint removal	Lead
Toxic hepatitis	Fumigators	Methyl bromide

Source: Adapted from Mullan R, Murthy L: Occupational sentinel health events: An updated list for physician recognition and public health surveillance. American Journal of Industrial Medicine 1991; 19: 775–799. Reprinted with permission from: Sullivan P, Moon Bank K, Hearl F, Wagner G. Respiratory risk in the construction industry. In: Ringen K, Englund A, Welch LS, et al. (eds.). Health and safety in construction. State of the Art Reviews in Occupational Medicine 1995; 10: 269–284.

(OSHA) lead standard applied only to general industry, not to construction. In 1992, blood lead levels (BLLs) in bridge construction workers ranged from 51 to 160 µg/dL, with 62% of elevated BLLs involving work in a containment structure. High-risk activities associated with lead dust and fumes among bridge and structural steelworkers include abrasive blasting, sanding, burning, cutting, and welding on steel structures coated with lead paint, while working in containment enclosures. In 1993, the OSHA lead standard was reversed, incorporating a presumption of exposure during specific high-risk tasks and requiring specific protections during these tasks—unless air monitoring demonstrates airborne lead exposure at a concentration below the permissible exposure limit (PEL). However, it is important to recognize that even the revised OSHA standard may not fully protect construction workers from lead toxicity. The standard requires monitoring every 2 months, but some tasks, such as burning lead-coated steel, can cause a rapid increase in BLL. Thus, more frequent monitoring and a lower threshold for mandated industrial hygiene inspection or medical removal of workers has been recommended in some circumstances.

Elevated BLLs are reported by 32 states to the national Adult Blood Lead Epidemiology and Surveillance (ABLES) program. In 2010, the construction industry accounted for 16% of the workers with BLLs at or above 25 µg/dL, while construction employment accounted for only about 7% of the total U.S. workforce. Among the top five construction subsectors with the most reported cases of BLLs above 25 and 40 µg/dL in this period were building finishing; highway, street, and bridge work; and other specialty trades. These minimal estimates indicated significant lead exposure occurring in the construction industry.

Construction workers can be exposed to manganese and chromium during welding; pipefitters, ironworkers, boilermakers, and sheet-metal workers routinely perform welding and related processes, such as arc cutting. This work often occurs in tanks, boilers, or other poorly ventilated settings. Fumes generated during welding contain fine and ultrafine particles from the base metal, the electrodes, fluxes, and the filler rods. In the United States, there are an estimated 398,000 full-time welders and more than 1 million intermittent welders who are exposed to welding fumes. The International Agency for Research on Cancer has determined that welding fumes cause cancer. Welders of stainless steel have higher rates of lung cancer than workers who weld using other metals.

Manganese, a known neurotoxin, is a component of nearly all types of steel and many welding rods and wires. Excessive exposure to manganese in other industries, such as manganese mining and smelting, causes symptoms and signs closely resembling those of Parkinson disease. Recent studies of welders suggest the level of manganese exposure in welding fumes can also cause these symptoms and signs.

Metal fumes from stainless steel welding contain hexavalent chromium and nickel, both of which cause lung cancer. The Occupational Safety and Health Administration estimates almost 200,000 construction workers in the United States are exposed to airborne hexavalent chromium and that a substantial proportion of these workers are exposed above the OSHA PEL.

NOISE

Occupational hearing loss frequently occurs in U.S. workers. Construction workers have a high risk of hearing loss due to excessively loud work environments. Chronic exposure to noise is the most common cause of work-related hearing loss, although it can also be caused by ototoxic chemicals or a single instantaneous high-noise exposure. (See Chapter 12A.)

From 1981 to 2010, the prevalence of hearing loss in the construction industry remained relatively stable, with 5-year prevalence estimates ranging from 21% to 28%.[7] Although the incidence of hearing loss trended downward for most U.S. industries during this time period, incidence in the construction industry increased in the early 2000s after having steadily declined from 1981 to 2000. The most recent estimates indicate a lower prevalence of hearing impairment among construction workers (16%), which may reflect improved preventive measures; however, hearing loss still results in 3.09 healthy years lost for every 1,000 construction workers, and 3% have moderate or severe impairment.[8] A person with moderate hearing impairment cannot hear and understand someone in a noisy place, such as a city street; has difficulty hearing people in a quiet place; and may also experience tinnitus. Tinnitus can also occur with mild hearing impairment, although not always.

Hearing loss can increase the risk of occupational injury. For example, a construction worker may not be able to hear oncoming vehicles or warning signals. In addition, hearing loss can impact both productivity and morale. U.S. businesses spend an estimated $242 million on workers' compensation for hearing loss annually.

U.S. regulations require a hearing conservation program for construction workers exposed to noise above the PEL of 90 dBA as an 8-hour time-weighted average (TWA). When exposures cannot be reduced below the PEL, hearing protection devices are required. The noise standard for general industry is stricter than that for construction: A hearing conservation program with specific components is required when the TWA exceeds 85 dBA. These requirements, which are not in the construction standard, include audiometric testing of workers, noise monitoring in the workplace, personal protective equipment, training, and recordkeeping.

When exposed to average daily noise levels at the current PEL of 90 dBA, approximately 25% of construction workers are expected to develop hearing impairment over a 40-year career.[9] On average, construction workers are exposed to noise levels above the general industry PEL for 73% of their work shifts; ironworkers, carpenters, and operating engineers are exposed above the PEL for a higher percentage of their work shifts.[10]

In some other countries, there is less noise exposure in the construction industry, compared with this industry in the United States. For example, since British Columbia implemented a hearing conservation program in construction, reported use of hearing protection by workers increased from 55% to 85%, and the proportion of 50- to 59-year-old construction workers with hearing impairment decreased from 36% to 25%. The National Institute for Occupational Safety and Health (NIOSH) has sponsored the Buy Quiet initiative, which encourages and facilitates contractors to purchase or rent tools and machinery that are less noisy. A demand for quieter products will likely motivate manufacturers to design quieter equipment.

MUSCULOSKELETAL DISORDERS

Soft-tissue musculoskeletal disorders (MSDs) make up a high proportion of all work-related injuries in construction (see Figure 32B-1). In 2010 in the United States, there were an estimated 74,950 injuries with lost workdays in construction; 34% of these injuries were attributable to strains and sprains. The rates for these injuries are considerably higher in construction than in all private industry combined.[3] Most lost-time MSDs in construction affect the back, and most are caused by overexertion. Other risk factors for MSDs include bending, twisting, and repetitive motion. Concrete and masonry contractors have an especially high risk for MSDs due to the type of work they perform. A brick mason handling an average of 200 masonry blocks per day, each weighing 38 pounds, would lift a combined weight of more than five pick-up trucks over the course of a week. (See Chapter 20.)

Musculoskeletal disorders are more serious for older workers. On average, construction workers

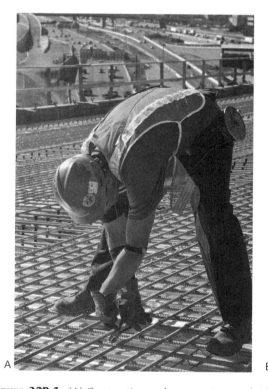
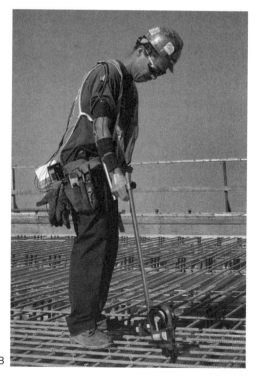

Figure 32B-1. (A) Construction workers are at increased risk of upper-extremity and back strain. (B) An ergonomically designed device decreases upper-extremity and back strain on construction workers who are tying rebar. (Photographs by Earl Dotter.)

retire 2 years earlier than other workers, often because of musculoskeletal conditions, such as arthritis and degenerative disc disease. Among sheetmetal workers, MSDs account for almost half of long-term work disability pensions, compared to less than 30% among the general working population.[11] Musculoskeletal disorders account for substantial medical expenses and impact quality of life after retirement. A cross-sectional study found that approximately 20% of male construction retirees reported having severe pain, compared to 3% of male nonconstruction retirees.[12] Controlling for other factors, longer job tenure and physically demanding jobs in construction are associated with increased risk of back disorders.[13]

Reducing the physical demands on construction workers will require changing the culture of construction, developing new task-specific ergonomic innovations, and promoting participatory ergonomics programs. The construction work environment changes as a project progresses. Both this dynamic nature of the construction process and the project-by-project nature of employment limits employers' incentives to prevent chronic MSDs. Effective interventions to reduce physical demands in construction include decreasing back stress in masons through adjusting work height, eliminating shoulder and neck strain during overhead drilling tasks with a drill support, and various approaches to reduce manual materials handling. Interventions that are more likely to succeed have a perceived relative advantage, are compatible with prevailing norms or practices, can be tried before being fully implemented, and have impacts that are readily observable.[14] (See Chapter 9.)

RESPIRATORY DISEASES

Construction workers are exposed to many respiratory hazards, including asbestos, crystalline silica, synthetic vitreous fibers, cadmium, chromates, formaldehyde, resin adhesives, cobalt, metal fumes, creosote, gasoline, oils, diesel fumes, paint fumes and dusts, pitch, sealers, solvents, wood dusts and wood preservatives, and extremes of temperature.[15] In 2014, the BLS reported 400 nonfatal work-related respiratory conditions among 9.8 million wage-and-salary construction workers in the United States—thought to

be a major underestimate. For comparison, the National Center for Health Statistics reported that, in 2004, approximately 21,000 people were hospitalized with asbestosis. (See Chapter 22.)

Asbestosis

Asbestos has been recognized as a respiratory hazard for several construction trades. Many construction workers are occupationally exposed to asbestos, especially insulators, plumbers and pipefitters, electricians, and sheetmetal workers. Any construction worker may be at risk for asbestos-induced disease from working near asbestos insulation. Although asbestos is no longer used in new residential or heavy construction, workers may continue to be exposed to previously installed asbestos during maintenance, renovation, addition, or demolition activities.

Silicosis

Occupational exposure to silica can occur among various types of construction workers, including those employed in concrete removal and demolition work, bridge and road construction, tunnel construction, and concrete or granite cutting, sanding, and grinding. Sandblasters are at increased risk from exposure to crystalline silica. Those working nearby on the same construction site may also be at risk from silica-related disease. In the United States, sand containing crystalline silica is still used in abrasive blasting operations for maintenance of structures, preparing surfaces for painting, and forming decorative patterns during installation of building materials; these uses of sand have been banned in many other countries. Silica exposures in the construction industry in the United States continue to exceed recommended limits, and silicosis continues to occur in construction workers worldwide. In addition, silica is a cause of chronic obstructive pulmonary disease (COPD), independent of the presence of radiological evidence of silicosis.

A major step toward the prevention of silica-related disease was the promulgation of a revised OSHA silica standard in 2016, which set forth a new PEL of 50 µg/m³ as an 8-hour TWA for general industry, maritime, and construction. This PEL is about half the prior PEL for general industry and one-fifth the prior PEL for construction. The new standard requires medical monitoring of highly exposed workers and sets forth requirements for reducing exposure.

Chronic Obstructive Pulmonary Disease and Asthma

Among construction workers, occupational exposures account for about 18% to 24% of COPD risk overall and 32% to 53% of COPD risk among workers without a history of smoking.[16,17] Exposure to vapors, gases, dusts, and fumes (VGDF), which occurs frequently in construction, is a strong predictor of COPD. Within exposures to VGDF, exposures to asbestos, welding fumes, silica, cement dust, engine exhausts, acids/caustics, metal cutting and grinding aerosols, isocyanates, organic solvents, wood dust, and molds or spores have all been associated with an increased risk of COPD. Asthma can be exacerbated among construction workers who are exposed to allergens, cold temperatures, particulates, dusts, fumes, or irritants.

DERMATITIS

Construction workers are exposed to many chemicals that cause irritant or allergic dermatitis. Portland cement, which is found in plaster and concrete mixes, is extremely alkaline. Wet plaster also contains slaked lime (calcium hydroxide), which is even more caustic. In addition, Portland cement contains trace amounts of hexavalent chromium, a strong sensitizing agent that causes allergic contact dermatitis in cement workers. Other sensitizing agents include epoxy adhesives, sealants, and chemicals mixed within cement and plaster. Rubber gloves also may cause allergic dermatitis. A free web resource (www.choosehandsafety.org) is available that offers guidance for construction workers to choose appropriate hand tools and gloves for working safely. Glove selection is based on the task to be performed, chemicals to be encountered, and the performance and characteristics of the glove itself. (See Chapter 25.)

For 2014, the BLS reported that skin diseases or disorders accounted for 24% of all occupational illnesses among construction workers. Experts have estimated that the actual number of occupational skin disorders is 10 to 50 times

Table 32B-3. Epidemiology of Lung Cancer in Construction Workers

Trade	Known Lung Carcinogens
Insulators	Asbestos
Painters and plasterers	Hexavalent chromium, cadmium, asbestos
Sheetmetal workers	Asbestos, welding fume
Welders	Welding fume, asbestos, hexavalent chromium
Masons	Asbestos, hexavalent chromium, silica
Electricians	Asbestos
Plumbers and pipefitters	Asbestos, welding fume
Roofers	Coal tar, bitumen, polycyclic aromatic hydrocarbons
Carpenters	Wood dust

higher than prior numbers reported by the BLS. One way to prevent allergic contact dermatitis in cement workers is to add ferrous sulfate to hexavalent chromium in cement, a process that forms, when water is added, an insoluble trivalent chromium compound that is not easily absorbed by the skin.

CANCER

Construction workers are exposed to many carcinogens (Table 32B-3). Insulators, painters and plasterers, sheet-metal workers, and other construction workers are at increased risk of lung cancer. Woodworkers, cabinetmakers, furniture makers, and carpenters and joiners have an increased risk of nasal cancer. Workers in many trades have had increased rates of mesothelioma after widespread exposure to asbestos from approximately 1940 to 1980. Given the long latency period for mesothelioma, asbestos-related cases are likely to occur for many years to come. (See Chapter 21.)

POTENTIAL HAZARDS OF NANOMATERIALS

The use of nanomaterials in the construction industry poses a variety of hazards. (See Chapter 8 for a discussion of nanomaterials and nanotechnology.)

In construction, engineered nanomaterials (those that are designed for a specific function or purpose) are being used in numerous materials and applications, including high-strength cement, scratch-resistant and self-cleaning coatings, and highly insulating materials. Based on available research, NIOSH has established recommended exposure limits for nanoscale titanium dioxide and carbon nanotubes or nanofibers, reflecting size-dependent health concerns.[18,19]

Engineered nanomaterials can be incorporated into solid materials, such as wood or cement, and also liquid materials, such as paints and coatings. Construction workers could potentially be exposed to engineered nanomaterials during installation, maintenance, renovation, and demolition activities. Additional research is needed to better characterize exposures to engineered nanomaterials in mixed aerosols among construction workers and to determine whether these exposures can induce adverse health effects. Research has demonstrated that engineering controls and respirators can effectively reduce exposure to engineered nanomaterials; doing so proactively may be prudent to protect the health of construction workers.

REGULATIONS AND HEALTH SERVICES FOR CONSTRUCTION WORKERS

Construction workers are often not covered by the OSHA regulations that cover most other workers. For example, the standard for noise exposure for the construction industry has no action level above which a hearing conservation program is required and no detailed requirements for training or recordkeeping. The rationale for separate OSHA standards for construction is that controls that work in general industry may not work in construction. Therefore, feasibility of a standard must be demonstrated specifically in construction before the standard can be applied to the construction sector. Although this is a reasonable consideration, leaving construction out of a standard until feasibility is demonstrated has led to decades of hazardous exposure for construction workers. Underreporting of injury and illness is prevalent in construction, in part because the construction industry is comprised mainly of small employers. A legal requirement

to report injuries by construction project, which could apply to many small employers, could help to better elucidate and focus more attention on the health and safety problems faced by construction workers.

In the United States, intermittent employment and the high cost of health insurance can leave construction workers and their families without insurance coverage for medical care. In 2010, 32% of construction workers had no health insurance, compared to 17% of all workers in the United States.[3] Because construction is a complex industry, there are proportionately fewer research and prevention activities in construction than in general industry. All of these factors leave the construction industry in great need for improvement in health and safety.

REFERENCES

1. Bureau of Labor Statistics. Census of Fatal Occupational Injuries (CFOI)—Current and revised data 2014. Washington, DC: BLS, 2016. Available at: http://www.bls.gov/iif/oshcfoi1.htm. Accessed September 12, 2016.
2. Bureau of Labor Statistics. Labor Force Statistics from the Current Population Survey: 2014 Annual Averages. Washington, DC: BLS, 2016. Available at: http://www.bls.gov/cps/cps_aa2014.htm. Accessed September 12, 2016.
3. Center for Construction Research and Training. The construction chart book: The US construction industry and its workers (5th ed.). Silver Spring, MD: CPWR, 2013. Available at: http://www.cpwr.com/rp-chartbook.html.
4. Center for Construction Research and Training. The construction chart book: The US construction industry and its workers (4th ed.). Silver Spring, MD: CPWR, 2007. Available at: http://www.cpwr.com/rp-chartbook.html.
5. Dong X, Ringen K, Men Y, Fujimoto A. Medical costs and sources of payment for work-related injuries among Hispanic construction workers. Journal of Occupational and Environmental Medicine 2007; 49: 1367–1375.
6. Levin SM, Goldberg M. Clinical evaluation and management of lead-exposed construction workers. American Journal of Industrial Medicine 2000; 37: 23–43.
7. Masterson EA, Deddens JA, Themann CL, et al. Trends in worker hearing loss by industry sector, 1981–2010. American Journal of Industrial Medicine 2015; 58: 392–401.

8. Masterson EA, Bushnell PT, Themann CL, Morata TC. Hearing impairment among noise-exposed workers—United States, 2003–2012. Morbidity and Mortality Weekly Report 2016; 65: 389–394.

9. National Institute for Occupational Safety and Health. Criteria for a recommended standard: Occupational noise exposure revised criteria. DHHS (NIOSH) Publication No. 98-126. Cincinnati, OH: NIOSH, June 1998.

10. Neitzel RL, Stover B, Seixas NS. Longitudinal assessment of noise exposure in a cohort of construction workers. Annals of Occupational Hygiene 2011; 55: 906–916.

11. West GH, Dawson J, Teitelbaum C, et al. An analysis of permanent work disability among construction sheet metal workers. American Journal of Industrial Medicine 2016; 59: 186–195.

12. LeMasters G, Bhattacharya A, Borton E, Mayfield L. Functional impairment and quality of life in retired workers of the construction trades. Experimental Aging Research 2006; 32: 227–242.

13. Dong XS, Wang X, Fujimoto A, Dobbin R. Chronic back pain among older construction workers in the United States: A longitudinal study. International Journal of Occupational and Environmental Health 2012; 18: 99–109.

14. Weinstein MG, Hecker SF, Hess JA, Kincl L. A roadmap to diffuse ergonomic innovations in the construction industry: There is nothing so practical as a good theory. International Journal of Occupational and Environmental Health 2007; 13: 46–55.

15. Sullivan PA, Bang KM, Hearl FK, Wagner GR. Respiratory disease risks in the construction industry. In: Ringen K, Englund A, Welch LS, et al. (eds.). Health and safety in construction. State of the Art Reviews in Occupational Medicine 1995; 10: 313–334.

16. Dement J, Welch L, Ringen K, et al. A case-control study of airways obstruction among construction workers. American Journal of Industrial Medicine 2015; 58: 1083–1097.

17. Toren K, Jarvholm B. Effect of occupational exposure to vapors, gases, dusts, and fumes on COPD mortality risk among Swedish construction workers: A longitudinal cohort study. Chest 2014; 145: 992–997.

18. National Institute for Occupational Safety and Health. Current Intelligence Bulletin 63: Occupational exposure to titanium dioxide. DHHS (NIOSH) Publication No. 2011–160. Cincinnati, OH: NIOSH, April 2011.

19. National Institute for Occupational Safety and Health. Current Intelligence Bulletin 65: Occupational exposure to carbon nanotubes and nanofibers. DHHS (NIOSH) Publication No. 2013-145. Cincinnati, OH: NIOSH, April 2013.

FURTHER READING

Center for Construction Research and Training. The construction chart book: The US construction industry and its workers (5th ed.). Silver Spring, MD: CPWR, 2013. Available at: http://www.cpwr.com/rp-chartbook.html.

An excellent compendium of statistics related to the safety and health of construction workers.

National Institute for Occupational Safety and Health website. Available at: http://www.cdc.gov/niosh/homepage.html.

The NIOSH website has a special section for construction workers. There is an electronic database of available materials that is periodically updated: the Electronic Library of Construction Safety and Health at http://www.cdc.gov/niosh/elcosh.html.

32C

Hazards for Healthcare Workers

Jane A. Lipscomb

In 2014, more than 15 million people were employed in healthcare in the United States.[1] About 80% of healthcare workers are women. The healthcare sector includes a greater percentage of African Americans and Asians but a slightly lower percentage of Hispanics than all industries combined. The number of workers in healthcare has grown dramatically over the past decade, with approximately 20% of newly created jobs in this sector. This growth is projected to continue in the 2020s but at a somewhat slower rate.[1]

Healthcare workers probably confront a greater range of significant workplace hazards (Table 32C-1) than workers in any other sector, including the following:

- Biological hazards associated with airborne and bloodborne exposures to infectious agents, including newly emerging infectious diseases (Chapter 13)
- Chemical hazards, such as hazardous drugs, industrial-strength disinfectants and cleaning compounds, and anesthetic gases (Chapter 11)
- Physical hazards, including lasers as well as ionizing and non-ionizing radiation (Chapters 12A through 12D)

- Safety and ergonomic hazards, which cause a variety of acute injuries and chronic musculoskeletal disorders (Chapters 9, 19, and 20)
- Violence, including physical assaults and threats of assaults (Chapter 19)
- Psychosocial and organizational factors, including work stress, compassion fatigue, short staffing, and shift work (Chapter 14)
- Health consequences associated with changes in the organization and financing of healthcare.

Some groups within the healthcare workforce are at increased risk of adverse effects of work-related exposures and demands. For example, registered nurses over the age of 50 are at increased risk of injuries due to the physical demands of patient care.

In 2014, the occupational injury and illness rate per 100 workers among hospital workers (6.2) was nearly double that of the overall private sector rate (3.2) and higher than rates for workers employed in mining (2.8), manufacturing (4.0), and construction (3.6). Workers in nursing and residential-care facilities had an even higher rate of occupational injuries and illnesses (7.1 per 100 full-time workers).[1] Although occupational injury

Table 32C-1. Illustrative Hazards, Health Effects, and Control Strategies in Healthcare

Hazards	Health Effects	Control Strategies
Biological		
Viral (hepatitis B virus, hepatitis C virus)	Acute febrile illness, liver disease	Safer needle devices, hepatitis B vaccine
Bacteria (*Mycobacterium tuberculosis*)	TB infection, TB illness, multiple drug resistance	Tuberculin skin testing, isolation of patients with suspected active TB
Emerging infectious diseases	Ebola virus disease	Strict patient screening to identify potential cases of Ebola viral disease, respiratory and dermal protection via PPE
Chemical		
Formaldehyde and glutaradehyde	Allergy, nasal cancer; Mucous-membrane irritation, sensitization, reproductive effects	Subsitution, local ventilation
Antineoplastic drugs	Cancer, mutagenicity, reproductive effects	Class 1 ventilation hoods, isolation of patient excreta
Waste anesthetic gases	Hepatotoxicity, neurologic effects, reproductive effects	Scavenging systems, substitution of toxic anesthetic gases
Physical		
Patient handling	Back pain, injury	Patient handling devices, lifting teams, training
Static postures	Musculoskeletal disorders	Rest breaks, exercise, support hose and shoes
Ionizing radiation	Cancer, reproductive disorders	Shielding and maintenance of equipment, radiation badges
Lasers	Eye and skin burns, inhalation of toxic chemicals and pathogens, fires	Local exhaust ventilation, equipment maintenance, respirators and face shields
Physical assault	Traumatic injuries	Comprehensive workplace violence prevention program, alarm systems, security personnel, training
Psychosocial/Organizational		
Threat of violence	Anxiety	Security personnel, training
Restructuring	Job strain, exacerbation of musculoskeletal disorders, traumatic injuries, burnout	Acuity-based staffing, employee involvement in restructuring activities; improved safety culture
Work stress	Job strain, burnout	Stress prevention and management programs; improved safety culture
Shift work and long work hours	Gastrointestinal disorders, sleep disorders	Forward, stable, and predictable shift rotation

Note. TB = tuberculosis; PPE = personal protective equipment.

and illness rates have been declining among all industry sectors over the past decade, the decline in the healthcare sector has been more modest. In 2014, healthcare and social assistance was one of three private-sector industries with more than 100,000 incidents involving lost workdays (days away from work).[1] The incidence rate for injuries and illnesses requiring lost workdays among nursing aides, orderlies, and attendants in healthcare was 4.4 per 100 full-time workers, almost four times the rate of all industries combined.[2]

The most common injuries resulting in lost workdays are sprains and strains, which account for 54% of injuries. Healthcare leads other sectors in the incidence of nonfatal workplace assaults; 32% involving lost workdays occur in healthcare. Exposure to infectious diseases tend to be undercounted as they often do not result immediately in affected workers missing work. In general, illnesses are greatly undercounted. Among reported illnesses in healthcare, skin disorders represent 10% of cases.[3]

The healthcare industry appears to be a decade or more behind other high-risk industries in ensuring safety.[1] There have long been deep-rooted beliefs that patient health and safety supersede worker health and safety and that it is acceptable for healthcare workers to have less than optimal protection against workplace hazards.[4] For example, infection-control practitioners often promote maximum patient protection while de-emphasizing appropriate measures to prevent worker infections. In many healthcare settings at high risk of patient assaults, such as psychiatric units, emergency departments, and long-term care facilities, staff assaults are often considered "part of the job." Both patient and worker hazards arise from the same sources—healthcare practices, products, and materials and the built environment. Therefore, development of effective approaches to control these hazards benefits from an integrated approach, which has been demonstrated to reduce injuries in both workers and patients.

MUSCULOSKELETAL DISORDERS

Musculoskeletal disorders (MSDs), especially back, neck, and shoulder injuries, continue to account for a significant proportion (32%) of all injuries and illness cases for all industries combined and account for 54% of cases occurring in nurses' assistants. Healthcare and social-assistance workers have a higher overall rate of MSDs involving lost workdays—121.3 per 10,000 full-time workers, compared with a rate of 107.1 for all private-sector industry workers.[1] Hazardous exposures include those involved with lifting, pulling, sliding, turning, and transferring patients; moving equipment; and standing for long periods. Among all categories of workers, hospital and nursing-home workers have the highest number of occupational injuries and illnesses involving lost workdays due to back injuries. Patient-handling injuries accounted for approximately 25% of all workers' compensation claims among healthcare workers.

Safe patient-handling programs have become more prevalent in healthcare over the past decade. Such programs include the use of permanent or portable lifts, sheets and other equipment for transfers, training on equipment use and maintenance, implementation of "minimal lift" policies that eliminate manual handling where possible, and use of a dedicated "lift team" of workers who move patients with proper equipment and technique. These programs, which are mandated in some states and voluntary in others, are highly cost-effective, with initial capital investments typically recovered within 5 years.[5] More importantly, safe patient-handling programs

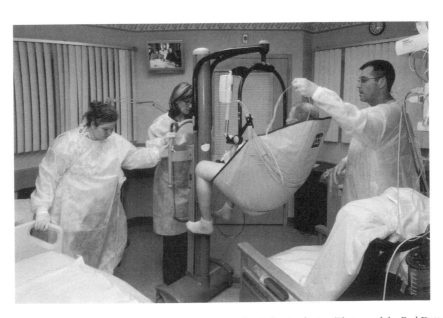

Figure 32C-1. Nurses' aides lift a patient by using a mechanical assist device. (Photograph by Earl Dotter.)

significantly reduce the number, severity, and rate of worker injuries. Patients also benefit from safe patient-handling, with lower rates of falls, skin tears, and pressure ulcers.[6] Patients report feeling significantly more comfortable and secure when a mechanical transfer device is used.[7] (See Figure 32C-1.)

Direct-care workers are not the only healthcare workers who face increased risks for MSDs. Laboratory workers are at increased risk for cumulative trauma disorders of the hand and wrist due to repetitive work. Operating-room workers, who must maintain static postures for long periods of time or hold instruments overhead during long operations, are at increased risks of neck and shoulder pain and injury. Workers who provide healthcare in patients' homes face risks related to assisting patients who have limited mobility, since few patients have mechanical lifting devices at home and a second person is often not available to assist with patient transfers.

Falls on the same level cause acute injuries among healthcare workers. In 2014, lost workday incident rates for falls on the same level was 26.8 per 10,000 full-time workers in healthcare and social assistance, compared with a rate of 18.8 for all workers combined.[1] The increased rate in healthcare is, in part, due to infection-control measures, which often leave surfaces wet and slippery.

WORKPLACE VIOLENCE

Healthcare leads other sectors in the incidence of nonfatal workplace assaults. Of all nonfatal assaults against workers resulting in lost workdays, 32% have occurred in the healthcare sector. Patients cause about half of nonfatal assault injuries. In 2014, the incidence rate of violence-related injuries in healthcare and social assistance was over three times the rate in all of private industry (14.4 vs 4.0 per 10,000 workers).[1]

From 1993 to 2009, 572,00 *violent victimizations*, such as simple and aggravated assault, rape, sexual assault, and robbery, occurred annually at work against persons age 16 or older.[8] Among all victims, 12% reported physical injuries, half of them requiring medical treatment. Less than half of incidents were reported to the police. The groups within healthcare with the highest

average annual rate of workplace violence were among mental health workers (20.5 assaults per 1,000 workers) and custodial-care workers in mental health (37.6 assaults per 1,000 workers). An average of 77% of psychiatric nurses surveyed reported experiencing physical violence during the previous year.[9]

Emergency department workers face a high risk of injuries from assaults by patients or patients' family members. Carrying weapons in emergency departments creates opportunities for severe or fatal injuries. Since no department in a healthcare setting is immune from workplace violence, all departments should have violence prevention programs.

Environmental and organizational factors have been associated with patient assaults, including understaffed situations (especially during times of increased activity), poor workplace security, unrestricted movement by the public around the facility, and the transport of patients. The presence of security personnel reduces the rate of assault; so does a system for identifying the charts of patients who have a history of violence. The rate of assault is increased when (a) administrators consider assault to be part of the job, (b) there is a high patient-to-worker ratio, and (c) work is primarily with patients with psychiatric disorders or with patients who have long hospital stays.

Many psychiatric settings now require that all care providers receive annual training in the management of aggressive patients, but few studies have examined the effectiveness of such training. Those that have done so have generally found improvement in nurses' knowledge, confidence, and safety after taking an aggressive behavior-management program.

Healthcare workplaces must be made safe for all workers through the development and implementation of a comprehensive workplace violence prevention program that includes strong employee involvement; comprehensive and ongoing risk analyses; use of engineering and administrative controls, such as security alarm systems; adequate staffing; and training and ongoing evaluation.[10]

NEEDLESTICK INJURIES

A prevalent and largely preventable serious risk that healthcare workers face arises from the use of needles and sharp devices, especially those that lack an engineered injury protection feature. Unsafe needles and other sharps continue to transmit bloodborne infections to healthcare workers employed in a wide variety of occupations. Injuries can be dramatically reduced by eliminating unnecessary sharp devices and using sharp devices with engineered injury-protection features.

After a needlestick injury, the risk for non-immune healthcare workers to develop occupationally acquired hepatitis B virus infection ranges from 2% to 40%, depending on the hepatitis B surface antigen status of the source patient. The risk of transmission from a positive source for hepatitis C virus is between 3% and 10%[11] and for HIV, 0.3%.[12] However, the risk of transmission increases if (a) the injury is caused by a device visibly contaminated with blood, (b) the device is used to puncture the vascular system, or (c) the stick causes a deep injury. All of these diseases are associated with significant morbidity and mortality. Only hepatitis B can be prevented by vaccine. Healthcare, laundry, and housekeeping workers are often engaged in tasks that create a potential for these high-risk needlestick injuries.

In addition to the risk of transmission of a serious or potentially fatal disease, there is a great emotional impact to a healthcare worker following a needlestick. Drug prophylaxis can be exhausting and debilitating with impacts on the daily lives of healthcare workers and their ability to perform their jobs, maintain stable relationships with their coworkers and family members, and have emotional balance.

The passage of the federal Needlestick Safety and Prevention Act in 2000 has afforded healthcare workers better protection from this unnecessary and potentially fatal hazard. Not only does the act amend the 1991 Bloodborne Pathogen Standard to require that safer needles be made available, but it requires employers to solicit the input of frontline healthcare workers when making decisions to purchase safe needles. Immediately after the passage of the act, there was a 33% decrease in the injury rate, based on a study of healthcare workers at 85 hospitals— probably due to an increase in use of safety-engineered needles and other devices. Nationwide, sharps injuries decreased by 100,000 annually, with a savings of $69 million to $415 million.[13] (See Chapter 13.)

EMERGING INFECTIOUS DISEASES

Within the past several years, emerging infectious diseases (EIDs) have been added to the list of biologic hazards to which healthcare workers are at increased risk. Emerging infectious diseases are defined as those whose incidence in humans has increased in the past two decades or threatens to increase in the near future. These infections, which know no national boundaries, include:

- New infections resulting from changes or evolution of existing organisms
- Known infections spreading to new geographic areas or populations
- Previously unrecognized infections appearing in areas undergoing ecologic transformation
- Old infections reemerging as a result of antimicrobial resistance in known agents or breakdowns in public health measures.

Ebola virus disease (EVD), probably the most well-recognized and feared of recent EIDs, is a severe and often fatal disease in humans. The 2014 Ebola outbreak was the largest one in history and the first in West Africa. During this outbreak, the Centers for Disease Control and Prevention (CDC) developed Ebola prevention and control recommendations for healthcare workers, laboratory workers, air medical transport, mortuary and funeral workers, and first responders such as firefighters, emergency medical technicians, and police officers. These guidelines direct all frontline healthcare facilities to ensure that facility-specific protocols and procedures are in place to rapidly identify and isolate persons with a travel or exposure history and signs and symptoms of EVD.[14] Some key points from these guidelines include:

- Healthcare workers caring for patients with EVD must have received comprehensive training and demonstrated competency in performing Ebola-related infection control practices and procedures.
- Personal protective equipment (PPE) that covers the clothing and skin and completely protects mucous membranes is required when caring for patients with EVD.

- Personnel providing care to patients with EVD must be supervised by an onsite manager at all times, and a trained observer must supervise each step of every PPE donning/doffing procedure to ensure established PPE protocols are completed correctly.
- Individuals unable or unwilling to adhere to infection control and PPE use procedures should not provide care for patients with EVD.

HAZARDOUS DRUGS AND OTHER CHEMICAL HAZARDS

Healthcare workers who prepare or administer hazardous drugs or who work in areas where these drugs are used may be exposed to these agents in the workplace. About 8 million U.S. healthcare workers are potentially exposed to hazardous drugs, including pharmacy and nursing personnel, physicians, operating-room personnel, environmental-services workers, workers in research laboratories, veterinary-care workers, and shipping and receiving personnel. Hazardous drugs include those used for cancer chemotherapy, antiviral drugs, hormones, and some bioengineered drugs.

Guidelines for the safe compounding, administration, and disposal of hazardous drugs have been developed by the National Institute for Occupational Safety and Health (NIOSH) and the Occupational Safety and Health Administration (OSHA).[15,16] Safe-handling guidelines address how to control dermal and inhalation exposures associated with the mixing and administration of these drugs. These guidelines state that these drugs should be prepared in a centralized area by trained individuals in a biological safety cabinet. Proper glove material designated for use with hazardous drugs should be used because most of these substances easily penetrate regular latex gloves. Aerosolized medications pose threats because of how these drugs are administered. Use of aerosolized medication requires use of engineering controls, such as specially designed booths, and worker respiratory protection, including compliance with all elements of the OSHA Respiratory Protection Standard.

Healthcare workers are also exposed to a wide range of chemical disinfectants used in large volumes for infection control, including those used to clean and disinfect diagnostic and surgical instruments. Healthcare workers in operating and postoperative recovery units may be exposed to anesthetic waste gases. Anesthetic agents, which are used in large amounts in hospitals, continue to pose a threat to healthcare workers when operating room scavenging systems are poorly maintained. Healthcare workers may also be exposed when patients are transferred to the recovery room and exhale anesthesia gases. Specially designed, nonrecirculating, general ventilation systems, with adequate room-air exchange, are necessary in these areas.

ORGANIZATION OF WORK

Organization of work refers to management and supervisory practices as well as production processes and their influence on the way work is performed. Perhaps no other single factor influences worker injury and illness rates more than the manner in which work is organized and staffing decisions are made. Healthcare in the United States has undergone sweeping changes in the organization of work over the past three decades. Macro-level changes have included organizational mergers, downsizing, increased contract work (workers employed part- or full-time by outside contractors), job restructuring and redesign, changes in worker–management relations, and a shift of many healthcare services from hospitals to subacute, outpatient, or home or community settings. (See Chapter 14.) These changes have contributed to increased acuity levels of patients treated in hospitals and decreased lengths of hospital admissions and a shift in the provision of many healthcare services from hospitals to community settings. This shift of healthcare services out of hospitals presents challenges for the health and safety of healthcare workers since regulations and health and safety research studies focus on hospitals. Long work shifts, use of temporary and contract workers, and inadequate staffing levels continue to contribute to high injury and illness rates among hospital-based nurses. Policies to ensure safe staffing levels have reduced injuries among nurses. For example, state-mandated minimum nurse-to-patient staffing ratios in California hospitals have been associated with a one-third reduction in the rate of occupational injuries and illnesses.[17]

Because many healthcare and supportive services that were traditionally provided in the hospital or other residential facilities are now being provided in the home, new risks have arisen for healthcare workers, home health aides, and personal care assistants who provide care outside of conventional work settings, often without hazard controls. In addition, these workers provide care in isolation, without the benefit of coworkers' support in performing tasks and providing assistance. To address these challenges, NIOSH has developed an online occupational safety and health curriculum for home care workers.[16]

Finally, the Affordable Care Act, while a major advancement in healthcare access and public health, included many provisions that impacted the way in which healthcare services are delivered and reimbursed.

LAWS, REGULATIONS, AND GUIDELINES TO PROTECT HEALTHCARE WORKERS

Laws, regulations, and voluntary guidelines to protect healthcare workers have been improving gradually over the past decade, but are still inadequate. In 1958, the American Medical Association and American Hospital Association issued a joint statement in support of worker health programs in hospitals. In 1977, NIOSH published criteria for effective hospital occupational health programs. In 1982, the CDC published the *Guideline for Infection Control in Hospital Personnel*, which focused on infections transmitted between healthcare workers and patients—not only healthcare workers' risks of contracting infectious diseases. Centers for Disease Control and Prevention guidelines for Blood and Body Fluid (BBP) Precautions (1983), Universal Precautions (1987), and Standard Precautions (2007), the latter of which combines the major features of Universal Precautions and Body Substance Isolation, were published to provide guidance to healthcare workers.

In 1984, OSHA promulgated its first healthcare worker–specific standard, covering the use of ethylene oxide. This regulatory action was followed by promulgation of the BBP Standard in 1991 and its revision in 2000. Standards addressing tuberculosis and ergonomics were also completed by OSHA but not implemented, and few new regulations are being proposed.

In the absence of federal legislation to protect healthcare workers, individual states have developed laws and regulations to protect healthcare workers from injuries related to patient handling and workplace violence. In addition, 14 states have passed legislation addressing safe staffing levels in healthcare directed at nurses' work environments and patient safety. Eleven states have enacted laws or promulgated regulations on safe patient handling. Ten of these states require a comprehensive program on safe patient handling in healthcare facilities, in which there is established policy, guidelines for securing appropriate equipment and training, collection of data, and evaluation.

In the absence of a federal standard that requires workplace violence protections, nine states have passed legislation mandating a comprehensive prevention program for healthcare workers and several others have passed legislation mandating increased penalties for those convicted of assaults of a nurse and/or other healthcare workers. In 2016, California OSHA (Cal/OSHA) promulgated the first workplace violence regulation in the United States, and a coalition of unions representing healthcare workers petitioned OSHA for a workplace violence standard.

In the absence of additional federal regulations, OSHA has used its existing authority to focus more of its compliance and enforcement efforts on healthcare. Between 2012 and 2015, OSHA conducted the National Emphasis Program in Nursing and Residential Care Facilities, during which it conducted 1,100 inspections of nursing and residential facilities with a focus on MSDs, bloodborne pathogens, tuberculosis, workplace violence, and slips, trips, and falls. In 2015, it extended the program to include hospitals.

During this same period, OSHA has used the General Duty Clause of the OSH Act to inspect and cite healthcare and social-assistance workplaces where workers are exposed to workplace violence. Between 2011 and 2016, OSHA inspected over 100 employers in response to complaints about workplace violence. However, OSHA has issued citations for only about 5% of these inspections, in part because of the challenge of developing support to issue a General Duty Clause citation in the absence of a hazard-specific standard.

Despite progress in decreasing exposure to bloodborne infections, unsafe patient transfers, and, to a lesser extent, workplace violence over the past decade, it is unlikely that the high rates of occupational injuries and illnesses among healthcare workers will be reduced without the adoption and strong enforcement of new federal regulations addressing the main hazards facing healthcare workers. All healthcare workers should work collectively to advocate for greater protection from the wide range of frequent and potentially fatal exposures that they face on the job.

REFERENCES

1. U.S. Bureau of Labor Statistics. Survey of occupational injuries and illnesses. Washington, DC: U.S. Department of Health and Human Services, 2015.
2. U.S. Bureau of Labor Statistics. Survey of occupational injuries and illnesses. Washington, DC: U.S. Department of Health and Human Services, 2012.
3. U.S. Bureau of Labor Statistics. Survey of occupational injuries and illnesses. Washington, DC: U.S. Department of Health and Human Services, 2013.
4. National Institute for Occupational Safety and Health. State of the sector | healthcare and social assistance—identification of research opportunities for the next decade of NORA. DHHS (NIOSH) Publication No. 2009-138. Cincinnati, OH: Author, June 2009.
5. Nelson AL, Collins J, Knibbe K, et al. Safe patient handling. Nursing Management 2007; 38: 26–33.
6. Facilities Guidelines Institute. Patient handling and movement assessments: A white paper. 2010 Health Guidelines Revision Committee Specialty Subcommittee on Patient Movement. Available at: http://www.wsha.org/wp-content/uploads/Worker-Safety_4-Equipment-needs-FGI_PHAMA_whitepaper_042810.pdf. Accessed January 19, 2017.
7. Pellino TA, Owen B, Knapp L, Noack J. The evaluation of mechanical devises for lateral transfer on perceived exertion and patient comfort. Orthopaedic Nursing 2006; 25: 4–10.

8. Duhart D. Violence in the workplace, 1993–1996: Special Report Bureau of Justice Statistics National Crime Victimization Survey (NCJ 190076). Washington, DC: Bureau of Justice, 2001.
9. Bowers L, Stewart D, Papadopoulos C, et al. Inpatient violence and aggression: A literature review. May 2011. Available at: http://www.kcl.ac.uk/ioppn/depts/hspr/research/ciemh/mhn/projects/litreview/LitRevAgg.pdf. Accessed January 19, 2017.
10. Lipscomb JA, London M. Not part of the job: How to take a stand against violence in the work setting. Silver Spring, MD: American Nurses Association, 2015.
11. Gerberding JL. Prophylaxis for occupational exposures to bloodborne viruses. New England Journal of Medicine 1995; 332: 444–455.
12. Centers for Disease Control and Prevention. Recommendations for preventing transmission of human immunodeficiency virus and hepatitis B virus to patients during exposure-prone invasive procedures. Morbidity and Mortality Weekly Report 1991; 40: 1–9.
13. Phillips EK, Conaway M, Parker G, et al. Issues in understanding the impact of the Needlestick Safety and Prevention Act on hospital sharp injuries. Infection Control and Hospital Epidemiology 2013; 34: 935–939.
14. Centers for Disease Control and Prevention. Guidance on personal protective equipment (PPE) to be used by healthcare workers during management of patients with confirmed Ebola or persons under investigation (PUIs) for Ebola who are clinically unstable or have bleeding, vomiting, or diarrhea in U.S. hospitals, including procedures for donning and doffing PPE. Available at: www.cdc.gov/vhf/ebola/healthcare-us/ppe/guidance.html. Accessed January 19, 2017.
15. Occupational Safety and Health Administration. Controlling occupational exposure to hazardous drugs. Available at: www.osha.gov/SLTC/hazardousdrugs/controlling_occex_hazardousdrugs.html. Accessed January 19, 2017.
16. National Institute for Occupational Safety and Health. Caring for yourself while caring for others (DHHS [NIOSH] Publication Number 2015-102). Available at: https://www.cdc.gov/niosh/docs/2015-102/. Accessed January 19, 2017.
17. Leigh JP, Markis CA, Iosif AM, Romano PS. California's nurse-to-patient ratio law and occupational injury. International Archives of Occupational and Environmental Health 2015; 88: 477–484.

33

Conducting Worksite Investigations

Bruce P. Bernard

Most workplaces in the United States do not have on-site occupational safety and health specialists, and the United States has not signed on to several International Labour Organization conventions requiring them. Employment of occupational health and safety specialists in the United States is projected to grow only 4% from now until 2024, slower than the average for all occupations.[1] Therefore, many workplaces will lack specialists capable of conducting onsite workplace investigations.

Proactive workplace investigations can generate knowledge, implement preventive interventions, and offer control of hazardous exposures. Despite best-practice recommendations by safety and health organizations, investigations at worksites generally are not done proactively. They are usually performed to fulfill legal requirements, to determine costs of injuries or illnesses after the fact, to determine compliance with applicable safety regulations, or to address specific workers' compensation claims. Occupational health and safety specialists are rarely consulted to conduct investigations because of new workplace processes/technologies or other newly introduced changes, at which time they would have the opportunity to identify the need for any new preventive measures.

Employees in small businesses have much higher fatal and nonfatal traumatic injury rates compared to larger worksites, but small businesses are least likely to have onsite safety and health capabilities. The Occupational Safety and Health Administration (OSHA) provides funding for no-cost worksite investigations through its On-Site Consultation Program for small businesses, which offers industrial hygiene and safety evaluations unrelated to enforcement (see https://www.osha.gov/dcsp/smallbusiness/consult.html for further information). These services are able to identify known hazards and provide recommendations based on existing standards. When new hazards or new health outcomes occur, or require new approaches to prevention, the National Institute for Occupational Safety and Health (NIOSH) Health Hazard Evaluation program offers an approach that offers assistance to the affected workers and worksites as well as generalizable new information for others.

This chapter describes the general principles of conducting workplace investigations, recognizing potential hazards, preparing for on-site investigations, conducting these investigations, making useful and practical recommendations, and proactively intervening to implement them. After identifying hazards, exposures, or working conditions, the goal is to control or reduce them to acceptable risk levels—or eliminate them entirely—and then to ensure that periodic reevaluations are done as part of routine operations. Cases 1 through 4 at the end of this chapter describe four worksite investigations that the NIOSH Health Hazard Evaluation Program has performed, illustrating the elements of this approach.

IMPORTANCE OF WORKSITE OBSERVATION

There is no substitute for being on-site and witnessing work processes and tasks in "real time." Direct observation leads to a better understanding of exposures and working conditions, and it assists in developing better strategies for intervention. It helps with formulating recommendations on (a) the occupational health and safety hierarchy of controls, such as eliminating a hazardous substance or substituting a less hazardous one; (b) specific engineering controls, such as local ventilation; and (c) administrative controls. It also enables a health and safety specialist to recognize hazards or unsafe conditions that may go unnoticed by workers or employers.

Evaluating a workplace often requires a multidisciplinary approach. Input by employees and employers, physicians, engineers, chemists, health physicists, and social scientists may be needed to successfully address hazards and unsafe work conditions. The most successful approaches coordinate many disciplines and incorporate effective communication between employees and employers for recognizing, evaluating, and controlling hazards and unsafe working conditions. A multidisciplinary approach may not be practical for many workplace situations. However, each person evaluating a workplace must be knowledgeable of possible contributions of other professionals in solving problems. For example, a physician studying a work environment should have not only knowledge of the health effects of specific chemical exposures but also a basic understanding

of the relevant chemistry, chemical-sampling techniques, and engineering requirements for control.

To recognize potential hazards at a workplace, one should become familiar with work processes, review a list of possible hazardous exposures, consider job activities and job conditions in work areas of interest, and determine possible control options for exposures or hazards that may be present. One also needs to determine how managers and direct supervisors respond to workers' reports of health concerns. Supervisors' or managers' responses to these reports and investigations of potential causative factors provide clues on how they approach workplace problems and how committed they are to prevention.

THE NIOSH HEALTH HAZARD EVALUATION PROGRAM

The NIOSH Health Hazard Evaluation (HHE) Program responds to requests for workplace evaluations from employees, unions, employers, and other governmental agencies. A *health hazard evaluation* is an investigation of a workplace to assess whether workers are exposed to hazards or harmful conditions. The NIOSH HHE program, using teams of various occupational health experts, including epidemiologists, industrial hygienists, occupational health specialists (physicians, nurses, and veterinarians), and psychologists, conducts about 250 investigations annually. Through this program, NIOSH identifies hazards and recommends practical, scientifically valid solutions for reducing exposures, controlling harmful conditions, and preventing disease, injury, and disability.

Preparing for a Workplace Investigation

Gathering Information

Investigators develop overall plans, collaboratively determine specific questions to be answered, and plan the investigative strategy. Initial telephone calls obtain information about workplace problems with those who requested the investigation, workers, managers, and other people. Initial information is obtained on workplace operations, the materials or chemicals used, hazards present, processes and work tasks, time sequence and duration of existing problems or concerns, previous actions taken to address the problems, recent process or materials changes, and the urgency of the situation. According to OSHA, emergency situations are those that are immediately hazardous. Investigators determine who might be aware of the potentially work-related health problem at the workplace. If there is a labor union that represents workers who may be affected or exposed, it is informed about the investigation and a representative is asked pertinent questions, including about whether the union has any additional relevant information and if the union provides any medical surveillance, special medical testing, or recordkeeping on its members.

At the time of the initial telephone call, determination is made about the parties who need to be included in the investigation: employers, workers, any worker representatives (from local and national unions), medical care providers, other health professionals, and local and state health department representatives. Critical to a successful investigation is involvement from the start of employees and their representatives, such as union stewards, as well as managers and other employer representatives.

Because employees have a unique understanding of job tasks and working conditions, information gained from them is especially valuable in determining whether hazards exist and assessing them. Involving employees from the start helps to improve the quality of the investigation, minimize oversights, and enable them to fully understand the need for the investigation and gain their cooperation.

Usually, with some background investigation, early clues help determine the scope of necessary work. For example, illness among many workers in different jobs in various departments likely indicates the need for a full-scale, workplace-wide investigation. Alternately, if suspected problems are confined to isolated tasks or relatively few workers, only a more limited, focused investigation may be necessary.

During the first encounter (by phone, e-mail, web-based conferencing, or a face-to-face meeting), one needs to determine what health and safety hazards might be encountered onsite

and what personal protective equipment (PPE) members of the investigative team might need during the initial investigation to the site. If respirators are required on-site, only personnel who have been medically cleared, trained, and fit-tested can use them.

Roles of the Investigative Team

For the industrial hygienist, preparation for a field investigation begins with identifying exposures of concern, determining whether there are appropriate sampling and analytical procedures that will need to be performed, determining analytical chemistry or microbiological services needed, determining proper instruments to be selected, and making an industrial hygiene equipment list. Determining appropriate sampling usually requires being on-site or having enough information beforehand to know exactly what needs to be sampled, where, and why; performing sampling in a rush and obtaining unneeded data points (because "it may be the only opportunity to sample") is rarely fruitful. Preparation for sampling includes arranging for equipment, supplies, and analytical services and knowing any shipment requirements for hazardous materials. It also requires preparing consent and notification forms for personal sampling.

For the occupational medicine physician, preparation involves searching the medical literature, reviewing medical records, and having the diagnostic and examination skills to sort out what may be work related in the workplace. Medical support staff responsibilities may include designing a study; developing the investigative protocol; obtaining necessary approval from an institutional review board; preparing consent forms, notification forms, questionnaires, and other data-collection forms; and arranging for field-study materials, personnel, and medical tests.

If biological testing is to be conducted, arrangements need to be made for clerical support, data-collection forms, supplies for venipuncture and collection of urine or other biological samples, as well as forms to request tests not routinely performed by clinical laboratories, such as those for metals, pesticides, volatile organic compounds, polychlorinated biphenyls, furans, dioxins, polycyclic aromatic hydrocarbons, phthalates, and flame-retardants. Plans also need to be made for special studies, such as pulmonary function tests, chest X-rays, neurological and neuropsychological tests, or other examinations that may require a consultant.

Obtaining Needed Information Before the Site Visit

Team members need to be informed about the worksite—exposures, products, and personnel with whom they will be interacting on-site. Many manufacturers have technical and other information on their websites on product lines, work processes, financial status, and managerial systems. Major unions also have useful information on their websites. Information on websites also includes research findings, technical experts, and survey instruments.

If the worksite is a manufacturing facility, investigators need to learn about goods produced, chemicals and other substances used, and intermediate products formed in the production processes. Much of this information can be obtained before the site visit through discussions with employees, employers, and technical experts or from the Internet.

Before the site visit, it is useful to obtain worksite records on exposure monitoring, purchasing, production, health and safety policies, and operating procedures, all of which can help in determining the exposures of greatest concern. Employee rosters, staffing lists, employee turnover rates, and floor plans may also provide useful information. Reviewing these documents prior to the site visit will help give investigators a better understanding of potential hazardous exposures and company procedures to respond to hazardous situations. The site visit will help to determine whether these procedures are actually operational or are only "on paper" and not performed.

Safety data sheets (SDSs) on hazardous substances, which are mandated at manufacturing plants by the OSHA Hazard Communication Standard, are useful documents to obtain from management. Workplaces in certain industries may not have SDSs; however, containers of hazardous substances that they use, such as cleaning products and insecticides, are required to have hazard warning labels that can provide some toxicity information.

OSHA Logs and Other Existing Records

Investigators can request to obtain (a) the logs of injuries and illnesses that are required by OSHA (OSHA's Form 300; Log of Work-Related Injuries and Illnesses) and (b) worksite medical records, workers' compensation claims, insurance claims, absentee records, and job-transfer applications, all of which can yield useful information on work-related injuries and illnesses. If workers in certain departments or processes have higher rates of health problems than others, especially if they have the same type of injuries or illnesses, this suggests specific areas for investigation. Jobs with increased rates of certain symptoms, such as lightheadedness or concentration problems, may also have higher risks for acute injuries.

The Occupational Safety and Health Administration mandates that each worksite it covers allows access to illness and injury log summaries; OSHA also has a new provision that mandates that employers electronically submit injury and illness data, in addition to keeping the same records on-site. Certain data must be posted to the OSHA website, which can provide valuable information for (a) other worksites with similar processes, (b) investigations of a specific worksite, and (c) comparison of rates within an industry. The Occupational Safety and Health Administration also still requires the posting of annual average number of employees and total hours worked during the calendar year, so that workplace injury and illness incidence rates can be calculated. Companies with no recordable injuries or illnesses must still post the form. All summaries must be certified by a company executive. Employers are also required to make a copy of the summary available to employees who move from worksite to worksite, such as construction workers, and employees who do not regularly report to any specific worksite.

Medical and First-Aid Records

Investigations of suspected work-related injuries and illnesses should also include review of first-aid and medical records to understand the magnitude and seriousness of such problems. The Health Insurance Portability and Accountability Act (HIPAA) requires that (a) specific medical-release authorization from individual workers be given before access to their medical records can be obtained and (b) employers and on-site healthcare providers protect individual health data. Public health officials are exempt from HIPAA requirements and are authorized by law to have access to individual health information for the purpose of preventing or controlling disease, injury, or disability—including for investigations and interventions. Examination of employee first-aid and medical records may offer clues to jobs or operations that may cause or contribute to other work-related problems. Review of electronic health data from first-aid stations or medical clinics at a worksite (without identifying information) may help identify trends or clusters of injuries or illnesses.

Performing a Worksite Investigation

The Initial Worksite Visit

The primary purposes of the worksite visit are to (a) determine, while on-site, the extent and severity of the problem; (b) identify possible causes; (c) determine if, at an early stage of the investigation, there may be possible solutions to the problem; and (d) ascertain whether further assessment is needed. An initial site visit can be usually completed in 1 or 2 days, but it may take longer if more time is needed to complete it without a follow-up visit.

A good way to start the site visit is with a meeting with all those involved, including the facility manager, the chief local union official (or other worker representative if employees are not represented by a union), healthcare professionals, engineering and maintenance workers familiar with the facilities, and consultants who are familiar with the facility. Employees from the area of concern must attend meetings. It is important to discuss plans for (a) assuring confidentiality of information from worker interviews and personnel and medical records and procedures for videotaping, photographing, and other recording and (b) sharing summary data (without personal identifying information) with all parties. Personal protective equipment requirements and any other relevant safety procedures to be used during the investigation should be reviewed.

Walkthrough Observational Survey

A walkthrough survey, which can be the most important part of the investigation, should include managers, employees, and their representatives, including the person who requested the workplace investigation, unless that person has requested confidentiality or has declined to participate (Figure 33-1). Usually, the main purposes of the walkthrough survey are to observe the facility in routine operation, to view worker activities, to identify any potential hazards, and to talk

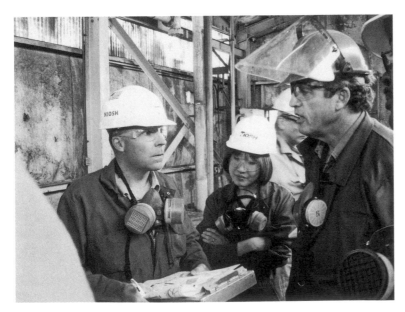

Figure 33-1. An industrial hygienist and an occupational medicine physician pause for questions from a worker during a workplace walkthrough survey. (Courtesy of the National Institute for Occupational Safety and Health.)

informally to employees, managers, and others about perceived exposure and health problems.

The walkthrough allows observation of workers performing job tasks, use of PPE or protective clothing, placement of materials, tools, physical layout of the workplace, and the organizational climate. Many potentially hazardous operations can be detected by observation during the walkthrough. Using lists obtained beforehand of chemicals, raw materials, products, and by-products assists in identifying hazardous inhalational and skin exposures. Knowledge of fuels used in burning processes assists in identifying air contaminants. Observation of ventilation systems helps to determine needs for improved control measures. The walkthrough can assist in understanding job tasks that place workers in specific jobs at risk and can help determine the need for additional industrial hygiene sampling, worker interviews, and medical testing.

The dirtiest, dustiest operations are not necessarily the most hazardous. For example, dust particles that cannot be seen by the unaided eye can be the most hazardous because they are of respirable size. The absence of a visible dust cloud does not necessarily mean that there is no airborne dust. Odors are not reliable indicators of exposure: odors one might not detect of vapors and gases present in concentrations considerably above their permissible levels, and one's ability to detect an odor often decreases as exposure continues.

Workers' Job Tasks

It is important to obtain a list of workers' routine job tasks and requirements in areas of the workplace being investigated. Changes in job requirements or modifications of work techniques or processes may have profoundly affected hazardous exposures. Shift work or overtime work requirements may contribute to prolonged exposure of workers, which may not occur on an 8-hour work schedule.

Most job tasks can be described in terms of (a) tools, equipment, and materials used; (b) workstation layout and physical environment; (c) task demands; and (d) organizational climate in which the work is performed. More definitive procedures for collecting information on job tasks can include the following:

- Videotaping to observe workers performing tasks for a time-activity analysis

- Photographing workstation layout, tools, materials, and chemicals used
- Recording workstation measurements and characteristics of work surfaces, including heights, edges, reach distances, and slip resistance
- Determining perceived exertion of workers.

While screening tools, such as checklists, have been widely used in many investigations, most have not been scientifically validated. Combining checklist observations with data on symptoms offers a way of reducing uncertainty.

Focusing on Jobs

Jobs associated with the most, or the highest rates of, occupational illnesses and injuries deserve the most attention. Jobs in which recent cases have occurred deserve priority attention. Priority for job analysis and intervention should be given to those jobs in which (a) the most people are affected or (b) changes in work exposures or processes are taking place or planned. Jobs associated with workers' complaints of fatigue and discomfort should be ranked next in priority for analysis and intervention. Finally, where screening suggests presence of significant risk factors or exposures for occupational illnesses or injuries, more-detailed job analyses should be done. Jobs with higher levels of exposure or multiple risk factors may indicate a need for control.

Selection of Instruments to Evaluate the Work Environment

Industrial hygiene sampling (Figure 33-2) is sometimes necessary on the initial site visit to determine the range of exposures to begin planning for more definitive sampling (Chapter 8). Direct reading instruments and/or detector tubes are generally used because of their portability and ease of use. In-depth quantitative air sampling is generally not done on the initial site visit.

Interviews

The lead investigator should establish a schedule to interview the following people:

- Managers and other employer representatives
- Workers (Although it is reasonable to interview specific workers at their request or the

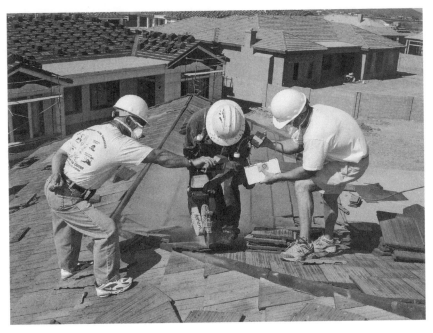

Figure 33-2. Industrial hygienists collect follow-up samples for a silica exposure among roofers. (Courtesy of the National Institute for Occupational Safety and Health.)

request of others, it is important to interview a cross-section of workers. Group interviews can supplement individual interviews, recognizing group dynamics may provide different perspectives than individual interviews.)

- Union representatives
- Physicians, nurses, and other health and safety personnel
- Representatives of the human resources department.

Conducting Symptom Surveys

Symptoms surveys may assist in focusing on specific concerns of workers and in identifying possible work-related disorders that might otherwise go unrecognized. These surveys provide information to narrow the focus of investigation. In addition to questions about workers' job titles, work history, job tasks, and past and present medical history, the location, frequency, duration, and intensity of symptoms will help to determine the focus of the investigation. By definition, symptom surveys rely on self-reports, a potential limitation. One has to be careful not to overanalyze information obtained from surveys based on small numbers of workers. An epidemiologist can assist with questionnaire design and data analysis. It is important to mention that any personal identifying information generated from surveys will be protected, and confidential information will be accessible only to authorized medical personnel.

Medical Examinations

One disadvantage of using OSHA logs or company-based medical information to identify possible cases of work-related injuries or illnesses is the lack of uniform case definitions. In the NIOSH HHE program, investigations have included limited physical examinations focused on specific organ systems or parts of the body. Information obtained can help establish the prevalence of possible work-related conditions. Using a comparison group of unexposed workers may be helpful in determining a work-related condition based on differences in prevalence. Screening medical examinations, performed periodically at some workplaces may provide valuable clues, but they are generally not designed for continuous surveillance of specific exposures.

Integration of Data

All team members involved in an on-site investigation should have prepared an integrated strategy to answer specific questions prior to data gathering. After the initial meeting with all parties, the observational walkthrough, and data-gathering, the team needs to meet on-site to discuss changes in the strategy and integration of their initial findings. This process will help formulation and planning of the next steps.

Summarizing On-Site Information and Holding a Closing Conference

This involves the following steps:

- Hold a closing conference before the initial worksite visit is completed to discuss what has been accomplished
- Invite those present at the opening conference and other key employees and managers
- New recommendations can be made, and previous ones can be modified
- Future activities and reports can be discussed.

Data Management and Information Security

A computer database is an excellent format with which to manage information and records from a site visit. In order to maintain privacy required by law and to facilitate communication among investigators, issues of information security must be addressed prior to the on-site visit. All records, notes, forms, and other data from the site visit need safeguards to prevent unauthorized access. This means preplanning for records that will be obtained and may involve information technology personnel who can assist with methods for secure transfer of electronic data and records.

Miscellaneous Activities After the Site Visit

Miscellaneous activities include the following:

- Check and decontaminate all equipment used for industrial hygiene monitoring
- Arrange for laboratory analysis of samples
- Review and check analytical results for reliability
- Arrange for coding, entry, analysis, storage, and maintenance of investigation data and records.

Conducting Follow-up Activities

Within a few days of the initial site visit, a letter should be sent to the manager and the employee representative summarizing the findings of the visit. The letter should use plain language and provide a clear understanding of possible health effects associated with the hazards encountered. A conference call with all parties involved can also communicate information on findings from the site visit. For hazards recognized during the site visit and mentioned in the closing conference, written documentation can facilitate timely implementation of control measures. Any results and recommendations reported by phone should be included in a subsequent written report. Preparation of the final report to employers and employees should integrate both the industrial hygiene/environmental and medical/epidemiological components of the investigation.

Considering Recommendations

An employee (labor)-management health and safety committee or working group should discuss the recommendations and develop an action plan. (If employees belong to a labor union, this committee should already exist.) Those involved in the work can best set priorities and assess the feasibility of the recommendations for the specific situation.

The occupational health and safety hierarchy of controls—widely accepted as an intervention strategy for controlling workplace hazards (Chapters 4 and 8)—is useful in outlining recommendations in the report:

- Elimination and substitution
- Engineering controls
- Administrative controls (changes in work practices and management policies)
- Use of PPE

Elimination and Substitution

Eliminating or substituting hazardous processes or materials reduces hazards and protects employees more effectively than other approaches. Eliminating a hazard in design or development of a project reduces the future need for additional controls.

Engineering Controls

Engineering controls reduce employees' exposures by removing the hazard from the process or by placing a barrier between the hazard and the employee. Engineering controls protect employees effectively without placing primary responsibility of implementation on the employee. Questions on existing engineering control strategies at a worksite should include the following:

- If elimination of a hazard is not possible, are work operations isolated or enclosed to reduce worker exposures?
- Are wet methods being used to reduce generation of dusts?
- Is general ventilation adequate?
- Is shielding from radiant heat, ultraviolet light, radiation, and other forms of energy used?
- Are parts on an assembly line presented in a way to ensure proper reach, hold, and use by the worker?
- Is equipment height-adjustable, are tools in adequate proximity to workers, and are objects handled of appropriate weight?

Administrative Controls

Administrative controls refer to employer-dictated work practices and policies to reduce or prevent hazardous exposures. Their effectiveness depends on both employer commitment and employee acceptance. Regular monitoring and reinforcement are necessary to ensure that policies and procedures are followed consistently. Administrative control recommendations can address issues such as the following:

1. Scheduling shifts and rest breaks
2. Rotating workers in and out of specific jobs
3. Evaluating production quotas and performance standards concerning their impact on workplace stress, work pace, and worker control
4. Providing meaningful light-duty jobs, as deemed appropriate, to allow injured or ill workers to maintain contact with fellow employees and gradual return to normal activities, while providing for specific medical needs

5. Providing periodic training of employees on work risk factors and recordkeeping
6. Implementing medical management and surveillance programs
7. Implementing workplace policies to prohibit smoking
8. Implementing appropriate procedures for housekeeping, waste disposal, eating and washing, and use of restrooms.

Many administrative recommendations should be seen as (a) temporary measures until engineering controls can be implemented or (b) measures to use when engineering controls are not technically feasible. Since administrative controls do not eliminate hazards, managers must ensure that practices and policies are diligently followed. Administrative controls are "stop-gap" measures—not permanent solutions.

Personal Protective Equipment

Personal protective equipment is the least effective means for controlling hazardous exposures. Proper use of PPE requires a comprehensive program and a high level of employee involvement and commitment. Appropriate PPE must be chosen for each hazard. Supporting programs and procedures, such as training, schedules for the changing of respirator cartridges, and medical assessment, may be needed. Personal protective equipment should not be the sole method for controlling hazardous exposures. PPE should be used only until effective engineering and administrative controls have been implemented.

Implementing and Evaluating Controls

Implementing controls normally consists of (a) initial testing of the selected measures, (b) modifying these measures based on initial testing, (c) implementing them on a large scale, and (d) evaluating their effectiveness. By testing and evaluating measures, one can determine whether they achieve the desired outcome and identify any necessary modifications. Workers can provide valuable input into testing and evaluation. Worker acceptance of changes is important to the success of the control measures. Workplace control measures often start by targeting problems clearly identified in the workplace investigation and those problems that appear easiest to solve. Early success can build confidence and experience needed later to solve more complex problems.

Implemented controls should be periodically evaluated to determine whether they have reduced hazards and/or decreased injuries or illnesses and to ensure that control measures have not introduced new risk factors. Follow-up evaluation should occur no sooner than 6 weeks after implementation of control measures to avoid discarding effective control measures that may not have yet demonstrated their benefits. Evaluation may also include a symptom survey, completion of a risk-factor checklist, and/or another job-analysis method. Results of a follow-up symptom survey can be compared with those of the initial symptom survey to determine the effectiveness of control measures in reducing symptoms. (One should be aware that some ergonomic control measures lead to changes in work methods, requiring workers to use different muscle groups, which may make them sore during the "break-in" period.)

PROACTIVE APPROACHES

To this point, the topics outlined in this chapter have represented *reactive* approaches for workplace investigations. In contrast, *proactive* approaches are geared to preventing problems from developing. Proactive measures emphasize designing work tasks and processes to avoid causes of occupational illnesses and injuries. They include design of operations that ensure proper selection and use of tools, job tasks and processes, workstation layouts, and materials that are unlikely to harm workers.

Ideally, workplace problems are identified and resolved in the planning process. In addition, general occupational health and safety knowledge, learned from an ongoing health and safety program, can be used to build an approach more oriented to prevention. Management commitment and employee involvement in planning are essential. For example, management can set policy to require health and safety considerations for any equipment to be purchased, and production employees can offer ideas on the basis of their experiences for alleviating potential problems.

Decision-makers who are planning new work processes, especially those involved in the design of job tasks, equipment, and workplace layout, must become more aware of health and safety factors and principles. Designers must have appropriate information and guidelines about risk factors for occupational illnesses and injuries and ways to control them. Studying past job designs can help determine what improvements are needed. (See Chapter 9.)

Because design strategies try to target the causes of potential occupational illnesses and injuries, engineering approaches are preferred over administrative approaches. They eliminate risk factors instead of only reducing exposure to them.

WORKSITE INVESTIGATIONS

Heat Stress Among Firefighters

Firefighters are exposed to heat from several sources, including heat generated by fire, ambient temperatures, physical exertion, and firefighting "turnout" gear. The weight of the turnout gear and firefighting equipment increases physical exertion and, in turn, increases overall heat load. Heat exposure can result in heat-related illness (Chapter 12C). The combination of heat accumulation and overexertion can also result in rhabdomyolysis, with breakdown of muscle tissue resulting in potentially fatal effects on the heart and kidneys.

NIOSH conducted a site visit in response to a request from a fire department to evaluate the risk of heat-related illness and rhabdomyolysis among firefighter cadets and instructors during training. Investigators conducted a 4-day investigation during a 10-week training course. Thirty-two firefighters completed questionnaires on work history, medical history, hydration, and symptoms of heat-related illness and rhabdomyolysis. Investigators tested for levels of creatine kinase (a marker of muscle damage). They monitored participants for signs of dehydration during and after the 8th week of the training course, measured their body weight before and after each training day, and monitored their work activities and fluid intake. They also determined ambient wet bulb globe temperature each day.

One participant had rhabdomyolysis and 16 others had elevated creatine kinase levels. Most firefighters met criteria for excessive heat strain at some point during the week. Environmental conditions often exceeded heat stress limits.

Recommendations were made to schedule training sessions during cooler parts of the day and year; include specific training and educational materials about the signs, symptoms, and risk of rhabdomyolysis; and instruct firefighters to carry wallet cards (a) to inform healthcare workers of their risk for both heat stress and rhabdomyolysis (an often missed diagnosis); (b) to refrain from taking energy/exercise supplements; and (c) to tell their supervisors immediately if they experienced early symptoms of heat-related illness (dizziness, nausea, rapid heart rate, cramping, or lightheadedness) or rhabdomyolysis (muscle pain or weakness, or abdominal pain) or if they noted these symptoms in other firefighters.

Hazards in Nail Salons

Nail salon employees are potentially exposed to hazardous chemicals, ergonomic hazards, and work organization and job stress factors, including work–family imbalance, nonstandard work arrangements, and long work hours.

The National Institute for Occupational Safety and Health received several HHE requests to evaluate employee exposures at nail salons. A walkthrough evaluation of these salons identified hazardous airborne chemicals and ergonomic risk factors and ways of reducing these problems. Ethyl methacrylate and methyl methacrylate in nail polish can cause contact dermatitis, asthma, and irritation of the eyes and respiratory tract.

Investigators collected general area air samples for total and respirable particulate matter during the application of artificial nails. They measured temperature, relative humidity, and carbon dioxide concentration at various locations in salons. They traced ventilation-system ducts to determine the source of outside air, and they conducted employee interviews. The investigators made recommendations that could be quickly and easily implemented, such as keeping all bottles of fingernail liquid tightly capped, putting soaked gauze pads in sealed bags before being thrown in the trash, changing trash-can liners daily, and pouring only needed amounts of fingernail liquid into dispenser bottles. They advised technicians (a) to wear long sleeves and gloves to protect their skin from acrylic dust; (b) to wash their hands, arms, and face with mild soap and water several times during the day to remove potentially irritating dust; and (c) to avoid eating, drinking, and smoking in work areas where artificial fingernails were applied. They instructed workers that methacrylates in nail dust can be carried accidentally to one's mouth on a cup or other utensil. They recommended posters with information and warnings in appropriate languages. They also recommended adjustable chairs and equipment, instituting rest breaks for workers, and reducing use of tools that require a pinch grip.

Coffee and Diacetyl

Workers at coffee-processing facilities may be at risk for bronchiolitis obliterans, an irreversible lung disease due to exposure to diacetyl or 2,3-pentanedione (both alpha-diketones). These chemicals, which are naturally produced when coffee beans are roasted, are added to flavored coffee. The National Institute for Occupational Safety and Health has been investigating coffee-processing facilities to introduce exposure monitoring and workplace interventions to reduce levels to these chemicals and prevent illness among workers.

The National Institute for Occupational Safety and Health received a confidential HHE request from employees at a coffee-processing facility, who were concerned about severe shortness of breath and eye irritation. The facility roasted green coffee beans. It also produced and packaged flavored and unflavored coffee—both whole beans and ground coffee. Physicians had diagnosed bronchiolitis obliterans in five employees who had worked at this facility. Flavored coffees often contain alpha-diketones, which can cause severe respiratory problems.

The National Institute for Occupational Safety and Health conducted an industrial-hygiene and medical evaluation at the facility. Air concentrations of diacetyl and 2,3-pentanedione were above proposed NIOSH recommended exposure levels. The combined alpha-diketone exposure during grinding/packaging *unflavored* coffee was comparable to the manufacture and processing of *flavored* coffee. Compared to the general population, workers had a 60% higher prevalence of shortness of breath on exertion and a 170% higher prevalence of obstructive pulmonary disease, based on spirometry. Workers at this facility were at risk of bronchiolitis obliterans. The National Institute for Occupational Safety and Health provided its best-practices document on engineering controls, work practices, and exposure monitoring for diacetyl and 2,3-pentanedione to the employer and workers at the plant.

Recycling of Electronic Materials

A substantial—and increasing—amount of electronic waste (e-waste) is produced daily in the United States. Only about 20% is recycled to recover valuable, but hazardous, materials, including lead, cadmium, other toxic metals, and flame retardants. Recycling workers can be exposed to these materials, as well as to noise and ergonomic hazards. Risk of occupational illness and injury is especially high at facilities that shred electronics and process cathode ray tube glass.

The National Institute for Occupational Safety and Health received a request from a manager at an electronic-scrap (e-scrap) recycling facility, who was concerned about exposures of employees who handled recycled computers, monitors, hard drives, televisions, printers, and light bulbs. Eighty workers sorted, disassembled, and shredded e-scrap, including cathode ray tubes from computer monitors and televisions, using pneumatic pistol-grip tools. Then they sorted metals and glass. The warehouse had no ventilation. Workers in the shred room were required to wear company-provided long-sleeve uniforms, safety glasses, half-mask cartridge respirators, hearing protectors, bump caps (lightweight hard hats), steel-toed safety boots, and cut-resistant gloves and sleeves. Most other employees wore hearing protectors, safety glasses, and steel-toed safety boots.

Before making the site visit, NIOSH investigators obtained and reviewed company health and safety records, noise and airborne-lead exposure records, employee blood lead levels (BLLs), and company respiratory protection, hearing conservation, and hazard communication programs. On-site, they observed workplace conditions, work processes, and practices. They held confidential employee medical interviews, asking about medical history, health issues, job duties, and PPE use. They collected various biological and environmental samples. Although results of biological sampling for all metals were below OSHA standards, two employees had BLLs above 10 µg/dL. Lead and other metals were found on the skin of employees, both at lunch and prior to their leaving the workplace. Metals were also found on nonproduction work surfaces.

The investigators saw good compliance with the use of required PPE but that voluntary-use respirators were used improperly (used with only one strap or used despite facial hair). They noticed several work practices that could result in unnecessary lead exposure, such as workers reusing dirty uniforms, not showering at the end of shifts, laundering workclothes at home, not removing uniforms or gloves upon leaving the shred room, and using compressed air to clean work. Lead and other metals were being tracked outside of the shred room and were found on surfaces in nonproduction areas, on the skin of employees, and on an employee's clothing on leaving the workplace. There was concern about contaminating cars and homes, thereby exposing family members to these metals.

The investigators recommended several engineering controls, such as extending the glass shredding conveyor so that the lead-containing cathode ray tubes would be transported directly to the shredder without breaking them. They suggested providing employees elevated work surfaces to reduce bending and risk of back injury. They recommended providing employees with their BLLs and providing "scrubs" to wear under work uniforms (both to be laundered by a contractor) as well as disposable shoe covers. They also recommended better workplace "housekeeping," no dry sweeping or use of compressed air to clean, improved hand hygiene with lead-removing soap, and preventing employees from taking potentially contaminated PPE from the production areas to nonproduction areas, including the lunchroom.

AUTHOR'S NOTE

The findings and conclusions in this chapter are those of the author and do not necessarily represent the views of the National Institute for Occupational Safety and Health.

REFERENCE

1. U.S. Department of Labor, Bureau of Labor Statistics. Occupational outlook handbook: Occupational health and safety specialists. Available at: http://www.bls.gov/ooh/healthcare/occupational-health-and-safety-specialists.htm. Accessed October 18, 2016.

FURTHER READING

Australian Queensland Government, Department of Education and Training. Health and safety incident investigation: Guideline to conducting an investigation into a health and safety incident, 2012. Available at: http://education.qld.gov.au/health/pdfs/healthsafety/investigation-guideline.pdf
An outline of an investigative process to carry out a health and safety investigations.

Centers for Disease Control and Prevention. Health hazard evaluations. Available at: http://www.cdc.gov/niosh/hhe/.
Provides the complete guide to the "nuts and bolts" of the NIOSH Health Hazard Evaluation Program.

Health and Safety Executive. Investigating accidents and incidents: A workbook for employers, unions, safety representatives and safety professionals, 2004. Available at: http://www.hse.gov.uk/pubns/hsg245.pdf.
A step-by-step guide for organizations, especially small businesses, to perform their own health and safety investigations.

National Research Council and Institute of Medicine of the National Academies. The Health Hazard Evaluation Program at NIOSH. Reviews of Research Programs of the National Institute for Occupational Safety and Health. Washington, DC: National Academies Press, 2009.
Remains a useful resource on the NIOSH Health Hazard Evaluation Program.

Occupational Safety and Health Administration. Screening and surveillance: A guide to OSHA standards. OSHA 3162-12R. Washington, DC: U.S. Department of Labor, 2009. https://www.osha.gov/Publications/osha3162.pdf.
Remains a good reference for locating and implementing the screening and surveillance requirements of OSHA standards.

SAFE Work Manitoba. Conducting a workplace incident investigation (Video). Available at: http://www.youtube.com/watch?v=hQilV-mOnC4. Accessed August 21, 2017.
An excellent 10-minute video on the basics of incident investigations.

34

Addressing the Built Environment and Health

Richard J. Jackson

When we consider health and the environment, we often focus on the microscopic (bioaccumulating chemicals or infectious organisms) and the macroscopic (the disappearing polar ice caps and the effects of war). But there is another environment that surrounds us and profoundly shapes our health nearly every minute of the day: the built environment—not just our homes and our highways, but also our parks and watersides and all the other places where we spend most of our lives.

The built environment is so pervasive and people are so adaptable that we scarcely notice it. Historically, our notion of the "adverse effects" of the built environment has brought visions of slums and crowded cities—visions that have seemed to vanish with major infrastructure improvements, such as water systems and air conditioning—as well as abundant cars and superhighways.

It is critical, however, to understand that how and what we build affects the quality of air and water, the occurrence of acute and chronic disease, social well-being and prosperity, and the health and well-being of generations to follow. In the 19th century, the United States improved the built environment by supplying clean water,

safe food, home heat, and lighting; creating transit; reducing crowding; removing biological and industrial waste; and developing healthier cities and trolley-car suburbs. In the 20th century, thanks to cheap and abundant fossil fuel and unparalleled prosperity, the United States was rebuilt for automobiles (Figures 34-1 through 34-3). As the population grew, small towns became cities. Farmlands and forests were turned into subdivisions, industrial parks, and highways. Many public transit systems were abandoned. Schools became larger and more distant. Commutes became longer, and traffic congestion became overwhelming. Freshwater became increasingly more precious, and the atmosphere became hotter and more polluted. Our bodies became less fit and fatter. And our social and mental stress increased. In the 21st century, we need to develop communities that once again foster and protect health.

For the first 125 years or so of U.S. history, cities were the nation's economic and cultural engine, but they were often squalid and dangerous places. Thomas Jefferson viewed cities as "pestilential to the morals, the health and the liberties of man."[1] Cities were frequently affected by epidemics, such as yellow fever and cholera. Nearly every family

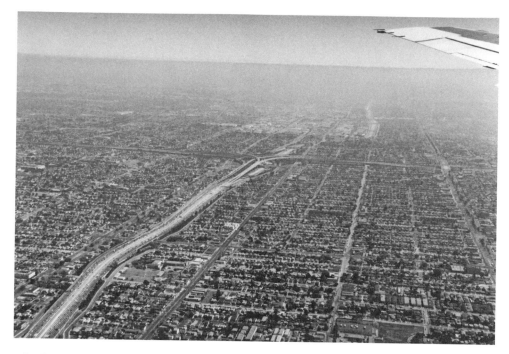

Figure 34-1. Urban sprawl in the Phoenix metropolitan area. (Photograph by Barry S. Levy.)

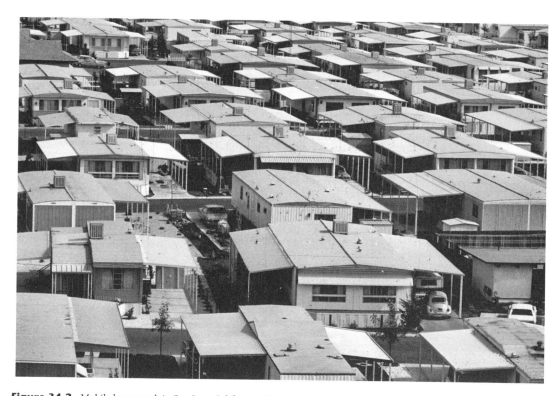

Figure 34-2. Mobile home park in San Jose, California. (Photograph by Earl Dotter.)

Suburban sprawl

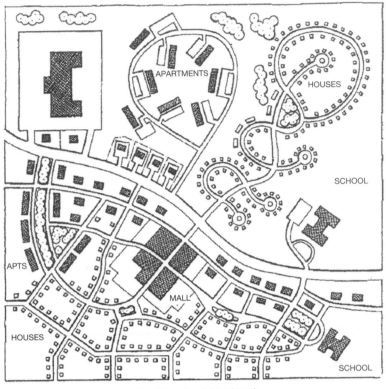

Traditional neighborhood

Figure 34-3. A schematic representation of streets and land use in both a sprawling suburb and a traditional neighborhood. Sprawling communities are characterized by being dispersed, dependent on automobiles, and having a low density, all of which makes walking and certain types of socializing challenging, in contrast to traditional neighborhoods, where shops and services are interspersed with residential areas and street networks are arranged in a highly connected grid. Sprawl necessitates the use of automobiles to travel between destinations and increases the risk of vehicle crashes, injuries, air pollution, and a sedentary lifestyle. (© DPZ. Printed with permission.)

lost a child to infectious diseases, such as measles and diphtheria, or lost friends and loved ones to tuberculosis. Household and animal wastes accumulated in the streets. Local water supplies were polluted. And crowding—especially among poor people—was the norm. "Noxious trades," including cloth dying, slaughtering, and tanning, all of which were frequent in cities, were located next to housing.[2] Industrial pollution, such as from gas works and steel mills, brought jobs, but it also made living in cities nearly unbearable. The leading causes of death were infectious diseases that were transmitted readily (Figure 34-4). Human waste, collected in privies and open trenches, bred flies and attracted pests. Housing for the poor was crowded, filthy, and poorly ventilated. More than 30% of all deaths were among children

under age 5—with pneumonia, tuberculosis, and gastrointestinal infections the main causes.[3]

Public health leaders began to develop partnerships with business leaders and social reformers to change the built environment in ways that focused largely on hygiene and sanitation. Clean water was brought in from rural areas to enable populations to discontinue use of contaminated wells.

It is easy to imagine the delight of the prospect of a detached home away from the unsafe city. The idea of a solo ride from work to a clean and uncrowded home in a comfortable air-conditioned vehicle would have been unimaginable. Understandably, the U.S. population welcomed the era of cheap fuel and abundant cars. Much of this progress came with

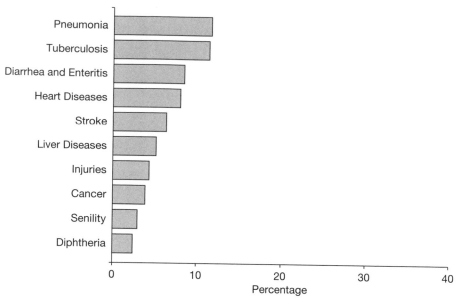

Figure 34-4. The 10 leading causes of death as a percentage of all deaths, United States, 1900. (Source: Centers for Disease Control and Prevention. Achievements in public health, 1900–1999—Control of infectious disease. Morbidity and Mortality Weekly Report 1999; 48: 621–629. Available at: http://www.cdc.gov/mmwr/preview/mmwrhtml/mm4829a1.htm#fig2. Accessed February 28, 2017.)

health benefits; 25 of the 30 years added to the average lifespan of U.S. residents in the 20th century (from 47 to 77 years) came from public health improvements, primarily immunizations and environmental health measures.

Zoning evolved to protect neighborhoods from nuisances. In the 1926 lawsuit, *Village of Euclid vs. Ambler Realty*, the Village of Euclid, Ohio, assigned zones to land owned by Amber Realty, which sued the Village for restraint of trade and the reduction of property value. The U.S. Supreme Court decided that the community had the right to zone for residential, commercial, industrial, and other uses—which became a precedent for increasing homogeny of communities in the United States. Zoning served well to prevent, for example, a tannery being operated next to residences, but, over time, it led to extreme exclusion of many uses from neighborhoods.

THE AUTOMOTIVE AND HOUSING TRANSFORMATIONS

The U.S. population's embrace of the automobile, which began early in the 20th century, coincided with—and was fueled by—a boom in

housing. Cars made new places accessible, but they required roads, stimulating governments to develop partnerships with builders. From 1906 to 1911, the Long Island Motor Parkway was built, greatly enabling habitation of the area. Automotive "destinations" were developed, including, in 1922, the first U.S. shopping mall: Kansas City's Country Club Plaza. During the Great Depression, with homelessness and unemployment increasing, the federal government made housing a national priority. After World War II, soldiers returned home to start new families, with education made accessible by the GI Bill and housing made accessible through Veterans Administration loans. Planned communities and subdivisions sprang up across the United States, further fueling a housing boom that increased homeownership from 44% in 1940 to 62% in 1960.[4]

This huge increase in housing required more roads, and car ownership was marketed as family destiny and part of the "American dream." The oil, rubber, asphalt, construction, automobile, home-finance, and other industries lobbied aggressively for a national highway system, which led to the Interstate Highway Act in 1956. Revenues for building this highway system came from gasoline taxes, which could not be used for other purposes—not even public transit. Every city wanted to be connected to the highway system; any town not connected feared, often correctly, that it would wither away.

What happened to cities? The results were mixed. Hartford, Connecticut, home to Frederick Law Olmsted, the father of landscape architecture, had a pleasant downtown on the Connecticut River. Hartford was prosperous and drew luminaries like Mark Twain in the late 1800s. But by the 1950s, it struggled to maintain its tax base, as wealthier residents moved to new suburbs that were accessible by car. The building of interstate highway I-91 along the river's west side dealt Hartford a devastating blow, destroying housing and neighborhoods and cutting off the city and its residents from the river, an environmental and social amenity. Construction of I-84 through the city resulted in loss of irreplaceable buildings. And the huge interchange of I-91 and I-84 paved over the historical original city center and crippled the potential growth of the downtown area.

Cities were not only damaged directly by highways, but they also bore the brunt of the movement of higher-income workers and their tax base to the suburbs. Federal grants and loans tended to devalue racially mixed and minority neighborhoods, exacerbating poor health status there. Developers sought to maximize land investments and rapid returns on investment by building as many homes as possible—often cheaply—on distant and less expensive land, preferably served by highways. To cut costs, these homes were often built with minimal energy efficiency and with little access to desirable amenities, such as sidewalks, parks, and nearby schools. Young families in car-dominated areas believed that their children were safer in dead-end cul de sacs.

As urban tax revenues and services decreased, cities needed to support more low-income and minority populations, which led to further attrition of tax revenues. One especially detrimental effect of this pattern was the closing of many fire stations in inner cities, which greatly contributed to increasing blight. The move of the higher-income population to suburban areas had a series of environmental impacts. With more people commuting long distances to work, the home became a place of refuge and recreation. For some, three-car garages became the

norm in new homes with game rooms and home theaters. With a garage that opened automatically, air conditioning, a large color TV, and a lawn service, one could live in a suburban home for years without meeting one's neighbors.

From 1950 to 2010, the average number of residents in a household in the United States decreased from 3.37 to 2.58.[5] Over a similar period, the average usable area in a new home increased from 1,000 to 2,400 square feet.[6] These changes were abetted by policies that used tax revenues to pay for the highways that commuters used and by a mortgage-interest tax deduction, which reduced the pain of large mortgage payments. Taxpayers in large homes with 37% marginal tax rates, in effect, had larger tax deductions than people less well off, who had a 15% marginal tax rate.

Changes in housing also impacted energy use. While energy use increases in a larger building, energy efficiency increases per unit of area, especially in multistory buildings. Detached housing is less energy-efficient than contiguous housing; however, throughout the 20th century, U.S. builders moved away from contiguous (row) houses in favor of single-family homes. Since energy efficiency represents long-term costs carried by the homeowner, there was little incentive for developers to add such amenities. In addition, more energy is lost the farther it is transmitted. Ten percent of all electricity produced in the United States is used to move it through transmission lines. Distant buildings also require more water, sewage, transport, and highway investments.

What happened to the countryside? As home building increased land valuations, taxes on agricultural land became very high and unsupportable. Prime agricultural land was lost, leading formerly self-sufficient agricultural counties to be used for residential and commercial purposes, with food and other goods brought from increasingly longer distances.

EFFECTS OF THE BUILT STRUCTURES ON THE OVERALL ENVIRONMENT

Roads supported housing sprawl, generating growing demands for services, causing increased driving and highway use, and requiring more

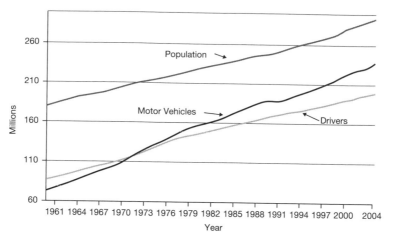

Figure 34-5. U.S. population, number of drivers, and number of motor vehicles from 1961 through 2004. (Source: https://www.fhwa.dot.gov/policyinformation/statistics/2010/dv1c.cfm. Accessed February 28, 2017.)

road surfaces. Today, roads in the United States feel crowded and congested because they are. From 1960 to 2011, the number of vehicles in the United States increased from 74 million to 242 million (Figure 34-5), and the number of licensed drivers from 87 million to 210 million.[7,8] The annual average miles driven by U.S. drivers increased from 10,043 to more than 16,000 in 2015.[9] Since each car requires a significant amount of pavement for roads and parking places, more than 60,000 square miles of land have been covered with asphalt and concrete—an area equal to the size of Georgia.[10]

EFFECTS OF THE BUILT ENVIRONMENT ON AIR QUALITY

Increased population growth, land development, and urbanization have led to the loss of natural land and habitats. Removal of trees has caused adverse health effects. More than aesthetic amenities, trees remove carbon dioxide and produce oxygen, as well as cool the local environment by as much as 2° to 9°F (3.6° to 16.2°C).[11] By reducing heat, they reduce ozone formation in the near-ground atmosphere. Cars counteract this effect. The burning of automotive fuel inherently generates heat and disperses particulate matter, oxides of nitrogen, and sulfur oxides as well as volatile organic

compounds, which, in the presence of sunlight and heat, lead to the formation of ozone. The higher the heat of combustion, the more oxides of nitrogen are produced. The more sulfur in fuel, the more sulfur oxides are produced. Incomplete fuel combustion and evaporation from fuel tanks during refueling increase volatile organic compounds. Catalytic convertors reduce, but do not eliminate, these emissions. Filters can reduce, but do not eliminate, particulates. Ozone is a highly reactive molecule and causes bronchial inflammation, asthma, pulmonary impairment, and other adverse effects. Children, people who are exercising, and people with impaired immunity are most susceptible to these effects. While the soot emitted from an old diesel truck is unsightly and unwanted, the smaller and near-invisible particles generated by newer cars can increase the risk of coronary heart disease, including myocardial infarction. (See Chapters 15, 22, and 26.)

Over the past 100 years, U.S. cities have become hotter. In Los Angeles, for example, annual maximum daytime temperatures have increased by 1.7°C (3.1°F) and minimum (nighttime) temperatures have increased by 4.0°C (7.2°F).[12] Heat presents significant health risks, most notably heat stroke. Elevated body temperature can cause death. A heat wave in Chicago in 1995 caused over 700 deaths, mainly among people without access to air conditioning who lived alone.[13] Most multiunit structures in

Chicago were built more for cold winters than for prolonged summer heat waves. Windows were small and frequently inoperable. Roofs were flat and had black tops, which absorb heat. And use of fans in overheated rooms *increased* risk of heat stroke by creating virtual convection ovens. Inadequate nighttime cooling was exacerbated by the loss of shade and the evaporation of groundwater into the atmosphere via trees and other plants, a process known as evapotranspiration.

THE BUILT ENVIRONMENT AND CLIMATE CHANGE

Ambient temperatures have increased from rising levels of greenhouse gases, including water vapor, carbon dioxide, methane, and other gases. From 1850 to 2016, the atmospheric carbon dioxide level increased from 280 to 404 ppm.[14] Two other important "climate-forcing" gases in the atmosphere are also rising at an increasing rate: from 1970 to 2015 methane increased from 1550 to 1825 ppm, and nitrous oxide increased from 320 to 340 ppm.[15] Planetary temperature levels have followed, increasing about 1.2°C over the past 100 years. (See Chapter 29.)

The burning of fossil fuels has accounted for about 80% of the increase in carbon dioxide and deforestation for about 20%. The built environment can accelerate deforestation. Most carbon dioxide emissions in the United States are related to buildings, and one-third are related to transportation. Building design that improves energy efficiency decreases waste of fossil fuels, and urban design, transit systems, and bulk shipping all reduce the use of fuel for transportation. Energy-inefficient homes have large "footprints," noncontiguous design, poorly insulated walls and windows, inadequate daylighting, and outdated illumination, heating and air-conditioning systems, and appliances.

THE BUILT ENVIRONMENT AND EFFECTS ON WATER QUANTITY AND QUALITY

Freshwater is essential for the survival of individuals and of entire civilizations and their economies. Human habitations were sited—and survived—based on water availability. Great cities flourished when large amounts of water were delivered and removed, along with wastes. Reservoirs, aqueducts, and water-removal systems have been essential to the growth and prosperity of communities—for potable water, hygiene and sanitation, and agriculture. In the United States, about one-half of drinking water comes from surface sources, and the remainder comes from groundwater wells. (See Chapter 16.)

The built environment profoundly affects water quality. The cholera outbreak in London in 1854, traced by John Snow to the Broad Street pump, illustrated the dangers of pit toilets and ponded waste overlying groundwater sources of drinking water. In general, the more layers of soil and the longer the residence time of water in soil, the better the quality of groundwater.

The built environment also affects water quantity. Moving water long distances is expensive in terms of human labor and use of fossil fuels. For soil moisture and groundwater to be recharged, rainwater and riverwater must percolate into the soil. Percolation also reduces the risk of flooding from storms; the more water captured on-site, the better. The *base flow* of a stream is the water that flows long after a rainstorm; it is the water that has been allowed to penetrate the earth and to seep slowly out to watercourses. As structures and paving cover the landscape, runoff of rainwater increases. In a forest, typically only 10% of rainwater runs off-site; in an urban area, about 55% runs off-site.[16] Sometimes the health effects of changing streets have late-appearing and indirect effects. Paving over cobblestones of streets in Lower Manhattan led to the death of street trees and loss of the shade and cooling that they provided.

To guard against disease, people in rural areas should carefully manage their water and waste systems. When human habitations become sprawled out and distant from each other, costly infrastructure for water supply and septic removal is required. To reduce these costs, many localities supply potable water through common systems but require on-site treatment by septic systems. These systems require homeowner diligence; however, thorough inspection and maintenance often occur only when the home is sold.

Between 5% and 40% of septic systems may fail, causing groundwater contamination.[17]

Water also provides an important source of recreation. People need respite on hot days and often seek park or shore lands for play and relaxation. Unfortunately, in many parts of the United States, these places are inaccessible, especially for poor people. New York City, for example, has 578 miles of waterfront, but only a fraction of it is accessible to pedestrians.

THE ADVERSE EFFECTS OF BUILDINGS ON HEALTH

People have always sought safe and secure dwelling places that afford climate protection, water, ventilation, and adequate light. The movement to assure decent housing for poor people and working people, especially children, did not arise from advanced understanding of disease processes but from an appreciation of the elements of a decent quality of life.

Science has since validated these basic human insights. Inadequate ventilation in buildings contributes to higher air levels of moisture, mold, smoke, volatile organic chemicals, radon, bacteria, allergens, and other noxious agents. Poorly insulated buildings do not mitigate outdoor heat and cold extremes and are hazardous to health. Structure, insulation, and windows can attenuate noxious outdoor noise, but, at the same time, inadequate light, including daylight, presents safety risks. All of these problems, which make reading, study, and socialization more challenging, are associated with depression. Buildings with inadequate exits and means of resisting fire are less safe, as are buildings with poor structural integrity to resist the impact of storms and earthquakes. Buildings with narrow, inaccessible, and sometimes locked stairways discourage the climbing of stairs, which can be a healthful physical activity.

Energy and Health

Structures that are single and unattached, one-story tall, and poorly designed, built, and insulated are less energy-efficient than dense, multistory, well-built structures. The longer the distance that energy—gas, oil, coal, or electricity—must be transported, the more expensive it becomes. The greater the distance that water and food, building materials, and other supplies must be transported, the more costly they become. The farther people must travel, the greater the cost of their work, school, or play. As more capital is directed to pay for inefficient use of space, less is available for education, healthcare, and other benefits.

The costs of transport are likely to change, in part because of changes in engineering, fuel-efficiency standards, and availability of energy sources. True costs of the associated environmental, social, political, and health impacts of energy production are not yet "priced" into the sale costs. The pressures of a growing global population and the depletion of natural resources will further increase demand. Renewable energy sources, such as solar and wind power, are countering some of these effects, especially as their costs become competitive with fossil fuels. As of early 2017, wind and solar power are at parity or less costly than fossil sources in several U.S. states and some countries. This trend is likely to accelerate, with the rapid development of more efficient and larger wind turbines and photovoltaic arrays, along with smaller and more powerful storage batteries. (See Chapter 29.)

Injuries

Virtually everyone knows someone who has been impacted by a car crash. The likelihood that any U.S. resident will ultimately die in a car crash is about 1 in 113.[18] Unintentional injuries are the leading cause of death for Americans age 1 to 44, with motor vehicle crashes being the first or second cause of fatal injuries in every age group above 12 months of age.[19] In 2015, more than 35,000 Americans were killed and at least 2.4 million were injured in motor vehicle crashes.[20] However, the per-mile car-related death rate in the United States decreased between 1965 and 2015, from 5.3 to 1.3 deaths per 100 million miles traveled, primarily due to laws restricting speed and alcohol use and laws requiring seat belts for vehicle passengers and helmets for cyclists.[20,21] Nevertheless, the annual cost associated with motor vehicle injuries and deaths in the United

Table 34-1. Passenger Fatality Rates, United States, 2000–2009

Type of Transit	Fatality Rate per Billion Passenger Miles
Car	7.28
Aircraft	0.07
Bus	0.11
Train	0.43
Motorcycle	213

Source: Savage I. Comparing the fatality risks in United States transportation across modes and over time. Research in Transportation Economics 2013; 43: 9–22.

States exceeds $260 billion with an additional societal harm estimated at over $870 billion.[22] While there has been major progress, average driving speeds and the number of motor vehicles have increased as enforcement has declined. The risk of car crashes increases dramatically with speed, doubling for each increase of 3 miles per hour above 35 miles per hour.[23]

Roadways are important to safety. Many roadways in the United States are designed and built to expedite movement of police cars, fire vehicles, and ambulances. Streets are wide, curves are rounded, and speed bumps minimized—all to enable rapid movement of emergency vehicles. Reducing injuries and deaths due to car crashes will require more use of improved public transit, lowering average speed, and better enforcement of laws and regulations. Table 34-1 illustrates the lifetime risks of death in the United States by car and other forms of transit.

Public transit is viable when there is population density around transit nodes sufficient to support its use. *Complete streets*, which are designed and operated to ensure safety and accessibility for pedestrians, cyclists, and public transit riders, serve to calm traffic. Features that make streets safer and more appealing to people on foot and bicycle include adequate sidewalks, bicycle lanes, pedestrian amenities, trees, and storefronts.

Chronic Disease

Obesity is a major risk factor for chronic disease.[24] From 1998 to 2009, the cost of medical treatment for obesity-related disease in the United States increased from $74 billion to over $140 billion annually. From 1998 to 2006, the prevalence

of obesity in the United States increased 37%. Obesity now accounts for more than 9% of medical expenses in the United States.[25]

People who reside in low-density areas are likely to drive more, walk less, and be overweight. Areas that have higher concentrations of fast-food restaurants have higher rates of obesity. Children whose schools are close to fast-food restaurants are more likely to eat high-calorie foods that are low in nutrients.

In the past, physical activity was woven into the activities of daily life. Getting to school or work, shopping for food, and cleaning one's home all required physical activity. Few U.S. residents were obese, and most would never have imagined joining a fitness club simply to exercise on machines. Fitness was taken somewhat for granted, and many working people longed to be free of backbreaking labor. While the lives of U.S. residents are now inundated with labor-saving devices, fast food, and instantaneous communication, we work harder, eat less healthy food, and seem to have less free time than ever before. Although fitness is essential to our health, 24% of U.S. adults report no leisure time physical activity at all.[26] In a study of thousands of nurses followed for over 25 years, those who were not physically active had a 20% to 25% higher rate of mortality than those who were.[27]

The built environment has significant impacts on physical activity. People who reside in denser areas use more public transit and have more physical activity than those who do not.[28,29] People who reside near parks and those who reside close to the places to which they travel frequently are more likely to walk or bicycle there.[30,31] Children who live close to schools are more likely to bicycle or walk to school.[32] Living in areas with walkable green spaces lengthens the life of older people in urban areas, independent of their age, gender, marital status, baseline functional status, and socioeconomic status.[33]

Mental Health

We drive up and down the gruesome, tragic suburban boulevards of commerce, and we're overwhelmed at the fantastic, awesome, stupefying ugliness of absolutely everything in sight—the fry pits, the big-box stores, the office units, the lube joints, the carpet warehouses, the parking lagoons, the jive plastic townhouse clusters, the uproar of signs, the highway itself clogged with cars—as though the whole thing had been designed by some diabolical force bent on making human beings miserable. And naturally this experience can make us feel glum about the nature and future of civilization.

—James Howard Kunstler, *Home from Nowhere*[34]

In the United States, the most prevalent mental disorder is depression, and the second-most prescribed group of medications is antidepressants. The costs of depression are substantial with losses of life, livelihood, happiness, and productivity. Stress and anxiety often coexist with and amplify depression. Nonclinical interventions for milder forms of depression, such as exercise, relate very much to the built environment. Exercise increases serotonin and alleviates depression. Contact and support from loved ones helps in managing acute depression, such as depression associated with death of a family member. Contact with nature and water revitalizes body and mind.

If one designed a depression-inducing environment, its key characteristics would include prevention of exercise, removal of interesting and pleasing natural features, and creation of social isolation and anxiety. Much of the built environment developed in the mid- to late 20th century in the United States succeeded in creating all of these characteristics. The built environment was designed for automobiles—not for salving the human mind and fostering relationships. Many U.S. residents spend hours commuting and driving long distances on high-speed, crowded roads, and many people report that their driving to and from work is more stressful than work itself.

EFFECTS ON FINANCIAL, SOCIAL, AND CULTURAL CAPITAL

In the United States, the average family income devoted to transportation has increased from about 12% in 1960 to 17% in 2015.[35] Families of lower income face an even greater burden as they allocate 30% of their average family income to transport-related expenses.[36] In some cities with substantial sprawl, the proportion is much higher.[37]

Most travel is not done for pleasure but to meet work needs and other needs of life. A need for affordable housing is a major factor. There is a maxim in the real-estate business that people drive (away from large cities) until they reach places where they can qualify for a mortgage. While some people seek a distant house in suburbia because they want or need a larger home with a lawn on a cul de sac, the primary determinant of where someone chooses to live is the cost of housing—and homes farther away from urban centers generally cost less.

This distance, however, creates perverse outcomes. Often children must be driven to schools and other activities, and many arrive home well before their commuting parents. The cost of a car is substantial, averaging $7,000 to $11,000 annually. If this amount were applied to a mortgage, the homeowner would be building assets over time rather than consuming them.[38] In addition, subdivision neighborhoods, built by developers, tend to be economically homogenous and lack economic engines. Children growing up in such places do not learn the lessons of living in a diverse community.

Social capital is the glue that holds communities together. People are healthier and live longer in communities with high social capital. After disasters, these communities recover more quickly. Long commute times to and from work and school reduce the level of community engagement and social capital. In a recent rating of best American cities, one of the measures was the level of cultural liveliness. A high prevalence of small local restaurants was recognized as an asset compared to an abundance of franchise restaurants. A vibrant cultural scene attracts most creative and productive workers, especially young workers, to an area.[39] Cities with lively cultural opportunities tend to generate more wealth during good times and to resist economic downturns better. Built environments can therefore enhance cultural life or stifle it.

EFFECTS ON VULNERABLE POPULATIONS

Children

While the built environment adversely affects all people, children are especially vulnerable. Children eat, drink, and breathe three to four times as much per unit of body weight than do adults. Children face greater hazards from air and water pollution, chemicals in food, and other environmental toxins. Because they have many years of life ahead of them, these adverse impacts last for a long time. (See Chapter 30.)

Air pollutants, especially ozone and particulate matter, cause both short- and long-term respiratory impairment in children. On days when ozone levels peak, children's school absenteeism, respiratory medication use, emergency department visits, and hospital admissions all increase. When children play outside, reside, or attend school in areas with heavy vehicle traffic, they are exposed to higher levels of air pollutants. (See Chapter 15.)

However, restricting children's exposure to the built or natural environment is also damaging. The built environment restricts children's opportunities for physical activity and contributes to childhood obesity.[40] Children who do not have opportunities for regular physical activity, such as walking or bicycling to school, are at risk for becoming overweight and developing diabetes, psychosocial problems, and other disorders. Young people spend much time in or near cars. In the United States in 2013, motor vehicle crashes were the second leading cause of death for children age 3 through 14—as passengers, pedestrians, and bicyclists.[41] About three children age 15 and younger are killed and about 500 are injured daily in motor vehicle crashes in the United States.[42]

Restricting children's exposure to the natural environment increases their risk of depression, isolation, and attention deficit hyperactivity disorder. There is a direct link between the lack of nature in children's lives—*nature-deficit disorder*—and childhood obesity, attention disorders, and depression; exposure to nature is essential for the healthy physical and emotional development of children.[43]

Older People

Older people also face health risks due to the built environment. Most U.S. communities are designed for driving, with few alternatives for older people who do not drive. Walking to stores, medical facilities, community centers, and places of recreation requires a safe pedestrian environment and a densely developed community, which is rare in much of the United States. As a result, many older people have little physical activity and social interaction and, as a result, become physically and socially isolated.

People with Physical Disabilities

The built environment must be designed to provide access to all community members, regardless of their level of physical ability. All too often, design of public transit systems, sidewalks, and crossing signals overlooks the unique needs of people with physical disabilities. People in wheelchairs require sidewalks that are wide and level and have appropriate cuts in the curb. People with visual impairment require signals that indicate safe crossing times at intersections.[44] In addition, traffic signals must be timed to allow people with disabilities sufficient time to safely cross streets.

Women

In sprawling communities, children and adults rely heavily on automobiles for transportation. Mothers, in particular, spend much time driving children to and from school, play, and athletic practice and driving older relatives to clinics and elsewhere. In 1995, the average married woman with school-age children in the United States made more than five automobile trips daily, 21% more than the average man.[45] Driving is a significant source of stress, and more time spent in cars leads to greater risk of crashes and more exposure to air pollutants. Low-density, sprawling communities do not encourage people, especially women who care for young children, elderly parents, and other family members, to perform their daily responsibilities by walking or bicycling.

Poor People and People of Color

Poor people and people of color have suffered the effects of systematic discrimination for many years. Loan and insurance policies created by the Federal Housing Administration, beginning in 1934, favored whites who purchased single-family homes, rather than members of racial and ethnic minorities who lived in multifamily, urban dwellings. For decades, these policies led to the migration of white, middle-class people out of inner cities, leading to racial segregation. With them went opportunities for employment, leading to economic segregation. Health indicators for people of color living in inner cities remain markedly worse than those of white people. A 1990 study conducted in Harlem in New York City, where at the time 96% of residents were black, found that life expectancy was lower than in Bangladesh. Harlem residents were found to die at three times the rate of white U.S. residents—mainly due to high rates of cardiovascular disease, cirrhosis, cancer, and homicide.[46] In addition, members of minority groups are more likely to live in areas with air pollution,[47] and black and Hispanic children have higher rates of asthma than do white children.[48] Exposure to air pollutants is concentrated disproportionately among poor people and people of color. (See Chapters 2 and 15.)

DEVELOPING HEALTHY COMMUNITIES

All of these descriptions of the built environment and its health consequences may seem very bleak. But nature maintains sustainability and enormous vitality by recycling. A forest, for example, does not create waste. It is critical that we, too, increase the sustainability and vitality of built-environment systems. We must move to reduce extraction and exploitation of limited natural resources and use innovative design to develop the built environment in concert with nature. In addition to sustaining our environment, we must sustain our rich cultural diversity. Many of the adverse health impacts of the built environment disproportionately affect vulnerable groups, including children, women, older people, poor people, and members of racial and ethnic minorities. We must meet the needs of these people and design and redevelop our communities to foster economic, social, and ethnic diversity—for the benefit of all people.

By 2100, the United States population is projected to almost double to 570 million.[49] To accommodate this growth in ways that are healthy, socially just, and environmentally stable, we need to design communities where people are able to move about safely on foot, bicycle, and public transit and where community members engage in the continuous process of healthy community development. It is unsustainable and irresponsible to continue using development practices that harm the public's health and that encourage people to drive cars, which emit nearly 20 pounds of carbon dioxide for each gallon of gasoline used.[50] (See Chapter 29.)

Public transit options that are clean, affordable, and accepted and utilized by local communities reduce use of fossil fuel and emissions. A major opportunity for healthy redevelopment of communities lies in the design of streets that have dense, mixed land use and are accessible and safe for all types of transit. These "complete streets" enable safe access for all users, including pedestrians, bicyclists, motorists, and transit riders of all ages and abilities.[51] Establishing and maintaining adequate bicycle lanes and bicycle paths promotes an alternative to automobile transport, and it enables people to engage in physical activity safely while moving about their communities. Bicycle paths encourage exercise, especially if they link to retail stores, schools, and public transit systems.

Urban redevelopment can promote health by decreasing the number of vacant properties and redesigning failed infrastructure projects. Redevelopment provides the opportunity to reduce urban blight, and it enables communities to have affordable housing, parks, schools, playgrounds, and other public facilities. The Embarcadero Freeway in San Francisco was originally intended to connect the Bay Bridge with the Golden Gate Bridge. It was partially constructed, but it was never completed. (If it had been fully completed, it would have cut the downtown area off from the waterfront.) More than 100,000 vehicles per day drove through local neighborhoods. The freeway was condemned after an earthquake in 1989; while the city weighed reconstruction options, the number of riders on public transit increased by 15%. City officials elected not to rebuild the freeway and instead, in 2002, redeveloped the area as a dynamic multiuse boulevard, accessible by car and public transit, with bicycle lanes, a waterfront promenade, a redeveloped historic building, and a new public plaza that hosts a farmers' market several times a week. Dense commercial development has lined nearby streets, housing in the area has increased by 51%, and jobs have increased by 23%.[52]

Another opportunity to enhance health and well-being through the built environment lies in improving architecture. Given that buildings account for 50% of the production of greenhouse gases in the United States,[53] the American Institute of Architects has asked its members to develop carbon-neutral buildings. Structures that are beautiful, quiet, and have good ventilation and lighting contribute to their surrounding areas and to the health of their occupants. Buildings with physically attractive and easily accessed stairways save electricity (because of less elevator use) and increase physical activity and socialization.

Third-party verification for green buildings, such as by Leadership in Energy and Environmental Design (LEED), can facilitate the development of environmentally sound buildings, ranging from homes to corporate headquarters. Certified buildings are resource efficient, using less water and energy and reducing greenhouse gas emissions.

Schools are a critically important element in the shift to healthier built environments. The number of schools in the United States decreased from 262,000 in 1930 to 91,000 in 2009, while average school size increased.[54] New schools are typically located on large sites on inexpensive land, distant from the neighborhoods that they serve. For many years, state and local governments had *minimum acreage standards*, which mandated that communities build schools on sites that met specific size requirements, depending on the type of school and the number of students. Although these standards are no longer nationally mandated, 27 states still have similar requirements.[54] Consequently, many schools are not located within walking or bicycling distance

for their students. Safety issues are a major concern for parents, who consistently cite traffic danger as a reason why they do not allow their children to bike or walk to school.[55] Children who are sedentary are at increased risk during their lifetimes for obesity, diabetes, and cardiovascular disease. In addition, decreases in walking and bicycling have had damaging effects on traffic congestion and air quality around schools.[56] A federal government program addresses these issues by providing funding and technical support to community programs that promote children safely and routinely walking and bicycling to school.[57]

Parks and green spaces are also essential parts of a healthy environment. Trees and other plants filter pollutants in the air and water, mitigate wind, reduce solar heat gain, stabilize soil to prevent or reduce erosion, create animal habitats, help filter and absorb stormwater runoff, and may help mitigate carbon emissions.[58] Parks are, by nature, public and recreational, and they provide opportunities for social interaction and community building. Parks that are well admired and frequented are community assets that can spur economic growth nearby; homes located close to parks often have higher resale value than those more distant.

The built environment has significant adverse impacts on water quality and availability, which are likely to intensify as global temperatures increase. For example, in the Los Angeles area, rainfall is very limited, and more than half of the water used by its 13 million residents comes from distant locations, such as the Colorado River. Transporting water there costs a lot of money and energy. Since the area is largely paved with impermeable materials, there are few places where rainwater can soak into the ground. Instead, it flows across hard surfaces, collecting oil, pesticides, animal waste, and garbage before flowing into storm drains and other channels that lead to the Pacific Ocean, squandering rainwater and polluting rivers, streams, and the ocean. A local organization advocates for residents to collect rainwater in order to reduce the need to import water, decrease runoff, and supply more water during dry months.[59]

The availability of food is another issue linking health with the built environment. Throughout the United States, urban farms and community gardens are producing more local food. For example, in 2009, San Francisco initiated an audit of all unused city land that could be developed into gardens or small-scale farms to create jobs and promote local production of fresh food. Another program in the area, which integrates science with gardening, uses school gardens to teach students about the importance of good nutrition, while producing the ingredients for student lunches, eliminating food transportation costs, and ensuring the freshness of food.

CONCLUSION

The World Health Organization defines health as "a state of complete physical, mental, and social well-being and not merely the absence of disease or infirmity."[60] The quality of our built environment affects our health and quality of life.

Academic institutions have major roles to play in developing healthy built environments. Academic courses and further research are needed to expand the body of knowledge on the relationship between the built environment and public health. Research on the association between economics, health, and development policy is especially important. We must develop metrics and methods to account for all of the financial, environmental, social, and health costs associated with development strategies. Our focus must shift away from getting a rapid return on investments to developing sustainable systems.

A *health impact assessment* (HIA) is a "combination of procedures, methods, and tools by which a policy, program, or project may be judged as to its potential effects on the health of a population, and the distribution of those effects within the population."[61] Using an HIA enables community planners to apply public health analysis to the built environment. By explicitly incorporating health into design and planning decisions, an HIA can be utilized to anticipate and quantify the health impacts of a specific development strategy.

This critical period for humankind and for the earth requires informed, holistic, and strong decision-making. Health practitioners, urban and rural planners, government officials, and community members must demonstrate leadership in developing and implementing sustainable approaches to the challenges in our natural and built environments.

ACKNOWLEDGMENTS

The author acknowledges the assistance of Rachel Cushing, Lisa Martin, and Tamanna Rahman in the development of this chapter.

REFERENCES

1. Jefferson T. Letter to Benjamin Rush, 1800. In: Lipscomb A, Bergh A, Johnston R (eds.). The writings of Thomas Jefferson, Vol. 10. Washington, DC: Thomas Jefferson Memorial Association of the United States, 1903–1904.
2. Duffy J. The sanitarians: A history of American public health. Urbana: University of Illinois Press, 1990.
3. Centers for Disease Control and Prevention. Control of infectious diseases, 1900–1999. Morbidity and Mortality Weekly Report 1999; 48: 621–629.
4. U.S. Bureau of the Census. Average population per household and family: 1940–Present. 2004. Available at: http://www.census.gov/population/socdemo/hh-fam/tabHH-6.pdf. Accessed January 5, 2017.
5. Lofquist D, Lugaila T, O'Connell M, Feliz S. Households and families: 2010. 2010 census briefs. Available at: https://www.census.gov/prod/cen2010/briefs/c2010br-14.pdf. Accessed January 5, 2017.
6. Dietz R. New single-family home size increases at the start of 2015. Available at: http://eyeonhousing.org/2015/05/new-single-family-home-size-increases-at-the-start-of-2015/. Accessed January 5, 2017.
7. Bureau of Transportation Statistics. Table 1-11: Number of U.S. aircraft, vehicles, vessels, and other conveyances. Available at: https://www.rita.dot.gov/bts/sites/rita.dot.gov.bts/files/publications/national_transportation_statistics/2011/html/table_01_11.html. Accessed January 5, 2017
8. U. S. Department of Transportation. Office of Highway Policy Information. Licensed drivers, vehicle registrations and resident population. Available at: https://www.fhwa.dot.gov/policyinformation/statistics/2010/dv1c.cfm. Accessed January 5, 2017.

9. U. S. Department of Transportation, Federal Highway Administration, Office of Highway Policy Information. Average annual miles per driver by age group. Available at https://www.fhwa.dot.gov/ohim/onh00/bar8.htm. Accessed January 5, 2017.

10. Brown L. Paving the planet: Cars and crops competing for land. Earth Policy Institute website. February 14, 2001. Available at: http://www.earth-policy.org/index.php?/plan_b_updates/2000/alert12. Accessed January 5, 2017.

11. U.S. Environmental Protection Agency. Reducing urban heat islands: compendium of strategies. Available at: http://www.epa.gov/heatisland/resources/pdf/TreesandVegCompendium.pdf. Accessed January 5, 2017.

12. LaDochy S, Medina R, Patzert W. Recent California climate variability: Spatial and temporal patterns in temperature trends. Climate Research 2007; 33: 159–169.

13. Semenza JC, Rubin CH, Falter KH, et al. Heat-related deaths during the July 1995 heat wave in Chicago. New England Journal of Medicine 1996; 335: 84–90.

14. NOAA Earth System Research Labortory Global Monitoring Division. Trends in atmospheric carbon dioxide. Available at: https://www.esrl.noaa.gov/gmd/ccgg/trends/. Accessed January 5, 2017.

15. NOAA Earth System Research Labortory Global Monitoring Division. NOAA's annual greenhouse gas index: An introduction. Available at: https://www.esrl.noaa.gov/gmd/aggi/. Accessed January 5, 2017.

16. Federal Interagency Stream Restoration Working Group. Stream corridor restoration: Principles, processes, practices. Available at: https://www.nrcs.usda.gov/Internet/FSE_DOCUMENTS/stelprdb1044574.pdf. Accessed January 5, 2017.

17. Schueler T. Microbes in urban watersheds: Concentrations, sources & pathways: The practice of watershed protection. Ellicott City, MD: Center for Watershed Protection, 2000, pp. 74–84. Available at http://owl.cwp.org/mdocs-posts/elc_pwp17/. Accessed January 5, 2017

18. National Safety Council. Odds of death due to injury, United States, 2016. Available at: http://www.nsc.org/learn/safety-knowledge/Pages/injury-facts-chart.aspx. Accessed January 5, 2017.

19. Centers for Disease Control and Prevention. Ten leading causes of injury deaths by age group highlighting unintentional injury deaths, United States, 2014 Available at: https://www.cdc.gov/injury/images/lc-charts/leading_causes_of_injury_deaths_unintentional_injury_2014_1040w740h.gif. Accessed January 5, 2017.

20. National Highway Traffic Safety Administration's National Center for Statistics and Analysis. 2008 traffic safety annual assessment—Highlights. June 2009. Available at: http://www-nrd.nhtsa.dot.gov/Pubs/811172.pdf. Accessed January 10, 2017.

21. NHTSA's National Center for Statistics and Analysis. Fatalities and fatality rate per 100 million VMT, by year, 1965–2015 per 100 million VMT. Available at: https://crashstats.nhtsa.dot.gov/Api/Public/ViewPublication/812318. Accessed January 5, 2017.

22. U.S. Department of Transportation, National Highway Traffic Safety Administration. The economic and societal impact of motor vehicle crashes, 2010 (revised 2015). Available at: https://crashstats.nhtsa.dot.gov/Api/Public/ViewPublication/812013. Accessed January 5, 2017.

23. Kloeden CN, McLean AJ, Glonek G. Reanalysis of traveling speed and the risk of crash involvement in Adelaide, South Australia. Australian Transport Safety Bureau, April 2002. Available at: http://casr.adelaide.edu.au/speed/RESPEED.PDF. Accessed January 5, 2017.

24. Finkelstein EA, Trogdon JG, Cohen JW, Dietz W. Annual medical spending attributable to obesity: Payer- and service-specific estimates. Health Affairs, July 27, 2009. Available at: http://content.healthaffairs.org/cgi/content/short/hlthaff.28.5.w822. Accessed January 5, 2017

25. Berenson T. Obesity now costs the world $2 trillion, November 20, 2014. Available at: http://time.com/3597407/obesity-global-cost-report/. Accessed January 5, 2017.

26. Centers for Disease Control and Prevention. 2014: Percent of adults who indulge in no leisure-time physical activity. Available at: https://nccd.cdc.gov/NPAO_DTM/IndicatorSummary.aspx?category=71&indicator=36. Accessed January 5, 2017.

27. Rockhill B, Willett WC, Manson JE, et al. Physical activity and mortality: A prospective study among women. American Journal of Public Health 2001; 91: 578–583.

28. Atkinson JL, Sallis JF, Saelens BE, et al. The association of neighborhood design and recreational environments with physical activity. American Journal of Health Promotion 2005; 19: 304–309.

29. Frank LD, Pivo G. Impacts of mixed use and density on utilization of three modes of

travel: Single-occupant vehicle, transit, and walking. Transportation Research Record 1995; 1466: 44–52.

30. Cohen DA, McKenzie TL, Sehgal A, et al. Contribution of public parks to physical activity. American Journal of Public Health 2007; 97: 509–514.

31. Roemmich JN, Epstein LH, Raja S, et al. Association of access to parks and recreational facilities with the physical activity of young children. Preventive Medicine 2006; 43: 437–441.

32. Ewing R, Schroeer W, Greene W. School location and student travel analysis of factors affecting mode choice. Transportation Research Record 2004; 1895: 55–63.

33. Takano T, Nakamura K, Watanabe M. Urban residential environments and senior citizens' longevity in megacity areas: The importance of walkable green spaces. Journal of Epidemiology and Community Health 2002; 56: 913–918.

34. Kunstler JH. Home from nowhere: Remaking our everday world for the 21st century. New York: Simon & Schuster Limited, 1996.

35. Bureau of Labor Statistics. Consumer expenditures in 2015. Available at: https://www.bls.gov/news.release/pdf/cesan.pdf. Accessed January 5, 2017.

36. Bureau of Labor Statistics. 100 years of U.S. consumer pending: Data for the nation, New York City, and Boston. Available at: http://www.bls.gov/opub/uscs/home.htm. Accessed January 5, 2017.

37. Surface Transportation Policy Project. Center for Neighborhood Technology. Driven to spend: A transportation and quality of life publication. Available at: http://transact.org/wp-content/uploads/2014/04/DriventoSpend.pdf. Accessed January 10, 2017.

38. Bureau of Labor Statistics. Consumer expenditures 2015. Available at: https://www.bls.gov/news.release/cesan.nr0.htm Accessed January 5, 2017.

39. Florida R. The rise of the creative class: And how it's transforming work, leisure, community and everyday life. New York: Basic Books, 2003.

40. Committee on Environmental Health. The built environment: Designing communities to promote physical activity in children. Pediatrics 2009; 123: 1591–1598.

41. National Highway Traffic Safety Administration. Traffic safety facts, 2013 data: Children. Washington, DC: National Highway Traffic Safety Administration, 2015.

42. National Highway Traffic Safety Administration. Traffic safety facts 2014: A compilation of motor vehicle crash data from the fatality analysis reporting system and the general estimates system. Washington, DC: National Highway Traffic Safety Administration, 2014, p. 106.

43. Louv R. Last child in the woods. Chapel Hill: Algonquin Books, 2006.

44. Barlow JM, Bentzen BL, Tabor LS. Accessible pedestrian signals: Synthesis and guide to best practice. Transportation Research Board, National Research Council, May 2003. Available at: http://onlinepubs.trb.org/onlinepubs/nchrp/nchrp_rrd_278/. Accessed January 5, 2017

45. Surface Transportation Policy Project. High mileage moms. Washington, DC, May 1999.

46. McCord C, Freeman HP. Excess mortality in Harlem. New England Journal of Medicine 1990; 322: 173–177.

47. Wernette DR, Nieves LA. Breathing polluted air: Minorities are disproportionately exposed. EPA Journal 1992; 18: 16–17.

48. Persky VW, Slezak J, Contreras A, et al. Relationships of race and socioeconomic status with prevalence, severity, and symptoms of asthma in Chicago school children. Annals of Allergy, Asthma and Immunology 1998; 81: 266–271.

49. U.S. Census Bureau. Annual projections of the total resident population as of July 1: Middle, lowest, highest, and zero international migration series, 1999 to 2100. Available at: http://www.census.gov/population/projections/data/national/natsum.html Accessed January 5, 2017.

50. Environmental Protection Agency. Emssions facts: Average carbon dioxide emissions resulting from gasoline and diesel fuel. Available at: https://energy.gov/eere/vehicles/fact-576-june-22-2009-carbon-dioxide-gasoline-and-diesel-fuel Accessed January 5, 2017.

51. Smart Growth America. National Complete Streets Coalition. https://smartgrowthamerica.org/program/national-complete-streets-coalition/. Accessed January 5, 2017.

52. Congress for the New Urbanism. San Francisco's Embarcadero Freeway. Available at: https://www.cnu.org/highways-boulevards/model-cities/embarcadaro. Accessed January 5, 2017.

53. American Institute of Architects. AIA 2030 commitment progress report. Available at: https://www.aia.org/resources/6676-aia-2030-commitment-progress-report. Accessed January 5, 2017.

54. Safe Routes to School. School siting: Location affects the potential to walk or bike. Available at: http://saferoutespartnership.org/state/bestpractices/schoolsiting. Accessed January 5, 2017.

55. Centers for Disease Control and Prevention. Barriers to children walking to or from school, United States, 2004. Available at: http://www.cdc.gov/mmwr/preview/mmwrhtml/mm5438a2.htm. Accessed January 5, 2017

56. Centers for Disease Control and Prevention. Health topics: Childhood obesity. Available at: http://www.cdc.gov/HealthyYouth/obesity/index.htm. Accessed January 5, 2017.

57. U. S. Department of Transportation Federal Highway Administration. Safe routes to school. Available at: http://www.fhwa.dot.gov/environment/safe_routes_to_school/. Accessed January 5, 2017.

58. American Society of Landscape Architects. Livable communities: Public policies: Vegetation in the built environment. Available at: https://www.asla.org/livable.aspx. Accessed January 5, 2017.

59. Tree People. Available at: http://www.treepeople.org/. Accessed January 5, 2017.

60. World Health Organization. Constitution of WHO: Principles. Available at: http://www.who.int/about/mission/en/. Accessed February 22, 2017.

61. Committee on Health Impact Assessment; National Research Council. Improving health in the United States: The role of health impact assessment. Washington, DC: National Academies Press, 2011. Available at: https://www.nap.edu/catalog/13229/improving-health-in-the-united-states-the-role-of-health. Accessed January 5, 2017.

35

A Global Perspective
on Occupational Health and Safety

Jorma H. Rantanen

Occupational hazards and resultant illnesses and injuries are serious and frequently occurring problems in the United States—as reflected by other chapters in this book—and in other high-income countries. However, these problems are generally far more serious and occur much more frequently in low- and middle-income countries (LMICs), many of which have been described as "developing countries" or "emerging economies." This chapter presents a global perspective on occupational health and safety, initially presenting a global overview of work and workers, then focusing on vulnerable workers and some industries and some issues of special concern. While not intended to comprehensively cover all important topics and issues of globalization, this chapter aims to provide some basic information and to stimulate the reader to become actively engaged in global and international aspects of occupational health and safety.

THE GLOBAL WORKFORCE

The global workforce comprises about 3.3 billion people, comprising 68% of all people from 15 to 64 years of age.[1] The International Labour Organization (ILO) has identified four main economic categories for employment: wage and salary workers, "own-account workers" (workers who work on their own account or with one or more partners in a self-employed job and have not engaged on a continuous basis any employees to work for them[2]), employers, and contributing family members. In North America and Europe, employment tends to be formal and relatively stable; however, in Africa and Asia, work is mainly informal and in Latin America almost half of all workers are in the informal sector. In industrialized countries (mainly in North America and Europe), 70% to 80% of workers are wage-earners, usually on permanent contracts. In contrast, about 70% of workers in sub-Saharan Africa and South Asia are own-account workers or "contributing family members"— who are informally employed[3-5] (Table 35-1).

Approximately 42 million workers are added to the global workforce each year. There are approximately 200 million unemployed workers, 75 million of whom are young. About one-fourth of workers (approximately 900 million) are considered the "working poor," whose families earn less than the equivalent of US$2 per day. The global workforce also includes

Table 35-1. Percentage of workers in the four major categories of employment in Africa, high-income countries, and globally, 2016.

Employment Status	Africa	High-income Countries	Globally
Employees*	34.8%	86.1%	54.8%
Employers	2.7%	3.9%	2.4%
Own-account workers	42.7%	9.1%	33.6%
Contributing family members	19.8%	0.9%	9.2%

* Wage and salary workers.
Source: International Labour Organization. Status in employment -- ILO modelled estimates, November 2016. Available at: http://www.ilo.org/ilostat/faces/oracle/webcenter/portalapp/pagehierarchy/Page3.jspx;ILOSTATCOOKIE=Af4qYnvgmVQjTlvLjB5xLIqrQ8hcGoytL-qiZ6hXFH29Fmnd07-M!-1311753266?MBI_ID=32&_adf.ctrl-state=18cwnin6q3_33&_afrLoop=306034437462395&_afrWindowMode=0&_afrWindowId=moat_callback#!%40%40%3F_afrWindowId%3Dmoat_callback%26_afrLoop%3D306034437462395%26MBI_ID%3D32%26_afrWindowMode%3D0%26_adf.ctrl-state%3D3n2y4yfp7_4. Accessed August 26, 2017.

approximately 150 million migrant workers, 100 million domestic workers, and 102 million workers 65 years of age and older (28% of men and 15% of women).[2,6]

Social protections are lacking for many workers. For example, there are approximately 1.9 billion workers (about 60% of the global workforce) who are not included in "old-age pension" programs. Many workers do not have unemployment protection; for example, in ILO member states, 68% of workers do not have this protection. In addition, more than 60% of workers (1.92 billion) are not covered by insurance for compensation for occupational injuries and diseases.[7]

In general, more informal and precarious employment is associated with more work instability and more job insecurity. Workers with lower socioeconomic status have higher risks of unemployment, poverty, and occupational illness and injury. Informal employment and job instability are associated with low income and poverty, lack of social protection, and little or no access to health services.[4,8,9]

SHIFTING EMPLOYMENT TRENDS

During the past 70 years, modes of work have changed substantially. In the second half of the 20th century, employment in industrialized countries evolved from primary production to manufacturing (secondary production) and then to services (tertiary production). In the past 20 years, there has been a global shift from agriculture and other primary production to services. Especially in industrialized countries, the combination of computerization, automation, and robotization have reduced the need for manual industrial workers and increased the need for workers with highly competent skills—leading to a "white collarization" of the workforce. Different parts of the world are in different stages of this evolution, with industrialized countries at a more advanced stage, followed by rapidly industrializing countries in Asia and Latin America. There has been rapid growth in the services sector, not only in North America and Europe but also in East Asia. Globally, close to 50% of all workers work in the services sector. While 43% of men work in services, 62% of women are employed in this sector—a marked increase since 1995, when 41% of women worked in this sector. In North America, 91% of women work in services, and in northern, southern, and western Europe, 86% work in this sector.[1,10]

During the second half of the 20th century, employment in agriculture declined in high- and middle-income countries but remained high in low-income countries, such as countries in Southeast Asia and sub-Saharan Africa, where most workers still work in agriculture. An increasing percentage of agricultural workers are female—about 25% globally.[8,9]

Long-term trends of automation, computerization, and expansion of the services sector have substantially reduced heavy physical and manual work and substantially increased the number of jobs in office-type environments—with important implications for psychosocial hazards at work. Simultaneously, differences in working conditions and workloads between workers in agriculture, forestry, and fisheries and those in the office and service sector have increased.

GLOBALIZATION

Globalization involves the free movement of capital, goods, technologies, and services across international borders. It has profound demographic and cultural, health and safety, economic and political, and ecological and ethical implications. Its impact may be positive or negative, depending on location, industry, individuals affected, and other factors.

Globalization has positively impacted global economic growth, trade, poverty, and, for many people, employment opportunities. It has also positively impacted distribution of new technologies and Internet access, thereby enhancing global connectivity.[11-13]

On the other hand, globalization has many negative impacts, including forced migration, unemployment for many people, widening gaps in income and wealth, increased transmission of some infectious diseases, ecological problems, spread of financial crises, and occupational and environmental health problems. The impacts of globalization have greatly varied among countries and among socioeconomic groups of people. The "winners" are middle-class people in China, India, and countries with emerging economies as well as extremely rich people in countries with advanced economies. The "losers" are middle-class people in industrialized countries and, generally to a greater degree, poor people in many countries in Africa, Asia, Latin America, and Eastern Europe. Many countries have had difficulty adapting to these impacts.[12,14,15]

In many LMICs, national governments have established *free enterprise zones*, in which multinational corporations have been encouraged, with reduced taxes and other incentives, to establish factories. At these factories, companies have often employed many workers for small-scale manufacturing, such as garment making and microelectronics assembly, and other types of jobs. Workers benefit from potentially steady employment, but, as the ILO and other

organizations have reported, in all countries with free enterprise zones, many workers face occupational health and safety hazards, lower minimum wages, and very long work shifts. Companies in these zones benefit from a potentially large number of available workers who are willing to work long hours, at low wages, with minimal benefits, without occupational safety services, and without social protection.[16]

Globalization has often facilitated the export of hazardous materials and hazardous industries from high-income countries to LMICs. For example, multinational corporations that produce pesticides that are banned or restricted in the high-income countries where they are based have sometimes exported these pesticides to LMICs, where their sale and use is not restricted. Often, agriculture and public health officials in the countries importing these hazardous pesticides have not been adequately informed about health risks associated with their use, and, as a result, serious health and environmental damage has often occurred.

The international community, under the leadership of the United Nations Environmental Programme and the Food and Agricultural Organization of the United Nations, has responded with the Rotterdam Convention (on the export and import of hazardous chemicals) and Stockholm Convention on Persistent Organic Pollutants, which minimize generation, require prior informed consent, regulate, and ban the transfer and use of hazardous chemicals and hazardous wastes. In view of the Sustainable Development Goals of the United Nations, more-coordinated international actions are being planned for the International Conference on Chemicals Management in 2020.[17,18]

In many ways, globalization has socially affected, often in adverse ways, agricultural workers (including family farmers), fishers and forestry workers, domestic workers, owners and workers in microenterprises, workers in traditional manufacturing industries, aging workers, female workers, workers with limited education, migrant workers, temporary and contingent workers, and those who are unemployed. Gaps between the rich and the poor have been widening. Financial crises and armed conflicts aggravate these situations. Simultaneously, social protection policies and social services have generally been declining.[7,11,12]

OCCUPATIONAL INJURIES AND ILLNESSES

Each day globally, an average of 86,000 workers are injured at work, 5,600 develop occupational illnesses, and about 6,300 die as a result of occupational causes. Each year, an estimated 313,000 workers die as a result of fatal occupational injuries and about 2 million as a result of fatal work-related diseases.[19] Injuries and illnesses related to work account for about 2% of all disability-adjusted life years lost. Occupational injuries and illnesses have a profound economic impact, equal to about 5% of gross domestic product of many countries.

The concept of occupational injury is clear and easy to understand.[20] Countries vary, however, in their practices of registering and reporting injuries, which may include all injuries, only severe or fatal injuries, or those associated with a minimum number of days away from work. (Most countries include [and compensate for] injuries incurred while commuting to or from work.) The registration and reporting of occupational diseases are less developed in most countries. Rates of fatal occupational injuries differ widely among countries. These rates are substantially higher in LMICs. However, even among high-income countries, rates of fatal occupational injuries differ widely. For example, in 2008, there was a wide (7.7-fold) variation in the rates of fatal injury among 29 countries (including 28 European Union [EU] countries and Switzerland). (See Figure 35-1.) Workers at especially high risk of injury at work are the

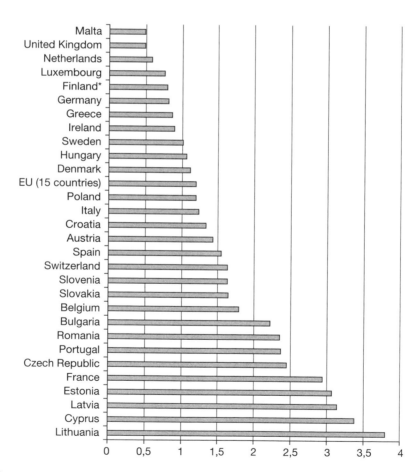

Figure 35-1. Rates per 100,000 of fatal occupational injuries in 29 European countries, including 28 European Union countries and Switzerland, 2008. (Source: Health and Safety Executive. Last updated November 2016. Available at: http://www.hse.gov.uk/statistics/tables/index.htm#europeancomparisons. Accessed March 1, 2017. Note: Data for Finland added by the author.)

Table 35-2. Estimated number of deaths attributed to hazardous substances at work, 2011.

Type of Disorder	Estimated Number of Deaths	Percentage of Total
Respiratory diseases	441,016	49.6%
Cancers	361,109	40.6%
Cardiovascular diseases	75,470	8.5%
Genitourinary diseases	10,186	1.1%
Neuropsychiatric conditions	1,112	0.1%
Total	888,893	100.0%

Source: International Labour Organization. Safety and health at work: A vision for sustainable prevention. 2014. Available at: http://www.ilo.org/wcmsp5/groups/public/---ed_protect/---protrav/---safework/documents/publication/wcms_301214.pdf. Accessed March 1, 2017.

1 billion people who work in agriculture, in the informal sector, or as domestic workers. Also at high risk are those who work without formal employment contracts and therefore often do not have legal occupational health and safety protection or workers' compensation insurance coverage. In general, their working conditions are hazardous, their employment insecure, and their income low. There are many other types of workers at high risk of fatal occupational injuries including emergency and rescue workers in major industrial and natural disasters.[20-22]

Although not done in the United States (or elsewhere in this book), the ILO and countries in the EU make a distinction between the following two categories of diseases.[21,22] *Occupational diseases* are those for which the causal association between work, workplace exposures, or other causal agents can be identified and associated with the onset of disease (usually 50% or higher attribution). In contrast, *work-related diseases* may be either (a) partially caused by work or (b) diseases in which work affects the symptoms or the course of the disease. Attributing multiple causes of work-related diseases may be difficult; while these diseases may not be compensable, identifying them may provide important information for prevention.[19-21] The causes of deaths due to work-related diseases are as follows:

Circulatory diseases: 35%
Malignant neoplasms: 29%
"Accidents" and violence: 15%
Communicable diseases: 10%
Respiratory diseases: 7%
Neuropsychiatric conditions: 2%
Digestive diseases: 1%
Genitourinary diseases: 1%.

Table 35-3. Distribution of occupational diseases, by cause, Finland, 2012

Cause	Number	Percentage
Chemical factors	2,034	46.2%
Physical factors	1,141	25.9%
Biological factors	596	13.5%
Ergonomic factors	476	10.8%
Other	157	3.6%
Total	4,404	100.0%

Source: Occupational diseases in Finland 2012: New cases of recognized and suspected occupational diseases. Available at: https://www.julkari.fi/bitstream/handle/10024/131563/Occupational_diseases_2012.pdf?sequence=1: Accessed March 1, 2017.

There are several classification systems for recording and analyzing occupational diseases. The ILO has identified 105 categories of occupational diseases, which have been grouped into broader categories for reporting the annual incidence of occupational diseases. (See Table 35-2.) In reporting occupational disease, countries provide data not only on diagnoses of affected workers but also on cause, degree of severity, possible loss of work ability, and possible disability.[23] (See Table 35-3.)

Chemical Exposures

The production and trade of chemicals is globalized with concentration in large multinational corporations. Global production and trade of chemicals has grown for decades due to the essential role of chemicals in production of almost all other industrial products. In 2015, global chemical production was valued at US$5 trillion, about 6% of the total global gross domestic product. The annual volume of global production of hazardous chemicals is not known; however, the annual generation of hazardous waste is estimated at 400 million tons (about 60 kg per capita). Chemical production, especially of bulk chemicals, is moving from industrialized high-income countries to LMICs, which generally have less capacity for addressing chemical health and safety hazards than high-income countries. China and countries in North America and Europe are the main producers of chemicals, but the role of other Asian countries is growing rapidly. Global employment in the chemical industry has been estimated at 10 million—about 1.3% of workers in manufacturing and about 0.3% of all workers throughout the world.[18,24]

Chemicals have a wide range of uses. Bulk chemicals are used as raw materials in industrial processes. Fertilizers, pesticides, and other agrochemicals are used in the growing production of food, feed, and other plant materials. (See Figure 35-2.) Pharmaceuticals are used in healthcare. Metals have many industrial uses. Petrochemicals are used as fuels and in production of polymers and many other synthetic materials. Newly emerging electrochemicals and nanomaterials have an incalculable number of potential uses.[17,18] (See Chapter 8 for a discussion of nanomaterials.)

While large-scale chemical production is concentrated in a relatively few countries, consumption of chemicals is global. International organizations, national governments, industries, and corporations work to improve chemical safety and product safety through a variety of approaches, including product standards, risk assessment, occupational and environmental regulations and guidelines, and programs to monitor workers' health and environmental protection.

The European Union's Registration, Evaluation, Authorisation and Restriction of Chemicals (REACH) program is an advanced system for chemical regulation in both global and domestic markets. There are about 30,000 potentially hazardous chemicals used in Europe, with about 300 new ones added each year. REACH includes all of the 28 member states of the EU as well as Iceland, Lichtenstein, and Norway. Established in 2007, REACH aims to improve protection of the health of workers, consumers, and the environment through a system in which chemicals are registered, evaluated, authorized, and, if necessary, restricted. Included is health risk assessment, for both toxic and socioeconomic impacts.[25]

REACH aims to assess and control the entire life cycle of new chemicals entering the market.

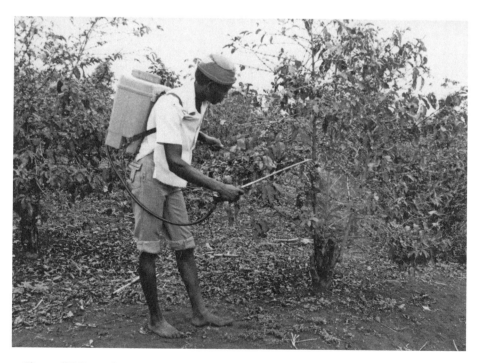

Figure 35-2. Worker spraying herbicide on coffee plants in Kenya. (Photograph by Barry S. Levy.)

It includes both the chemicals produced in EU member states as well as the import of chemicals into the EU area. It also aims to control export of chemicals from the EU area. All substances manufactured, exported, or imported in quantities totaling over 1 ton per year must be registered in the REACH database. Substances not registered may not be manufactured or imported.

The ILO and the United Nations Environmental Programme have helped to spread the concepts and underlying philosophy of REACH to many countries. In addition, the Organisation of Economic Co-operation and Development (OECD) in partnership with other international organizations has developed a system for harmonized labeling and marking of chemicals and premarketing risk assessment. The OECD and the ILO have developed guidance for control of exposure through occupational exposure limits (OELs). Participating countries have implemented OELs for 500 to 1,500 hazardous workplace chemicals.[18,26-28]

In all economic sectors, workers are exposed to chemicals. In the EU, 18% of workers handle hazardous substances and 11% are exposed to vapors and fumes at work. In addition, 11% of workers are exposed to tobacco smoke at work.[28] If the European data are extrapolated to the world, the total number of workers handling hazardous substances at work is 600 million, which likely is an underestimate.

Beyond the chemical industry, workers are exposed to hazardous chemicals in:

- Primary extraction industries (mining, quarrying, and oil and gas drilling)
- Manufacturing industries, including food production
- Agriculture
- Service industries
- Healthcare
- Construction
- Waste disposal and recycling.

Psychosocial Burdens of Work

An increasing number of workers suffer from psychosocial stress at work because of increasing pressures in their jobs, work environment, organization of work, and employment policies and practices. (See Chapter 14.) Psychological stressors in the work environment have been recognized and intensively studied in high-income countries, but they are likely more intensive and burdensome in LMICs, though less recognized and studied in these countries. Globalization has increased these stressors in several ways, including:

- Application of new technologies that require increased knowledge and skills
- Increased work intensity, including high pace of automated production
- Outsourcing and "offshoring" of work
- Loss of traditional manufacturing jobs in high-income countries, with pressure to find new jobs in other industries and/or new locations along with the increased risk of unemployment
- Changes in job tasks and necessary skills, leading to needs for retraining, especially difficult for older workers
- Introduction of "immature" technologies, equipment, and procedures, with adaptation made more difficult because they are new and not previously tested or refined
- Changes in organization of work
- Growing time pressures to produce along with pressures for productivity, while maintaining high standards of quality
- New management methods, making wages and continuing employment dependent on quantitative and qualitative work output
- Increased need to maintain work abilities and functional capacity, especially given the other challenges at work.[29-31]

A recent study identified the leading causes of work-related stress in countries of the EU (listed here in order of frequency reported by workers studied):

Job reorganization or job insecurity
Hours worked or workload
Subjected to unacceptable behavior, bullying, and/or harassment
Lack of clarity on roles and responsibilities
Limited opportunities to manage one's own work patterns
Working at high speed
Working with tight deadlines.[29]

Psychological health and well-being at work are increasingly recognized not only as occupational health and safety issues but also as important factors related to productivity and quality of products and services.[29]

Vulnerable Workers

An estimated 1.5 billion workers are especially vulnerable to occupational health and safety hazards because of their position in the labor market (economically and socially vulnerable workers), risks specific to their jobs, or personal health–related factors. The percentage of workers who are considered vulnerable varies by country. (See Figure 35-3.) Since there are different causes of vulnerability for different groups of workers, different types of actions are needed to protect their health and safety and to prevent occupational illnesses and injuries.[32-34]

European researchers and those from the ILO have categorized vulnerable workers into the following three slightly overlapping groups:

1. *Economically and socially vulnerable workers:* This group includes own-account workers and unpaid family workers, young workers, unemployed workers, migrants,

the working poor, precarious workers, temporary-agency workers, and informal-sector workers. The relationship between health and poverty is multifaceted. Poor health and associated poor ability to work lowers one's potential for employment and therefore increases the likelihood of poverty. In addition, the high costs of healthcare in LMICs may lead to *health poverty* from which hundreds of millions of people, including the working poor, suffer. Protecting these workers requires improved labor and social policies by governments and better provision of occupational health and safety services for them.[6,32,34]

2. *Workers vulnerable because of health and safety risks specific to their jobs:* These workers are vulnerable because of occupational health and safety hazards as well as poor access to occupational health services, including measures to reduce these hazards and measures to prevent illnesses and injuries. This group of vulnerable workers includes those in construction, agriculture, and small-scale enterprises, as well as self-employed workers and informal-sector and domestic workers. These workers need protective health and safety measures at their

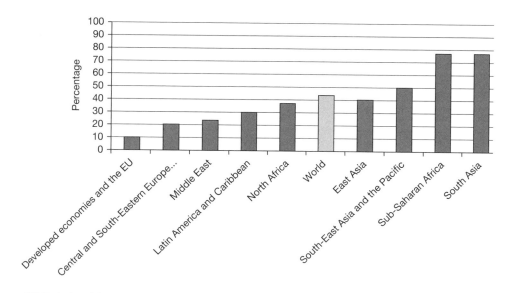

Figure 35-3. Vulnerable employment as a percentage of total employment in various "developing economies" in low- and middle-income countries by region, 2007–projected to 2019. (Source: International Labour Organization. World employment and social outlook: Trends 2015. Available at: http://www.ilo.org/wcmsp5/groups/public/@dgreports/@dcomm/@publ/documents/publication/wcms_337069.pdf. Accessed March 1, 2017.)

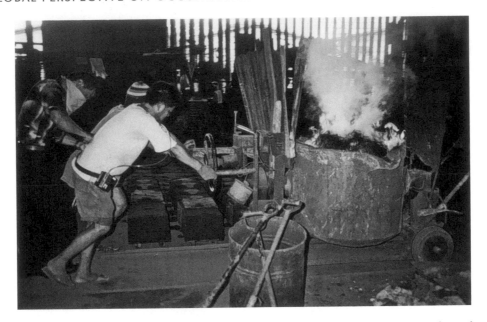

Figure 35-4. A worker pouring molten metal into molds in an iron foundry in Manila, the Philippines. The employer provided no protective clothing or equipment. (Photograph by Aaron Sussell.)

workplaces as well as government policies and programs, including health and safety inspections.[34-36] (See Figures 35-4 and 35-5.)

3. *Workers with health-related vulnerabilities*: These workers include workers with chronic medical conditions, disabilities, and learning difficulties, as well as female workers, child and young adult workers, and older workers, who are vulnerable because of physiological factors. These workers require accommodations by their employers in work and in the work environment and increased access to both preventive and curative occupational health services and general medical services.[32-34,36,37]

Female Workers

More than 1.3 billion women work, accounting for about 40% of the global workforce. Female workers face additional burdens at work,[37,38] for reasons that include the following:

- More often than men, they are in part-time or precarious jobs, or jobs in the informal sector.
- On average, they receive less pay than men for equal work.

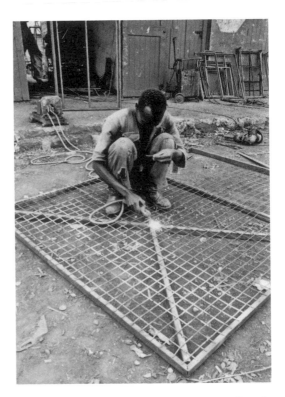

Figure 35-5. Welder making bed frame at small workshop in Kenya, without adequate eye protection against ultraviolet radiation. (Photograph by Barry S. Levy.)

- They are not paid for domestic work in their own households and often not paid for other work performed.
- Given their "nonoccupational" family responsibilities, including raising children, obtaining and preparing food, and, especially in LMICs, obtaining water, they shoulder increased physical and psychosocial burdens—often double or triple the total workload of males. An estimated 70% of the total workload, in both paid and unpaid work, is shouldered by women. (See Figure 35-6.)
- They are often exposed to reproductive health hazards, including those that may adversely affect pregnancy outcome.
- They face more ergonomic hazards than men because tools and equipment, including safety equipment, are often designed primarily, if not exclusively, for use by men.
- They are often physically, psychologically, and sexually harassed at work.
- About 1 billion women work outside formal economic systems. Therefore, they have less independence and low income. In addition, they and their communities and countries do not benefit from their full work potential.[39]

The percentage of female workers in many sectors has led to changes in needs, demands, and expectations at work and changes in policies, such as for ergonomics, chemical safety, and better work hours. Globally, in 2015, one-fourth of female workers were in agriculture. Although women's employment in this sector has decreased over the past 20 years, agriculture remains the most important source of employment for women in most LMICs. In Southern Asia and sub-Saharan Africa, over 60% of working women work in this sector. In many of these countries, women are concentrated in time- and labor-intensive agricultural work that is poorly remunerated.[37,39,40] In contrast, only 2.6% of working women in high-income countries work in agriculture. Between 1995 and 2015, the percentage of women employed in agriculture decreased by 15% and that of men by 12%. The decline in women's employment in agriculture during this 20-year period was most evident in East Asia (31%). Between 1995 and 2015, most women who left agriculture shifted to services, while men who left agriculture found employment in both services and industry; during this period, male employment in industry increased by 5.3%, while female employment in industry decreased by 5.6%.

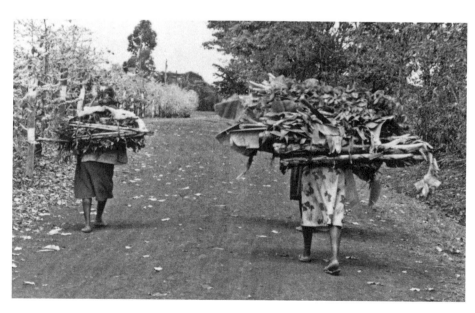

Figure 35-6. Women in rural area of Kenya carrying heavy loads. (Photograph by Barry S. Levy.)

Child Workers

Although the international conventions and trade agreements prohibit child labor, many children are forced to work, often in hazardous jobs.[41] However, both the total number of children working and the number working in hazardous jobs have substantially decreased in recent years. (See Figure 35-7.) For 2016, the number of child workers was estimated at 134 million, with 65 million of them in the worst forms of child labor.[42] This is remarkable progress over a short period of time, which needs to continue until all child labor is eliminated. Approximately 60% of children work in farming and related activities, 30% in service work, and 11% in industrial work. Millions of children work in hazardous jobs in crop agriculture, fishing and aquaculture, domestic work, manufacturing, mining and quarrying, construction, service industries, and street work. (See Figures 35-8 through 35-10.)

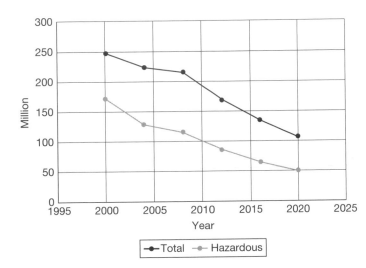

Figure 35-7. Total numbers of child workers and child workers performing hazardous work. (Source: International Programme on the Elimination of Child Labor. Marking progress against child labour: Global estimates and trends 2000-2012. 2013. Available at: http://www.ilo.org/wcmsp5/groups/public/@ed_norm/@ipec/documents/publication/wcms_221513.pdf. Accessed August 26, 2017.)

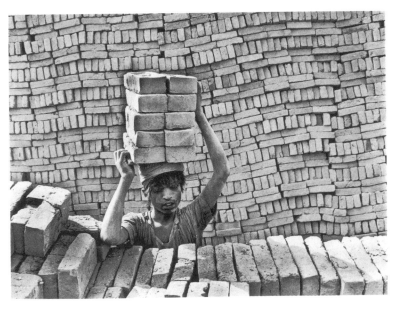

Figure 35-8. Young boy carrying fired bricks for storage in Nepal, 1993. Thousands of children are forced to work in brick kilns, rock quarries, or mines. (Photograph by David L. Parker.)

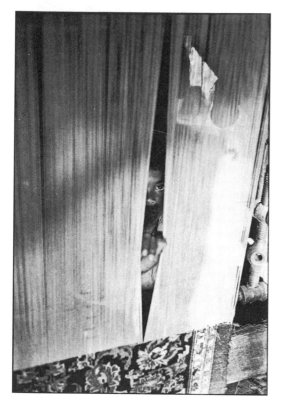

Figure 35-9. Young girl working as a carpet weaver in India. (Photograph by David L. Parker.)

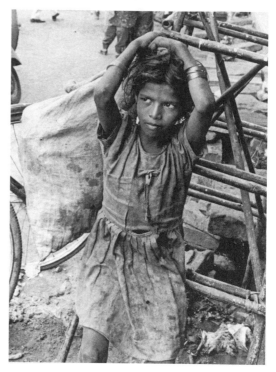

Figure 35-10. Child laborers, such as this girl working as a garbage picker in India, are exploited and exposed to many serious occupational health and safety hazards. (Photograph by David L. Parker.)

Children are exposed to many chemicals, including pesticides, solvents, heavy metals, hazardous dusts, and toxic gases. They often work long hours in physically demanding jobs in poor ergonomic conditions. Child workers face many safety risks and, as a result, have higher rates of occupational injuries than adults. Today about 65 million children are working in hazardous jobs, the worst forms being prostitution and de facto slavery.[32,42] Children are more vulnerable to environmental exposures than adults because, compared to adults, they have thinner skin, breathe faster and more deeply, more easily absorb and retain heavy metals and other hazardous chemicals, and do not have fully developed neurological, endocrine, and other systems. They may face substantial psychosocial stressors at work. In addition, many child workers do not receive adequate education. The ILO has worked, since its founding in 1919, to protect children from occupational hazards and,

since the 1970s, to reduce and ultimately eliminate child labor. (See Chapter 30.)

Older Workers

The global workforce is aging rapidly. The proportion of workers between 45 and 64 years of age will increase by 41% by 2030.[43] The aging of the workforce causes many challenges, including stress related to the following:

- Maintenance of work skills and abilities
- Demand for greater productivity
- Need to learn new skills and work procedures
- Need to adapt to continuous changes
- Managing chronic diseases that can adversely affect work.

Aging workers may also have limitations in heavy physical activity and face increased health and safety hazards from shift work, noise, and extremes of temperature.

One-third of workers over age 50 have at least one chronic disease. Their most common chronic diseases are musculoskeletal disorders, mental health problems, cardiovascular disorders, respiratory diseases, diabetes, and neurological disorders.

Even without disease, physical work ability declines with age by about 1% to 2% a year. Nevertheless, older workers have several strengths, including experience that fosters good judgment, high levels of work engagement and employment stability, low rates of absenteeism due to illness, good social skills, and abilities to train younger workers in good work practices and serve as role models for them.

To meet the needs of aging workers, workplace policies need to do the following:

- Adjust work procedures and organization of work
- Prevent chronic diseases and promote health, starting as early as possible during workers' careers
- Detect disease early and intervene with effective treatment
- Limit long working shifts
- Reduce or eliminate work at night and shift work
- Moderate physical workloads, heavy moving and lifting tasks, and repetitive work
- Avoid extremes of temperature
- Ensure rest breaks, according to physiological needs
- Develop programs for maintenance and promotion of work abilities
- Maintain functional capacities with health promotion, nutrition, and physical fitness programs.[45]

In many countries, national and local programs aim to maintain the work ability, the physical and psychological performance, and the competence of older workers so they can fully participate in the workforce.[46] These programs attempt to eliminate obstacles to participation of older workers—obstacles that are related to health, work, the work environment, and/or competence to perform work (lifelong learning). These programs improve functional capacities of aging workers, promote their health, provide training

and education, and, most importantly, adjust the working environment and working practices to the needs of aging workers, including facilitating their return to work after sick leave.[45,47]

Countries throughout the world have responded in different ways to the aging of the workforce. The European 2020 Strategy of the EU proposes smart, sustainable, and inclusive growth and emphasizes the need to promote active-aging policies, which the EU defines "as growing old in good health and as a full member of society, feeling more fulfilled at work, more independent in daily life and more involved as citizens." No matter how old, older people can play a part in society and enjoy a good quality of life. The challenge is to make the most of the enormous potential that older people have, even at a more advanced age. Promotion and maintenance of work ability of workers plays a central role in the EU strategy.

A new innovation is the Active Ageing Index (AAI) for measurement of countries' and communities' status in active-aging programs. The AAI groups 22 indicators into four main domains: employment, social participation, healthy living, and capabilities and enabling environments. Countries and communities can benefit with the help of the AAI benchmark and receive status reports and information for further development.[45]

Agricultural Workers

Over 1 billion workers are employed in agriculture, more than half of whom are informally employed. They represent almost one-third of the total global workforce. In sub-Saharan Africa, over 60% of the workforce is employed in agriculture. In the rural areas, most other workers are employed in jobs that are closely related or dependent on agriculture. Many of these workers are seasonally employed in jobs that pay low wages and do not offer opportunities to learn new skills or gain upward mobility.[6,9]

Globalization has had both positive and negative impacts on agriculture-related work and agricultural workers. There has been rapid growth of nonfarming jobs, especially in large cities, which has heightened rural-to-urban migration and often marginalized family farmers and other workers in rural areas. As a result, a greater percentage of workers are employed in non-farming sectors—a contributing factor to the 50% reduction in the global poverty rate between 2000 and 2015. During the same period, in many countries income disparities widened. Part of the reason for these widening disparities has been increased control (up to 80%) and concentration by large multinational corporations of the global agricultural market. Those corporations typically pay workers low wages and sometimes utilize bonded labor and child labor. The ILO has estimated that there are 21 million forced-labor workers, 26% of whom are children and 55% of whom are women or girls. The ILO estimated that the rates of forced-labor workers per 1,000 residents are 4.2 in Asia, 4.0 in Africa, 3.4 in the Middle East, 3.3 in Asia and the Pacific, 3.1 in Latin America and the Caribbean, and 1.5 in the "developed economies," including the EU.

Because most of these workers are employed by large agricultural corporations that exploit cheap labor, small farmers, especially those in LMICs, are placed at a significant disadvantage in this "distorted market." Small farmers have also suffered from global climate change, with increased ambient temperature and extremes of precipitation, accompanied by droughts and floods. (See Chapter 29.)

Many health and safety issues associated with economic globalization and climate change have increasingly enhanced international organizations to allocate more resources and develop new or improved policies and programs to address these issues. Under the international pressures by consumers, transnational corporations have initiated programs for corporate social responsibility and decent work in their respective sectors. The ILO, the Food and Agriculture Organization, OECD, and other international organizations have developed policies and programs to address the human rights, health, and safety of workers throughout the global supply chain; improve occupational health and safety overall; address climate change; reduce poverty; and promote sustainable employment and decent work.[48]

International Migrant Workers

Between 1950 and 2015, North America, Europe, and Oceania were net receivers of international migrant workers from Africa, Asia, and Latin America and the Caribbean, with annual net migration averaging 2.8 million. From 2000 to 2015, all high-income countries received from LMICs an annual net migration averaging 4.1 million.[9,49]

Migration is projected to continue to be a major contributor to population growth in many high-income countries. Between 2015 and 2050, total births in high-income countries are projected to exceed deaths by 20 million, while net gain from migration is projected to be 91 million. Therefore, net migration is projected to account for 82% of population growth in high-income countries.

According to recent ILO estimates, among the 232 million migrants, there are about 150 million international migrant workers currently employed or seeking employment, 11.5 million of whom are employed as migrant domestic workers. In addition, there are many illegal international migrant workers, "paperless" workers who are in a country illegally and therefore without legal and social protections. They are highly vulnerable to occupational health and safety hazards and exploitation.

The vast majority of international migrant workers are low-skilled. Most are young, with little or no work experience in jobs and work environments in their new countries of residence. Most of them work in low-wage and unsafe jobs that are not favored by workers in their new countries. Language barriers and cross-cultural differences make working conditions even more challenging.

Migrant workers are frequently exploited and discriminated against. Their human rights are frequently violated. Female and child migrants are at risk of human trafficking and related severe hazards.

There is some, but not conclusive, evidence that international migrant workers face higher risks of occupational injuries than native-born workers. International migrant workers may have endemic diseases from their home countries, such as chronic parasitic infestations. Despite their needs, they underutilize health services and often do not apply for social services for which they would be eligible.

International migrant workers contribute positively to the gross domestic product and economic growth of host countries that have inclusive labor policies. Their 60% to 80% employment rates in the 35 OECD countries are about the same as those of citizens of their host countries. Their high rates of employment may be due in part to their willingness to accept hazardous and demanding jobs and poorer working conditions.

The ILO, the EU, and other organizations have proposed improving the health and safety of international migrant workers by the following measures:[49,50]

- Ensuring coverage and implementation of occupational safety and health law and providing technical advice
- Facilitating access to labor markets
- Strengthening institutional capacity and coordination mechanisms to combat unacceptable forms of work and child labor
- Supporting inclusive employment policies and decent work principles
- Recognizing the skills of the migrant workers
- Developing enterprises, job opportunities, and workplaces
- Formalizing informal work
- Protecting workers' rights
- Promoting employment-intensive investments.

The same measures are also valid for domestic workers.

Unemployment

Although globalization has substantially increased formal employment, many high-income countries have experienced higher rates of unemployment because of multinational corporations moving operations and often entire factories to LMICs where wages are lower, labor laws less strict, occupational and environmental regulations weaker, and labor unions less powerful or nonexistent. Low-wage and unskilled workers, especially in manufacturing in these high-income countries, have suffered disproportionately. However, unemployment rates in high-income countries are generally much lower than unemployment rates in LMICs. For example, some LMICs in Africa and Asia have unemployment rates that are more than double those in Europe. Some of this gap may be due to the high proportion of informal workers in LMICs who are not included in surveys of formally employed workers.

Unemployment is associated with many adverse health consequences, including negative impacts on personal and community mental health. In addition, people with mental health problems are more likely than others to become unemployed. These associations add to the urgency of helping laid-off workers find new jobs quickly and providing services to assist workers in managing occupational stress. These associations also highlight the importance of governments providing unemployment insurance benefits to unemployed workers.[51-53]

SELECTED INTERNATIONAL ORGANIZATIONS

This section provides brief summaries of important international organizations in both occupational health and safety as well as environmental health.

The *International Labour Organization* (ILO) advances opportunities for women and men to obtain decent and productive work in conditions of freedom, equity, security, and human dignity. Its main aims are to promote rights at work, encourage decent employment opportunities, enhance social protection, and strengthen dialogue in addressing work-related issues. In promoting social justice as well as human rights and labor rights, the ILO pursues its founding mission that labor peace is essential to prosperity. The ILO helps advance the creation of decent jobs and economic and working conditions that give workers and employers a stake in lasting peace, prosperity, and progress. (For more information, see http://www.ilo.org/public/english/download/glance.pdf.)

The *World Health Organization* (WHO) is the directing and coordinating authority for health within the United Nations system. WHO aims to strengthen national systems to respond to the needs of populations (including working populations), establish basic levels of health protection for all workers, and ensure all workers access to basic and comprehensive occupational health services. Occupational health experts at WHO's Geneva headquarters and its regional offices operate a network of collaborating centres that actively participate in the WHO's Global Plan of Action on Workers' Health. The Department of Public Health and Environment of WHO aims to promote a healthier environment, intensify primary prevention, and influence public policies in all sectors so as to address the root causes of environmental threats to health. The Pan American Health Organization is the regional organization of WHO for North and South America as well as the Caribbean region. (For more information, see http://www.who.int/occupational_health/about/en/.)

The *International Agency for Research on Cancer* (IARC), which is part of WHO, coordinates and conducts research on the causes of human cancer and the mechanisms of carcinogenesis, and develops scientific strategies for cancer prevention and control. IARC performs and supports epidemiological and laboratory research and disseminates scientific information through publications (including its *Monographs on the Evaluation of Carcinogenic Risks to Humans*) meetings, courses, and fellowships. The IARC list of established carcinogenic substances and agents guides recognition of cancer risks. (For more information, see https://www.iarc.fr/en/about/index.php.)

The *United Nations Environment Programme* (UNEP) provides leadership and encourages partnership in caring for the environment by inspiring, informing, and enabling nations and peoples to improve their quality of life without compromising that of future generations. (For more information, see http://web.unep.org/about/who-we-are/overview.)

The *Intergovernmental Panel on Climate Change* (IPCC) is the leading global body for the assessment of climate change. It was established by UNEP and the World Meterological Organization to provide a clear scientific view of the current state of climate change and its potential environmental and socioeconomic consequences. (See Chapter 29.) (For more information, see https://www.ipcc.ch.)

The *International Commission on Occupational Health* (ICOH) is an international nongovernmental professional society that aims to foster the scientific progress, knowledge, and development of occupational health and safety in all its aspects. Its numerous scientific committees hold regular symposia and publish scientific monographs on important issues. (For more information, see http://www.icohweb.org.)

The *European Trade Union Institute* (ETUI) is the independent, nonprofit, research and training center of the European Trade Union Confederation, which brings together European trade unions into one organization. It receives financial support from the EU. ETUI conducts studies on socioeconomic topics and industrial relations. It established bridges between academia, the research community, and the trade union movement. ETUI provides technical assistance in occupational health and safety. (For more information, see https://www.etui.org.)

REFERENCES

1. International Labour Organization. World employment social outlook: Trends 2017. Available at: http://www.ilo.org/wcmsp5/groups/public/---dgreports/---dcomm/---publ/documents/publication/wcms_541211.pdf. Accessed August 26, 2017.
2. International Labour Office. World social security report: Providing coverage in times of crisis and beyond. 2010/2011. Available at: http://www.ilo.org/wcmsp5/groups/public/---dgreports/---dcomm/---publ/documents/publication/wcms_146566.pdf. Accessed August 26, 2017.
3. International Labour Office. Non-standard forms of employment: Report for discussion at the Meeting of Experts on Non-Standard Forms of Employment (Geneva, February 16–19, 2015). Available at: http://www.ilo.org/wcmsp5/groups/public/---ed_protect/---protrav/---travail/documents/meetingdocument/wcms_336934.pdf. Accessed February 27, 2017.
4. International Labour Office. Decent work and the informal economy. 2002. Available at: http://www.ilo.org/wcmsp5/groups/public/---ed_emp/---emp_policy/documents/publication/wcms_210442.pdf. Accessed February 27, 2017.
5. International Labour Organization. Status in employment - - ILO modelled estimates, November 2016. Available at: http:// www.ilo.org/ ilostat/ faces/ oracle/ webcenter/ portalapp/ pagehierarchy/ Page3.jspx?MBI_ID=32&_ adf.ctrl state=3x7aujuti_9&_ afrLoop=1492954121896304&_afrWindowMode=0&_ afrWindowId=3x7aujuti_6#!. Accessed July 25, 2017.

6. International Labour Office. Global employment trends 2012: Preventing a deeper jobs crisis. Available at: http://www.ilo.org/global/research/global-reports/global-employment-trends/WCMS_171571/lang--nl/index.htm. Accessed February 27, 2017.

7. International Labour Organization. World social protection report: Building economic recovery, inclusive development and social justice 2014/15. Available at: http://www.ilo.org/wcmsp5/groups/public/---dgreports/---dcomm/documents/publication/wcms_245201.pdf. Accessed February 27, 2017.

8. International Labour Organization. Global employment trends 2014: Risk of a jobless recovery? Available at: http://www2.warwick.ac.uk/fac/soc/pais/research/researchcentres/csgr/green/foresight/demography/2014_ilo_global_employment_trends_2014.pdf. Accessed February 27, 2017.

9. Food and Agriculture Organization of the United Nations. Sustainable Agriculture and Rural Development (SARD) Policy Brief 1: SARD and agricultural workers. 2006. Available at: http://www.fao.org/docrep/015/i2490e/i2490e01b.pdf. Accessed March 1, 2017.

10. International Labour Office. Women in labour markets: Measuring progress and identifying challenges. 2010. Available at: http://www.ilo.org/wcmsp5/groups/public/---ed_emp/---emp_elm/---trends/documents/publication/wcms_123835.pdf. Accessed March 1, 2017.

11. World Commission on the Social Dimension of Globalization. A fair globalization: Creating opportunities for all. 2004. Available at: http://www.ilo.org/public/english/wcsdg/docs/report.pdf. Accessed March 1, 2017.

12. Bhorat H, Lundall P. Employment and labour market effects of globalization: Selected issues for policy management. 2004. Available at: http://ilo.org/wcmsp5/groups/public/---ed_emp/---emp_elm/documents/publication/wcms_114330.pdf. Accessed March 1, 2017.

13. International Telecommunication Union. ICT facts and figures 2016. Available at: http://www.itu.int/en/ITU-D/Statistics/Pages/facts/default.aspx. Accessed March 1, 2017.

14. International Labour Organization. ILO global estimate of forced labour 2012: Results and methodology. 2012. Available at: http://www.ilo.org/wcmsp5/groups/public/---ed_norm/---declaration/documents/publication/wcms_182004.pdf. Accessed March 1, 2017.

15. Milanovic B. The real winners and losers of globalization: Globalization has radically changed global income dynamics. So who has won and who has lost? October 25, 2012. Available at: https://www.theglobalist.com/the-real-winners-and-losers-of-globalization/. Accessed March 1, 2017.

16. Milberg W, Amengual M. Economic development and working conditions in export processing zones: A survey of trends. 2008. Available at: http://citeseerx.ist.psu.edu/viewdoc/download?doi=10.1.1.490.1514&rep=rep1&type=pdf. Accessed March 1, 2017.

17. Honkonen T, Khan SA. Chemicals and waste governance beyond 2020: Exploring pathways for a coherent global regime. TemaNord 2017: 502. Available at: https://norden.diva-portal.org/smash/get/diva2:1061911/FULLTEXT01.pdf. Accessed on March 1, 2017.

18. United Nations Environment Programme. Global chemicals outlook—Towards sound management of chemicals. 2013. Available at: https://sustainabledevelopment.un.org/content/documents/1966Global%20Chemical.pdf. Accessed March 1, 2017.

19. International Labour Organization. Safety and health at work: A vision for sustainable prevention. 2014. Available at: http://www.ilo.org/wcmsp5/groups/public/---ed_protect/---protrav/---safework/documents/publication/wcms_301214.pdf. Accessed March 1, 2017.

20. International Labour Office. Programme on Safety and Health at Work and the Environment (SafeWork). National system for recording and notification of occupational diseases: Practical guide. 2013. Available at: http://www.ilo.org/wcmsp5/groups/public/---ed_protect/---protrav/---safework/documents/publication/wcms_210950.pdf. Accessed March 1, 2017.

21. European Commission. Report on the current situation in relation to occupational diseases' systems in EU member states and EFTA/EEA countries, in particular relative to Commission Recommendation 2003/670/EC concerning the European Schedule of Occupational Diseases and gathering of data on relevant related aspects. 2003. Available at: https://osha.europa.eu/fi/legislation/guidelines/commission-recommendation-concerning-the-european-schedule-of-occupational-diseases. Accessed March 1, 2017.

22. Health and Safety Executive. Standardised incidence rate of fatal accidents at work, excluding road traffic accidents and accidents on board transport in the course of work. Updated November 2016. Available at: http://www.hse.gov.uk/statistics/tables/index.

htm#europeancomparisons. Accessed March 1, 2017.

23. Finnish Institute of Occupational Health. Occupational diseases in Finland in 2012: New cases of recognized and suspected occupational diseases. 2014. Available at: https://www.julkari.fi/bitstream/handle/10024/131563/Occupational_diseases_2012.pdf?sequence=1. Accessed March 1, 2017.

24. European Chemical Industry Council. The European Chemical Industries: Facts & Figures. 2016. Available at: http://www.cefic.org/Facts-and-Figures/. Accessed March 1, 2017.

25. European Chemicals Agency. Understanding REACH. Available at: https://echa.europa.eu/regulations/reach/understanding-reach. Accessed March 1, 2017.

26. Organisation of Economic Cooperation and Development. Classification and labelling of chemicals. Available at: http://www.oecd.org/chemicalsafety/risk-ma. Accessed March 1, 2017.

27. International Labour Organization. C170—Chemicals Convention, 1990 (No. 170): Convention concerning safety in the use of chemicals at work (Entry into force: 04 Nov 1993). Available at: http://www.ilo.org/dyn/normlex/en/f?p=NORMLEXPUB:12100:0::NO::P12100_ILO_CODE:C170. Accessed March 1, 2017.

28. European Agency for Health and Safety at Work. OSH WIKI. Dangerous substances (chemical and biological). Available at: https://oshwiki.eu/wiki/Dangerous_substances_(chemical_and_biological). Accessed on March 1, 2017.

29. Eurofound and European Agency for Health and Safety at Work. Psychosocial risks in Europe: Prevalence and strategies for prevention. 2014. Available at: https://osha.europa.eu/en/publications/reports/psychosocial-risks-eu-prevalence-strategies-prevention/view. Accessed March 1, 2017.

30. European Agency for Health and Safety at Work. E-guide to managing stress and psychosocial risks. Available at: https://osha.europa.eu/en/tools-and-publications/e-guide-managing-stress-and-psychosocial-risks. Accessed March 1, 2017.

31. Siegrist J, Wahrendorf M (eds.). Work stress and health in a globalized economy: The model of effort-reward imbalance. Geneva: Springer Verlag, 2016.

32. International Labour Organization. World employment and social outlook: Trends 2015. Available at: http://www.ilo.org/wcmsp5/groups/public/@dgreports/@dcomm/@publ/documents/publication/wcms_337069.pdf. Accessed March 1, 2017.

33. World Health Organization. The world health report. Health systems financing: The path to universal coverage. 2010. Available at: http://apps.who.int/iris/bitstream/10665/44371/1/9789241564021_eng.pdf. Accessed March 1, 2017.

34. Belin A, Zamparutti T, Tull K, et al. Occupational health and safety risks for the most vulnerable workers. 2011. Available at: http://www.europarl.europa.eu/RegData/etudes/etudes/join/2011/464436/IPOL-EMPL_ET(2011)464436_EN.pdf. Accessed March 1, 2017.

35. Lay M, Smith PM, Saunders R, et al. The relationship between individual, occupational and workplace factors and type of occupational health and safety vulnerability among Canadian employees. American Journal of Industrial Medicine 2015; 59: 119–128.

36. Lindbohm M-L, Sallmén M. Reproductive effects caused by chemical and biological agents. Finnish Institute of Occupational Health and EU OSHA, May 29, 2017. Available at: https://oshwiki.eu/wiki/Reproductive_effects_caused_by_chemical_and_biological_agents. Accessed August 26, 2017.

37. Institute for Work & Health. Vulnerable workers and risk of work injury. Available at: https://www.iwh.on.ca/system/files/documents/vulnerable_workers_ib_-_nov-2016-final.pdf. Accessed March 1, 2017.

38. International Labour Office. Programme on Safety, Health and the Environment. Safety and health in agriculture. 2000. Available at: http://www.ilo.org/wcmsp5/groups/public/---ed_protect/---protrav/---safework/documents/publication/wcms_110193.pdf. Accessed March 1, 2017.

39. Strategy&. Empowering the third billion: Women and the world of work. 2012. Available at: http://www.strategyand.pwc.com/media/file/Strategyand_Empowering-the-Third-Billion_Full-Report.pdf. Accessed March 1, 2017.

40. Food and Agriculture Organization of the United Nations. The state of food and agriculture: Social protection and agriculture: Breaking the cycle of rural poverty. 2015. Available at: http://www.fao.org/3/a-i4910e.pdf. Accessed March 1, 2017.

41. International Labour Office. C182—Worst Forms of Child Labour Convention, 1999 (No. 182): Convention concerning the Prohibition and Immediate Action for the Elimination of the Worst Forms of Child Labour (Entry into

force: 19 Nov 2000). Available at: http://www.ilo. org/dyn/normlex/en/f?p=NORMLEXPUB:121 00:0::NO::P12100_INSTRUMENT_ID:312327. Accessed March 1, 2017.

42. International Labour Office. Marking progress against child labour: Global estimates and trends 2000–2012. 2013. Available at: http://www.ilo. org/wcmsp5/groups/public/---ed_norm/---ipec/ documents/publication/wcms_221513.pdf). Accessed March 1, 2017.

43. Global Age Watch. Global ageing—Its implications for growth, decent work and social protection beyond 2015. May 2012. Available at: http://www.beyond2015.org/sites/ default/files/Global%20AgeWatch%20PB2%20-%20Growth.pdf. Accessed March 1, 2017.

44. Harbers MM, Achterberg PW. Europeans of retirement age: Chronic diseases and economic activity. December 2012. Available at: http:// ec.europa.eu/health//sites/health/files/major_ chronic_diseases/docs/rivm_report_retirement_ en.pdf. Accessed March 1, 2017.

45. Eurofound. Living longer, working better: Active ageing in Europe. November 2012. Available at: http://www.eurofound.europa.eu/ resourcepacks/activeageing.htmr. Accessed March 1, 2017.

46. European Commission and the United Nations Economic Commission for Europe. Active Ageing Index. Available at: http:// www1.unece.org/stat/platform/display/AAI/ Active+Ageing+Index+Home. Accessed March 1, 2017.

47. Ilmarinen J. Promoting active ageing in the workplace. Available at: https://osha.europa.eu/ en/tools-and-publications/publications/articles/ promoting-active-ageing-in-the-workplace. Accessed March 1, 2017.

48. Organisation for Economic Co-operation and Development. OECD-FAO guidance for responsible agricultural supply chains. Available at: http://www.oecd.org/daf/inv/investment-policy/rbc-agriculture-supply-chains.htm. Accessed March 1, 2017.

49. International Labour Organization. ILO global estimates on migrant workers: Results and methodology: Special focus on migrant domestic workers. 2015. Available at: http://www.ilo.org/ wcmsp5/groups/public/---dgreports/---dcomm/ documents/publication/wcms_436343.pdf. Accessed March 1, 2017.

50. International Labour Organization. Decent work for migrants and refugees [Brochure]. 2016. Available at: http://www.ilo.org/wcmsp5/groups/ public/---dgreports/---dcomm/documents/ publication/wcms_524995.pdf. Accessed March 1, 2017.

51. Möller H. Health effects of unemployment. August 2012. Available at: http://info.wirral. nhs.uk/document_uploads/Short-Reports/ Unemployment-2%20Sept%2012.pdf. Accessed March 1, 2017.

52. van der Noordt M, IJzelenberg H, Droomers, M Proper KI. Health effects of employment: A systematic review of prospective studies. Occupational and Environmental Medicine 2014; 71: 730–736.

53. Waddell G, Burton K. Is work good for your health and well-Being? 2006. Available at: http:// iedereen-aandeslag.nl/wp-content/uploads/2016/ 07/hwwb-is-work-good-for-you.pdf. Accessed March 1, 2017.

Appendix: Illustrative Organizations

Please note that clinically oriented organizations are listed in Chapter 4 and selected international organizations are listed in Chapter 35.

Professional Organizations

Occupational and Environmental Medicine

American College of Occupational and Environmental Medicine
http://www.acoem.org
An association of physicians and other healthcare professionals who specialize in occupational and environmental medicine. It is dedicated to promoting the health of workers through preventive medicine, clinical care, research, and education.

American Thoracic Society
http://www.thoracic.org
A professional society of physicians, research scientists, nurses, and other allied healthcare professionals in such specialties as pulmonology, critical care, sleep medicine, infectious disease, pediatrics, and environmental and occupational medicine. Programs developed by its Environmental & Occupational Health Assembly are featured on its website. In addition to publishing journals and sponsoring educational activities, it establishes, through the publication of statements, workshop reports, and clinical guidelines, the latest standards of care for a variety of adult and pediatric respiratory, critical care, and sleep disorders.

Occupational Health Nursing

American Association of Occupational Health Nurses
http://www.aaohn.org
An association whose mission is to advance the profession of occupational and environmental health nursing through education and research, professional practice/ethics, communications, governmental issues, and alliances.

Industrial Hygiene

American Industrial Hygiene Association
http://www.aiha.org
An association that serves the needs of occupational and environmental health and safety professionals practicing industrial hygiene in industry, government, labor, academic institutions, and independent organizations.

International Occupational Hygiene Association
http://ioha.net
An association of occupational hygiene organizations throughout the world, which promotes, develops, and improves occupational hygiene to provide safe and healthy working environments.

Safety and Injury Prevention

American Society of Safety Engineers

http://www.asse.org

The oldest and largest professional safety society, which is committed to protecting people, property, and the environment. It provides information and services concerning occupational safety, health, and environmental issues and practices.

National Safety Council

http://www.nsc.org

A nonprofit organization that aims to eliminate preventable deaths at work, at home, in communities, and on the road through leadership, research, education, and advocacy. A leading source of occupational safety information and resources, it shares research and best practices widely.

Society for Advancement of Violence and Injury Research

https://savir.wildapricot.org

A professional organization that provides leadership and fosters excellence in the prevention of violence and injuries. It promotes collective, educational, and scholarly activity in developing the field of injury prevention and control research, policy and program development, teaching, and related activities.

Ergonomics

Chartered Institute of Ergonomics & Human Factors

http://www.ergonomics.org.uk

A professional society for ergonomic specialists that is based in the United Kingdom.

International Ergonomics Association

http://www.iea.cc

A federation of ergonomics and human factor societies throughout the world whose mission is to elaborate and advance ergonomic science and practice and to expand the application or ergonomics and its contribution to society.

Toxicology

Society of Toxicology

http://www.toxicology.org

A professional and scholarly organization of scientists from academic institutions, government, and industry, representing the great variety of scientists who practice toxicology in the United States and elsewhere. Its mission is to create a safer and healthier world by advancing the science and increasing the impact of toxicology.

Epidemiology

EPICOH Scientific Committee on Epidemiology in Occupational Health

http://www.epicoh.org

This organization, one of the scientific committees of the International Commission on Occupational Health (see below), focuses on problems unique to the study of health and work. With membership open to occupational epidemiologists and other scientists worldwide, EPICOH offers discussions, critical reviews, collaborations, and education on issues of occupational exposures and their human health effects.

International Society for Environmental Epidemiology

http://www.iseepi.org

An international organization that provides a variety of forums for discussions, critical reviews, collaboration, and education on issues of environmental exposures and their human health effects.

Occupational Health Psychology

American Psychological Association

http://www.apa.org

Its Work, Stress and Health Office promotes research, training, practice, and policy to examine the impact of the changing organization of work on stress, health, safety, and productivity in the workplace.

International Occupational Health

International Commission on Occupational Health

http://www.icohweb.org/site/homepage.asp

Aims to foster the scientific progress, knowledge, and development of occupational health and safety in all its aspects. Presents a triennial World Congress on Occupational Health. Has 37 scientific committees, most of which have regular symposia, publish scientific monographs, and review abstracts submitted to international congresses.

Public Health

American Public Health Association

http://www.apha.org.

The oldest and largest professional association for public health workers in a wide variety of disciplines and work settings, including occupational and environmental health. Its primary sections devoted to this field are the Occupational Health and Safety Section, the Environment Section, and the Injury Prevention and Emergency Health Services Section.

Illustrative Labor Organizations

American Federation of Labor and Congress of Industrial Organizations
http://www.aflcio.org

The Change to Win Strategies Organizing Center
http://www.changetowin.org

National Education Association
http://www.nea.org

Service Employees International Union
http://www.seiu.org

American Federation of State, County, and Municipal Employees
http://www.afscme.org

International Brotherhood of Teamsters
http://www.teamster.org

United Food and Commercial Workers
http://www.ufcw.org

American Federation of Teachers
http://www.aft.org

United Steel, Paper and Forestry, Rubber, Manufacturing, Energy, Allied Industrial and Service Workers International Union
http://www.usw.org

International Brotherhood of Electrical Workers
http://www.ibew.org

Laborers' International Union of North America
http://www.liuna.org

International Association of Machinists and Aerospace Workers
http://www.goiam.org

Illustrative Environmental Nongovernmental Organizations

American Council for an Energy-Efficient Economy
http://www.aceee.org
Advances energy efficiency as a means of promoting economic prosperity, energy security, and environmental protection.

Center for Health, Environment, & Justice
http://www.chej.org
Provides technical information and training to grassroots community environmental activists on how to organize and on the rights of local communities.

Center for a Livable Future
http://www.jhsph.edu/clf

Engages in research, education outreach, and community action in farming, eating, and living for our future.

Clean Water Network
http://www.clean-water-network.org
Works as a national coalition of more than 1,200 nonprofit public-interest organizations to protect the health, safety, and quality of U.S. water resources.

Earth Island Institute
http://www.earthisland.org
Supports people who are creating solutions to protect the planet.

Environmental Defense Fund
http://www.edf.org
Links science, economics, and law to create innovative, equitable, and cost-effective solutions to environmental problems.

Environmental Working Group
http://www.ewg.org
Uses the power of public information to protect public health and the environment.

Friends of the Earth
http://www.foe.org
Supports clean energy and solutions to global warming, protects people from new and potentially harmful technologies, and promotes low-pollution transportation alternatives.

Greenpeace
http://www.greenpeace.org
Uses nonviolent confrontation to raise the level and quality of public debate on environmental issues.

Health Care Without Harm
https://noharm.org
Works to transform healthcare worldwide so that it reduces its environmental footprint and becomes a community anchor for sustainability and a leader in the global movement for environmental health and justice.

League of Conservation Voters
http://www.lcv.org
Advocates for sound environmental policies and to elect pro-environmental candidates who will adopt and implement such policies.

Natural Resources Defense Council
http://www.nrdc.org
Works to protect wildlife and wild places and to ensure a healthy environment for all life on earth.

Renewable Energy Policy Project
http://www.repp.org

Aims to accelerate the use of renewable energy by providing credible information, insightful policy analysis, and innovative strategies.

Sierra Club

http://www.sierraclub.org

Works as a grassroots environmental organization, to protect communities, wild places, and the planet.

Union of Concerned Scientists

http://www.ucsusa.org

Combines independent scientific research and citizen action to develop innovative, practical solutions and to secure responsible changes in government policy, corporate practices, and consumer choices.

World Resources Institute

http://www.wri.org

Works, as an environmental think tank, to find practical ways to protect the earth and improve people's lives.

Student Organizations

American Medical Student Association

http://www.amsa.org

A student-governed, national organization that represents the concerns of physicians-in-training.

Its action committees and interest groups help expose medical students to information on subjects not generally covered in traditional curricula. Its Community and Environmental Health Action Committee helps medical and premedical students educate their schools and communities about important public health issues, enables medical and premedical students to influence debate about and achieve progress related to these issues, empowers chapters to develop and execute local public health projects, and provides guidance and training in public health and public health careers.

Student Assembly of the American Public Health Association

https://www.apha.org/apha-communities/student-assembly

As the largest student-led public health organization in the United States, it furthers the development of students in public health and health-related disciplines. Its members include not only students but also young professionals in a variety of health professions. It connects people who are interested in working together on public health and student-related issues.

Index